## Quick Reference to
## Pediatric Nursing Care Plans

# Introduction to
# Maternity
# and
# Pediatric
# Nursing

# Introduction to Maternity and Pediatric Nursing

## SECOND EDITION

**Eleanor Dumont Thompson, MS, RNC, APR**
Clinical Nurse Specialist
Columbia/HCA Portsmouth Regional Hospital
Portsmouth, New Hampshire

**W.B. SAUNDERS COMPANY**
*A Division of Harcourt Brace & Company*
Philadelphia    London    Toronto    Montreal    Sydney    Tokyo

**W.B. SAUNDERS COMPANY**
*A Division of Harcourt Brace & Company*

The Curtis Center
Independence Square West
Philadelphia, PA 19106

**Library of Congress Cataloging-in-Publication Data**

Thompson, Eleanor Dumont.
    Introduction to maternity and pediatric nursing / Eleanor D.
Thompson.—2nd ed.
      p.    cm.
    Includes bibliographical references.
    ISBN 0-7216-4828-2
    1. Maternity nursing.  2. Pediatric nursing.  I. Title.
    [DNLM:  1. Maternal-Child Nursing.  WY 157.3 T469i 1995]
RG951.T46  1995
610.73'62—dc20
DNLM/DLC                                  94-18065

INTRODUCTION TO MATERNITY AND
PEDIATRIC NURSING, 2nd edition             ISBN 0-7216-4828-2

Printed in the United States of America

9    8    7    6    5    4    3    2    1

*To the student, who is also our teacher.*

*To the nursing instructor, whose wisdom and perseverance will help guide future generations of nurses to care for children and their families.*

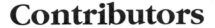

# Contributors

**Joan M. Croteau, MSN, MS, RN**

Director of Staff Development
M.I. Nursing/Restorative Center
Lawrence, Massachusetts
Formerly, Instructor, Maternal-Newborn Nursing
St. Joseph Hospital/Rivier College, School of Nursing
Nashua, New Hampshire

*Human Reproduction; Fetal Development; Prenatal Care and Adaptations to Pregnancy*

**Emily Slone McKinney, MSN, RNC**

Associate Professor of Nursing
Tarrant County Junior College
Fort Worth, Texas

*Nursing Care of Women with Complications During Pregnancy; Nursing Care During Labor and Birth; Nursing Management of Pain During Labor and Birth; Nursing Care of Women with Complications During Labor and Birth; Nursing Care of Women with Complications Following Birth*

# Preface

Dear Reader:

Welcome to the second edition of *Introduction to Maternity and Pediatric Nursing!* I thank you for the wonderful reception you gave to my first combined book. This edition features many exciting changes while building on the successful themes and organization of the first edition. Every chapter has been completely revised and updated. Perhaps the easiest way for you to recognize these changes would be to compare this edition chapter by chapter with the first edition.

## MATERNITY NURSING

In addition to the revision of Joan M. Croteau's chapters (Chapters 2, 3, and 4), Chapters 5, 6, 7, 8, and 10 have been rewritten by Emily Slone McKinney, a coauthor of *Foundations of Maternal-Newborn Nursing* (Gorrie, T. M., McKinney, E. S., & Murray, S. S. [1994]. Philadelphia: W.B. Saunders.)

You will enjoy the readability of these chapters as well as the logical thought progression. As you read, note the emphasis on the nursing process, both within the text and in the many new nursing care plans. Basic knowledge and theory based on sound physiology and pathophysiology are presented. New line drawings help you to understand complex information.

At the heart of the material lies the individual pregnant woman and her family. The authors ask you to think about how culturally diverse needs can be met and provide suggestions. They stress the need for safety for the nurse and for the family. Because of the brevity of hospital stays, client teaching is incorporated and emphasized throughout the text. The family's experience of pregnancy, birth, and the postpartum period is stressed. The nurse's role and interventions that contribute to a successful outcome for the family are also stressed.

Important current topics include trauma during pregnancy, communicating with families experiencing pregnancy loss, reassuring and nonreassuring fetal heart rates and uterine activity patterns, how childbirth pain differs from other pain, the epidural block, and nursing care related to operative procedures. Procedures are carefully outlined. Information is highlighted in blocks to reinforce student comprehension. Appendices at the end of the book include tables such as Some Factors with Known or Possible Teratogenic Effects on the Fetus; Drugs Used During Antepartum, Intrapartum, Postpartum, and Neonatal Care; Effects of Drugs During Breast Feeding; and Drugs Commonly Used in Pediatric Nursing.

Chapter 11, the Nurse's Role in Reproductive Health, is new. We conceived this chapter as the ideal way to assist the nurse in expanding the mother's health care by assessing her contraceptive needs and by teaching her how to prevent certain gynecologic problems. This chapter includes family planning, toxic shock syndrome, fertility counseling, and breast self-examination. I expanded the material to include physical changes surrounding menopause, the final phase of the reproductive cycle in the female. This section should provide an excellent resource for the nurse both professionally and personally.

## PEDIATRIC NURSING

**Normal Growth and Development.** Chapters 16 through 21 summarize important aspects of normal growth and development. Developmental milestones are depicted usually, and anticipatory guidance is stressed. A comparison summary of import theorists such as Maslow, Erickson, Freud, Piaget, Kohlberg, and Sullivan is presented. Accident prevention is discussed by age group and stresses awareness both in the hospital and in the home. Nutrition counseling is discussed for each age group, and culturally diverse food patterns are summarized. The National Cholesterol Education Program recommendations for detection and management of hypercholesterolemia in children and adolescents are summarized. Topics new in the second edition include communicating love and respect to the child, and expanded topics include the family as part of the community, the divorced family, the abused family, suggested nursing diagnoses for children and families from diverse sociocultural backgrounds, developmental dental hygiene, and effective approaches to problems experienced by teenagers.

**The Hospitalized Child.** Chapter 22, The Child's Experience of Hospitalization, presents the emotional impact of hospitalization on the child at various ages. In Chapter 23, Health-Care Adaptations for the Child and Family, all pediatric procedures are grouped for students' and instructors' convenience. Chapters on pediatric disease conditions use a system approach. Each chapter starts with an illustration depicting the child's developing system and how it differs from the adult system. Every chapter briefly summarizes the particular system being covered and also reviews the child's development of the system during fetal life. This nicely emphasizes the interdependence of obstetrics and pediatrics. It also lists the common diagnostic tests that might be performed on a patient with a condition related to the body system being discussed.

All of the chapters on disorders contain updated and new nursing care plans based on the latest NANDA-approved diagnoses. A list of nursing diagnoses is also provided in Appendix H. On the recommendations of reviewers, I have included the following additional conditions: conjunctivitis, hyphema, cataracts, retinoblastoma, osteosarcoma, Ewing's sarcoma, torticollis, rheumatic fever, gastroesophageal reflux, rotavirus infection, Meckel's diverticulum, constipation, Hirschsprung's disease, hypospadias, exstrophy of the bladder, obstructive uropathy, folliculitis, fungal infection, scabies, herpes simplex, maple syrup urine disease, galactosemia, Tay-Sachs disease, and hypothyroidism. There is a continued emphasis on the prevention of AIDS and other sexually transmitted diseases as well as on the use of universal precautions.

**Color Inserts.** A color insert in Chapter 31, The Child with a Skin Condition, will assist the student to recognize specific skin conditions and conditions related to the more common communicable diseases. Many new photographs enhance the textbook's appeal and express visually that which is difficult to describe in words.

## SPECIAL FEATURES

Features that enhance learning include vocabulary terms, chapter outlines, objectives, nursing briefs, study questions, and multiple choice review questions. New to this edition are key points at the end of each chapter. Tables are used to summarize or compare complex information. A glossary appears at the end of the book. Quick Reference to Emergencies in Maternity Nursing and Quick Reference to Maternity Nursing Care Plans are found inside the front cover. Quick Reference to Emergencies in Pediatric Nursing and Quick Reference to Pediatric Nursing Care Plans are found inside the back cover. This material expands material found in the first edition.

## STUDY GUIDE

The Study Guide to Accompany Introduction to Maternity and Pediatric Nursing, written by Emily McKinney, MSN, RNC, and Jean Ashwill, MSN, RN, CPNP, has been revised to correspond with this new edition. It is intended to help the student master the content of the textbook. Every chapter in the Study Guide coincides with the chapter of the same name in the text.

Traditional learning methods, such as matching and completion questions, help reinforce factual material related to maternity and pediatric nursing. In addition, Thinking Critically exercises, Case Studies, and Other Learning Activities help the student apply factual material to the clinical setting.

Multiple choice review questions appear at the end of each chapter. The questions have a dual purpose: to help students review chapter content and to help them become more comfortable in answering typical test items.

## INSTRUCTOR'S MANUAL

I have written a new instructor's manual to accompany the text. Selected objectives, course outlines, and lesson plans are included. Suggestions for clinical site activities are numerous. An annotated bibliography of audiovisual supplements is included, as well as a test bank and transparency masters.

As you might guess, I am excited about this new edition. I hope that it serves you well and that you will complete your rotation through maternity and pediatric nursing with an increased appreciation of the uniqueness, beauty, and frailty of life. God Bless.

Sincerely,

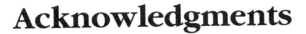

# Acknowledgments

**REVIEWERS.** I would like to thank the following educators and clinicians who carefully reviewed the first edition and offered many excellent suggestions for improvement.

Sylvia Austin, MEd, BS, RN
Department Head, Department of
   Practical Nursing
Bay Area Technical School
Ft. Walton Beach, Florida

Tracey A. Bergeron, MS, RNC
Maternal Child Health
Columbia/ HCA Portsmouth Regional
   Hospital
Portsmouth, New Hampshire

Veronica K. Casey, MA, RNC
School of Practical Nursing
J.M. Wright Technical School
Stamford, Connecticut

Eileen J. Colon, BSN, RN
School of Practical Nursing
Isothermal Community College
Spindale, North Carolina

JoAnne Jacobson, BSN, RN
Southern State Community College
Hillsboro, Ohio

Kathleen Jesiolowski, BSN, RN
School of Practical Nursing
Lebanon County Area Vocational-Technical
   School
Lebanon, Pennsylvania

Priscilla P. LaHann, BS, RN
School of Practical Nursing
Idaho State University
Pocatello, Idaho

Mary Patricia Norrell, BSN, RNC
School of Practical Nursing
Indiana Vocational Technical College
Columbus, Indiana

Bernice Rudolph, BS, RN, PHN
School of Vocational Nursing
Casa Loma College
Lake View Terrace, California

Mary P. Schapper, MS, RNC, PHN
School of Vocational Nursing
Hartnell College
Salinas, California

Sondra Smith, RN
School of Practical Nursing
Northwest Technical Institute
Springdale, Arkansas

Ann C. Stewart, BA, RNC
School of Practical Nursing
Washington State Community College
Marietta, Ohio

Judith M. Young, MSN, RN
Senior Staff Development Coordinator
Family and Ambulatory Services
Lankenau Hospital
Philadelphia, Pennsylvania

**CONTRIBUTORS.** I would also like to express my appreciation to Joan M. Croteau, MSN, MS, RN, for her contributions to both the first and second editions. I extend my appreciation to Emily Slone McKinney, MSN, RNC, our new contributor, for her thoroughness and careful attention to detail. I had the good fortune to be able to use line drawings from Emily's new book, *Foundations of Maternal-Newborn Nursing*. I would like to thank her coauthors, Trula Myers Gorrie, MN, RNC, and Sharon Smith Murray, MSN, RNC, as well as Emily for their care in making these drawings so remarkably easy to understand and follow.

**COLUMBIA/HCA PORTSMOUTH REGIONAL HOSPITAL.** To the many persons at Columbia/HCA Portsmouth Regional Hospital who were always happy to answer my questions, direct me to resources, and provide encouragement. Stanley Plodzik, Jr., MEd, RN, Assistant Administrator of Patient Services, gave permission to use photographs taken within the hospital. Darryl Hamson, Health Sciences Librarian, was an enormous help in obtaining articles for research and for searching out hard-to-find information. Jeanne Smallwood, RN, pediatric nurse; Tracey Bergeron, MS, RNC, maternity nurse; and Philip Hosmer, RRT, respiratory therapist, graciously helped me to meet my photography needs. Tracey also provided photographs from her work in the Dominican Republic.

**NURSE PRACTITIONER.** Geraldine DePrey, ARNP, nurse practitioner, Planned Parenthood of Northern New England, reviewed the section on contraceptives in Chapter 11.

**NUTRITIONIST.** Donna Sienknecht Larson, MS, RD, LD, Mercy Hospital Medical Center, Des Moines, Iowa, reviewed the nutrition segments. The Mercy Hospital Nutrition Specialists also provided permission for the use of the food plans for pregnant and lactating women.

**W.B. SAUNDERS COMPANY.** My first textbook published by W.B. Saunders Company, *Pediatrics for Practical Nurses*, came out in 1965. The release of this one marks over 30 years of writing! I would not have predicted such longevity. Ilze Rader, senior nursing editor, and Marie Thomas, editorial assistant, have accompanied and guided me since my fifth edition published in 1985. Many thanks for their expertise and cooperation.

My current developmental editor Leslie Fenton was also my copyeditor. We spent many hours on the telephone arranging and rearranging and coordinating materials. She was patient and friendly and did a great job of smoothing out the manuscript and getting things ready for production.

Jacqui Brownstein was the production manager. Time is of the essence when a book reaches production. There is a great deal of checking and proofreading of galleys and pages as the textbook begins to take shape.

Amy Norwitz, project supervisor, oversaw the book to completion.

The illustrations created by Melissa Walter, Marie Dean, and Gene Floersch add to the clarity and appeal of the material. Terri Wood was in charge of the Instructor's Guide.

**FAMILY.** My daughters, Justine and Julie, who posed for photographs as infants and children, are now adults. They grew up with "Mom working on her book." Little fingers that poked at typewriter keys now run their own computers. We have one 4-year-old grandson, Chad, who has replaced our daughters as a model and keeps us current on developmental issues. My husband Carl, who has been a continuous support throughout the years, makes a wonderful grandfather. From that very first day when I told him I was thinking about writing a textbook, he believed in my abilities. Everyone needs someone like that.

**INSTRUCTORS AND PRACTICAL NURSING STUDENTS.** Finally, I appreciate the confidence in the first edition of *Introduction to Maternity and Pediatric Nursing* shown by so many. Your enthusiasm and encouraging remarks provided the stimulus for the updating of this text.

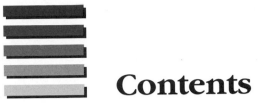

# Contents

# Unit 2   The Growing Child and Family

369

# Unit 1

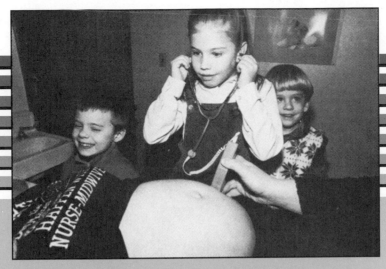

*Courtesy of Woman Care, Des Moines BirthPlace, Des Moines, IA.*

# Maternal-Newborn Nursing

# Part 1 Introduction

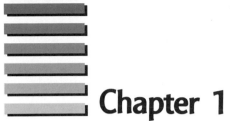

## Chapter 1

# History and Trends in Family-Centered Childbearing

## OBJECTIVES

*On completion and mastery of Chapter 1, the student will be able to*

■ Define each vocabulary term listed.
■ Discuss the contributions Ignaz Semmelweis made to maternal and child health care.
■ List two historical developments that affected maternity care.
■ State the medical contribution of Karl Credé.
■ Contrast present-day concepts of maternity care with those of the past.
■ Name three different health-care personnel who deliver babies.
■ List three environmental stresses on the childbearing family.
■ List four reasons why statistics are an important consideration in modern maternity care.
■ Discuss how one's culture affects childbirth.
■ List the five steps of the nursing process.

## History (Fig. 1–1)

The word *obstetrics* is derived from the Latin term *obstetrix*, which means "midwife." It is the branch of medicine that pertains to care of women during pregnancy, childbirth, and the postpartum period (puerperium). Maternity nursing is the care given by the nurse to the expectant family before, during, and following birth.

A physician specializing in the care of women during pregnancy, labor, birth, and the postpartum period is an *obstetrician*. These physicians perform cesarean deliveries and treat women with known or suspected obstetric problems as well as attend normal deliveries. Many family physicians and certified nurse-midwives also deliver babies. The skill and knowledge related to obstetrics have evolved over centuries.

### EUROPE

The earliest records concerning childbirth are in the Egyptian papyruses (circa 1550 BC). Later advances were made by Soranus, a Greek physician who practiced in 2nd-century Rome and who is known as the father of obstetrics. He instituted the practice of podalic version, a procedure used to rotate a fetus to a breech, or feet-first, position. Podalic version is important in delivering the second baby in a set of twins. In this procedure, the physician reaches into the uterus and grasps one or both of the baby's feet to facilitate delivery. Planned cesarean birth is safer and used more often today. Such scientific exploration halted with the decline of the Roman Empire and the ensuing Dark Ages.

During the 18th century, Karl Credé (1819–1892) and Ignaz Semmelweis (1818–1865) made contributions that have improved the safety and health of mother and child during and after childbirth. In 1884, Credé recommended instilling 2% silver nitrate to prevent blindness caused by gonorrhea in the newborn. This procedure has basically stayed the same, except that 1% silver nitrate is administered or antibiotic ointments are used. Credé's innovation has saved the eyesight of incalculable numbers of babies.

The classic story of Semmelweis is interesting and tragic. In the 1840s, he worked as an assistant professor in the maternity ward of the Vienna general hospital. There he discovered a

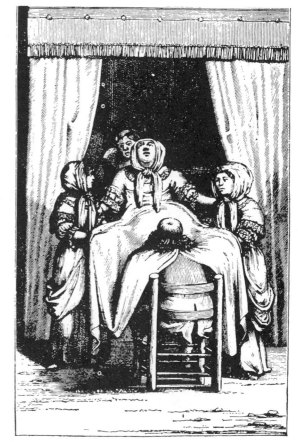

**Figure 1–1.** Doctor delivering under a sheet for modesty's sake.

relationship between the incidence of puerperal fever (or "childbed fever"), which caused many deaths among women in lying-in wards, and the examination of new mothers by student doctors who had just returned from dissecting cadavers. At that time, coincidentally, a colleague died of an infected cut from a contaminated scalpel. Semmelweis deduced that puerperal fever was septic, contagious, and transmitted by the *unwashed hands* of physicians and medical students.

By insisting on aseptic measures, such as handwashing with a chlorinated lime solution before examining patients, he reduced the maternal mortality rate due to puerperal fever at the Vienna hospital from 12.24% to 1.27% in 2 years. Nevertheless, he encountered great opposition and ridicule. Eventually he went into private practice, discouraged by his failure to convince the medical community of his innovative findings. His health failed, and he died in 1865 from a septic disease caused by infection from a cut on his hand.

Semmelweis' outstanding work, written in 1861, is titled *The Causes, Understanding, and Prevention of Childbed Fever*. Not until 1890 was his teaching finally accepted.

Louis Pasteur (1822–1895), a French chemist, confirmed that puerperal fever was caused by bacteria and could be spread by improper handwashing and contact with contaminated objects. The simple but highly effective procedure of handwashing continues to be one of the most important means of preventing the spread of infection in the hospital and home today. Joseph Lister (1827–1912), a British surgeon influenced by Pasteur, experimented with chemical means of preventing infection. He revolutionized surgical practice by introducing antiseptic surgery.

### UNITED STATES

The immigrants who reached the shores of America brought a wide variety of practices and beliefs about the birth process. Many practices were also contributed by the Native American nations. Most deliveries in the early United States were attended by a midwife or relative. One midwife, Samuel Bard, who was educated outside the United States, is credited with writing the first American textbook in obstetrics.

Oliver Wendell Holmes (1809–1894), when a young Harvard physician, wrote a paper detailing the contagiousness of puerperal fever, but

## Nursing Brief

Two nursing journals focusing on maternal and child health are the *Journal of Obstetric, Gynecologic, and Neonatal Nursing (JOGNN)* and the *American Journal of Maternal Child Nursing (MCN)*.

he, like Semmelweis, was widely criticized by his colleagues. Eventually, the "germ theory" became accepted, and more mothers and babies began to survive childbirth in the hospital.

Before the 1900s, most babies were born at home. Only very ill patients were cared for in lying-in hospitals. Maternal and child morbidity and mortality rates were high in such institutions because of crowded conditions and unskilled nursing care. Hospitals began to develop training programs for nurses. As the medical profession grew, physicians developed a closer relationship with hospitals. This, along with the advent of obstetric instruments and anesthesia, caused a shift to hospital care during childbirth. By the 1950s, hospital practice in obstetrics was well established. By 1970 more than 90% of births in the United States occurred in hospitals.

Organizations concerned with setting standards for maternity nursing developed. These include the American College of Nurse-Midwives (ACNM), the Association of Women's Health, Obstetric, and Neonatal Nurses (AWHONN), formerly the Nurses' Association of the American College of Obstetricians and Gynecologists (NAACOG), and the Division of Maternal Nursing within the American Nurses' Association.

## Current Trends

Significant changes have occurred in maternity care. In family-centered childbearing, the family is recognized as a unique system. Every family member is affected by the birth of a child. Family involvement during pregnancy and birth is seen as constructive and, indeed, necessary for bonding and support. To accommodate family needs, alternative birth centers, birthing rooms, rooming-in units, and mother-baby coupling have been developed. The whole sequence of events may take place in one suite of rooms. These arrangements are alternatives to the previously standard, separate areas of labor and delivery, which made it necessary to transport a mother from one area to another and fragmented her care.

Current maternity practice focuses on a high-quality family experience. *Childbearing is seen as a normal and healthy event.* Parents are prepared for the changes that take place during pregnancy, labor, and delivery. They are also prepared for the changes in family dynamics. Treating each family according to their individual needs is considered paramount.

During the 1950s, the hospital stay was 1 week. The current stay in uncomplicated cases is 2–3 days or less. Routine follow-up of the newborn takes place in about 2 weeks. A nurse visits the homes of infants and mothers who appear to be at high risk.

Procedural modifications for the nurse include the institution of universal precautions during delivery, during umbilical cord care, and in the nursery. More emphasis on data entry and retrieval makes it necessary for personnel to be computer-literate. The widespread use of per diem staffing may disrupt continuity of patient care, flow of information, and integration of the nurse as a team member. This pattern and the trend toward brief patient stays make communication among nurses and between nurses and families particularly essential. Spross notes that "in addition to being one minute managers, health care providers are now one minute nurses, doctors, social workers, and chaplains" (Hamric & Spross, 1989).

Sociologically, families have become smaller, the number of single parents is increasing, child and spouse abuse is rampant, and more mothers must work to help support the family. These developments present special challenges to maternal and child health nurses. Careful assessment and documentation to detect abuse are necessary, and nurses must be familiar with community support services for women and children in need. Nurses must also be flexible and promote policies that make health care more available for working parents. Teaching must be integrated into care plans and individually tailored to the family's needs and its cultural and ethnic background.

## MIDWIVES

Throughout history, women have played an important role as birth attendants or midwives. The first school of nurse-midwifery opened in New York City in 1932. There are now 35 accredited programs across the United States, all located in or affiliated with institutions of higher learning. They graduated over 400 new nurse-midwives in 1993, more than double the number in 1990 (American College of Nurse-Midwives, 1993). The certified nurse-midwife (CNM) is a registered nurse who has graduated from an accredited midwife program and is nationally certified by the American College of Nurse-Midwives (Fig. 1–2).

The CNM attends uncomplicated deliveries. Each patient must have a back-up physician who will accept her should a problem occur. CNMs attended 148,728 births in 1990, 139,229 in hospitals. Up to 70% of the care provided by CNMs is to women from traditionally underserved communities, and they play a major role in solving access problems in perinatal health-care services (American College of Nurse-Midwives, 1993).

## Nursing Brief

According to standards recommended by the American College of Obstetricians and Gynecologists, pregnant women should ideally make about 13 visits for prenatal care during the course of a normal, full-term pregnancy.

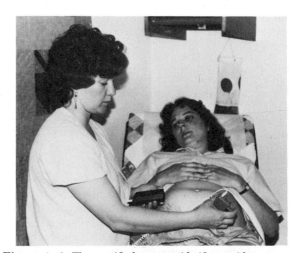

**Figure 1–2.** The certified nurse-midwife provides comprehensive maternity care for her clients.

## ROLE OF THE CONSUMER

Consumerism has played an important part in family-centered childbirth. In the early 1960s, the natural childbirth movement awakened expectant parents to the need for education and involvement. Prepared childbirth, La Leche League (breast feeding advocates), and Lamaze classes gradually became accepted. Parents began to question the routine use of anesthesia and the exclusion of fathers from delivery.

Today, a father's attendance at birth is commonplace. Visiting hours are liberal, and extended contact with the newborn is encouraged. The consumer continues to be an important instigator of change. Consumer groups, with the growing support of professionals, are helping to revise restrictive policies once thought necessary for safety. It has been demonstrated that informed parents can make wise decisions about their own care during this period if they are adequately educated and given professional support.

## CROSS-CULTURAL CONSIDERATIONS

The cultural background of the expectant family strongly influences its adaptation to the birth experience. In the United States, there are many diverse cultures, such as Asian (Chinese, Korean, Laotian, Vietnamese, and Cambodian), Mexican, Native American, Hawaiian, and African American. Table 1–1 depicts some childbearing patterns of several cultures. Each comes with its own heritage of beliefs, customs, religions, and health practices. Generalizing about cultural groups can lower the quality of care. This approach is often simplistic and does not account for individual differences within the group or the rate of an individual's assimilation into the mainstream. Nursing Care Plan 1–1 lists nursing interventions for selected diagnoses that pertain to cultural diversity.

One way in which the nurse gains important information about an individual's culture is to *ask the pregnant woman* what she considers normal practice. A summary of assessment questions might be

- How does the woman view her pregnancy (as an illness, a vulnerable time, or a healthy time)?
- Does she view the birth process as dangerous? Why?
- Is birth a public or private experience for her?
- In what position does she expect to deliver (i.e., squatting, lithotomy, or some other position)?
- What type of help does she need before and after delivery?
- What role does her immediate or extended family play in relation to the pregnancy and birth?

Such information helps promote understanding and individualizes patient care. It also increases the satisfaction of patient and nurse with the quality of care provided. Food preferences for various ethnic groups are given in Table 16–6.

## FINANCIAL AND GEOGRAPHIC CONSIDERATIONS

The ability of the pregnant woman to pay for services has a profound effect on the quality of services she receives. Private care providers, such as physicians and CNMs, usually work on a fee-for-services basis. They are usually eligible for insurance reimbursement (often referred to as "third-party pay"). Health maintenance organizations and other prepaid health plans offer a wide variety of services. The woman is provided care by a designated physician or clinic. Public health agencies and city and county hospitals, which depend on federal funding, usually treat, among others, persons with limited resources.

The geographic location of the pregnant woman has an important influence on the type of care received. Private care providers tend to be in urban areas rather than in rural or remote areas. Metropolitan areas offer a wide variety of services to those who can pay. However, the urban poor are often limited to a few clinics or to the city hospital; thus, the high-risk populations have fewer options. Private caregivers may lose money when reimbursed by federal health and welfare programs, as the lower rate of reimbursement frequently does not cover the expense of treatment. This creates many moral, ethical, and fiscal dilemmas.

## STATISTICS

*Statistics* refers to the process of gathering and analyzing numeric data. Health-related statistics, such as the number of births, deaths, and diseases (morbidity), provide valuable in-

**Table 1–1.** PERCENTAGE OF BIRTHS WITH SELECTED CHARACTERISTICS, BY RACE AND HISPANIC ORIGIN OF MOTHER: UNITED STATES, 1990

| Race/Ethnicity of Mother | Births to Mothers Aged <20 Years | Births to Mothers Aged ≥30 Years | Fourth and Higher-Order Births | Births to Unmarried Mothers | Mothers with ≥12 Years of School — All Ages | Mothers with ≥12 Years of School — Aged ≥20 Years | Mothers Born in U.S. | Mothers Who Began Prenatal Care in 1st Trimester | Mothers Who Had Late/No Prenatal Care | LBW[†] Infants | Preterm Infants[‡] |
|---|---|---|---|---|---|---|---|---|---|---|---|
| **Non-Hispanic** | | | | | | | | | | | |
| White | 9.6 | 33.5 | 8.0 | 16.9 | 84.8 | 89.6 | 95.8 | 83.3 | 3.4 | 5.6 | 8.5 |
| Black | 23.2 | 20.5 | 15.2 | 66.7 | 69.9 | 80.6 | 93.2 | 60.7 | 11.2 | 13.3 | 18.9 |
| **Hispanic§** | | | | | | | | | | | |
| Mexican American | 17.7 | 22.0 | 17.2 | 33.3 | 38.6 | 42.6 | 38.2 | 57.8 | 13.2 | 5.5 | 10.6 |
| Puerto Rican‖ | 21.7 | 19.0 | 13.2 | 55.9 | 57.2 | 66.4 | 56.7 | 63.5 | 10.6 | 9.0 | 13.4 |
| Cuban American | 7.7 | 34.0 | 6.0 | 18.2 | 82.1 | 86.5 | 20.6 | 84.8 | 2.8 | 5.7 | 9.8 |
| Central and South American | 9.0 | 32.0 | 12.5 | 41.2 | 55.8 | 58.8 | 4.4 | 61.5 | 10.9 | 5.8 | 10.9 |
| **Asian/Pacific Islander** | | | | | | | | | | | |
| Chinese American | 1.2 | 57.5 | 3.4 | 5.0 | 84.2 | 84.7 | 10.4 | 81.3 | 3.4 | 4.7 | 7.3 |
| Japanese American | 2.9 | 59.3 | 3.9 | 9.6 | 96.5 | 97.6 | 52.5 | 87.0 | 2.9 | 6.2 | 7.7 |
| Hawaiian | 18.4 | 21.6 | 15.8 | 45.0 | 80.7 | 87.9 | 96.0 | 65.8 | 8.7 | 7.2 | 11.3 |
| Filipino American | 6.1 | 46.3 | 7.3 | 15.9 | 89.7 | 92.1 | 15.4 | 77.1 | 4.5 | 7.3 | 11.4 |
| Other¶ | 6.3 | 39.4 | 14.6 | 12.6 | 73.1 | 76.0 | 6.3 | 71.9 | 7.1 | 6.6 | 10.6 |
| **American Indian/ Alaskan Native** | 19.5 | 21.3 | 22.6 | 53.6 | 63.6 | 71.3 | 96.5 | 57.9 | 12.9 | 6.1 | 11.8 |
| All** | 12.8 | 30.2 | 10.5 | 28.0 | 76.2 | 82.4 | 84.4 | 75.8 | 6.1 | 7.0 | 10.6 |

*Excludes data for New York (exclusive of New York City) and Washington state, which did not require reporting of educational attainment of mother.
†Low birth weight (≤2500 gm [5 lb, 8 oz]).
‡Born before 37 completed weeks of gestation.
§Persons of Hispanic origin may be of any race.
‖ Comprising persons of Puerto Rican origin residing in the 50 states and the District of Columbia.
¶ Comprising primarily Southeast Asian and Asian Indian Americans.
**Includes persons for whom origin was not stated.
From Childbearing patterns among selected racial/ethnic minority groups, United States, 1990. (1993). *Morbidity and Mortality Weekly Report, 42,* 401.

| NURSING CARE PLAN 1–1 | | |
|---|---|---|
| **Selected Nursing Diagnoses: Care of Childbearing Families Related to Potential or Actual Stress Caused by Cultural Diversity** | | |
| Goals | Nursing Interventions | Rationale |

**Nursing Diagnosis:** Communication, impaired verbal related to language barriers.

| Goals | Nursing Interventions | Rationale |
|---|---|---|
| Woman will have an opportunity to share information and states she understands what is explained to her | 1. Arrange for a family or staff member interpreter as needed | 1. Interpreter can provide support for woman and help lessen her anxieties; poor communication can result in time delays, errors, and misunderstanding of intent |
|  | 2. Clearly define instructions in woman's language of origin | 2. A shared language is necessary for communication to take place |
|  | 3. Provide written instructions in woman's language wherever possible | 3. Written instructions can be reviewed at less stressful time by client; in some cases it is necessary to determine if person can read |
|  | 4. Explain the use and purpose of all instruments and equipment, along with the effects or possible effects on the mother and fetus | 4. Education of family lessens anxiety and provides family with a sense of control |
|  | 5. Provide opportunities for clarification and questions | 5. Learning takes time; repetition of important material promotes learning; nurse can determine woman's understanding of information and clarify misconceptions |

**Nursing Diagnosis:** Family coping; compromised related to isolation, different customs, attitudes, or beliefs.

| Goals | Nursing Interventions | Rationale |
|---|---|---|
| Family members will state that they feel welcome and safe in the environment provided | 1. Encourage prenatal classes and a visit to the maternity unit before delivery | 1. Families who have clear, accurate information can better participate in labor and delivery; viewing the delivery setting before using it decreases anxiety about the unknown |
|  | 2. Inform families about routines, visiting hours, significant persons who can assist in labor and delivery, and location of newborn after delivery | 2. Families have different expectations of the health-care system; they may hesitate to ask questions because of shyness or fear of "losing face" |
|  | 3. Determine and respect practices and values of family and incorporate them into nursing care plans as much as possible | 3. Clarification of culturally specific values and practices will avoid misunderstanding and conflict with the nurse's value system; nursing care plans promote organization of care and communication among staff members |

formation for determining or projecting the needs of a population or subgroup and for predicting trends. In the United States, vital statistics are compiled for the country as a whole by the National Center for Health Statistics and are published in its annual report, *Vital Statistics of the United States*, and in the pamphlet *Monthly Vital Statistics*. Reports in this field are also issued by the various state bureaus of vital statistics. Other independent agencies also supply statistics on various specialties.

Lists and tables are compiled into graphs to clarify and consolidate information. An example of a birth rate graph is shown in Figure 1–3. A maternity nurse may use statistical data to become aware of reproductive trends, to determine populations at risk, to evaluate the quality of prenatal care, or to compare relevant information from state to state and country to

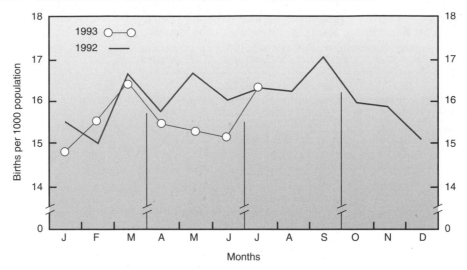

**Figure 1–3.** Provisional birth rates per 1000 population by month: United States, 1992–1993. (Redrawn from National Center for Health Statistics. [1994]. Births, marriages, divorces and deaths for July 1993. *Monthly Vital Statistics Report, 42.*)

country. Box 1–1 lists some terms used in gathering vital statistics.

**Birth Rate.** According to provisional reports, an estimated 4,043,000 births occurred in the 12-month period ending with July 1993, a decline of 2% for the same period 1 year earlier. The birth rate of 15.7 per 1000 was 3% lower than the rate of 16.2 per 1000 for the preceding 12 months (Table 1–2).

**Maternal Mortality Rate.** The *maternal mortality rate* in the United States for 1991 was 7.9 deaths per 100,000 live births, compared with a rate of 8.2 per 100,000 in 1990. African-American (black) women have a higher mortality rate than do Caucasian (white) women (Table 1–3).

Factors influencing the decrease include the development of obstetrics and gynecology as a medical specialty, hospitalization, advent of antibiotics to control infection, improvements in medical and surgical techniques, development of high-risk centers for mother and baby, and improvements in anesthesia.

**Infant Mortality Rate.** The *infant mortality rate* refers to the number of deaths of infants under 1 year of age per 1000 live births. The infant mortality rate of a country indicates the general health of its people. In the United States, the infant mortality rate for the 12 months ending with June 1993 was 8.4 (Fig. 1–4). It is inconsistent from state to state, and the decline for

Caucasians is higher than for African Americans. Improvements in the infant mortality rate have been slower than improvements in maternal mortality. Table 1–4 ranks the causes of infant mortality for children under 1 year of age. The mortality rates of children older than 1 year of age are depicted in Table 1–5.

The United States infant mortality rate continues to lag behind several nations that record

---

**BOX 1–1** | **Common Vital Statistics Terms**

**Birth rate:** The number of births per 1000 population

**Fertility rate:** The number of births per 1000 women ages 15–44 yr in a given population

**Maternal mortality rate:** The number of maternal deaths per 100,000 live births that occurs as a direct result of pregnancy (includes the 42-day postpartum period)

**Neonatal mortality:** The number of deaths of infants less than 28 days of age per 1000 live births

**Fetal mortality:** The number of fetal deaths (fetuses weighing 500 gm or more) per 1000 live births

**Perinatal mortality:** Includes both fetal and neonatal deaths per 1000 live births

**Table 1–2.** PROVISIONAL VITAL STATISTICS FOR THE UNITED STATES

| Item | July Number 1993 | July Number 1992 | July Rate 1993 | July Rate 1992 | January to July Number 1993 | January to July Number 1992 | January to July Rate 1993 | January to July Rate 1992 | 12 Months Ending with July Number 1993 | 12 Months Ending with July Number 1992 | 12 Months Ending with July Rate 1993 | 12 Months Ending with July Rate 1992 |
|---|---|---|---|---|---|---|---|---|---|---|---|---|
| Live births | 357,000 | 352,000 | 16.3 | 16.3 | 2,333,000 | 2,375,000 | 15.6 | 16.0 | 4,043,000 | 4,107,000 | 15.7 | 16.2 |
| Fertility rate | — | — | 71.2 | 70.5 | — | — | 68.0 | 69.2 | — | — | 68.5 | 69.6 |
| Deaths | 184,000 | 180,000 | 8.4 | 8.3 | 1,344,000 | 1,294,000 | 9.0 | 8.7 | 2,227,000 | 2,179,000 | 8.7 | 8.6 |
| Infant deaths | 2,800 | 2,800 | 7.8 | 8.1 | 19,900 | 20,500 | 8.5 | 8.6 | 33,800 | 35,000 | 8.4 | 8.6 |
| Natural increase | 173,000 | 172,000 | 7.9 | 8.0 | 989,000 | 1,081,000 | 6.6 | 7.3 | 1,816,000 | 1,928,000 | 7.0 | 7.6 |
| Marriages | 236,000 | 228,000 | 10.8 | 10.5 | 1,295,000 | 1,313,000 | 8.7 | 8.8 | 2,343,000 | 2,368,000 | 9.1 | 9.3 |
| Divorces | 103,000 | 109,000 | 4.7 | 5.1 | 697,000 | 715,000 | 4.7 | 4.8 | 1,196,000 | 1,206,000 | 4.7 | 4.7 |
| Population base (in millions) | — | — | 257.9 | 255.1 | — | — | — | — | — | — | 256.7 | 253.9 |

Rates for infant deaths are deaths under 1 year per 1000 live births; fertility rates are live births per 1000 women aged 15–44 years; all other rates are per 1000 total population.

From National Center for Health Statistics. (1994). Births, marriages, divorces, and deaths for July 1993. *Monthly Vital Statistics Report, 42,* 1.

**Table 1–3.** MATERNAL DEATHS AND MATERNAL
MORTALITY RATES BY RACE:
UNITED STATES, 1991

| Race | Rate |
| --- | --- |
| All races | 7.9 |
| White | 5.8 |
| All other | 15.6 |
| Black | 18.3 |

Maternal deaths are those assigned to complications of pregnancy, childbirth, and the puerperium, category numbers 630–676 of the *Ninth Revision International Classification of Diseases*, 1975. Rates per 100,000 live births.
From National Center for Health Statistics. (1993). Advance report of final mortality statistics, 1991. *Monthly Vital Statistics Report, 42* (Suppl. 2).

statistics, particularly the Scandinavian countries and Japan. Figure 1–5 compares infant mortality rates for Canada, Japan, the United Kingdom, and the United States. It is disturbing that many other countries, often with fewer resources, have progressed more rapidly in decreasing infant mortality. Four factors contributing to this discrepancy are the high rate of adolescent pregnancy, unequal access to care, premature births, and poverty. The nation is on the brink of health-care reform at this writing.

Nurses must become involved in supporting policies that will promote better, more accessible, and fairer distribution of health care.

In many developing nations children who do not die at birth are still at high risk during their early years. UNICEF's "The State of the World's Children, 1992" (Grant, 1992) directs attention not only to infant mortality but to the very high death rates among preschool children in developing countries. "Forty-two percent of the world's births are estimated to have occurred in countries with under-5 mortality rates of more than 140 per 1000. The median under-5 mortality rate for those countries in 1990 was 189 per 1000, meaning that almost 20% of their infants that were born alive died before their fifth birthday, mortality levels not seen in the U.S. in this century." (Wegman, 1993). Nurses and other medical personnel often participate in international programs to assist in improving health-care conditions in impovished countries (see Figs. 1–6 to 1–8).

## ROLE OF THE MATERNITY NURSE

The maternity nurse is a team member who assists and provides safe, confidential, and

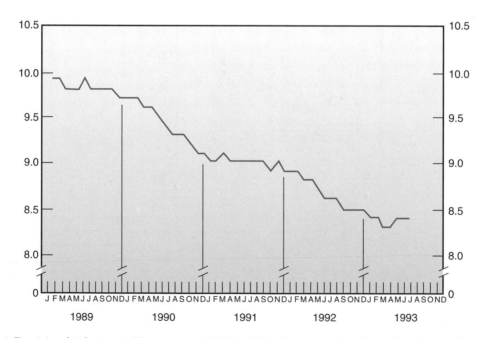

**Figure 1–4.** Provisional infant mortality rates per 1000 live births for successive 12-month periods ending with month indicated: United States, 1989–1993. (Redrawn from National Center for Health Statistics. [1994]. Births, marriages, divorces and deaths for July 1993. *Monthly Vital Statistics Report, 42.*)

**Table 1–4.** TEN LEADING CAUSES OF DEATHS IN INFANTS UNDER 1 YEAR: ALL RACES

Congenital anomalies
Sudden infant death syndrome
Prematurity and low birth weight
Respiratory distress syndrome
Maternal complications of pregnancy affecting newborn
Complications of placenta, cord, and membranes
Accidents
Infections
Pneumonia and influenza
Intrauterine hypoxia and birth asphyxia

From National Center for Health Statistics. (1993). Advance report of final mortality statistics, 1991. *Monthly Vital Statistics Report, 42* (Suppl. 2).

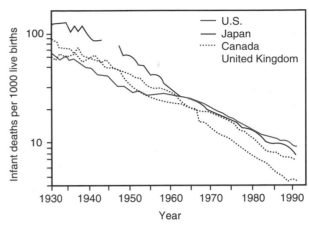

**Figure 1–5.** Comparison of infant mortality rates: Canada, Japan, United Kingdom, United States, 1930–1991. (Redrawn from Wegman, M.E. [1993]. Annual summary of vital statistics—1992. *Pediatrics, 92*, 743.)

state-of-the-art care to childbearing families. Health promotion and anticipatory guidance are of particular value in interacting with very young parents. Maternity nurses are especially active in teaching. Determining the resources of the family and the community is important in planning discharge. Nurses collaborate with physicians, other nurses, social workers, and numerous other professionals and nonprofessionals. This requires flexibility.

The complexities of the modern hospital are a challenge to even the most experienced nurse. *Nurses must support and assist one another.* Ongoing education is necessary to keep abreast of rapid developments in technology and in legal and ethical issues. Accountability is essential as the role of the maternity nurse continues to expand. Involvement in state and national organizations helps extend the nurse's horizons, provides for exchange of information with peers, and promotes growth in the profession.

**Table 1–5.** LEADING CAUSES OF DEATH AGES 1–24 YEARS, 1991: ALL RACES, BOTH SEXES*

| Cause | 1–4 Years | 5–14 Years | 15–24 Years |
|---|---|---|---|
| All causes | 47.4 | 23.6 | 100.1 |
| Accidents and adverse effects | 17.5 | 10.2 | 42.0 |
| Motor vehicle | 5.9 | 5.6 | 32.0 |
| All other | 11.6 | 4.6 | 9.9 |
| Congenital anomalies | 5.7 | 1.4 | 1.2 |
| Malignant neoplasms | 3.5 | 3.1 | 5.0 |
| Homicide | 2.8 | 1.4 | 22.4 |
| Suicide | | 0.7 | 13.1 |
| Heart disease | 2.2 | 0.8 | 2.7 |
| Pneumonia and influenza | 1.4 | 0.4 | 0.7 |
| Human immunodeficiency virus | 1.0 | 0.3 | 1.7 |
| Perinatal conditions | 0.9 | | |
| Septicemia | 0.6 | | |
| Chronic obstructive pulmonary disease | | 0.3 | 0.6 |
| Cerebrovascular disease | | 0.2 | 0.6 |

*Rate per 100,000.
Data from National Center for Health Statistics. (1993). Advance report of final mortality statistics, 1991. *Monthly Vital Statistics Report, 42.*

## NURSING PROCESS

The nursing process is a method of identifying and solving problems that includes five steps: assessment, diagnosis, planning, implementation, and evaluation. In maternity nursing, the mother and family are the focus. In the assessment stage, subjective and objective data are gathered from the mother and family. The nursing diagnosis is determined by analyzing the gathered data. Each nursing diagnosis describes actual or potential health problems. These direct the nursing care plan. Diagnoses approved by the North American Nursing Diagnosis Association (NANDA) are found in Appendix H. Table 1–6 differentiates between

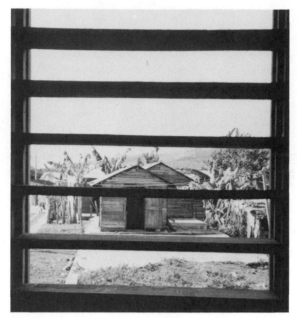

**Figure 1–6.** A view from a rural clinic in a third-world country.

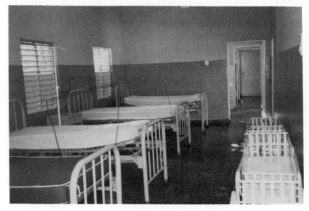

**Figure 1–8.** The maternity unit of a third-world country. Patients provide their own bed linens. There is no running water.

medical and nursing diagnoses. In many hospitals, the defining characteristics ("evidenced or manifested by . . .") are not recorded on the care plan as they are in the patient's chart. Goals are developed and prioritized in the planning stage. During the implementation stage, interventions specify the nursing care to be carried out. Many skills used in maternity care are specific, but some are common to other areas of nursing (such as blood pressure measurement). Finally, the nurse evaluates what has been accomplished in relation to the goals set. Although this is a logical end step, the nurse actually evaluates throughout the nursing process by asking, "Is this working? If not, should I reassess?"

## NURSING CARE PLAN

The nursing care plan is developed as a result of the nursing process. It is a written instrument of communication among staff members that focuses on individualized patient care. Sample care plans for maternity and pediatric nursing are provided throughout the text.

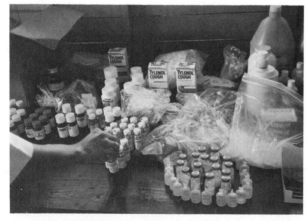

**Figure 1–7.** Having traveled for many hours into the mountainous regions, the maternal-child nurse organizes medications for distribution.

**Table 1–6.** COMPARISON OF MEDICAL AND NURSING DIAGNOSES

| Medical Diagnosis | Nursing Diagnosis |
| --- | --- |
| AIDS | Nutrition: Less than body requirements related to (R/T) anorexia and evidenced by weight loss |
| Gestational Diabetes | Knowledge deficit (R/T) effects of diabetes mellitus on pregnant woman and fetus, manifested by crying, anxious effect. |
| Cystic Fibrosis | Ineffective airway clearance (R/T) mucus accumulation manifested by rales, fatigue |

## KEY POINTS

- In 1840, Semmelweis suggested that handwashing was an important concept in preventing infection. This simple procedure is still a cornerstone of nursing care.
- The certified nurse-midwife is a registered nurse who has advanced education and is nationally certified by the American College of Nurse-Midwives.
- The cultural background of the expectant family plays an important role in their adaptation to the birth experience.
- The educational focus for the childbearing family is that childbirth is a normal and healthy event.
- *Statistics* refers to gathering and analyzing numeric data.
- *Birth rate* refers to the number of births per 1000 population.
- *Maternal mortality rate* refers to the number of maternal deaths per 100,000 live births that occur as a direct result of pregnancy.
- In the United States, vital statistics are compiled for the country as a whole by the National Center for Health Statistics.
- Nurses must be concerned for the families of the world. In many countries, mothers still deliver babies under impoverished conditions.
- The nursing process consists of five steps: assessment, nursing diagnosis, planning, implementation, and evaluation. It is an organized method of nursing practice and a means of communication among staff members.

# Study Questions

1. What was Karl Credé's contribution to obstetrics?
2. Name two factors that contributed to the shift from home deliveries to hospital deliveries.
3. What role has the consumer played in maternity care practices?
4. Of what importance are statistics to the field of maternal-child health care?

# Multiple Choice Review Questions

*Choose the most appropriate answer.*

1. Which of the following persons advocated handwashing to reduce puerperal fever?
   a. Credé
   b. Semmelweis
   c. Lister
   d. Hippocrates
2. A physician specializing in the care of the woman during pregnancy is called
   a. an obstetrician
   b. a pediatrician
   c. a cardiologist
   d. a dermatologist
3. The number of deaths of infants younger than 28 days of age per 1000 live births is termed
   a. birth rate
   b. neonatal mortality rate
   c. fertility rate
   d. maternal mortality rate

4. The quality of care a mother receives is influenced mainly by
   a. relationships
   b. ethnic background
   c. ability to pay
   d. cultural beliefs

5. The focus of today's maternity care is on the
   a. patient
   b. family
   c. neonate
   d. hospital

## BIBLIOGRAPHY

American College of Nurse-Midwives. (1993). *Educating nurse-midwives*. Washington, DC. By American College of Nurse Midwives.

Black, J.M., & Matassarin-Jacobs, E. (1993). *Luckmann and Sorensen's medical-surgical nursing: A psychophysiologic approach* (4th ed.). Philadelphia: W.B. Saunders.

Centers for Disease Control. (1993). Childbearing patterns among selected racial/ethnic minority groups, United States, 1990. *Morbidity and Mortality Weekly Report, 42,* 20.

Grant, J. (1992). *The state of the world's children*. New York: UNICEF.

Hamric, A.B., & Spross, J.A. (1989). *The clinical nurse specialist in theory and practice* (2nd ed.). Philadelphia: W.B. Saunders.

Ladewig, P.W., London, M.L., & Olds, S.B. (1994). *Essentials of maternal-newborn nursing* (3rd ed.). Reading, MA: Addison-Wesley Nursing.

National Center for Health Statistics. (1992, September). Annual summary of births, deaths, marriages and divorces, United States, 1991. *Monthly Vital Statistics Report.*

National Center for Health Statistics (1993). Advanced report of final mortality statistics, 1991. *Monthly Vital Statistics Report, 42.*

Olds, S.B., London, M.L., & Ladewig, P.W. (1992). *Maternal-newborn nursing* (4th ed.). Reading, MA: Addison-Wesley.

Pillitteri, A. (1992). *Maternal and child health nursing*. Philadelphia: J.B. Lippincott.

Wegman, M. (1993). Annual summary of vital statistics—1992. *Pediatrics, 92.*

# Chapter 2

# Human Reproduction

## OBJECTIVES

Human reproduction is a phenomenon that may follow sexual intercourse between a woman and a man. This chapter describes the anatomy and physiology of the male and female reproductive systems and how a new life develops within the uterus.

## Puberty

Puberty is a period of rapid change in the lives of boys and girls during which the reproductive systems mature and become capable of reproduction.

This transition from childhood to adulthood has been identified and often celebrated by various rites of passage. Some cultures have required demonstrations of bravery, such as hunting wild animals or displays of self-defense. Ritual circumcision has been another rite of passage. In the United States today, some adolescents participate in religious ceremonies such as bar/bat mitzvah or confirmation, but for others, these ceremonies are unfamiliar. The lack of a "universal rite of passage" to identify adulthood has led to confusion for many adolescents.

Before and during the development of sexual characteristics, adolescent boys and girls experience sudden increases in height and weight. In the boy, this growth spurt begins at about 12 years of age, when the genitals start to increase in size and the shoulders begin to broaden and become muscular. In the girl between 9 and 11 years of age, the hips start to broaden, and feminine curves begin to appear. Adipose (fatty) tissue is formed, especially at the breasts (see Fig. 21–4B).

Secondary sexual characteristics develop as testosterone in the boy and estrogen in the girl are released. Boys develop secondary sexual characteristics more slowly and later than girls do. In addition to pubic and axillary (armpit) hair, the boy experiences an increase in size of penis and testes, voice changes, facial hair, erections, and nocturnal emissions; the girl experiences breast development, vaginal secretions, and menarche. (See Chapter 21, pp. 519–522, for further discussion of puberty.)

## Male Reproductive System

The male reproductive system is made of external and internal organs (Fig. 2–1). The male and female systems must be anatomically and physiologically functional in order for healthy sperm to fertilize a mature ovum.

### EXTERNAL GENITALIA

There are two external male organs, the penis and the scrotum.

**Penis.** The penis, made of the glans and the body, is the organ of copulation. The glans is the round, most distal end of the penis. It is visible on a circumcised penis but is not readily seen on an uncircumcised one. At the tip of the glans is an opening called the urethral meatus. The body of the penis contains the urethra (the passageway for sperm and urine), which lies within the corpus spongiosum, and two corpora cavernosa.

The cavernosa muscles contract in response to sexual stimulation. This action traps venous blood within the rich network of blood vessels of the corpora cavernosa, and the engorgement results in erection of the penis. The penis has two functions. One function is to deposit sperm into the vagina for fertilization. Its other function is to expel urine through the urethra and its meatus.

**Scrotum.** The scrotum is a sac that protects the male gonads (testes). The scrotum is suspended from the perineum, keeping the testes away from the body and thereby lowering their

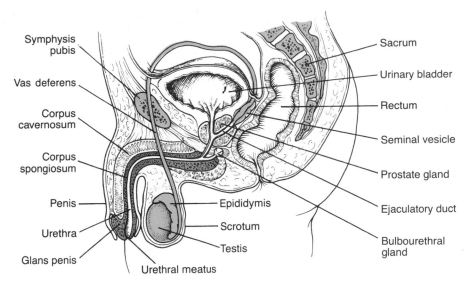

**Figure 2–1.** The male reproductive organs.

temperature. This cooling is necessary to the production of sperm (spermatogenesis).

## INTERNAL GENITALIA

The internal genitalia include the testes, ducts, and accessory glands.

**Testes.** The testes (testicles) are a pair of oval, compound organs housed in the scrotum. They have two important functions: manufacture of male reproductive germ cells (spermatozoa, or sperm) and secretion of male hormones (androgens).

The production of sperm, called spermatogenesis, occurs by means of a special type of cell division and is further described in Chapter 3. Sperm are made in the convoluted semen-producing (seminiferous) tubules that make up the 250–400 lobules of the testes. Sperm production begins at puberty and continues throughout the life span of the male.

The production of *testosterone*, the most abundant male hormone, begins with the anterior pituitary gland. Under the "direction" of the hypothalamus, it secretes follicle-stimulating hormone (FSH) and luteinizing hormone (LH). FSH and LH initiate the production of testosterone in the Leydig cells of the testes. Testosterone increases muscle mass, promotes strength and growth of long bones, and enhances production of red blood cells, which result in the greater strength and stature and higher hematocrit level in males, compared with females. Testosterone also increases pro-

duction of sebum, a fatty secretion of the sebaceous glands of the skin, and may contribute to development of acne. Male hormonal activity continues throughout life.

**Ducts.** An epididymis, one from each testicle, is the beginning of the duct system that stores and carries the sperm. The sperm may remain in the epididymis for 2–10 days, where they mature, and then move on to the vasa deferens (ductus deferens). Each vas deferens is approximately 40 cm (16 inches) long. As seen in Figure 2–1, each vas deferens passes upward into the body, goes around the symphysis pubis, circles the bladder, and passes downward to form, with the ducts from the seminal vesicles, the ejaculatory ducts. The ejaculatory ducts then enter the back of the prostate gland and end in the upper part of the urethra.

**Accessory Glands.** The accessory glands produce seminal plasma (secretions) that provides for both protection and motility of the sperm. The accessory glands are the *seminal vesicles*, the *prostate gland*, and the *bulbourethral glands*. The seminal vesicles are two glands between the bladder and rectum and above the prostate; they secrete a yellow fluid rich in fructose, amino acids, and prostaglandins. The prostate gland lies just below the bladder and surrounds the upper part of the urethra. It secretes a thin, milky, alkaline fluid that aids sperm mobility and helps protect sperm from the acidic vaginal environment. The bulbourethral (Cowper's) glands are two small glands just below the prostate, one on each side of the middle part of the urethra; they secrete a mucinous substance.

The seminal plasma and sperm together are called *semen*. Semen may be secreted during sexual intercourse before ejaculation. Therefore, pregnancy may occur even if ejaculation takes place outside the vagina.

# Female Reproductive System

The female reproductive system consists of external genitalia, internal genitalia, and accessory structures, namely the bony pelvis and mammary glands (breasts).

### EXTERNAL GENITALIA

The female external genitalia are called the *vulva* or *pudenda*. They include the mons pubis, labia majora, labia minora, fourchette, clitoris, vaginal vestibule, urethral meatus, vaginal introitus, and perineum (Fig. 2–2).

The *mons pubis* (mons veneris) is a pad of fatty tissue covered by coarse skin. It protects the symphysis pubis and contributes to the rounded contour of the female body. Short curly hair, called the pubic escutcheon, develops on the skin at puberty.

The *labia majora* are two protective folds of adipose tissue on each side of the vaginal vestibule. Many small glands are located on the moist interior surface. At puberty, the skin develops hair.

The *labia minora* are two thin, soft folds of erectile tissue that are seen when the labia majora are separated. The connective tissue that makes up the labia minora contains sebaceous glands that open directly onto the skin's surface. The secretions from these glands are bactericidal, and they also lubricate and protect the skin of the vulva.

The *fourchette* is a fold of tissue just below the vagina, where the labia majora and the labia minora meet. Lacerations during childbirth often occur in that area.

The *clitoris* is a small erectile body in the most anterior portion of the labia minora. It is similar in structure to the penis. Functionally, it is the most erotic, sensitive part of the female genitalia, and it produces smegma. Smegma is a cheeselike secretion of the sebaceous glands and has a characteristic, sensual odor.

The vaginal vestibule is the area seen when the labia minora are separated. There are four

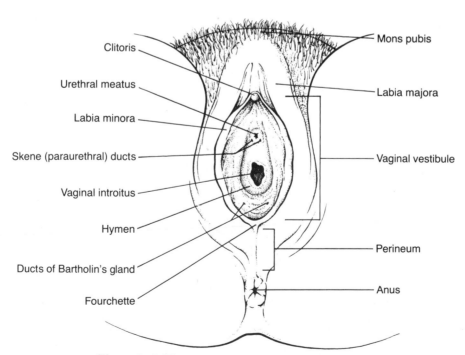

**Figure 2–2.** The external female reproductive organs.

Clitoris

Urethral meatus

Labia minora

Skene (paraurethral) ducts

Vaginal introitus

Hymen

Ducts of Bartholin's gland

Fourchette

Mons pubis

Labia majora

Vaginal vestibule

Perineum

Anus

openings: urethral meatus, vaginal introitus, and two ducts of Bartholin glands. The *urethral meatus* is approximately 2 cm below the clitoris. It has a foldlike appearance with a slit-type opening, and it serves as the exit for urine. On either side of the urethra are *Skene's ducts* (paraurethral ducts), which provide lubrication for the urethra and may be sites for infection. The *vaginal introitus* is the external portion of the vagina. The external vagina is separated from the internal vagina by the hymen. The *hymen* is a thin elastic membrane that is normally open to permit entry of a tampon or a fingertip without pain or bleeding. The ducts of Bartholin glands (vulvovaginal glands) open into the vaginal introitus. They produce clear, viscid (sticky) mucous secretions. The alkaline pH of these secretions enhances viability and motility of sperm deposited in the vaginal vestibule (Olds et al., 1992). They may also be the site of bacterial infection.

The *perineum* is a strong, muscular area below the vaginal opening and in front of the anus. The elastic fibers and connective tissue within the muscles allow for generous stretching to permit delivery of a full-term infant. The perineum is the site of the episiotomy (surgical incision) or tears during delivery. Correct repair is essential; otherwise, pelvic weakness or painful intercourse (dyspareunia) may result.

## INTERNAL GENITALIA

The internal organs are the vagina, uterus, fallopian tubes, and ovaries. Figure 2–3 illustrates the side view of these organs, and Figure 2–4 illustrates the frontal view.

**Vagina.** The vagina, beyond the hymen, is a tubelike structure made of muscle and membrane tissue that connects the external genitalia to the midpelvis. Because it meets at a right angle with the cervix, the anterior wall is about 2.5 cm (1 inch) shorter than the posterior wall, which varies from 7 to 10 cm (approximately 2.8 to 4 inches). The marked stretching of the vagina during delivery is made possible by the *rugae* or transverse ridges of the mucous membrane lining. The vagina is self-cleansing and, during the reproductive years, maintains a normal pH of 4–5. Within this range, the pH is lowest at midcycle and highest premenstrually. The self-cleansing activity may be altered by antibiotic therapy, by frequent douching and indiscriminate use of vaginal sprays, or by deodorant sanitary pads or deodorant tampons.

The vagina (1) functions as an organ for intercourse, (2) provides for the drainage of menstrual fluids and other secretions that protect the woman from infection, and (3) provides a passageway for delivery of the newborn.

**Uterus.** The uterus (womb) is a hollow muscular organ in which a fertilized ovum is implanted, an embryo develops, and a fetus is nourished. It is shaped like a pear or lightbulb. In a mature, nonpregnant female, it weighs approximately 60 gm (2 ounces) and is 7.5 cm (3 inches) long, 5 cm (2 inches) wide, and 1–2.5 cm (0.4–1 inch) thick. The uterus is in the center of the pelvic cavity, between the bladder and

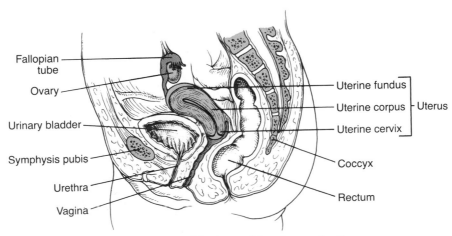

**Figure 2–3.** Side view of the internal female reproductive organs.

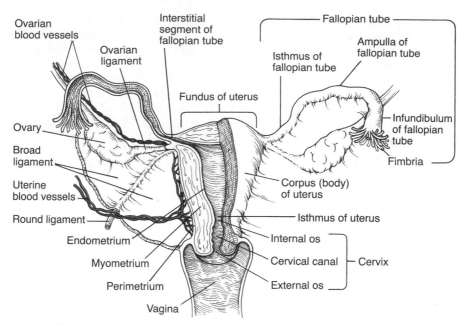

**Figure 2–4.** Frontal view of the internal female reproductive organs.

the rectum. It is supported by ligaments, two major ones being the round and broad ligaments. When these become stretched during pregnancy, discomfort and backache may result.

***Blood and Nerve Supply.*** The chief supply of blood to the uterus is the bilateral uterine arteries, which branch off the hypogastric (internal iliac) arteries, and the ovarian arteries, which branch off the descending aorta. A unique and highly oxygenated vascular network supplies the entire uterus.

The autonomic nervous system innervates the entire uterus. During labor, pain from the cervix and upper vagina passes to the central nervous system through the ilioinguinal and pudendal nerves. The 11th and 12th thoracic nerve roots carry the pain of the uterine contractions to the central nervous system.

***Anatomy.*** The uterus is separated into three parts: fundus, corpus, and cervix.

The *fundus* (upper part) is broad and flat. The fallopian tubes enter the uterus on each

## Nursing Brief

The self-cleansing function of the vagina is emphasized in teaching women about feminine hygiene.

side of the fundus. The *corpus* (body) is the middle portion, and it plays an active role in menstruation and pregnancy. The *cervix* (lower part) is narrow and tubular and opens downward into the distal end of the vagina, where it is permanently anchored. The portion of the uterus that joins the corpus to the cervix is called the isthmus and during pregnancy is referred to as the lower uterine segment.

The fundus and corpus have three distinct layers: the perimetrium (the outermost or serosal layer), the myometrium (the middle muscular layer), and the endometrium (the inner or mucosal layer). The perimetrium envelops the entire uterus. The myometrium, the functional unit in pregnancy and labor, has three involuntary muscle layers: a longitudinal outer layer, a figure-eight interlacing middle layer, and circular inner muscle fibers that form sphincters at the fallopian tube attachments and at the internal opening of the cervix. These muscles function as a single unit to efface and dilate the cervix and to expel the fetus through the pelvis and vaginal canal. The endometrium, the functional unit in menstruation and implantation (conception), is governed by cyclic hormonal changes.

The cervix connects the vagina and the uterus. It consists of a cervical canal with an in-

## Nursing Brief

An excellent opportunity for the nurse to reinforce women's learning about the protective functions of the cervix is during examinations such as the Papanicolaou (Pap) smear and while discussing family planning.

ternal opening near the corpus, called the internal os, and an opening at the distal end of the vagina (visible during gynecologic examination), called the external os. The mucosal lining of the cervix has four functional activities: (1) it lubricates the vagina; (2) it acts as a bacteriostatic agent; (3) it provides an alkaline environment to shelter deposited sperm from the acidic pH of the vagina; and (4) it produces a mucous plug in the cervical canal during pregnancy. At ovulation, cervical mucus is clear, viscous, and alkaline.

**Fallopian Tubes.** The Fallopian tubes, also called uterine tubes or oviducts, are slender, multilayered tubes extending laterally from the uterus, one to each ovary (see Fig. 2–4). They vary in length from 8 to 13.5 cm (3 to 5.3 inches) and link the peritoneal cavity to the outside of the female body.

Each tube comprises four parts: interstitial portion, isthmus, ampulla, and infundibulum. The isthmus is a thick, muscular area, nearest to the uterus. It is the usual site for tubal ligation (a sterilization technique). The ampulla, a thin, stretchable tubal muscle, makes up two-thirds of the tube and is the usual site of fertilization. The funnel-like enlarged distal end of the tube is called the infundibulum. The moving, finger-like projections are called *fimbriae*. They hover over each ovary and "capture" the egg as it is released by the ovary at ovulation. It takes approximately 5 days for the ovum to reach the uterus.

The four functions of the fallopian tubes are to provide (1) a passageway in which sperm meet the ovum, (2) a site of fertilization, (3) a safe, nourishing environment for the ovum or zygote (fertilized egg), and (4) a means of transporting the ovum or zygote to the corpus of the uterus.

The four functions are made possible by the muscular and mucosal layers. The muscular layer provides peristaltic movement of each

tube, which is affected by hormonal action during the menstrual cycle. The mucosal layer is activated by (1) cells with cilia that constantly move to create a current toward the uterus, and (2) nonciliated cells, called goblet cells, which secrete protein-rich fluid to nourish the ovum.

**Ovaries.** The ovaries are two almond-shaped glands, each about the size of a walnut. They are in the lower abdominal cavity, one on each side of the uterus. The two ovarian ligaments connect the ovaries to the lateral uterine walls (see Fig. 2–4). The functions of the ovaries are ovulation and secretion of hormones, chiefly estrogen and progesterone. Each ovary has three layers: (1) the tunica albuginea—the dense, dull white protective layer; (2) the cortex—the major functional layer, containing follicles in various stages of development and degeneration; and (3) the medulla—the innermost layer surrounded by cortex. It contains nerves, blood vessels, and lymph vessels.

At birth, every baby girl has all the egg cells (oocytes) that will be available during her reproductive years (approximately 2 million cells). These degenerate significantly so that by adulthood the remaining oocytes number in the thousands. Of these, only a small percentage are actually ovulated. Oogenesis (formation and development of the ovum) does not occur after fetal development. Almost 400 mature ova are extruded during the reproductive years.

### FEMALE PELVIS

The pelvis is the lower portion of the trunk of the body. It is formed by four bones: two innominate bones (os coxae), sacrum, and coccyx. Each innominate bone is made up of an ilium, pubis, and ischium, which are separate during childhood and fused by adulthood. The ilium is the lateral, flaring portion of the hip bone; the pubis is the anterior hip bone. These two bones join to form the symphysis pubis. The ischium is inferior to the ilium—its significant feature is the ischial spine (Fig. 2–5). An ischial spine, one from each ischium, juts inward, toward the pelvic outlet, and forms the shortest diameter of the pelvic cavity.

The posterior segment of the pelvis consists of the sacrum and coccyx. Five fused, triangular vertebrae at the base of the spine are called the sacrum. Below the sacrum is a small bone formed by the union of four rudimentary vertebrae; this is called the coccyx.

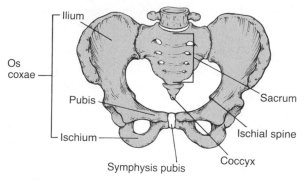

**Figure 2–5.** Frontal view of the female pelvis.

linea terminalis, has three obstetrically important diameters—anteroposterior, transverse, and right and left oblique. The anteroposterior diameter is between the symphysis pubis and the sacrum. It is the shortest one, and it can hinder fetal entry into the inlet if it is inadequate. Transverse diameter is measured across the linea terminalis and is the largest diameter. Right oblique diameter is measured from the right sacroiliac joint to the prominence of the linea terminalis. Left oblique diameter is measured in the same way on the other side.

Functionally, the pelvis supports and distributes body weight, supports and protects pelvic viscera, and forms the birth passageway. The strong muscles of the pelvic floor stabilize and support the internal and external reproductive organs. The most important of these muscles is the levator ani, which supports the three structures that penetrate it: the urethra, vagina, and rectum.

**Types of Pelves.** There are four basic types of pelves: gynecoid, android, anthropoid, and platypelloid (Fig. 2–6). Gynecoid pelvis is the typical female pelvis, with rounded anterior and posterior segments providing adequate space for the passage of a baby. Android pelvis has a wedge-shaped inlet with a narrow anterior segment; it is typical of the male anatomy. Anthropoid pelvis has an anteroposterior diameter that equals or exceeds its transverse diameter—the shape is a long, narrow oval. Platypelloid pelvis has a shortened anteroposterior diameter and a flat, transverse oval shape. This type often encourages a transverse lie for the fetus and is a poor risk for vaginal delivery.

**True and False Pelves.** The pelvis is divided into the false and true pelves by an imaginary line, called the linea terminalis, which proceeds from the sacroiliac joint to the anterior iliopubic prominence. The upper, or false, pelvis supports the enlarging uterus and guides the fetus into the true pelvis. The lower, or true, pelvis consists of the inlet, pelvic cavity, and outlet, and it determines the direction of the fetus during labor.

**Pelvic Diameters.** The diameters of the pelvis are important to consider for a successful vaginal delivery (Fig. 2–7).

***Pelvic Inlet.*** The pelvic inlet, just below the

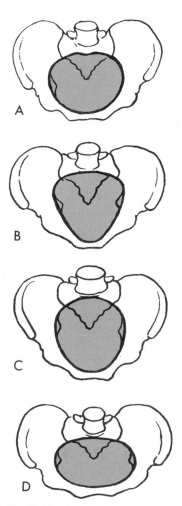

**Figure 2–6.** The Caldwell-Moloy classification of pelves. *A,* Gynecoid. *B,* Android. *C,* Anthropoid. *D,* Platypelloid. (Modified from Moore, M. [1983]. *Realities in childbearing* [2nd ed., p. 69]. Philadelphia: W.B. Saunders.)

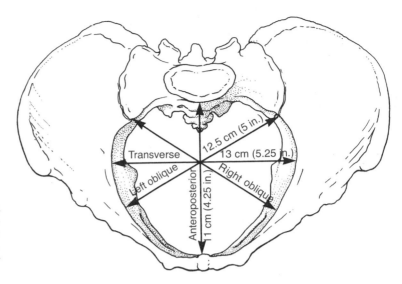

**Figure 2–7.** Three obstetrically important pelvis diameters, just below the linea terminalis. (Modified from *Illustrated Stedman's medical dictionary* [25th ed., p. 1156]. [1990]. © 1990. The Williams & Wilkins Co., Baltimore.)

*Pelvic Cavity.* The pelvic cavity has a number of diameters, the most important being the interspinous transverse diameter. The distance between the ischial spines is 10.5 cm (4.13 inches) and is the shortest pelvic diameter. The diameters of the pelvic outlet are the anteroposterior, intertuberous transverse, and anterior and posterior sagittals. The anteroposterior diameter is adaptable during passage of the fetus, since the coccyx can be displaced posteriorly at the sacrococcygeal joint. The intertuberous transverse diameter is measured between the ischial tuberosities and is the shortest of the outlet diameters. The sagittal diameters are measured from the middle of the transverse diameter to the suprapubic bone anteriorly and to the sacrococcygeal joint posteriorly.

## BREASTS

Female breasts (mammary glands) are accessory organs of reproduction. They produce milk following childbirth, thus providing nourishment and maternal antibodies to the infant (Fig. 2–8). The nipple, in the center of each breast, is surrounded by a pigmented areola. Montgomery's glands (tubercles of Montgomery), which are small sebaceous glands in the nipple and areola, secrete a lipoid (fatlike) substance that lubricates and protects the breasts during lactation.

Each breast is made of 15–24 radially arranged lobes separated by adipose and fibrous tissues. The fibrous tissues are called Cooper's ligaments, and they support the breasts. The

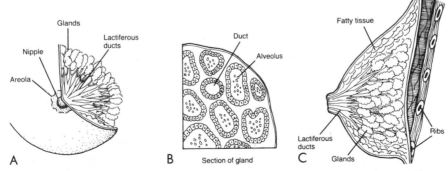

**Figure 2–8.** Details of breast tissue that are important in lactation. *A,* Partially dissected breast showing milk-forming glands and lactiferous ducts leading into the nipple. *B,* Microscopic cross-section of a milk-producing gland. *C,* Side view of the breast, illustrating fatty tissue. (From O'Toole, M. [1992]. *Miller-Keane encyclopedia & dictionary of medicine, nursing, & allied health* [5th ed., p. 216]. Philadelphia: W.B. Saunders.)

adipose tissue affects size and firmness and gives the breasts a smooth outline.

The glandular tissues that produce milk are ducts and lobules. About 20 separate lactiferous (milk-carrying) ducts empty into each nipple. Each duct comes from alveoli, called lobules, within the breast, where the milk is secreted. Milk is stored in widened areas of the ducts, called ampullae or lactiferous sinuses.

## MENSTRUAL CYCLE

The menstrual cycle is a periodic build-up and discharge of blood mixed with fluid from the endometrial lining of the uterus, which demonstrates a response to hormonal changes.

The beginning of menstruation, called *menarche*, occurs at about 12 years of age. Early cycles occur irregularly and may be anovulatory. A young woman establishes her own regular cycle within 6 months to 2 years. In an average cycle, the flow (menses) occurs every 28 days, plus or minus 5–10 days. Stress, fatigue, or illness may interfere with the cycle. The flow itself lasts from 2 to 8 days with a blood loss of 50–100 ml.

The interrelationship of hormones and the menstrual cycle is best illustrated by the female reproductive cycle (Fig. 2–9). The anterior pituitary gland, in response to the hypothalamus, secretes follicle-stimulating hormone (FSH) and luteinizing hormone (LH). The FSH is primarily responsible for the maturation of a follicle, a spherical cavity on an ovary that contains a single ovum. The ovary produces increasing amounts of estrogen, which leads to rebuilding of the endometrium. The follicle does not mature into the graafian follicle

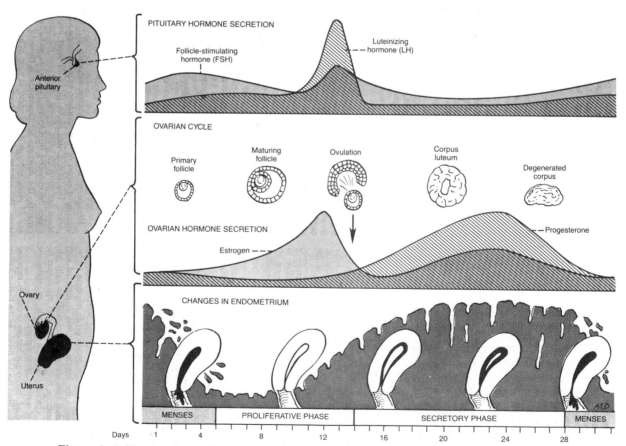

**Figure 2–9.** Menstrual cycle. Note hormonal control of the menstrual cycle and the effects on ovaries (*center*) and endometrium (*bottom*). (From Black, J.M., & Matassarin-Jacobs, E. [1993]. *Luckmann and Sorensen's medical-surgical nursing: A psychophysiologic approach* [4th ed.]. Philadelphia: W.B. Saunders.)

without the enhancing action of LH. LH also affects ovulation and the formation of the corpus luteum.

Ovulation occurs when a mature egg is released from the follicle. The corpus luteum is the empty follicle, which turns yellow immediately after ovulation. Once the luteinizing action occurs, ovarian estrogen production decreases and progesterone production continues in larger amounts. About 10 days after ovulation, the corpus luteum begins to degenerate, and progesterone and estrogen levels decrease. Within a few more days, the anterior pituitary gland starts secreting FSH, beginning a new ovarian cycle. Meanwhile the menstrual phase of the endometrium is in progress.

## PREMENSTRUAL SYNDROME

Because of the abrupt reduction of progesterone secretion and a decreased progesterone-to-estrogen ratio, 30–40% of all ovulating women experience a condition known as premenstrual syndrome (PMS). Symptoms and signs occur several days before menstruation and often spontaneously disappear when the flow begins. The following may be present: pelvic fullness, abdominal weight gain, bloating, headache, irritability, anxiety, depression, fatigue, exhaustion, food craving, nausea, vomiting, diarrhea, and constipation. It is less well-known that just before menstruation, some women have heightened creativity and better

## Nursing Brief

Although PMS is seldom seen in a hospital setting, a nurse often receives queries from women in the community. Accurate information on this subject dispels superstitions and myths.

powers of concentration and are more productive, physically and mentally.

Specific criteria necessary for diagnosis of PMS include the following: (1) symptoms are present only after ovulation; (2) symptoms must be charted as they occur, not by recall; and (3) symptoms are cyclic and severe enough to alter the woman's life style. Calendar diaries are available for charting the time and severity of signs and symptoms.

Recommendations to prevent PMS include (1) restrict intake of salt and sugar; (2) increase intake of complex carbohydrates; and (3) maintain a balanced lifestyle that includes adequate rest and sleep and regular, vigorous, aerobic exercise. The physician may prescribe medications including progesterone supplements, spironolactone (a progesterone agonist), or pyridoxine (vitamin $B_6$). For women who are more seriously affected or kept from their normal activities by PMS, counseling is often recommended. Nursing Care Plan 2–1 specifies nursing interventions for PMS.

| NURSING CARE PLAN 2–1 | | |
|---|---|---|
| **Selected Nursing Diagnoses for Premenstrual Syndrome (PMS)** | | |
| **Goals** | **Nursing Interventions** | **Rationale** |
| **Nursing Diagnosis:** Knowledge deficit related to syndrome and symptom management. | | |
| Woman will verbalize understanding of PMS and report a decrease in symptoms | 1. Provide suggestions for a diet low in sodium and refined sugars and high in complex carbohydrates | 1. Reduction in sodium decreases abdominal bloating; low intake of refined sugars may decrease irritability; complex carbohydrates reduce fatigue and exhaustion |
| | 2. Encourage moderation in daily activities and a balance of exercise and rest | 2. Fluctuations in the circulating levels of estrogen and progesterone are better tolerated with a balanced lifestyle |
| | 3. Reinforce the necessity of taking medications if prescribed by health-care provider | 3. Prescribed medications have improved physical well-being of some PMS patients |
| | 4. Provide information for professional counseling as requested | 4. Seeking help from family and friends as well as competent counselors helps provide coping strategies |

## KEY POINTS

- The scrotum is a sac suspended from the perineum that protects the testes.
- Two important functions of the testes are the manufacture of sperm and the secretion of male hormones (androgens).
- Testosterone is the principal male hormone responsible for the changes that occur at puberty. Estrogen is the principal female hormone that causes pubertal changes.
- Semen consists of seminal plasma and sperm. It is secreted during ejaculation.
- The external organ of the female reproductive system is termed the vulva.
- The clitoris is a structure of the female genitalia. It corresponds to the male penis and is the most erotic and sensitive of the female organs.
- The uterus is made up of three parts: the fundus, corpus, and cervix.
- The myometrium, the middle muscular layer of the uterus, is the functional unit in pregnancy and labor.
- The four functions of the fallopian tubes are (1) to provide a passageway for sperm to meet the ovum (egg), (2) to act as the site of fertilization, (3) to provide a safe nourishing environment for the fertilized egg (zygote), and (4) to transport the ovum or zygote to the corpus of the uterus.
- The pelvic cavity has a number of diameters important for a successful vaginal delivery. The most significant is the interspinous transverse diameter.

# Study Questions

1. Compare puberty in the developing male and female.
2. What are the four functional activities of the cervical mucosa?
3. Name and describe the four basic types of pelves.
4. List and identify the obstetric significance of the diameters of the pelvic inlet, the pelvic cavity, and the pelvic outlet.
5. Briefly describe the mammary glands and their function during lactation.
6. What is the function of the follicle-stimulating hormone and luteinizing hormone during the menstrual cycle?
7. What is the corpus luteum?
8. List two measures the nurse might suggest for women experiencing premenstrual syndrome.

# Multiple Choice Review Questions

*Choose the most appropriate answer.*

1. Spermatozoa are produced in the
   a. vas deferens
   b. seminiferous tubules
   c. prostate gland
   d. Leydig cells
2. Before ovulation, the production of estrogen from the ovaries is made possible by the secretion of
   a. luteinizing hormone
   b. growth hormone
   c. adrenocorticotropic hormone
   d. follicle-stimulating hormone
3. The hormones that interact to regulate the female reproductive cycle are produced by the
   a. posterior pituitary gland and adrenal gland
   b. adrenal gland and hypothalamus
   c. anterior pituitary gland and hypothalamus
   d. posterior pituitary gland and hypothalamus

4. The name for the typical female pelvis that is best suited for vaginal delivery is the
   a. gynecoid
   b. android
   c. anthropoid
   d. platypelloid

5. The muscular layer of the uterus that is the functional unit in pregnancy and labor is the
   a. perimetrium
   b. myometrium
   c. endometrium
   d. cervix

## BIBLIOGRAPHY

Black, J.M., & Matassarin-Jacobs, E. (1993). *Luckmann and Sorensen's Medical-surgical nursing: A psychophysiologic approach* (4th ed.). Philadelphia: W.B. Saunders.

Guyton, A.C. (1991). *Textbook of medical physiology* (8th ed.). Philadelphia: W.B. Saunders.

Ladewig, P.W., London, M.L., & Olds, S.B. (1994). *Essentials of maternal-newborn nursing.* (3rd ed.). Redwood City, CA: Addison-Wesley.

Moore, M. (1983). *Realities in childbearing* (2nd ed.). Philadelphia: W.B. Saunders.

Olds, S.B., London, M., & Ladewig, P. (1992). *Maternal-newborn nursing* (4th ed.). Reading, MA: Addison-Wesley.

O'Toole, M. (1992). *Miller-Keane encyclopedia & dictionary of medicine, nursing, & allied health* (5th ed.). Philadelphia: W.B. Saunders.

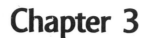

# Chapter 3

# Fetal Development

## VOCABULARY
amniotic sac (36)
chorion (35)
decidua (35)
embryo (35)
fertilization (32)
fetus (35)
gametogenesis (32)
germ layers (36)
placenta (36)
zygote (35)

# OBJECTIVES

*On completion and mastery of Chapter 3, the student will be able to*

- Define each vocabulary term listed.
- Describe the process of gametogenesis in human reproduction.
- Explain human fertilization and implantation.
- Describe embryonic development.
- Describe fetal development and maturation of body systems.
- Describe the development of the placenta and umbilical cord.
- Identify the unique structures of fetal circulation.
- Compare fetal circulation during prenatal life and circulation shortly after birth.
- Define the two types of twins.

Each human being is unique, even though each consists of the same organ systems functioning in more or less the same manner. One's uniqueness results from the interaction of three factors. First, a person's particular combination of features is determined by the 46 chromosomes contained in each cell of the body. Chromosomes are the bearers of genes, which are the units of heredity and contain the information necessary for expression of specific features, traits, and body functions. Second, the passing on of familial traits that are uniquely blended in a new person begins when male and female reproductive cells (ovum and sperm) form in the process known as gametogenesis. Third, the uterine environment also influences the developing embryo and fetus. This environment is affected by the mother's nutritional status and her use of drugs, alcohol, and cigarettes.

## Cell Division

Cell division is the basic mechanism of human growth and regeneration. The division of a cell begins in its nucleus, which contains the gene-bearing chromosomes. The genes contain the information necessary for the inheritance of familial traits. There are two types of cell division: mitosis and meiosis.

*Mitosis* occurs in somatic (body) cells and is chiefly responsible for the body's growth, development, and replenishment throughout its life.

The number of chromosomes in a somatic cell is 46, known as the *diploid number*. A cell divides mitotically by first replicating each chromosome in its nucleus; each of the 46 pairs of chromosomes then separates to form two identical "daughter" cells, each containing 46 single chromosomes with the same genetic material as the "parent" cell.

*Meiosis* occurs only in sexual reproduction, during a process known as gametogenesis (see following discussion). In gametogenesis, there are two successive meiotic divisions that result in four cells, each containing 23 chromosomes; this is known as the *haploid number* of chromosomes. These cells are called *gametes*: In the male, the gamete is called a *sperm*; in the female, an *ovum*.

## Gametogenesis

Gametogenesis is the process by which cells divide, by meiosis, to form gametes. Male gametogenesis occurs in the seminiferous tubules of the testes (see p. 19) and is called *spermatogenesis*. This process involves two meiotic divisions and results in four sperm, each with 22 single chromosomes and either an X or a Y sex chromosome, for a total of 23 (see discussion of sex determination, p. 34).

Female gametogenesis, called *oogenesis*, also involves two meiotic divisions but results in one ovum and three small structures known as polar bodies. Oogenesis begins with the first meiotic division of an oocyte in the graafian follicle on the ovary. The second meiotic division is completed if the ovum is fertilized (penetrated) by a sperm.

The mature ovum contains the haploid number of chromosomes: 22 single chromosomes and always the X sex chromosome. In oogenesis, the extra chromosomes produced by each meiotic division are carried away by the polar bodies, which eventually disintegrate. This process is illustrated in greater detail in Figure 3–1.

## Fertilization

Fertilization occurs when a sperm penetrates an ovum and unites with it. The time during which fertilization can occur is brief because of the short lifespan of mature gametes. The ovum

# NORMAL GAMETOGENESIS

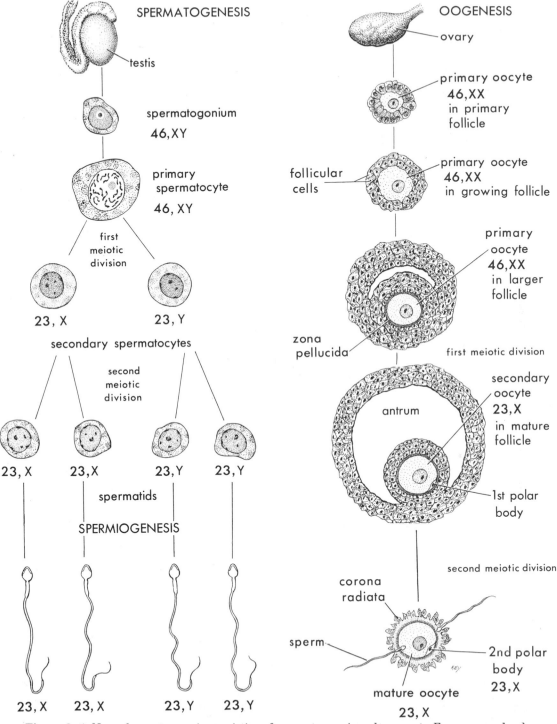

**Figure 3–1.** Normal gametogenesis, consisting of spermatogenesis and oogenesis. Four sperms develop from one primary spermatocyte, but only one mature oocyte (ovum) results from maturation of a primary oocyte. (From Moore, K.L., & Persaud, T.V.N. [1993]. *The developing human: Clinically oriented embryology* [5th ed., p. 16]. Philadelphia: W.B. Saunders.)

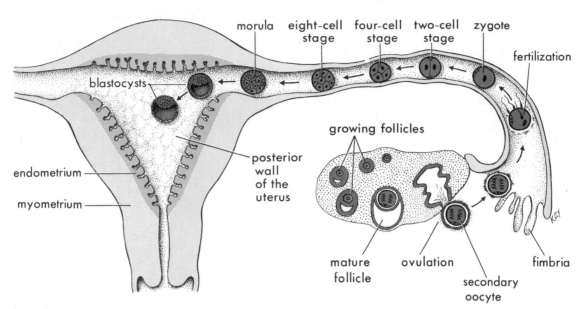

**Figure 3-2.** Ovulation and fertilization, which initiate human development. The zygote passes through the fallopian tube and enters the uterus in the blastocyst stage, where normally it implants in the center of the posterior uterine wall. (From Moore, K.L., & Persaud, T.V.N. [1993]. *The developing human: Clinically oriented embryology* [5th ed., p. 37]. Philadelphia: W.B. Saunders.)

survives for up to 24 hours after ovulation—sometimes for only 1 hour. The sperm remains viable for at least 24 hours after being ejaculated into the area of the cervix, and it sometimes survives for up to 72 hours.

The amount of semen in a normal ejaculation is 2–5 ml, and the number of sperm ranges from 200 million to 600 million. The sperm pass through the cervix and uterus and into the fallopian tubes by means of the flagellar (whiplike) activity of their tails.

Fertilization takes place in the outer third of the fallopian tube, which is closest to the ovary (Fig. 3–2). The high estrogen levels that exist at ovulation facilitate movement of the ovum through the fallopian tube and produce a cervical mucus that is favorable for the passage of sperm. (See p. 287 for a discussion of in vitro fertilization.)

## SEX DETERMINATION

The sex of human offspring is determined at fertilization. The ovum always contributes an X chromosome, whereas the sperm can carry an X *or* a Y chromosome. When a sperm carrying the larger, X chromosome fertilizes the X-bearing ovum, a female child (XX) results. When a smaller, Y-bearing sperm fertilizes the ovum, a male child (XY) is produced.

Because his sperm can carry *either* an X or a Y chromosome, the male partner determines the gender of the child. However, the pH of the female reproductive tract and the estrogen levels of the woman's body affect the survival rate of the X- and Y-bearing sperm and the speed of their movement through the cervix and fallopian tubes. Thus, the mother has some influence on which sperm fertilizes the mature ovum.

## Nursing Brief

During sexuality counseling, the nurse emphasizes that the survival time of sperm ejaculated into the area of the cervix may be up to 72 hours.

## Nursing Brief

Both mother and father influence the sex of their offspring. This fact may reduce blame when the child is not of the sex preferred by the parents.

# Development

Each new human being passes through three stages of prenatal development: zygote, embryo, and fetus. The *zygote* is the primary stage, which begins when the oocyte is fertilized by the sperm and continues for 15 days. During this time, its cells rapidly divide to create a suitable environment for growth during the next stage. The *embryo*, the second stage of development, begins at day 15 and continues until the 8th week of gestation. During this stage, cells differentiate to form specific internal organ systems and discrete external body parts. The *fetus*, the third stage of prenatal development, begins at the end of the 8th week and continues until the 40th week of gestation or until birth. It is characterized by the continuing growth of organs and body parts and the development of the capability to function in extrauterine life.

## TUBAL TRANSPORT OF THE ZYGOTE

The fertilized ovum, called the *zygote*, becomes impenetrable to other sperm. It now must be transported through the fallopian tube and into the uterus, where it will become implanted into the uterine wall. During the estimated 7-day transport, the zygote undergoes rapid mitotic division, or *cleavage*. This cleavage begins with two cells, which subdivide into four and then eight cells to form the *blastomere*. The size of the zygote does not increase; rather, the individual cells become smaller as they continue to divide and eventually form a solid cellular cluster called the *morula* (see Fig. 3–2).

The morula enters the uterus and floats there while other changes occur. The cells form a cavity, and two distinct layers evolve. The inner layer is a solid mass of cells called the *blastocyst* (see Fig. 3–2), which develops into the embryo and embryonic membranes. The outer layer of cells, called the *trophoblast*, develops into an embryonic membrane, the *chorion* (see Fig. 3–3 for more detail on the chorion). Occasionally, the zygote does not move through the fallopian tube and instead becomes implanted into the lining of the tube, resulting in a tubal ectopic pregnancy (see pp. 82–84).

## IMPLANTATION OF THE ZYGOTE

The trophoblast layer of cells chooses the implantation site, usually in the upper section of the posterior uterine wall. The cells burrow into the prepared lining of the uterus, called the endometrium, until the entire blastocyst is covered. On implantation, the endometrium is called the *decidua* (Fig. 3–3). The decidua over the blastocyst is called the decidua capsularis; the area under the blastocyst is called the decidua basalis and gives rise to the maternal portion of the placenta; the remaining uterine lining is called the decidua vera (parietalis).

## CELL DIFFERENTIATION

From initial fertilization to implantation, the cells within a zygote are identical to one another. At implantation, the cells begin to differentiate and adopt special functions; the chorion, amnion, yolk sac, and primary germ layers appear.

**Chorion.** The chorion, which develops from the trophoblast (outer layer of cells of the morula), envelops the amnion, embryo, and yolk sac (see Fig. 3–3). It is a thick membrane with finger-like projections called *villi* on its outermost surface. The villi immediately below the embryo extend into the decidua basalis on the uterine wall and form the embryonic portion of the placenta (see pp. 36–37).

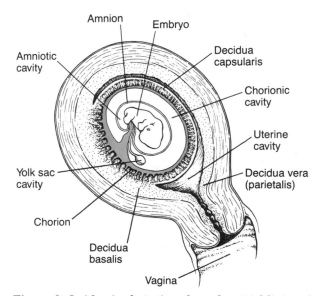

**Figure 3–3.** After implantation, the endometrial lining of the uterus is known as the decidua. The cells of the zygote begin to differentiate into the chorion, amnion, yolk sac, and embryo.

**Amnion.** The second embryonic membrane, the amnion, is a thin membrane that envelops and protects the embryo. It forms the boundaries of the amniotic cavity, and its outer aspect meets the inner aspect of the chorion (see Fig. 3–3).

The chorion and amnion together form an amniotic sac filled with fluid (bag of waters) that permits the embryo to float. Amniotic fluid is slightly alkaline and contains albumin, uric acid, urea, lecithin, creatinine, sphingomyelin, bilirubin, fat, fructose, leukocytes, epithelial cells, enzymes, and lanugo hair; *lanugo hair* is a fine, downy hair that appears on the skin of the fetus during gestation.

The volume of amniotic fluid steadily increases from about 30 ml at 10 weeks of pregnancy to 350 ml at 20 weeks (Moore, 1992). After 20 weeks, the amount of fluid increases to 500 ml and then to 1000 ml, until the last few weeks of pregnancy, when it gradually diminishes in volume. In the latter part of the pregnancy, the fetus may swallow up to 400 ml of amniotic fluid per day and normally excretes urine into the fluid. The functions of amniotic fluid are as follows:

- Maintains an even temperature
- Prevents the amniotic sac from adhering to delicate embryonic skin
- Provides for freedom of movement during all stages of prenatal development
- Acts as a cushion to protect the fetus from injury

**Yolk Sac.** At about the time of implantation, on the 9th day after fertilization, a cavity called the yolk sac forms in the blastocyst. It functions only during embryonic life and initiates the production of red blood cells. This function continues for about 6 weeks, until the embryonic liver takes over. The umbilical cord then encompasses the yolk sac, and the yolk sac degenerates.

**Primary Germ Layers.** Subsequent to implantation, the zygote in the blastocyst stage transforms its *embryonic disc* into three primary germ layers known as *ectoderm, mesoderm,* and *endoderm* (Fig. 3–4). Each germ layer develops into a different part of the growing embryo. The specific body parts that develop from each layer are listed in Box 3–1.

## ACCESSORY STRUCTURES OF PREGNANCY

As embryonic development progresses, the accessory structures of pregnancy, namely the placenta, umbilical cord, and circulation, are established. These structures provide continuing support for the fetus as it completes prenatal life and prepares for birth.

### Placenta

The placenta is a temporary organ of pregnancy that provides for fetal respiration, nutrition, and excretion. It also functions as an endocrine gland. Maternal-placental-fetal circulation is complete at about 22 days after conception, when the embryonic heart begins to function.

The placenta begins to form when the chorionic villi of the embryo extend into the blood-filled spaces of the mother's decidua basalis (see earlier discussion of the chorion, p. 35). The maternal part of the placenta arises from the decidua basalis, and because of the large number of arterioles and venules, that side has a "beefy" red appearance. The fetal side of the placenta develops from the chorionic villi and the chorionic blood vessels. The amniotic fetal membrane covers this side and gives it a grayish, shiny appearance at term.

A thin membrane separates the maternal and fetal blood, and the two blood supplies do not, normally, intermingle. However, the separation of the placenta at delivery may allow some fetal blood to enter the maternal circulation. The placenta is divided by septa (partitions) into 15–20 segments called *cotyledons*. Each contains complex vascular systems through which

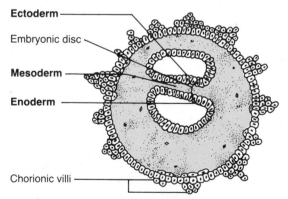

**Figure 3–4.** The primary germ layers of the zygote. The location of the embryonic disc and the three germ layers (*bold type*) is shown, together with the beginning of the chorionic villi. (Modified from Reeder, S.J., & Martin, L.L. [1992]. *Maternity nursing* [17th ed., p. 149]. Philadelphia: J.B. Lippincott.)

---

## BOX 3–1   Body Parts That Develop from the Primary Germ Layers

### Ectoderm

Outer layer of skin
Oil glands and hair follicles of skin
Nails and hair
External sense organs
Mucous membrane of mouth and anus

### Mesoderm

True skin
Skeleton
Bone and cartilage
Connective tissue
Muscles
Blood and blood vessels
Kidneys and gonads

### Endoderm

Lining of trachea, pharynx, and bronchi
Lining of digestive tract
Lining of bladder and urethra

---

fetal respiration, nutrition, and excretion occur. The arrangement of placental blood vessels is shown in detail in Figure 3–5.

In the early months of pregnancy, the placenta stores glycogen and iron, to be supplied, as needed, to the growing fetus. Eventually the fetal liver assumes this function.

Placental transport is vital for the health and growth of the fetus. The deoxygenated blood leaves the fetus by way of the umbilical arteries and passes into the placenta through the branch of a main stem villus. Oxygenated blood from the mother flows, in funnel-shaped spurts, into the intervillous space from the spiral-shaped endometrial arteries.

As mentioned, maternal and fetal blood streams flow close to each other but do not mix in the placenta. The circulations are separated by a very thin layer of tissues known as the placental membrane. At this time, fetal blood is able to pick up oxygen and nutrients from the maternal blood. The placental membrane provides some protection but is no longer considered a "placental barrier." Many harmful substances, such as drugs, nicotine, and viral infectious agents, are known to be transported to the fetal circulation and result in fetal drug addiction, congenital anomalies, and fetal infection. However, the placenta can also be used to deliver therapeutic medications to the fetus, such as to deliver digitalis to the fetus with heart failure (Gorrie et al, 1994).

### Placental Hormones

The hormones produced by this temporary endocrine gland are progesterone, estrogen, human chorionic gonadotropin (hCG), and human placental lactogen (HPL).

**Progesterone.** Progesterone, the pregnancy hormone, provides these vital functions for a successful pregnancy:

- Increases tubal and uterine nourishing secretions in order to provide nutrition for the morula and blastocyst stages.
- At high levels, converts the endometrial lining into decidual cells in order to permit implantation of the blastocyst.
- Reduces contractibility of the uterus to prevent spontaneous abortion.
- Prepares mammary glands for secretion of milk.

**Estrogens.** Estrogens chiefly provide for the expansion, needed during pregnancy, of the uterus, breasts, and breast glandular tissue. They play a role in the increasing vascularity and vasodilation of the villous capillaries of the placenta.

**Human Chorionic Gonadotropin.** hCG has a direct influence on the corpus luteum. When fertilization occurs, hCG is immediately secreted and prevents involution (degeneration, or shriveling) of the corpus luteum. The corpus luteum increases its production of estrogen and progesterone and continues doing so until the 11th week, when the placenta takes over. hCG is detectable in maternal blood as soon as implantation occurs, usually 8–10 days after fertilization.

**Human Placental Lactogen.** HPL is also known as human chorionic somatomammotropin. The HPL stimulates adjustments in the mother's metabolism, so that adequate protein, glucose, and minerals are available for the developing fetus.

### Umbilical Cord

The umbilical cord forms simultaneously with the placenta and is the lifeline between mother and fetus. Early in the embryonic stage, the body stalk, which contains blood ves-

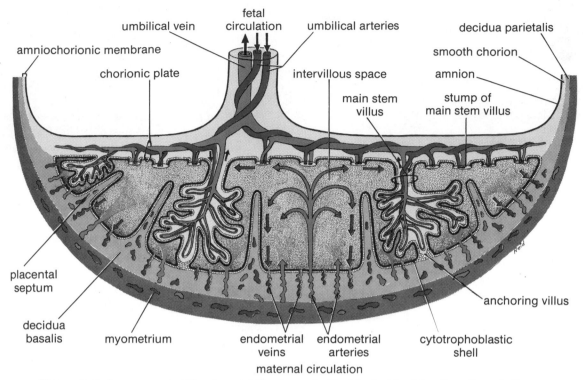

**Figure 3–5.** Arrangement of the placental blood vessels. The blood of the fetus flows through the umbilical arteries into the fetal capillaries in the villi and then back to the fetal circulation through the umbilical vein. Maternal blood is transported by the uterine arteries to the intervillous space, and it leaves by the uterine veins to return to the maternal circulation. (From Moore, K.L., & Persaud, T.V.N. [1993]. *The developing human: Clinically oriented embryology* [5th ed., p. 117]. Philadelphia: W.B. Saunders.)

sels, elongates to form the cord. The multiple vessels in the body stalk become one large vein and two small arteries. Occasionally, only one vein and one artery form, and this occurrence may be associated with congenital abnormalities.

Surrounding and separating the vessels is a whitish connective tissue called *Wharton's jelly*. This substance provides the space needed for growth of the umbilical vessels along with the fetus, and it keeps the vessels separate so as not to compromise circulation. The large volume of blood moving through the vessels prevents compression of the cord. In addition, the vessels are somewhat coiled within the Wharton's jelly to allow for movement and stretching without compromising circulation.

Usually, the umbilical cord is inserted into the center of the placenta. Insertion of the cord into the periphery of the placenta is known as battledore insertion. A rare insertion, called velamentous placenta, is the insertion of the umbilical cord away from the placenta so that the vessels are seen along the membranes adjacent to the placental surface.

The umbilical cord is usually 55 cm (22 inches) long and 2 cm (0.8 inch) wide at term. The normal range of length for the cord is 30–90 cm (12–36 inches). A cord much longer or much shorter may interfere with a successful labor and delivery.

### Fetal Circulation

After week 4 of gestation, circulation of blood through the placenta to the fetus is established (Fig. 3–6). Fetal circulation provides oxygen and nutrients to the fetus and disposes of carbon dioxide and other waste products from it. The umbilical vein transports richly oxygenated blood from the placenta to the fetus. The umbilical vein enters the fetus's body through the

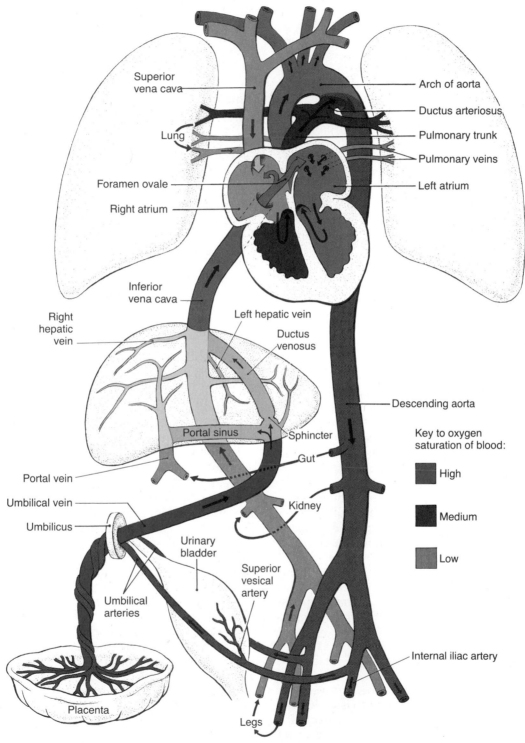

**Figure 3–6.** Fetal circulation. (From Moore, K.L., & Persaud, T.V.N. [1993]. *The developing human: Clinically oriented embryology* [5th ed., p. 344]. Philadelphia: W.B. Saunders.)

umbilical cord in the abdominal fetal wall. It travels up toward the fetal liver, where it branches.

The first branch, the portal sinus, carries some of the oxygenated blood to the portal circulation and empties, via the hepatic vein, into the inferior vena cava. The second branch, the *ductus venosus*, carries most of the blood directly into the inferior vena cava, where it mixes with the blood returning from the lower limbs, abdomen, and pelvis of the fetus to the fetal heart.

The mixed blood enters the right atrium and passes through the *foramen ovale* (septal opening) into the left atrium. The blood flows into the left ventricle and pumps into the aorta, so that the blood with the highest oxygen concentration is made available to the fetal brain and upper extremities, and empties into the right atrium. From there, the blood enters the right ventricle, where it is pumped into the pulmonary artery. Another fetal branching occurs at this artery, permitting a small amount of blood to enter the pulmonary circulation to nourish the lungs. The larger volume of blood passes through the *ductus arteriosus* into the descending aorta.

The blood continues its passage, nourishing the abdominal viscera and lower extremities. Eventually, it flows into the iliac arteries to the hypogastric arteries (internal iliac arteries), which join the two umbilical arteries to return to the placenta. At birth, the baby breathes and the cord is clamped, thus terminating fetal circulation.

The foramen ovale closes within 2 hours after birth, and permanent closure normally occurs by 3 months of age. The ductus arteriosus closes functionally within 15 hours and closes permanently in about 3 weeks. The ductus venosus closes functionally when the cord is cut and closes permanently in about 1 week. After permanent closure, the ductus arteriosus and ductus venosus become nonfunctional ligamentous tissue.

## THE EMBRYO

**Week 3.** At the beginning of the 3rd week after fertilization (day 15), the zygote is called the embryo (Table 3–1). The embryo measures 2 mm (0.08 inch) from crown to rump (CR), and its weight is negligible. The primary germ layers evolve into organ systems. The embryonic disc is pear-shaped, having a wide cephalic (head) end and a narrow caudal (tail) end. The primitive streak and primitive node, the earliest evidence of the spinal cord and brain, are visible. The gastrointestinal tract is evolving from the endoderm and is in close proximity to the yolk sac. A major development is the heart, which is single-chambered and tubular at this stage.

**Week 4.** During this week, the embryo continues growing in the cephalocaudal axis and grows to 5 mm (0.2 inch) CR in length. It weighs about 0.4 gm (0.01 ounce). The neural tube closes anteriorly to form the brain, and posteriorly to form the spinal cord. The primitive structure of the eyes, ears, jaws, limb buds, and kidneys has been established. Division of the esophagus and trachea is noted. At day 28, the heart is able to pump its own blood through its own main blood vessels.

The major feature of the 4th week is the formation of 42 *somites*. Somites are paired segments along the neural tube, formed by the thickened mesoderm, that develop into the vertebral column and muscles of the body.

**Week 5.** During the 5th week, the embryo grows to 8 mm (0.3 inch) CR. The eyes and nose continue noticeable development. The embryo assumes a C-shape, and a large head and a tail are seen. The brain establishes five distinct areas, and 10 pairs of cranial nerves are present. The heart has two atrial chambers.

**Week 6.** The embryo is now 12 mm (0.5 inch). The limb buds are extending, and the primitive skeletal and muscle systems are developing. The beating heart now has all four chambers and is pumping blood that the liver is beginning to produce. The external, middle, and internal ears appear. The trachea, bronchi, and lung buds of the respiratory system are evolving. The upper lip along with the oral and nasal passages is forming.

**Week 7.** At 7 weeks, the embryo is 18 mm (0.7 inch) CR and weighs less than 2 gm (0.07 ounce). The face is formed, the tongue is a separate structure within the mouth, and the palate folds. The diaphragm is complete and separates the thoracic cavity from the abdominal cavity. The optic nerve is formed, and fused eyelids are apparent. Differentiation of internal male and female reproductive organs occurs.

**Week 8.** In this last week of embryonic development, the embryo's length is 2.5–3 cm (1–1.18 inches) CR and its weight is 2 gm (0.07 ounce). Fingers and toes are formed, as is the structure of the ear. Heart function and fetal circulation are established.

## THE FETUS

At the end of week 8, the embryo becomes known as the fetus (see Table 3–1). The body form is easily recognized as human, with all the necessary external features and internal organ systems in place. Because fetal growth proceeds cephalocaudally (from head to foot), the head is somewhat large, compared with the rest of the body.

**Week 10.** The fetus is now about 6 cm (2.4 inches) in length CR and weighs 14 gm (0.5 ounce). Fingernails and toenails begin growing, the intestines are enclosed in the abdomen, urine forms and enters the bladder, and the lacrimal (tear) ducts have developed.

**Week 12.** The fetus is now 11.5 cm (4.5 inches) crown to heel (CH) and weighs 45 gm (1.6 ounces). The fetal liver gradually decreases production of red blood cells, and the spleen begins to produce them. Bile begins to form in the liver, and the gallbladder starts to form. Lungs have a definite shape, and the skin is a delicate pink. Bones and muscles continue growing and developing, and the fetus has been moving around for 4 weeks, although the mother will not feel it for another 4 weeks.

**Week 16.** The length of the fetus has increased to 15 cm (5.9 inches) CH, and weight has dramatically increased to approximately 200 gm (7 ounces). Fetal heart tones are heard with a *fetoscope*, which is a specially adapted stethoscope for listening to the fetal heart. Teeth begin to form, and the digestive tract begins to function with the collection of *meconium*, which is a mixture of amniotic fluid and secretions of the intestinal glands (shortly after birth it is a dark green sticky material, the first stool a newborn expels). Scalp hair and lanugo hair appear, and sweat glands develop. Blood vessels are visible through the now-transparent skin. The sex of the fetus is externally discernible.

**Week 20.** The fetus reaches a milestone in development, the midpoint of the gestational period. Weight is about 450 gm (15.9 ounces), and length is 25 cm (10 inches) CH. Incisors, canine, and first molar teeth are all developing. The fetus can suck its thumb and swallow amniotic fluid. The cellular structure of the alveoli of the lungs is complete.

*Brown fat* begins to form. Also called "brown adipose tissue," brown fat has a dark brown hue that is due to its density, enriched blood supply, and abundant nerve supply. It forms around the kidneys, adrenals, and neck; between the scapulas; and behind the sternum. Because of its greater heat-generating activity compared with normal fat, brown fat becomes the primary source of heat for the cold-stressed newborn. By the end of week 20, lanugo hair also is fully present, covering the fetus's body except for the palms of the hands and soles of the feet.

**Week 24.** Growth continues at a rapid pace, with the fetus now weighing 750–950 gm (1.6–2 pounds) and measuring 30 cm (12 inches) CH. The eyes are structurally complete. The skin is wrinkled, and much *vernix caseosa* is present. Vernix caseosa is a greasy cheeselike mixture of fatty secretion from the fetal sebaceous glands and dead epidermal cells. It protects the delicate fetal skin from abrasions, chapping, and hardening that could result from the constant immersion in amniotic fluid.

Also during week 24, the nostrils open, respiratory movements occur, and alveoli begin to produce *surfactant*. Surfactant is a complex mixture of lipids that covers the internal walls of the alveoli of the lungs; it enables the alveoli to stay open so that air can enter the lungs at birth and adequate expansion of the lungs will occur.

**Week 28.** Adipose tissue quickly accumulates, and fetal weight increases to 1250 gm (2.75 pounds). Length increases to 35 cm (13.8 inches) CH. Eyebrows and eyelashes are present, and the eyelids are open. The nervous system begins some regulatory functions, and in males the testes descend into the scrotum.

**Week 32.** The fetal nervous system continues to mature, so that rhythmic respirations and regulation of body temperature are possible if delivery of the fetus occurs at this time. The fully developed skeletal system is soft and flexible, permitting the fetus to position itself for passage through the pelvis. Muscle and fat accumulate, and the fetus weighs about 2000 gm

(4 pounds, 7 ounces) and measures 37–44 cm (14.5–17.3 inches) CH.

**Week 36.** The fetus has now filled out its wrinkled skin with subcutaneous fat, so that it weighs somewhere between 2600 and 2750 gm (5 pounds, 12 ounces, to 6 pounds, 1 ounce). Its length has increased to 42–48 cm (16.5–18.9 inches). The identifying characteristics of this age are soft ear lobes, few creases on the soles of the feet, ample vernix caseosa, and diminishing lanugo.

**Week 40.** The fetus has been ready for 2 weeks to enter the next stage of life—birth and extrauterine life. Its weight averages between 3000 and 3600 gm (6 pounds, 10 ounces, and 7 pounds, 15 ounces), and the length varies from 48 to 52 cm (18.9 to 20.4 inches). The skin is pink and smooth with vernix caseosa present only in skin folds. Some lanugo may persist on the shoulders and upper back. Identifying characteristics of the mature fetus include firm ear lobes, many creases over the soles of the foot, and either rugae in the scrotum or well-developed labia majora.

**Table 3–1.** EMBRYONIC AND FETAL DEVELOPMENT

| Age | Length | Weight | Body systems |
|-----|--------|--------|--------------|
| **Embryo**<br>Week 3<br> | 2 mm<br>(0.08 in) | n/c* | *Cardiovascular*: single tubular heart and major blood vessels appear<br>*Nervous*: embryonic disc and primitive spinal cord and brain appear<br>*Gastrointestinal*: GI tract is close to yolk sac |
| Week 4<br> | 5 mm<br>(0.2 in) | 0.4 gm<br>(0.01 oz) | *Musculoskeletal*: somites (42) appear along neural tube (will develop into vertebral column and muscles); primitive jaw and limb develop<br>*Nervous*: neural tube closes: anterior—brain; posterior—spinal cord<br>*Gastrointestinal*: esophagus and trachea division occurs<br>*Genitourinary*: primitive kidney appears<br>*Respiratory*: trachea is noted<br>*Skin / senses*: primitive eyes and ears appear |
| Week 5<br> | 8 mm<br>(0.3 in) | | *Musculoskeletal*: limbs begin to lengthen<br>*Cardiovascular*: heart has two atrial chambers and pumps its own blood<br>*Nervous*: five distinct areas of brain exist, and 10 pairs of cranial nerves<br>*Skin / senses*: eyes and nose are noticeable |

**Table 3–1.** EMBRYONIC AND FETAL DEVELOPMENT *Continued*

| Age | Length | Weight | Body systems |
|---|---|---|---|
| **Embryo** | | | |
| Week 6 | 12 mm (0.5 in) | | *Musculoskeletal*: limbs continue to extend; primitive skeleton, skull, and jaws begin to ossify<br>*Cardiovascular*: heart has all four chambers and pumps its own blood<br>*Gastrointestinal*: oral and nasal cavities and upper lip are forming<br>*Genitourinary*: sex glands appear<br>*Respiratory*: trachea, bronchi, and lung buds are evolving<br>*Skin/senses*: external, middle, and internal ear is forming |
| Week 7 | 18 mm (0.7 in) | <2 gm | *Musculoskeletal*: limbs continue to extend<br>*Cardiovascular*: heart continues to pump fetal blood, which liver begins to make<br>*Nervous*: optic nerve is formed<br>*Gastrointestinal*: abdominal cavity separates from thoracic cavity; tongue is separate in mouth; palate folds<br>*Genitourinary*: male and female reproductive organs differentiate<br>*Skin/senses*: face is formed; eyelids fuse |
| Week 8 | 2.5–3.0 cm (1–1.8 in) | 2 gm (0.07 oz) | *Musculoskeletal*: fingers and toes are formed<br>*Cardiovascular*: heart function and fetal circulation are complete<br>*Skin/senses*: ears are complete |
| **Fetus**<br>Week 10 | 6 cm (2.4 in) | 14 gm (0.5 oz) | *Musculoskeletal*: growth continues<br>*Cardiovascular*: fetal circulation is functioning<br>*Nervous*: fetus moves about<br>*Gastrointestinal*: intestines are enclosed in abdomen<br>*Genitourinary*: urine forms and enters bladder<br>*Skin/senses*: Tear ducts form; fingernails and toenails grow |
| Week 12 | 11.5 cm (4.5 in) | 45 gm (1.6 oz) | *Musculoskeletal*: growth and development continue<br>*Cardiovascular*: fetal liver produces red blood cells<br>*Gastrointestinal*: bile is stored in gallbladder<br>*Respiratory*: lungs have definite shape<br>*Skin/senses*: skin is delicate pink |

*Continued*

**Table 3–1.** EMBRYONIC AND FETAL DEVELOPMENT *Continued*

| Age | Length | Weight | Body systems |
|---|---|---|---|
| Week 16 | 15 cm (5.9 in) | 200 gm (7 oz) | *Musculoskeletal*: acceleration of growth<br>*Cardiovascular*: fetal heart is heard with fetoscope; blood vessels are visible under skin<br>*Nervous*: mother feels movement of fetus<br>*Gastrointestinal*: teeth form; digestive tract begins to function and collects meconium<br>*Genitourinary*: sex of fetus is externally noted<br>*Skin/senses*: scalp hair, lanugo hair, and sweat glands develop; skin is transparent |
| Week 20 | 25 cm (10 in) | 450 gm (15.9 oz) | *Musculoskeletal*: midpoint of gestation; brown fat begins to form<br>*Nervous*: fetus is able to suck thumb<br>*Gastrointestinal*: incisors, canine, and first molar teeth are developing; fetus swallows amniotic fluid<br>*Respiratory*: structure of alveoli of lungs is complete |
| Week 24 | 30 cm (12 in) | 750–950 gm (1.6–2 lb) | *Respiratory*: nostrils open; respiratory movements occur<br>*Skin/senses*: eyes are complete; skin is red and wrinkled; vernix caseosa is present |
| Week 28 | 35 cm (13.8 in) | 1250 gm (2.75 lb) | *Musculoskeletal*: adipose tissue increases<br>*Nervous*: regulatory function noted<br>*Genitourinary*: testes descend into scrotum in male<br>*Skin/senses*: eyebrows and eyelashes are present; eyelids are open |
| Week 32 | 37–44 cm (14.5–17.3 in) | 2000 gm (4 lb, 7 oz) | *Musculoskeletal*: skeletal system is fully developed and flexible for passage at birth<br>*Nervous*: continues to mature; fetus regulates body temperature<br>*Respiratory*: rhythmic respirations |
| Week 36 | 42–48 cm (16.5–18.9 in) | 2600–2750 gm (5 lb, 12 oz– 6 lb, 1 oz) | *Musculoskeletal*: few creases on soles of feet<br>*Skin/senses*: ear lobes are soft; skin is filled out with subcutaneous fat; vernix caseosa is ample; lanugo hair is diminishing |
| Week 40 | 48–52 cm (18.9–20.4 in) | 3000–3600 gm (6 lb, 10 oz– 7 lb, 15 oz) | *Musculoskeletal*: many creases are seen over soles of feet<br>*Genitourinary*: rugae in scrotum (males) or labia majora (females) are well developed<br>*Skin/senses*: skin is pink and smooth; vernix caseosa remains only in skin folds; lanugo hair remains on shoulders and upper back; ear lobes are firm |

*Not calculable.

Drawings after Moore, K. (1988). *The developing human* (4th ed.). Philadelphia, W.B. Saunders.

# Twins

Twins occur once in every 90 pregnancies in North America. When hormones are given to assist with ovulation, twinning and other multiple births (triplets, quadruplets, and quintuplets) increase.

About two-thirds of all twins are *dizygotic* (DZ) (Fig. 3–7). DZ twins are fraternal, may or may not be of the same sex, and develop from two separate ova fertilized by two separate sperm. DZ twins always have two amnions and two chorions (placenta). If the blastocysts implant close to each other, the placentas may fuse. DZ twins are distinctly different from each other. DZ twins tend to repeat in families, and the incidence increases with maternal age.

About one-third of twins are *monozygotic* (MZ) (Fig. 3–8). MZ twins are genetically identical, have the same sex, and look alike.

Physical differences between MZ twins are caused by prenatal environmental factors involving variations in the blood supply from the placenta. Most MZ twins begin to develop at the end of the 1st week after fertilization. The result is two identical embryos, each with its own amniotic sac but with a common placenta and some common placental vessels. If the embryonic disc does not divide completely, various types of conjoined (formerly called Siamese) twins may form. They are named according to the regions that are joined (e.g., thoracopagus indicates an anterior connection of the thoracic regions).

Most twins, both DZ and MZ, are born prematurely, because the uterus becomes overdistended and the twins become crowded inside the uterus. This crowding interferes with growth in the last trimester. The placenta may not be able to supply sufficient nutrition to both fetuses, resulting in one twin's being smaller. Birth defects are more common in twins.

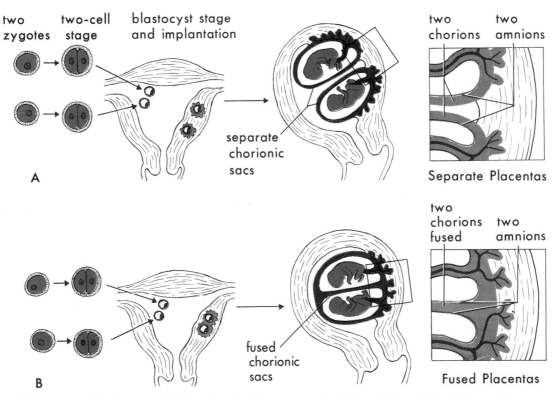

**Figure 3–7.** Development of dizygotic twins from two zygotes. The relations of the fetal membranes and placentas are shown. *A*, The blastocysts implant separately. *B*, The blastocysts implant close together. In both cases there are two amnions and two chorions, and the placentas may be separate or fused. (From Moore, K.L., & Persaud, T.V.N. [1993]. *The developing human: Clinically oriented embryology* [5th ed., 133]. Philadelphia: W.B. Saunders.)

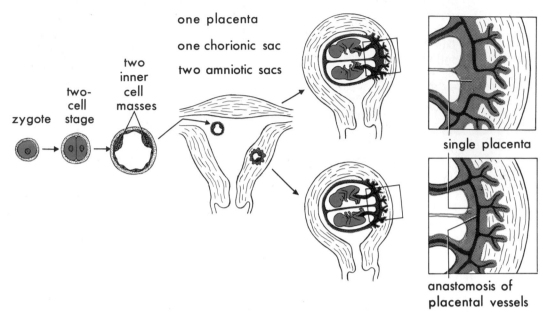

one placenta
one chorionic sac
two amniotic sacs

single placenta

anastomosis of
placental vessels

**Figure 3–8.** Development of about 65% of monozygotic twins: one zygote undergoes division of its inner cell mass (embryoblast) toward the end of the first week. Such twins always have separate amnions, a single chorion, and a common placenta. (From Moore, K.L., & Persaud, T.V.N. [1993]. *The developing human: Clinically oriented embryology* [5th ed., p. 133]. Philadelphia: W.B. Saunders.)

## KEY POINTS

- The uniqueness of each individual results from the interaction of the 46 chromosomes (diploid number) contained in each somatic (body) cell, the inheritance of these chromosomes during gametogenesis, and the physiologic environment of the embryo and the fetus, from conception through birth.
- Gametogenesis in the male is called spermatogenesis, occurs in the seminiferous tubules of the testes, and results in four sperm. Each has 22 single chromosomes plus either an X or a Y sex chromosome, for a total of 23 chromosomes (haploid number). Gametogenesis in the female is called oogenesis. It begins in the graafian follicle, continues at ovulation, and is not completed until fertilization occurs. The mature ovum has 22 chromosomes plus the X sex chromosome, equaling the haploid number of 23 chromosomes.
- When the oocyte is fertilized by an X-bearing sperm, the child will be female; when it is fertilized by a Y-bearing sperm, the child will be male. The pH of the female reproductive tract and the estrogen levels of the woman affect the survival rate of the X- and Y-bearing sperm and the speed of their movement through the cervix and into the tubes. Therefore, both mother and father play a role in sex determination.
- After fertilization in the fallopian tube, the zygote travels for about 7 days to reach the uterus, where implantation occurs and the accessory structures of pregnancy develop. If the zygote fails to move through the tube, implantation occurs there and a tubal ectopic pregnancy results.
- When implantation occurs in the uterine lining, the cells of the zygote differentiate and develop into the following structures: chorion, amnion, yolk sac, and primary germ layers. The chorion develops into the embryonic portion of the

placenta; the amnion encloses the embryo and the amniotic fluid; the primary germ layers develop into different parts of the growing fetus; and the yolk sac —which functions only during embryonic life—begins to form red blood cells.

- The primary germ layers of the embryo are called the ectoderm, mesoderm, and endoderm. From these, all the structures of the individual will develop.
- By 6 weeks after fertilization, all the unique features of the embryo have developed. The internal organs are formed; the limb buds are developing and are functional; and the heart has all four chambers.
- The accessory structures of pregnancy are the placenta, umbilical cord, and fetal circulation. These structures continuously support the fetus throughout prenatal life in preparation for birth.
- One of the placenta's functions is as a temporary endocrine gland that produces progesterone, estrogen, human chorionic gonadotropin (hCG), and human placental lactogen (HPL).
- Fetal circulation provides oxygen and nutrients to the fetus and disposes of carbon dioxide and other waste products from the fetus. The temporary structures within the fetal circulatory system are the foramen ovale, ductus arteriosus, and ductus venosus.

# Study Questions

1. Compare the two types of cell division.
2. Describe gametogenesis in the male and female.
3. Describe the process of human fertilization.
4. How is the sex of human offspring determined?
5. Identify and describe the three stages of human prenatal development.
6. What is the function of the yolk sac in the embryo?
7. Describe the function of each accessory structure of pregnancy.
8. List and identify the functions of the four placental hormones.
9. Explain how the umbilical cord functions.
10. Compare monozygotic and dizygotic twins.
11. What are the temporary structures in fetal circulation?
12. Define crown-to-rump and crown-to-heel measurements of the developing embryo and fetus.
13. Describe the fetus at the midpoint of the gestational period, and explain why the fetus is described as "reaching a milestone in development."

# Multiple Choice Review Questions

*Choose the most appropriate answer.*

1. Following ovulation, the human ovum survives for up to
   a. 1 hour
   b. 12 hours
   c. 24 hours
   d. 2 days

2. Fertilization of the human ovum occurs in the
   a. corpus of the uterus
   b. outer third of the fallopian tube
   c. fimbriae of the fallopian tube
   d. uterine fundus

3. After implantation of the zygote, the endometrium is called the
   a. decidua
   b. myometrium
   c. blastocyst
   d. chorion
4. The child's sex is determined by the
   a. union of the X chromosomes from the ovum and sperm
   b. ovary, which releases a mature gamete
   c. ovum, which contributes either an X or a Y chromosome
   d. sperm, which contains either an X or a Y chromosome
5. The umbilical cord normally contains
   a. one artery, one vein, and Wharton's jelly
   b. two arteries and two veins
   c. two arteries, one vein, and Wharton's jelly
   d. two veins and Wharton's jelly
6. The foramen ovale, a temporary structure of fetal circulation, closes shortly after birth and normally closes permanently by
   a. 3 weeks
   b. 6 weeks
   c. 3 months
   d. 6 months
7. How many chromosomes does the mature ovum have?
   a. 23
   b. 24
   c. 46
   d. 48

## BIBLIOGRAPHY

Blackburn, S.T., & Loper, D.L. (1992). *Maternal, fetal, and neonatal physiology: A clinical perspective*. Philadelphia: W.B. Saunders.

Burroughs, A. (1992). *Maternity nursing* (6th ed.). Philadelphia: W.B. Saunders.

Danforth, D. (1990). *Obstetrics and gynecology* (6th ed.). Philadelphia: J.B. Lippincott.

Gorrie, T., McKinney, E., & Murray, S. (1994). *Foundations of maternal newborn nursing*. Philadelphia: W.B. Saunders.

Guyton, A. (1991). *Textbook of medical physiology* (8th ed.). Philadelphia: W.B. Saunders.

Hacker, N.F., & Moore, J.G. (1992). *Essentials of obstetrics and gynecology* (2nd ed.). Philadelphia: W.B. Saunders.

Knuppel, R.A., & Drukker, J.E. (1993). *High-risk pregnancy: A team approach* (3rd ed.). Philadelphia: W.B. Saunders.

Ladewig, P.W., London, M.L., & Olds, S.B. (1994). *Essentials of maternal-newborn nursing* (3rd ed.). Redwood City, CA: Addison-Wesley.

Moore, K.L. (1992). *Clinically oriented anatomy* (3rd ed.). Baltimore: Williams & Wilkins.

Moore, K.L., & Persaud, T.V.N. (1993). *The developing human: Clinically oriented embryology* (5th ed.). Philadelphia: W.B. Saunders.

Thompson, M.W., McInnes, R.R., & Willard, H.F. (1991). *Thompson and Thompson's genetics in medicine* (5th ed.). Philadelphia: W.B. Saunders.

# Part 2 The Expectant Family

## Chapter 4

# Prenatal Care and Adaptations to Pregnancy

## VOCABULARY

**Antepartum (51)**
**Braxton Hicks' contractions (54)**
**Chadwick's sign (53)**
**Goodell's sign (53)**
**gravida (51)**
**lightening (58)**
**multigravida (51)**
**para (51)**
**pica (66)**
**trimester (52)**

Goals of Prenatal Care
   Prenatal Visits
   Definition of Terms
   Determining Due Date
Signs of Pregnancy
   Presumptive Signs
   Probable Signs
   Positive Signs
Normal Physiologic Changes in Pregnancy
   Reproductive System
   Respiratory System
   Cardiovascular System
   Gastrointestinal System
   Urinary System
   Integumentary and Skeletal Systems
Nutrition
   Weight Gain
   Nutritional Requirements
   Other Nutritional Considerations
Common Discomforts in Pregnancy
Emotional Considerations in Pregnancy
   General Considerations
   Impact on the Mother
   Impact on the Father
   Impact on the Single Mother
   Impact on the Single Father
   Impact on the Adolescent

## OBJECTIVES

*On completion and mastery of Chapter 4, the student will be able to*

■ Define each vocabulary term listed.
■ List the goals of prenatal care.
■ Discuss prenatal care for a normal, uncomplicated pregnancy.
■ Describe nursing interventions significant to the pregnant woman during each trimester.
■ Calculate the expected date of delivery and duration of pregnancy using Nägele's rule.
■ Differentiate among the presumptive, probable, and positive signs of pregnancy.
■ Describe the normal physiologic adaptations of each body system during pregnancy.
■ Identify specific nutritional needs during pregnancy and lactation.
■ List several nourishing fast foods that might appeal to the pregnant teenager.
■ Identify frequently experienced discomforts of pregnancy and their causes.
■ Discuss three emotional changes that may occur in a family during pregnancy.

Pregnancy is an eventful period in a woman's life. It is a *normal*, temporary, physiologic process that affects the woman physically and emotionally. All systems of the body adapt in a miraculous way to accommodate the growing fetus. The focus of nursing is teaching self-care to maintain the mother's good health or, in the case of a mother with a predisposing condition, to maximize her health. This chapter reviews prenatal care, the physiologic and psychological changes of pregnancy, and the nurse's interventions to meet the needs of mothers and families during this transitional period.

## Goals of Prenatal Care

Care during pregnancy is essential to ensure a healthy pregnancy and a healthy baby. For optimal results, prenatal care should begin early in, or even before, the pregnancy. Obstetricians, certified nurse-midwives (CNMs), and family practice physicians provide prenatal care in both inpatient and outpatient clinics. The CNM and the nurse practitioner perform in-depth prenatal assessments. The office or clinic nurse often is the one who provides assistance, education, and counseling and assesses the expectant family's psychological needs. The nurse also promotes a relaxed environment to enhance communication with the family. Some goals of prenatal care include

- Providing physical care
- Educating in self-care
- Teaching health habits that may be continued after pregnancy
- Providing a safe delivery for mother and baby
- Providing an environment that is caring, aware of cultural diversity, and supportive of the family
- Providing psychological care, particularly when complications in the mother or baby arise
- Preparing parents for the responsibilities of parenthood

### PRENATAL VISITS

Prenatal care should begin as soon as a woman suspects that she is pregnant. A complete past and present history is obtained at the first visit. The history emphasizes the woman's past gynecologic and obstetric experience. After the health history is obtained, the woman is given a physical examination. A body systems review is completed, and baseline weight and vital signs are obtained. A pelvic examination is performed to evaluate the size, adequacy, and condition of the pelvis and organs. The expected due date is established. Risk assessment is done during the first visit and updated at subsequent visits.

Other procedures and tests include drawing blood for complete blood count (CBC), ABO and Rh typing, and antibody titers for rubella and hepatitis B (HBsAg). Women of African or Mediterranean descent should be screened for sickle cell trait. Women at high risk for human immunodeficiency virus (HIV) infection are asked if they would like screening tests. A tuberculin skin test may also be appropriate. Urinalysis, Papanicolaou's (Pap) smear, and *Neisseria* and *gonorrhoeal* cultures are also performed. The health-care provider uses universal precautions for protection when collecting and handling body fluids (see Appendix E and Fig. 23–31).

Psychosocial and family medical profiles are taken. These include information about cultural

## Nursing Brief

The major role of the nurse during prenatal care includes physical assessment of the pregnant woman, education in self-care, nutrition counseling, monitoring of blood values, evaluating risk factors, and providing emotional support.

## Nursing Brief

The nurse utilizes routine prenatal visits to listen to and answer questions from the expectant family. This is a prime time for teaching good health habits, as the woman is highly motivated.

and ethnic beliefs that may affect the pregnancy. Important information can be elicited by having the woman describe her typical day. The nurse asks her how she would like to be addressed (e.g., first name, last name, nickname) and records this information on the chart. The woman and her partner are encouraged to attend all prenatal appointments. They are educated about health-care options and encouraged to participate in decision-making.

Monthly visits are continued up to the 5th month, at which time visits are scheduled for every 2–3 weeks through the 8th month. In the 9th month, the visits are scheduled weekly until delivery. Frequency of antepartal visits is increased if abnormal changes are noted.

The prenatal visits provide for continuing assessment of the pregnant woman in the following areas: weight gain; blood pressure; height of the uterus; fetal heartbeat; swelling of ankles, face, or hands; and urinalysis and antibody screening.

Nutrition is reviewed, and risk factors are continually assessed. High-risk factors, such as smoking, drug use, alcohol consumption, being overweight or underweight, and socioeconomic problems, are identified, and goals are established. The nurse establishes rapport with the expectant family by conveying concern for their needs, listening to their concerns, and directing them to appropriate resources.

### DEFINITION OF TERMS

The following terms are used in describing the obstetric history of a pregnant patient:

**Ante:** Before
**Antepartum:** Before delivery
**Gravida:** Any pregnancy, regardless of duration
**Nulligravida:** A woman who has never been pregnant
**Primigravida:** A woman pregnant for the first time
**Multigravida:** A woman who was previously pregnant
**Para:** A woman who has borne offspring who reached the age of viability (approximately 20 weeks of gestation); this does not include the number of fetuses delivered
**Primipara:** A woman who has given birth to her first child (past the point of viability), regardless of whether that child is living or was alive at birth
**Multipara:** A woman who has had more than one pregnancy in which the fetus lived
**Nullipara:** A woman who has not delivered a live fetus
**Abortion:** The end of pregnancy before 20 weeks of gestation, either spontaneously or electively
**Gestational age:** The number of complete weeks of fetal development calculated in weeks from the first day of the last menstrual period

The gravida number increases by one each time a woman is pregnant, whereas the para number increases only when a woman delivers an infant of 20 weeks of gestation or more. For example, a woman who has had two spontaneous abortions (miscarriages) at 12 weeks of gestation, has a 3-year-old son, and is now 32 weeks pregnant would be described as gravida 4, para 1.

## Nursing Brief

Early, regular, prenatal care is important in reducing the number of low-birth-weight babies born and in reducing mortality and morbidity rates for mothers and newborns.

The TPAL system of identifying gravida and para (Box 4–1) is used on antepartal charts to provide detailed information about a woman's obstetric history.

### DETERMINING DUE DATE

A woman's pregnancy lasts 40 weeks (280 days) after the last menstrual period, plus or minus 2 weeks. To determine the expected date of confinement or expected date of delivery (EDD), Nägele's rule is used. To calculate the EDD, one identifies the first day of the last menstrual period, counts backward 3 months, and then adds 7 days (Box 4–2). This is an *estimated* date, as many normal deliveries occur before and after the exact date. The due date may also be determined by a gestation calculator or "wheel" (Fig. 4–1), physical examination, or ultrasound.

The pregnancy is divided into three *trimesters*, each of which is a 3-calendar month period of time. They are simply termed first, second, and third. Within a specific trimester certain predictable developments take place within the mother and the fetus. The knowledge of these developments assists in providing anticipatory guidance.

# Signs of Pregnancy

The signs of pregnancy are divided into three general groups: presumptive, probable, and positive.

### PRESUMPTIVE SIGNS

The presumptive signs of pregnancy, sometimes referred to as "subjective," are those from which a definite diagnosis of pregnancy cannot be made. These signs may result from illness or other bodily changes. The presumptive signs are amenorrhea, nausea and vomiting, breast changes, urinary disturbances, fatigue, and quickening.

*Amenorrhea*, the cessation of menses, in a healthy, sexually active female is often the first sign of pregnancy. However, strenuous exercise, changes in metabolism, endocrine dysfunction, certain medications, or serious psychological disturbances may be the cause.

*Nausea* and sometimes vomiting occurs in at least half of all pregnancies. These symptoms are commonly referred to as "morning sick-

---

**BOX 4–1**  **TPAL System of Identifying Gravida and Para**

**T**—number of *term* infants born (infants having at least 37 weeks of gestation)
**P**—number of *preterm* infants born (infants having less than 37 weeks of gestation)
**A**—number of pregnancies *aborted* (spontaneously or therapeutically)
**L**—number of children now *living*

**Example:**

| Name | Gravida | Term | Preterm | Aborted | Living |
|---|---|---|---|---|---|
| Katie Field | 3 | 1 | 0 | 1 | 1 |
| Anna Luz | 4 | 1 | 1 | 1 | 2 |

Katie Field: gravida 3, para 1011
Anna Luz: gravida 4, para 1112

---

ness," although they may occur at any time of day. A distaste for certain foods or even their odors occurs soon after fertilization and persists until the end of the 1st trimester. The high level of human chorionic gonadotropin (hCG) secreted from the fertilized ovum is the major factor in the development of these symptoms. Emotional problems or gastrointestinal upsets may also result in nausea and vomiting.

*Breast changes* frequently occur premenstrually, especially in women with chronically cystic breasts. During pregnancy the action of progesterone from the corpus luteum and the placenta results in swelling and tenderness.

*Urinary disturbances* are common and often annoying in the early months of pregnancy. The enlarging uterus, along with the increased blood supply to the pelvic area, exerts pressure on the bladder. Frequency and urgency of uri-

---

**BOX 4–2**  **Nägele's Rule**

Identify last menstrual period (LMP) (day 1; count backward 3 mo and add 7 days; result = expected date of delivery

**Example:**  1st day of LMP — Jan 27
Count backward 3 mo — Oct 27
Add 7 days — Nov 3 = expected date of delivery

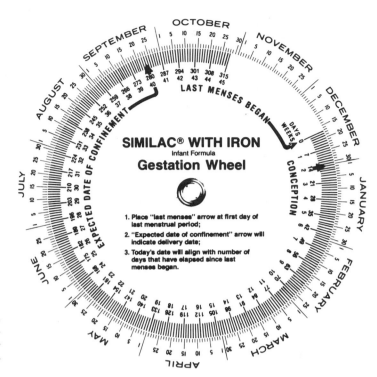

**Figure 4–1.** The EDD wheel can be used to calculate due date. The arrow is placed on the date the woman's last menstrual period began. The estimated date of delivery (EDD) is read at the arrow labeled "40." (Courtesy of Ross Laboratories, Columbus, OH.)

nation occur in the 1st trimester until the uterus expands and becomes an abdominal organ in the 2nd trimester. Again in the 3rd trimester, the pregnant woman experiences frequency of urination when the presenting part engages in the pelvis. Causes of urinary disturbances other than pregnancy are urinary tract infections and pelvic masses.

*Fatigue* is an early symptom of pregnancy that may suddenly become noticeable after the first missed menstrual period. It is believed to be caused by increased metabolic needs of the body. Urinary frequency may also interrupt sleep. In an otherwise healthy young woman, fatigue may be a significant sign of pregnancy.

*Quickening*, the first fetal movement felt by the mother, occurs at 18–20 weeks after the last menstrual period (LMP) and is described as a faint abdominal fluttering. This is an important symptom to record, because it marks the first half of the pregnancy and is a good reference point in identifying gestational age.

## PROBABLE SIGNS

The probable signs of pregnancy are termed "objective signs," as they are observable by the physician or CNM during physical and obstetric examination. The probable signs are Goodell's sign, Chadwick's sign, uterine enlargement, Hegar's sign, Braxton Hicks' contractions, ballottement, enlargement of the abdomen, presence of a fetal outline, abdominal striae (stretch marks), skin pigmentation, and positive results of pregnancy tests. Like the presumptive signs, the probable signs may be the result of other conditions, such as vascular congestion in the pelvic area due to, for example, tumors, myomas, or obesity.

*Goodell's sign* is the softening of the cervix and the vagina caused by increased vascular congestion.

*Chadwick's sign* is the purplish or bluish discoloration of the cervix, vagina, and vulva also caused by increased vascular congestion.

*Uterine enlargement* occurs rather irregularly at the onset of a pregnancy. By the end of the 12th week, the uterine fundus may be felt just above the symphysis pubis, and it expands to the umbilicus between the 20th and 22nd weeks (Fig. 4–2).

*Hegar's sign* is a softening of the lower uterine segment, which makes it easily compressed by the health-care provider. The wall feels as thin as tissue paper. This sign is present during

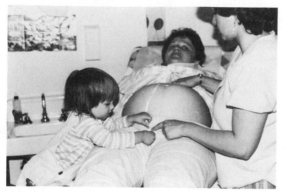

**Figure 4-2.** In the second half of the pregnancy, the height of the fundus is regularly checked to ascertain continuing fetal growth. Siblings are encouraged to participate actively in prenatal care of the expanding family. Here, "big sister" holds the tape measure. (Courtesy of Woman-Care, Des Moines BirthPlace, Des Moines, IA.)

the 2nd and 3rd months of pregnancy. Because of the softening it is easy to flex the body of the uterus against the cervix (*McDonald's sign*).

*Braxton Hicks'* contractions are irregular, painless uterine contractions that may occur throughout pregnancy.

*Ballottement* is a palpatory maneuver by which the fetal part is displaced by a light tap of the examining finger through the vagina and then rebounds quickly.

*Enlargement of the abdomen* in the sexually active female during childbearing years is usually a sign of pregnancy when it is continuous and accompanied by amenorrhea.

*Fetal outline* may be identified by palpation after the 24th week. It is possible to mistake a tumor for a fetus.

*Abdominal striae* (stretch marks) are fine, pinkish-white or purplish-gray lines that some women develop when the elastic tissue of the skin has been stretched to its capacity. Increased amounts of estrogen cause a rise in adrenal gland activity. This change plus the stretching is believed to cause a breakdown and atrophy of the underlying connective tissue in the skin. Striae are seen on the breasts, thighs, abdomen, and buttocks. After pregnancy the striae lose their bright color and become thin, silvery lines. Striae are depicted in Figure 4-3.

*Skin pigmentation changes* occur in most pregnant women because of the hormonal changes during pregnancy. The nipples and areola of the breasts may darken, particularly in a dark-skinned woman. The abdomen may develop a pink or brown midline, which is called the *linea nigra*. This line extends from the umbilicus or above to the symphysis pubis (see Fig. 4-3). Some women may develop *chloasma gravidarum* (mask of pregnancy), which is a brownish pigmentation on the face and around the eyes. Exposure to strong sunlight may deepen the color. The skin changes usually fade after the pregnancy.

*Pregnancy tests* are done using maternal urine or blood in order to determine the presence of hCG. hCG is a hormone produced by the chorionic villi of the placenta. It is detected shortly after the first missed menstrual period. One blood test considered highly reliable is the *radioimmunoassay (RIA)*. About 1 hour is needed to complete the RIA, which can determine pregnancy a few days after fertilization. It is useful in the diagnosis of pregnancies outside the uterus (see discussion of ectopic pregnancy, pp. 82–84.) Laboratory tests are considered probable signs, because there is always a risk of inaccuracy.

Urine tests are seldom used in health-care settings but are popular in *home testing kits*. They are fairly accurate when done properly.

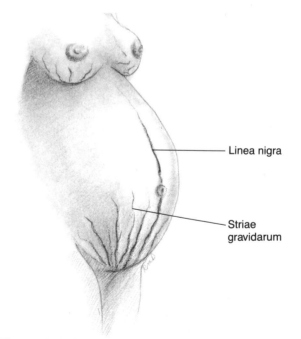

Linea nigra

Striae gravidarum

**Figure 4-3.** Abdominal striae are fine, pinkish-white or purple-gray lines that occur later in pregnancy. They may be found on the breasts, abdomen, and thighs. The brownish-black line at the midline is the linea nigra.

Women using these kits are instructed to follow the directions carefully. The first voided specimen of the day is required because hCG levels are highest at that time. Antianxiety medications and oral contraceptives may cause false-positive results (Pillitteri, 1992).

Women who test for their own pregnancy may independently improve self-care or postpone seeing a health-care provider unless they have bothersome symptoms. To prevent postponement of care, the nurse explains to women the importance of scheduling an appointment for prenatal care shortly after tests results are positive.

## POSITIVE SIGNS

Positive signs of pregnancy, also called "diagnostic signs," are the only absolute indicators of a developing fetus. The three positive signs of pregnancy are fetal heartbeat, fetal movements felt by the examiner, and identification of a fetus by ultrasound.

*Fetal heartbeat* may be detected as early as 10 weeks of pregnancy by using an ultrasound Doppler device (Fig. 4–4). The traditional fetoscope can detect the fetal heartbeat between the 18th and 20th weeks of pregnancy. With ultrasound, movement of the fetal heart can now be *seen* as early as 7 weeks. The fetal heart rate at term ranges between a low of 110–120 beats/min and a high of 150–160 beats/min (NAACOG, 1990; Gorrie et al., 1994) and tends to be higher earlier in gestation.

Additional sounds heard while assessing the fetal heartbeat are the uterine and funic souffles. *Uterine souffle* is a soft blowing sound heard over the uterus during auscultation. The sound is synchronous with the mother's pulse and is caused by blood entering the dilated arteries of the uterus. The *funic souffle* is a soft swishing sound heard as the blood passes through the umbilical cord vessels.

*Fetal movements* are palpable by a trained examiner in the 2nd trimester. Fetal activity must be distinguished by the examiner, because to a prospective mother, normal intestinal movements can appear similar to fetal movements. Ultrasound observation of fetal movements may be detected earlier.

*Identification of the embryo or fetus* by means of ultrasound observation and photography of the gestational sac is possible as early as 5–6 weeks of gestation with 100% reliability. This

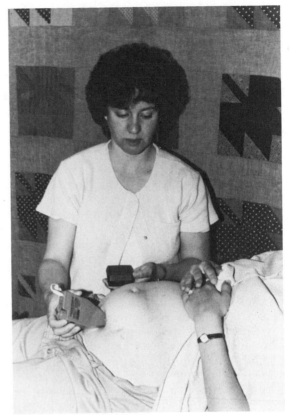

**Figure 4–4.** The fetal heart rate is checked at each prenatal visit. Hearing the baby's heartbeat is reassuring to the mother-to-be. (Courtesy of WomanCare, Des Moines Birth-Place, Des Moines, IA)

method is noninvasive and is the earliest positive sign of a pregnancy. Figure 4–5 shows a CNM, later in the pregnancy, checking for the location of the fetal head.

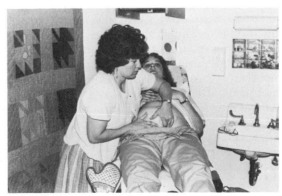

**Figure 4–5.** In the 3rd trimester, the certified nurse-midwife checks location of the fetal head. (Courtesy of WomanCare, Des Moines BirthPlace, Des Moines, IA.)

# Normal Physiologic Changes in Pregnancy

Nursing Care Plan 4–1 lists nursing interventions for selected diagnoses pertaining to normal physiologic changes during pregnancy.

## REPRODUCTIVE SYSTEM

### Uterus

The uterus undergoes the most obvious changes in pregnancy. Before pregnancy it is a small, pear-shaped pelvic organ that weighs approximately 60 gm (2 ounces) and measures 7.5 cm (3 inches) × 5 cm (2 inches) × 2.5 cm (1 inch). The uterus expands gradually during the pregnancy, chiefly by increasing the size of the individual cells of the myometrium.

At the end of the 1st trimester, the uterus becomes a temporary abdominal organ. At term, its weight has increased approximately 20 times, so that it weighs 1000 gm (2.2 pounds), its size has increased to approximately 28 cm (11 inches) × 24 cm (9.4 inches) × 21 cm (8.2 inches). Its capacity increases from 10 ml to 5 liters or more. (Ladewig et al., 1994).

Braxton Hicks' contractions are stimulated by increased estrogen production and enlargement of the uterus. These painless, intermittent contractions can be felt through the abdominal wall, beginning in the 2nd trimester. They prepare the cervix for labor and are sometimes mistaken for true labor.

### Cervix

Following conception, the cervix changes in color and consistency. Chadwick's and Goodell's signs appear. The endocervical glands of the cervical mucosa increase in number and activity. These combined changes prepare for uterine effacement (thinning) and cervical dilation (enlargement) when the baby is born.

An increased cervical discharge (mucorrhea) of thick, tenacious mucus leads to the formation of a *mucous plug* that seals the cervical canal. This seal prevents the ascent of any organisms into the uterus; normally, the vagina is not sterile. With the beginning of cervical dilation in the first stage of labor, the plug is loosened and expelled.

### Ovaries

The ovaries cease to produce ova (eggs) during pregnancy. The *corpus luteum* (empty graafian follicle; see p. 27) remains on the ovary and produces progesterone during the first 10–12 weeks of the pregnancy. Proges-terone maintains the *decidua* (uterine lining) until the placenta is established. The corpus luteum diminishes in size and disappears by the 20th week of pregnancy.

### Vagina

Vascularization of the vagina increases, and Chadwick's sign appears. Estrogen levels increase to prepare the vagina for the passage of the baby. Estrogen directly acts on the vaginal mucosa to cause a thickening of the mucosa and a loosening of the connective tissue. At term, the vaginal wall and perineum become sufficiently relaxed for delivery. Along with these temporary physical changes, the secretions of the vagina increase. In addition, the pH becomes more acidic to protect the vagina and uterus from pathogenic microorganisms.

### Breasts

Hormone-induced breast changes occur early in pregnancy. High levels of estrogen and progesterone prepare the breasts for lactation (breast feeding). The areolae of the breasts usually become deeply pigmented, and nodules called tubercles of Montgomery become prominent. Striae may become visible.

In the last few months of pregnancy, a yellow protein and mineral secretion called colostrum may be expressed from the breasts. This "premilk" is low in fat and sugar and contains the mother's antibodies to diseases. Colostrum is converted to milk 3–4 days after delivery.

## RESPIRATORY SYSTEM

The pregnant woman breathes more deeply and more rapidly (18–20 breaths/min), which allows for increased exchange of oxygen and carbon dioxide at the cellular level. She is, in effect, "breathing for two." An increase in progesterone levels relaxes ligaments, allowing the chest cage to expand and the diaphragm to move more easily. During the pregnancy, the

## Selected Nursing Diagnoses for Normal Physiologic Changes During Pregnancy

| Goals | Nursing Interventions | Rationale |
|---|---|---|
| **Nursing Diagnosis:** Health-seeking behaviors related to normal pregnancy. | | |
| Woman will communicate her understanding of changes that take place in her body during pregnancy<br>Woman will verbalize telephone number to call as questions arise | 1. Encourage woman to write down questions to ask her health-care provider | 1. Many women are nervous during early prenatal visits, and they often forget to ask questions; if there are language barriers, they need to be addressed |
| | 2. Answer questions during prenatal visits | 2. Answers to questions reduce a woman's anxiety and promote a more relaxed and enjoyable pregnancy |
| | 3. Clearly identify problems about which woman should immediately call | 3. Not all changes during pregnancy are normal, and the woman should clearly understand danger signals that require immediate attention (see Box 5–1) |
| | 4. Provide printed material for woman to take home for reference and to share with "significant other" | 4. Printed material needs to be in native language of client; this provides reference if woman forgets and/or for review later if questions arise |
| **Nursing Diagnosis:** Knowledge deficit related to common discomforts of pregnancy | | |
| Woman is able to identify causes of discomfort | 1. Explain physiologic causes of discomforts according to knowledge level of woman | 1. Woman will not interpret normal discomforts as dangerous; she is able to distinguish between normal and abnormal |
| Woman states appropriate measures to alleviate problems:<br>Nasal stuffiness and epistaxis | 2. Provide suggestions for self-help measures to reduce discomforts:<br>a. Teach woman to improve humidity in house by cool-air vaporizor | a. Humidity reduces drying nasal mucosa, which alleviates some causes of epistaxis |
| | b. Teach woman to blow nose gently | b. This prevents trauma to membranes and vessels of nose |
| | c. When bleeding occurs, instruct woman to apply pressure to nostrils and to place ice over nose | c. Most epistaxis occurs in anterior part of the septum; pressure and ice compresses produce vasoconstriction, which may decrease bleeding |
| | d. Instruct woman to call health-care provider if bleeding continues for longer than 5 min | d. These measures generally stop bleeding; however, nasal packing may be required |
| Increased blood volume | a. Explain that dizziness or a clammy feeling that may occur when lying flat on the back is relieved by rolling onto left side | a. Enlarging uterus may cause pressure on vena cava, which interferes with returning blood flow and cardiac output; this produces a marked decrease in blood pressure, termed *supine hypotensive syndrome* |
| Constipation | a. Instruct woman to increase daily fluid intake by 4–6 glasses | a. Delay in emptying time of intestine, due to decreased muscle tone, allows more water to be absorbed from the bowel; during pregnancy, peristaltic action of gastrointestinal tract is reduced because of increase in progesterone |
| | b. Teach woman to eat a well-balanced diet with whole grains, fruits, and vegetables | b. Roughage promotes peristalsis |
| | c. Encourage woman to respond immediately to urge to defecate | c. This helps to promote regularity |

*Continued*

## Selected Nursing Diagnoses for Normal Physiologic Changes During Pregnancy

| Goals | Nursing Interventions | Rationale |
|---|---|---|
| **Nursing Diagnosis:** Knowledge deficit related to common discomforts of pregnancy. | | |
| Heartburn | a. Teach woman to eat small meals at more frequent intervals throughout day | a. Cardiac sphincter of stomach relaxes, causing gastric contents to enter esophagus; small meals prevent further pressure |
| | b. Instruct to sit up for 30 min following meals | b. Sitting up may prevent reflux |
| Frequency in urination | a. Explain to woman that pressure on bladder during 1st trimester is due to expansion of uterus in pelvic area; in 3rd trimester, pressure is due to developing fetus | a. As long as other symptoms of urinary tract infection are not present, frequency is considered normal during 1st and 3rd trimesters |
| | b. Teach woman signs and symptoms of actual infection, i.e., burning, pain, and fever | b. Early detection prevents complications |
| | c. Teach woman to avoid caffeine, which can be found in tea, coffee, cocoa, chocolate, some over-the-counter drugs such as Anacin, Excedrin, and No Doz, and in some prescription drugs | c. Caffeine is a stimulant that increases urination; its half-life triples during pregnancy because of impeded caffeine clearance; the fetus faces a higher risk of exposure because of this. Pregnant woman consults with health-care provider *before* taking any over-the-counter or previously prescribed medications |
| Skin changes | a. Reassure woman that darkened skin areas are temporary and will gradually disappear after birth of baby | a. Changes in skin pigmentation are stimulated by elevated levels of melanocyte-stimulating hormone, which may be caused by increased levels of estrogen and progesterone; these include chloasma, linea nigra, spider nevi, striae, darkened nipples and areolae, and increased pigmentation of palms of hands |
| | b. Softening oils and creams may reduce stretch marks but do not completely prevent them | b. Applying softeners together may enhance closeness of couple |
| Backache | a. Advise woman to wear low-heeled shoes | a. Joints of pelvis relax during pregnancy as a result of hormonal changes, causing lumbosacral lordosis; changes in posture also occur as a result of shifts in woman's center of gravity due to enlarging uterus. Excessive weight gain also puts strain on back |
| | b. Demonstrate good body mechanics | b. Good posture and good body mechanics prevent additional strain |

expanding uterus exerts pressure on the sternum so that the diaphragm rises and the rib cage flares, increasing the diameter of the chest about 5 cm (2 inches). The greater chest diameter compensates for the elevated diaphragm, so there is no significant loss of lung capacity. This change is normal and is explained to the expectant mother. Some dyspnea may occur until the fetus descends into the pelvis, a process referred to as *lightening*.

Increased estrogen levels during pregnancy are responsible for edema or swelling of the nasal mucosa. This swelling may cause nasal stuffiness and epistaxis (nosebleeds).

## CARDIOVASCULAR SYSTEM

The pressure of the growing uterus displaces the heart upward and to the left. This makes the heart appear enlarged on x-ray films. The most significant normal change is the gradual increase of blood volume, called *hypervolemia*, beginning in the 1st trimester and reaching at term a 30–50% increase over that of the prepregnant state. This increase provides adequate exchange of nutrients in the placenta and compensates for blood lost at delivery. To accommodate the increase, the heart works harder and more blood is pumped out of the heart. This shortens the diastolic or relaxation period. The pulse rate increases by 10–15 beats/min.

Blood pressure does not increase because the increase in heart rate accommodates hypervolemia. An elevation in blood pressure above that of the woman's prepregnant state requires careful attention.

*Palpitations* may occur from increases in thoracic pressure, particularly if the woman moves suddenly. Orthostatic (*ortho*, "straight," and *statikos*, "to stand") hypotension may occur whenever a woman stands from a recumbent position. This may result in faintness or lightheadedness. Cardiac output decreases because of reduced venous return from the lower body.

Although both plasma (fluid) and red blood cells increase during pregnancy, they are disproportionate. A dilutional or pseudoanemia often occurs because the total red blood cell increase is only half of the blood plasma volume increase (there is more fluid than red blood cells). As a result, the normal prepregnant hematocrit level (38–47%) may fall. Although not true anemia, it is carefully followed. The white blood cell (leukocyte) count likewise increases (Box 4–3).

As pregnancy continues, the weight of the distended uterus exerts pressure on the vessels returning blood from the lower extremities. Pooling of venous blood results in dependent edema and varicosities in the legs, vulva, and rectum. When a woman is lying flat on her back, the weighty uterus may rest heavily on the vena cava and cause *supine hypotension syndrome*. The woman feels dizzy and clammy and is pale. Her blood pressure drops. Rapid relief is promoted by having the woman turn onto her left side or sit, or by raising the head of the bed.

## GASTROINTESTINAL SYSTEM

The larger uterus displaces the stomach and intestines toward the back and sides of the abdomen. In early pregnancy, the increased hCG levels cause nausea and vomiting (morning sickness). There may be increased salivary secretions (ptyalism), which in turn affect taste and smell. The gums may become tender and bleed more easily. This is believed to be caused by increases in estrogen.

The demands of the growing fetus increase the woman's appetite and thirst. The acidity of gastric secretions is decreased; emptying of the stomach and motility (movement) of the intestines are slower. Women often feel bloated and may experience constipation and hemorrhoids. Pyrosis (heartburn), a frequent complaint, is caused by the relaxation of the cardiac sphincter of the stomach, which permits reflux (backward flow) of the acid secretions into the lower esophagus.

## URINARY SYSTEM

The urinary system excretes the waste products of the mother and fetus during pregnancy. The glomerular filtration rate of the kidneys

---

| BOX 4–3 | Standard Blood Values in Pregnant Women* |
|---|---|

Hemoglobin: 11.5–14 gm/dl (higher in high altitudes)
Hematocrit: 32–46%
Complete blood count (higher in high altitudes)
  Red blood cells: 4.2–5.4 million/mm³
  White blood cells: 5000–15,000/mm³
Differential
  Neutrophils: 50–70%
  Eosinophils: 1–3%
  Lymphocytes: 20–40%
  Bands: up to 5%
  Basophils: up to 1%
  Monocytes: 4–8%

---

*These standards vary somewhat among references.

rises. The renal tubules increase their reabsorption. Water is retained because it is needed for increased blood volume and for dissolving nutrients for the fetus. The diameter of the ureters and bladder capacity increase because of increased levels of progesterone.

The renal pelvis and ureters lose tone, which causes a decrease in peristalsis to the bladder and stasis of urine. Thus the woman is more susceptible to urinary infection during pregnancy. Therefore, a fluid consumption of 8 glasses a day is recommended. Although the bladder can hold up to 1500 ml of urine, the pressure of the enlarging uterus causes frequency of urination, especially in the 1st and 3rd trimesters.

### INTEGUMENTARY AND SKELETAL SYSTEMS

The high levels of hormones produced during pregnancy cause a variety of temporary changes in the integument (skin) of the pregnant woman. Skin darkens in the nipple and areola of the breast. Darkened areas, called chloasma gravidarum, may appear on the forehead, cheeks, and nose. The sweat and sebaceous glands of the skin become more active.

Small red elevations of skin with lines radiating from the center, called *spider nevi*, may also occur. The palms of the hands may become deeper red. All these skin pigmentation changes are reversed shortly after delivery.

The skeletal system undergoes some temporary posture changes because of the gradual change in the contour of the body as the baby grows within the uterus. The uterus increases in weight in the anterior portion of the body, and there is a more noticeable curve in the dorsal lumbar spine. The woman frequently experiences low backaches, and in the last few months of pregnancy, rounding of the shoulders may occur along with aching in the cervical spine and upper extremities.

The joints of the pelvis relax somewhat because of the hormonal changes as well as the entry of the presenting fetal part into the pelvic brim in the last trimester. Often, especially in her first pregnancy, a woman demonstrates a "waddling gait" in the last few weeks of pregnancy because of a slight separation of the pubic joint. These pelvic changes are reversed, usually within the 6-week postpartum period.

## Nutrition

Nutrition is the single most important factor both in establishing and maintaining a healthy pregnancy and in the successful delivery of a healthy baby. Good nutritional habits maintained before conception, and continued during pregnancy, permit an easy adaptation to the accelerated metabolic needs of pregnancy. The food guide pyramid presents a healthy guide to daily food choices for the public (Fig. 4–6). Women who follow this food plan when they are not pregnant will be well-nourished at the time of conception.

*Careful reading of food labels* is important to obtaining nutritional rather than empty calories. The Food and Drug Administration (FDA) along with the U.S. Department of Agriculture has developed new food labels that manufacturers must follow (Fig. 4–7). This will help to inform the pregnant women and other consumers of the contents of packages and canned goods.

### WEIGHT GAIN

The acceptable amount of weight gain has fluctuated over the years. The National Academy of Sciences (NAS) recommends a weight gain of 25–35 pounds for women of normal weight, 28–40 pounds for underweight women, and 15–25 pounds for overweight women (Table 4–1). Women with multiple fetuses should gain more weight. The distribution of weight gain in pregnancy is depicted in Table 4–2. Weight gain in the adolescent should be in the upper part of the range currently recommended for adults.

Little if any weight is gained in the 1st trimester, usually because of nausea and vomiting and some transient food dislikes. If nausea and vomiting are minimal, any lost weight is regained. Weight gain continues at an average of 1 pound/week; approximately 3, 12, and 12

## Nursing Brief

There is a high correlation between maternal diet and fetal health. To ensure that deficiencies do not occur early in pregnancy (the first 6 weeks), the nurse explains to women of childbearing age the value of eating well-balanced meals.

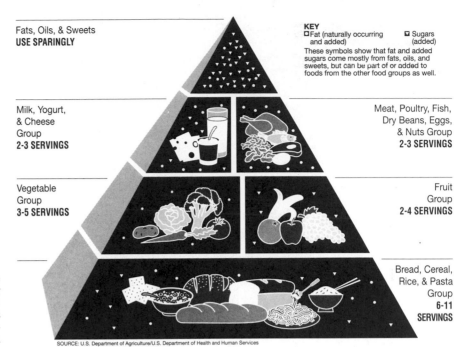

**Figure 4–6.** The food guide pyramid. This is a chart listing healthy foods to eat each day. (Courtesy of U.S. Department of Agriculture and U.S. Department of Health and Human Services).

In the image:

Fats, Oils, & Sweets
**USE SPARINGLY**

KEY
□ Fat (naturally occurring and added)    ☑ Sugars (added)
These symbols show that fat and added sugars come mostly from fats, oils, and sweets, but can be part of or added to foods from the other food groups as well.

Milk, Yogurt, & Cheese Group
**2-3 SERVINGS**

Meat, Poultry, Fish, Dry Beans, Eggs, & Nuts Group
**2-3 SERVINGS**

Vegetable Group
**3-5 SERVINGS**

Fruit Group
**2-4 SERVINGS**

Bread, Cereal, Rice, & Pasta Group
**6-11 SERVINGS**

SOURCE: U.S. Department of Agriculture/U.S. Department of Health and Human Services

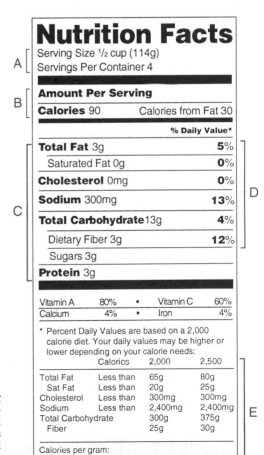

**Figure 4–7.** The new food label is headed "Nutrition Facts." *A*, Serving sizes are now standardized for varying products and are given in common measures. *B*, Calories from fat should be under 30% of one's total caloric intake. *C*, Nutrients are listed. *D*, Percentage of daily value is given for each nutrient. This can be used to compare foods for a balanced diet. *E*, Daily values are listed for people who eat 2000 calories (most women, children, and men over 50 years of age) and 2400 calories (most teenage boys, younger men, and very active people). (Courtesy of Food and Drug Administration, U.S. Department of Agriculture).

**61**

**Table 4–1.** RECOMMENDED WEIGHT GAIN FOR PREGNANT WOMEN BASED ON BODY MASS INDEX*

| Weight Category Based on BMI[†] | Total Weight Gain[‡] | | 1st-Trimester Gain | | 2nd- and 3rd-Trimester Weekly Gain | |
|---|---|---|---|---|---|---|
| | lb | kg | lb | kg | lb | kg |
| Underweight (BMI < 19.8) | 28–40 | 12.5–18 | 5 | 2.3 | 1.07 | 0.49 |
| Normal weight (BMI = 19.8–26) | 25–35 | 11.5–16 | 3.5 | 1.6 | 0.97 | 0.44 |
| Overweight (BMI > 26–29) | 15–25 | 7–11.5 | 2 | 0.9 | 0.67 | 0.3 |
| Obese (BMI > 29) | ≥15 | 6 | | | | |

*Data from Subcommittee on Nutritional Status and Weight Gain During Pregnancy and Subcommittee on Dietary Intake and Nutrient Supplements During Pregnancy, Food and Nutrition Board, National Academy of Sciences. (1990). *Nutrition during pregnancy, parts I and II.* Washington, DC: National Academy Press.
[†]BMI, body mass index; metric BMI, weight (kg)/height (m)$^2$.
[‡]Young adolescents and African-American women should strive for gains at the upper end of the recommended range. Short women (<62 inches or <157 cm) should strive for gains at the lower end of the range.
From Mahan, L.K., & Arlin, M.T. (1992). *Krause's food, nutrition & diet therapy* (8th ed.). Philadelphia: W.B. Saunders.

pounds are gained in the first, second, and third trimesters, respectively.

## NUTRITIONAL REQUIREMENTS

To provide for the growth of the fetus, fetal support tissue, and maternal support systems, an increase in caloric intake of 300 kcal/day is vital. Caloric intake must be nutritious. Four important nutrients in pregnancy are protein, calcium, iron, and folic acid. The amounts are specified in Table 4–3.

**Protein.** The best sources of protein are meat, fish, poultry, and dairy products. Because excessive protein intake in the form of animal and dairy products has been related to high cholesterol and saturated fat in the diet, adequate amounts of protein can alternatively be obtained from plant sources (Poleman & Peckenpaugh, 1991). Beans, lentils, and other legumes; breads and cereals; and seeds and nuts, complemented with another plant or animal protein, provide all the protein (amino acids) needed to build and repair body tissues. They also provide protein for the developing fetus.

Examples of complementary plant protein sources are corn and beans, lentils and rice, and peanut butter and bread. Plant proteins are also complemented with animal proteins, for example, in grilled cheese sandwiches, cereal with milk, and chili made of meat and beans. The complementary foods must be eaten together, because all the amino acids necessary for building tissues must be present at the same time.

This information should be given to women who are vegetarians, to ensure that their protein needs are met. The information can also help reduce the family's food budget, because many plant protein sources are less expensive than animal sources.

**Calcium.** Pregnancy and lactation increase calcium requirements by nearly 50%. The recommended daily allowance of calcium for pregnant women is 1200 mg. Milk (or other dairy products) is the single most important source of this nutrient. Other sources of calcium include enriched cereals, cheese, and green leafy veg-

**Table 4–2.** DISTRIBUTION OF WEIGHT GAIN IN PREGNANCY

| Source of Weight Gain | Weight Gain |
|---|---|
| Uterus | 2.5 lb (1.1 kg) |
| Fetus | 7.0–7.5 lb (3.2–3.4 kg) |
| Placenta | 1.0–1.5 lb (0.5–0.7 kg) |
| Amniotic fluid | 2.0 lb (0.9 kg) |
| Breasts | 1.5–3.0 lb (0.7–1.4 kg) |
| Blood volume | 3.5–4.0 lb (1.6–1.8 kg) |
| Extravascular fluids | 3.5–5.0 lb (1.6–2.3 kg) |
| Maternal stores | 4.0–9.5 lb (1.8–4.3 kg) |
| Total | 25.0–35.0 lb (11.4–15.9 kg) |

Data from Gorrie, T.M., McKinney, E.S., & Murray, S.S. (1994). *Foundations of maternal newborn nursing.* Philadelphia: W.B. Saunders.

**Table 4–3.** RECOMMENDED DIETARY ALLOWANCES FOR WOMEN

| | 15–18 Years | 19–24 Years | 25–50 Years | Pregnant | Lactating 1st 6 Months | Lactating 2nd 6 Months |
|---|---|---|---|---|---|---|
| Energy (kcal) | 2200 | 2200 | 2200 | +0 1st tri +300 2nd tri +300 3rd tri | +500 | +500 |
| Protein (gm) | 44 | 46 | 50 | 60 | 65 | 62 |
| Vitamin A ($\mu$g RE) | 800 | 800 | 800 | 800 | 1300 | 1200 |
| Vitamin D ($\mu$g) | 10 | 10 | 5 | 10 | 10 | 10 |
| Vitamin E (mg $\alpha$-TE) | 8 | 8 | 8 | 10 | 12 | 11 |
| Vitamin K ($\mu$g) | 55 | 60 | 65 | 65 | 65 | 65 |
| Vitamin C (mg) | 60 | 60 | 60 | 70 | 95 | 90 |
| Thiamin (mg) | 1.1 | 1.1 | 1.1 | 1.5 | 1.6 | 1.6 |
| Riboflavin (mg) | 1.3 | 1.3 | 1.3 | 1.6 | 1.8 | 1.7 |
| Niacin (mg NE) | 15 | 15 | 15 | 17 | 20 | 20 |
| Vitamin $B_6$ (mg) | 1.5 | 1.6 | 1.6 | 2.2 | 2.1 | 2.1 |
| Folate ($\mu$g) | 180 | 180 | 180 | 400 | 280 | 260 |
| Vitamin $B_{12}$ ($\mu$g) | 2 | 2 | 2 | 2.2 | 2.6 | 2.6 |
| Calcium (mg) | 1200 | 1200 | 800 | 1200 | 1200 | 1200 |
| Phosphorous (mg) | 1200 | 1200 | 800 | 1200 | 1200 | 1200 |
| Magnesium (mg) | 300 | 280 | 280 | 320 | 355 | 340 |
| Iron (mg) | 15 | 15 | 15 | 30 | 15 | 15 |
| Zinc (mg) | 12 | 12 | 12 | 15 | 19 | 16 |
| Iodine ($\mu$g) | 150 | 150 | 150 | 175 | 200 | 200 |
| Selenium ($\mu$g) | 50 | 55 | 55 | 65 | 75 | 75 |

Adapted with permission from RECOMMENDED DIETARY ALLOWANCES: 10th edition. Copyright 1989 by the National Academy of Sciences. Courtesy of the National Academy Press, Washington, D.C.

tri, trimester; RE, retinol equivalent; TE, tocopherol equivalent; NE, niacin equivalent.

etables. For women who, for whatever reason, do not drink milk (or eat sufficient amounts of equivalent products), calcium supplementation is necessary. Alternatives for women with lactose intolerance are given on page 66.

**Iron.** Pregnancy causes a heavy demand for iron, because the fetus must store an adequate supply to meet the needs of the first 5 months of life. In addition, the pregnant woman must increase her production of red blood cells because of the increase in hemoglobin and blood volume needed to support the fetus. A nutritional assessment of dietary iron should be considered for each pregnant woman. The recommended dietary allowance (RDA) is 15 mg/day for nonpregnant adult women and 30+ mg/day for pregnant women.

Iron comes in two forms: *heme*, found in red and organ meats, and *nonheme*, found in plant products. Heme iron is readily absorbed by the body. Nonheme high-iron plant foods, such as molasses, whole grains, iron-fortified cereals and breads, dark-green leafy vegetables, and dried fruits, are poorly absorbed by the body unless vitamin C foods or meat is consumed at the same meal (Poleman & Peckenpaugh, 1991).

Nutritional teaching by the nurse during prenatal visits is important for maintaining the health of the mother and ensuring a healthy baby. Many American women do not meet the minimum iron requirement in their daily diet, and iron supplementation is recommended during pregnancy in order to prevent iron-deficiency anemia. Ferrous sulfate or ferrous gluconate, 30–60 mg three times/day, is widely recommended, along with a well-balanced diet.

**Folic Acid.** Folic acid (folacin) is a water-soluble B vitamin essential for the formation and maturation of both red and white blood cells in bone marrow. The 1989 RDA for a pregnant woman is 400 $\mu$g during pregnancy. The most effective dietary sources are liver; kidney and lima beans; fresh, dark-green leafy vegetables; lean beef; potatoes; whole-wheat bread; dried beans; and peanuts.

The March of Dimes Foundation recommends that all women in their childbearing years obtain sufficient amounts of folic acid to reduce neural tube defects, which can occur in the fetus before the woman realizes she is pregnant. Nursing Care Plan 4–2 lists nursing diagnoses for nutrition during pregnancy and lactation, and Table 4–4 is a daily food guide for the pregnant woman.

## OTHER NUTRITIONAL CONSIDERATIONS

**Pregnant Teenager.** *Gynecologic age* is the number of years between the onset of menses and the date of conception. The teenager who

---

| NURSING CARE PLAN 4–2 | | |
| --- | --- | --- |
| **Selected Nursing Diagnoses for Nutrition During Pregnancy and Lactation** | | |
| Goals | Nursing Interventions | Rationale |

**Nursing Diagnosis:** Knowledge deficit related to importance of nutrition in pregnancy and lactation.

| | | |
| --- | --- | --- |
| Woman verbalizes need for good nutrition in pregnancy and lactation | 1. Assess age, parity, prepregant nutritional status, food preferences and dislikes, food intolerances and general health of pregnant woman | 1. Many factors influence nutritional status of woman during pregnancy and lactation; they must be considered on an individualized basis to guide woman in verbalizing her own specific needs |
| | 2. Assess socioeconomic and cultural factors that may influence food choices, and make recommendations to fit specific needs | 2. Socioeconomic and cultural factors affect family's nutritional status; it is vital that these be individually considered and specific adaptations be made |
| | 3. Review specific nutritional requirements and food sources for optimum outcome of pregnancy and lactation | 3. If woman understands specific nutritional needs of pregnancy and food sources to meet these needs, she is more likely to meet dietary needs |
| | 4. Provide written information on nutrition for use as reference in preparation of meals | 4. Written information reinforces verbal teaching and helps woman recall forgotten information |
| | 5. Encourage questions and provide appropriate answers | 5. Allows nurse to identify areas of inadequate knowledge or misunderstanding |
| | 6. Suggest options to decrease cost of food | 6. Refer to Women, Infants and Children nutrition program, as appropriate |
| Woman implements good nutrition during pregnancy and lactation, as evidenced by food diary | 1. Review a 24-hour diet intake and make appropriate recommendations for improvement | 1. Analysis of specific meals and snacks enables the nurse to identify adequate and inadequate intake of specific nutrients |
| | 2. Provide written guidelines for dietary intake | 2. Written guidelines provide reinforcement |
| | 3. Instruct woman about food guide pyramid and proper reading of labels | 3. Choices on food guide pyramid provide essential nutrients on a daily basis   Reading labels is important in aiding consumer to select more nutritious items |
| Woman demonstrates a gradual weight gain consistent with her specific needs | 1. Maintain a chart to show actual weight of woman at each visit | 1. Weight chart is a visual display of actual weight changes |
| | 2. Review progress of weight with woman at each visit, and arrange for specific nutritional counseling as needed | 2. Reviewing the progress demonstrates support and determines areas that need reinforcement; weight gain in pregnancy should be gradual over 9-mo period; women of average weight should gain 25–35 lb; overweight women should gain less; underweight women should gain more; those experiencing multifetal gestation also need to gain more weight |

**Table 4-4.** A DAILY FOOD GUIDE DURING PREGNANCY

| Food Group | Serving Size | Recommended Number of Servings | Foods to Avoid If the Woman Has Problems with Nausea and Vomiting | Sample Menu Plan for 1 Day |
|---|---|---|---|---|
| ***Milk Products*** * | | | Chocolate milk | **Breakfast** |
| Fluid milk | 8-oz cup | 3–4 | | 1 cup milk |
| Yogurt | 8-oz cup | | | 1 toasted English muffin, 1 teaspoon margarine |
| Hard cheese | 1½ oz | (Note: Age 18 and under—4 servings per day) | | ¾ cup shredded wheat |
| | | | | ½ sliced banana |
| | | | | ½ cup orange juice |
| Cottage cheese | 2 cups | | | **Snack** |
| Dry milk powder | ⅓ cup | | | ½ cup rice pudding with raisins |
| Ricotta cheese | ½ cup | | | **Lunch** |
| ***Meat and Protein Substitutes*** | | | | 1 cup milk |
| | | | | Sandwich |
| Lean beef, pork, poultry, fish, lamb, veal | 2 oz | 3–4 | Meats seasoned with strong spices such as garlic, chili powder, taco seasoning, pizza seasoning | 2 slices wheat bread |
| | | | | 2 oz tuna |
| | | | | 1 tablespoon mayonnaise |
| | | | | Sliced tomato and lettuce |
| | | | | ½ cup three-bean salad |
| | | | | 1 small apple |
| Eggs | 2 | | | **Snack** |
| Dried peas and beans | 1 cup | | | Fresh pear |
| Peanut butter | 4 tablespoons | | | **Dinner** |
| ***Fruits and Vegetables*** | | | | Tomato soup with ⅓ cup nonfat dry milk added and 6 crackers |
| Good vitamin A sources: dark green or deep yellow vegetables (spinach, mustard, turnip or dandelion greens, chard, sweet potatoes, winter squash, broccoli) | ½ cup | 1 or more | Gas-forming vegetables, such as cabbage, onions, cauliflower, broccoli | 1 cup milk |
| | | | | 4 oz chicken breast |
| | | | | 1 medium baked potato |
| | | | | Asparagus spears |
| | | | | Tossed salad: spinach, lettuce, celery, carrots, radishes, tomatoes, 1 tablespoon salad dressing |
| | | | | Angelfood cake with ½ cup sliced strawberries |
| Good vitamin C sources: citrus fruit, such as oranges and grapefruits and their juices; tomatoes; strawberries; cantaloupes | ½ cup | 2 or more | | **Snack** |
| | | | | ½ toasted bagel with ¼ cup ricotta cheese and 1 teaspoon jelly |
| Other fruits and vegetables | ½ cup | 3–5 | | |
| ***Breads and Cereals (Enriched or Whole-Grain)*** | | | | |
| Breads | 1 slice | 6–8 | | |
| Cereals | ½–¾ cup | (Note: Age 18 and under—8 servings per day or more) | | |
| Rice, pasta | ½ cup | | | |
| ***Others*** | | | | |
| Fats, oils, salad dressing | Use sparingly | | Chocolate, greasy and fried foods, rich desserts | |
| Sweets, desserts, candy, jam | Use moderate amounts only | | | |

*Portion sizes for milk products provide the same amount of calcium as one 8-oz portion of milk.
Courtesy of Mercy Nutrition Specialists, Mercy Hospital Medical Center, Des Moines, IA.

conceives soon after having her first period has greater nutritional needs than one who is more sexually mature. In any nutritional intervention for the pregnant teenager, one must consider the teenager's characteristics of resistance, ambivalence, and inconsistency.

Even a moderate change in diet to ensure compliance is helpful. Fast foods with poor nutritional content are often the teenager's foods of choice. However, the nurse can advise the teenager that many fast food restaurants offer salads, muffins, chicken, tacos, baked potatoes, and pizza. These foods provide many important nutrients and allow her to socialize with her peers at mealtime. A cheeseburger and a glass of milk are also nutritious.

Nutritional intervention is necessary early in prenatal care to ensure a healthy mother and baby. Many communities offer programs for adolescents that provide social support, education about prenatal care, and nutritional advice. Teenagers often respond well in peer groups. The nurse is often the advocate for these young women and may encourage them to apply for programs such as Women, Infants, and Children and food stamps. Pregnant teenagers, whether or not they need financial assistance, need frequent review and reinforcement of nutritional information during prenatal visits.

**Sodium Intake.** The salt (sodium chloride) intake of pregnant women has been restricted in the past in an attempt to prevent edema and pregnancy-induced hypertension. It is now accepted that sodium should not be restricted during pregnancy. Sodium intake is essential for maintaining normal sodium levels in plasma, bone, brain, and muscle, because both tissue and fluid expand during the prenatal period.

Taking diuretics during pregnancy to rid the body of excess fluids is no longer recommended because they reduce fluids necessary for the fetus. The excess fluid may also support blood volume in the mother should hemorrhage occur.

**Pica.** The craving for and ingestion of nonfood substances such as clay, starch, raw flour, and cracked ice is known as pica. Ingestion of small amounts of these substances may be harmless, but frequent ingestion in large amounts may result in complications. Starch may interfere with iron absorption, and ingestion of large amounts of clay may cause fecal impaction. Any other nonfood substance ingested in large quantities may be harmful to the mother and developing fetus, because necessary nutrients for healthy development will not be available.

Pica is an extremely difficult habit to break, and the nurse often becomes aware of the practice when discussing nutrition, food cravings, and myths with the pregnant woman. The nurse should take the time to educate the pregnant woman about the importance of good nutrition, so that the pica habit can be eliminated or at least decreased.

**Lactose Intolerance.** Some women cannot digest milk or milk products. Intolerance to lactose is caused by a deficiency of lactase, the enzyme that digests the sugar in milk. African Americans, Native Americans, and persons of Asian heritage tend to have a high incidence of lactose intolerance. Symptoms include abdominal distention, nausea, vomiting, and loose stools. In such cases a daily calcium substitute can be taken.

Food substitutions for milk or dairy products are calcium-fortified tofu, soy milk, and canned salmon with bones. Green leafy vegetables are also high in calcium. The woman needs to check with her health-care provider before taking the enzyme lactase. This is available in tablet form or as a liquid to add to milk. Lactase-treated milk is also available commercially and should be used under a physician's direction.

**Gestational Diabetes.** Gestational diabetes refers to diabetes first diagnosed during pregnancy (see p. 100). Diet control generally entails three healthy meals a day, planned with the food pyramid as a guide, and three snacks. Calories should be evenly distributed during the day to maintain adequate blood glucose levels. Pregnant diabetic women are susceptible to hypoglycemia during the night, because the fetus continues to use glucose while the mother sleeps. It is suggested that the final bedtime snack be one of protein and complex carbohydrate to counteract this effect. Ideally, dietary management is supervised by a nutritionist. Nausea and vomiting during the 1st trimester can complicate regulation of the diabetes.

**Nutrition During Lactation.** Lactation is a natural occurrence following childbirth. With proper maternal nutritional intake, breast feeding promotes the health and growth of a baby throughout the 1st year of life. The intake during lactation should be about 500 cal more than the nonpregnant woman's RDA. A guide to adequate caloric intake is a stable maternal weight and a gradually increasing infant weight.

The protein intake should be increased over that of the prepregnant state, so that the growing baby will have adequate protein. Calcium and iron intake is the same as that during pregnancy to allow for the infant's demand on the mother's supply. To maintain sufficient milk production, the mother is advised to drink at least 4–5 glasses of milk daily and more during hot weather and physical exertion. Vitamin supplementation is often continued during lactation. The pediatrician should be notified when vitamins are discontinued by the mother. Vitamins will then be recommended for the baby. Table 4–5 is a daily food plan for the nursing mother.

Some foods may need to be omitted during lactation, especially if they cause gastric upset in the mother. These same foods may affect the baby in a similar way. The most common "gassy" foods are cabbage, onions, and strong spices. Chocolate may cause diarrhea and should be avoided. Lactating mothers should be instructed that ingested drugs are secreted in varying amounts in the breast milk. Drugs should be taken only with the doctor's advice, and breast feeding may be discontinued if harmful side effects are known or suspected (see Appendix C).

## Common Discomforts in Pregnancy

Table 4–6 illustrates the more frequently encountered discomforts of pregnancy. Recognizing that the discomforts are temporary helps the mother cope with them. The nurse should be familiar with measures to relieve these discomforts in order to educate the patient.

*Nausea* is a problem chiefly in the 1st trimester. Despite its popular name, "morning sickness," nausea and vomiting may occur throughout the day and may affect the same woman in different ways with each pregnancy. The increased levels of hormones during pregnancy alter the functioning of the gastrointestinal system, and most women do experience some nausea. Recommendations for relief may include the following:

- Eat dry toast or crackers before getting out of bed in the morning
- Drink fluids between meals instead of with meals
- Eat small, frequent meals
- Check with medical care provider about the use of B-complex vitamins
- Never use over-the-counter or prescription drugs to control nausea

*Vaginal discharge* is more noticeable because of the increased blood supply to the pelvic area. If the discharge is yellow or has a foul odor or is accompanied by itching and inflammation, vaginal infection may be present and must be treated immediately by the health-care provider. Douching is not done during pregnancy (unless specifically ordered to manage infection), mainly because the mucous plug in the cervix may be disturbed. A daily bath or shower is most effective in keeping the vaginal discharge odor-free. Other important practices include wearing loose-fitting cotton panties, wiping the perineal area from front to back after toileting, and, if desired, powdering with cornstarch after the daily bath or shower.

*Fatigue* may be difficult to control, especially in the early months of the pregnancy, if the mother is working or has other small children. The body is using tremendous energy in order to establish the support system—the placenta—to maintain the pregnancy, and the mother finds herself extremely exhausted all day.

The nurse reassures the mother at prenatal visits that planning for 8–10 hours of sleep at night is beneficial for both mother and baby. If possible, naps during the day are also helpful. The working mother may use such measures as relaxation techniques, meditation, or a change of scenery at lunch to increase energy levels. The extreme exhaustion is usually relieved in the 2nd trimester, and often women then feel exhilarated and full of energy. The tired feeling may return again during the last 4–6 weeks of the pregnancy. Again, daytime naps and plenty of restful nighttime sleep help provide the energy needed for labor.

*Backache* occurs frequently because of the spine's adaptation to the back's changing contour as the uterus grows. Simple measures such as good posture, sensible footwear, warm showers, swimming, and bending from the knees, instead of at the waist, all noticeably relieve backaches.

*Constipation* occurs because of the slowing of peristalsis, use of iron supplements, and pressure of the growing uterus on the lower in-

**Table 4–5.** A DAILY FOOD PLAN FOR THE NURSING MOTHER

| Food Group | Serving Size | Recommended Number of Servings | Foods That May Produce "Off" Flavors in Milk or Increased Gas in Infants | Sample Menu Plan for 1 Day |
|---|---|---|---|---|
| *Milk Products\** | | | | *Breakfast* |
| Fluid milk | 8-oz cup | 4–5 | Chocolate milk | 1 cup milk |
| Yogurt | 8-oz cup | | | 1 toasted English muffin, 1 teaspoon margarine |
| Hard cheese | 1½ oz | (Note: Age 18 and under—5 or 6 servings per day) | | ¾ cup shredded wheat |
| | | | | ½ sliced banana |
| | | | | ½ cup orange juice |
| Cottage cheese | 2 cups | | | *Lunch* |
| Dry milk powder | ⅓ cup | | | 1 cup milk |
| Ricotta cheese | ½ cup | | | Sandwich |
| *Meat and Protein Substitutes* | | | | 2 slices wheat bread |
| | | | | 2 oz tuna |
| Lean beef, pork, poultry, fish, lamb, veal | 2 oz | 3–4 | Meats seasoned with strong spices, such as garlic, chili powder, taco seasoning, pizza seasoning | 1 tablespoon mayonnaise |
| | | | | Sliced tomato and lettuce |
| | | | | ½ cup three-bean salad |
| | | | | 1 small apple |
| | | | | ½ cup rice pudding with raisins |
| Eggs | | 2 | | *Snack* |
| Dried peas and beans | 1 cup | | | ½ cup plain yogurt with sliced fresh pear and 1 teaspoon vanilla |
| Peanut butter | 4 tablespoons | | | *Dinner* |
| *Fruits and Vegetables* | | | | Tomato soup with ⅓ cup nonfat dry milk added and 6 crackers |
| | | | | 1 cup milk |
| Good vitamin A sources: dark green or deep yellow vegetables (spinach, mustard, turnip or dandelion greens, chard, sweet potatoes, winter squash, broccoli) | ½ cup | 1 or more | Gas-forming vegetables, such as cabbage, onions, cauliflower, broccoli | 4 oz chicken breast |
| | | | | 1 medium baked potato |
| | | | | Asparagus spears |
| | | | | Tossed salad: spinach, lettuce, celery, carrots, radishes, tomatoes, 1 tablespoon salad dressing |
| | | | | Angelfood cake with ½ cup sliced strawberries |
| Good vitamin C sources: citrus fruits, such as oranges and grapefruits, and their juices; tomatoes; strawberries; cantaloupes | ½ cup | 2 or more | | *Snack* |
| | | | | 2 toasted bagel halves with ½ cup ricotta cheese and 2 teaspoons jelly |
| Other fruits and vegetables | ½ cup | 3–5 | | |
| *Breads and Cereals (Enriched or Whole-Grain)* | | | | |
| Breads | 1 slice | 6–10 | | |
| Cereals | ½–¾ cup | (Note: Age 18 and under— 8 servings per day or more) | | |
| Rice, pasta | ½ cup | | | |
| *Others* | | | | |
| Fats, oils, salad dressing | Use sparingly | | Chocolate | |
| Sweets, desserts, candy, jam | Use moderate amounts only | | | |

\*Portion sizes for milk products provide the same amount of calcium as one 8-oz portion of milk.
Courtesy of Mercy Nutrition Specialists, Mercy Hospital Medical Center, Des Moines, IA.

testines. The most efficient measures that provide relief are increasing the intake of fluids by at least 4–6 glasses daily, using a stool softener as recommended by a health-care provider, including regular exercise (such as walking) in daily activities, increasing dietary fiber, and responding without delay to the urge to defecate.

*Varicose veins* are frequently seen in the pregnant woman. They appear because the large uterus impedes venous return, causing the blood to pool in the veins. This pooling may eventually break down the competence of the valves within the veins. Varicose veins are seen most often on the back of the calves and behind the knees. Excessive weight gain and genetic predisposition may affect the occurrence of varicosities and their persistence after the pregnancy.

Effective measures to relieve the discomfort of varicosities include support hosiery and regular exercise, especially walking. The woman is instructed to wear low-heeled, sturdy shoes; to avoid crossing the legs; and to lie on the left side when she rests during the day. Varicosities may occur on the vulva, especially after the 20th week of pregnancy. They are usually temporary and subside after the delivery.

*Hemorrhoids*, varicosities of the rectum and anus, are dilated veins that become more severe with constipation and with descent of the baby's head into the pelvis. They generally decrease or disappear after birth, when pressure is relieved. Treatment for hemorrhoids may include anesthetic ointments, witch hazel pads, rectal suppositories, and sitz baths.

*Heartburn* causes discomfort chiefly in the last 6 weeks of the pregnancy, when the fundus of the large uterus presses against the esophagus where it enters the stomach. This pressure may cause a reflux of gastric acids into the esophagus, resulting in a burning feeling in the chest and a bitter taste in the mouth. Suggestions that frequently help reduce the occurrence of heartburn include eating small, more frequent meals that are not spicy or fried; drinking adequate fluids; avoiding coffee; and raising the head and shoulders when lying down. The woman should avoid antacids and use them only when recommended by her health-care provider.

*Dyspnea* is a discomfort frequently encountered in late pregnancy as the enlarging uterus exerts pressure on the diaphragm. Even with mild exercise, many women are unable to

**Table 4–6.** COMMON DISCOMFORTS OF PREGNANCY: ONSET AND NURSING CARE

| Discomfort | Trimester | Nursing Interventions |
|---|---|---|
| Nausea | 1st | Encourage eating small frequent meals and dry carbohydrates, and drinking fluids before meals |
| Nasal stuffiness or nosebleeds | 1st | Instruct to avoid nasal sprays and use cool-air vaporizer |
| Vaginal discharge | 1st | Instruct to take a daily shower or bath and wear a peripad |
| Fatigue | 1st and end of 3rd | Encourage sleeping 8–10 hr at night and napping during day; working mothers elevate legs on chair during lunch break, rest before beginning dinner, and ask for help from partner or other family members |
| Backache | 2nd and 3rd | Encourage good posture and use of low-heeled, sturdy shoes; instruct in good body mechanics for bending and lifting |
| Constipation | 2nd and 3rd | Instruct to increase fluid intake and fiber; increase regular exercise |
| Varicose veins | 2nd and 3rd | Encourage wearing support hosiery and avoiding crossing legs; encourage elevating feet and legs when sitting |
| Hemorrhoids | 2nd and 3rd | Instruct to avoid constipation |
| Heartburn | 2nd and 3rd | Instruct to avoid coffee and spicy foods and not to lie down right after eating |
| Dyspnea | 2nd and 3rd | Instruct to rest with head elevated |
| Leg cramps | 3rd | Encourage to stretch legs, dorsiflex foot, avoid pointing toes, and avoid excess milk but get enough calcium |
| Edema of lower extremities | 2nd and 3rd | Encourage elevating legs when seated and avoiding standing in one position |

breathe deeply. Suggestions for relief include resting with the upper torso propped up and avoiding exertion. When the presenting part of the fetus enters the pelvic brim (lightening) about 2 weeks before delivery, most women feel a dramatic change to easier breathing.

*Leg cramps* may occur in the first 6 weeks of pregnancy but are more often experienced during the 3rd trimester. The superficial calf muscles of the legs involuntarily contract, causing severe pain. Increased uterine weight, increased circulatory load, inadequate rest, and imbalance of the calcium-to-phosphorus ratio may be implicated as causes. Excessive intake of phosphorus may exceed the calcium intake, resulting in a calcium-to-phosphorus imbalance.

Phosphorus intake can easily be reduced by avoiding snack foods, processed meats, and cola drinks. Adequate intake of vitamin D and magnesium, which are found in milk, may help maintain a proper calcium-to-phosphorus ratio. The mother is instructed to avoid drinking more than 1 quart of milk per day.

Stretching of the leg in spasm by dorsiflexion of the foot, along with application of warm packs and massage, provides relief. Pointing the toes should be avoided.

*Edema of the lower extremities* is not uncommon, especially after the 20th week of pregnancy. It is caused by the increased circulatory load and slower venous return of blood from the legs. Temporary relief is obtained by elevating the legs when sitting, lying down when resting, and avoiding tight restrictive bands around the legs. Edema in the face and hands may be a sign of complications and is reported to the health-care provider (see discussion of pregnancy-induced hypertension, pp. 88–98).

# Emotional Considerations in Pregnancy

Reva Rubin, a registered nurse, is considered an expert in identifying maternal behaviors during pregnancy. Some of her findings are summarized in the following discussion.

## GENERAL CONSIDERATIONS

Pregnancy creates a variety of confusing and conflicting feelings in all members of the family. It does not matter whether the pregnancy is wanted or unwanted. Frequently, there is ambivalence about the desire for a child and about one's ability to be a successful parent. In the case of a first-born child, parents may be anxious about how the new baby will affect their relationship as a couple. Because of these confusing and disarming feelings, pregnancy may indeed be considered a crisis, and each woman and her family need to resolve the crisis in their own ways. Nursing Care Plan 4–3 lists nursing interventions for selected diagnoses pertaining to emotional considerations in pregnancy.

## IMPACT ON THE MOTHER

The developmental task faced by mothers in early pregnancy involves accepting the pregnancy and integrating it into the self. This is termed *resolution*. Resolution is affected by the social, religious, and moral beliefs of the woman's cultural background. Much of this is accomplished by "role playing" and "fantasy" (Rubin, 1984). The mother-to-be observes other mothers caring for their children, and she looks for opportunities to hold, feed, and change the diapers of newborns to prepare for her new role in life.

In the 1st trimester, the baby is not perceived as an individual, so fantasy provides the opportunity to imagine the baby's hair and eye color, body features, and sex. During this time, mothers often worry about whether the baby will be defective, especially if there have been previous miscarriages or if genetic defects have occurred in either parent's family.

In the 2nd trimester, the pregnancy is more evident as the uterus rises out of the pelvic area and becomes a progressively enlarging, but temporary, abdominal organ. During this time, the fetal heartbeat is heard for the first time, and quickening is felt by the mother. The task is one of differentiation, in which the woman begins to distinguish herself from, and to accept, the fetus.

The mother becomes totally involved with her developing baby and her changing body image.

## Nursing Brief

Ambivalence about becoming a mother is a characteristic of early pregnancy in most women. Mood swings are common throughout pregnancy.

| NURSING CARE PLAN 4–3 | | |
|---|---|---|
| **Selected Nursing Diagnoses for Emotional Considerations During Pregnancy** | | |
| **Goals** | **Nursing Interventions** | **Rationale** |

**Nursing Diagnosis:** High risk for altered family processes related to emotional experience of the pregnancy.

| | | |
|---|---|---|
| Couple identifies two concerns of becoming parents | 1. Listen and provide anticipatory guidance | 1. Becoming new parents is a crisis; listening helps nurse to identify major concerns |
| | 2. Discuss woman's mood swings as being normal | 2. Mood swings are caused by sustained increase in estrogen as well as mother's focus on herself; discussion helps clarify causes and promotes understanding |
| | 3. Refer mother and partner to prenatal and parenting classes | 3. Prenatal classes help develop an accurate picture of developing fetus, provide support and socialization, and educate parents in responsibilities in care of newborn and growing child |
| Prospective parents verbalize problems and seek guidance | 1. Assess family structure and roles | 1. Correctly identifying family structure provides means for nurse to assist in identifying usual roles and provides a basis for identifying and intervening to solve problems |
| | 2. Identify and reinforce strengths of family relationships | 2. Knowing strengths of family fosters a positive outlook and foundation on which the family can build |
| | 3. Refer to family counseling as needed | 3. Professional family counseling provides for objective appraisal of family problems and suggests means of dealing with problems at hand |

**Nursing Diagnosis:** Health-seeking behaviors related to fear of pregnancy outcome.

| | | |
|---|---|---|
| Couple will voice decreased fear of pregnancy outcome | 1. Listen to couple's concern | 1. Providing for open communication in a supportive, professional manner assists couple in coping with fears |
| | 2. Provide accurate information | 2. There is much misinformation about childbearing practices |

This focus on herself can become difficult for her husband and family to accept. She may experience frequent and dramatic mood swings. The family that tries to understand and accept these temporary behavior changes helps the mother to overcome them. It is also beneficial to reinforce a mother's positive feelings about herself and her ability to weather motherhood.

In the 3rd trimester, as her body changes even more dramatically, a mother alternates from feeling "absolutely beautiful" and "productive" to feeling "as big as a house" and "totally unloved" by her husband. These feelings are normal and transient. Toward the end of this trimester, much introspection occurs about the challenge of labor and the outcome of delivery. The mother begins to separate herself from the pregnancy and to commit herself to the care of her newborn by preparing for the arrival. The minor discomforts of pregnancy can become tiresome. Again, a woman benefits from the gentle understanding of the people near and dear to her. During the last trimester, she develops the inner strength to accomplish the tasks of labor and delivery.

## IMPACT ON THE FATHER

The emotional impact of pregnancy on the father needs to be considered. He is often asked to provide emotional support to his partner while struggling with the issue himself. It is important to praise and encourage the father during childbirth preparation classes and during labor and delivery. Many fathers look forward to being present at the birth of their child. With preparation and encouragement, the father can actively participate and provide much assistance to his wife. Sometimes a father is uncomfortable with participating and seeing his wife in labor. The nurse acknowledges this and supports whatever decision he reaches.

### IMPACT ON THE SINGLE MOTHER

The single mother, often still in her adolescent years, presents special emotional considerations, especially when the father has left her or does not acknowledge the pregnancy. Sometimes single mothers are able to turn to their parents or siblings for acceptance and encouragement. At other times, close friends provide that support. Whatever the source, the pregnant woman needs love, patience, and understanding during her pregnancy in order to accomplish the developmental tasks that prepare her for the role of mother.

### IMPACT ON THE SINGLE FATHER

The single father, who may be an adolescent, has been given little consideration over the years. Some young men take an active interest in and financial responsibility for the child. Marriage may be planned but is often delayed a few years for economic reasons. A single father may provide emotional support for the mother of his child during the pregnancy, labor, and delivery. He may have an opportunity to bond with his newborn child. He often has strong feelings of surprise and accomplishment when he becomes aware of his partner's pregnancy. He may want to participate in plans for the new baby, but he may be rejected by the mother.

Situations such as these require sensitive intervention by the nurse. It is necessary to consider the well-being of the mother and baby as paramount while providing support to the sin-

## Nursing Brief

The nurse educating the adolescent mother must anticipate resistive behavior, ambivalence, and inconsistency, which are normal behaviors for this age group. Building on the adolescent mother's achievements acknowledges her efforts to cope with the pregnancy and may help increase self-esteem.

gle father. The nurse does this by building on the strengths of each individual. This may help create an environment of cooperation between the parents.

### IMPACT ON THE ADOLESCENT

Pregnant adolescents often have to struggle with fears they find difficult to express. They are fraught with conflict about how to handle the unplanned pregnancy. Initially, they must face the anxiety of breaking the news to their parents. There may be financial problems, shame, guilt, relationship problems with the baby's father, and feelings of low self-esteem. There may be problems of alcoholism or drug abuse.

Areas of assessment by the nurse include taking a thorough history and determining the adolescent's developmental level and support system. A primary intervention is to establish trust and to assist the teenage girl in completing the developmental tasks of adolescence while assuming the new role of motherhood. Cyndi Roller (1992), a childbirth nurse educator, integrated "art class" into the curriculum of a residential adolescent pregnancy program. She found that drawing was a vehicle for expressing concerns about changing body image and fears and concerns about labor and birth. Prenatal classes need to be adapted to fit the special physical and emotional needs of this age group.

## Nursing Brief

Throughout the pregnancy, there is a need for sensitivity to the partner and other family members who have their own fears and concerns.

## Nursing Brief

The pregnant teenager has to cope with two of life's most stress-laden transitions, adolescence and parenthood.

## KEY POINTS

- One main goal of prenatal care is the safe delivery of a healthy baby at full term to a healthy mother.
- The nurse instructs the mother that prenatal care is the most important method of ensuring a healthy mother and baby.
- The length of a pregnancy is 40 weeks after the last menstrual period plus or minus 2 weeks. The expected date of delivery is determined by using Nägele's rule.
- The signs of pregnancy are divided into three groups: presumptive (subjective), probable (objective), and positive.
- Quickening, a presumptive sign of pregnancy that occurs at 18–20 weeks, marks the first half of the pregnancy and is a good reference point for identifying the gestational age of the developing fetus.
- All systems of the woman's body adapt to provide for the developing fetus.
- The uterus undergoes the most obvious changes in pregnancy: it increases in weight from approximately 60 gm (2 ounces) to 1000 gm (2.2 pounds); it increases in size from approximately $7.5 \times 5 \times 2.5$ cm to $28 \times 24 \times 21$ cm; and its circulation increases to contain about one-sixth of the total maternal blood volume.
- Nutrition is a vital factor in the development of a healthy baby. To provide for the growth of the fetus, fetal support tissue, and maternal support systems, the mother's calorie intake must increase from an average of 2200 to 2500 cal. Important nutrients that must increase are protein, calcium, iron, and folic acid.
- Single mothers, who may be adolescents, need creative nursing interventions to resolve their unique problems. The single father also requires sensitive interventions by the nurse. Building on the strengths of each individual may foster cooperation between the mother and father. The developmental tasks of pregnancy include accepting the pregnancy (resolution), differentiating the fetus from self, and committing oneself to the child.

# Study Questions

1. List the goals of prenatal care and describe how each goal can be met.
2. Calculate the estimated date of delivery for these dates, which represent the first day of the last menstrual period: March 10th, November 26th, and August 4th.
3. List the presumptive (subjective) signs of pregnancy and give a brief description of each.
4. List the probable (objective) signs of pregnancy and briefly describe each.
5. List the positive (diagnostic) signs of pregnancy and briefly describe each.
6. Briefly describe prenatal care provided for an uncomplicated pregnancy by an obstetrician, certified nurse-midwife, or family practice physician.
7. Describe how the nurse would explain to the mother the purpose of the mucous plug in the cervix?
8. What interventions would the nurse employ to help 17-year-old Rosa improve her nutrition during pregnancy?
9. Why does a primigravida demonstrate a "waddling gait" in the last few weeks of pregnancy?

10. Describe nursing interventions provided during prenatal care for the following minor discomforts of pregnancy: backache, varicose veins, constipation, vaginal discharge, leg cramps, and nausea.

11. Describe how the nursing care of the pregnant adolescent differs from that of the pregnant adult.

# Multiple Choice Review Questions

*Choose the most appropriate answer.*

1. The length of a normal pregnancy is within the range of
   a. 32–35 weeks
   b. 36–37 weeks
   c. 38–42 weeks
   d. 43–44 weeks

2. Hegar's sign, a probable sign of pregnancy, is elicited on the lower uterine segment during the 2nd and 3rd months of the pregnancy because
   a. the uterus is a temporary abdominal organ at that time
   b. the developing fetus does not fill the uterine cavity
   c. the uterus has softened and has become very thin
   d. the fetus rebounds quickly when tapped

3. The palpation of the fetal outline by a trained examiner is a probable sign of pregnancy that is determined after the
   a. 16th week
   b. 20th week
   c. 24th week
   d. 32nd week

4. The normal fetal heart rate
   a. 80–100 beats/min
   b. 100–140 beats/min
   c. 110–160 beats/min
   d. 140–180 beats/min

5. A woman may develop varicose veins in her legs or vulva area because of
   a. increased cardiac load
   b. pressure from the enlarging uterus impeding venous return
   c. decrease in maternal blood pressure
   d. pressure from the enlarging vena cava impeding venous return

6. The nurse should instruct the pregnant woman to relieve morning sickness by
   a. not eating breakfast and having a large lunch
   b. eating some dry, absorbent food, such as crackers, before arising
   c. avoiding food with roughage
   d. drinking large amounts of clear fluids between meals

7. The best source of iron from the following food list is
   a. bran
   b. white potatoes
   c. beef liver
   d. lima beans

8. As pregnancy progresses, the normal changes in hemoglobin and hematocrit include which one of the following?
   a. both become slightly lower because of increased blood volume
   b. both become slightly higher because of increased blood volume
   c. hematocrit increases slightly while hemoglobin decreases
   d. hematocrit decreases slightly while hemoglobin increases

9. Braxton Hicks' contractions are defined as
   a. first fetal movement felt by the mother
   b. false labor pains
   c. severe contractions of early labor
   d. irregular uterine contractions that may occur throughout pregnancy

10. Leg cramps, one of the common discomforts in pregnancy, may be decreased by reducing an excessive intake of

a. calcium
b. sodium
c. iron
d. phosphorus

## BIBLIOGRAPHY

American Academy of Pediatrics & American College of Obstetricians and Gynecologists. (1992). Maternal and newborn nutrition. In *Guidelines for perinatal care* (3rd ed.). Elk Grove Village, IL: American Academy of Pediatrics.

Bishop, B.E. (1992). Congratulations Reva! [Editorial]. *MCN: American Journal of Maternal-Child Nursing, 17.*

Bushy, A. (1992, March). Preconception health promotion: Another approach to improve pregnancy outcomes. *Public Health Nursing.*

Carpenito, L. (1993). *Handbook of nursing diagnosis* (5th ed.). Philadelphia: J.B. Lippincott.

Cunningham, F.G., et al. (1989). *Williams obstetrics* (18th ed.). Norwalk, CT: Appleton & Lange.

Gizis, F.C. (1992, December). Nutrition in women across the life span in women's health. *Nursing Clinics of North America.* Philadelphia: W.B. Saunders.

Gorrie, T.M., McKinney, E.S., & Murray, S.S. (1994). *Foundations of maternal-newborn nursing.* Philadelphia: W.B. Saunders.

Hacker, N.F., & Moore, J.G. (1992). *Essentials of obstetrics and gynecology* (2nd ed.). Philadelphia: W.B. Saunders.

Ladewig, P.W., London, M.L., & Olds, S.B. (1994). *Essentials of maternal-newborn nursing.* Redwood City, CA: Addison-Wesley.

Mahan, L.K., & Arlin, M.T. (1992). *Krause's food, nutrition & diet therapy* (8th ed.). Philadelphia: W.B. Saunders.

NAACOG. (1990). *OGN nursing practice resource: Fetal heart rate auscultation.* Washington, DC: Author.

Pillitteri, A. (1992). *Maternal and child health nursing.* Philadelphia: J.B. Lippincott.

Poleman, C., & Peckenpaugh, N. (1991). *Nutrition essentials and diet therapy* (6th ed.). Philadelphia: W.B. Saunders.

Roller, C. (1992). Drawing out young mothers. *MCN: American Journal of Maternal-Child Nursing, 17,* 254.

Rubin, R. (1984). *Maternal identity and the maternal experience.* New York: Springer.

Rubin, R. (1975). Maternal tasks in pregnancy. MCN: American Journal of Maternal-Child Nursing, 4, 143.

U.S. Department of Health and Human Services. (1988). *Surgeon General's report on nutrition and health: Summary and recommendations.* (DHHS Publication No. PHS 88-50311). Washington, DC: U.S. Government Printing Office.

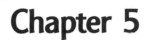

# Chapter 5

# Nursing Care of Women with Complications During Pregnancy

Pregnancy-Related Complications
   Hyperemesis Gravidarum
   Bleeding Disorders of Early Pregnancy
   Bleeding Disorders of Late Pregnancy
   Hypertension During Pregnancy
   Blood Incompatibility Between the Pregnant
      Woman and Fetus
Pregnancy Complicated by Medical Conditions
   Diabetes Mellitus
   Heart Disease
   Anemia
   Infections
Environmental Hazards During Pregnancy
   Substances Harmful to the Fetus
   Treatment
   Nursing Care
Trauma During Pregnancy
   Manifestations of Battering
   Treatment
   Nursing Care
Effects of High-Risk Pregnancy on the Family
   Disruption of Usual Roles
   Financial Difficulties
   Delayed Attachment to the Baby
   Loss of Expected Birth Experience

# OBJECTIVES

*On completion and mastery of Chapter 5, the student will be able to*

- Define each vocabulary term listed.
- Describe each antepartum complication and its therapy.
- Identify methods to reduce a woman's risk for antepartum complications.
- Discuss management of concurrent medical conditions during pregnancy.
- Describe environmental hazards that may adversely affect the outcome of pregnancy.
- Describe how pregnancy affects care of the trauma victim.
- Explain nursing care for each antepartum complication.
- Describe psychosocial nursing interventions for the woman who has a high-risk pregnancy and her family.
- Explain use of fetal diagnostic tests in women with complicated pregnancies.

Most women have uneventful pregnancies that are free of complications. However, others have complications that threaten their well-being and that of their babies. Many problems can be anticipated during prenatal care and thus prevented or made less severe. Others occur without warning.

Early and regular prenatal care allows the physician or nurse-midwife to identify a woman's risk factors. Women who have no prenatal care or begin care late in pregnancy may have complications that are severe because they were not identified early. Box 5–1 describes danger signs that should be taught to every pregnant woman and reinforced on each prenatal visit.

Complications may originate in the pregnancy itself; they may occur because the woman has a medical condition or injury unrelated to the pregnancy; or they may result from environmental hazards.

## Pregnancy-Related Complications

Complications of pregnancy include hyperemesis gravidarum, bleeding, hypertension, and blood incompatibility between the woman and fetus.

## HYPEREMESIS GRAVIDARUM

Mild nausea and/or vomiting are common and easily managed during pregnancy (see p. 67). In contrast, the woman with hyperemesis gravidarum has excessive nausea and vomiting, which significantly hinder her nutritional status.

**Manifestations.** Hyperemesis gravidarum is different from "morning sickness" of pregnancy in one or more of these ways:

- Persistent nausea and vomiting, often with complete inability to retain food and fluids
- Significant weight loss
- Dehydration, evidenced by a dry tongue and mucous membranes, by decreased turgor (elasticity) of the skin, and by scant and concentrated urine
- Electrolyte and acid-base imbalances
- Psychological factors, such as unusual stress, emotional immaturity, passivity, or ambivalence about the pregnancy

**Treatment.** The primary medical treatment is to correct dehydration and electrolyte or acid-base imbalances with oral or intravenous fluids. Antiemetic drugs may be prescribed after the physician informs the woman about potential harm to the developing baby. The condition is self-limiting in most women.

**Nursing Care.** Factors that trigger nausea and vomiting should be reduced. The woman's room should be located away from food odors, such as tray carts and the nurses' lounge. The emesis basin is kept out of sight so that it is not

| BOX 5–1 | Danger Signals in Pregnancy |
|---|---|

Sudden gush of fluid from vagina
Vaginal bleeding
Abdominal pain
Persistent vomiting
Epigastric pain
Edema of face and hands
Severe, persistent headache
Blurred vision or dizziness
Chills with fever over 38.3°C (101°F)
Painful urination or less urine excreted

a visual reminder of vomiting. It is emptied at once if the woman vomits.

The nurse records the woman's intake and output to assess her fluid balance. Frequent, small amounts of food and fluid keep her stomach from becoming too full. Easily digested carbohydrates, such as crackers or baked potatoes, are tolerated best. Many women have less nausea if they take liquids between meals instead of at the same time as solid foods. Food should be served attractively and without negative comments such as "I hope you will be able to hold this down."

Stress may contribute to hyperemesis gravidarum; it may also result from this complication. Emotional support can be provided by listening to the woman's feelings about pregnancy, childrearing, and living with constant nausea. Although psychological factors may play a role in some cases of hyperemesis gravidarum, the nurse should not assume that every woman with this complication is adjusting poorly to her pregnancy.

## BLEEDING DISORDERS OF EARLY PREGNANCY

Several bleeding disorders can complicate early pregnancy, such as spontaneous abortion, ectopic pregnancy, or hydatidiform mole. This section also includes a discussion of therapeutic abortion.

### Spontaneous Abortion

Abortion is the intentional or nonintentional ending of a pregnancy before 20 weeks' gestation. Spontaneous abortion occurs in at least 15% of pregnancies. Lay people often use the word "miscarriage" to describe spontaneous abortion and to distinguish it from therapeutic or elective abortion. In most cases, the developing baby or placenta (products of conception) is abnormal; this is nature's way to prevent the birth of an abnormal infant.

**Manifestations.** There are six categories of spontaneous abortion. Four are based on the extent of cervical dilation and amount of tissue

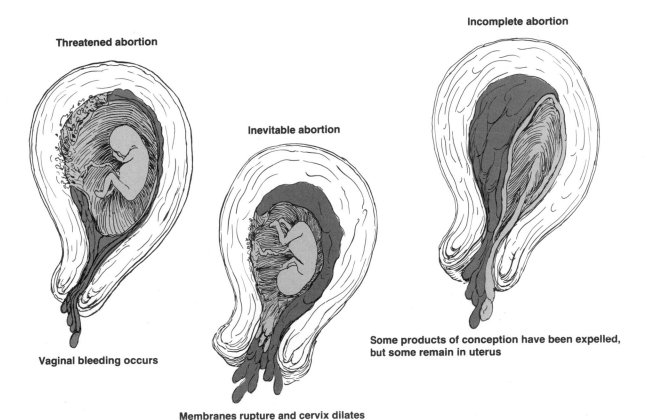

**Threatened abortion**

**Vaginal bleeding occurs**

**Inevitable abortion**

**Membranes rupture and cervix dilates**

**Incomplete abortion**

**Some products of conception have been expelled, but some remain in uterus**

**Figure 5–1.** Three types of spontaneous abortion.

passed (Fig. 5–1). Two others describe special situations related to spontaneous abortion.

*Threatened Abortion.* The woman has intermittent light bleeding ("spotting"). The cervix is closed, and no tissue is passed. In about half of the women with threatened abortion, inevitable abortion develops.

*Inevitable Abortion.* The woman has increased bleeding and cramping, and the cervix dilates. The membranes (bag of waters) may rupture, but no tissue is passed.

*Incomplete Abortion.* Signs and symptoms are similar to those of inevitable abortion, but some tissue is passed.

*Complete Abortion.* All products of conception are passed. Bleeding and cramping decrease, and the cervix closes.

*Missed Abortion.* The fetus dies within the uterus during the first half of pregnancy, but is not expelled for several weeks.

*Recurrent Abortion.* Three or more consecutive spontaneous abortions are a commonly recognized standard. Genetic factors, a cervix that fails to remain closed until the end of pregnancy (incompetent cervix), or medical conditions such as diabetes mellitus or infections contribute to recurrent abortions.

**Treatment.** A vaginal ultrasound examination is done to determine if the fetus is living. If the process has not advanced beyond threatened abortion, the woman is advised to stop sexual activity until the bleeding has stopped for 2 weeks. Bed rest at home may be recommended for 48 hours after each bleeding episode.

If the woman has an inevitable or incomplete abortion, her uterus is emptied by vacuum (suction) aspiration or by dilation and curettage (D & C). See Table 5–1 for description of these procedures. Missed abortion may be managed by awaiting spontaneous expulsion of the fetus, which usually occurs within a few weeks.

Therapy for the woman who has recurrent spontaneous abortion depends on whether a treatable cause is identified. Incompetent cervix is managed with a surgical procedure (cerclage), which reinforces the cervix, allowing the fetus to mature. A pursestring suture (similar to a drawstring on a bag) is placed around the circumference of the cervix and drawn tight to hold it closed.

**Table 5–1.** PROCEDURES USED IN SPONTANEOUS AND THERAPEUTIC ABORTION

| Procedure and Description | Comments |
| --- | --- |
| *Vacuum curettage (vacuum aspiration)*: cervical dilation with metal rods or laminaria (a substance that absorbs water and swells, thus enlarging the cervical opening) followed by controlled suction through a plastic cannula to remove all products of conception (POC) | Used for 1st-trimester abortions (primary method used in the United States); also used to remove remaining POC following spontaneous abortion; may be followed by curettage (see dilation and curettage); paracervical block (local anesthesia of the cervix) or general anesthesia needed; conscious sedation with midazolam (Versed) may be used |
| *Dilation and curettage (D & C)*: Dilation of the cervix as in vacuum curettage followed by scraping of the uterine walls to remove POC | Used for 1st-trimester abortions and to remove all POC following a spontaneous abortion; greater risk of cervical or uterine trauma and excessive blood loss than with vacuum curettage; paracervical block or general anesthesia needed |
| *Dilation and evacuation (D & E)*: similar to vacuum curettage but requires more cervical dilation and a large-diameter aspirating cannula; may require use of crushing instruments | Used primarily in 2nd-trimester therapeutic abortions (13–16 wk); paracervical block or general anesthesia needed |
| *Prostaglandin*: may be given as a vaginal suppository or injected into the uterine cavity; induces uterine contractions, which expel the fetus; may be supplemented with oxytocin (Pitocin) to intensify contractions | Used for 2nd-trimester therapeutic abortions; side effects are nausea, vomiting, diarrhea, elevated temperature, excessive blood loss; may be contraindicated in the woman with asthma because it causes bronchial constriction; a live fetus may be born; often requires follow-up aspiration or D & C to remove all fetal tissue |
| *Hypertonic sodium chloride*: withdrawal of 150–250 ml of amniotic fluid followed by instillation of hypertonic sodium chloride into the uterus; uterine contractions expel the fetus within 24 hr | Used for 2nd-trimester therapeutic abortions; may require oxytocin to intensify contractions; complications include infection, clotting disorders, hypernatremia (excess blood sodium), or embolism; uncommon in the United States |
| *Hypertonic urea*: instilled into the amniotic cavity; contractions later expel the fetus | Used for 2nd-trimester therapeutic abortions; contractions often weak, requiring augmentation with prostaglandin; uncommon in the United States |

Oxytocin (Pitocin) controls blood loss before and after curettage. Rh immune globulin (RhoGAM [300 μg] or the lower-dose MIC-RhoGAM [50 μg]) is given to Rh-negative women to prevent development of antibodies that might harm the fetus during a subsequent pregnancy. The dose ordered depends on duration of gestation.

### Nursing Care

*Physical Care.* The nurse documents the amount and character of bleeding and saves anything that looks like clots or tissue. A pad count and an estimate of how much each is saturated (e.g., 50%, 75%) more accurately documents blood loss. The woman having a threatened abortion is taught to report increased bleeding or passage of tissue.

After vacuum aspiration or curettage, the amount of vaginal bleeding is observed (see p. 221 for a useful method to describe the amount of bleeding on perineal pads). The blood pressure, pulse, and respirations are checked every 15 minutes for 1 hour, then every 30 minutes until discharge from the recovery area to identify hypovolemic shock resulting from blood loss.

Many women are discharged directly from the recovery room to their home after curettage. Rh immune globulin is given to the Rh-negative woman before she leaves. Guidelines for self-care at home include

- Report increased bleeding. Do not use tampons, which may cause infection.
- Take temperature every 8 hours for 3 days. Report signs of infection (temperature of 38°C [100.4°F]; foul odor or brownish color of the vaginal drainage). The woman is taught to use a thermometer, if needed.
- Resume sexual activity as recommended by the physician (usually after the bleeding has completely stopped).
- Return to the physician at the recommended time for a checkup and contraception information. Pregnancy can occur before the first menstrual period.

*Emotional Care.* Our society often underestimates the emotional distress spontaneous abortion causes the woman and her family. Even if the pregnancy was not planned or not suspected, they often grieve for what might have been. Their grief may last longer and be deeper than they or other people expect. The nurse listens to the woman and acknowledges the grief

## Nursing Brief

Supporting and encouraging the grieving process in families that suffer a pregnancy loss, such as a spontaneous abortion or ectopic pregnancy, allow them to resolve their grief.

she and her partner feel. Table 5–2 contains information about communicating with the family experiencing pregnancy loss. Spiritual support of the family's choice and community support groups, such as RTS Bereavement Services (formerly known as Resolve Through Sharing), may help the family work through the grief of spontaneous abortion. Nursing Care Plan 5–1 suggests interventions for families experiencing early pregnancy loss.

### Therapeutic (Elective) Abortion

Therapeutic abortion is an issue heavily laden with legal, social, moral, and ethical conflicts. Women terminate a pregnancy for a variety of reasons, such as preservation of their health, prevention of the birth of an abnormal infant, social or economic factors, or prevention of birth in cases of rape or incest.

Although abortion is currently legal in the United States, there are circumstances in which it is not legal. If the abortion is performed in an inappropriate facility and/or by an unqualified person, it is illegal. Some women who cannot afford a legal abortion and cannot get public funding for one may resort to "back-alley" abortionists. They are more likely to suffer life-threatening hemorrhage or infection (septic abortion).

**Treatment.** The physician chooses the most appropriate method (see Table 5–1) to end the pregnancy. The choice depends on gestational age and the woman's physical condition.

### Nursing Care

*Physical Care.* Nursing care of the woman depends on the method of therapeutic abortion. Care after the procedure is similar to that following spontaneous abortion. Rh immune globulin should be administered to the Rh-negative woman.

*Recognizing Personal Beliefs and Values.* The nurse who cares for women having a therapeutic abortion must examine personal beliefs

**Table 5–2.** COMMUNICATING WITH A FAMILY EXPERIENCING PREGNANCY LOSS

| Effective Techniques | Ineffective Techniques |
| --- | --- |
| Keep the family together | Do not give the woman/family any information |
| Wait quietly with family: "being there" | Separate family members |
| Say "I'm sorry," or "I'm here if you need to talk" | Discourage expressions of sadness; for example, expecting the father to be strong for the mother's sake |
| Touch (may not be appreciated by some people or in some cultures) | Avoid interacting with the family and talking about their loss |
| Refer to spontaneous abortion as "miscarriage" rather than the harsher-sounding "abortion" | Act uncomfortable with the family's expressions of grief |
| Provide mementoes as appropriate (lock of hair, photograph, footprint); save mementoes for later retrieval if the family does not want them immediately | Minimize the importance of the pregnancy by comments such as, "You're young—you can always have more children," "At least you didn't lose a real baby," "It was for the best—the baby was abnormal," or "You have another healthy child at home" |
| Alert other hospital personnel to the family's loss to prevent hurtful comments or questions | Say, "I know how you feel" (unless you have had a truly similar experience); self-disclosure must be used very carefully and only if it is likely to be therapeutic to the client |
| Allow the family to see the fetus if they wish; prepare them for the fetus's appearance | Encourage the family not to cry |
| Reduce the number of staff with whom the family must interact | |
| Summon a chaplain, minister, or rabbi | |
| Make referrals to support groups in the area | |

and biases so that they do not interfere with the woman's care. The woman needs nonjudgmental, compassionate care. The nurse who has ethical or moral objections to caring for a woman undergoing therapeutic abortion must make this fact known before being employed in an agency that provides these services. It is unethical to wait until being assigned to care for a client who is having any procedure that violates the nurse's moral, ethical, or religious beliefs, then to refuse to care for that client, if the situation could have been foreseen.

### Ectopic Pregnancy

Ectopic pregnancy occurs when the fertilized ovum (zygote) is implanted outside the uterine cavity (Fig. 5–2). Of all ectopic pregnancies, 95% occur in the fallopian tube (tubal pregnancy). An obstruction or other abnormality of the tube prevents the zygote from being transported into the uterus. Scarring or deformity of the fallopian tubes or inhibition of normal tubal motion to propel the zygote into the uterus may result from

- Hormonal abnormalities
- Inflammation
- Infection
- Adhesions
- Congenital defects
- Endometriosis (uterine lining outside the uterus)

Use of an intrauterine device for contraception may contribute to ectopic pregnancy, because these devices promote inflammation and infection within the uterus.

A zygote that is implanted in a fallopian tube cannot survive, because the blood supply and size of the tube are inadequate. The zygote/embryo may die and be reabsorbed by the woman's body, or the tube may rupture with bleeding into the abdominal cavity.

**Manifestations.** The woman often complains of lower abdominal pain, sometimes accompanied by light vaginal bleeding. If the tube ruptures, she may have vaginal bleeding and signs of hypovolemic shock (Box 5–2). The amount of vaginal bleeding may be minimal because most blood is lost into the abdomen rather than externally. Shoulder pain is a symptom that often accompanies bleeding in the abdomen.

**Treatment.** A sensitive pregnancy test for human chorionic gonadotropin (hCG) is done to determine if the woman is pregnant. Transvaginal ultrasound examination determines whether the embryo is growing within the uterine cavity. Culdocentesis (puncture of the upper posterior vaginal wall with removal of peritoneal fluid) may be done to identify blood in the woman's pelvis, which suggests tubal rupture. A laparoscopic examination is sometimes needed to view the damaged tube with an endoscope (lighted instrument for viewing internal organs).

| NURSING CARE PLAN 5–1 | | |
|---|---|---|
| **Selected Nursing Diagnoses for the Family Experiencing Early Pregnancy Loss** | | |
| **Goals** | **Nursing Interventions** | **Rationale** |

**Nursing Diagnosis:** Grieving related to loss of anticipated infant.

| | | |
|---|---|---|
| Woman and family will express grief to significant others<br>Woman and family will complete each stage of the grief process within individual time frames | 1. Promote expression of grief by providing privacy, eliminating time restrictions, allowing support persons of choice to visit, and recognizing individualized grief expressions and cultural norms<br>2. Use the four stages of grief as a basis for nursing interventions:<br>  a. Stage 1: shock and disbelief at loss; characterized by numbness, apathy, impaired decision-making<br>  b. Stage 2: seeking answers for why loss happened; characterized by crying, tears, guilt, loss of appetite, insomnia, blame-placing<br>  c. Stage 3: disorganization; characterized by feelings of purposelessness and malaise; gradual resumption of normal activities<br>  d. Stage 4: reorganization; characterized by sad memories, but daily functioning returns<br>3. Use open communication techniques, such as<br>  a. Quiet presence<br>  b. Expression of sympathy ("I'm sorry this happened")<br>  c. Open-ended statements ("This must be really sad for you")<br>  d. Reflection of client's expressed feelings ("You feel guilty because you didn't stay in bed constantly?")<br>4. Reinforce explanations given by the physicians or others (e.g., what the problem was, why it occurred); use simple language | 1. Grief is an individual process and people react to it in different ways; these measures encourage woman and family to express grief and begin resolving it<br><br>2. Knowledge of normal stages of grieving helps nurse identify whether it is progressing normally or if there is dysfunctional grieving in any family member; stages help nurse better interpret clients' behavior; for example, blame-placing is a normal part of grieving and is not necessarily directed at the nurse or caregivers; allows nurse to reassure client that feelings are normal without diminishing intensity of their feelings<br><br><br>3. These examples of open communication encourage family to express feelings about the loss, which is the first step in resolving them<br><br><br>4. Grieving people often do not hear or understand explanations the first time they are given because their concentration is impaired |

The physician attempts to preserve the tube if the woman wants other children, but this may not be possible in all cases. The priority medical treatment is to control blood loss. Blood transfusion may be required for massive hemorrhage. One of three courses is chosen, depending on the gestation and the amount of damage to the fallopian tube:

- No action if the pregnancy is being reabsorbed by the woman's body

- Medical therapy with methotrexate, which inhibits cell division in the embryo and allows it to be reabsorbed
- Surgery to remove the pregnancy from the tube if damage is minimal; severe damage requires removal of the entire tube and occasionally the uterus

**Nursing Care.** Nursing care includes observing for hypovolemic shock. Vaginal bleeding is assessed, although most lost blood may enter

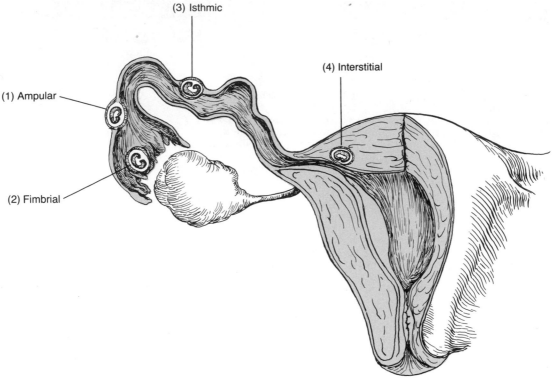

**Figure 5–2.** Four possible locations of tubal ectopic pregnancy.

the abdomen. The nurse should report increasing pain, particularly shoulder pain, to the physician.

If the woman has surgery, postoperative care is similar to that for other abdominal surgery (see a medical-surgical nursing text). The nurse provides emotional support, because the woman

and her family may experience grieving similar to that accompanying spontaneous abortion (see Table 5–2). Loss of a fallopian tube threatens future fertility and is another source of grief.

### Hydatidiform Mole

Hydatidiform mole (gestational trophoblastic disease) occurs when the chorionic villi (fringe-like structures that form the placenta) develop vesicles (small sacs) that resemble tiny grapes (Fig. 5–3). Hydatidiform mole may cause hemorrhage, hypertension, and later development of cancer (choriocarcinoma).

**Manifestations.** The woman has signs associated with normal early pregnancy, but her uterus grows more rapidly than expected as the vesicles enlarge. An ultrasound examination reveals a distinctive "snowstorm" pattern caused by the fluid-filled vesicles but shows no developing baby within the uterus. Levels of hCG are unusually high. Bleeding may range from spotting to profuse hemorrhage; cramping may be present. Many women display signs and symptoms of hyperemesis gravidarum (see p. 78) or

| BOX 5–2 | Signs and Symptoms of Hypovolemic Shock |
|---|---|

Fetal heart rate changes (increased, decreased, less fluctuation)
Rising, weak pulse (tachycardia)
Rising respiratory rate (tachypnea)
Shallow, irregular respirations; air hunger
Falling blood pressure (hypotension)
Decreased or absent urine output, usually less than 30 ml/hr
Pale skin or mucous membranes
Cold, clammy skin
Faintness
Thirst

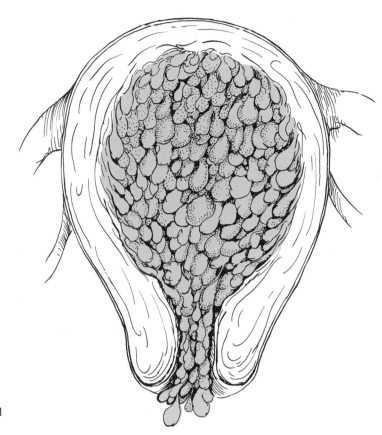

**Figure 5–3.** Hydatidiform mole of gestational trophoblastic disease.

preeclampsia (see p. 88). The woman may have respiratory distress if vesicles enter her circulation and lodge in the blood vessels of the lungs.

Some women have a partial hydatidiform mole, in which only part of the placenta has the characteristic vesicles. A fetus develops and may be born alive, depending on the extent of the problem.

**Treatment.** The uterus is evacuated by vacuum curettage and sharp curettage (D & C). The level of hCG is monitored weekly for 6 months, then every 6 months for another year, or longer for women with a higher risk for choriocarcinoma. hCG should be nondetectable by 16 weeks. Persistent or rising levels suggest that vesicles remain or that malignant change

has occurred. The woman should delay conceiving until follow-up care is complete because a new pregnancy would confuse tests for hCG. Rh immune globulin is prescribed for the Rh-negative woman.

**Nursing Care.** The nurse observes for bleeding and shock; care is similar to that given in spontaneous abortion and ectopic pregnancy. If the woman also experiences hyperemesis or preeclampsia, the nurse incorporates care related to those conditions as well. The need for follow-up examinations is reinforced, as is the need to avoid pregnancy during this time. Prescribed Rh immune globulin is administered to the Rh-negative woman. The woman is taught how to use contraception (see Chapter 11).

## Nursing Brief

The nurse should teach the woman to report promptly any danger signs that occur during pregnancy.

### BLEEDING DISORDERS OF LATE PREGNANCY

Bleeding in late pregnancy is often caused by placenta previa or abruptio placentae (Table 5–3).

**Table 5–3.** COMPARISON OF PLACENTA PREVIA AND ABRUPTIO PLACENTAE

| Placenta Previa | Abruptio Placentae |
|---|---|
| Abnormal implantation of the placenta in the lower uterus<br>  Marginal: approaches, but does not reach, the cervical<br>    opening<br>  Partial: partially covers the cervical opening<br>  Total: complete covers the cervical opening | Premature separation of the normally implanted placenta<br>  Partial: detachment of part of the placenta<br>  Total: complete detachment of the placenta<br>  Marginal: detachment at the edge of the placenta<br>  Central: detachment of the central surface of the placenta;<br>    edges stay attached |
| Bleeding: obvious vaginal bleeding, usually bright; may be<br>  profuse | Bleeding: visible dark vaginal bleeding and/or concealed<br>  bleeding within the uterus; enlargement of uterus<br>  suggests that blood is accumulating within the cavity |
| Painless | Gradual or abrupt onset of pain and uterine tenderness; pos-<br>  sibly low back pain |
| Uterus soft; no abnormal contractions or irritability | Uterus firm and boardlike; may be irritable, with frequent,<br>  brief contractions |
| Fetus may be in an abnormal presentation, such as breech<br>  or transverse lie (see p. 121) | Fetal presentation usually normal |
| Blood clotting normal | Often accompanied by impaired blood clotting<br>More likely to occur if the woman recently ingested cocaine |
| Postpartum complications<br>  Infection: placental site is near the nonsterile vagina<br>  Hemorrhage: lower uterine segment does not contract as<br>    effectively to compress bleeding vessels | Postpartum complications<br>  Infection: bleeding into uterine muscle fibers predisposes<br>    to bacterial invasion<br>  Hemorrhage: bleeding into uterine muscle fibers damages<br>    them, inhibiting uterine contraction after birth |
| Signs of fetal compromise if maternal shock or extensive<br>  placental detachment occur | Signs of fetal compromise, depending on amount and<br>  location of the placental surface that is disrupted |
| Fetal/neonatal anemia may occur because some lost blood<br>  may be fetal | Fetal/neonatal anemia may occur because some lost blood<br>  may be fetal |

## Placenta Previa

Placenta previa occurs when the placenta develops in the lower part of the uterus rather than in the upper part. There are three degrees of placenta previa, depending on the location of the placenta in relation to the cervix (Fig. 5–4):

- Marginal: placenta reaches the edge of the cervical opening
- Partial: placenta partly covers the cervical opening
- Total: placenta completely covers the cervical opening

A low-lying placenta is implanted near the cervix, but it does not cover any of the opening. This variation is not a true placenta previa and may or may not be accompanied by bleeding. The low-lying placenta may be discovered during a routine ultrasound examination in early pregnancy. It also may be diagnosed during late pregnancy, because the woman has signs and symptoms similar to those of a true placenta previa.

**Manifestations.** Vaginal bleeding without pain is the main characteristic of placenta previa. The woman's risk of hemorrhage increases as term approaches and the cervix begins to efface (thin) and dilate (open). These normal prelabor changes disrupt the placental attachment. Diagnosis is made by ultrasound examination, which reveals the abnormal placement of the placenta. The fetus is often in an abnormal presentation, such as breech or transverse lie (see p. 125), because the placenta occupies the lower uterus, which prevents the fetus from assuming the normal head-down presentation.

The fetus or neonate may have anemia or hypovolemic shock because some of the blood lost may be fetal blood. Fetal hypoxia may occur because disruption of the placental surface reduces transfer of oxygen and nutrients.

The woman with placenta previa is more likely than others to have an infection or hemorrhage after birth (see Chap. 10). Infection is more likely to occur because vaginal organisms can easily reach the placental site, which is a good growth medium for microorganisms. Postpartum hemorrhage may occur because the lower segment of the uterus, where the placenta was attached, has fewer muscle fibers than the upper uterus. Weak contraction of the lower uterus does not as effectively compress open vessels at the placental site.

**Treatment.** Medical care depends on the gestation and amount of bleeding. Bed rest reduces downward pressure on the cervix, which might increase bleeding. If bleeding is extensive or the gestation is close to full term, cesarean delivery is done for partial or total placenta previa. The woman with a low-lying placenta or marginal placenta previa may be able to deliver vaginally unless blood loss is excessive.

**Nursing Care.** The priorities of nursing care include observation of vaginal blood loss and for signs and symptoms of shock. Vital signs are taken every 15 minutes if the woman is actively bleeding. Vaginal examination is *not* done, because it may precipitate bleeding. The fetal heart rate is monitored, usually with continuous electronic monitoring (see p. 141). The nurse implements care for cesarean delivery, as needed (see p. 195). Postpartum care is routine, although the nurse is especially watchful for hemorrhage or infection (see pp. 252 and 261).

## Abruptio Placentae

Abruptio placentae is the premature separation of a placenta that is normally implanted. It usually accompanies other complications rather than occurring alone:

- Hypertension
- Cocaine use by the mother
- Rupture of the membranes when the uterus was overdistended with fluid (hydramnios [polyhydramnios])
- Blows to the abdomen, as might occur in battering or accidental trauma
- Short umbilical cord, which pulls the placenta from the uterine wall as the fetus descends during late pregnancy or labor

Abruptio placentae may be partial or total (Fig. 5–5); it may be marginal or central. Bleeding may be visible or concealed behind the partially attached placenta.

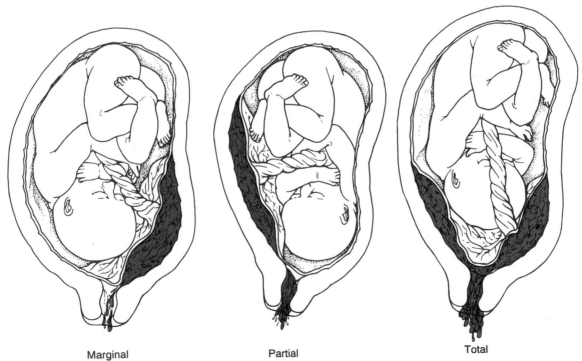

Marginal                    Partial                    Total

**Figure 5–4.** Placenta previa may be marginal, partial, or total, depending on the placental position in relation to the cervical opening.

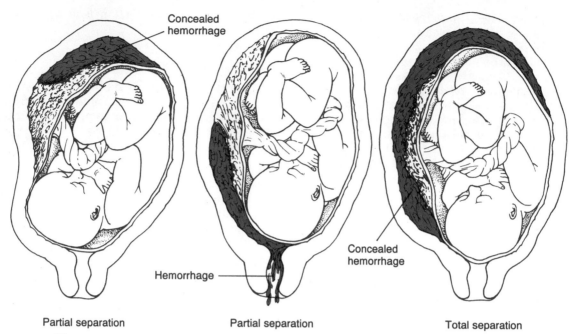

**Figure 5–5.** Abruptio placentae may be partial or total; bleeding may be visible or concealed.

**Manifestations.** Bleeding accompanied by abdominal or low back pain is the typical characteristic of abruptio placentae (see Table 5–3). Unlike bleeding in placenta previa, most or all of the bleeding may be concealed behind the placenta. Obvious dark-red vaginal bleeding occurs when blood leaks past the edge of the placenta. The woman's uterus is tender and unusually firm (boardlike) because blood leaks into its muscle fibers. Frequent cramplike uterine contractions often occur (uterine irritability).

The fetus may or may not have problems, depending on how much placental surface is disrupted. As in placenta previa, some of the blood lost may be fetal, and the fetus or neonate may have anemia or hypovolemic shock.

Disseminated intravascular coagulation (DIC) is a complex and confusing disorder that may complicate abruptio placentae. Clot formation and anticoagulation (destruction of clots) occur simultaneously throughout the body in the woman with DIC. She may bleed from her mouth, nose, incisions, or venipuncture sites because her clotting factors are depleted.

Postpartum hemorrhage may occur because the injured uterine muscle does not contract effectively to control blood loss. Infection is more likely to occur because the damaged tissue is susceptible to microbial invasion.

**Treatment.** In most cases, immediate cesarean delivery is done because of the risk for maternal shock, clotting disorders, and fetal death. Blood and clotting factor replacement is often needed because of DIC. The mother's clotting quickly returns to normal after birth.

**Nursing Care.** The nurse observes for and reports signs and symptoms of abruptio placentae, especially if a woman has any of the conditions described. Observation for shock and for bleeding from the nose, gums, or other unexpected sites allows prompt medical intervention. The fetus is monitored, as with placenta previa. Rapid increase in the size of the uterus suggests that blood is accumulating within it. Care after birth is similar to that with placenta previa.

The fetus sometimes dies before delivery (see p. 229 for nursing care related to fetal death [stillbirth] and support of the grieving family). Many therapeutic communication techniques outlined in Table 5–2 are also appropriate.

## HYPERTENSION DURING PREGNANCY

Hypertension may exist before pregnancy (chronic hypertension), but it usually develops as a pregnancy complication (pregnancy-induced hypertension [PIH]). A woman with chronic hypertension may develop PIH in addition to her chronic condition. Others develop hypertension in late pregnancy, without other signs of PIH (transient hypertension). Table 5–4 compares different types of hypertension during pregnancy. This section focuses on PIH because it is a common complication, occurring in 7% of pregnancies. One sometimes hears the word *toxemia,* an old word for PIH.

The cause of PIH is unknown, but birth is its cure. It usually develops during late pregnancy but can develop during the intrapartum or even the early postpartum period. Vasospasm (spasm of the arteries) is the main characteristic of PIH. Although the cause is unknown, any of several risk factors increases a woman's chance of developing PIH (Box 5–3).

PIH is divided into two categories, preeclampsia and eclampsia. Preeclampsia is further divided into mild and severe forms. Eclampsia is an extension of severe preeclampsia to include one or more generalized seizures (convulsions).

## Manifestations

Vasospasm impedes blood flow to the mother's organs and placenta, resulting in one

| BOX 5–3 | Risk Factors for Pregnancy-Induced Hypertension (PIH) |
|---|---|

First baby
Non-Caucasian race
Age under 18 or over 35 yr
Multifetal pregnancy (e.g., twins)
Hydatidiform mole
History of PIH with previous pregnancy
Family history (mother or sister) of PIH
Malnutrition
Inadequate prenatal care
Chronic hypertension
Chronic renal disease
Diabetes mellitus

or more of these signs: (1) hypertension, (2) edema, and (3) proteinuria (protein in the urine). PIH can also affect the central nervous system, eyes, urinary tract, liver, gastrointestinal system, and blood clotting function.

**Hypertension.** Blood pressure normally de-

**Table 5–4.** HYPERTENSIVE DISORDERS OF PREGNANCY

| | |
|---|---|
| Pregnancy-induced hypertension (PIH) | Elevation of blood pressure (BP) in a previously normotensive woman after 20 weeks of gestation: 30 mmHg systolic or 15 mmHg diastolic over the baseline; systolic of 140 mmHg or diastolic of 90 mmHg, regardless of baseline |
| Preeclampsia | Hypertension as above, accompanied by edema and/or proteinuria |
|   Mild preeclampsia | BP lower than 160 mmHg systolic and 110 mmHg diastolic |
| | Edema of hands and/or face |
| | Proteinuria 1+ to 2+ |
| | Fetal compromise possible because of impaired placental circulation |
|   Severe preeclampsia | BP greater than 160 mmHg systolic and/or 110 mmHg diastolic |
| | Edema of hands and/or face |
| | Proteinuria 3+ or 4+ |
| | Other signs and symptoms: |
| |   Urine output less than 400 ml/24 hr |
| |   Central nervous system alterations, such as altered consciousness, headache |
| |   Visual disturbance, such as spots or flashes of light |
| |   Epigastric or right upper abdominal pain |
| |   Clotting disorders |
| |   Abnormal liver function tests |
| |   Pulmonary edema, with breathing difficulty and "wet" lung sounds |
| | Fetal compromise more likely because of reduced placental circulation |
| Eclampsia | Progression of preeclampsia to include one or more seizures |
| Transient hypertension | Development of hypertension (BP elevation as above) without other signs of preeclampsia, such as edema or proteinuria |
| Chronic hypertension | Documented hypertension existing before 20 weeks' gestation |
| Preeclampsia superimposed on chronic hypertension | Worsening of preexisting hypertension, accompanied by other signs and symptoms of PIH |

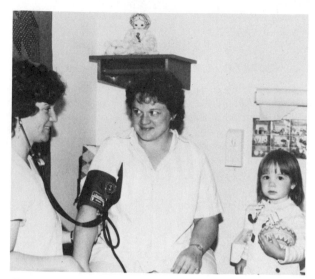

**Figure 5–6.** Blood pressure is checked at every prenatal visit to detect early signs of pregnancy-induced hypertension. (Courtesy of WomanCare, Des Moines BirthPlace, Des Moines, IA.)

creases slightly during the 2nd trimester of pregnancy, returning to prepregnancy levels by the end of pregnancy (Fig. 5–6). Therefore, a specific blood pressure cannot be used to diagnose hypertension. Hypertension during pregnancy is defined as an increase of 30 mmHg in the systolic pressure or 15 mmHg in the diastolic pressure *over the woman's baseline reading*. A systolic pressure of 140 mmHg or a diastolic pressure of 90 mmHg indicates hypertension, regardless of the baseline reading.

Identifying mild PIH is difficult if the woman did not have early prenatal care, because her baseline blood pressure is not known. For example, her blood pressure might be 130/75, which is usually normal. However, if her typical pressure is 100/60, the elevation is significant.

**Edema.** Edema occurs because fluid leaves the blood vessels and enters the tissues. Although total body fluid is increased, the amount within the blood vessels is reduced (hypovolemia), further decreasing blood flow to the maternal organs and placenta.

*Sudden* excessive weight gain is the first evidence of fluid retention. Visible edema follows the weight gain. Edema of the feet and legs is common during pregnancy, but edema above the waist suggests PIH. The woman may notice facial swelling or stop wearing rings because

they are hard to remove. Edema is severe ("pitting") if a depression remains after the tissue is compressed.

Edema resolves quickly after birth as excess tissue fluid returns to the circulation and is excreted in the urine. Urine output may reach 6 liters daily and often exceeds fluid intake.

**Proteinuria.** Proteinuria develops later in pregnancy as reduced blood flow damages the kidneys. This damage allows protein to leak into the urine. A clean-catch or catheterized urine specimen is used to check for proteinuria, because vaginal secretions might give a false-positive result.

**Other Manifestations.** Other signs and symptoms occur with severe preeclampsia. All are related to decreased blood flow and edema of the organs involved.

*Central Nervous System.* A severe, unrelenting headache may occur because of brain edema and small cerebral hemorrhages. Deep tendon reflexes become hyperactive because of central nervous system irritability.

*Eyes.* Visual disturbances such as blurred or double vision, or "spots before the eyes" occur because of arterial spasm and edema of the retina.

*Urinary Tract.* Decreased blood flow to the kidneys reduces urine production. The kidneys respond to low blood flow as they do to shock, by releasing substances to raise the blood pressure. This aggravates hypertension.

*Liver.* Liver enzymes are elevated because of reduced circulation, edema, and small hemorrhages.

*Gastrointestinal System.* Epigastric pain or nausea occurs because of liver edema. *These symptoms often precede a convulsion.*

*Blood Clotting.* HELLP syndrome is a variant of preeclampsia, typified by *h*emolysis (breakage of erythrocytes), *e*levated *l*iver enzymes, and *l*ow *p*latelets. Low platelets cause abnormal blood clotting.

**Eclampsia.** Progression to eclampsia occurs when the woman has one or more tonic-clonic seizures. Facial muscles twitch; this symptom is followed by generalized contraction of all muscles (tonic phase), then alternate contraction and relaxation of muscles (clonic phase). *An eclamptic seizure may result in cerebral hemorrhage, abruptio placentae, fetal compromise, or death of the mother or fetus.*

**Effects on Fetus.** PIH reduces maternal blood flow through the placenta and decreases oxygen available to the fetus. Fetal hypoxia may result in meconium (first stool) passage into the amniotic fluid or in fetal distress. The fetus may have growth retardation and at birth may be long and thin with peeling skin. Fetal death sometimes occurs.

## Medical Care

Medical care focuses on prevention and early detection of PIH and on treatment. Drugs are often needed to prevent convulsions and to reduce a dangerously high blood pressure.

**Prevention.** Studies of therapy to prevent PIH in women at risk are under way. These involve taking calcium supplements or low-dose aspirin. The safety and effectiveness of these treatments are not yet known.

Correction of some risk factors reduces the risk for PIH. For example, improving the diet, particularly of the adolescent, may prevent PIH and promote normal fetal growth. Other risk factors, such as family history, cannot be changed. However, early and regular prenatal care allows PIH to be diagnosed promptly, so that it is more effectively managed.

**Treatment.** If PIH occurs, medical care focuses on (1) maintaining blood flow to the woman's vital organs and the placenta and (2) preventing convulsions. Birth is the cure for PIH. If the fetus is mature, pregnancy is ended by labor induction (see p. 189) or cesarean birth (see p. 195). If the fetus is immature, medical management depends on the severity of PIH. Fortunately, most women are near term when PIH occurs. If PIH is severe, the fetus is often in greater danger from being in the uterus than from being born prematurely.

Most women are hospitalized because their condition, or that of the fetus, may rapidly deteriorate. Some are managed at home if they can comply with treatment and if frequent home nursing visits are possible. Specialized agencies offer nursing care that allows some women with mild PIH or other pregnancy complications to remain at home, rather than being hospitalized.

## Nursing Brief

Bed rest on the side, particularly the left side, helps improve blood flow to the placenta and more effectively provides oxygen and nutrients to the fetus.

Bed rest is essential in PIH care. Bed rest allows blood that would be circulated to skeletal muscles to be conserved for circulation to the mother's vital organs and the placenta. The woman should spend as much time as possible on her left side to improve blood flow to the placenta. She may walk to the bathroom and to the shower if PIH is mild.

Diuretics and sodium restriction are not prescribed for PIH. They are not effective for treatment of PIH and may aggravate it because they further deplete the woman's blood volume. Salt is not restricted, but intake of high-salt foods is discouraged. The woman's diet should have adequate calories, protein, and sodium (see Chap. 4 for prenatal dietary guidelines).

Fetal diagnostic tests (Table 5–5) that may be done are

- Amniocentesis to determine if the fetal lungs are mature before labor induction or cesarean birth (Fig. 5–7)
- Evaluations of placental function and its ability to provide oxygen and waste removal for the fetus, such as biophysical profile (Fig. 5–8), nonstress test, and contraction stress test

***Magnesium Sulfate.*** Magnesium sulfate is an anticonvulsant given to prevent seizures. It may slightly reduce the blood pressure, but its main use is as an anticonvulsant. It is usually given by intravenous infusion (controlled with an infusion pump). It may be given intramuscularly, but this is painful and the injections must be given every 4 hours. Administration continues for 12–24 hours or longer after birth because the woman remains at risk for seizures.

Magnesium is excreted by the kidneys. Poor urine output (<30 ml/hr) allows serum levels of magnesium to reach toxic levels. Excess magnesium first causes loss of the deep tendon reflexes, which is followed by depression of respirations; if levels rise further, collapse and death can occur. *Calcium gluconate* reverses the effects of magnesium and should be available for immediate use when a woman receives magnesium sulfate.

The therapeutic serum level of magnesium is 3–8 mg/dl, an abnormal level in a person not receiving this therapy. The woman with this serum level is slightly drowsy but retains all her reflexes and has normal respiratory function; the level is high enough to prevent convulsions.

Magnesium inhibits uterine contractions.

**Table 5–5.** FETAL DIAGNOSTIC TESTS

| Tests and Description | Uses During Pregnancy |
|---|---|
| *Ultrasound examination*: use of high-frequency sound waves to visualize structures within the body; the examination may use a transvaginal probe or an abdominal transducer; abdominal ultrasound during early pregnancy requires a full bladder for proper visualization (have the woman drink 1–2 quarts of water before the examination) | Visualize a gestational sac in early pregnancy to confirm the pregnancy<br>Identify site of implantation (uterine or ectopic)<br>Verify fetal viability or death<br>Identify a multifetal pregnancy, such as twins or triplets<br>Diagnose some fetal structural abnormalities<br>Provide guidance for other procedures, such as chorionic villous sampling, amniocentesis, percutaneous umbilical blood sampling<br>Determine gestational age of the embryo or fetus<br>Locate the placenta<br>Determine the amount of amniotic fluid<br>Observe fetal movements |
| *Doppler ultrasound blood flow assessment*: use of high-frequency sound waves to study the flow of blood through vessels | Determine adequacy of blood flow through the placenta and umbilical cord vessels in women in whom it is likely to be impaired (such as those with pregnancy-induced hypertension or diabetes mellitus) |
| *Alpha-fetoprotein testing*: determining the level of this fetal protein in the pregnant woman's serum or in a sample of amniotic fluid; correct interpretation requires an accurate gestational age | Identify high levels, which are associated with open defects, such as spina bifida (open spine), anencephaly (incomplete development of the skull and brain), or gastroschisis (open abdominal cavity)<br>Identify low levels, which are associated with chromosome abnormalities or gestational trophoblastic disease (hydatidiform mole) |
| *Chorionic villous sampling*: obtaining a small part of the developing placenta to analyze fetal cells at 9–12 wk gestation | Identify chromosome abnormalities or other defects that can be determined by analysis of cells. Results of chromosome studies are available 24–48 hr later. Cannot be used to determine spina bifida or anencephaly (see alpha-fetoprotein testing). Higher rate of spontaneous abortion following procedure than after amniocentesis. Rh immune globulin (RhoGAM) is given to the Rh-negative woman |
| *Amniocentesis*: insertion of a thin needle through the abdominal and uterine walls to obtain a sample of amniotic fluid, which contains cast-off fetal cells and various other fetal products; standard genetic amniocentesis is done at 16–20 wk gestation; early genetic amniocentesis is done at 10–15 wk gestation for some disorders | Early pregnancy: Identify chromosome abnormalities, biochemical disorders (such as Tay-Sachs' disease), and level of alpha-fetoprotein. A fetus cannot be tested for every possible disorder. Spontaneous abortion following the procedure is the primary risk<br>Late pregnancy: Identify severity of maternal-fetal blood incompatibility and assess fetal lung maturity. Rh immune globulin is given to the Rh-negative woman |
| *Nonstress test (NST)*: evaluation of the fetal heart rate response to fetal movement using an electronic fetal monitor. The expected response is an acceleration of 15 beats/min lasting 15 sec with at least two fetal movements | Identify fetal compromise in conditions associated with poor placenta function, such as hypertension, diabetes mellitus, or postterm gestation. Adequate accelerations of the fetal heart rate with movement are reassuring that the placenta is functioning properly and the fetus is well oxygenated |
| *Vibroacoustic stimulation test*: procedure is similar to the NST; in addition, an artificial larynx device is used to stimulate the fetus with sound; expected response is acceleration of the fetal heart rate, as in the NST | Clarify, if the NST is questionable, whether the fetus is well oxygenated, thereby reducing the need for more complex testing<br>Clarify, during labor, questionable fetal heart rate patterns |
| *Contraction stress test (CST)*: evaluation of the fetal heart rate response to mild uterine contractions by using an electronic fetal monitor; contractions may be induced by self-stimulation of the nipples, which causes the woman's pituitary gland to release oxytocin, or by intravenous oxytocin (Pitocin) infusion | Purposes are the same as the NST; the CST may be done if the NST results are abnormal (the fetal heart does not accelerate) or if they are questionable |

**Table 5–5.** FETAL DIAGNOSTIC TESTS *Continued*

| Tests and Description | Uses During Pregnancy |
|---|---|
| *Biophysical profile (BPP)*: a group of five fetal assessments: fetal heart rate and reactivity (the NST), fetal breathing movements, fetal body movements, fetal tone (closure of the hand), and the volume of amniotic fluid; some physicians omit the NST from this profile | Identify reduced fetal oxygenation in conditions associated with poor placental function, but with greater precision than the NST alone. As fetal hypoxia gradually increases, fetal heart rate changes occur first, followed by cessation of fetal breathing movement, gross body movements, and finally loss of fetal tone. Amniotic fluid volume is reduced when placental function is poor |
| *Percutaneous umbilical blood sampling*: obtaining a fetal blood sample from a placental vessel or from the umbilical cord; may be used to give a blood transfusion to an anemic fetus | Identify fetal conditions that can be diagnosed only with a blood sample<br>Blood transfusion for fetal anemia caused by maternal-fetal blood incompatibility, placenta previa, or abruptio placentae |
| *Maternal assessment of fetal movement (kick counts)*: the mother counts the number of fetal movements in a period of 30–60 min three times a day. Another technique is the "count to ten" method, in which the mother begins counting at a specific time of day, then records the time when she feels 10 fetal movements | Identify, inexpensively and noninvasively, the fetus that may be having slight hypoxia or other compromise. The woman should report a change in the movements or fewer than four movements per hour |
| *Tests of fetal lung maturity*: tests a sample of amniotic fluid (obtained by amniocentesis or from the pool of fluid in the vagina) to determine substances that indicate fetal lungs are mature enough to adapt to extrauterine life:<br>• Lecithin-to-sphingomyelin (L:S) ratio: A 2:1 ratio indicates fetal lung maturity (3:1 ratio desirable for diabetic mother); fluid usually obtained by amniocentesis<br>• Presence of phosphatidylglycerol (PG)<br>• Presence of phosphatidylinositol (PI)<br>• Foam stability index (FSI, or "shake test"): persistence of a ring of bubbles for 15 min after shaking together equal amounts of 95% ethanol, isotonic saline, and amniotic fluid | Evaluate whether the fetus is likely to have respiratory complications in adapting to extrauterine life. May be done to determine if the fetal lungs are mature before performing an elective cesarean birth or inducing labor if the gestational age is questionable. Also used to evaluate whether the fetus should be promptly delivered or allowed to mature further when the membranes rupture and the gestation is less than about 37 wk or if the gestation is questionable |

Most women receiving the drug must also receive oxytocin to strengthen labor contractions (see p. 189). They are at risk for postpartum hemorrhage because the uterus does not contract firmly on bleeding vessels after birth (see p. 252). This effect of magnesium makes it useful to stop preterm labor (see p. 206).

***Antihypertensive Drugs.*** Antihypertensive drugs reduce blood pressure if it reaches a level that might cause a stroke, usually higher than 160/100. Severe hypertension can harm the fetus by causing abruptio placentae or placental infarcts (death of placental tissue). Hydralazine (Apresoline) is usually prescribed, although newer drugs, such as nifedipine (Procardia), may be used.

### Nursing Care

Nursing care focuses on (1) assisting women to obtain prenatal care, (2) helping them cope with therapy, (3) caring for acutely ill women, and (4) administering medications, primarily magnesium sulfate. Nursing Care Plan 5–2 specifies interventions for women with PIH.

**Promoting Prenatal Care.** Nurses can promote awareness of how prenatal care allows risk identification and early intervention if complications arise. Nurses can help the woman feel like an individual, especially in busy clinics, which often seem impersonal, thus encouraging her to return regularly.

**Coping with Therapy.** Daily weight assessments identify sudden gain. The weight should be checked early in the morning, after urination, and in similar clothes each day.

The nurse helps the woman understand the importance of bed rest and find ways to manage it. Activity diverts blood from the placenta, reducing her baby's oxygen supply. The nurse helps her find quiet activities if she must be on

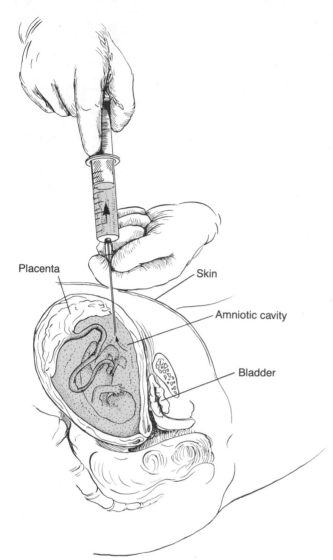

Placenta

Skin

Amniotic cavity

Bladder

**Figure 5–7.** Amniocentesis may be done to obtain a sample of amniotic fluid for a variety of studies, such as genetic studies and tests of fetal lung maturity.

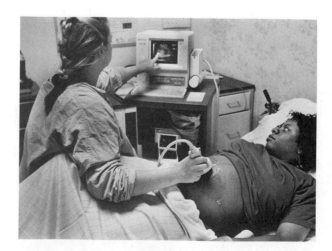

**Figure 5–8.** The biophysical profile is done to evaluate the condition of the fetus in the woman who has a problem that may result in impaired placental blood flow.

## Selected Nursing Diagnoses for the Woman with Pregnancy-Induced Hypertension

| Goals | Nursing Interventions | Rationale |
|---|---|---|

**Nursing Diagnosis:** Knowledge deficit: home care of mild pregnancy-induced hypertension (PIH).

| | | |
|---|---|---|
| Woman will restate correct home care measures related to PIH<br>Woman will keep prescribed prenatal appointments | 1. Ask woman what she knows about hypertension during pregnancy; include family members if present<br>2. Teach woman importance of keeping prenatal appointments, which will be more frequent (2–3/wk) because she has mild PIH | 1. Allows nurse to build on woman's existing knowledge, reinforcing it and correcting any misunderstandings<br>2. PIH can quickly become more severe between frequent prenatal care visits; many signs of worsening PIH can be detected only at prenatal visits, and some (such as edema) are considered normal by many women; if woman understands why she should keep appointments, she is more likely to do so |
| | 3. Reinforce prescribed measures to care for herself at home:<br><br>a. Remain on bed rest, spending most of the time on the left side (may walk to the bathroom and eat meals at table in most cases)<br>b. Eat a well-balanced, high-protein diet; limit high-sodium foods, such as potato chips, salted nuts, pickles, and many snack foods; include high-fiber foods and at least eight glasses of noncaffeine drinks each day; consider food preferences and economic restraints when helping woman choose appropriate foods<br><br>c. Discuss quiet activities the woman enjoys that can be done while she is on bed rest<br><br>4. Teach woman to report signs that indicate worsening PIH promptly: headache; visual disturbances (blurring, flashes of light, "spots" before the eyes); gastrointestinal symptoms (nausea, pain); worsening edema, especially of the face and fingers; noticeable drop in urine output | 3. If woman understands these measures to limit severity of PIH, she may be more motivated to maintain them:<br>a. Bed rest reduces flow of blood to skeletal muscles, thus making more available to placenta; this enhances fetal oxygenation<br>b. Women with PIH lose protein in their urine, which must be replaced to maintain nutrition and fluid balance; severe sodium restriction may increase severity of PIH, but a high sodium intake may worsen hypertension and decrease the woman's blood volume; fiber and fluids help reduce constipation, which is more likely when activity is restricted<br>c. Bed rest can lead to boredom, and the woman may not maintain the prescribed activity if she is bored<br>4. PIH can worsen despite careful home management and client compliance; if the woman has these symptoms, she needs to be evaluated and hospitalized to prevent progression to eclampsia |

**Nursing Diagnosis:** Altered tissue perfusion (maternal vital organs and placenta) related to constriction of small blood vessels.

| | | |
|---|---|---|
| Woman will not have a seizure<br>Rate and pattern of the fetal heart will remain reassuring (see p. 145) | 1. Assist with fetal heart rate monitoring according to facility's protocol (see pp. 140–145 for more information about fetal heart rate assessments)<br>2. Keep room quiet and lights dimmed; limit number of personnel and visitors who enter room; side rails should be pulled up and the woman should maintain strict bed rest on her left side; maintain continuous nursing observation | 1. Generalized vasoconstriction in PIH reduces blood flow to the placenta, thus compromising fetal oxygenation; fetal heart rate patterns may reflect reduced placental blood flow<br>2. Environmental stimulants may precipitate a seizure; if a woman has severe preeclampsia, she could unexpectedly have a seizure, and the nurse must intervene to minimize injury |

*Continued*

| NURSING CARE PLAN 5–2 *Continued* | | |
|---|---|---|
| **Selected Nursing Diagnoses for the Woman with Pregnancy-Induced Hypertension** | | |
| Goals | Nursing Interventions | Rationale |

**Nursing Diagnosis:** Altered tissue perfusion (maternal vital organs and placenta) related to constriction of small blood vessels.

| Goals | Nursing Interventions | Rationale |
|---|---|---|
| | 3. Keep an emergency tray in her room (often called a "toxemia tray" or a "PIH tray") | 3. Contains emergency drugs and equipment that may be needed quickly; equipment often includes airways, Ambu bag, and suction and oxygen equipment; drugs usually include magnesium sulfate, calcium gluconate (to reverse the effects of magnesium sulfate), and hydralazine (for severe hypertension) |
| | 4. Assist the experienced registered nurse with magnesium sulfate administration according to facility protocol; typical care includes<br> a. Deep tendon reflexes (DTRs)<br> b. Maternal blood pressure, pulse, and respirations; report respiration rate of under 12/min<br> c. Urine output; report output of less than 30 ml/hr<br> d. Monitor serum magnesium levels according to protocol | 4. Magnesium sulfate is a central nervous system depressant given to prevent convulsions; inadequate magnesium may not prevent seizures, whereas excess drug levels may cause respiratory depression or cardiopulmonary collapse |
| | 5. Observe for signs that may indicate an imminent seizure: twitching of facial muscles, hyperactive DTRs, epigastric or right upper abdominal quadrant pain, nausea or vomiting; try to prevent injury if woman has a seizure, but do not forcibly restrain her; after seizure, an airway is inserted to facilitate suctioning and oxygen administration; after she awakens following the seizure, reorient her to surroundings | 5. Early intervention can reduce maternal injuries if a seizure occurs; forcible restraint may cause greater injury; the woman is likely to be confused and possibly combative after a seizure; continuous oxygenation restores oxygen delivery to the fetus |

bed rest for a prolonged time. See preterm labor (p. 208) for more information about bed rest.

**Caring for the Acutely Ill Woman.** The acutely ill woman requires intensive nursing care directed by an experienced registered nurse. A quiet, low-light environment reduces the risk of convulsions. Bed side rails should be padded and raised to prevent injury if a convulsion occurs. There should be no loud noises or bumping of the bed. Visitors are limited, usually to one or two support persons. An emergency tray ("toxemia tray") containing drugs and emergency equipment is placed in the room. Suction equipment is available for immediate use.

If a seizure occurs, the nursing focus is to prevent injury and restore oxygenation to the mother and fetus. If possible, the mother is turned on her side before the seizure begins. The nurse does not forcibly hold the woman's body but prevents her from striking hard surfaces.

Breathing stops during a seizure. An oral airway, inserted *after* the seizure, facilitates breathing and suctioning of secretions. Oxygen by face mask improves fetal oxygenation. The fetus is monitored continuously (see p. 141). The woman is reoriented to the environment when she regains consciousness. Labor may progress rapidly after a seizure (see p. 138 for signs of impending birth).

**Administering Medications.** Magnesium sulfate is administered by an experienced registered nurse. A practical nurse may assist.

Hospital protocols provide specific guidelines for care when magnesium sulfate is given. Common protocols include

- Blood pressure, pulse, respirations hourly; temperature every 4 hours
- Deep tendon reflexes every 1–4 hours (Fig. 5–9).
- Intake and output (sometimes hourly); an indwelling Foley catheter may be ordered
- Check urine protein with a reagent strip (dipstick) at each voiding

The registered nurse reports deteriorating of the maternal or fetal condition:

- Increasing hypertension, particularly if blood pressure is 160/100 or higher
- Signs of central nervous system irritability, such as facial twitching or hyperactive deep tendon reflexes
- Decreased urine output, especially if less than 30 ml/hr
- Abnormal fetal heart rates (see p. 145)
- Symptoms such as severe headache, visual disturbances, or epigastric pain, which often immediately precede a convulsion

The registered nurse reports signs of possible magnesium toxicity to the physician and

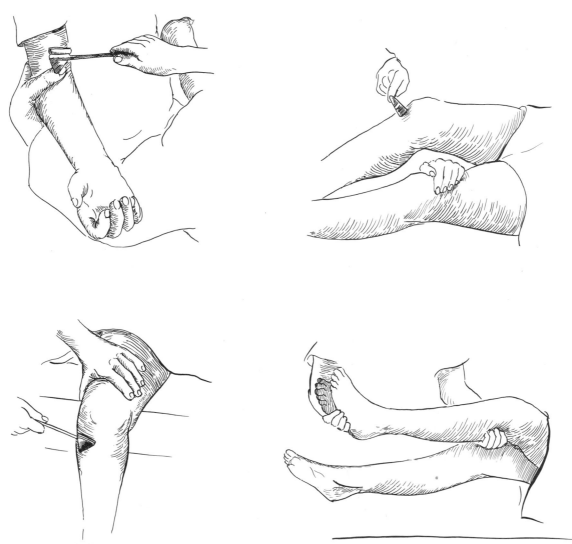

**Figure 5–9.** Assessment of the deep tendon reflexes is essential to determine whether the woman is receiving too much or too little magnesium sulfate and to identify the woman likely to have a convulsion.

prepares calcium gluconate to reverse this toxicity:

- Absent deep tendon reflexes
- Respiration rate of under 12/min
- Urine output less than 30 ml/hr
- Serum magnesium levels above 8 mg/dl

PIH can develop after birth, and the risk for convulsions remains for up to 24 hours. Nursing care continues after birth until magnesium sulfate is stopped. The woman must be carefully observed for postpartum hemorrhage (see p. 252) in addition to being given usual postpartum care.

## BLOOD INCOMPATIBILITY BETWEEN THE PREGNANT WOMAN AND FETUS

The placenta allows maternal and fetal blood to be close enough for exchanging oxygen and waste products without actually mixing (see p. 36). However, small leaks may occur during pregnancy, allowing fetal blood to enter the mother's circulation. Larger amounts of fetal blood enter the mother's circulation when the placenta detaches at birth.

If maternal and fetal blood types are compatible, no problem occurs, just as deliberate transfusion of compatible blood is not harmful. However, if the maternal and fetal blood types differ, the mother's body may produce antibodies to destroy fetal red blood cells (RBCs, or erythrocytes). There are two types of blood incompatibility during pregnancy, Rh incompatibility and ABO incompatibility.

### Rh Incompatibility

People either have the Rh blood factor on their erythrocytes or they do not. If they have the factor, they are Rh-positive; if not, they are Rh-negative. Rh-negative blood type is an autosomal recessive trait, which means that a person must receive a gene for this characteristic from both parents. The Rh-positive person may have inherited two Rh-positive genes or may have one Rh-positive and one Rh-negative gene. This explains why two Rh-positive parents can conceive a baby that is Rh-negative. About 15% of Caucasians and 5% of African Americans are Rh-negative.

A person with Rh-negative blood is not born with antibodies against the Rh factor and does not immediately react to Rh-positive blood that enters the circulation. However, exposure to Rh-positive blood causes the person to make

## Nursing Brief

Most cases of Rh incompatibility between an Rh-negative mother and an Rh-positive fetus can be prevented with administration of Rh immune globulin (RhoGAM) every time it is indicated.

antibodies (sensitization), which destroy Rh-positive erythrocytes that enter the circulation later. Thus, Rh incompatibility between the woman and fetus can occur only if the woman is Rh-negative and the fetus is Rh-positive.

If fetal Rh-positive blood leaks into the mother's circulation, her body may respond by making antibodies to destroy the Rh-positive erythrocytes. Because this response usually occurs at birth, the first Rh-positive baby is rarely affected. However, each time the woman is "exposed" to more Rh-positive blood (in subsequent pregnancies with Rh-positive fetuses), her body produces antibodies more rapidly. Antibodies against Rh-positive blood are small enough to cross the placenta and destroy the fetal Rh-positive erythrocytes.

**Manifestations.** The woman has no obvious effects if her body produces anti-Rh antibodies. However, increased levels of these antibodies in her blood are revealed by rising antibody titers in laboratory tests.

The fetus will have erythroblastosis fetalis if maternal anti-Rh antibodies cross the placenta and destroy fetal erythrocytes. The fetus becomes anemic, and accumulated bilirubin from the broken RBCs causes jaundice that is obvious at birth. In severe cases, the fetus has heart failure and severe edema (hydrops fetalis). A sample of amniotic fluid shows high bilirubin levels. (See p. 356 for care of the infant with erythroblastosis fetalis.)

**Treatment.** The primary management is to prevent manufacture of anti-Rh antibodies by giving Rh immune globulin to the Rh-negative woman at 28 weeks of gestation and within 72 hours after birth of an Rh-positive infant or abortion (see p. 227). It is given after amniocentesis and to women who have bleeding during pregnancy, because fetal blood may leak into the mother's circulation at these times. Rh immune globulin has greatly decreased the incidence of infants with Rh incompatibility problems. However, some women are still sensitized, usually because they did not receive Rh immune globulin after childbirth or abortion.

The woman who already has antibodies against Rh-positive blood is carefully monitored during pregnancy to determine if too many fetal erythrocytes are being destroyed. Several diagnostic tests may be used, including the Coombs test (see p. 355), amniocentesis, or percutaneous umbilical blood sampling (see Table 5–5).

An intrauterine transfusion may be done for the severely anemic fetus. Group O-negative red blood cells are injected into the fetal peritoneal cavity, where they are absorbed into the circulation or into one of the fetal umbilical vessels. O-negative blood is transfused because it is compatible with all blood types (universal donor).

The infant is jaundiced at birth because of high blood bilirubin levels. Phototherapy (see p. 356) reduces the infant's bilirubin level. In severe cases, exchange transfusion is done to replace the infant's blood with compatible blood that has no anti-Rh antibodies and has a normal bilirubin level.

### ABO Incompatibility

ABO incompatibility can occur if the woman has group O blood and the fetus has group A, group B, or group AB blood. Unlike anti-Rh antibodies, anti-A and anti-B antibodies are already in the woman's body. However, fewer of these antibodies cross the placenta than those associated with Rh problems. The fetus does not usually have severe problems.

The infant may develop jaundice within the first 24 hours, and bilirubin levels may rise rapidly. Phototherapy is usually sufficient to reduce the bilirubin level in ABO incompatibility.

### Nursing Care for Pregnancy-Related Blood Incompatibilities

Giving Rh immune globulin *every* time it is indicated prevents nearly all cases of Rh incompatibility. The chart should be checked for a woman's Rh factor after birth, abortion (spontaneous or elective), episodes of bleeding, or amniocentesis. The physician or nurse-midwife is notified if the Rh factor is not documented or if there is no order for Rh immune globulin for an Rh-negative woman when the drug is indicated.

Care of the infant involves observing for jaundice, especially during the first 24 hours of life. Early jaundice or rapidly increasing jaundice is reported to the physician so that serum bilirubin levels can be obtained. (See Chaps. 13 and 14 for discussion of nursing care related to neonatal jaundice and phototherapy.)

# Pregnancy Complicated by Medical Conditions

Medical conditions may require special management during pregnancy. Many become harder to diagnose or control. Others have more adverse effects for the woman or fetus than at other times. Four disorders are discussed in this section: (1) diabetes mellitus, (2) heart disease, (3) anemia, and (4) infections.

## DIABETES MELLITUS

A woman may have either of two types of diabetes mellitus:

- Preexisting diabetes mellitus, which includes insulin-dependent (type I) and non-insulin-dependent (type II) diabetes
- Gestational diabetes mellitus (GDM), which occurs only during pregnancy

Of all pregnant diabetic women, 90% have gestational diabetes mellitus. See a medical-surgical nursing text for a more detailed discussion of diabetes in the nonpregnant person.

### Pathophysiology of Diabetes Mellitus

Diabetes mellitus is a disorder in which there is inadequate insulin to move glucose from the blood into body cells. It occurs because the pancreas produces no insulin or insufficient insulin, or because cells resist the effects of insulin.

In the woman with diabetes, cells are essentially starving because they cannot use glucose. To compensate, the body metabolizes protein and fat for energy, which causes ketones and acids to accumulate (ketosis). The person loses weight despite eating large amounts of food (polyphagia). Fatigue and lethargy accompany cell starvation. To dilute excess glucose in the blood, thirst increases (polydipsia) and fluid moves from the tissues into the blood. This results in dehydration and excretion of large amounts (polyuria) of glucose-bearing urine (glycosuria).

Diabetes also may cause obstruction of small blood vessels and loss of nerve function. These effects can cause delayed wound healing, blindness, heart disease, or kidney failure. These problems are more likely if the diabetes is poorly controlled. (See a medical-surgical nursing text and pp. 836–851 of this book for detailed discussion of diabetes.)

### Effect of Pregnancy on Glucose Metabolism

Pregnancy affects a woman's metabolism, whether or not she has diabetes, to make ample glucose available to the growing fetus. Hormones (estrogen and progesterone) and an enzyme (insulinase) produced by the placenta have two effects:

- Increase resistance of cells to insulin
- Increase speed of insulin breakdown

Most women respond to these changes by secreting extra insulin to maintain normal carbohydrate metabolism while still providing plenty of glucose for the fetus. If the woman cannot increase her insulin production, she will have periods of hyperglycemia as glucose accumulates in the blood.

Women who are diabetic before pregnancy must alter the management of their condition. In the past, women with diabetes often had poor outcomes, such as abnormal fetal growth, stillbirth, and congenital abnormalities. Today, with careful management, most diabetic women can have successful pregnancies and healthy babies. Nevertheless, the woman and fetus or newborn have many potential complications of diabetes (Box 5–4).

### Gestational Diabetes Mellitus

GDM is common and resolves quickly after birth. Affected women do not have all the classic signs and symptoms of diabetes. They are not usually affected by blood vessel and nerve damage as are people who have diabetes independent of pregnancy. However, they are more likely to develop overt diabetes within the next 15 years.

Several factors in a woman's history are linked to gestational diabetes:

- Large infant, over 9 pounds (Fig. 5–10)
- Previous unexplained stillbirth or infant having congenital defects
- Excess amniotic fluid (hydramnios)
- Recurrent candidiasis (monilial, or "yeast," vaginal infections)

---

**BOX 5–4    Effects of Diabetes in Pregnancy**

**Maternal Effects**

Spontaneous abortion
Pregnancy-induced hypertension (preeclampsia and eclampsia)
Preterm labor
Hydramnios (excessive amniotic fluid; also called polyhydramnios)
Infections of all kinds, particularly
  Vaginitis
  Urinary tract infections
Cesarean or forceps-assisted birth

**Fetal and Neonatal Effects**

Congenital abnormalities
Macrosomia (large size) or growth retardation
Delayed lung maturation
Neonatal hypoglycemia
Neonatal hyperbilirubinemia and jaundice
Neonatal polycythemia (excess erythrocytes)
Learning disabilities
Later development of diabetes during childhood or adulthood

---

- Glycosuria on two successive prenatal visits
- Fetal macrosomia (large size) on ultrasound examination
- Family history
- Ethnic group with higher risk: Navajo Indian, Hispanic, Chinese, Saudi Arabian, African American

Nursing Care Plan 5–3 lists specific interventions for the pregnant woman with GDM.

### Treatment

The nonpregnant person is treated with a balance of insulin or an oral hypoglycemic drug (agent that reduces blood sugar), diet, and exercise. Some people with mild diabetes do not need drugs and control their condition by diet alone. Medical therapy during pregnancy includes identification of gestational diabetes, diet, monitoring of blood glucose levels, insulin, exercise, and selected fetal assessments.

**Identification of Gestational Diabetes Mellitus.** If the woman does not have preexisting diabetes, the American Diabetes Association

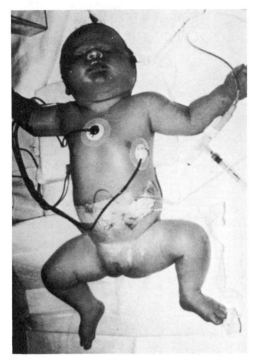

**Figure 5-10.** Newborn with macrosomia due to maternal diabetes mellitus during pregnancy. Despite the large size, the infant of a diabetic mother is likely to have problems similar to those of a preterm infant. (From La Franchi, S. [1987]. Hypoglycemia of infancy and childhood. *Pediatric Clinics of North America*, *34*, 969.)

recommends that a prenatal screening test to identify GDM be done between 24 and 28 weeks of gestation. The woman drinks 50 gm of an oral glucose solution (fasting is not necessary). One hour later, a blood sample is analyzed for glucose. If the blood glucose level is 140 mg/dl or higher, a more complex 3-hour glucose tolerance test is done.

**Diet.** The diet is similar to that for any pregnant woman. Carbohydrate, protein, and fat are balanced to provide for growth and energy needs and to provide adequate calories, vitamins, and minerals. Food intake is divided among three meals and two snacks throughout the day to maintain stable blood glucose levels.

**Monitoring of Blood Glucose Levels.** To ensure a successful pregnancy, the woman must keep her blood glucose levels as close to normal as possible. The pregnant diabetic woman monitors her blood glucose levels four to six times a day. Blood glucose self-monitoring is discussed on page 841. Urine testing for glucose is not useful during pregnancy because the sugar easily passes into the urine. Urine testing for ketones is done two to four times per day.

**Insulin.** Oral hypoglycemics are *not* used during pregnancy because they can cross the placenta, possibly resulting in fetal birth defects or hypoglycemia. Insulin is the only drug prescribed to lower blood glucose during pregnancy because it does not cross the placenta. GDM may be controlled by diet and exercise alone, or the woman may require insulin injections.

The woman with preexisting diabetes may need less insulin during early pregnancy because nausea and vomiting reduce her food intake. Insulin needs increase steadily after the 1st trimester in either preexisting or GDM. During the second half of pregnancy, a woman may need two or three times her nonpregnant insulin dose to maintain normal blood glucose levels. After birth, her insulin requirements fall dramatically, usually below prepregnancy needs. GDM resolves promptly after birth, when the insulin-antagonistic (diabetogenic) effects of pregnancy cease.

A combination of short-acting (regular) and intermediate-acting (neutral protamine Hagedorn [NPH]) insulin is prescribed to keep glucose levels stable and near normal throughout the day. Most women with preexisting diabetes need several injections per day to achieve good glucose control. The woman with GDM who needs insulin may be well controlled with a single injection each day. An insulin pump provides a constant level of insulin plus doses at mealtimes to maintain steady blood glucose levels. (See pp. 844–846 for discussion of insulin administration and the insulin pump.)

**Exercise.** Mild exercise, such as walking, is encouraged during pregnancy because it decreases insulin requirements and enhances the body's use of glucose. Women who have additional complications may have to stop exercising and stay on bed rest. If so, their insulin requirements may increase. When they resume activity after a period of bed rest, their insulin needs fall and they may have episodes of hypoglycemia.

**Fetal Assessments.** Assessments (see Table 5-5) may be done to identify fetal growth and the placenta's ability to provide oxygen and nutrients. Ultrasound examinations identify intrauterine growth retardation, macrosomia, and the amount of amniotic fluid that may be excessive in the poorly controlled diabetic woman.

## Selected Nursing Diagnoses for the Pregnant Woman with Gestational Diabetes Mellitus

| Goals | Nursing Interventions | Rationale |
|---|---|---|

**Nursing Diagnosis:** High risk for ineffective management of therapeutic regimen related to lack of knowledge about new diagnosis.

| Goals | Nursing Interventions | Rationale |
|---|---|---|
| Woman identifies appropriate and inappropriate food choices<br>Woman demonstrates correct self-care techniques for assessing blood glucose and administering insulin<br>Woman verbalizes symptoms of hypoglycemia and hyperglycemia, including correct self-care | 1. Assess knowledge of diabetes and its management, including family members if appropriate | 1. Allows nurse to identify correct and incorrect information and relate new knowledge to what woman already knows, thus promoting individualized teaching |
| | 2. Assist registered nurse to teach prescribed diet; provide written information; have woman identify appropriate foods and the best time to eat them; general guidelines are<br>• Avoid simple sugars, such as cakes, candies, and ice creams because they are quickly converted to glucose, causing wide fluctuations in the blood glucose levels<br>• Eat complex, high-fiber carbohydrates, such as grains, breads, and pasta, because these foods are converted to glucose slowly, thus maintaining stable blood glucose levels<br>• Eat three meals a day plus a mid-afternoon and an evening snack to balance insulin and provide sustained release of glucose to prevent hypoglycemia during late afternoon and evening | 2. A woman who understands diet requirements is more likely to follow them carefully; written information helps refresh her memory if she forgets verbal teaching; verbalizing food choices allows the nurse to determine if she has correctly learned the information |
| | 3. Refer woman to a dietitian if she has difficulty accepting or tolerating foods permitted on her diet | 3. A dietitian specializes in foods and nutrition and can help woman select foods that are acceptable within her dietary limits and that meet her preferences and cultural needs |
| | 4. Assist registered nurse to teach how to perform blood glucose monitoring; have her perform a return demonstration and/or verbalize the regimen; common teaching includes testing frequency, accurate technique, and responses to low or high levels | 4. Insulin requirements fluctuate during pregnancy, generally increasing as pregnancy progresses; frequent blood glucose monitoring allows adjustment of insulin, thus maintaining stable blood glucose levels; stable blood glucose levels are associated with better outcomes for mother and baby; return demonstration of skills or verbalizing information helps the nurse determine if the woman has learned information |
| | 5. Assist registered nurse to teach insulin self-administration (see pp. 844–848 for additional information); have woman give a return demonstration and/or verbalization of each step; teaching includes when to take insulin and how to administer it | 5. Correct insulin administration maintains the most stable blood glucose levels; see #4 for rationale for return demonstration and verbalization |

*Continued*

| NURSING CARE PLAN 5–3 *Continued* | | |
| --- | --- | --- |
| **Selected Nursing Diagnoses for the Pregnant Woman with Gestational Diabetes Mellitus** | | |
| **Goals** | **Nursing Interventions** | **Rationale** |
| **Nursing Diagnosis:** High risk for ineffective management of therapeutic regimen related to lack of knowledge about new diagnosis. | | |
|  | 6. Teach signs and symptoms of hypoglycemia and hyperglycemia (see Table 5–6); teach appropriate responses to these signs and symptoms | 6. Abnormally low or high blood glucose levels require adjustment of insulin dose and/or food intake; additionally, hyperglycemia may be an early sign of infection in diabetic woman; woman who understands signs, symptoms, and corrective actions is likely to seek care needed to maintain optimal blood glucose levels |
|  | 7. Explain that gestational diabetes usually resolves quickly after birth but that it may recur in future pregnancies or in mid-life | 7. Short-term nature of gestational diabetes makes its management easier to tolerate; advance information about possible future diabetes improves ongoing health monitoring |
| **Nursing Diagnosis:** Knowledge deficit: complications of diabetes during pregnancy. | | |
| Woman verbalizes correct responses to potential complications of gestational diabetes | 1. Teach danger signs in pregnancy (Box 5–1) and reinforce them at each prenatal visit | 1. Increases likelihood that woman will seek prompt treatment for all pregnancy complications, including those relating to diabetes |
|  | 2. Teach signs and symptoms of urinary tract infection and vaginal infection, especially candidiasis (see p. 109) | 2. Candidiasis is common in women with diabetes mellitus; urinary tract infections are common and also can lead to maternal sepsis or preterm labor |
|  | 3. Teach woman to report signs of onset or worsening pregnancy-induced hypertension (PIH) (severe headache, vision disturbances, abdominal pain); explain importance of keeping prenatal care appointments | 3. PIH is more likely to occur in diabetic pregnant woman; regular prenatal visits at prescribed intervals can prevent or allow early intervention for complications, including PIH |
|  | 4. Teach about fetal diagnostic tests done; for example, biophysical profile evaluates how well placenta is delivering oxygen and nutrients to baby. | 4. Fetal diagnostic tests allow for early identification and prompt intervention for problems; knowledge decreases woman's anxiety related to the unknown; if woman does not understand reason for doing diagnostic tests, she may incorrectly assume that she or her baby is in danger |

Diabetes may affect the blood vessels that supply the placenta, impairing transport of oxygen and nutrients to the fetus and removal of fetal wastes. The nonstress test, contraction stress test, and biophysical profile provide information about how the placenta is functioning. Tests of fetal lung maturity are common if early delivery is considered.

**Care During Labor.** Labor is work (exercise) that affects the amount of insulin and glucose needed. Some women receive an intravenous infusion of a dextrose solution plus regular insulin as needed. (Regular insulin is the *only* type given intravenously.) Blood glucose levels are assessed every 2 hours and the insulin dose is adjusted accordingly. The woman usually has continuous electronic fetal monitoring (see p. 141).

**Care of the Neonate.** Infant complications after birth may include hypoglycemia, respiratory distress, and injury due to macrosomia. Some infants have growth retardation because the placenta functions poorly. Neonatal nurses and a neonatologist (a physician specializing in care of newborns) are often present at the birth. (See Chap. 14 for discussion of these neonatal problems.)

### Nursing Care

Nursing care of the pregnant woman with diabetes mellitus involves helping her learn to care for herself and providing emotional care to meet the demands imposed by this complication. Care during labor primarily involves careful monitoring for signs of fetal distress (see p. 142).

**Self-Care.** Most women with preexisting diabetes already know how to check their blood sugar and administer insulin. They should be taught why management changes during pregnancy. The woman with GDM must be taught these self-care skills.

The woman is taught how to select appropriate foods for the prescribed diet. She is more likely to maintain the diet if her caregivers are sensitive to her food preferences and cultural needs. A dietitian can determine foods to meet her needs and find solutions to problems in adhering to the diet.

The woman who is taking insulin may experience episodes of hypoglycemia (low blood sugar) or hyperglycemia (high blood sugar). These two conditions are summarized in Table 5–6. The woman is taught to recognize and respond to each condition. A family member is included in teaching, because the woman's thinking and responses may be altered (e.g., confused, combative, lethargic) in either hypoglycemia or hyperglycemia.

**Emotional Support.** Pregnant women with diabetes often find that living with the close management, diet control, and frequent insulin administration is trying. The expectant mother may be anxious about the outcome for herself and her baby. Therapeutic communication helps her express her frustrations and fears. For example, to elicit her feelings about her condition the nurse might say, "Many women find that all the changes they have to make are demanding. How has it been for you?" It may help to emphasize that the close management is usually temporary, especially if she has GDM.

As she learns to manage her care, liberal praise motivates the woman to maintain her therapy. She can be encouraged to find alternative exercise or foods to meet her prescribed therapy. Referral to diabetes management centers is often helpful, if these are available. A woman who is actively involved in her care is more likely to maintain the prescribed therapy.

### HEART DISEASE

Heart disease affects a small percentage of pregnant women. Most heart disease during pregnancy is a result of rheumatic fever or congenital heart defects. Mitral valve prolapse is a benign condition in which the leaflets of the mitral valve bulge into the left atrium when the ventricles contract.

**Table 5–6.** COMPARISON OF HYPOGLYCEMIA AND HYPERGLYCEMIA IN THE DIABETIC WOMAN

| Hypoglycemia | Hyperglycemia |
|---|---|
| Caused by excess insulin, excess exercise, and/or inadequate food intake | Caused by inadequate insulin, reduced activity, and/or excessive food intake; more likely if the woman has an infection because this increases her need for insulin |
| Blood glucose level low (usually under 60 mg/dl)<br>Urine glucose absent | Blood glucose above normal (greater than 120 mg/dl)<br>Glucosuria (glucose in the urine); possibly ketonuria (ketones in the urine) |
| Behavioral and physiologic manifestations: hunger; trembling; weakness; faintness; lethargy; headache; irritability; sweating; pale, cool, moist skin; blurred vision; loss of consciousness | Behavioral and physiologic manifestations: fatigue; headache; flushed, hot skin; dry mouth; thirst; dehydration; frequent urination; weight loss; nausea and vomiting; rapid, deep respirations (Kussmaul's respirations); acetone odor to the breath; depressed reflexes |
| Measures to correct: drink a glass of milk or juice; eat a piece of fruit or 2 crackers; recurrent hypoglycemia requires adjustment of insulin or food intake | Measures to correct: evaluate food intake; emphasize that client be honest if she "cheats," to avoid inappropriate adjustment of insulin dose; identify and treat infections; insulin dose often adjusted throughout pregnancy to maintain normal glucose levels |

**Manifestations.** If its existence is not known, heart disease is difficult to diagnose during pregnancy, because normal changes mimic cardiac problems. For example, palpitations and heart murmurs are common in uncomplicated pregnancy but may also occur with heart disease.

A woman with heart disease may not tolerate the demands of pregnancy well. The blood volume and cardiac output increase to supply the placenta and enlarged maternal organs, but they also impose a greater burden on her impaired heart. Increased levels of clotting factors predispose her to thrombosis (formation of clots in the veins). If her heart cannot meet these demands, congestive heart failure (CHF) results. The fetus suffers from reduced placental blood flow if the mother's heart fails. See Box 5–5 for signs and symptoms of CHF.

Body fluid rapidly returns to the circulation after birth, predisposing the woman to circulatory overload. She is at risk for CHF after birth until her circulating blood volume returns to normal levels.

**Treatment.** The woman with heart disease needs frequent antepartum visits. Excessive weight gain must be avoided because it adds to the demands on her heart. Sodium is limited to prevent pulmonary edema. Preventing anemia with adequate diet and supplemental iron prevents a compensatory rise in the heart rate, which may strain her heart. Frequent rest periods decrease the heart's workload. However, the woman on prolonged bed rest has a greater risk for forming venous thrombi (blood clots).

Drug therapy may include heparin to prevent

---

| BOX 5–5 | Signs of Congestive Heart Failure During Pregnancy |
|---|---|

Persistent cough, often with expectoration of mucus that may be blood-tinged
Moist lung sounds due to fluid within lungs
Fatigue or fainting on exertion
Difficulty breathing on exertion
Orthopnea (having to sit upright to breathe more easily)
Severe pitting edema of the lower extremities or generalized edema
Palpitations
Fetus: hypoxia or growth retardation if placental blood flow is reduced

---

## Nursing Brief

The nurse should observe the woman with heart disease for signs of congestive heart failure, which can occur before, during, or after birth.

---

clot formation. Anticoagulants, such as warfarin (Coumadin), may cause birth defects and are not given during pregnancy. Other drugs may include antiarrhythmics to control abnormal heart rhythms. Antibiotics are usually given during the intrapartum period to prevent infection of the heart (bacterial endocarditis) due to organisms that enter the blood during birth. The woman who has mitral valve prolapse usually needs only prophylactic antibiotics at delivery.

Vaginal birth is preferred over cesarean delivery, because it carries less risk for infection or respiratory complications that would further tax the impaired heart. Forceps may be used to decrease the need for maternal pushing (see Chap. 8).

**Nursing Care.** A woman with heart disease may be familiar with its management. She will be taught needed changes, such as the change from warfarin anticoagulants to heparin. She is taught to inject the drug and told when to have her clotting time checked. She should promptly report signs of excess anticoagulation, such as bruising without reason, petechiae (tiny red spots on the skin), nosebleeds, or bleeding from the gums when brushing her teeth.

The woman is taught signs that may indicate CHF, so that she can promptly report them. The nurse helps her identify how she can obtain rest to minimize the demands on her heart.

The woman may need help to plan her diet, so that she has enough calories to meet her needs during pregnancy but without gaining too much weight. She should be taught about foods that are high in iron, such as dark-green vegetables, to prevent anemia. She should avoid foods high in sodium, such as smoked meats, potato chips, and many snack foods.

### ANEMIA

Anemia is a reduced ability of the blood to carry oxygen to the cells. Hemoglobin levels under 10 gm/dl indicate anemia during pregnancy. Three anemias are significant during pregnancy: two nutritional anemias, iron-deficiency anemia and folic acid–deficiency anemia, and one anemia resulting from sickle cell disease, a genetic disorder.

## Nutritional Anemias

Many women with anemia have no symptoms or have vague ones. The anemic woman may fatigue easily and have little energy. Her skin and mucous membranes are pale. Shortness of breath, a pounding heart, and a rapid pulse may occur with severe anemia. The woman who develops anemia gradually has fewer symptoms than the woman who becomes anemic abruptly, such as through blood loss.

**Iron-Deficiency Anemia.** The pregnant woman needs additional iron for her own increased blood volume, for transfer to the fetus, and for a cushion against the blood loss expected at birth. The red blood cells are small (microcytic) and pale (hypochromic) in iron-deficiency anemia.

*Prevention.* Iron supplements (30–60 mg three times/day) are commonly used to meet the needs of pregnancy and maintain iron stores. Vitamin C enhances absorption of iron. Iron should not be taken with milk or antacids because they impair absorption. Women who take iron supplements have dark-green or black stools. They may have mild gastrointestinal distress, diarrhea, or constipation.

*Treatment.* The woman with iron-deficiency anemia needs extra iron to correct the anemia and replenish her stores. She is treated with 180–200 mg/day plus vitamin C.

**Folic Acid–Deficiency Anemia.** Folic acid, or folate, deficiency is characterized by large, immature red blood cells (megaloblastic anemia). Iron-deficiency anemia is often present at the same time. The woman sometimes complains of a sore tongue.

*Prevention.* Folic acid is essential for normal growth and development of the fetus. A supplement of 300 μg (0.3 mg)/day ensures adequate folic acid.

*Treatment.* Treatment of folate deficiency is with folic acid, 0.7–1.0 mg/day, approximately two or three times the level of the preventive supplement.

## Sickle Cell Disease

Unlike nutritional anemias, people with sickle cell disease have abnormal hemoglobin that causes their erythrocytes to become dis-torted in a sickle (crescent) shape during hypoxia or acidosis. The abnormally shaped blood cells do not flow smoothly, and they clog small blood vessels. The sickle cells are destroyed faster, resulting in chronic anemia. (See pp. 724–727 for further discussion of sickle cell disease.)

Pregnancy may cause a sickle cell crisis with massive erythrocyte destruction and occlusion of blood vessels. Pregnant women with sickle cell disease are more likely to have infections, heart disease, and PIH. The main risk to the fetus is occlusion of vessels that supply the placenta, leading to preterm birth, growth retardation, and fetal death.

The woman will have frequent evaluation and treatment for anemia during prenatal care. Fetal evaluations concentrate on fetal growth and placental function. Oxygen and fluids are given continuously during labor to prevent sickle cell crisis.

## Nursing Care for Anemia During Pregnancy

The woman is taught which foods are high in iron and folic acid (Box 5–6) to prevent or treat anemia. She is taught how to take the supplements so that they are optimally effective. For example, the nurse emphasizes that iron is best absorbed if taken with a juice or food high in vitamin C. The nurse also explains that although milk is good to drink during pregnancy, it should not be taken at the same time as the

---

| BOX 5–6 | Foods That Prevent Anemias in Pregnancy |
|---|---|

**Foods High in Iron**

Meats, chicken, fish, liver, legumes, green leafy vegetables, whole or enriched grain products, nuts, blackstrap molasses, tofu, eggs, dried fruits, foods cooked in cast-iron pans

**Foods High in Folic Acid**

Green leafy vegetables, asparagus, green beans, fruits, whole grains, liver, legumes, yeast

**Foods High in Vitamin C (enhanced absorption of iron)**

Citrus fruits and juices, strawberries, cantaloupe, cabbage, green and red peppers, tomatoes, potatoes, green leafy vegetables

## Nursing Brief

To prevent or correct nutritional anemias, such as iron and folic acid deficiencies, the nurse should teach all women good food sources of those nutrients.

iron supplement or the iron will not be well absorbed.

The woman is taught that when she takes iron, her stools will be dark-green to black and mild gastrointestinal discomfort may occur. She should contact her physician or nurse-midwife if these side effects trouble her; another iron preparation may be better tolerated. She should not take antacids with iron.

The woman with sickle cell disease requires close medical and nursing care. She should be taught to seek care for infections promptly, as they may lead to a sickle cell crisis. She is taught about iron and other supplements that are part of her therapy.

### INFECTIONS

Infections may jeopardize the life of the pregnant woman or fetus, or both. Some infections are relatively harmless at other times. Infections covered in this section include

- TORCH infections
- Hepatitis B
- Varicella
- Group B streptococcus
- Sexually transmitted diseases
- Vaginal infections
- Urinary tract infections
- Acquired immunodeficiency syndrome

Table 12–2 lists the signs of infection in the newborn.

### TORCH Infections

The acronym *TORCH* stands for the first letters of these four infections and infectious agents: *t*oxoplasmosis, *r*ubella, *c*ytomegalovirus, and *h*erpes simplex virus. TORCH infections do not seriously affect the mother's general health but can be devastating for the fetus or newborn. Rubella is particularly significant, because it is a cause of birth defects that are usually preventable if the woman is immunized before pregnancy. Table 5–7 summarizes the TORCH infections.

### Hepatitis B

The virus that causes hepatitis B infection can be transmitted by blood, saliva, vaginal secretions, semen, and breast milk, and it can cross the placenta. The person may be asymptomatic or acutely ill with chronic low-grade fever, anorexia, nausea, and vomiting. About 10% of those infected develop chronic hepatitis. The fetus is most likely to be infected transplacentally if the mother has hepatitis B during the 3rd trimester. The infant may contract the disease by contact with blood or vaginal secretions at birth. The infant is more likely than an adult to become a chronic carrier and a continuing source of infection. Box 5–7 lists those who are at greater risk of having hepatitis B infection.

All women should be screened for hepatitis B during prenatal care, and the screening should be repeated during the 3rd trimester for women in high-risk groups. Infants born to women who are positive for hepatitis B should receive a single dose of hepatitis B immune globulin (for temporary immunity right after birth) followed by hepatitis B vaccine (for long-term immunity). The Centers for Disease Control and Prevention recommends routine immunization with hepatitis B vaccine for all newborns (those born to carrier mothers and to noncarrier mothers) at birth, 1–2 months, and 6–18 months (see pp. 434 and 435). Immunization during pregnancy is contraindicated.

**Nursing Care.** If possible, injections should be delayed until after the infant's first bath, so that blood and other potentially infectious secretions are removed to avoid introducing them under the skin. Nurses, because they have occupational exposure to blood, should have hepatitis B immunizations.

### Varicella Infection

Varicella (chickenpox) is usually a mild infection during childhood. Most women are immune from childhood infection, but about 5–10% of pregnant women are not immune. Varicella

## Nursing Brief

Rubella is a cause of birth defects almost completely preventable by immunization before childbearing age. The nurse should check each postpartum woman's chart for rubella immunity and notify her physician or nurse-midwife if she is not immune.

**Table 5–7.** TORCH INFECTIONS

| Transmission and Maternal Effects | Fetal and Neonatal Effects | Prevention and Treatment |
|---|---|---|
| *Toxoplasmosis*: caused by *toxoplasma gondii* (protozoon); often asymptomatic; self-limiting infection accompanied for a few days by mild fatigue, muscle pains, and swollen lymph nodes | Low birth weight, enlarged liver and spleen, jaundice, anemia, and chorioretinitis (inflammation within the eye); may show later neurologic damage | Wash hands after handling raw meat; wash kitchen surfaces and equipment that have contacted raw meat; thoroughly cook all meat; avoid uncooked eggs or unpasteurized milk; wash fresh fruits and vegetables; avoid cat feces or litter; wear gloves when gardening; pyrimethamine and sulfadiazine may be used during pregnancy (not widely accepted) |
| *Rubella*: caused by rubella virus; transmitted by droplet or direct contact; may cause mild fever, general malaise, and a rash | Effects vary according to when the infection occurs—most serious during the 1st trimester; may cause spontaneous abortion, deafness, mental retardation, congenital cataracts, heart defects, growth retardation, and microcephaly (small head); newborn is infectious because excretion of the virus continues for many months after birth | Immunization of all women and girls can prevent virtually all infection during pregnancy; should not become pregnant for at least 3 months after immunization; if pregnant woman is not immune, she should avoid situations in which she is likely to encounter the virus, such as day care centers or care of infected infants; nonimmune postpartum woman is immunized before discharge |
| *Cytomegalovirus (CMV)*: caused by one of the herpes virus group; transmitted by contamination with body fluids containing the virus, such as saliva, urine, blood, cervical mucus, semen, breast milk, and feces; usually asymptomatic | Mental retardation, blindness, epilepsy, deafness; petechiae ("blueberry muffin" rash) | No immunization or effective treatment; isolate infected infants because they can continue to shed the virus in urine and saliva, possibly infecting a pregnant woman |
| *Herpes*: caused by herpes simplex virus; transmitted by direct contact with infected lesions; painful blisters appear in the lower reproductive tract, on the vulva, and in the perineal area; virus becomes latent in the nerves and re-activated later | Fetus or infant infected by organisms that ascend into the amniotic cavity after the membranes rupture or by direct contact with lesions during birth; spontaneous abortion, growth retardation, or preterm labor may occur if the mother has her first infection during pregnancy; infections at birth may result in generalized infection, with a 60% mortality rate; infant may have unstable temperature, lethargy, poor feeding, jaundice, seizures, and lesions that resemble those of the adult | Acyclovir (oral or topical ointment) reduces severity and duration of outbreaks, but the benefits of its use are weighed against potential fetal harm; cesarean birth allows the fetus to bypass the infected vagina and thus avoid the infection; the woman's privacy must be respected if family members are not aware of the reason for the cesarean delivery |

may be severe during adulthood, particularly during pregnancy. Preterm labor, encephalitis, and maternal varicella pneumonia may occur. Immunization is now available for children and high-risk individuals.

### Group B Streptococcus Infection

This organism is normally found in the gastrointestinal tract, but it may be found in the urine, vagina, cervix, throat, and skin. The woman is healthy, but the infant may be infected through contact with vaginal secretions at birth. The risk is greater if the woman has a long labor or premature rupture of membranes. Group B streptococcus infection is the most common cause of neonatal sepsis in the United States. It is also associated with postpartum maternal infection.

### Sexually Transmitted Diseases

Sexually transmitted diseases (STDs) are those for which the most common mode of transmission is sexual intercourse, although some can be transmitted in other ways (Table

5–8). Herpes simplex infection was presented with the TORCH infections. Five other infections that are typically transmitted sexually are syphilis, gonorrhea, chlamydia, trichomoniasis, and condylomata acuminata (genital warts). Syphilis and gonorrhea are persistent public health problems, despite effective antibiotic treatment.

All sexual contacts of persons infected with a disease that can be sexually transmitted should be informed and treated; otherwise, the cycle of infection and reinfection will continue. Consistent use of a latex condom, including the female condom, helps reduce sexual spread of infections.

### Vaginal Infections

Vaginal infections besides those in other categories are candidiasis and bacterial vaginosis.

**Candidiasis (Monilial Vaginitis).** The fungus *Candida albicans* causes most cases of candidiasis, or "yeast infection." Candidiasis is more likely if there is a change in the vaginal environment that favors its growth, such as pregnancy, diabetes mellitus, systemic antibiotic therapy, or oral contraceptive use in the nonpregnant woman. It is more likely if the woman is obese, eats a diet high in sugar, or has impaired immune function. Occasionally, it is transmitted sexually.

Candidiasis causes intense itching of the vagina, vulva, and perirectal area. Urination and sexual intercourse may be painful because of inflammation. The discharge has a curdlike, or "cottage cheese" appearance. Miconazole (Monistat) or clotrimazole (Gyne-Lotrimin) are treatments available over the counter.

The neonate may acquire the organism in the mouth during passage through the birth canal (thrush). The mouth has white patches that resemble milk curds but that bleed if removal is attempted. Oral nystatin (Mycostatin) is the usual treatment for thrush; gentian violet solution may sometimes be used.

**Bacterial Vaginosis.** *Gardnerella vaginalis* causes profuse vaginal discharge that has a fishy odor. The fetus is usually unaffected. Metronidazole (Flagyl) is an effective treatment, but it should not be used until after the 1st trimester because of the potential for causing birth defects. Ampicillin is an alternate treatment. Antibiotics for the woman's sexual partner are often prescribed, although not universally.

---

| BOX 5–7 | Persons at Higher Risk for Hepatitis B Infection |
| --- | --- |

Intravenous drug users
Prostitutes
Persons with multiple sexual partners
Repeated infection with sexually transmitted diseases
Health-care workers with occupational exposure to blood products and needle sticks
Hemodialysis patients
Recipients of multiple blood transfusions
Workers or residents of institutions for the mentally handicapped
Household contact with hepatitis carrier or hemodialysis patient
Persons of Haitian, Central African, Southeast Asian, Middle Eastern, Pacific Island, and Alaskan descent

---

**Nursing Care.** The client is taught measures to reduce the discomfort of vaginal infections. Warm sitz baths followed by dry heat from a hair dryer on a low setting wash away the discharge and are comforting. Cotton underwear promotes air circulation and makes the vaginal environment less favorable for growth of the organisms. Tampons and sanitary pads with plastic backing or deodorant should not be used.

### Urinary Tract Infections

The urinary tract is normally self-cleaning, because acidic urine inhibits growth of microorganisms and flushes them out of the body with each voiding. Pregnancy alters the self-cleaning action, because pressure on urinary structures keeps the bladder from emptying completely. Urine that is retained (urinary stasis) becomes more alkaline and provides a favorable environment for growth of microorganisms.

Some women have excessive microorganisms in their urine but no symptoms (asymptomatic bacteriuria). The asymptomatic infection may ascend to cause cystitis or pyelonephritis. The woman with cystitis (bladder infection) complains of burning, increased frequency, and urgency of urination; her temperature is usually normal or slightly elevated. If not treated, cystitis can ascend in the urinary tract and cause pyelonephritis.

Pyelonephritis (kidney infection) is a serious infection in pregnancy and is accompanied by acute signs and symptoms (high fever, chills, flank pain or tenderness, nausea, and vomiting).

**Table 5–8.** SEXUALLY TRANSMITTED DISEASES DURING PREGNANCY

| Maternal Effect | Fetal and Neonatal Effects | Treatment in Pregnancy and Nursing Considerations |
|---|---|---|
| *Syphilis*: caused by bacterium *Treponema pallidum*; a chancre (painless, persistent sore) is the first manifestation; a generalized rash, which appears on the palms and soles as well as on the body, follows 4–6 wk later; low fever may accompany the rash; in untreated patients, syphilis may attack the heart and central nervous system | Transmitted transplacentally; may produce spontaneous abortion, preterm labor, stillbirth, and congenital defects; exposure during the 3rd trimester produces milder effects, such as enlarged liver and spleen, rash, and jaundice | Screening during prenatal care is standard; treatment with penicillin (erythromycin if patient is allergic) before 16 wk can prevent fetal infection; follow-up visits are essential to be sure the infection has been eradicated; sexual partners should be notified; reinfection during pregnancy is possible |
| *Gonorrhea*: caused by bacterium, *Neisseria gonorrhoeae*; vaginal discharge, which may be profuse and purulent; itching of vulva; painful urination; may be asymptomatic; may cause infertility by blocking the fallopian tubes | Transmitted to the infant during birth by direct contact with the mother's infected birth canal, resulting in eye infection that can cause blindness (ophthalmia neonatorum); may also cause premature rupture of the membranes or preterm birth | Screening during prenatal care is standard; treatment is with ceftriaxone, spectinomycin, amoxicillin, or aqueous procaine penicillin; probenecid is given to increase blood levels of the antibiotics and effectiveness of treatment; prophylactic eye treatment with erythromycin or tetracycline ointment is standard for all neonates; infected neonates will have additional antibiotics |
| *Chlamydia*: caused by bacterium *Chlamydia trachomatis*; increased yellow vaginal discharge; painful, frequent urination; patient may be asymptomatic; may cause infertility by blocking the fallopian tubes | Transmitted to the infant's eyes during birth by direct contact with the mother's infected birth canal, resulting in conjunctivitis; associated with preterm labor, premature rupture of the membranes, growth retardation | Treated during pregnancy with erythromycin; tetracycline is effective but should not be taken during pregnancy; doxycycline is used post partum; eye prophylactic antibiotic ointment is used as discussed under gonorrhea; silver nitrate eye prophylaxis is not effective against chlamydia |
| *Trichomoniasis*: caused by protozoon *Trichomonas vaginalis*; frothy, gray-green, foul vaginal discharge; perineal itching; reddened skin | Does not cross the placenta; neonatal infection is short-lived | Avoid treatment until after the 1st trimester to prevent adverse drug effects on fetus; clotrimazole (Gyne-Lotrimin) can be given during the 1st trimester, and metronidazole (Flagyl) can be given during the 2nd and 3rd trimesters; woman taking metronidazole should avoid alcohol for 48 hr after she stops taking the drug |
| *Condylomata acuminata*: caused by virus, human papillomavirus (HPV); genital warts: cauliflower-like growths accompanied by itching, vulva pain, and vaginal discharge; woman often has a candidiasis (yeast) infection or other sexually transmitted disease; associated with development of genital cancer | Laryngeal papillomas causing abnormal cry, voice change, hoarseness, or airway obstruction; appear between 2 and 5 yr of age | Trichloroacetic acid applied topically to the growths; cryotherapy in the 2nd and 3rd trimesters; laser or electrocautery |

Maternal septic shock and preterm birth may occur. The high maternal fever is dangerous for the fetus because it increases fetal oxygen needs, which the mother cannot readily supply.

**Treatment.** Urinary tract infections (UTIs) are treated with antibiotics, often ampicillin. Asymptomatic bacteriuria is treated with oral antibiotics for 10 days, cystitis for 10–14 days. Pyelonephritis is treated with multiple antibiotics, initially administered intravenously.

## Nursing Brief

The nurse should teach all women measures to reduce their risk for urinary tract infections.

**Nursing Care.** All women and girls should be taught how to reduce introduction of rectal microorganisms into the bladder. For example, a front-to-back direction should be used when wiping after urination or a bowel movement, or when doing perineal cleansing or applying perineal pads.

Adequate fluid intake promotes frequent voiding. At least eight glasses of liquid per day, excluding caffeine-containing beverages, helps flush urine through the urinary tract regularly. Although evidence of its benefit is inconclusive, cranberry juice may make the urine more acidic and therefore less conducive to growth of infectious organisms. In any case, cranberry and other juices add to the woman's fluid intake.

Sexual intercourse mildly irritates the bladder and urethra, which promotes UTI if a woman is prone to it. Urinating before intercourse reduces irritation; urinating afterward flushes urine from the bladder. Using water-soluble lubricant can also reduce periurethral irritation related to intercourse.

Pregnant women should be taught signs and symptoms of cystitis and pyelonephritis, so that they will know to seek treatment at once. Prompt treatment of urinary tract infections reduces the risk for preterm labor and birth (see p. 206).

### Acquired Immunodeficiency Syndrome

Acquired immunodeficiency syndrome (AIDS) is caused by the human immunodeficiency virus (HIV). The virus cripples the immune system, making the person susceptible to infections, which eventually result in death. There is no immunization (to prevent infection) or curative treatment. (See pp. 360–365 or a medical-surgical text for further discussion of AIDS, infections associated with the syndrome, and treatment.)

Although first identified in homosexual males, the incidence of HIV infection and AIDS continues to rise in women, particularly African-American women. In fact, death from AIDS is one of the leading causes of death among women of childbearing age. Pneumonia caused by *Pneumocystis carinii* is the principal infection that kills HIV-positive women and children (Hammill & Murtagh, 1993).

HIV infection is acquired one of three ways: (1) sexual contact with an infected person, (2) parenteral or mucous membrane exposure to infected blood or tissue, and (3) through perinatal exposure (infants). Women of childbearing age are most likely to acquire the virus by contaminated needles used in intravenous drug abuse or through heterosexual contact.

The infant may be infected (1) transplacentally, (2) through contact with infected maternal secretions at birth, and (3) occasionally, through breast milk. The infected woman has a 25–35% chance of transmitting the virus to her fetus perinatally (Ricci, 1992a). Cesarean birth does not reduce transmission of the virus to the infant during birth. Infants born to HIV-positive women will be HIV-positive at birth because maternal antibodies to the virus pass through the placenta to the infant. Three to six months are needed to identify the infants who are truly infected. Infected infants have a short survival time, about 4 years. (See pp. 362–365 for care of children with AIDS.)

**Treatment.** Pregnant women are questioned about high-risk behaviors for HIV infection (Box 5–8). They are evaluated for symptoms associated with HIV infection and AIDS, such as weight loss, loss of appetite, nausea, vomiting, diarrhea, fever, night sweats, cough, shortness of breath, and sore throat. Physical examination and laboratory studies are done to determine the status of the woman's immune system, presence of infections associated with AIDS, and presence of STDs.

| BOX 5–8 | High-Risk Factors for Human Immunodeficiency Virus (HIV) |
|---|---|

Intravenous drug abuse
Multiple sexual partners
Prostitution
Blood transfusion before 1985
History of sexually transmitted diseases
Immigration from area where infection is endemic, such as Haiti or Central Africa
Sexual partner being a person in a high-risk group
Sexual partner being a person with HIV infection

Treatment during pregnancy involves prevention and care of the various infections that occur. Women are more likely to have complications during pregnancy that are unrelated to their infection, because of adverse social situations such as poverty, malnutrition, and chronic stress. Regular prenatal care identifies these problems as early as possible. Unfortunately, many women with HIV infection do not have prenatal care.

**Nursing Care.** Nursing care has two major dimensions: (1) educating the public, including children, about AIDS; and (2) consistent use of universal precautions to prevent transmission of blood-borne and other infections from the patient to the nurse and between patients.

Nurses should seize opportunities to educate others about the problem of AIDS and how to prevent it. Prevention involves either complete avoidance of high-risk behaviors or measures to make transmission of the virus less likely. For example, drug abuse is discouraged because of its many adverse effects; however, if a person continues using intravenous drugs, avoiding shared needles reduces the risk of acquiring HIV infection. Use of a latex condom (not those made from sheep intestines, or "skins") reduces, but does not eliminate, the risk of acquiring the virus through coitus. Oral sex is also a risk factor because infectious secretions can enter small tears in the mucous membranes.

Universal precautions apply to body substances likely to carry blood-borne infections such as HIV and hepatitis B. Broadening the use of protective wear to avoid contact with *all* body secretions reduces transmission of blood-borne and other pathogenic organisms. A good rule of thumb is "If it's wet and it's not yours, wear protective equipment." (See Appendix F for universal precautions.)

# Environmental Hazards During Pregnancy

Substance abuse is widespread in the United States. It affects every group of people, including pregnant women. The actual prevalence of drug use during pregnancy is difficult to determine because many women hide or underreport it, especially illicit drug use. Women rarely consider legal substances, such as nicotine (smoking) or alcohol, to be drugs; they may not report them unless specifically asked.

## Nursing Brief

The nurse should wear protective equipment, such as gloves, with *every* potential exposure to a patient's body secretions. This practice protects one from many pathogens, not just the HIV.

Evaluating the effects of both legal and illicit substances on the woman and fetus is difficult, because women often ingest several substances and illicit drugs often contain impurities that alter their properties. The woman and fetus may be affected directly; an example is the vasoconstriction caused by nicotine and cocaine. Indirect effects include inadequate diet, late or absent prenatal care, and infections, such as STDs, hepatitis B, and HIV.

Several substances are metabolized and eliminated slowly during pregnancy, which prolongs their effects. Many drugs are concentrated in the amniotic fluid, which the fetus drinks. Thus, the substance-exposed fetus, who has a tiny body, is exposed to high levels of the drug(s) for a longer time.

### SUBSTANCES HARMFUL TO THE FETUS

Several legal and illicit substances are well-established as harmful to the developing baby. A substance that causes an adverse physical effect on the embryo or fetus is a teratogen. The best policy is to abstain entirely from unnecessary substance use during pregnancy, including therapeutic drugs that can be delayed. Many environmental substances are most harmful to the developing baby early in pregnancy, before the woman even knows she is pregnant.

**Smoking.** Smoking, including passive smoking, can cause intrauterine growth retardation (IUGR). Tobacco use during pregnancy has been linked to abruptio placentae, preterm birth, stillbirth, increases in neonatal death, and sudden infant death syndrome. It is not clear whether smoking causes malformations.

**Alcohol.** Alcohol is the drug most commonly abused by women of childbearing age. The fetal alcohol syndrome (FAS) is well documented: prenatal and postnatal growth retardation; mental retardation; and facial abnormalities, including a flat, thin upper lip border and downslanting eyes (Fig. 5–11).

No "safe" level of alcohol intake during pregnancy is known. These amounts arc known to increase the risk of alcohol-related defects:

- Three cans of beer per day
- Three glasses of wine or mixed drinks per day
- Repetitive binge drinking

Women should abstain from alcohol use when pregnant. A woman trying to get pregnant should avoid alcohol because it can damage the fetus before she knows she is pregnant.

**Marijuana.** Harmful effects of marijuana during pregnancy have not been clearly identified, but they cannot be ruled out. Many marijuana users also ingest other substances that may themselves be harmful or that may exert harmful effects when combined with marijuana.

**Cocaine.** Cocaine is a local anesthetic and a powerful central nervous system stimulant. It is highly addictive, and it causes euphoria

(sense of well-being) and vasoconstriction that may harm the woman and/or the fetus. Potential effects include tachycardia, hypertension, seizures, stroke, myocardial infarction, and sudden death.

The fetus is affected by vasoconstriction. Spontaneous abortion, abruptio placentae, IUGR, and preterm birth are more likely. Abnormalities of the heart, urinary tract, and abdominal wall have also been linked to cocaine use.

**Heroin.** Heroin is an opiate drug related to morphine. The heroin-addicted woman is particularly likely to be exposed to HIV infection because the drug is taken intravenously. She becomes physically dependent on the drug, and an abstinence syndrome (withdrawal) results if she does not have it regularly:

- Agitation
- Tearing, rhinorrhea (runny nose)

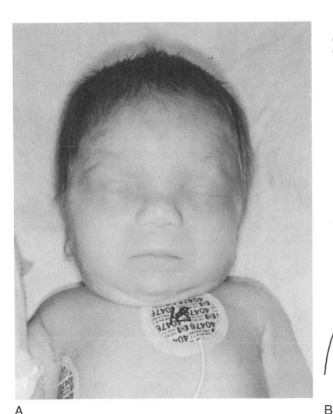

A

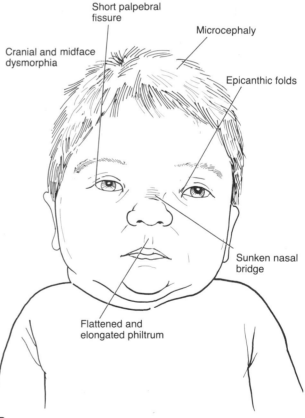

B

**Figure 5-11.** *A,* Infant with fetal alcohol syndrome (FAS). (Courtesy of Trish Beachy, MS, RN, Perinatal Program Coordinator, University of Colorado Health Sciences, Denver, Colorado). *B,* Diagram of facial malformations associated with FAS. (*B* is adapted from Gorrie, T.M., McKinney, E.S., & Murray, S.S. [1994]. *Foundations of maternal newborn nursing.* Philadelphia: W.B. Saunders.)

- Yawning
- Perspiring
- Abdominal and uterine cramps
- Diarrhea
- Muscle pain

Fetal effects include spontaneous abortion in early pregnancy, hyperactivity, hypoxia, passage of meconium into the amniotic fluid, and stillbirth. Neonatal abstinence syndrome occurs within 24 hours of birth: high-pitched crying, high need for sucking, tremulousness, seizures, hyperactivity, and disrupted sleep-wake cycles. Maintaining the pregnant woman on methadone (another opiate) can prevent serious effects to the fetus during pregnancy and lessen, but not eliminate, neonatal abstinence effects.

**Anticonvulsants.** Several anticonvulsants, such as diphenylhydantoin (Dilantin), are linked to birth defects during pregnancy. However, the mother may have seizures if the drug is stopped. The physician prescribes the anticonvulsant that is least teratogenic to the fetus while controlling the mother's seizures. Phenobarbital has a lower risk than other anticonvulsants.

**Anticoagulants.** Heparin cannot cross the placenta to affect the fetus. However, drugs such as warfarin (Coumadin) cross the placenta. Warfarin may cause growth retardation, a small and abnormally shaped head, mental retardation, minor eye abnormalities, depressed bridge of the nose, and hand abnormalities.

**Acne Medications.** Isotretinoin (Accutane) is a form of vitamin A that can cause serious fetal defects: microcephaly, ear abnormalities, cardiac defects, and central nervous system abnormalities. Acne medications are not essential and a pregnant woman should not take them. The woman of childbearing age must use reliable birth control during isotretinoin therapy and for a time afterward to allow the drug to leave the body. A related drug (etretinate [Tegison]) requires a long time for elimination; it may affect a fetus 11 months after the woman stops using it.

## TREATMENT

Care focuses on identifying the woman who uses drugs or other harmful substances early in pregnancy, educating her about their effects, and encouraging her to reduce or eliminate their use. Unfortunately, many drug-abusing

## Nursing Brief

When questioning about substance use during pregnancy, focus on how the information will help nurses and physicians provide the safest and most appropriate care to the pregnant woman and her baby.

pregnant women first enter care when they are admitted to the hospital in active labor. They often leave the hospital quickly after birth to resume drug ingestion.

Women are screened for infections that are more likely among drug users, such as hepatitis, HIV infection, and STDs. Dietary support and monitoring of their weight gain promote better health for the infant. Methadone may be prescribed for the heroin-dependent woman because it is safer and prevents maternal abstinence syndrome.

The woman is referred for specific treatment of substance abuse, as indicated. She may have care in outpatient or residential facilities. See a psychiatric text for more information about treatment of substance abuse.

## NURSING CARE

Educating women and girls about effects of drugs on a developing baby is best done before pregnancy, since many hazards are most harmful during early pregnancy. Women should be taught to eliminate use of any unnecessary substance before becoming pregnant. A woman is encouraged to tell any health-care provider if she thinks she is pregnant (or is trying to conceive) before having a nonemergency x-ray examination or being prescribed a drug.

A trusting, therapeutic relationship makes it more likely that a woman will be truthful about use of substances, both legal and illicit. The nurse who collects data must use a nonjudgmental approach and regard the problem as a health problem rather than a moral problem. The nurse acknowledges personal feelings about drug use, especially in a pregnant woman. Nursing inservice education and support from peers increase the nurse's effectiveness in helping the substance-abusing person.

Screening for drug use begins in a nonthreatening way by questioning about over-the-counter drugs. Next, the nurse asks about regularly taken prescription drugs. Smoking and alcohol use are then assessed. Use of illicit drugs is discussed last. If the woman acknowledges using any substances, legal or illicit, the type, amount, route of ingestion, and frequency of drug use are clarified.

To reduce defensiveness, the nurse might say, "We need to know everything that may affect you or your baby. Some questions may be uncomfortable for you, but we can give you better care if we have honest answers." Reveal an awareness of drugs commonly abused in the community. For example, say, "Do any of your friends have problems with crack cocaine? Is there a lot of drug use in your school or neighborhood?"

If a woman acknowledges using drugs, follow with specific questions about how much she uses and how often. Use terms that are familiar to the drug user. For example, if a woman says she uses cocaine (including "crack"), the nurse might ask these questions:

- How often do you use cocaine?
- Do you snort? Smoke crack? Shoot cocaine? Freebase?
- How many lines or rocks do you use?
- How long do you stay high?
- Do you use other drugs at the same time?
- What do you use to cut your cocaine?

Support the woman who is trying to reduce her drug use. Recognize her efforts to improve her health and that of her baby. For example, acknowledge that avoiding her drug(s) of choice requires great self-control, even if she has been drug-free for only a short time. Avoid adding to her guilt if she relapses.

Praise her efforts to improve her overall health and to have a successful pregnancy. For example, praise her weight gain when it is normal. Give her positive feedback when she tries to maintain a healthful diet.

## Trauma During Pregnancy

There is a high incidence of trauma during the childbearing years. Automobile accidents, homicide, and suicide are the three leading causes of death. Although pregnant women usually are more careful to protect themselves from harm, increased stress from pregnancy may lead to injury both in and out of the home. Frequently, couples are remodeling a room to prepare for the new baby. In the 3rd trimester, falls from stepstools or ladders are not uncommon owing to the woman's altered sense of balance. The pregnant woman also needs to be especially careful when stepping in and out of the bathtub.

The automobile is another potential hazard. The woman needs to wear a seat belt every time she is in an automobile, both as a driver and as a passenger. The lap portion of the belt is placed low, just below her protruding abdomen. The pregnant woman and her fetus are more likely to suffer severe injury or death because of not being restrained during a crash than they are to be injured by the restraint itself. Air bags are a supplemental restraint, intended for use in addition to seat belts. The woman should not ride with anyone who has been drinking alcohol or whose judgment is impaired for other reasons.

Physical trauma is usually blunt trauma (that caused by falls or blows to the body) but may be penetrating trauma (such as knife or gunshot wounds). Battering, also called spouse abuse, domestic violence, wife battering, marital rape, or intimate violence, is a significant cause of trauma.

The fetus may be injured directly, such as by a skull fracture, or indirectly by disruption of placental blood flow from abruptio placentae, uterine rupture, or maternal hypovolemic shock. The most common cause of fetal death is death of the mother. The fetus who survives trauma may have neurologic deficits.

Battering occurs in all ethnic groups and all social strata. It often begins or becomes worse during pregnancy. One in five teenagers and one in six adults are likely to be abused during pregnancy. The abuser is usually her male partner, but he may be another male, such as the father of the pregnant adolescent. Men who abuse women are also likely to abuse children in the relationship.

Women abused during pregnancy are more likely to have miscarriages, stillbirths, and low-birth-weight babies. They often enter prenatal care late, if at all. The risk of homicide escalates during pregnancy. The time of greatest danger to the abused woman occurs when she leaves her abuser.

Abuse during pregnancy, as at other times, may take many forms. It is not always physical abuse—many women are abused emotionally. Emotional abuse makes leaving the relationship especially difficult, because it lowers the woman's self-esteem and isolates her from sources of help.

## MANIFESTATIONS OF BATTERING

In addition to having late or erratic prenatal care, the battered woman may have bruises or lacerations in various stages of healing. An x-ray examination may reveal old fractures. The woman tends to minimize injury, or "forget" its severity. She may assume responsibility for the trauma, as evidenced by remarks such as, "If I had only kept the children quiet, he wouldn't have gotten so mad." Her abuser is often unusually solicitous after the battering episode.

## TREATMENT

Pregnancy is a good time to assess the woman for battering, because then she may have more regular contact with a health-care provider and may face increased danger. She must be interviewed for possible battering in private, away from the person who is abusing her. If the woman admits to being battered, further assessment should be done to determine the level of danger to her.

Care of the mother's life-threatening injuries, regardless of their cause, has priority. Management of the fetus depends on the gestational age and whether the fetus is still living. Cesarean birth may be done to save the life of a fetus mature enough to survive outside the uterus. If the fetus is too immature to survive or is already dead, cesarean birth is done if it will improve the woman's status or save her life.

## NURSING CARE

Nurses must be aware that any woman may be in an abusive relationship. Therapeutic, nonjudgmental communication helps establish a trusting relationship. Nonabused women, including nurses, often cannot understand why a woman would stay in a harmful relationship. The abuser has usually isolated the woman by controlling who she sees, where she goes, and how she spends money. Emotional abuse often supplements physical abuse, making the woman feel that she is "stupid" or "no good" and that she is "lucky that he loves her because no one else would ever love her." She usually feels that she has no choice but to stay in the abusive relationship. She may assume part of the blame, believing that her abuser will stop hurting her if she tries harder.

## Nursing Brief

If a woman confides that she is being abused during pregnancy, this information must be kept absolutely confidential. Her life may be in danger if her abuser learns that she has told anyone. She should be referred to local shelters, but the decision to leave her abuser is hers alone.

The woman being assessed for abuse is taken to a private area. The nurse determines whether there are factors that increase the risk for severe injuries or homicide, such as drug use by the abuser, a gun in the house, use of a weapon, or violent behavior by the abuser outside the home. The nurse also ascertains whether the children are being hurt. It is vital that the abuser *not* find out that the woman has reported the abuse or that she intends to leave.

Nurses can refer women to shelters and other services if they wish to leave the abuser. The decision about whether to end the relationship rests with the woman, however. Abuse of children must be reported to appropriate authorities (see p. 896).

Nursing care for the pregnant trauma victim supplements medical management: the focus is on stabilizing the mother's condition when life-threatening injuries occur. Placing a small pillow under the right side tilts the heavy uterus off the inferior vena cava to improve blood flow throughout the woman's body and to the placenta. An assessment of vital signs and urine output reflects blood circulation to the kidneys. Urine output should average at least 30 ml/hr. Bloody urine may indicate damage to the kidneys or bladder.

The nurse assesses for uterine contractions or tenderness, which may indicate onset of labor or abruptio placentae. Continuous electronic fetal monitoring (see p. 141) is often instituted if the fetus is viable and near maturity.

# Effects of High-Risk Pregnancy on the Family

Normal pregnancy is a crisis because it is a time of significant change and growth. The woman with a complicated pregnancy has stressors beyond those of the normal pregnancy. Her family is also affected by her problem.

## DISRUPTION OF USUAL ROLES

The woman who has a difficult pregnancy must often continue bed rest at home or in the hospital, sometimes for several weeks. Others must assume her usual roles in the family, in addition to their own obligations. Care of young children is difficult if the woman provides most of their supervision. Placing them in day care may not be an option because the woman must usually stop working.

Nurses can help families adjust to these disruptions by identifying sources of support to help maintain reasonably normal household function. Remind the family that the disruptions in their lives are temporary.

## FINANCIAL DIFFICULTIES

Many women work outside the home, and their salary may stop if they cannot work for an extended period. At the same time, their medical costs are rising. Social service referrals may help the family cope with their expenses.

## DELAYED ATTACHMENT TO THE BABY

Pregnancy normally involves gradual acceptance of and emotional attachment to the fetus, especially after the woman feels movement. Fathers feel a similar attachment, although at a slower pace than that of the pregnant woman. The woman who has a high-risk pregnancy often halts planning for the baby and may withdraw emotionally to protect herself from pain and loss if the outcome is poor.

## LOSS OF EXPECTED BIRTH EXPERIENCE

Couples rarely anticipate problems when they begin a pregnancy. Most have specific expectations about how their pregnancy, particularly the birth, will proceed. A high-risk pregnancy may result in the loss of their expected experience. They may be unable to attend childbirth preparation classes or to have a vaginal birth. Nurses can help incorporate as many of the couple's plans as possible, particularly at the time of birth.

## KEY POINTS

- Hyperemesis gravidarum is persistent nausea and vomiting of pregnancy, often accompanied by weight loss, dehydration, and metabolic imbalances. Psychological factors may play a role.
- The most common reason for early spontaneous abortion is abnormality of the developing baby or placenta.
- If a woman has a rupture from an ectopic pregnancy, the nurse should observe for shock due to hemorrhage into the abdomen. Vaginal blood loss may be minimal, whereas intraabdominal blood loss can be massive.
- The woman who has gestational trophoblastic disease (hydatidiform mole) should have follow-up medical care for 1–2 years to detect possible development of choriocarcinoma. She should not get pregnant during this time.
- Placenta previa is abnormal implantation of the placenta in the lower part of the uterus. Abruptio placentae is premature separation of the placenta that is normally implanted.
- The three main manifestations of pregnancy-induced hypertension are hypertension, edema, and proteinuria. The greatest risk to the fetus is reduced blood flow through the placenta, which impairs oxygenation and nutrition. Eclampsia occurs if the woman has one or more generalized seizures.
- Pregnancy promotes development of diabetes (gestational diabetes) or aggravates preexisting diabetes, because it increases resistance to insulin and breaks down insulin more quickly.
- TORCH infections are relatively mild in the adult but often severe or fatal to the fetus or newborn.
- Urinary tract infections are more common during pregnancy because compression and dilation of the ureters result in urine stasis. Preterm labor is more likely to occur if a woman has pyelonephritis.
- The fetus of the woman who takes drugs (legal or illicit) or alcohol is exposed to higher levels for a longer time, because the substances become concentrated in the amniotic fluid and the fetus ingests the fluid.

# Study Questions

1. How does hyperemesis gravidarum differ from common "morning sickness" of pregnancy? How can the nurse provide psychological support to the woman who has this condition?
2. Your friend is about 6 weeks pregnant and calls to say she is having some light bleeding. What is the best advice to give her?
3. What other pregnancy complications are more common when a woman has a hydatidiform mole?
4. A woman is hospitalized for placenta previa and begins to have heavy bleeding. What signs and/or symptoms might indicate hypovolemic shock?
5. Explain disseminated intravascular coagulation.
6. What are the typical changes in a pregnant woman who develops preeclampsia? Severe preeclampsia? Eclampsia? How do these disorders affect the fetus?
7. Why might percutaneous umbilical blood sampling be done if there is incompatibility between the Rh factor of the maternal and fetal bloods?
8. What are the main differences between preexisting diabetes mellitus during pregnancy and gestational diabetes mellitus?
9. A pregnant woman has iron-deficiency anemia. She says she "hates vegetables" and "can't afford much meat." Identify foods that increase her iron intake and meet her food preferences and budget restrictions.
10. How does sickle cell disease cause anemia? How is this disease different from the nutritional anemias?
11. What is the best way to counsel a pregnant woman who asks if one or two alcoholic drinks will hurt her baby? Give a reason for your answer.

# Multiple Choice Review Questions

*Choose the most appropriate answer.*

1. Most spontaneous abortions during early pregnancy occur because
   a. the developing baby or placenta is abnormal
   b. maternal illness alters the hormones needed to maintain pregnancy
   c. the woman does not want to be pregnant
   d. maternal substance abuse damages the developing baby

2. A woman has an incomplete abortion, followed by vacuum aspiration. She is now in the recovery room and is crying softly with her husband. Select the most appropriate nursing action:
   a. leave the couple alone, except for necessary recovery room care
   b. tell the couple that most abortions are for the best because the baby would be abnormal
   c. tell the couple that spontaneous abortion is very common and does not mean they cannot have other children
   d. express your regret at their loss and remain nearby if they want to talk about it

3. A woman is admitted with a diagnosis of "possible ectopic pregnancy." Select the nursing assessment that should be promptly reported:
   a. absence of vaginal bleeding
   b. complaint of shoulder pain
   c. stable pulse and respiratory rate; rise in blood pressure of 10 mmHg systolic
   d. temperature of 99.6°F (37.6°C)

4. It is important to emphasize that a woman who has gestational trophoblastic disease (hydatidiform mole) continue to have follow-up medical care after initial treatment because
   a. choriocarcinoma sometimes occurs after the initial treatment
   b. she has lower levels of immune factors and is vulnerable to infection
   c. anemia complicates most cases of hydatidiform mole
   d. permanent elevation of her blood pressure is more likely

5. What additional complications are more likely to occur with both placenta previa and abruptio placentae?
   a. blood clotting abnormalities and small hemorrhages
   b. hypertension and excessive vomiting
   c. venous thrombosis and altered glucose metabolism
   d. postpartum infection and hemorrhage

6. Select the primary difference between the symptoms of placenta previa and abruptio placentae:
   a. fetal presentation
   b. presence of pain
   c. abnormal blood clotting
   d. presence of bleeding

7. The action of Rh immune globulin (RhoGAM) is to
   a. prevent maternal antibody production against Rh-positive erythrocytes
   b. enhance production of maternal hemoglobin
   c. reduce mixing of incompatible maternal and fetal erythrocyte-santibodies against Rh-positive erythrocytes
   d. suppress production of fetal antibodies against Rh-positive erythrocytes

8. Pregnancy alters a woman's glucose metabolism because
   a. the woman produces additional insulin and is prone to recurrent episodes of hypoglycemia
   b. fetal glucose uptake is blocked until late pregnancy
   c. maternal cells become more resistant to insulin than when the woman is not pregnant
   d. the placenta produces insulin in addition to that produced by the woman's pancreas, leading to hyperglycemia

9. The safest policy is for the nurse to use protective barrier equipment when coming in contact with
   a. blood or blood products
   b. all body secretions
   c. intact skin surfaces
   d. secretions of persons at high risk for HIV infection

10. The battered pregnant woman is at greatest risk for homicide when she
    a. reports the abuse to the authorities
    b. tells her abuser that she is pregnant
    c. attempts to leave her abuser
    d. goes to prenatal appointments

## BIBLIOGRAPHY

American Academy of Pediatrics (AAP) and American College of Obstetricians and Gynecologists (ACOG). (1992). *Guidelines for perinatal care* (3rd ed.). Washington, DC: Author.

Archie, C.L. (1992). Licit and illicit drug use in pregnancy. In N.F. Hacker & J.G. Moore (Eds.), *Essentials of obstetrics & gynecology* (2nd ed., pp. 189–196). Philadelphia: W.B. Saunders.

Bendell, A., & Efantis-Potter, J. (1992). Acquired immune deficiency syndrome in pregnancy. In L. Mandeville & N. Troiano (Eds.), *High-risk intrapartum nursing* (pp. 237–254). Philadelphia: J.B. Lippincott.

Bennett, M.J. (1992). Abortion. In N.F. Hacker & J.G. Moore (Eds.), *Essentials of obstetrics & gynecology* (2nd ed., pp. 415–424). Philadelphia: W.B. Saunders.

Campinha-Bacote, J., & Bragg, E. (1993). Chemical assessment in maternity care. *MCN: American Journal of Maternal-Child Nursing, 18,* 24–28.

Crawford, N.G., & Pruss, A.M. (1993). Preventing neonatal hepatitis B infection during the perinatal period. *JOGNN: Journal of Obstetric, Gynecologic, & Neonatal Nursing, 22,* 491–497.

Daddario, J., & Johnson, G. (1992). Trauma in pregnancy. In L. Mandeville & N. Troiano (Eds.), *High-risk intra-*

*partum nursing* (pp. 255–279). Philadelphia: J.B. Lippincott.

Gilbert, E., & Harmon, J. (1993). *Manual of high risk pregnancy & delivery*. St. Louis: Mosby.

Gorrie, T., McKinney, E., & Murray, S. (1994). *Foundations of maternal-newborn nursing*. Philadelphia: W.B. Saunders.

Hammill, H.A., & Murtagh, C. (1993). AIDS in pregnancy. In R.A. Knuppel & J.E. Drukker (Eds.), *High-risk pregnancy: A team approach* (pp. 139–148). Philadel-phia: W.B. Saunders.

Hayashi, R.H., & Castillo, M.S. (1993). Bleeding in pregnancy. In R.A. Knuppel & J.E. Drukker (Eds.), *High-risk pregnancy: A team approach* (pp. 539–560). Philadelphia: W.B. Saunders.

House, M. (1990). Cocaine. *American Journal of Nursing, 90*, 41–45.

Ingardia, C., & Pitcher, E. (1993). Additional medical complications in pregnancy. In R.A. Knuppel & J.E. Drukker (Eds.), *High-risk pregnancy: A team approach* (pp. 597–618). Philadelphia: W.B. Saunders.

Knuppel, R.A., & Drukker, J. (1993). Hypertension in pregnancy. In R.A. Knuppel & J.E. Drukker (Eds.), *High-risk pregnancy: A team approach* (pp. 468–517). Philadelphia: W. B. Saunders.

Lone, P. (1991). Silencing crack addiction. *MCN: American Journal of Maternal-Child Nursing, 16*, 202–207.

Mandeville, L. Diabetes in pregnancy. In L. Mandeville & N. Troiano (Eds.), *High-risk intrapartum nursing* (pp. 165–186). Philadelphia: J.B. Lippincott.

McFarlane, J., Parker, B., Soeken, K., & Bullock, L. (1992). Assessing for abuse during pregnancy: Severity and frequency of injuries and associated entry into prenatal care. *JAMA: Journal of the American Medical Association, 267*, 3176–3179.

Newman, V., Fullerton, J.T., & Anderson, P.D. (1993). Clinical advances in the management of severe nausea and vomiting during pregnancy. *JOGNN: Journal of Obstetric, Gynecologic, & Neonatal Nursing, 22*, 483–490.

Parker, B., & McFarlane, J. (1991). Identifying and helping battered pregnant women. *MCN: American Journal of Maternal-Child Nursing, 16*, 161–164.

Parker, B., McFarlane, J., Soeken, K., Torres, S., & Campbell, D. (1993). Physical and emotional abuse in pregnancy: A comparison of adult and teenage women. *Nursing Research, 42*, 173–178.

Ricci, J.M. (1992a). AIDS and infectious diseases in pregnancy. In N.F. Hacker & J.G. Moore (Eds.), *Essentials of obstetrics & gynecology* (2nd ed., pp. 175–188). Philadelphia: W.B. Saunders.

Ricci, J.M. (1992b). Antepartum hemorrhage. In N.F. Hacker & J.G. Moore (Eds.), *Essentials of obstetrics & gynecology* (2nd ed., pp. 154–162). Philadelphia: W.B. Saunders.

Rotondo, L., & Coustan, D. (1993). Diabetes mellitus in pregnancy. In R.A. Knuppel & J.E. Drukker (Eds.), *High-risk pregnancy: A team approach* (pp. 518–538). Philadelphia: W.B. Saunders.

Surratt, N. (1993). Severe preeclampsia: Implications for critical care obstetrical nursing. *JOGNN: Journal of Obstetric, Gynecologic, & Neonatal Nursing, 22*, 500–507.

Tillman, J. (1992). Syphilis: An old disease, a contemporary perinatal problem. *JOGNN: Journal of Obstetric, Gynecologic, & Neonatal Nursing, 21*, 209–213.

Troiano, N. (1992). Cardiac diseases in pregnancy. In L. Mandeville & N. Troiano (Eds.), *High-risk intrapartum nursing* (pp. 187–206). Philadelphia: J.B. Lippincott.

# Part 3 Labor and Birth

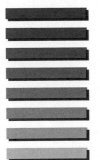

## Chapter 6

# Nursing Care During Labor and Birth

# OBJECTIVES

*On completion and mastery of Chapter 6, the student will be able to*

■ Define each vocabulary term listed.
■ Describe the four components ("four Ps") of the birth process: the powers, the passage, the passenger, and the psyche.
■ Describe how the four Ps of labor interrelate to result in the birth of a baby.
■ Explain the normal processes of childbirth: premonitory signs, mechanisms of birth, stages and phases of labor.
■ Explain how false labor differs from true labor.
■ Compare advantages and disadvantages for each type of childbearing setting: hospital, freestanding birth center, and home.
■ Determine appropriate nursing care for the intrapartum client, including the woman in false labor and the woman having a vaginal birth after cesarean delivery (VBAC).
■ Explain common nursing responsibilities during the birth.
■ Determine nursing care of the mother during the immediate postbirth period.

Caring for women and their families during the hours of labor is one of the most challenging of nursing roles. The intrapartum nurse must use many skills when caring for the family at this time—psychosocial, medical, surgical, and pediatric nursing skills. Good communication skills, effective problem-solving, sharp observation, empathy, and common sense are valuable assets for the intrapartum nurse.

Childbirth is a normal process, but one word describes the intrapartum unit: *unpredictable.* The number and status of women needing care can change dramatically in a few minutes. Intrapartum nurses must remain flexible to accommodate these changing client needs.

Nursing students are often apprehensive because intrapartum care seems different from nursing care they have given before. For example, pain is an expected and normal part of the birth process, but it may be distressing for the student who had negative experiences related to pain during her own births. Other students feel intrusive because of the intimate nature of intrapartum care.

The nursing student who has no children may feel inadequate to give good care to these women; yet the same student probably would not hesitate to care for a client whose gallbladder was removed. Men are particularly apprehensive about caring for women in the maternity setting. The ideal approach for both men and women nursing students is a professional approach that emphasizes the nurse's caregiving role. Above all, laboring women need compassionate, competent caregivers, regardless of their previous experience or gender.

## Components of the Birth Process

Four interrelated components, often called the "four Ps," constitute the process of labor and birth. They are (1) the powers, (2) the passage, (3) the passenger, and (4) the psyche.

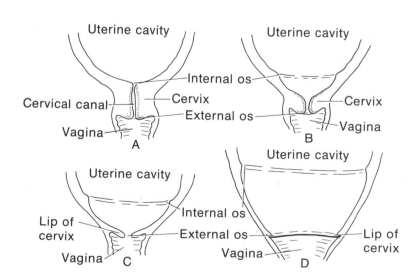

**Figure 6–1.** Changes in the cervix during labor. *A,* Before labor, the cervix is a tubular structure, about 2 cm long. *B,* The cervix is about 50% effaced (thinned), because it is about half its original length. No cervical dilation has occurred. *C,* The cervix is now completely (100%) effaced and feels like a thin membrane during vaginal examination. Note how the cervix is pulled upward into the lower part of the uterus. Little dilation has occurred. *D,* The cervix is now completely effaced (100%) and dilated (10 cm). (From Moore, M.L. [1983]. *Realities in childbearing* [2nd ed.]. Philadelphia: W.B. Saunders, p. 448.)

## THE POWERS

The powers of labor are forces that cause the cervix to open and that propel the fetus downward through the birth canal. The two powers are (1) the uterine contractions and (2) the mother's pushing efforts.

### Uterine Contractions

Uterine contractions are the primary power of labor during the first stage (from onset until full dilation of the cervix). Uterine contractions are involuntary smooth muscle contractions; the woman cannot consciously cause them to stop or start. However, their intensity and effectiveness are influenced by a variety of factors, such as walking, drugs, maternal anxiety, and vaginal examinations.

**Effect of Contractions on the Cervix.** Contractions cause the cervix to efface (thin) and dilate (open) to allow the fetus to descend in the birth canal (Fig. 6–1). Before labor begins, the cervix is a tubular structure about 2 cm long. Contractions simultaneously push the fetus downward as they pull the cervix upward, an action similar to pushing a small ball out the cuff of a sock. This causes the cervix to become thinner and shorter. Effacement is described as a percentage. Thus, if the cervix is 75% effaced, it is about one-quarter of its original length. When the cervix is 100% effaced, it feels like a thin, slick membrane over the fetus.

Dilation of the cervix is determined during a vaginal examination. Dilation is described in centimeters, full dilation being 10 cm (Fig. 6–2). Both dilation and effacement are estimated by touch rather than being precisely measured.

**Phases of Contractions.** Each contraction has three phases (Fig. 6–3):

- Increment, the period of increasing strength
- Acme, or peak, the period of greatest strength
- Decrement, the period of decreasing strength

Contractions are also described by their average frequency, duration, intensity, and interval.

*Frequency.* Frequency is the elapsed time from the beginning of one contraction until the beginning of the next contraction. Frequency is described in minutes, such as "contractions every 5 minutes."

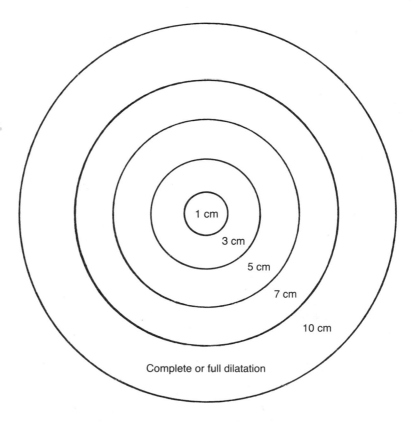

1 cm

3 cm

5 cm

7 cm

10 cm

Complete or full dilatation

**Figure 6–2.** Cervical dilation in centimeters; 10 cm is full dilation.

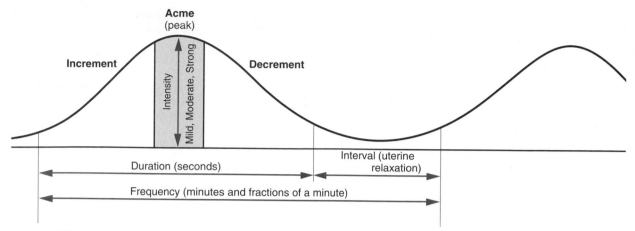

**Figure 6–3.** Contraction cycle. Each contraction can be likened to a bell shape, with an increment, acme (peak), and decrement. The frequency of contractions is the average time from the beginning of one to the beginning of the next. The duration is the average time from the beginning to the end of one contraction. The interval is the period of uterine relaxation between contractions.

*Duration.* Duration is the elapsed time from the beginning of a contraction until the end of the same contraction. Duration is described as the average number of seconds for which contractions last, such as "duration 45–50 seconds." *Persistent contraction durations longer than 90 seconds may reduce fetal oxygen supply.*

*Intensity.* Intensity is the approximate strength of the contraction. In most cases, intensity is described in words such as "mild," "moderate," or "strong." Contractions are mild if the uterus is easily indented with the fingertips; it feels similar to the tip of the nose. During moderate contractions, the uterus can be indented with the fingertips but with more difficulty; it feels similar to the chin. During firm contractions the uterus is not readily indented with the fingertips; it feels similar to the forehead. An internal uterine activity monitor (see p. 141) allows recording of the actual pressure within the uterus.

*Interval.* The interval is the amount of time the uterus relaxes between contractions. Blood flow from the mother into the placenta, which essentially ceases during contractions, resumes during each interval. The placenta refills with freshly oxygenated blood for the fetus and removes fetal waste products. *Persistent contraction intervals shorter than 60 seconds may reduce fetal oxygen supply.*

## Maternal Pushing

When the woman's cervix is fully dilated, she adds voluntary pushing to involuntary uterine contractions. The combined powers of uterine contractions and voluntary maternal pushing propel the fetus downward through the pelvis.

Most women feel a strong urge to push or bear down when the cervix is fully dilated and the fetus begins to descend. However, factors such as maternal exhaustion or epidural anesthesia (see p. 174) may reduce or eliminate the natural urge to push. Some women feel a premature urge to push before the cervix is fully dilated, because the fetus pushes against the rectum.

## THE PASSAGE

The passage consists of the mother's bony pelvis and the soft tissues (cervix, muscles, ligaments, fascia) of her pelvis and perineum (see pp. 23–25 for a review of the structure of the bony pelvis).

**Bony Pelvis.** The pelvis is divided into two major parts: (1) the false pelvis (upper, flaring part) and (2) the true pelvis (lower part). The true pelvis is directly involved in childbirth. The true pelvis is further divided into the inlet at the top,

## Nursing Brief

Report contractions that last longer than 90 seconds or that have intervals shorter than 60 seconds to the registered nurse.

the midpelvis in the middle, and the outlet near the perineum. It is shaped somewhat like a curved cylinder or a wide, curved funnel.

**Soft Tissues.** Women who have had previous vaginal births generally deliver more quickly than women having their first births, primarily because their soft tissues yield more readily to the forces of contractions. This advantage is not present if the woman's prior births were cesarean. Soft tissue may yield less readily

- In older mothers
- After cervical procedures that have caused scarring
- After many years between births

## THE PASSENGER

The passenger is the fetus, along with the placenta (afterbirth) and membranes. Because the fetus usually enters the pelvis head-first (cephalic presentation), the nurse should understand the basic structure of the fetal head.

**Fetal Head.** The fetal head is composed of several bones linked by tough connective tissue, the sutures (Fig. 6–4). A wider area called a fontanel is formed where the sutures meet. Two fontanels are important in obstetrics:

- The anterior fontanel, a diamond-shaped area formed by the intersection of four sutures (frontal, sagittal, and two coronal)
- The posterior fontanel, a tiny triangular depression formed by the intersection of three sutures (the sagittal and two lambdoid)

The sutures and fontanels of the fetal head allow it to change shape as it passes through the pelvis (molding). They are important landmarks in determining how the fetus is oriented within the mother's pelvis during birth.

The main transverse diameter of the fetal head is the biparietal diameter, measured between the points of the two parietal bones on each side of the head. The anteroposterior diameter of the fetal head can vary, depending on how greatly the head is flexed or extended.

**Lie.** Lie describes how the fetus is oriented to the mother's spine (Fig. 6–5). The most common one is the longitudinal lie (over 99% of births), in which the fetus is parallel to the mother's spine. The fetus in a transverse lie is at right angles to the mother's spine. The transverse lie may also be called a shoulder presentation. In an oblique lie, the fetus is between a longitudinal and a transverse lie.

**Attitude.** The fetal attitude is normally one of flexion, with the head flexed forward and the arms and legs flexed. The flexed fetus is compact and ovoid and most efficiently occupies the space in the mother's uterus and pelvis. Extension of the head, arms, and/or legs sometimes occurs.

**Presentation.** Presentation refers to the fetal part that enters the pelvis first. The cephalic presentation is the most common one, occurring in about 95% of births at term. Any of four variations of cephalic presentations can occur, depending on the extent to which the fetal head is flexed (Fig. 6–6). The vertex presentation, with the fetal head fully flexed, is the most favorable cephalic variation because the smallest possible diameter of the head enters the pelvis.

The next most common presentation is the breech (about 3–4% of term births). There are three variations of the breech presentation (Fig. 6–7). The frank breech, with the fetal legs flexed at the hips and extending toward the shoulders, is the most common.

Many women with a fetus in the breech presentation have cesarean births because the head, which is the largest single fetal part, is the last to be born and may be too big to pass through the pelvis. After the fetal body is born, the head must be delivered quickly so that the fetus can breathe, because at this point the umbilical cord is outside and subject to compression.

When the fetus is in a transverse lie, the fetal shoulder enters the pelvis first. A fetus in this orientation is born by cesarean delivery because it cannot pass through the pelvis.

**Position.** Position refers to how a reference point on the fetal presenting part is oriented within the mother's pelvis. The occiput is used to describe how the head is oriented if the fetus is in a cephalic vertex presentation. The sacrum is used to describe how a fetus in a breech presentation is oriented within the pelvis. The shoulder and back are reference points if the fetus is in a shoulder presentation.

The pelvis is divided into four imaginary quadrants: right and left anterior, and right and left posterior. If the fetal occiput is in the left front quadrant of the mother's pelvis, it is described as left occiput anterior. If the sacrum of a fetus in a breech presentation is in the mother's right posterior pelvis, it is described as right sacrum posterior. See Figure 6–8 for various fetal presentations and positions.

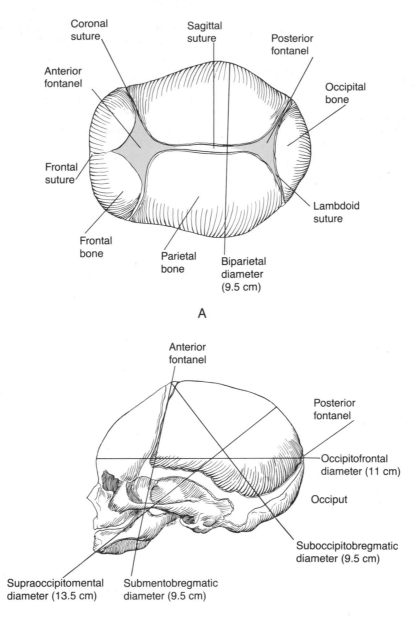

**Figure 6–4.** *A,* Bones, sutures, and fontanels of the fetal head. Note that the anterior fontanel has a diamond shape; the posterior fontanel is triangular. *B,* Side view of the fetal head. Note how the anteroposterior diameter will change as the fetal head becomes less flexed.

Abbreviations describe the fetal presentation and position within the pelvis (Box 6–1). Three letters are used for most abbreviations:

- First letter: Right or left side of the woman's pelvis. This letter is omitted if the fetal reference point is directly ante-

rior or posterior, such as occiput anterior (OA).

- Second letter: Fetal reference point (occiput for vertex presentations; mentum [chin] for face presentations; and sacrum for breech presentations).
- Third letter: Front or back of the mother's

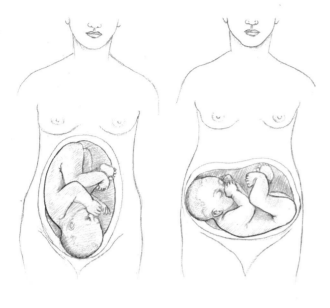

**Longitudinal lie**          **Transverse lie**

**Figure 6–5.** Lie. In the longitudinal lie, the fetus is parallel to the mother's spine. In the transverse lie, or shoulder presentation, the fetus is at right angles to the mother's spine.

pelvis (anterior or posterior). Transverse (T) denotes a fetal position that is neither anterior nor posterior.

The bregma (brow) may be specified when the fetal head is partly extended in the brow presentation, but it is not usually important to abbreviate this position because it tends to convert to either a vertex or a face presentation. Four-letter abbreviations exist for shoulder presentations, but they have little use because the position requires a cesarean delivery.

## THE PSYCHE

Childbirth is more than a physical process; it involves the woman's entire being. Women do not recount the births of their children in the same manner that they do surgical procedures. They describe births in emotional terms like those they use to describe marriages, anniversaries, religious events, or even deaths. Families are having fewer children, and they often have greater expectations about the birth

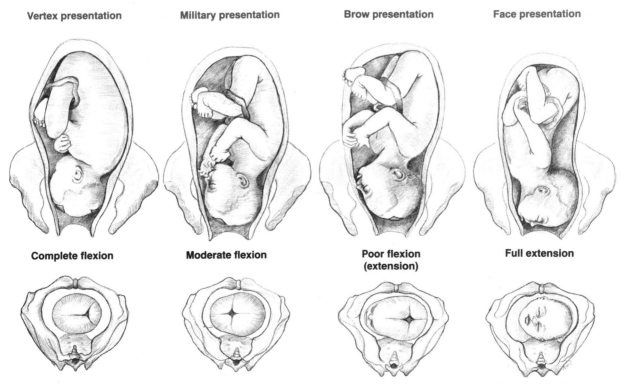

| Vertex presentation | Military presentation | Brow presentation | Face presentation |

| Complete flexion | Moderate flexion | Poor flexion (extension) | Full extension |

**Figure 6–6.** Four types of cephalic presentation. The vertex presentation, in which the fetal chin is flexed on the chest, is the most favorable for vaginal birth because it allows the smallest diameter of the head to go through the pelvis. Note how the anterior and posterior fontanels can be used during vaginal examination to determine the fetal presentation and position in the pelvis.

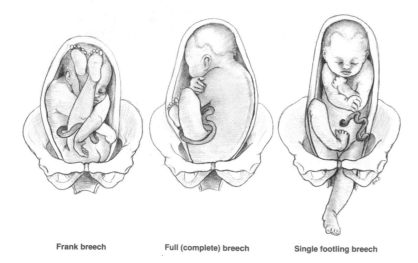

Frank breech          Full (complete) breech          Single footling breech

**Figure 6–7.** Three variations of the breech presentation. Frank breech is the most common variation. Footling breeches may be single, with one foot presenting, or double, with both feet presenting.

*experience*. The nurse can promote a positive childbearing experience by incorporating as many of the family's birth expectations as possible.

A woman's mental state can influence the course of her labor. For example, the woman who is relaxed and optimistic during labor is better able to tolerate discomfort and work with the physiologic processes. By contrast, marked anxiety can increase her perception of pain and reduce her tolerance of it. Anxiety and fear also cause secretion of stress compounds from the adrenal glands. These compounds, called catecholamines, inhibit uterine contractions and divert blood flow from the placenta.

A woman's cultural and individual values influence how she views and copes with childbirth. For example, the father's presence is encouraged in most birth facilities in the United States. However, if the family's culture is one in which childbirth is truly "woman's work," the father may feel uncomfortable at her side during labor. The woman would probably not welcome his nearness at this time either.

Culture influences, but does not dictate, how a woman behaves in labor. For example, in cultures that value stoicism, a woman may quietly endure labor pain without complaint. Other cultural groups express their feelings openly; women from these groups may respond loudly and vigorously to labor.

## Normal Childbirth

The specific event that triggers the onset of labor remains a mystery. Labor normally begins when the fetus is mature enough to adjust easily to life outside the uterus yet is still small enough to fit through the mother's pelvis. This point is usually reached between 38 and 42 weeks after the mother's last menstrual period.

### SIGNS OF IMPENDING LABOR

Signs and symptoms that labor is about to begin may occur from a few hours to a few weeks before the actual onset of labor.

**Braxton-Hicks Contractions.** Braxton-Hicks contractions are irregular contractions that begin during early pregnancy and intensify as full term approaches. They often become regular and somewhat uncomfortable, leading many women to believe labor has started (see discussion of true and false labor, p. 130).

**Increased Vaginal Discharge.** Fetal pressure causes an increase in clear and nonirritating mucous secretions. Irritation or itching with the increased secretions is not normal and should be reported to the physician or certified nurse-midwife (CNM).

## Nursing Brief

Provide emotional support to the laboring woman so that she is less anxious and fearful. Excessive anxiety or fear can cause greater pain, inhibit progress of labor, and reduce blood flow to the placenta.

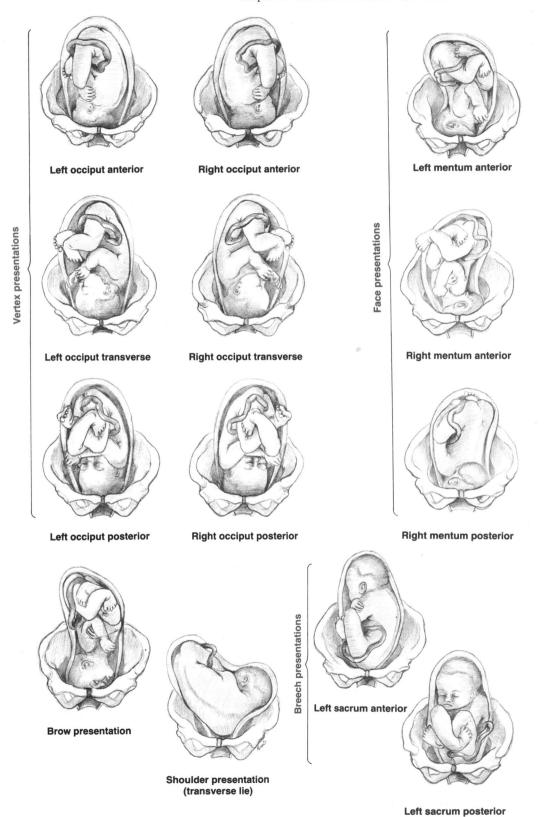

**Figure 6–8.** Fetal presentations and positions. The left and right occiput anterior positions are most common.

| BOX 6–1 | Classifications of Fetal Presentations and Positions |
|---------|------------------------------------------------------|

**Cephalic Presentations**

| Vertex | LOA | Left occiput anterior |
| | ROA | Right occiput anterior |
| | ROT | Right occiput transverse |
| | LOT | Left occiput transverse |
| | OA | Occiput anterior |
| | OP | Occiput posterior |
| Face | LMA | Left mentum anterior |
| | RMA | Right mentum anterior |
| | LMP | Left mentum posterior |
| | RMP | Right mentum posterior |

**Breech Presentations**

| | LSA | Left sacrum anterior |
| | RSA | Right sacrum anterior |
| | LSP | Left sacrum posterior |
| | RSP | Right sacrum posterior |

Abbreviations that designate brow, military, and shoulder presentations are not included here because these presentations occur infrequently.

**Bloody Show.** As the time for birth approaches, the cervix undergoes changes in preparation for labor. It softens ("ripens"), effaces, and dilates slightly. When this occurs, the mucous plug that has sealed the uterus during pregnancy is dislodged from the cervix, tearing small capillaries in the process. Bloody show is thick mucus mixed with pink or dark-brown blood. It may begin a few days before labor, or a woman may not have bloody show until labor is under way. Bloody show may also occur if the woman has had a recent vaginal examination or sexual intercourse.

**Rupture of the Membranes.** The amniotic sac (bag of waters) sometimes ruptures before labor begins. Infection is more likely if many hours elapse between rupture of membranes and birth, because the amniotic sac seals the uterine cavity against organisms from the vagina. Additionally, the fetal umbilical cord may slip down and become compressed between the mother's pelvis and fetal presenting part. For these two reasons, women should go to the birth facility when their membranes rupture, even if they have no other signs of labor.

**Energy Spurt.** Many women have a sudden burst of energy shortly before the onset of labor ("nesting"). The nurse should teach women to conserve their strength, even if they feel unusually energetic.

**Weight Loss.** An occasional woman may notice that she loses 1–3 pounds shortly before labor begins as hormone changes cause her to excrete extra body water.

## TRUE AND FALSE LABOR

Many women have contractions and other symptoms that make them think they are in labor. However, when they go to the birth facility, their cervix does not efface or dilate within a short observation period (about 1 or 2 hours).

True labor is characterized by progress (i.e., cervical change). Change in the cervix (effacement and/or dilation) is the essential distinction between false labor and true labor. See Table 6–1 for other characteristics that distinguish true labor from false labor.

## MECHANISMS OF LABOR

As the fetus descends into the pelvis, it undergoes several positional changes so that it adapts optimally to the changing pelvic shape and size. Many of these mechanisms, also called cardinal movements, occur simultaneously (Fig. 6–9).

**Descent.** Descent is required for all other

**Table 6–1.** COMPARISON OF TRUE LABOR AND FALSE LABOR

| False Labor | True Labor |
|-------------|------------|
| Contractions are irregular or do not increase in frequency, duration, and intensity | Contractions gradually develop a regular pattern and become more frequent, longer, and more intense |
| Walking tends to relieve or decrease contractions | Contractions become stronger and more effective with walking |
| Discomfort is felt in the abdomen and groin | Discomfort is felt in the lower back and lower abdomen; often feels like menstrual cramps at first |
| No change in effacement or dilation of the cervix occurs | Progressive effacement and dilation of the cervix occur |

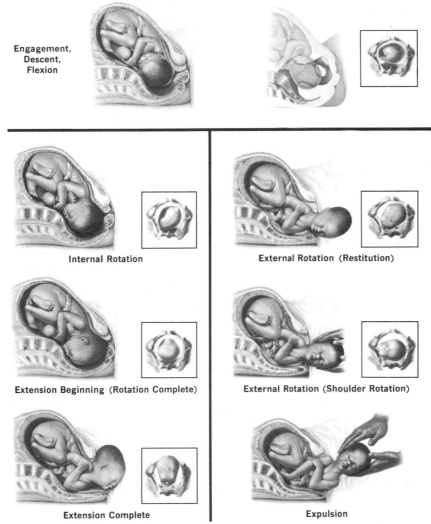

**Figure 6–9.** The mechanisms of labor, also called cardinal movements. The positional changes allow the fetus to fit through the pelvis with the least resistance. (From *Clinical education aid no. 13, G169*. [1979]. Columbus, OH: Ross Laboratories. Reprinted with permission of Ross Laboratories.)

mechanisms to occur and for the baby to be born. Station describes the level of the presenting part, usually the head, in the pelvis. Station is measured from the level of the ischial spines in the mother's pelvis (a zero station). Minus stations are above the ischial spines; plus stations are below the ischial spines (Fig. 6–10). As the fetus descends, the minus numbers get smaller (e.g., −2, −1) and the plus numbers get higher (+1, +2, etc.).

**Engagement.** Engagement occurs when the fetal presenting part is at a zero station or lower. Engagement often occurs before labor's onset in the woman who has not given birth (a nullipara); it may not occur until well after labor begins if the woman has had prior births (a multipara).

**Flexion.** To pass most easily through the pelvis, the fetal head should be flexed. As labor progresses, uterine contractions increase the amount of fetal head flexion until the fetal chin is on the chest.

**Internal Rotation.** When the fetus enters the pelvis, the head is usually oriented so that the occiput is toward the mother's right or left side. As the fetus is pushed downward by contractions, the curved, cylindrical shape of the pelvis causes the head to turn until the occiput is di-

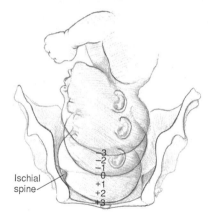

**Figure 6–10.** Station describes the level of the fetal presenting part in relation to the ischial spines of the mother's pelvis. It is determined with vaginal examination. "Minus" stations are above the ischial spines; "plus" stations are below the ischial spines.

rectly under the symphysis pubis (occiput anterior, or OA).

**Extension.** As the fetal head passes under the mother's symphysis pubis, it must change from flexion to extension so that it can properly negotiate the curve. To do this, the fetal neck stops under the symphysis, which acts as a pivot. The head swings anteriorly as it extends with each maternal push until it is born.

**External Rotation.** When the head is born in extension, the shoulders are crosswise in the pelvis and the head is somewhat twisted in relation to the shoulders. The head spontaneously turns to one side as it realigns with the shoulders (restitution). The head then turns further toward one of the mother's thighs. As the head rotates, the shoulders turn within the pelvis so that they can be born.

**Expulsion.** The anterior shoulder and then the posterior shoulder are born, quickly followed by the rest of the body.

## STAGES AND PHASES OF LABOR

Childbirth consists of four stages, each having typical physical and behavioral characteristics. Women who have epidural anesthesia during labor may not exhibit the behaviors and sensations associated with each stage and phase. Table 6–2 summarizes the stages and phases of labor.

### First Stage

The first stage of labor is the *stage of dilation*. It describes the time from the onset of

**Table 6–2.** STAGES AND PHASES OF LABOR

| Stage | Characteristics | Nursing Care |
|---|---|---|
| *First Stage (Stage of Dilation)* | Average duration: nullipara, 8–10 hr; multipara, 6–8 hr; onset of labor until full dilation of cervix | |
| Latent Phase | Onset of labor until about 4 cm of cervical dilation | Orient woman and her partner to the labor area |
| | Cervix effaces almost completely in the nullipara; may remain thick in the multipara | Review parents' birth plan, if they have made one; ask if they have any specific requests about how labor and birth are conducted |
| | Contractions mild and infrequent at first; gradually increase to moderate intensity, about every 5 min | Monitor fetus by intermittent auscultation or with fetal monitoring (continuous or intermittent) |
| | Woman is usually relatively comfortable | Monitor woman's vital signs (temperature every 4 hr, or every 2 hr after membranes rupture); assess pulse, respirations, and blood pressure hourly |
| | Woman is sociable and excited, although somewhat anxious | Teach or review coping skills, such as breathing techniques |
| | | Encourage walking if there is no contraindication |
| | | Sign permits |
| | | Initiate procedures such as laboratory examinations, shave prep, and enema |

**Table 6–2.** STAGES AND PHASES OF LABOR *Continued*

| Stage | Characteristics | Nursing Care |
|---|---|---|
| Active Phase | Cervix dilates from 5 to 7 cm; effacement is completed<br>Membranes may rupture<br>Contractions intensify until about 3 min apart, duration 45 sec or longer; intensity is moderate to firm<br>Woman concentrates inwardly, although still cooperative<br>May need analgesia or epidural anesthesia during this phase | Continue fetal and maternal assessments<br>Observe amniotic fluid for color, quantity, and odor when the membranes rupture<br>Provide general comfort measures, such as attention to her environment, hygiene<br>Encourage changes of position about every half hour; avoid the supine position<br>Watch for bladder distention<br>Assist the woman to use breathing and relaxation techniques (see Chap. 7)<br>Provide reassurance, praise, and support for both the laboring woman and her partner |
| Transition Phase | Cervix dilates from 8 to 10 cm<br>Intense contractions, firm, 2–3 min apart; duration of some may be as long as 90 sec<br>Woman becomes uncooperative and irritable | Continue maternal and fetal assessments<br>Continue comfort measures, but do not disturb the woman unnecessarily<br>Reassure woman and her partner that this is a short, intense phase and that she will regain control |
| *Second Stage*<br>*(Stage of Expulsion)* | Average duration: nullipara, 1.5 hr; multipara, 20–45 min<br>Cervix fully dilated (10 cm)<br>Rectal pressure as fetus descends results in urge to push with contractions; women with epidural anesthesia may not have characteristic urge to push<br>Contractions are still intense but may be slightly less so than in transition phase | Continue comfort measures, reassurance, support, maternal and fetal assessments<br>Observe for perineal bulging and crowning of the fetal head<br>Coach woman in effective pushing techniques; advise her to exhale while pushing or hold her breath for no longer than 5–6 sec<br>Make final preparations for birth (multiparas are prepared earlier than nulliparas) |
| *Third Stage*<br>*(Placental Stage)* | Average duration: 5–10 min; up to 30 min<br>Woman may feel a slight cramp when placenta detaches<br>Uterus must contract firmly to control bleeding<br>Woman is fatigued and excited; wants to see baby | Give medications as ordered and as appropriate within scope of practice<br>Observe for blood loss<br>Give initial care to the infant, focusing on respirations and temperature maintenance |
| *Fourth Stage*<br>*(Immediate Postbirth Recovery)* | First 1–4 hr after birth<br>Uterus should remain firmly contracted, about halfway between the woman's umbilicus and symphysis pubis<br>Bleeding (lochia rubra) should saturate no more than one pad per hour<br>Afterpains (uterine cramping) may occur | Assess woman's temperature at beginning of recovery period<br>Assess pulse, respirations, blood pressure every 15 min the first hour, every 30 min the second hour, then hourly<br>Assess uterine fundus for firmness, height, and deviation from the midline with each blood pressure check; massage if not firm<br>Have woman try to urinate if bleeding is excessive or if the uterus is high or not in the midline of the abdomen; catheterize her if she cannot urinate<br>Provide analgesia if needed; place ice compresses to her perineum as needed |

labor until full dilation of the cervix. The first stage is usually the longest for both nulliparas and for multiparas. Duration of the first stage averages 8–10 hours for the nullipara and 6–8 hours for the multipara.

Three phases occur within first stage labor: (1) latent phase; (2) active phase; and (3) transition phase. Each phase has specific characteristics that distinguish it from the others.

**Latent Phase.** The latent phase of labor is often completed before the woman enters the birth facility. It extends from the onset of labor until about 4 cm of cervical dilation. The cervix effaces almost completely during the latent phase of a nullipara's labor; the multipara's cervix often remains thicker, even during advanced labor.

During the latent phase of labor, contractions gradually increase in strength and intensity. They are mild and infrequent in the early part of this phase, increasing to moderate intensity with a frequency of about 5 minutes during the later part.

The woman is usually sociable and excited. She is cooperative but somewhat anxious. She is relatively comfortable, although many women describe sensations similar to menstrual cramps or lower back discomfort.

**Active Phase.** The pace of labor picks up during the active phase as the cervix dilates from about 5 to 7 cm. Effacement is completed during the active phase. Contractions intensify until they are about 3 minutes apart, last about 45 seconds or longer, and are moderate to firm.

The expectant mother becomes less sociable, although she is still cooperative. Mentally, she turns inward and concentrates on the task of giving birth. Most women who take analgesia request it during this phase.

**Transition Phase.** Transition is an intense, short phase of labor during which the cervix dilates from 8 to 10 cm. Contractions are firm, 2–3 minutes apart; the duration of some may be as long as 90 seconds.

The mother often feels as if she is losing control and thinks that labor will never be over. She often becomes uncooperative and even hostile to her partner and caregivers. The partner and nurse should not be offended by the mother's apparent hostility because it is normal behavior during this phase and means that labor will soon end.

## Second Stage

The second stage of labor is the *stage of expulsion*, extending from the time of full cervi-

## Nursing Brief

If a woman suddenly loses control and becomes irritable, suspect that she has progressed to the transition phase of labor.

---

cal dilation (10 cm) until the baby's birth. The average duration of the second stage is 1.5 hours in the nullipara, although it may last 2 hours or longer. The multipara usually has a second stage of 20–45 minutes. Contractions are firm, although they may be slightly less frequent and slightly shorter than during transition.

The woman who has not had regional anesthesia describes an involuntary urge to push, or bear down with each contraction as the fetal presenting part presses on her rectum. She may say, "I have to push," or "I need to have a bowel movement" when this occurs. Epidural anesthesia depresses the woman's natural urge to push and can prolong the second stage of labor.

The expectant mother usually regains control during the second stage and often says that pushing feels good or makes her feel useful. She may push intensely during contractions yet seem oblivious to her surroundings when each contraction ends. She is simultaneously tired and excited as the second stage ends with her baby's birth.

## Third Stage

The third stage of labor is the *placental stage*, extending from the birth of the baby until the placenta detaches and is expelled. It is the shortest stage, lasting an average of 5–10 minutes, although 30 minutes is also normal.

The placenta may be expelled in one of two ways. If the shiny fetal side of the placenta exits first, the placenta is expelled in the more common Schultze mechanism. The Duncan mechanism describes the exit of the placenta with the rough maternal side presenting (see Fig. 6–22).

The uterus must promptly contract and remain contracted after placental expulsion, to control bleeding from the vessels that supplied the placenta before birth. Oxytocin (Pitocin) is usually given in the mother's intravenous fluid; it may also be given intramuscularly or by intravenous push. The infant's suckling at the mother's breast stimulates uterine contractions because it causes her posterior pituitary gland to release natural oxytocin.

Pain is usually minimal during the third stage. The mother feels brief cramping as the placenta detaches and is expelled. She is tired and excited and wants to see her baby.

### Fourth Stage

The fourth stage of labor is the first 1 to 4 hours following birth. The uterus should be easily felt through the abdominal wall as a round, firm object abut the size of a grapefruit. It should be centered in the midline, about halfway between the umbilicus and the symphysis pubis.

The woman often has a chill for about 20–30 minutes after birth. The cause is unknown, but it stops spontaneously. Discomfort is usually minimal during the fourth stage. Perineal discomfort from bruising, lacerations, or an episiotomy (surgical opening to enlarge the vaginal outlet) is usually felt as a burning or throbbing pain. Some women, especially multiparas or those who had a large baby, have afterpains, or cramping, as the uterus alternately contracts and relaxes.

The woman's bladder fills rapidly after birth because of intravenous fluids given during labor and because fluid retained in her tissues quickly returns to her circulation for excretion. A full bladder can cause excessive bleeding because it pushes the uterus upward and interferes with contraction.

The woman is tired, but eager to see and hold her baby. The fourth stage of labor is an ideal time to promote bonding between the family and the new baby.

### VAGINAL BIRTH AFTER CESAREAN BIRTH

It was once thought that a woman who had a cesarean delivery for one infant must have a surgical birth for every subsequent infant. Today, physicians carefully select women who are appropriate candidates for vaginal birth after cesarean (VBAC). Of women who have previous cesarean births, 50–80% can deliver vaginally (American Academy of Pediatrics & American College of Obstetricians and Gynecologists, 1992) (see p. 195 for more information about cesarean birth and subsequent vaginal births).

## Nursing Brief

The woman having a vaginal birth after cesarean delivery needs special emotional support. She is often anxious, and a cesarean may seem like the easiest way to end her pregnancy.

Nursing care for women who plan a VBAC is similar to that for women who have had no cesarean births. The main concern is that the uterine scar will rupture (see p. 210), which can disrupt the placental blood flow and cause hemorrhage. Observation for signs of uterine rupture should be part of the nursing care for all laboring women, regardless of whether they have had a cesarean delivery.

Women having VBAC often need more support than other laboring women. They are often anxious about their ability to cope with labor's demands and to deliver vaginally. If their cesarean birth occurred during labor, rather than before labor started, they may become anxious at the same point in the current labor. The nurse must provide empathy and support to help the woman cross this psychological barrier.

## Settings for Childbirth

Depending on facilities available in their area and whether complications are likely, a woman can choose among three settings in which to deliver her baby. Most women give birth in the hospital, whereas others choose free-standing birth facilities. A few women choose home.

### HOSPITALS

Hospital births can take place in a traditional setting, in a birthing room, or in a single-room maternity care setting. The woman who chooses a hospital birth may have a "traditional" setting, in which she labors, delivers, and recovers in three separate rooms. After the recovery period, she is transferred to the postpartum unit.

An increasingly popular option for hospital maternity care is the birthing room, often called an LDR (labor-delivery-recovery) room. The woman labors, delivers, and recovers in this room. She is then transferred to the post-partum unit for continuing care.

The birthing room has a more homelike appearance. The fully functional birthing bed has wood trim that hides its utilitarian purpose. When the time of birth is near, the foot of the bed is detached or rolled away to reveal foot supports. Stirrups may also be used on birthing beds. They can be used as operating tables in an emergency, although they are wider than conventional operating room tables. A birthing chair is available in some settings. The mother's position is similar to that in a birthing bed.

Another hospital birth setting is a single-room maternity care arrangement, often called an LDRP (labor-delivery-recovery-postpartum) room. It is similar to the LDR, but the mother and infant remain in the same room until discharge.

Advantages of hospital-based birth settings are

- Easy access to sophisticated services and specialized personnel if complications develop
- Ability to provide family-centered care to the woman who has a complicated pregnancy

Disadvantages include

- Higher overall costs because the hospital must provide expensive services such as emergency, anesthesia, and critical care departments
- Limited choice of birth attendants (i.e., physician or CNM)

### FREE-STANDING BIRTH CENTERS

Some communities have birth centers that are separate from, although geographically close to, hospitals. These settings are similar to outpatient surgical centers. Many birth centers are operated by full-service hospitals and are close enough for easy transfer if the mother, fetus, or newborn develops complications. CNMs often attend the births.

Advantages of free-standing birth centers are

- A homelike setting for the low-risk woman
- Lower costs because the free-standing center does not require expensive departments, such as emergency or critical care

Disadvantages include

- A slight, although significant, delay in emergency care if the mother or baby develops life-threatening complications

### HOME

Some women have their babies at home. Many factors enter their decision, and most families have carefully weighed the pros and cons of their choice.

Advantages of a home birth include

- Control over persons who will or will not be present for the labor and birth, including children
- No risk of acquiring microorganisms from other clients
- A low-technology birth, which is important to some families

Disadvantages include

- Limited choice of birth attendants. Most physicians will not attend home births, and many nurse-midwives will not, either. In many communities, only lay midwives, whose training and abilities vary widely, attend home births.
- Significant delay in reaching emergency care if the mother or baby develops life-threatening complications
- No preestablished relationship with a physician if the woman or newborn must be transferred to the hospital

# Admission to the Hospital or Birth Center

Intrapartum nursing care begins before admission by educating the woman about the appropriate time to come to the facility. Nursing care includes admission assessments and initiation of needed procedures. Many women have false labor and are discharged after a short observation period; nursing care of these clients is included.

### WHEN TO GO TO THE HOSPITAL OR BIRTH CENTER

During late pregnancy, the woman should be instructed about when to go to the hospital or birth center. This is not an exact time, but general guidelines are as follows:

- *Contractions.* The woman should go when the contractions have a pattern of increasing frequency, duration, and intensity. The woman having her first baby is usually advised to enter the facility when contractions are regular (every 5 minutes) for 1 hour. Women having second or later babies should go sooner, when regular contractions are 10 minutes apart for 1 hour.
- *Ruptured membranes.* The woman should go to the facility if her membranes rupture or if she thinks they may have ruptured.
- *Bleeding, other than bloody show.* Bloody show is a mixture of blood and thick mucus.
- *Decreased fetal movement.* If the fetus is moving less than usual, the woman should be evaluated. Many fetuses become quiet shortly before labor, but decreased fetal activity can also be a sign of fetal compromise or fetal demise (death).
- *Any other concern.* Because these guidelines cannot cover every situation, the woman should go to the birth facility for evaluation if she has any other concerns.

## INFECTION CONTROL IN THE INTRAPARTUM AREA

The nurse must observe appropriate infection control measures when providing care in any clinical area. Although universal precautions apply to specific substances, many of these are encountered during childbirth: blood, amniotic fluid, and vaginal secretions. Additionally, many drugs are parenterally (intramuscularly or intravenously) administered, and sharp instruments are used, thus increasing the nurse's risk for injury and infection.

Individual facilities vary in specific guidelines and policies for protection of staff and clients from infection. However, general guidelines include the following:

- Wear clean gloves (or sterile ones, if appropriate) when contact with any body substance is anticipated. Examples of these situations would be when doing shave preps or enemas, changing disposable underpads or linens, giving perineal care, and changing perineal pads. The newborn infant should be handled with gloves until after the first bath.
- Wear a water-repellent covergown when exposure to larger amounts of body substances is likely. The nurse wears a water-repellent covergown during birth to avoid contact when handling the infant.
- Wear mask and eye shields if splashing of mucous membranes is likely, such as when "scrubbed in" for vaginal or cesarean birth.

See Appendix E for more information about universal precautions.

## ADMISSION ASSESSMENTS

When the woman is admitted, the nurse establishes a therapeutic relationship by welcoming her and her family members (Fig. 6–11). The nurse continues developing the therapeutic relationship during labor by determining her expectations about birth and trying to help her achieve these expectations. Her partner and other family members whom she wants to be part of her care are included. From the first encounter, the nurse conveys confidence in the woman's ability to cope with labor and give birth to her baby.

Three major assessments are done promptly on admission: (1) fetal condition, (2) maternal condition, and (3) nearness to birth.

**Fetal Condition.** The fetal heart rate (FHR) is assessed with a fetoscope (stethoscope for listen-

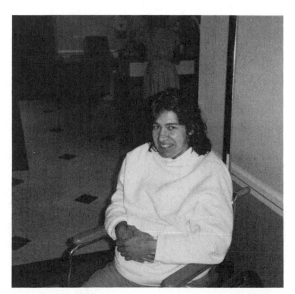

**Figure 6–11.** This expectant mother arrives at the hospital birth center by wheelchair. Greeting her and her partner warmly helps make them feel welcome. (Courtesy of John and Sue Croteau, taken at Brigham and Women's Hospital, Boston, MA.)

ing to fetal heart sounds), a hand-held Doppler transducer, or the external fetal monitor (see p. 141). An older guideline for a normal FHR in a term baby was 120–160 beats/min. The newer guidelines state that the normal average FHR at term is 110–160 beats/min (NAACOG, 1990). A preterm fetus usually has a faster FHR. The FHR is somewhat irregular, fluctuating within a range of about 5–15 beats/min. It may slow during contractions but should return to its baseline by the end of each contraction.

When the membranes are ruptured, the color, amount, and odor of the fluid are assessed. Amniotic fluid should be clear, possibly with flecks of white vernix (fetal skin protectant). Green-stained fluid means that the fetus passed the first stool (meconium) before birth and is sometimes associated with fetal compromise or newborn respiratory problems after birth. The amount expelled is variable, ranging from a small, intermittent trickle to a large gush. The odor is distinctive but not offensive. Foul- or strong-smelling amniotic fluid suggests infection, as does cloudy or yellow fluid.

If it is not clear whether the mother's membranes have ruptured, a Nitrazine or a fern test may be done. Nitrazine paper is a pH paper; amniotic fluid turns it dark blue-green or dark blue. In the fern test, a sample of amniotic fluid is spread on a microscope slide and allowed to dry. It is then viewed under the microscope; the crystals in the fluid look like tiny fern leaves.

**Maternal Condition.** The temperature, pulse, respirations, and blood pressure are assessed for signs of infection or hypertension. A temperature over 38°C (100.4°F) is to be reported. Blood pressure elevations of 30 mmHg systolic or 15 mmHg diastolic over the prenatal baseline are significant, as is a blood pressure of 140 mmHg systolic or 90 mmHg diastolic, regardless of baseline.

**Impending Birth.** The nurse constantly observes the woman for behaviors that suggest she is about to give birth. Examples of these behaviors are

- Sitting on one buttock
- Making grunting sounds
- Bearing down with contractions
- Stating "The baby's coming"
- Bulging of the perineum

If it appears that birth is imminent, the nurse does not leave the woman but summons help with the call bell. Gloves should be applied in case the infant is born quickly. Emergency de-

| BOX 6–2 | Assisting with an Emergency ("Precip") Birth |

Find the emergency delivery tray ("precip" tray).
Priorities of care are to prevent injury to the mother and baby.
Do not leave the woman if she exhibits any signs of imminent birth, such as grunting, bearing down, perineal bulging, or a statement that the baby is coming. Instead, summon the experienced nurse with the call bell and remain calm.
Put on gloves. Either clean or sterile is acceptable, because the baby is only being caught and no invasive procedures will be done. Gloves are used primarily to protect the nurse from secretions.
Support the infant's head and body as it emerges. Wipe secretions from the face. Use a bulb syringe to remove secretions from the mouth and nose.
Dry the infant quickly and wrap in blankets. Skin-to-skin contact with the mother will help maintain the infant's temperature.
Observe the infant's color and respirations. The cry should be vigorous, and the color pink (bluish hands and feet are acceptable).
Observe for placental detachment and bleeding. After the placenta detaches, observe for a firm fundus. If the fundus is not firm, massage it. The infant can suckle at the mother's breast to cause release of oxytocin, which causes uterine contraction.

livery kits (called "precip trays" for "precipitous birth") containing essential equipment are in all delivery areas. These trays should be promptly found at the beginning of a clinical experience in the intrapartum area. See Box 6–2 for emergency delivery procedures.

**Additional Assessments.** If the maternal and fetal conditions are normal and if birth is not imminent, other data can be gathered in a more leisurely way. Most birth facilities have a

## Nursing Brief

It is unlikely that a nursing student must "catch" a baby during an unexpected birth, but the process should be reviewed in case it does occur.

preprinted form to guide admission assessments.Examples of data needed are as follows:

- Basic information, such as woman's reason for coming to the facility, the name of her physician or CNM, medical and obstetric history, allergies, food intake, any recent illness, and medications (including illicit substances)
- Woman's plans for birth
- Status of labor: a vaginal examination is done by the registered nurse, CNM, or physician to determine cervical effacement and dilation, fetal presentation, position, and station; contractions are assessed for frequency, duration, and intensity
- General condition: a brief physical examination is done to evaluate this; any edema, especially of the fingers and face, and abdominal scars should be further explored; fundal height is measured (or estimated by an experienced nurse) to determine if it is appropriate for her gestation

## ADMISSION PROCEDURES

Several procedures may be done when a woman is admitted to a birth facility. Some common ones are described.

**Permits.** The mother may sign permits for care of herself and her infant during labor, delivery, and the postbirth period. Permission for emergency cesarean delivery is usually included. The woman signs these permits, except in rare instances, such as if she has a mental or physical handicap.

**Laboratory Tests.** Blood for hematocrit and a midstream urine specimen for glucose and protein are obtained. The woman who did not have prenatal care will have additional tests, often including those for sexually transmitted diseases and a drug screen.

**Intravenous Infusion.** An intravenous (IV) line allows administration of fluids and drugs. The woman may have a constant fluid infusion, or venous access may be maintained with a heparin lock to permit greater mobility.

**Perineal Shave.** A perineal shave prep is sometimes done to remove pubic hair that would interfere with the repair of a laceration or episiotomy. Its use has declined because it does not prevent infection, as once thought. If done, it is usually restricted to the perineal area (a "mini-prep"). The woman who has a cesarean birth will have an abdominal shave prep.

**Enema.** An enema is sometimes administered if the woman has been constipated or if the nurse notes a significant amount of stool in the rectum when doing a vaginal examination. Small-volume enemas, such as the Fleets, are most commonly used. Extra lubrication of the enema tip avoids irritating hemorrhoids (varicose veins in the rectum), which are common in pregnant and postpartum women.

## NURSING CARE OF THE WOMAN IN FALSE LABOR

Many women are observed for a short while (1–2 hours) if their initial assessment suggests that they are not in true labor and their membranes are intact. The mother and fetus are assessed during observation as if labor were occurring. Most facilities run an electronic fetal monitor strip of at least 20 minutes to document fetal well-being (see p. 141). The woman can usually walk about when not being monitored. If she is in true labor, walking often helps intensify the contractions and cause cervical effacement and dilation.

After the observation period, the experienced nurse, CNM, or physician reevaluates the woman's labor status by doing a vaginal examination. If there is no change in the cervical effacement or dilation, the woman is usually sent home to await true labor. Sometimes, if it is her first baby and she lives nearby, the woman in very early labor is sent home because the latent phase of most first labors is quite long.

Each woman in false labor (or early latent-phase labor) is evaluated individually. Factors to be considered include

- Number and duration of previous labors
- Distance from the facility
- Availability of transportation

If her membranes are ruptured, she is admitted because of the risk for infection or a prolapsed umbilical cord (see p. 209).

The woman in false labor is usually frustrated because she believes pregnancy is finally almost over, only to be told this is not the "real thing" after all. She needs generous reassurance that her "warming up" symptoms will eventually change to true labor. Guidelines for coming to the facility should be reinforced before she leaves. Some women gradually make the transition from false labor to true labor and are reluctant to return. They should be reas-

## Nursing Brief

Encourage the woman in false labor to return when she thinks she should. It is better to have another "trial run" than to wait at home until she is in advanced labor.

sured that they are not foolish for coming to the facility to be examined, no matter how many times they do so.

# Continuing Nursing Care During Labor

After admission, nursing care consists of regularly assessing fetal and maternal status and helping the woman cope with labor.

## OBSERVING THE FETUS

Intrapartum care of the fetus includes assessment of FHR patterns and the amniotic fluid. Additionally, several observations of the mother's status, such as vital signs and contraction pattern, are closely related to fetal well-being because they influence fetal oxygen supply.

### Fetal Heart Rate Assessment

The FHR can be assessed by intermittent auscultation, using a fetoscope or Doppler transducer (usually called simply a "Doppler"), or with continuous electronic fetal monitoring. See the procedure for assessing fetal heart rate. Electronic fetal monitoring is more widely used in the United States, but intermittent auscultation is a valid method of intrapartum fetal assessment (American Academy of Pediatrics & American College of Obstetricians and Gynecologists, 1992; NAACOG, 1988, 1990).

**Intermittent Auscultation.** Intermittent auscultation allows the mother greater freedom of movement, which is helpful during early labor. It is the only method possible if the mother is using a whirlpool or shower during labor and is the method used during home births and in most birth centers. However, intermittent ausculta-

## PROCEDURE FOR ASSESSING FETAL HEART RATE

1. Identify where the fetal heart sounds will most likely be found. This is over the fetal back, and is usually found in the lower abdomen. (The nurse may use a procedure called Leopold's maneuvers to feel the approximate location of the fetal head, back, arms, and legs.)
2. *Fetoscope.* Place the head attachment (if there is one) over your head and the earpieces in your ear. Place the bell in the approximate area of the fetal back and press firmly while listening for the muffled fetal heart sounds. When they are heard, count the rate for 1 min. It is acceptable to count for 15 sec and multiply by 4, but continue to listen for slowing or other substantial changes in the rate for at least 1 min. Check the mother's pulse if uncertain whether the fetal heart sounds are being heard; the rates and rhythms will be different.
3. *Doppler transducer.* Put water-soluble gel over the head of the hand-held transducer. Put the earpieces in your ear, or connect the transducer to a speaker. Turn the switch on and place the head over the approximate area of the fetal back. Count as instructed in step #2.
4. *External fetal monitor.* Connect cable to color-coded socket on monitor unit. Put water-soluble gel on the transducer and apply as instructed in step #3. Either belts or a wide band of stockinette is used to secure the transducers for external fetal monitoring. The rate is calculated by the monitor and displayed on an electronic panel. The displayed number will constantly change as the machine recalculates the rate.
5. Chart the rate. Promptly report rates below 110 beats/min or above 160 beats/min for a full-term fetus. Report slowing of the rate that lingers after the end of a contraction.

tion is used to collect data about the fetus during a small part of labor. It does not provide a written recording as continuous monitoring does.

Intermittent auscultation of the FHR should be performed as noted in Box 6–3. Figure 6–12 shows the approximate location of the fetal heart sounds when the fetus is in various

## BOX 6–3 When to Assess and Document the Fetal Heart Rate

Use these guidelines for charting the fetal heart rate when the woman has intermittent auscultation or continuous electronic fetal monitoring.

### Low-Risk Women

Every hour in latent phase
Every 30 min in active phase
Every 15 min in second stage

### High-Risk Women

Every 30 min in latent phase
Every 15 min in active phase
Every 5 min in second stage

### Other Assessment Time

When the membranes rupture (spontaneously or artifically)
Before and after ambulation
Before and after medication or anesthesia administration or change in medication
At time of peak action of analgesic drugs
After vaginal examination
After expulsion of enema
After catheterization
If uterine contractions are abnormal or excessive

---

Adapted from NAACOG.* (1990). *Fetal heart rate auscultation*. Washington, DC: Author.
With permission of the Association of Women's Health, Obstetric and Neonatal Nurses.
*Now AWHONN

presentations and positions. *Any FHR outside the normal limits or slowing of the FHR that persists after the contraction ends is promptly reported.*

**Continuous Electronic Fetal Monitoring.** Continuous electronic fetal monitoring (EFM) allows the nurse to collect more data about the fetus than intermittent auscultation. Except during periods of ambulation, the FHR and uterine contraction pattern are continuously recorded. Most hospitals use continuous EFM because more data are obtained and because the permanent written recording becomes part of the mother's chart.

One disadvantage of EFM is that it hampers ambulation. Some monitors have telemetry, al-

lowing the woman to walk while a transmitter sends the data back to the monitor at her bedside for recording (like a cordless telephone). Intermittent monitoring is a variation that promotes walking during labor. An initial recording of at least 20 minutes is obtained, then the fetus is remonitored for 15 minutes at regular intervals of 30–60 minutes.

EFM can be done with external or internal devices (Fig. 6–13). Internal devices require that the membranes be ruptured and the cervix be dilated 1–2 cm. External and internal devices may be combined, usually as an internal FHR sensor and an external uterine contraction sensor. Internal devices are available as disposable items to reduce transmission of infection.

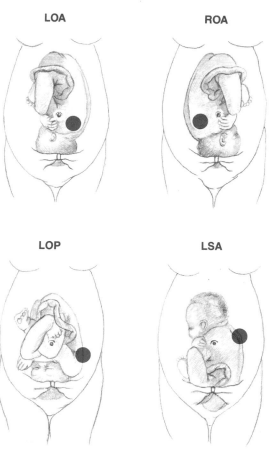

**Figure 6–12.** Approximate location of the fetal heart sounds when the fetus is in various presentations and positions. Note that the fetal heart sounds in breech presentations are higher on the mother's abdomen. (LOA, left occiput anterior; ROA, right occiput anterior; LOP, left occiput posterior; and LSA, left sacrum anterior.)

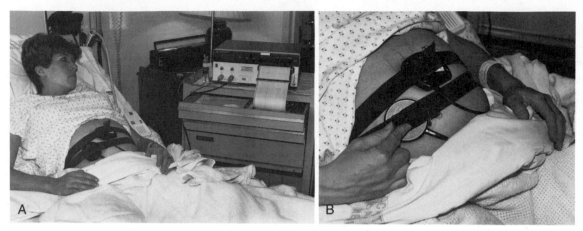

**Figure 6–13.** *A,* External fetal monitoring is being used on this mother during labor. The sensors are held in place with either belts, as in this picture, or a wide band of stockinette. *B,* The upper sensor (tocotransducer) has a pressure-sensitive button that is placed over the area of the uterine fundus, where the contraction is most easily felt. The lower sensor, a Doppler transducer, is placed where the fetal heart sounds are clearest. Water-soluble gel is applied to the Doppler transducer.

External fetal heart monitoring is done with a Doppler transducer, which uses sound waves to detect motion of the fetal heart and calculate the rate, just as the hand-held model does. A small spiral electrode applied to the fetal presenting part allows internal FHR monitoring.

Contractions are sensed externally with a tocotransducer (a "toco"), with a pressure-sensitive button. The toco is positioned over the mother's upper uterus (fundus), about where the nurse would palpate contractions by hand (see p. 146). Either of two types of devices is used for internal contraction monitoring. One uses a fluid-filled catheter connected to a pressure-sensitive device on the monitor. The other uses a solid catheter with an electronic pressure sensor in its tip.

***Evaluating Fetal Heart Rate Patterns.*** The FHR is recorded on the upper grid of the paper; the uterine contraction pattern is recorded on the lower grid (Fig. 6–14). Both grids must be evaluated together for accurate interpretation of FHR patterns.

The FHR is evaluated for baseline, variability, and periodic changes. The baseline rate is the rate between contractions and between periodic changes. Normal baseline at term is 110–160 beats/min, although some full-term fetuses have a rate between 100 and 110 beats/min without problems.

Variability describes fluctuations, or constant changes, in the baseline rate (Fig. 6–15). Variability causes the recording of the FHR to have a fine sawtooth appearance with larger, undulating wavelike movements. Variability is desirable, but it may be depressed by narcotics given to the woman and may not be evident if the fetus is preterm.

Periodic changes are temporary changes in the baseline rate. Periodic changes include accelerations (rate increases) or one of three types of decelerations (rate decreases).

***Accelerations.*** Accelerations are rate increases of at least 15 beats/min lasting for at least 15 seconds. They suggest a fetus that is well-oxygenated.

***Early Decelerations.*** Early decelerations are rate decreases during contractions; they always return to the baseline rate by the end of the contractions. They result from compression of the fetal head and are normal.

***Variable Decelerations.*** Variable decelerations begin and end abruptly; they are V-, W-, or U-shaped (Fig. 6–16). They do not always exhibit a consistent pattern in relation to contractions. Variable decelerations suggest that the umbilical cord is being compressed, often because it is around the fetal neck (a nuchal cord) or because there is inadequate amniotic fluid to cushion it well.

***Late Decelerations.*** Late decelerations look similar to early decelerations, except that they do not return to the baseline FHR until after the contraction ends (Fig. 6–17). Late decelerations suggest that the placenta is not delivering enough oxygen to the fetus (uteroplacental insufficiency).

***Nursing Response to Monitor Patterns.*** An

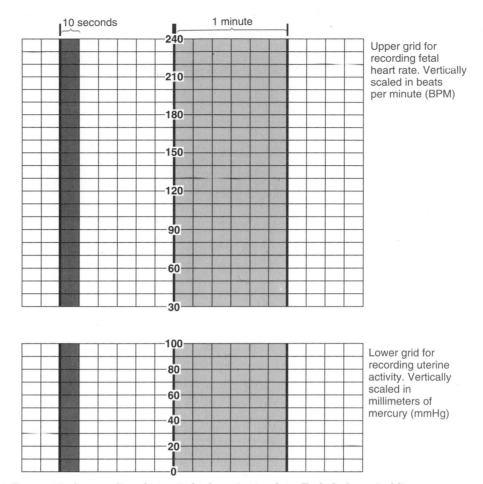

**Figure 6-14.** Paper strip for recording electronic fetal monitoring data. Each dark vertical line represents 1 minute. Each lighter vertical line represents 10 seconds.

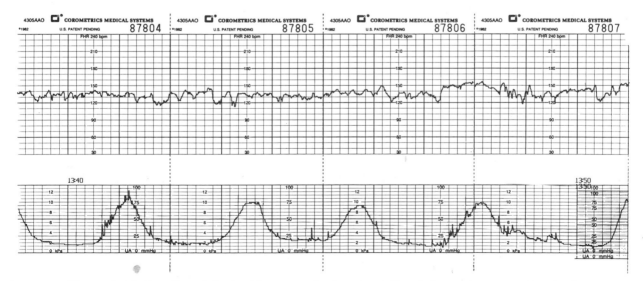

**Figure 6-15.** Recording of the fetal heart rate in the upper grid and the uterine contractions in the lower grid. Note the sawtooth appearance of the fetal heart rate tracing due to the constant changes in the rate (variability). (Courtesy of Corometrics Medical Systems, Inc., Wallingford, CT. Redrawn with permission.)

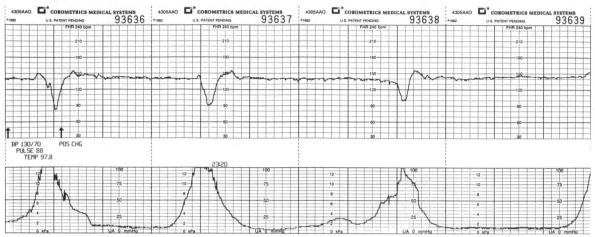

**Figure 6–16.** Variable decelerations, showing their typically abrupt onset and offset. They are caused by umbilical cord compression. The first response to this pattern is to reposition the mother to relieve pressure on the cord. (Courtesy of Corometrics Medical Systems, Inc., Wallingford, CT. Redrawn with permission.)

experienced registered nurse with additional education directs the nursing response to EFM patterns. The nursing response depends on the pattern identified (Box 6–4). Accelerations and early decelerations are reassuring of fetal well-being and thus require no intervention other than continued observation.

Repositioning the woman is usually the first response to a pattern of variable decelerations.

Changing the mother's position relieves pressure on the umbilical cord and improves blood flow through it. The woman is turned to her side, or to the other side if she is already on her side. Other positions, such as the knee-chest or a slight Trendelenburg (head-down) may be tried if the side-lying positions do not restore the pattern to a reassuring one.

Late decelerations are initially treated by

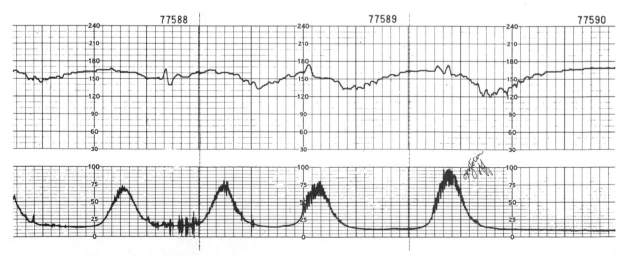

**Figure 6–17.** Late decelerations, showing their pattern of slowing, which persists after the contraction ends. The usual cause is reduced blood flow to the placenta (uteroplacental insufficiency [UPI]). Measures to correct this include repositioning the woman, giving oxygen, increasing the nonmedicated intravenous fluid, and stopping administration of oxytocin if it is being given. (Courtesy of Corometrics Medical Systems, Inc., Wallingford, CT. Redrawn with permission.)

## Nursing Brief

Report any questionable fetal heart rate or contraction pattern to the experienced labor and delivery nurse for complete evaluation.

measures to increase maternal oxygenation and blood flow to the placenta. The specific measures depend on the most likely cause of the pattern:

- Repositioning to prevent supine hypotension (see p. 59)
- Giving oxygen by face mask to increase the amount in the mother's blood
- Increasing the nonadditive IV fluid to expand the blood volume and make more available for the placenta
- Stopping oxytocin (Pitocin) infusion because the drug intensifies contractions and reduces placental blood flow

The CNM or physician is notified of any nonreassuring pattern (see Box 6-4).

### Assessment of Amniotic Fluid

The membranes may rupture spontaneously or the physician or CNM may rupture them artificially in a procedure called an amniotomy. The color, odor, and amount of fluid are charted. The amount of amniotic fluid is usually estimated as scant (only a trickle), moderate (about 500 ml), or large (about 1000 ml or more). Green-stained, cloudy, or yellowish amniotic fluid, and fluid that has a strong odor should be reported.

The FHR should be assessed for at least one full minute following rupture of membranes. Marked slowing of the rate or variable decelerations suggest that the fetal umbilical cord may have come down with the fluid gush and is being compressed.

### OBSERVING THE WOMAN

Intrapartum care of the woman includes assessment of her vital signs, contractions, progress of labor, intake and output, and responses to labor.

**Vital Signs.** The temperature is checked every 4 hours, and every 2 hours if it is elevated or if the membranes have ruptured. A temperature

---

| BOX 6–4 | Reassuring and Nonreassuring Fetal Heart Rate and Uterine Activity Patterns |
|---|---|

**Reassuring Patterns**

Stable rate 110–160 beats/min
Variability present
Accelerations of rate with fetal movement
Contraction frequency greater than every 2 min; duration less than 90 sec; relaxation interval of at least 60 sec

**Nonreassuring Patterns**

Tachycardia: rate over 160 beats/min for 10 min or longer
Bradycardia: rate under 110 beats/min for 10 min or longer
Decreased or absent variability: little fluctuation in rate
Late decelerations: begin after the contraction starts, and persist after the contraction is over
Variable decelerations: rate abruptly falls when deceleration occurs, returns abruptly to the baseline; may or may not occur in a consistent relationship with contractions

---

of 38°C (100.4°F) or higher should be reported. If the temperature is elevated, the amniotic fluid is assessed for signs of infection, as noted in fetal assessments.

The pulse, blood pressure, and respirations are assessed every hour. Maternal hypotension, particularly if below 90 mmHg systolic, or hypertension (see p. 88) can reduce blood flow to the placenta.

**Contractions.** Contractions can be assessed by palpation (touch) or by continuous EFM. Some women have sensitive abdominal skin, especially around the umbilicus. When palpation is used to evaluate contractions, the fingers are placed lightly on her uterine fundus. They should not be palpated for longer than required.

**Progress of Labor.** The registered nurse, CNM, or physician periodically does a vaginal examination to determine how labor is progressing. The cervix is evaluated for effacement and dilation. The descent of the fetus is determined in relation to the ischial spines (station). There is no set interval for doing vaginal exam-

## PROCEDURE FOR ASSESSING CONTRACTIONS BY PALPATION

1. Place fingertips of one hand lightly on the upper uterus. Keep the fingers relatively still, but move them occasionally so that mild contractions can be felt.
2. Palpate at least 3–5 contractions for a more accurate estimate of their average characteristics.
3. Note the time when each contraction begins and ends. Calculate the frequency by counting the elapsed time from the beginning of one contraction to the beginning of the next. Calculate the duration by determining the number of seconds from the beginning to end of each contraction.
4. Estimate the intensity by trying to indent the uterus at the contraction's peak. If it is easily indented, the contraction is mild; if harder to indent, it is moderate; if nearly impossible to indent, it is firm.
5. Chart the average frequency (in minutes), duration (in seconds), and intensity.
6. Report contractions lasting longer than 90 sec or intervals of relaxation shorter than 60 sec.

inations. The observant nurse watches for physical and behavioral changes associated with progression of labor to reduce the number of vaginal examinations needed. Vaginal examinations are limited to prevent infection, especially if the membranes are ruptured.

**Intake and Output.** Most women in labor do not need strict measurement of intake and output, but the time and approximate amount of each urination are recorded. The woman may not sense a full bladder; she should be checked every 1–2 hours for a bulge in front of her uterus. A full bladder is a source of vague discomfort and can impede fetal descent.

Policies about oral intake vary among birth facilities. Ice chips are usually allowed, unless it is likely that the woman will have a cesarean delivery. Many facilities allow fruit juices, Popsicles, or hard candy.

**Response to Labor.** The nurse assesses the woman's response to labor, including her use of breathing and relaxation techniques, and supports adaptive responses. Nonverbal behaviors

that suggest difficulty coping with labor include a tense body posture and thrashing in bed. The physician or CNM is notified if the woman requests pain-relieving drugs.

Signs that suggest rapid labor progress are promptly addressed. Bloody show may increase markedly, and the perineum may bulge as the fetal head stretches it. The student or inexperienced nurse should summon an experienced nurse with the call signal if bloody show or perineal bulging increases or if the woman exhibits behaviors typical of imminent birth that were listed earlier.

### HELPING THE WOMAN COPE WITH LABOR

In addition to consistent assessment of the fetal and maternal conditions, the nurse helps the woman cope with labor by comforting, positioning, teaching, and encouraging her. Another aspect of intrapartum nursing is care of the woman's partner. Nursing Care Plan 6–1 lists selected nursing diagnoses and interventions for the woman in uncomplicated labor.

**Promoting Comfort.** In addition to specific nonpharmacologic and pharmacologic comfort measures discussed in Chapter 7, attention to her environment and hygiene reduces irritants that contribute to the woman's overall discomfort. Positioning makes her more comfortable and helps the progress of labor.

***Making the Environment More Comfortable.*** The nurse adjusts the temperature for comfort. Many women are hot during labor, and a fan circulates the air. Although they are hot, their feet are often cold, so they may want to wear socks. If they are cold, a warmed blanket relieves this discomfort. Soft, indirect lighting, or even semidarkness, promotes relaxation. Bright overhead lights are annoying.

***Hygienic Measures.*** Bloody show and amniotic fluid constantly leak from the woman's vagina. Regularly changing disposable underpads keeps her somewhat dry. Several underpads are placed beneath her hips at one time so that they can be removed one by one as they are soiled. A folded towel absorbs large amounts of fluids. The absorbent pads should be placed from her mid-back to her knees.

Oral fluids are provided, as permitted. If oral intake is prohibited, a lemon-glycerine swab is used to moisten the woman's mouth. Lip balm makes her lips more comfortable when they become dry from mouth breathing.

If there is no contraindication, a bath or a

**NURSING CARE PLAN 6–1**

## Selected Nursing Diagnoses for the Woman in Uncomplicated Labor

| Goals | Nursing Interventions | Rationale |
|---|---|---|

**Nursing Diagnosis:** Anxiety related to unfamiliarity with hospital birth environment.

| Goals | Nursing Interventions | Rationale |
|---|---|---|
| Woman will express reduced anxiety after interventions<br><br>Woman will have a relaxed body posture and facial expression after interventions | 1. Greet woman and her partner/family warmly on arrival, and escort them to the assigned birthing room<br>2. Briefly orient woman/couple to birthing room; place call signal within easy reach and tell her how to use it; explain any equipment that is used, including its purpose and how it will feel and sound<br>3. Talk with woman/couple about what they expect of the birth experience; for example, ask who they plan on having present at (or immediately after) birth and type of medications or anesthesia anticipated | 1. Makes family feel welcome and that staff will be considerate of their needs and desires<br>2. Teaching helps decrease anxiety related to the unknown and increases a sense of personal control over the situation<br>3. Enables nursing staff to help woman/couple achieve their expected experience more closely, which promotes their satisfaction; even if all their expectations are not met, they will probably be less anxious if they believe staff cares about their desires |

**Nursing Diagnosis:** Altered comfort related to effect of uterine contractions and pressure from fetal descent.

| Goals | Nursing Interventions | Rationale |
|---|---|---|
| Woman will state that she is able to manage and tolerate the discomfort of labor | 1. Encourage woman to assume any position she finds comfortable, other than supine<br>2. Assist woman to assume specific positions for special situations in labor:<br>  a. Upright positions (sitting, walking, standing) facilitate fetal pressure against cervix, favoring effacement, dilation, and descent<br>  b. Back labor may be lessened by sitting or standing while leaning forward or by hands-and-knees position because they shift fetal head away from mother's back<br>  c. Squatting can increase the pelvic diameters slightly, straighten the pelvic curve, and promote fetal descent by gravity<br>3. Adjust temperature with a fan if woman is hot, or a warm blanket if she is cool; have her wear socks if her feet are cold<br>4. Change disposable underpads when they become wet or soiled; use a folded towel between her legs if a large quantity of amniotic fluid is draining<br>5. Give woman ice chips, Popsicles, hard candy, or fruit juices as permitted; if she must remain NPO, use lemon-glycerin swabs to moisten her mouth; a wet washcloth can also be used | 1. Promotes comfort; supine position can reduce placental blood flow and compromise fetal oxygenation<br>2. Many women are not aware that position can significantly improve comfort during labor; position can also facilitate normal processes of labor. Although any position except supine is usually acceptable, these positions may be more comfortable for the mother in the situations described<br><br>3. Environmental comfort promotes relaxation, which decreases pain perception and increases pain tolerance<br>4. Hygienic measures promote comfort and make the environment less favorable for growth of microorganisms<br>5. Relieves discomfort of a dry mouth; fruit juices, hard candies, and Popsicles also provide some calories for energy |

## Nursing Brief

Regular changes of position make the laboring woman more comfortable and promote the normal processes of labor.

shower promotes relaxation and comfort. To avoid overheating the mother, which increases fetal oxygen needs, the water should not be too hot.

**Positioning.** The woman should regularly change position, avoiding the supine (flat-on-her-back) position. In the supine position, the heavy uterus may compress the large blood vessels that supply the placenta and return blood to the woman's heart. This compression may result in *supine hypotensive syndrome* (see p. 59). The main risk of this syndrome is reduction of the placental blood flow, which decreases fetal oxygen supply.

Upright positions, such as walking or sitting in a chair or rocker, add the force of gravity to uterine contractions. Upright positions are good during early labor because they promote pressure of the fetal presenting part against the cervix.

Leaning forward while sitting or standing helps make the woman who has "back labor" more comfortable, because it shifts the fetus away from her lower spine. A variation is to kneel on the bed facing the raised head end. The hands-and-knees position has the same effect of shifting the fetus away from her spine; it also favors internal rotation to a more optimal position.

The side-lying position is favored by many women who stay in bed. The woman should regularly change sides to reduce pressure and constant strain on her muscles. Her back and extremities are supported with pillows as she desires. A side-lying position can be used when she is pushing during second-stage labor. The woman who remains in bed may prefer the semi-sitting position. This position can also be useful when she pushes during the second stage.

Squatting while being supported by two people on either side or gripping a "squat bar" improves the ability to push because it makes use of gravity and straightens the pelvic curve. Squatting increases the pelvic diameters slightly, which may provide the extra room needed to push her baby out.

**Teaching.** Teaching the laboring woman and her partner is an ongoing task of the intrapartum nurse. Even women who had prepared childbirth classes often find that the measures they learned are inadequate or that they need to be adapted. Positions or breathing techniques different from those learned in class can be tried. A woman should usually try a change in technique or position for two or three contractions before abandoning it.

Many women are discouraged when their cervix is about 5 cm dilated, because it took many hours to reach that point. They think that they are only halfway through labor (full dilation is 10 cm). However, 5 cm signifies that about two-thirds of the labor is over, because the rate of progress increases. Laboring women often need support and reassurance to overcome their discouragement at this point.

The nurse must often help the woman avoid pushing before her cervix is fully dilated. She can be taught to blow out in short puffs when the urge to push is strong before the cervix is fully dilated. Pushing before full dilation can cause the cervix to swell, slowing progress rather than speeding it.

The nurse teaches or supports effective pushing techniques when the cervix is fully dilated. The woman takes a deep breath and exhales at the beginning of a contraction. She takes another deep breath and pushes with her abdominal muscles while exhaling. Prolonged breath-holding impairs blood circulation; she should not push longer than 5 or 6 seconds with her breath held. When she pushes down with a contraction, she should pull back on her knees, behind her thighs, or using hand-holds on the bed.

**Providing Encouragement.** Encouragement is a powerful tool for intrapartum nursing care, because it helps the woman summon inner strength and gives her courage to continue. After a vaginal examination, she is told of cervical change or fetal descent. Liberal praise is given if she successfully uses techniques to cope with labor. Her partner needs encouragement as well; labor coaching is a demanding job.

The nurse's caring presence cannot be overlooked as a source of support and encouragement for the laboring woman and her partner. Many women feel dependent during labor and are more secure if the nurse is in their room or nearby. Just being present helps, even if no specific care is given.

**Supporting the Partner.** Partners, or coaches, vary considerably in how much involvement they are comfortable with. The labor partner

Support the woman's partner so that he or she can be the most effective coach possible during labor.

If a laboring woman says her baby is coming, *believe her.*

is most often the baby's father but may be the woman's mother or friend. Some partners are truly coaches and take a leading role in helping the woman cope with labor. Others are willing to assist if they are shown how, but they will not take the initiative. Still other couples are content with the partner's encouragement and support and do not expect him or her to have an active role. The partner is allowed to provide the kind of support comfortable for the couple. The nurse does not take the partner's place but remains available as the couple needs.

The partner should be encouraged to take a break and periodically eat a snack or meal. Many are reluctant to leave the woman's bedside, but they may faint during the birth if they have not eaten. The partner is laboring, too, and needs energy to do so. A chair or stool near the bed allows the partner to sit down as much as possible.

## Nursing Care During Birth

As birth draws near, the nurse must decide when to make final preparations for delivery. Specific nursing responsibilities during and immediately after the birth promote the safety and well-being of the mother and baby.

### MAKING FINAL PREPARATIONS FOR DELIVERY

There is no exact time when the woman should be prepared for birth. It depends on the number of babies the woman has had, the length of previous labors, and the overall speed of labor and rate of fetal descent. In general, the woman having her first baby is prepared when about 3–4 cm of the fetal head is visible (crowning) at the vaginal opening. The multipara is usually prepared when her cervix is fully dilated but before crowning has occurred. If the woman must be transferred to a delivery room rather than give birth in a birthing room,

she should be moved early enough to avoid a last-minute rush.

The risk for muscle strains is reduced by moving the woman's legs to foot supports or stirrups simultaneously and not separating her legs too widely. The area behind the knee should be well padded if stirrups are used to avoid compression, which might result in development of a blood clot. These measures are especially important if she has a regional anesthetic, such as an epidural, because she does not have normal sensation or movement. The woman should not be in a supine position during delivery.

### RESPONSIBILITIES DURING BIRTH

During the birth, most physicians or CNMs do not need a scrub nurse. The registered nurse who cares for the woman during labor usually continues to do so in a "circulating" capacity in the birthing room. Typical delivery and birthing room responsibilities include

- Preparing the delivery instruments and infant equipment (Fig. 6–18)
- Doing the perineal scrub prep (Fig. 6–19)
- Giving drugs to the mother or infant
- Providing initial care to the infant, such as suctioning the airway with a bulb syringe, drying the skin, and placing the infant in a radiant warmer to maintain body heat
- Assessing the infant's Apgar score (see p. 231)
- Assessing the infant for obvious abnormalities; a note is made if the infant has a stool or urinates
- Identifying the mother and infant with like-numbered identification bands; the father or other support person often receives a band as well; infant footprints and the mother's fingerprints are often done
- Promoting parent-infant bonding by encouraging parents to hold and explore their newborn while maintaining the temperature; observe for eye contact, fingertip

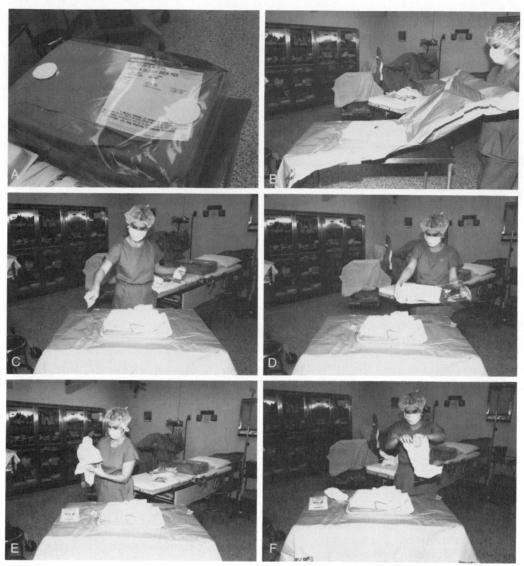

**Figure 6–18.** *A,* Sterile delivery packs are prepackaged for hospitals and birth centers. They are stored in clear plastic, airtight wraps and dated to ensure sterility. *B,* Nurse opens the sterile pack on a movable table and uses the inside of wrap as a sterile field. *C,* Before the nurse puts on sterile gloves, packages are opened and the sterile contents are dropped onto the sterile field. Extra packets of sterile gauze pads are opened and dropped onto the sterile field. *D,* Sterile forceps are dropped from the package in which they were sterilized and onto the sterile table. *E,* A set of clamps and forceps, double-wrapped and sterilized, is opened, and the inside wrapped set is placed on the sterile field. *F,* Sterile-wrapped sharp scissors for use if episiotomy is needed are opened from wrapping and dropped onto the sterile field. *G,* Note that the nurse wears sterile gloves and that the table is arranged with equipment set up for the physician or CNM who will be doing the delivery. *H,* Sterile-wrapped individual packets of suture kits are placed in a readily accessible area for the physician or CNM. *I,* The nurse checks each of the instruments, counts them, and places them in a readily accessible area on the sterile field while wearing sterile gloves. The sterile table is set up for the delivery. *J,* The scale for weighing the newborn is kept in the delivery room. Note that the four sides are raised to provide security and safety for the baby. The scale measures weight in both grams and pounds/ounces in a digital read-out. (Courtesy of St. Joseph Hospital, Nashua, NH.)

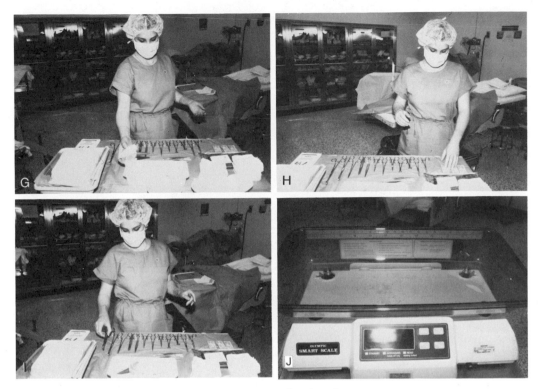

**Figure 6–18.** *Continued*

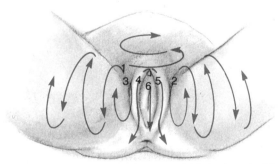

**Figure 6–19.** Perineal scrub prep, which is done just before birth. Numbers and arrows indicate the order and direction of each stroke.

or palm touch of the baby, and talking in high-pitched tones, all of which are associated with initial bonding; these observations continue throughout the postpartum period

The newborn is covered with blood and amniotic fluid, which are potentially infectious fluids. Use gloves, waterproof covergowns, and any other appropriate protective equipment to avoid contact with these secretions. Gloves should be used when caring for the infant until after the first bath.

Figure 6–20 shows an infant being born in the vertex presentation in a spontaneous vaginal birth. Note that the mother has a right mediolateral episiotomy (from her vagina toward her right buttock). This episiotomy provides more room for a large infant to be born than does the median, or midline, episiotomy (from the vagina directly toward, but not into, her rectum). See Chapter 8 for more information on operative procedures.

Figure 6–21 shows an infant being born vaginally in the frank breech presentation. Most fetuses in the breech presentation are born by cesarean delivery to prevent the larger head from being trapped in the mother's pelvis. However, some breech vaginal births are planned, and they may occur unintentionally if a mother enters the birth facility in advanced labor.

Figure 6–22 shows the appearance of the placenta after delivery.

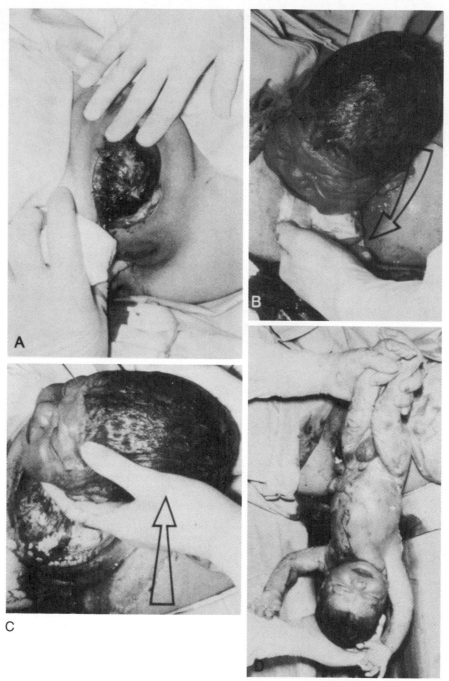

**Figure 6–20.** Vaginal birth of a fetus in a vertex presentation. *A,* The fetal head is crowning. An episiotomy has been done to enlarge the vaginal opening. *B,* Birth of the fetal head and restitution as the head realigns with the shoulders. *C,* The fetal head has externally rotated, the anterior shoulder has been brought under the mother's symphysis pubis, and the posterior shoulder is now being brought over her perineum. *D,* The physician or nurse-midwife firmly grasps the baby as it slips from the mother's vagina. (From Beischer, N., & Mackay, E. [1986]. *Obstetrics and the newborn.* Philadelphia: W.B. Saunders.)

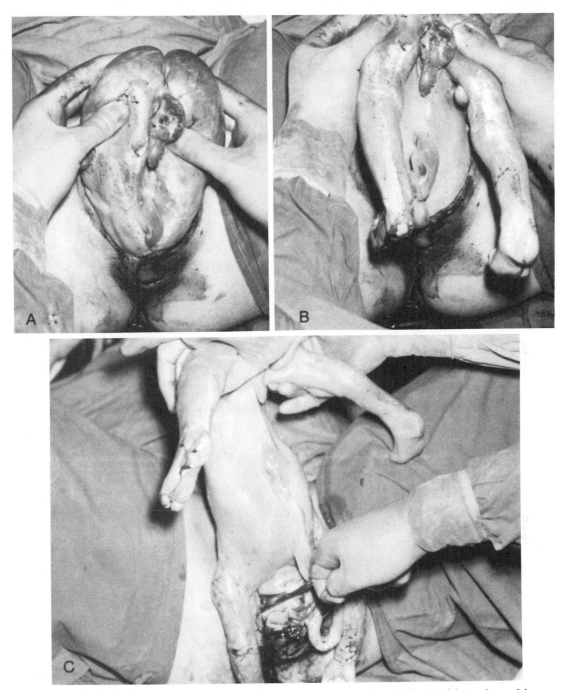

**Figure 6-21.** Delivery of a male fetus in a frank breech presentation. *A,* The fetal buttocks and legs emerge. *B,* The fetal legs, abdomen, and most of the chest have emerged. Note that the fetus's umbilical cord is now out and can be compressed between the fetal head and the mother's pelvis. Thus, the head must be delivered quickly. *C,* An assistant holds the fetal legs while the obstetrician assists birth of the fetal head with forceps. (From Beischer, N., & Mackay, E. [1986]. *Obstetrics and the newborn.* Philadelphia: W.B. Saunders.)

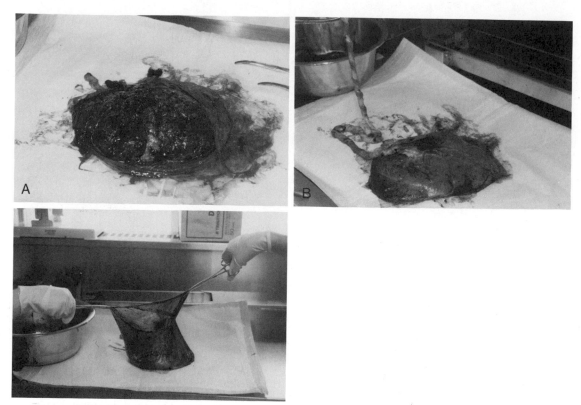

**Figure 6–22.** The placenta after delivery. *A*, Maternal side (Duncan delivery). *B*, Fetal side (Schultze delivery). *C*, The amniotic sac, which housed the fetus during intrauterine life.

# Nursing Care Immediately After Birth

During the immediate post-birth period (fourth stage), the nurse is responsible for observing the mother's condition and promoting her comfort. If the infant remains with her, the nurse also maintains the infant's safety and observes for complications. This is a good time for the parents to celebrate their new arrival with family and friends (Fig. 6–23).

### CARE OF THE MOTHER

Care of the mother in the recovery room includes observation for hemorrhage and promotion of comfort (see Chap. 9 for additional care).

**Observing for Hemorrhage.** The new mother is assessed for signs associated with hemorrhage, which may occur if the uterus relaxes or if lacerations bleed. A common schedule for these assessments is every 15 minutes for 1

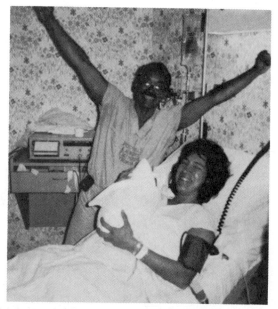

**Figure 6–23.** Birth is often full of emotion even for the obstetrician. (Courtesy of John and Sue Croteau, taken at Brigham and Women's Hospital, Boston, MA.)

hour, every 30 minutes during the second hour, then hourly until she is stable and her recovery period ends.

The uterine fundus is assessed for firmness, height in relation to the umbilicus, and position (midline or deviated to one side). Vaginal bleeding should be dark red (lochia rubra). No more than one pad should be saturated within an hour, and she should not pass large clots. A continuous trickle of bright red blood suggests a bleeding laceration. The blood pressure, pulse, and respirations are taken to identify a rising pulse or falling blood pressure, which suggest shock. An oral temperature is taken hourly, unless it is elevated to 38°C (100.4°F) or higher.

The bladder is assessed for distention, which may occur soon after birth. The woman often does not feel the urge to urinate because of lingering anesthesia effects, perineal trauma, and loss of fetal pressure against the bladder. If her bladder is full, the uterus will be higher than expected and often displaced to one side. A full bladder inhibits uterine contraction and may lead to hemorrhage. Catheterization will be needed if the woman cannot urinate.

**Promoting Comfort.** Most women have a shaking chill after birth. They may be shaking yet deny that they are cold. A warm blanket or portable radiant warmer over the woman often makes her feel more comfortable until the chill subsides.

An ice pack is placed on the mother's perineum. A glove can be filled with ice and wrapped in a wash cloth. Chemical ice packs may also be used. Perineal pads that incorporate a chemical cold pack are often used. These pads do not absorb as much lochia as those without the cold pack, which must be considered in evaluating the quantity of bleeding. A warm pack pad is often used after the first 12–24 hours. Women who do not have an episiotomy or perineal laceration may not need cold or heat applications.

Afterpains, rhythmic uterine contractions that feel like menstrual cramps, are common in women who have had several babies or whose babies are large. They are often worse if the mother's bladder is full. Afterpains increase during breast feeding because infant suckling stimulates the mother's pituitary gland to secrete oxytocin, causing uterine contractions. Analgesics effectively reduce most afterpains.

The mother can have ordered analgesics when she is uncomfortable and desires them. Mild oral analgesics are usually sufficient for postbirth discomfort. Most analgesics used in postpartum care have little effect on the breast-fed infant.

## CARE OF THE INFANT

The infant often stays with the parents during recovery, especially when birth occurs in a birthing room (LDR or LDRP). The priority care involves promoting respiratory function and maintaining the temperature (see pp. 231–237 for information about care of the infant at birth).

## KEY POINTS

- The four components, or "four Ps," of the birth process are the powers, the passage, the passenger, and the psyche. All interrelate during labor to either facilitate or impede birth.
- True labor and false labor have several differences. However, the conclusive difference is that true labor results in cervical change (effacement and/or dilation).
- The woman should go to the hospital if she is having persistent, regular contractions (every 5 minutes for nulliparas, every 10 minutes for multiparas), if her membranes rupture, if she has bleeding other than normal bloody show, if fetal movement decreases, or for other concerns not covered by the basic guidelines.
- The woman having false labor is usually sent home after a short observation period. The nurse reassures her that she is not foolish for coming to the birth facility and emphasizes guidelines for returning.

- Three key assessments on admission are fetal condition, maternal condition, and nearness to birth.
- Four stages of labor have unique characteristics. The first stage is the stage of dilation, lasting from labor's onset to full (10 cm) cervical dilation. First-stage labor is subdivided into three phases: latent, active, and transition. Second-stage labor, the stage of expulsion, extends from full cervical dilation until birth of the baby. The third stage, the placental stage, is from the birth of the baby until the birth of the placenta. The fourth stage is the immediate postbirth recovery period and includes the first 1–4 hours after placental delivery.
- The main risk during first- and second-stage labor is fetal compromise due to interruption of the fetal oxygen supply. The main maternal risk during fourth-stage labor is hemorrhage due to uterine relaxation.
- Nursing care during the first and second stages focuses on observing the fetal and maternal conditions and on assisting the woman to cope with labor.
- Continuous electronic fetal monitoring is most common in hospital births, but intermittent auscultation is a valid method of fetal assessment.
- Laboring women can assume many positions. Upright positions add gravity to promote fetal descent. Hands-and-knees or leaning-forward positions promote normal internal rotation of the fetus if "back labor" is a problem. Squatting facilitates fetal descent during the second stage. The supine position should be discouraged because it causes the heavy uterus to compress the mother's main blood vessels, which can reduce fetal oxygen supply.

# Study Questions

1. Describe the contraction cycle. Why is it important that the contractions not last too long? Why is the interval important?
2. Why is it best if the fetal head is flexed, with the chin on the chest, during labor?
3. What is meant by engagement? What station designates that engagement has occurred?
4. What are the four stages of labor? What occurs during each? How do the three phases of first stage labor differ from one another?
5. Your friend wonders how she will know if labor is "real." What should you tell her? What signs and symptoms signify that she should go to the birth facility?
6. Describe normal and abnormal characteristics of the fetal heart rate, amniotic fluid, and maternal temperature and blood pressure.
7. What is the significance of variability on the electronic fetal monitor? Accelerations?
8. What initial nursing responses are expected if the fetus shows a pattern of late decelerations on the fetal monitor? Variable decelerations?
9. What nursing interventions help make the woman more comfortable and better able to cope with labor?
10. Describe nursing observations of the mother immediately after birth.

# Multiple Choice Review Questions

*Choose the most appropriate answer.*

1. The best description of effacement is when the cervix
   a. opens to allow the fetus to pass
   b. becomes shorter and thinner
   c. becomes softer near the end of pregnancy
   d. is pushed downward into the bony pelvis

2. Full cervical dilation is about
   a. 2 cm
   b. 4 cm
   c. 8 cm
   d. 10 cm

3. To determine the frequency of uterine contractions, the nurse should note the time from the
   a. beginning to end of the same contraction
   b. end of one contraction to the beginning of the next contraction
   c. beginning of one contraction to the beginning of the next contraction
   d. contraction's peak until the contraction begins to relax

4. The fetus in a breech presentation is often born by cesarean delivery because the
   a. large head comes last, and might be too big to fit through the pelvis
   b. fetal legs and feet are more likely to be injured
   c. placental blood flow is inadequate for normal fetal oxygenation
   d. emergency staff can be more easily assembled if the time of birth is predictable

5. Choose the abbreviation that describes the situation if the fetal occiput is in the left posterior quadrant of the mother's pelvis.
   a. LOO
   b. LOP
   c. LSA
   d. LSP

6. Excessive anxiety and fear during labor may result in
   a. an ineffective labor pattern
   b. abnormal fetal presentation or position
   c. release of oxytocin from the pituitary gland
   d. a rapid birth

7. The woman is most likely to first need pharmacologic pain relief, such as analgesia or anesthesia, in which part of labor?
   a. latent phase
   b. active phase
   c. second stage
   d. third stage

8. Which maternal behavior best characterizes the transition phase?
   a. sociable and excited, yet a little anxious
   b. focusing on her inward sensations
   c. irritable and somewhat out of control
   d. excited and tired

9. A woman who is pregnant with her first baby telephones an intrapartum facility and says her "water broke." She should be instructed to
   a. wait until she has contractions every 5 minutes for 1 hour.
   b. take her temperature every 4 hours, and come to the facility if it is over 38°C (100.4°F).
   c. come to the facility promptly, but safely
   d. call an ambulance to bring her to the facility

10. A laboring woman suddenly begins making grunting sounds and bearing down during a strong contraction. The most appropriate immediate nursing action is to
    a. ask the experienced nurse to do a vaginal examination
    b. look at her perineum for increased bloody show or perineal bulging
    c. ask her if she needs pain medication
    d. tell her that these are common sensations in late labor

11. To assess contractions by palpation, the nurse should palpate the
    a. fetal head
    b. mother's cervix
    c. uterine fundus
    d. lower abdomen

## BIBLIOGRAPHY

American Academy of Pediatrics (AAP) & American College of Obstetricians and Gynecologists (ACOG). (1992). *Guidelines for perinatal care* (3rd ed.). Elk Grove Village, IL, and Washington, DC: Authors.

Andrews, C.M., & Chrzanowski, M. (1990). Maternal position, labor, and comfort. *Applied Nursing Research, 3,* 7–13.

Bauer, B., & Kenney, J. (1993). Adverse exposures and use of universal precautions among perinatal nurses. *Journal of Obstetric, Gynecologic, & Neonatal Nursing, 22,* 429–435.

Berry, L.M. (1988). Realistic expectations of the labor coach. *Journal of Obstetric, Gynecologic, & Neonatal Nursing, 17,* 354–355.

Chapman, L.L. (1992). Expectant fathers' roles during labor and birth. *Journal of Obstetric, Gynecologic, & Neonatal Nursing, 21,* 114–120.

Church, L. (1989). Water birth: One birthing center's observations. *Journal of Nurse-Midwifery, 34,* 165–170.

Cosner, K., & deJong, E. (1993). Physiologic second-stage labor. *MCN: American Journal of Maternal-Child Nursing, 18,* 38–43.

Goff, K.J. (1993). Initiation of parturition. *MCN: Journal of Maternal-Child Nursing, 18*(Suppl.), 7–13.

Gorrie, T.M., McKinney, E.S., & Murray, S.S. (1994). *Foundations of maternal-newborn nursing.* Philadelphia: W.B. Saunders.

Kilpatrick, S., & Laros, R. (1989). Characteristics of normal labor. *Obstetrics & Gynecology, 74,* 85–87.

Kintz, D.L. (1987). Nursing support in labor. *Journal of Obstetric, Gynecologic, & Neonatal Nursing, 16,* 126–130.

Lowe, N.K. (1991). Maternal confidence in coping with labor: A self-efficacy concept. *Journal of Obstetric, Gynecologic, & Neonatal Nursing, 20,* 457–463.

Murray, M. (1988). *Antepartal and intrapartal fetal monitoring.* Washington, DC: NAACOG.

NAACOG. (1988). *Nursing responsibilities in implementing fetal heart rate monitoring.* Washington, DC: Author.

NAACOG. (1990). *OGN Nursing practice resource: Fetal heart rate auscultation.* Washington, DC: Author.

Nelsson-Ryan, S. (1988). Positioning: Second stage labor. In F. Nichols & S. Humenick (Eds.), *Childbirth education: Practice, research, and theory* (pp. 256–274). Philadelphia: W.B. Saunders.

Pavlik, M. (1988). Positioning: First stage labor. In F. Nichols & S. Humenick (Eds.), *Childbirth education: Practice, research, and theory* (pp. 234–255). Philadelphia: W.B. Saunders.

Rooks, J., Weatherby, N., Ernst, E., Stapleton, S., Rosen, D., & Rosenfield, A. (1989). Outcomes of care in birth centers: The national birth center study. *New England Journal of Medicine, 321,* 1804–1811.

Ross, T., & Dickason, E. (1992). Nursing alert: Vertical transmission of HIV and HBV. *MCN: American Journal of Maternal-Child Nursing, 17,* 192–195.

Stolte, K. (1987). A comparison of women's expectations of labor with the actual event. *Birth, 14,* 99–103.

Wilson, B. (1989). Delivery outcomes of low risk births: Comparison of certified nurse midwives and obstetricians. *Journal of the American Academy of Nurse-Practitioners, 1,* 9–13.

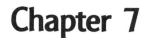

## Chapter 7

# Nursing Management of Pain During Labor and Birth

**VOCABULARY**

aspiration pneumonitis (178)
blood patch (177)
cleansing breath (169)
cricoid pressure (178)
effleurage (168)
endorphins (161)
focal point (168)
pain threshold (160)
pain tolerance (160)
systemic drug (170)

# OBJECTIVES

*On completion and mastery of Chapter 7, the student will be able to*

- Define each vocabulary term listed.
- Describe factors that influence a woman's comfort during labor.
- List common types of classes offered to childbearing families.
- Describe methods of childbirth preparation.
- Discuss advantages and limitations of nonpharmacologic methods of pain management during labor.
- Discuss advantages and limitations of pharmacologic methods of pain management.
- Explain nonpharmacologic methods of pain management for labor, including the nursing role for each.
- Explain each type of pharmacologic pain management, including the nursing role for each.

Pregnant women are usually interested in how labor will feel and want to know how they can manage the experience, especially the pain they expect. Women manage labor pain by using nonpharmacologic (nondrug) methods alone or with pharmacologic (drug) methods. Most women use a combination of the two. Because preparation for childbirth is an important part of nonpharmacologic pain management, it is also discussed in this chapter. General labor comfort measures, such as adjustment of the environment and maternal positioning, were discussed in Chapter 6.

# Childbirth and Pain

Pain is an unpleasant and distressing symptom that is personal and subjective. No one can feel another's pain, but empathic nursing care helps alleviate pain and helps the client cope with it.

## HOW CHILDBIRTH PAIN DIFFERS FROM OTHER PAIN

Childbirth pain differs from other types of pain in several ways:

- It is part of a normal body process.
- The woman has several months to prepare for pain management.
- The pain is self-limiting and rapidly declines after birth.

- The pain of labor ends with the birth of a baby.

Pain is usually a symptom of injury or illness; yet pain during labor is almost a universal part of this normal body process. Although excessive pain is detrimental, labor pain may cause a woman to feel vulnerable and seek shelter and help from others. Additionally, it often motivates her to assume different body positions, which can facilitate the normal descent of the fetus (see p. 148).

Labor pain occurs after several months' warning. There is time to prepare for it and develop knowledge and skills for best managing it when birth begins.

Unlike many other kinds of pain, childbirth pain is self-limiting. It lasts for hours, as opposed to days or weeks. Labor ends with the birth of a baby, followed by a rapid and nearly total cessation of pain.

## FACTORS THAT INFLUENCE LABOR PAIN

Several factors cause pain during labor and influence the amount of pain a woman experiences. Other factors influence a woman's response to and ability to tolerate labor pain.

### Pain Threshold and Pain Tolerance

Two terms are often used interchangeably to describe pain, although really they have different meanings. *Pain threshold*, also called pain perception, is the least amount of sensation that a person perceives as painful. Pain threshold is fairly constant, and it varies little under different conditions. *Pain tolerance* is the amount of pain one is willing to endure. Unlike the pain threshold, one's pain tolerance can change under different conditions. A primary nursing responsibility is to modify as many factors as possible so that the woman can tolerate the pain of labor.

# Nursing Brief

Laboring women often tolerate more pain than usual because they have high levels of endorphins and because they are concerned about the baby's well-being.

## Sources of Pain During Labor

Four physical factors contribute to pain during labor:

- Dilation and stretching of the cervix
- Reduced uterine blood supply during contractions
- Pressure of the fetus on pelvic structures
- Stretching of the vagina and perineum

See Chapter 6 for discussion of these labor processes. Additional physical and psychosocial factors alter the sensations a woman feels during labor and modify her pain.

## Physical Factors That Modify Pain

Several physical factors influence the amount of pain a woman feels or is willing to tolerate during labor.

### CENTRAL NERVOUS SYSTEM FACTORS

**Gate Control Theory.** The gate control theory explains how pain impulses reach the brain for interpretation. It supports several nonpharmacologic methods of pain control. According to this theory, pain is transmitted through small-diameter nerve fibers. However, stimulating large-diameter nerve fibers temporarily interferes with conduction of impulses through small-diameter fibers. Techniques to stimulate large-diameter fibers and "close the gate" to painful impulses include firm massage, palm and fingertip pressure, and heat and cold applications.

**Endorphins.** Endorphins are natural body substances that are similar to morphine. Levels of endorphins increase during pregnancy and reach a peak during labor. Endorphins may explain why laboring women often need smaller doses of analgesia or anesthesia than might be expected in a similar painful experience.

### MATERNAL CONDITION

**Cervical Readiness.** The mother's cervix normally undergoes changes that facilitate efface-

# Nursing Brief

Firm stroking or massage, palm- or foot-rubbing, or gripping a cool bed rail stimulates nerve fibers that interfere with transmission of pain impulses to the brain.

ment and dilation in labor (see p. 130). If her cervix does not make these changes ("ripening"), more contractions are needed to cause effacement and dilation.

**Pelvis.** The size and shape of the pelvis significantly influence how readily the fetus can descend through it. Pelvic abnormalities can result in a longer labor and greater maternal fatigue. Additionally, the fetus may remain in an abnormal presentation or position, which interferes with the mechanisms of labor (see p. 131).

**Labor Intensity.** The woman who has a short, intense labor often experiences more pain than the woman whose birth process is more gradual. Contractions are intense and frequent. The cervix, vagina, and perineum stretch more abruptly than in a gentler labor.

**Fatigue.** Fatigue reduces pain tolerance and a woman's ability to use coping skills. Many women are tired when labor begins because sleep during late pregnancy is difficult. The active fetus, frequent urination, and shortness of breath when lying down all interrupt sleep.

### FETAL PRESENTATION AND POSITION

The fetal presenting part acts as a wedge to efface and dilate the cervix as each contraction pushes it downward. The fetal head is a smooth, rounded wedge that most effectively causes cervical effacement and dilation. The fetus in an abnormal presentation or position applies uneven pressure to the cervix, resulting in less effective effacement and dilation.

The fetus usually turns during early labor so that the occiput is in the front left or right quadrant of the mother's pelvis (occiput anterior positions; see p. 125). If the fetal occiput is in a posterior pelvic quadrant, each contraction pushes it against the mother's sacrum, resulting in persistent and poorly relieved back pain (back labor). Labor is often longer with this fetal position.

### INTERVENTIONS OF CAREGIVERS

Although they are intended to promote maternal and fetal safety, several common interventions may add to pain during labor. Some examples are

- Intravenous lines
- Continuous fetal monitoring, especially if it hampers mobility

- Amniotomy (artificial rupture of the membranes)
- Vaginal examinations

### Psychosocial Factors That Modify Pain

Several psychosocial variables alter the pain a woman experiences during labor. Many of these variables interrelate with one another and with physical factors.

**Culture.** Culture influences how a woman feels about pregnancy and birth and how she reacts to pain during childbirth. Some cultures encourage loud and vigorous expressions of distress as a way of coping with pain, whereas others value stoicism and "silent suffering." The nurse must accept each woman's individual expression of pain and realize that some women "labor loudly."

**Anxiety and Fear.** Moderate anxiety can motivate a woman to learn techniques that increase her pain tolerance. However, excessive anxiety or fear raises her sensitivity to pain and reduces her ability to tolerate it. Additionally, excessive anxiety reduces uterine blood flow, makes uterine contractions less effective, and results in muscle tension that counteracts the expulsion powers of contractions and maternal pushing. The woman who learns about expected sensations of labor is less likely to interpret them as dangerous or as a symptom of something wrong.

**Previous Experiences.** Labor is not a woman's first painful experience. During other painful experiences she may have learned skills that increase her ability to cope with labor, including the first labor.

Experience with previous births influences a woman's reactions to her current labor. A woman who had a normal birth before is less likely to interpret the intense sensations with injury or abnormality. The woman who had an epidural block (see p. 174) may have little experience in coping with labor pain. If an epidural is not possible during a subsequent labor, she may be distressed because she compares the painful labor with the "painless" one.

The woman who had a long and difficult labor is often apprehensive during the next labor. If her difficult labor required a cesarean delivery, she may be uneasy about attempting vaginal birth. Repeat cesarean birth may seem like the easier and quicker option. If a repeat cesarean birth is planned and she begins labor before the surgery, she may be upset because she did not expect to experience labor at all.

**Childbirth Preparation.** Women who prepare for labor through classes, self-study, or other means usually have less anxiety and fear about the unknown. They learn a variety of skills for coping with labor pain. The preparation should be *realistic*, promoting reasonable expectations about pain and the effectiveness of both nonpharmacologic and pharmacologic pain relief methods.

**Support of Significant Others.** A woman's labor partner is usually her husband or the baby's father, although the partner may be her mother or a friend. A well-prepared partner is a valuable teammate during labor, encouraging the woman and helping her use different coping skills.

Friends and family members with children can provide support to the expectant mother if they convey accurate information about the discomfort of labor. It is most distressing to hear that labor is intolerable, but it is equally wrong for others to lead the woman to expect a painless labor. Every labor is different, even in the same woman.

## Education for Childbearing

A variety of classes are offered by most hospitals and free-standing birth centers to help women adjust to pregnancy, cope with labor, and prepare for life with a baby (Fig. 7–1). Women who plan home birth usually prepare intensely because they typically want to avoid medications and other interventions associated with hospital births.

### TYPES OF CLASSES AVAILABLE

Classes during pregnancy focus on topics that contribute to good outcomes for the mother and baby (Box 7–1). Special classes prepare other family members for the birth and new infant.

## Nursing Brief

It is easy to miss important cues about impending birth or development of a complication if a laboring woman is either very stoic or very vocal.

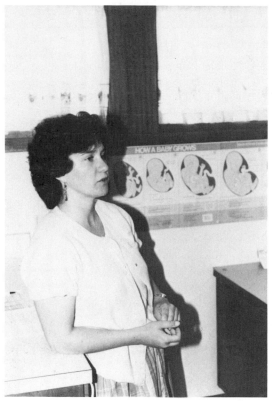

**Figure 7–1.** The certified nurse-midwife teaches childbirth preparation classes to expectant parents. (Courtesy of WomanCare, Des Moines BirthPlace, Des Moines, IA.)

Examples of classes that may be available include

- Early pregnancy classes
- Exercise classes for pregnant women
- Sibling classes
- Grandparent classes
- Breast-feeding classes
- Infant care classes

Because this chapter focuses on pain management during labor, techniques of prepared childbirth are discussed most extensively.

## PREPARATION FOR CHILDBIRTH

The time to prepare for labor is before it begins. Prepared childbirth classes teach the woman and her partner skills to manage labor effectively. Related classes prepare women planning a vaginal birth after cesarean (VBAC) or those expecting a cesarean birth. Classes for adolescents are sometimes available (Fig. 7–2).

### Methods of Childbirth Preparation

Most childbirth preparation classes are based on one of several methods. The basic method is often extensively modified to meet the specific needs of the women who attend.

**Dick-Read Method.** Grantly Dick-Read was an English physician who introduced the concept of a fear-tension-pain cycle during labor. He believed that fear of childbirth contributed to tension, which resulted in pain. His methods include education and relaxation techniques to interrupt the cycle.

**Bradley Method.** This method was originally called "husband-coached childbirth," and was the first to include the father as an integral part of labor. It emphasizes slow abdominal breathing and relaxation techniques.

**Lamaze Method.** The Lamaze method, also called the psychoprophylactic method, is the basis of most prepared childbirth classes in the United States. It uses mental techniques that condition the woman to respond to contractions with relaxation. Other mental and breathing techniques occupy her mind and limit the brain's ability to interpret labor sensations as painful.

### Content of Prepared Childbirth Classes

Regardless of the specific method taught, most classes are similar in basic content. Because the Lamaze method is popular in most areas of the United States, it is the focus of this chapter.

**Education.** The woman who learns about changes during pregnancy and childbirth is less likely to respond with fear and tension to labor. Information about cesarean birth is usually included, since 20–25% of births in the United States occur by this method.

**Exercises.** Conditioning exercises, such as the pelvic rock, tailor stretch, and tailor reach (Fig. 7–3), prepare the woman's muscles for the demands of birth. These exercises also relieve the back discomfort common during late pregnancy.

The Kegel exercise increases control of the muscles that support the pelvic organs. It reduces stress incontinence (loss of urine during straining), improves control of pelvic muscles during birth, recovers pelvic muscle tone after birth, and increases sexual sensitivity. To do the Kegel exercise, the woman contracts the muscles that stop her urine flow in the middle of voiding. The exercise is repeated five times; she gradually works up to about 100 repetitions each day.

---

| BOX 7–1 | **Types of Prenatal Classes** |
| --- | --- |

**Early Pregnancy Classes**

Changes of pregnancy
Fetal development
Prenatal care
Hazardous substances to avoid
Good nutrition for pregnancy
Relieving common pregnancy discomforts
Working during pregnancy and parenthood
Care of the new baby, such as feeding methods, choosing a pediatrician, and selecting clothing and equipment
Early growth and development

**Exercise Classes**

Maintaining woman's fitness during pregnancy
Possible availability after birth for toning and fitness
Special considerations for exercise during pregnancy:

■ Exercises should be low-impact
■ Woman's heart rate should be no more rapid than 140 beats/min; her temperature should be no higher than 38°C (100.4°F)
■ Woman should not lie in supine position (flat on her back) or use the Valsalva maneuver (similar to straining to have a bowel movement)

**Sibling Classes**

Helping children prepare realistically for their new brother or sister
Helping children understand that feelings of jealousy and anger are normal
Giving parents tips about helping older children adjust to the new baby after birth

**Grandparent Classes**

Changes in childbirth and parenting
Importance of grandparents to a child's development
Reducing conflict between the generations

**Breast-feeding Classes**

Processes of breastfeeding
Feeding techniques
Solving common problems
Possibility of continuing classes after birth

**Infant Care Classes**

Care of new baby
Needed clothing and equipment

---

**Relaxation Techniques.** The ability to release tension is a vital part of the expectant mother's "tool kit." Relaxation techniques require concentration, thus occupying the mind while reducing muscle tension. All require practice to be most effective during labor. Examples of relaxation techniques include

■ Progressive relaxation: the woman contracts, then consciously relaxes different muscle groups until all muscles are relaxed
■ Neuromuscular dissociation: the woman tenses a single muscle group while relaxing all others
■ Relaxing to touch: the woman relaxes tense muscles when they are touched or massaged; her partner learns how to identify signs of muscle tension
■ Relaxing in the presence of pain: the partner squeezes a large muscle in her arm or leg to simulate a labor contraction; the woman practices relaxing all muscles in response to this mild pain

See Box 7–2 for prenatal relaxation exercises.

**Pain Control Methods for Labor.** The woman and her partner learn a variety of techniques that may be used during labor as needed. Examples of these include

■ Skin stimulation
■ Mental stimulation
■ Breathing techniques

These techniques are most effective if learned before labor begins. They can also be used by the woman who has not attended classes and are discussed with nonpharmacologic pain management (see p. 166).

## Variations of Basic Prepared Childbirth Classes

**Refresher Classes.** Refresher classes consist of one to three sessions to review material learned during a previous pregnancy. Ways to help siblings adjust to the new baby and a review of breast feeding are often included.

**Cesarean Birth Classes.** Classes for women who expect cesarean birth help the woman and her support person understand the reasons for this method of delivery and anticipate what

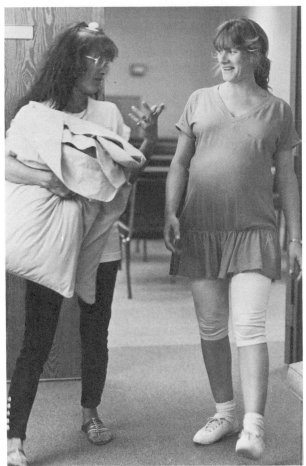

**Figure 7-2.** This expectant mother has asked her friend to be her labor partner. They are attending prepared childbirth classes together.

is likely to occur during and after surgery. Women who had previous cesarean births may recall little of their experience if it was done after a prolonged and exhausting labor or under emergency conditions. They may need to express their feelings about their past experiences so they can resolve them and better deal with the present pregnancy.

**Vaginal Birth After Cesarean Classes.** VBAC is desirable whenever it is possible. Women in VBAC classes may need to express unresolved feelings about their previous cesarean birth. Depending on the reason for the cesarean delivery, they may be more anxious about the forthcoming labor. In addition to teaching techniques for coping with labor, these women and their partners need ample time to discuss their experiences and feelings.

**Adolescent Prepared Childbirth Classes.** A pregnant adolescent's needs are different from an adult's needs. Adolescents are therefore usually uncomfortable in regular prepared childbirth classes. They are often single mothers and have a more immature perception of birth and childrearing. Some are not old enough to drive and may not be able to attend classes that target working adults. The content of classes for adolescents is tailored to their special needs. Because acceptance by their peer group is vitally important to teenagers, the girls are a significant source of support to each other. Classes may be held during school. Expectant fathers may be included.

# Nonpharmacologic Pain Management

Nonpharmacologic pain control methods are important, even if the woman has medication or anesthesia. Most pharmacologic methods cannot be instituted until labor is well established, because they tend to slow progress. Nonpharmacologic methods help the woman cope with labor before it has advanced far enough to give her medication. Also, medications do not always *eliminate* pain, and the woman will need nonpharmacologic methods to manage discomfort that remains. Nonpharmacologic methods are usually the only realistic option if the woman comes to the hospital in advanced labor.

## ADVANTAGES OF NONPHARMACOLOGIC METHODS

There are several advantages to nonpharmacologic methods *if pain control is adequate.* Poorly relieved pain increases fear and anxiety, thus diverting blood flow from the uterus and impairing the normal labor process. It also reduces the pleasure of this extraordinary experience.

Nonpharmacologic methods do not harm the mother or fetus. They do not slow labor if they provide adequate pain control. They carry no risk for allergy or adverse drug effects.

## LIMITATIONS OF NONPHARMACOLOGIC METHODS

For best results, nonpharmacologic methods should be rehearsed before labor begins. They

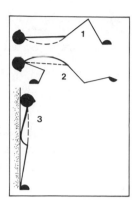

## PELVIC ROCK

### Purpose

- Improves muscle tone.
- Relieves backache.

### Instructions

1. Lie on your back with your knees bent, exhale, rolling your waist upward, toward your chest. Then inhale as you relax back to the starting position.
2. On your hands and knees, exhale as you pull your stomach up. Inhale as you relax.
3. Stand against a wall, pull your stomach in, and roll your hips forward and upward, tucking your buttocks under. Practice pressing the small of your back against the wall.

### Tips for performing this exercise

- Do not exaggerate the curve of your back when relaxing.
- Gradually increase from 10 to 30 repetitions daily.

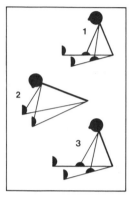

## TAILOR STRETCH

### Purpose

- Stretches the muscles that pull the legs together.
- Loosens the perineum.
- Reduces back strain.

### Instructions

1. Sit on the floor with your legs spread comfortably apart.
2. Exhale as you stretch your hands down toward your ankles.
3. Inhale as you relax back to the starting position.

### Tips for performing this exercise

- Keep your head and back straight.
- Keep your knees flat against the floor.
- Do slowly up to 10 repetitions daily.

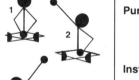

## TAILOR REACH

### Purpose

- Relieves fatigue in the upper back.
- Increases lung capacity.
- Aids rib cage expansion.

### Instructions

1. Sit in the tailor position with your arms in your lap.
2. Reach for the ceiling with your right hand, then relax.
3. Reach for the ceiling with your left hand, then relax.
4. Reach for the ceiling with both hands, then relax.
5. Inhale as you reach up to expand your lungs and ribs. Exhale as you relax.

### Tips for performing this exercise

- Do not arch your back—look straight ahead.
- Begin with 5 repetitions daily and work up to 10.

**Figure 7–3.** These conditioning exercises prepare the woman's muscles for labor and relieve some of the discomforts of late pregnancy.

can be taught to the unprepared woman, preferably during early labor, when she is anxious enough to be interested but comfortable enough to learn.

Many women will not have adequate pain control by using these methods alone. No matter how much a woman has practiced, the many factors that influence labor pain often require drug intervention.

## NONPHARMACOLOGIC TECHNIQUES

The nurse may help the woman use several techniques of nondrug pain control during labor. They include relaxation, skin stimulation, mental stimulation, and breathing techniques. If the woman and her partner attended prepared childbirth classes, the nurse builds on their knowledge during labor.

| BOX 7–2 | **Relaxation Exercises** |
| --- | --- |

**Phase I: Tension Release in Large Muscles**

*Technique*

Tense one large muscle area at a time
Feel the tension spread
Release the tension gradually and smoothly
Count to 10 during release

*Muscle areas*

Do each of these separately:

1. Face, neck, shoulders
2. Upper back
3. Lower back
4. Abdomen
5. Buttocks
6. Pelvic floor
7. Legs
8. Arms

*Practice positions*
Use different positions to provide for good circulation and body weight distribution:

Chaise lounge—lie flat on back with shoulders and head elevated to comfort with pillows; legs slightly apart, arms at sides, elbows bent, palms down, head to one side
Sims lateral—lie on side with pillows under head; place one pillow under bent, upper leg; make arms comfortable

**Phase II: Tension Release in Small Muscles**

*Technique*

Use slow, comfortable, natural breathing rate
Allow one complete breath for each activity
For each of the exercises listed below, follow these steps:

1. Inhale
2. Exercise
3. Exhale
4. Release tension

*Exercises*
Do the following exercises in sequence; *concentrate* on release of *all tension*

1. Pull toes downward, upward
2. Turn ankles inward, outward
3. Bend knees slightly
4. Straighten knees
5. Stretch, extend left leg from hip
6. Repeat with right leg
7. Squeeze thighs together
8. Tighten buttocks
9. Tighten pelvic floor
10. Roll legs inward, outward
11. Make fists
12. Extend fingers
13. Bend wrist downward, backward
14. Bend elbows slightly
15. Straighten elbows
16. Raise shoulder toward left ear
17. Repeat with right shoulder
18. Squeeze chest (shoulders forward)
19. Squeeze shoulder blades (shoulders back)
20. Expand chest
21. Arch lower back slightly
22. Erase curve in lower back slowly
23. Bend neck forward, chin to chest
24. Bend neck backward, erase curve

On completion of exercises, take several deep breaths and get up slowly.

## Relaxation

Promoting relaxation underlies all other methods, both nonpharmacologic and pharmacologic. The nurse should adjust the woman's environment and help her with hygienic measures as discussed in Chapter 6. Water in a tub or shower helps refresh her and promotes relaxation.

To reduce anxiety and fear, the woman is taught about the labor area, any procedures that are done, and what is happening in her body. The nursing focus should be on the normality of birth. For example, calling the woman by her first name, if that is her preference, promotes an atmosphere of wellness. A partnership style of nurse-client-labor partner relationship is usual in maternity settings.

Looking for signs of muscle tension and teaching her partner to do so help the woman who is not aware of becoming tense. She can change position or guide her partner to massage the area where muscle tension is noted. The laboring woman is guided to release the tension specifically, one muscle group at a time, for example, by saying, "Let your arm relax; let the tension out of your neck . . . your shoulders." Specific instructions are repeated until she relaxes.

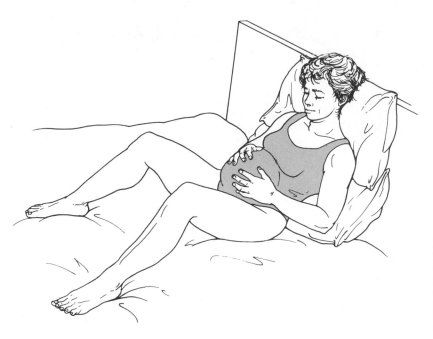

**Figure 7–4.** Effleurage is a technique for stimulating the large-diameter nerve fibers, thus interfering with pain transmission. Fingertip pressure should be firm enough to avoid a tickling sensation and sufficient to interrupt pain. Very light touch tends not to block pain.

### Skin Stimulation

Several variations of massage are often used during labor. Most can be taught to the woman and partner who did not attend prepared childbirth classes. Massage tends to become less effective unless varied periodically.

**Effleurage.** The woman strokes her abdomen in a circular movement during contractions (Fig. 7–4). If fetal monitor belts are on her abdomen, she can massage between them or on her side. Effleurage is best done by applying firm pressure, which stimulates the large-diameter nerve fibers that inhibit painful stimuli traveling through the small-diameter fibers. Very light fingertip stroking, once taught as the best way to do effleurage, stimulates small-diameter fibers and may increase pain rather than reduce it.

**Sacral Pressure.** Firm pressure against the lower back helps relieve some of the pain of back labor. The woman should tell her partner where to apply the pressure and how much pressure is helpful. Another method uses two or more tennis balls inserted into a man's sock; the woman lies on this firm wedge to apply sacral pressure. A plastic disposable bottle of warm sterile water can be used to apply heat and pressure to the woman's back. If it is not opened, the solution can be used for the scrub prep at birth.

**Thermal Stimulation.** In addition to the warm bottle of solution already described, heat can be applied with a warm blanket or glove filled with warm water. Most women appreciate a cool cloth on the face. Two or three moistened washcloths are kept at hand and changed as they become warm. Do not apply heat or cold to anesthetized areas because the woman will not be able to feel tissue injury that might occur.

### Positioning

Various positions were described in Chapter 6. Changing position every 30–60 minutes relieves muscle fatigue and strain and decreases constant pressure on one area of the body. Additionally, position changes promote normal mechanisms of labor. When the woman changes position, she may be more uncomfortable at first but is often more comfortable after a few contractions.

### Mental Stimulation

Several methods may be used to stimulate the woman's brain, thus limiting her ability to perceive sensations as painful. All methods direct her mind away from the pain.

**Focal Point.** The woman fixes her eyes on a picture, an object, or simply a particular spot in the room. Some women prefer to close their eyes during contractions and focus on an internal focal point.

**Imagery.** The woman learns to create a tranquil mental environment by imagining that she is in a place of relaxation and peace. Preferred mental scenes often involve warmth and sunlight, although some women imagine themselves in a cool environment. During labor, the woman can imagine her cervix opening and allowing the baby to come out, as a flower opens from bud to full bloom. The nurse can help create a tranquil mental image, even in the unprepared woman.

**Music.** Favorite music or relaxation recordings divert the woman's attention from pain. Sounds of rainfall, wind, or the ocean contribute to relaxation and block disturbing sounds. Headphones help the woman concentrate and minimize external sounds. For best results when music is used, the sound on the fetal monitor should be lowered or turned off.

**Television.** Especially during early labor, women often enjoy the diversion of television. The woman may not watch the program, but it provides background noise that reduces intrusive sounds. Some labor rooms have videotape players, and the woman can bring her own tapes to watch during and after birth.

## Breathing

Like other techniques, breathing techniques are most effective if practiced before labor. The woman should not use them until she needs them, generally when she can no longer walk or talk through a contraction. She may become tired if she uses them too early or if she moves to a more advanced technique sooner than she must. If the woman has had no prepared childbirth classes, each technique is taught as she needs it.

Each breathing pattern begins and ends with a cleansing breath, which is a deep inspiration and expiration. The cleansing breaths help the woman relax and focus on relaxing.

### FIRST-STAGE BREATHING

**Slow-Paced Breathing.** The woman begins with a technique of slow-paced breathing. She starts the pattern with a cleansing breath, then breathes slowly, as during sleep (Fig. 7–5A). A cleansing breath ends the contraction. An exact rate is not important, but about six to nine breaths a minute is average. The rate

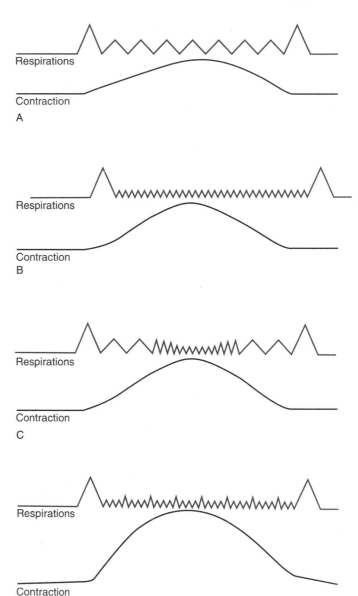

**Figure 7–5.** *A,* Slow-paced breathing. The pattern starts with a cleansing breath as the contraction begins. The woman breathes slowly, at about half her usual rate, ending with a second cleansing breath at the end of the contraction. *B,* As labor intensifies, the woman may need to use modified paced breathing. The pattern begins and ends with a cleansing breath. The woman breathes rapidly, no faster than twice her usual respiratory rate, during the peak of the contraction. She ends with another cleansing breath. *C,* In this variation of modified paced breathing, the woman begins with slow paced breathing at the first of the contraction, switching to faster breathing during its peak. A cleansing breath also begins and ends this pattern. *D,* Patterned paced breathing begins and ends with a cleansing breath. During the contraction, the woman emphasizes the exhalation of some breaths. She may use a specific pattern or may randomly emphasize the blow.

should be at least half her usual rate to ensure adequate fetal oxygenation.

**Modified Paced Breathing.** This pattern begins and ends with a cleansing breath. During the contraction, the woman breathes more rapidly and shallowly (Figs. 7–5B and C). The rate should be no more than twice her usual rate. She may combine slow-paced with modified paced breathing. In this adaptation, she begins with a cleansing breath and breathes slowly until the peak of the contraction, when she begins rapid, shallow breathing. As the contraction abates, she resumes slow, deep breathing and ends with a cleansing breath.

Hyperventilation is sometimes a problem when the woman is breathing rapidly. She may complain of dizziness, tingling, and numbness around her mouth and may have spasms of her fingers and feet. Measures to combat hyperventilation include breathing into her cupped hands or a paper bag, breathing with a washcloth over her face, or holding her breath for a few moments (Box 7–3).

**Patterned Paced Breathing.** Patterned paced breathing is more difficult to teach the unprepared laboring woman because it requires her to focus on the pattern of her breathing. It begins with a cleansing breath, which is followed by rapid breaths punctuated with an intermittent slight blow (Fig. 7–5D), often called pant-blow, or "hee hoo" breathing. The woman may maintain a constant number of breaths before the blow or may vary the number in a specific pattern:

---

- Constant pattern: pant-pant-pant-BLOW, pant-pant-pant-BLOW, etc.
- Stairstep pattern: pant-BLOW, pant-pant-BLOW, pant-pant-pant-BLOW, pant-pant-BLOW, pant-BLOW

In another variation, her partner calls out random numbers to indicate the number of pants to take before a blow.

If she feels an urge to push before her cervix is fully dilated, she is taught to blow in short breaths to avoid bearing down. Pushing before full cervical dilation may cause cervical edema or lacerations.

### SECOND-STAGE BREATHING

When it is time for her to push, the woman takes a cleansing breath, then takes another deep breath and pushes down while exhaling to a count of 10. She blows out, takes a deep breath, and pushes again. Intense breath-holding while pushing (Valsalva maneuver) can reduce uterine blood flow and reduce the fetal oxygen supply. Breath-holding, if necessary during pushing, should be limited to brief periods.

## Pharmacologic Pain Management

Pharmacologic pain management methods include analgesics, adjunctive drugs to improve the effectiveness of analgesics, and anesthetics. Analgesics are systemic drugs (affecting the entire body) that reduce pain without loss of consciousness. Anesthetics cause loss of sensation, especially to pain. Regional anesthetics block sensation from a localized area without causing loss of consciousness. General anesthetics are systemic drugs that cause loss of consciousness. Tables 7–1 and 7–2 summarize intrapartum analgesics and anesthetic methods.

Anesthetics are administered by a variety of clinicians, depending on the type of drug. Local anesthetics are given by the physician or nurse-

---

| BOX 7–3 | How to Recognize and Correct Hyperventilation |
|---|---|

**Signs and Symptoms**

Dizziness
Tingling of hands and feet
Cramps and muscle spasms of hands
Numbness around nose and mouth
Blurring of vision

**Corrective Measures**

Breathe slowly, especially in exhalation
Breathe into cupped hands
Breathe into small paper bag
Hold breath for a few seconds before exhaling

**Table 7–1.** INTRAPARTUM ANALGESICS AND RELATED DRUGS

| Drug/Common Dose/Route of Administration | Nursing Implications |
|---|---|
| *Narcotics*<br>Meperidine (Demerol), 12.5–50 mg IV every 2–4 hr | *Reduce pain*<br>Infant's respirations may be depressed; prepare for respiratory support at birth; continue observing respirations after birth for rate <30/min |
| Butorphanol (Stadol), 0.5–2.0 mg IV every 3–4 hr | Has mixed narcotic and narcotic-antagonist effects; should not be given to the opiate-dependent (heroin) woman or after giving a pure narcotic such as meperidine or morphine; less likelihood for infant respiratory depression, but interventions are the same as for meperidine |
| Nalbuphine (Nubain) 10 mg IV every 3–6 hr | Same as butorphanol |
| *Adjunctive drugs*<br>Promethazine (Phenergan), 12.5–25 mg IM or IV every 4–6 hr | *Enhance effects of narcotics; reduce nausea and vomiting*<br>Increases risk for infant respiratory depression (see meperidine); action is longer than narcotics |
| Propiomazine (Largon), 10–40 mg IM or IV every 3–4 hr | Same as promethazine |
| Diphenhydramine (Benadryl), 25–50 mg IV (dose interval varies) | Relieves itching from epidural narcotics; dries mouth and mucous membranes; provide fluids, if permitted |
| *Narcotic antagonists*<br>Naloxone (Narcan)<br>Adult: 0.4–2 mg IV<br>Neonate: 0.1 mg/kg IV (umbilical vein) or through endotracheal tube during resuscitation | *Reverse adverse effects of narcotics*<br>Action of naloxone is shorter than most narcotics it reverses; observe for recurrent respiratory depression |
| Naltrexone (Trexan): 6 mg PO | Relieves itching from epidural narcotics |

**Table 7–2.** TYPES OF ANESTHESIA FOR CHILDBIRTH

| Anesthetic Method | Nursing Implications |
|---|---|
| *Local infiltration:* injection of the perineum with local anesthetic drug just before vaginal birth; administered by nurse-midwife or physician | Injection may burn until area becomes numb; adverse effects rare |
| *Pudendal block:* injection of the pudendal nerves with local anesthetic just before vaginal birth; local infiltration of the perineum is usually done also; may be used for some forceps births; administered by nurse-midwife or physician | Similar to local infiltration; observe for hematoma (collection of blood within tissues), which may become evident during the recovery period and is evidenced by excessive perineal or pelvic pain; pelvic infection sometimes occurs, but is uncommon |
| *Epidural block:* injection of local anesthetic drug into the epidural space, which blocks transmission of pain impulses to brain; used for pain relief during labor and vaginal birth (including forceps-assisted)—also for cesarean birth; administered by physician (obstetrician or anesthesiologist), or by nurse-anesthetist | Observe for hypotension and urinary retention; assist woman to maintain position as needed by anesthesia clinician; record blood pressure every 5 min after the block is begun and after each reinjection until stable; record fetal heart rates, usually with an electronic fetal monitor; a full bladder often requires catheterization if the woman cannot feel the urge to void |
| *Subarachnoid (spinal) block:* injection of local anesthetic drug under the dura and arachnoid membranes to block transmission of pain impulses to brain; used primarily for cesarean birth; usually administered by anesthesiologist | Observe for hypotension and urinary retention, as in epidural block—interventions are the same; suspect post-spinal headache (usually during postpartum period) if woman complains of a headache that is worse when she is in an upright position; oral fluids and analgesics (as ordered) may relieve mild headache; more severe post-spinal headache will probably require a blood patch (see p. 177) |
| *General anesthesia:* uses a combination of IV and inhalational drugs to produce loss of consciousness; rarely used for vaginal births; used for cesarean birth under some conditions:<br>• Woman's refusal of regional block<br>• Contraindication for regional block<br>• Emergency cesarean when there is not time to establish a regional block | Regurgitation, with aspiration of gastric contents is primary risk; expect order for a clear oral antacid, such as sodium citrate with citric acid (Bicitra); IV drugs to reduce gastric acidity or speed emptying of the stomach may also be given by the anesthesia clinician; assistant gives cricoid pressure until woman is intubated to prevent any regurgitated stomach contents from reaching her trachea because anesthesia is light, woman may move on operating table |

midwife at the time of birth. Other anesthetics may be given by the birth attendant or by a specialist in anesthetic administration.

There are two types of anesthesia clinicians: anesthesiologists and certified registered nurse anesthetists (CRNAs). An anesthesiologist is a physician who specializes in giving anesthesia. A CRNA is a registered nurse who has advanced training in anesthetic administration. State licensing laws and individual facility policies affect what anesthetic methods each clinician may administer.

## ADVANTAGES OF PHARMACOLOGIC METHODS

Methods that employ drugs are among the most effective for reducing pain during birth and can relieve much of it. Many methods help the woman to be a more active participant in birth. They help her relax and work with contractions.

## LIMITATIONS OF PHARMACOLOGIC METHODS

Pharmacologic methods are effective, but they do have limits. One important limitation is that two persons are medicated—the mother and her fetus. Any drug given to the mother can affect the fetus, and the effects may be prolonged in the infant after birth. The drug may directly affect the fetus, or it may cause effects in the mother (such as hypotension) that indirectly affect the fetus.

Several pharmacologic methods may slow labor's progress if used early in labor. Also, some complications during pregnancy limit the pharmacologic methods that are safe to use. For example, a method that requires infusion of large amounts of intravenous fluids might overload the woman's circulation if she has heart disease. If she takes other medications (legal or illicit), they may interact with drugs used to relieve labor pain.

## ANALGESICS AND ADJUNCTIVE DRUGS

### Narcotics

Injectable narcotics are the analgesics most commonly used during labor. Common narcotics for intrapartum use are butorphanol (Stadol), nalbuphine (Nubain), and meperidine (Demerol).

Butorphanol and nalbuphine have mixed narcotic and narcotic-counteracting (antagonistic) effects. Meperidine is a pure narcotic, without mixed effects. Butorphanol and nalbuphine should not be given after a dose of a pure narcotic, or the effects of the first drug will be partly reversed. They should not be given to the woman who abuses opiate drugs, such as heroin, or they may cause withdrawal effects.

The primary risk of narcotic analgesics is that they cross the placenta and can cause the infant's breathing at birth to be sluggish. This is most likely if the drug is given shortly before birth. Meperidine has a prolonged action in the newborn and may depress respirations for several hours after birth. Butorphanol and nalbuphine cause less respiratory depression and are more popular for intrapartum use.

Narcotics are given in small, frequent doses in labor, usually by the intravenous route. This allows the mother to have a fairly stable level of pain relief and limits the amount of drug the fetus receives.

In general, narcotics are avoided if birth is expected within an hour. However, small doses are sometimes given in late labor if the fetus has no problems. The nurse must be prepared to support the respiratory efforts of all infants at birth, especially if the mother received narcotics during labor.

### Narcotic Antagonist

Naloxone (Narcan) is used to reverse respiratory depression caused by narcotics. Naloxone can be given to the infant or to an adult, but the narcotic dose is rarely enough to cause the mother to have respiratory depression. It can be given by the intravenous route, or it may be given through the endotracheal tube during resuscitation. Intravenous naloxone is given to the neonate immediately after birth via the umbilical cord vein.

Naloxone has a shorter duration of action than most of the narcotics it reverses. The nurse should observe for recurrent respiratory depression after each dose of naloxone until the narcotic effects completely cease.

### Adjunctive Drugs

Adjunctive drugs enhance the pain-relieving action of narcotics and reduce nausea. They also intensify the tendency of narcotics to cause respiratory depression.

Promethazine (Phenergan) is a common narcotic adjunct for labor. Promethazine is active longer than most narcotics, and it may not be given with every narcotic dose. Propiomazine (Largon) may be used; its effects are similar to those of promethazine.

## REGIONAL ANESTHETICS

Regional anesthetics block most sensation, and the area is generally numb. However, the woman still feels pressure and may feel some pain. The major advantage of regional anesthetics is that they allow the woman to be awake and participate in birth, yet have satisfactory pain relief.

Local and pudendal blocks are given in the vaginal-perineal area. Epidural and subarachnoid blocks are given by injecting anesthetic drugs so that they bathe the nerves as they emerge from the spinal cord. The spinal cord and nerves are not directly injected in these blocks.

Regional anesthesia uses any of several local anesthetic agents. The agents vary in time needed to become effective and in duration of their anesthetic action. The clinician chooses the agent based on the type of regional block and on the desired onset and duration. The names of most agents end in the suffix *-caine.* Common regional agents in obstetrics are bupivicaine, chloroprocaine, lidocaine, and mepivacaine.

Local anesthetic agents for childbirth are related to those for dental work. On admission, the nurse should ask each woman if she is allergic to or if she has had problems with dental anesthesia. If so, her physician or nurse-midwife should be alerted to enable her to have the most appropriate pain relief measures.

### Local Infiltration

Injection of the perineal area for an episiotomy is done just before birth, when the fetal head is visible (Fig. 7–6). It may also be done after birth to repair a perineal laceration. There is a short delay between injection of the anesthetic agent and loss of pain sensation. The physician or nurse-midwife allows the anesthetic to become effective before beginning the episiotomy. There are virtually no risks if the woman is not allergic to the drug.

### Pudendal Block

The pudendal block is popular for vaginal births. It provides adequate anesthesia for an

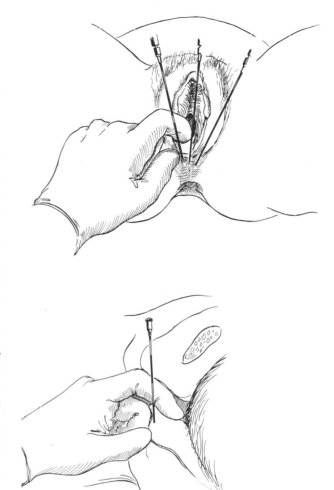

**Figure 7–6.** Local infiltration anesthesia. The physician or nurse-midwife injects a local anesthetic agent into the perineal tissues to numb them.

episiotomy and for most low forceps births (see p. 194). It does not block pain from contractions and, like local infiltration, is given just before birth. There is a delay of a few minutes between injection of the drug and onset of numbness.

The physician or nurse-midwife injects the pudendal nerves on each side of the mother's pelvis (Fig. 7–7). The nerves may be reached

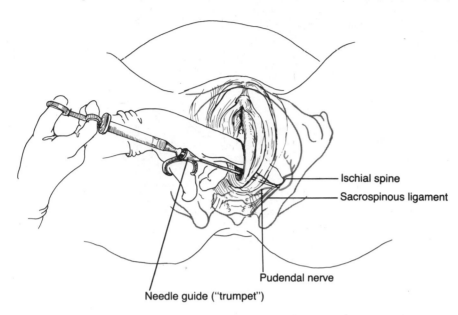

Ischial spine

Sacrospinous ligament

Pudendal nerve

Needle guide ("trumpet")

**Figure 7–7.** Pudendal block anesthesia. The two pudendal nerves on each side of the pelvis are injected to numb the lower two-thirds of the vagina. In addition, local infiltration of the perineum is usually done, because the pudendal block does not always numb this area fully.

through the vagina or by injection directly through her perineum. A long needle (13–15 cm or 5–6 inches) is needed to reach the pudendal nerves, which are near the mother's ischial spines (see Fig. 7–7). If the injection is done through the vagina, a needle guide ("trumpet") is used to protect the mother's tissues. The perineum is also infiltrated because the pudendal block alone may not anesthetize the perineum.

**Adverse Effects of Pudendal Block.** The pudendal block has few adverse effects if the woman is not allergic to the drug. A vaginal hematoma (collection of blood within the tissues) is the most common complication. An abscess may develop, but this is not common.

### Epidural Block

The epidural block, also called a lumbar epidural block, relieves pain of labor and birth. It also can be used for cesarean birth and for postdelivery tubal ligation (see p. 281). It is begun after active labor is established (about 4 cm of cervical dilation) or just before a cesarean birth. The woman may retain some movement and can feel the urge to push if a low concentration of anesthetic agent is used. Higher anesthetic concentrations and a higher level on the woman's body (see Fig. 7–9) are used for cesarean birth or postpartum tubal ligation.

The epidural space is a small space just outside the dura (outermost membrane covering the brain and spinal cord). The woman is in a sitting or side-lying position for the epidural block. Her back is relatively straight, rather than being sharply curved forward, to avoid compressing the tiny epidural space.

The physician or nurse anesthetist penetrates the epidural space with a large needle having a slight curve at the end (16-gauge Tuohy needle). A fine catheter is threaded into the epidural space through the bore of the needle (Fig. 7–8). A test dose (about 3 ml) of local anesthetic agent is injected through the catheter. The woman is *not* expected to have effects from the test dose if the catheter is in the right place. Numbness or loss of movement following the small test dose suggests that her dura mater was punctured and the drug was injected into the subarachnoid space, as in subarachnoid block.

If the test dose is normal (no effects), a larger amount of anesthetic agent is injected to begin the block. A few minutes are needed before the onset of anesthesia. If the block is being used for surgery, such as cesarean delivery or tubal ligation, the anesthesiologist or CRNA will test for the level of numbness before surgery begins (Fig. 7–9).

The woman lies relatively flat, with her head elevated slightly, immediately after the epidural block is begun to promote even dispersion of the anesthetic drug. A roll under her right hip displaces her heavy uterus off the large blood vessels (see discussion of supine hypoten-

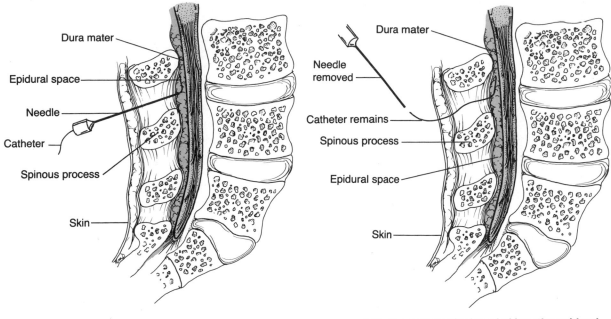

**The epidural space is entered with a needle below where the spinal cord ends. A fine catheter is threaded through the needle.**

**After the catheter is threaded into the epidural space, the needle is removed. Medication can then be injected into the epidural space intermittently or by continuous infusion for pain relief during labor and birth.**

**Figure 7–8.** Epidural block. A needle is inserted into the epidural space, just outside the dura mater. A small catheter is threaded into the space to allow repeated injections of anesthetic agent. The epidural block can eliminate sensations from both contractions and perineal stretching, and it can be used for cesarean birth or postdelivery sterilization.

sive syndrome, p. 59). After the block is established and anesthesia is adequate, she is repositioned about every 30 minutes to maintain anesthesia on both sides of her body.

To maintain pain relief during labor, the anesthetic drug is constantly infused into the catheter. Alternatively, repeat intermittent injections of the drug may be given.

Local anesthetic agents may be used alone in the epidural block, or they may be combined

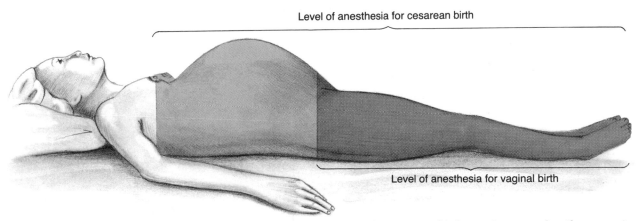

**Figure 7–9.** Levels of anesthesia for epidural or subarachnoid blocks. For cesarean birth, numbness reaches the woman's nipple level. For vaginal birth, the level is about at the hips.

with a narcotic such as fentanyl (Sublimaze). The combined medications provide quicker onset of pain relief, with a lower dose of local anesthetic agent. The woman is more likely to feel the urge to push with contractions during second-stage labor. She also retains more movement.

Long-acting epidural narcotics may be used after cesarean birth to give prolonged postoperative pain relief (up to 24 hours). The woman may need no other analgesia if she receives epidural narcotics, or she may need only mild oral analgesics. Long-acting epidural narcotics can cause respiratory depression that may occur many hours after they are injected. They may also cause intense pruritus (itching), which can be relieved with diphenhydramine (Benadryl) or naltrexone (Trexan).

**Dural Puncture.** The dura lies just below the small epidural space. This membrane is sometimes punctured accidentally with the epidural needle or the catheter that is inserted through it. If dural puncture occurs, a relatively large amount of spinal fluid leaks from the hole and may result in a headache.

**Limitations of Epidural Block.** Although it is a popular method of intrapartum pain relief, epidural block is not used if the woman has

- Defective blood clotting
- An infection in the area of injection or a systemic infection
- Hypovolemia (inadequate blood volume)

**Adverse Effects of Epidural Block.** The most common side effects are maternal hypotension, which can compromise fetal oxygenation, and urinary retention. To counteract hypotension, a large quantity (500–1000 ml or more) of warmed intravenous solution such as Ringer's lactate is infused rapidly before the block is begun. Solutions are warmed because rapid administration of room-temperature intravenous fluids will chill the woman.

The large quantity of intravenous fluids combined with loss of sensation often results in

urinary retention. The woman usually needs urinary catheterization, often several times, before and after birth.

The woman may not feel rectal pressure that gives her the urge to push in the second stage of labor. Therefore, this stage is often longer if a woman has an epidural block. There is no arbitrary time limit for the second stage if the maternal and fetal conditions are normal.

## Subarachnoid (Spinal) Block

Three membranes cover the brain and spinal cord: the dura mater, arachnoid mater, and pia mater membranes. The dura and arachnoid membranes are so close together that they are like a single membrane. The pia mater is a fragile membrane that tightly covers the nerve tissue. Cerebrospinal fluid circulates between the dura-arachnoid membranes and the pia membrane.

The woman's position for a subarachnoid block is similar to that for the epidural block, except that her back is curled around her uterus in a C-shape. The dura is punctured with a thin (25- to 26-gauge) spinal needle. A few drops of spinal fluid confirms entry into the subarachnoid space (Fig. 7–10). The local anesthetic drug is then injected. A much smaller quantity of drug is needed to achieve anesthesia in the subarachnoid block than in the epidural block. Anesthesia occurs quickly, and the woman loses movement and sensation below the block.

The subarachnoid block is a "one-shot" block, since it does not involve placing a catheter for reinjection of the drug. It is not often used for vaginal births today. It remains common for cesarean births. Its limitations are essentially the same as those for epidural block.

**Adverse Effects of Subarachnoid Block.** Hypotension and urinary retention are the main adverse effects of subarachnoid block, as in the epidural block. They are managed as in the epidural block. Hypotension is often more severe.

A postspinal headache sometimes occurs, most likely because of spinal fluid loss. The woman usually remains flat for 4 hours or longer after the block to decrease the chance of postspinal headache.

Postspinal headache is worse when the woman is upright and often disappears entirely when she lies down. Bed rest, analgesics, and oral and intravenous fluids help relieve the

## Nursing Brief

Assess the woman for bladder distention regularly if she has epidural or subarachnoid block. A full bladder can delay birth and can cause hemorrhage after birth.

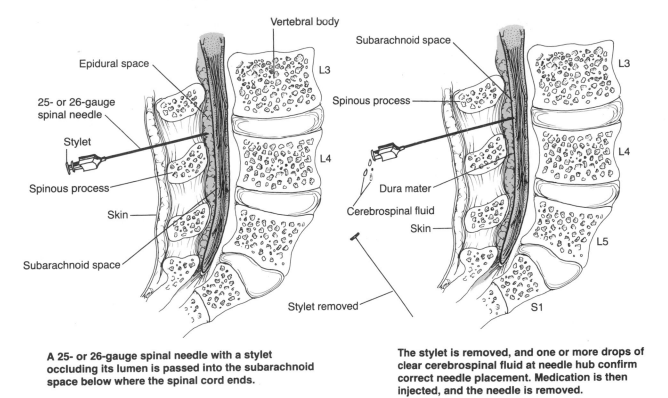

A 25- or 26-gauge spinal needle with a stylet occluding its lumen is passed into the subarachnoid space below where the spinal cord ends.

The stylet is removed, and one or more drops of clear cerebrospinal fluid at needle hub confirm correct needle placement. Medication is then injected, and the needle is removed.

**Figure 7–10.** Subarachnoid block. A fine-gauge hollow needle with a stylet to plug it is inserted into the subarachnoid space. The stylet is removed, and a few drops of cerebrospinal fluid confirm that the needle is in the correct space. Local anesthetic agent is injected. Unlike the epidural, repeat injections are not possible with this method.

headache. A *blood patch*, done by the nurse-anesthetist or anesthesiologist, may give dramatic relief from postspinal headache. The woman's blood (10–15 ml) is withdrawn from her vein and injected into the epidural space in the area of the subarachnoid puncture (Fig. 7–11). The blood clots and forms a gelatinous seal that stops spinal fluid leakage. The clot later breaks down and is reabsorbed by the body.

### Older Regional Blocks

Several regional blocks were once popular but have mostly been abandoned. Their use is uncommon today because of their limitations or adverse effects, or because others (such as epidural block) have become more popular.

**Caudal Block.** The caudal block, a variation of the lumbar epidural, is given in the sacral area. It is more difficult to insert and requires more anesthetic drug than the lumbar epi-

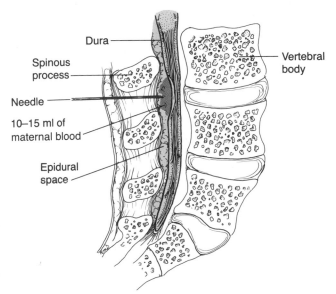

**Figure 7–11.** An epidural blood patch may give dramatic relief from postspinal headache.

dural, thereby increasing the risk that the woman will have an adverse reaction. Injection is also close to the fetal head, which increases the chance of injuring the fetus.

**Paracervical Block.** A paracervical block is done by injecting the cervix itself with a local anesthetic agent during labor. It does not relieve pain during the second stage or during birth. The paracervical block can cause fetal bradycardia (slow heart rate). There is a greater risk for maternal or fetal drug toxicity with this block, especially if several injections are needed.

**Saddle Block.** The saddle block is a subarachnoid block that anesthetizes the lower pelvis and upper legs (the "saddle" area, as in horseback riding). It provides anesthesia for vaginal birth only and is done just before birth. The woman loses all sensation to push. Forceps can be used.

### GENERAL ANESTHESIA

General anesthesia is rarely used for vaginal births and is not used for most cesarean births. Regional blocks are preferred for cesarean births, if possible. General anesthesia is used in these circumstances:

- Emergency cesarean birth, when there is not time to establish either an epidural or a subarachnoid block
- Cesarean birth in the woman who refuses or has a contraindication to epidural or subarachnoid block

Combinations of anesthetic drugs allow quick onset of anesthesia, minimal fetal effects, and prompt maternal wakening.

### Adverse Effects in the Mother

The major adverse effect of general anesthesia is the same during birth as at any other time: regurgitation with aspiration (breathing in) of the acidic stomach contents. This results in a chemical injury to the lungs, aspiration pneumonitis. It can be fatal.

Many women begin labor with a full stomach, and their gastric action slows during labor. Essentially, every pregnant woman is considered to have a full stomach for purposes of general anesthesia.

Several drugs are used to reduce gastric acidity. A clear oral antacid, such as sodium citrate with citric acid (Bicitra), 15 ml, is commonly given before surgery. Ranitidine (Zantac) or cimetidine (Tagamet) may be given intravenously to reduce gastric acidity.

A woman who plans to have epidural or subarachnoid block may unexpectedly need general anesthesia. Therefore, it is usual to give the woman one or more drugs to reduce gastric acidity, even if she plans regional block anesthesia for surgery.

An assistant (often the circulating nurse) gives cricoid pressure (Sellick's maneuver) by compressing the esophagus between the rigid trachea and spine. If regurgitation occurs, the gastric contents cannot pass the area of pressure. After the endotracheal tube is in place, stomach contents cannot enter the trachea, and the pressure is released.

General anesthesia can cause the uterus to relax. This is an advantage when uterine inversion occurs (see p. 210), but it may result in hemorrhage after birth (see p. 219 for assessment of the uterine fundus after birth and p. 252 for nursing care in postpartum hemorrhage).

### Adverse Effects in the Neonate

Respiratory depression is the main neonatal risk, because drugs given to the mother may cross the placenta. To reduce this risk, the time from induction of anesthesia to clamping of the umbilical cord is kept as short as possible. The woman is prepped and draped for surgery, and all personnel are scrubbed, gowned, and gloved before anesthesia begins. Additionally, the anesthesia is kept as light as possible until the cord is clamped. Because the anesthesia is light, the woman may move during surgery, although she does not recall the experience. Respiratory depression can occur in the woman, but this is less common than in the neonate because minimal doses of anesthetic drugs are used.

# The Nurse's Role in Pain Management

The nurse has many responsibilities in both nonpharmacologic and pharmacologic pain management during the intrapartum period. Nursing care reduces factors that hinder a woman's pain control and enhances factors that benefit it. Nursing Care Plan 7–1 is an exam-

| NURSING CARE PLAN 7–1 |
| --- |

## Selected Nursing Diagnoses for the Woman Needing Pain Management During Labor

| Goals | Nursing Interventions | Rationale |
| --- | --- | --- |

**Nursing Diagnosis:** Pain related to uterine contractions and descent of fetus in pelvis.

| | | |
| --- | --- | --- |
| Woman will relate that her discomfort is manageable during labor using techniques learned in prepared childbirth classes<br><br>Woman will have a relaxed facial and body appearance between contractions | 1. Assess for presence and character of pain continuously during labor:<br>  a. Statement of pain (assess nature of pain, such as location, intensity, whether intermittent or constant)<br>  b. Crying, moaning during and/or between contractions<br>  c. Tense, guarded body posture or thrashing with contractions<br>  d. "Mask of pain" facial expression | 1. These are common verbal and nonverbal signs of pain; assessment enables nurse to identify whether pain is normal for woman's labor status; assessment also helps nurse identify best interventions for pain relief (nonpharmacologic and/or pharmacologic measures); evaluating nonverbal and verbal communication helps nurse evaluate need for pain relief in women who may not directly communicate their need for pain relief or who do not speak prevailing language |
| | 2. Provide general comfort measures, such as<br>  a. Adjust the room temperature and light level for comfort<br>  b. Reduce irritants, such as wet underpads<br>  c. Provide ice chips, Popsicles, or juices to relieve dry mouth, if medical orders permit<br>  d. Avoid bumping her bed | 2. These general measures reduce outside irritants that make it harder for woman to use prepared childbirth techniques; they are also a source of discomfort themselves |
| | 3. Encourage woman to assume positions she finds most comfortable, other than the supine (see Chap. 6 for more information) | 3. Position changes promote comfort and help fetus adapt to size and shape of woman's pelvis; supine position can result in supine hypotensive syndrome (see p. 59), which may reduce placental blood flow and fetal oxygenation |
| | 4. Observe for a full bladder every 1–2 hr, or more often if the woman receives large amounts of PO or IV fluids | 4. A full bladder is a source of discomfort and can prolong labor by inhibiting fetal descent; it may cause pain that persists after epidural anesthesia is begun |
| | 5. Promote use of prepared childbirth techniques, including labor partner as appropriate:<br>  a. Do not stand in front of her focal point<br>  b. Offer a back rub or firm sacral pressure; ask the best location and amount of pressure; use baby powder to prevent skin irritation<br>  c. Encourage woman to switch to more complex patterns only when simpler ones are no longer effective<br>  d. Breathe along with woman if she has trouble maintaining patterns; make eye contact | 5. These are examples of how to assist woman and her partner in using methods they learned most effectively; use of nonpharmacologic pain relief techniques avoids problems associated with pharmacologic interventions and supplements any drug therapy used; they also give woman and partner a sense of control and mastery, which enhances perception of birth as a positive experience |

*Continued*

| NURSING CARE PLAN 7–1 *Continued* |
|---|

## Selected Nursing Diagnoses for the Woman Needing Pain Management During Labor

| Goals | Nursing Interventions | Rationale |
|---|---|---|

**Nursing Diagnosis:** Pain related to uterine contractions and descent of fetus in pelvis.

| | 6. If woman has signs of hyperventilation (dizziness, numbness or tingling sensations, spasms of the hands and feet), have her breathe into her cupped hands, a small bag, or a washcloth placed over her mouth and nose; or instruct her to hold her breath briefly | 6. Hyperventilation often occurs when woman uses rapid breathing patterns because she exhales too much carbon dioxide; these measures help her conserve carbon dioxide and rebreathe it to correct excess loss |
|---|---|---|
| | 7. Tell woman and her partner when labor progresses; for example, if she is pushing and her baby's head becomes visible, let her see or feel it | 7. Labor does not last forever; knowing that her efforts are having desired results gives her courage to continue and helps her tolerate pain |

**Nursing Diagnosis:** Knowledge deficit: procedures and expected effects of epidural block.

| After explanations, woman will state that she understands what will happen during and after epidural block is begun | 1. Explain what to expect as the epidural block is begun (reinforcing explanations of anesthesiologist or nurse-anesthetist):<br>a. An IV will be started and she will receive fluids to offset the tendency of her blood pressure to fall<br>b. Fetus will be monitored by electronic fetal monitoring<br>c. Nurse-anesthetist or anesthesiologist will position her; she should remain still in this position<br>d. A small plastic catheter will be taped to her back to allow constant infusion of medication (or reinjection, depending on the anesthesia clinician's preference)<br>e. Her blood pressure will be checked every 5 min when block is first begun | 1. This list reflects a common sequence of events for starting an epidural block; anesthesia clinician explains the procedure and expected effects; nurse reinforces explanations as needed; knowledge reduces anxiety and fear of the unknown; if woman understands that these procedures are a normal part of epidural block anesthesia, she is less likely to interpret them as abnormal |
|---|---|---|
| | 2. Explain that she will lie relatively flat for a short period but that a small pillow will be placed under her right hip. After she is numb, she should regularly turn from side to side | 2. These methods allow even dispersion of anesthetic drug to prevent a one-sided block; pillow under hip avoids supine hypotensive syndrome |
| | 3. Explain that she will feel less pain but that she may still feel pressure; she may be able to move her legs normally, or she may not be able to move them | 3. Helps woman understand that epidural block is not expected to completely eliminate pain; leg movement is affected in varying amounts; if she understands variation in effects, she is less likely to interpret them as abnormal or as evidence that block is not working |

| NURSING CARE PLAN 7–1 *Continued* | | |
|---|---|---|
| **Selected Nursing Diagnoses for the Woman Needing Pain Management During Labor** | | |
| **Goals** | **Nursing Interventions** | **Rationale** |

**Nursing Diagnosis:** High risk for injury related to loss of sensation.

| Goals | Nursing Interventions | Rationale |
|---|---|---|
| Woman will not have an injury, such as muscle strain or fall, during the time her epidural is in effect<br>Fetus will not be born in uncontrolled delivery | 1. Keep woman in bed while block is in effect; check for movement and sensation before ambulating after birth; ambulate cautiously, with an assistant, after her sensation returns<br>2. Observe for signs that birth may be near:<br>　a. Increase in bloody show<br>　b. Statement of pressure or need to push (may *not* be present, depending on individual response to block)<br>　c. Bulging of the perineum or appearance of head | 1. Woman is likely to fall if she does not have sensation and full control over her movements; there is considerable variation in time required for sensation and movement to return<br>2. Loss of sensation varies considerably among women; with her pain relieved, woman's labor may progress more rapidly than expected; these are signs associated with imminent birth that should be evaluated by the experienced nurse, nurse-midwife, or physician |

ple of nursing measures related to intrapartum comfort.

## THE NURSE'S ROLE IN NONPHARMACOLOGIC TECHNIQUES

When a woman is admitted, the nurse determines if she had preparation for childbirth and works with what the woman and her partner learned. The nurse may need to suggest variations in the methods they learned if what they are doing is ineffective. The nurse helps them identify signs of tension so that the woman can be guided to release it.

If the woman did not have childbirth preparation, the nurse teaches her the simple breathing techniques discussed earlier in the chapter. If the woman is extremely anxious and out of control, she will not be able to comprehend verbal instructions. It may be necessary to make close eye contact with her and breathe with her through each contraction until she can regain control.

The nurse minimizes environmental irritants as much as possible. The lights should be lowered and the woman kept reasonably dry by regularly changing her disposable underpads. The temperature should be adjusted; the nurse provides a warm blanket if that provides most comfort. See Chapter 6 for other general comfort measures during labor.

The nurse should be cautious not to overestimate or underestimate the amount of pain a woman is having. The quiet, stoic woman may need analgesia, yet be reluctant to ask. A tense body posture or grimacing may indicate she needs additional pain relief measures.

The vocal woman who complains bitterly about her distress in labor is also difficult to assess. It is difficult to evaluate pain relief needs in the woman who moans and cries most of the time. She may need additional pain relief measures, or she may simply be a person who is vocal during labor.

## THE NURSE'S ROLE IN PHARMACOLOGIC TECHNIQUES

The nurse's responsibility in pharmacologic pain management begins at admission. The woman should be closely questioned about allergy to drugs, including dental anesthetics, to identify pain relief measures that may not be advisable.

## Nursing Brief

Important admission assessments related to pharmacologic pain management are last oral intake (time and type), adverse reactions to drugs—especially dental anesthetics, and other medications taken.

The nurse keeps the side rails up if the woman takes pain relief drugs. Narcotics may cause drowsiness or dizziness. Regional anesthetics block sensation and movement to varying degrees, so the woman will have impaired control over her body.

The nurse ambulates the woman cautiously after birth if she had an epidural or subarachnoid block. She may be able to move her legs yet not be able to feel her feet, which would make her likely to fall.

If the woman receives narcotic drugs, the nurse observes her respiratory rate for depression. Because respiratory depression is more likely to occur in the neonate than in the mother, the neonate is observed after birth. Narcotic effects in the infant may persist for longer than in an adult. The nurse has naloxone on hand in case it is needed to reverse respiratory depression in the mother or infant.

The nurse observes the woman for late-appearing respiratory depression if she had epidural narcotics. This may be up to 24 hours for drugs given after cesarean birth. The woman's respiratory status is monitored with hourly respiratory rate assessment, a pulse oximeter, and/or an apnea monitor. Additional analgesics are given cautiously, and strictly as ordered. If mild analgesics do not relieve the pain, the physician is contacted for additional orders. Analgesics in addition to the epidural narcotic can increase respiratory depression.

The nurse reinforces explanations given by the anesthesia clinician about procedures and expected effects of the selected pain management method. Women often receive these explanations when they are very uncomfortable and do not remember everything they were told.

The woman is helped to assume and hold the position for the epidural or subarachnoid block. The nurse tells the anesthesia clinician if the woman has a contraction because it might prevent her from holding still. Also, the anesthetic drug is usually injected between contractions.

The woman is observed for hypotension if an epidural or subarachnoid block is given. Hospital protocols vary, but the blood pressure is usually taken every 5 minutes after the block is begun (and with each reinjection) until her blood pressure is stable. At the same time, the nurse observes the fetus for signs associated with fetal compromise (see p. 145), since maternal hypotension can reduce placental blood flow.

The epidural block is given during labor and may eliminate the mother's sensation of rectal pressure. The nurse coaches her about the right time to start and stop pushing with each contraction. The nurse also observes for signs of imminent birth, such as increased bloody show and perineal bulging, since she may not be able to feel the sensations clearly.

Nursing responsibilities related to general anesthesia include assessment and documentation of oral intake and administration of medications to reduce gastric acidity. The woman should be told that all preparations for surgery will be done *before* she is put to sleep. The nurse reassures her that she will be asleep before any incision is done. A familiar nurse in the operating room is reassuring to the woman before surgery.

The woman who has general anesthesia is usually awake enough to move from the operating table to her bed after surgery. Her respiratory status is observed every 15 minutes for 1–2 hours. A pulse oximeter provides constant information about her blood oxygen level. She may receive oxygen by face tent or other means until she is fully awake. See a medical-surgical nursing text for more information about postanesthesia nursing care. Her uterine fundus and vaginal bleeding are observed as for any other postpartum woman.

## KEY POINTS

- Pain during birth is different from other types of pain because it is part of a normal process that results in the birth of a baby. The woman has time to prepare for it, and the pain is self-limiting.
- A woman's pain threshold is fairly constant. Her pain tolerance varies, and nursing actions can increase her ability to tolerate pain.
- Prepared childbirth classes give the woman and her partner pain management tools they can use during labor. Some tools, such as breathing techniques, can be taught to the unprepared woman.

- The nurse should do everything possible to promote relaxation during labor because it enhances the effectiveness of all other pain management methods, nonpharmacologic and pharmacologic.
- Any drug that the expectant mother takes may cross the placenta and affect the fetus. Effects may persist in the baby much longer than in an adult.
- Observe the mother and/or infant for respiratory depression if she received narcotics, including epidural narcotics, during the intrapartum period.
- Regional anesthetics are the most common for birth because they allow the mother to remain awake, including for cesarean birth.
- Closely question the woman about drug allergies when she is admitted. Because drugs used for regional anesthesia are related to those used in dentistry, ask her about reactions to dental anesthesia.
- Observe the mother's blood pressure and the fetal heart rate after epidural or spinal block to identify hypotension or fetal compromise. Urinary retention is also likely.
- Be prepared to administer a drug to reduce gastric acidity if surgery is anticipated, since general anesthesia may unexpectedly be needed.

# Study Questions

1. What nursing measures can reduce a laboring woman's anxiety?
2. How can excessive pain, anxiety, or fear adversely affect labor?
3. A laboring woman uses breathing techniques she learned in prepared childbirth classes. She complains of feeling "tingly" and says her fingers are stiff. What is the most likely reason for her symptoms? What nursing measures relieve them?
4. Why should a woman's addiction to heroin be reported to her experienced intrapartum nurse?
5. A newborn is given naloxone (Narcan) because the mother received a narcotic 30 minutes before birth. What is the purpose of naloxone, and what should the nurse observe for in relation to this drug?
6. Why is bladder assessment, before and after birth, particularly important if the woman has epidural anesthesia?
7. Why should the woman receiving epidural block anesthesia be regularly repositioned?
8. A woman had a subarachnoid block for a cesarean birth. When the nurse gets her up the following day, she complains about a sudden severe headache. What is the most likely reason for her symptoms?
9. How should the nurse prepare a woman planning to have general anesthesia for a cesarean birth?

# Multiple Choice Review Questions

*Choose the most appropriate answer.*

1. Specify which of the following situations best describes a woman's use of the gate control theory to manage pain. She
   a. breathes slowly at the beginning and end of a contraction but more rapidly at its peak
   b. rubs the palms of her hands on the bed's side rails during each contraction
   c. focuses intently on a photograph that she brought to the birth center
   d. listens to tapes of rain and waterfalls through headphones

2. The most common method of child-birth preparation in the United States is the
   a. Dick-Read method to reduce fear, tension, and pain
   b. Bradley method of husband-coached childbirth
   c. Lamaze method of psychoprophylaxis
3. Which exercise is useful to reduce urine stress incontinence?
   a. neuromuscular dissociation
   b. tailor stretching
   c. pelvic rock
   d. Kegel exercise
4. Which technique is likely to be most effective for "back labor?"
   a. stimulating the abdomen by effleurage
   b. applying firm pressure in the sacral area
   c. blowing out in short breaths during the most intense part of each contraction
   d. rocking side to side at the peak of each contraction
5. A woman is dilated 7 cm and feels that she must push with each contraction. The most appropriate action at this time is to
   a. coach her to blow out in short bursts whenever she feels the urge to push
   b. encourage her to push when she feels the urge, but not to hold her breath
   c. give her a paper bag and have her breathe into it during each contraction
   d. have her take deep, slow breaths at the beginning of the contraction, then push briefly when she has a strong urge
6. Butorphanol (Stadol) should not be given to which of these laboring women?
   a. a primigravida whose cervix is dilated 5 cm
   b. a heroin-dependent primigravida
   c. a multipara whose cervix is dilated 4 cm
   d. a multipara who has pregnancy-induced hypertension
7. The usual route of administration for narcotics during labor is
   a. subcutaneous
   b. intramuscular
   c. intravenous
   d. intratracheal
8. What drug should be immediately available when a woman receives narcotics?
   a. fentanyl (Sublimaze)
   b. diphenhydramine (Benadryl)
   c. lidocaine (Xylocaine)
   d. naloxone (Narcan)
9. What order should be anticipated for a woman who expects to have an epidural block?
   a. antinausea drug
   b. intravenous infusion
   c. heat applications
   d. naltrexone (Trexan)
10. Choose the most important nursing assessment immediately after a woman has an epidural block.
    a. bladder distention
    b. intravenous site
    c. respiratory rate
    d. blood pressure
11. A woman will have general anesthesia for a repeat cesarean delivery. What order related to this anesthetic should the nurse expect?
    a. clear antacid
    b. narcotic premedication
    c. 500 ml oral fluids
    d. naloxone (Narcan) injection

## BIBLIOGRAPHY

Abboud, T.K., Afrasiabi, A., Davidson, J., Zhu, J., Reyes, A., Khoo, N., & Steffens, Z. (1990). Prophylactic oral naltrexone with epidural morphine: Effect on adverse reactions and ventilatory responses to carbon dioxide. *Anesthesiology, 72*, 233–237.

Abboud, T.K., Lee, K., Zhu, J., Reyes, A., Afrasiabi, A., Mantilla, M., Steffens, Z., & Chai, M. (1990). Prophylactic oral naltrexone with intrathecal morphine for cesarean section: Effects on adverse reactions and analgesia. *Anesthesia and Analgesia, 71*, 367–370.

American Academy of Pediatrics and American College of Obstetricians and Gynecologists. (1992). *Guidelines for perinatal care* (3rd ed.). Elk Grove Village, IL: Author.

Blackburn, S., & Loper, D. (1992). *Maternal, fetal and neonatal physiology: A clinical perspective.* Philadelphia: W.B. Saunders.

Bowes, W.A. (1989). Clinical aspects of normal and abnormal labor. In R.K. Creasy & R. Resnik (Eds.), *Maternal-fetal medicine: Principles and practice* (pp. 510–546). Philadelphia: W.B. Saunders.

Butler, M., Luther, D., & Frederick, E. (1988). Coaching: The labor companion. In F.H. Nichols & S.S. Humenick (Eds.), *Childbirth education: Practice, research and theory* (pp. 275–290). Philadelphia: W.B. Saunders.

Chung, D.C., & Lam, A.M. (1990). *Essentials of anesthesiology.* Philadelphia: W.B. Saunders.

Conklin, K. (1992). Obstetric analgesia and anesthesia. In N.F. Hacker & J.G. Moore (Eds.), *Essentials of obstetrics and gynecology* (2nd ed., pp. 134–146). Philadelphia: W.B. Saunders.

Eakes, M. (1990). Economic considerations for epidural anesthesia in childbirth. *Nursing Economics, 8,* 329–332.

Geden, E.A., Lower, M., Beattie, S., & Beck, N. (1989). Effects of music and imagery on physiologic and self-report of analogued labor pain. *Nursing Research, 38,* 37–40.

Gennaro, S. (1988). The childbirth experience. In F.H. Nichols & S.S. Humenick (Eds.), *Childbirth education: Practice, research and theory* (pp. 52–68). Philadelphia: W.B. Saunders.

Gorrie, T. (1989). *A guide to the nursing of childbearing families.* Baltimore: Williams & Wilkins.

Gorrie, T., McKinney, E., & Murray, S. (1994). *Foundations of maternal-newborn nursing.* Philadelphia: W.B. Saunders.

Hetherington, S.E. (1990). A controlled study of the effect of prepared childbirth classes on obstetric outcomes. *Birth, 17,* 86–90.

Isenor, L. & Penny-MacGillivray, T. (1993). Intravenous meperidine infusion for obstetric analgesia. *JOGNN: Journal of Obstetric, Gynecologic, and Neonatal Nursing, 22,* 349–356.

Jimenez, S.L.M. (1988). Supportive pain management strategies. In F.H. Nichols & S.S. Humenick (Eds.), *Childbirth education: Practice, research and theory* (pp. 95–117). Philadelphia: W.B. Saunders.

Nakahata, A. (1988). Exercise. In F.H. Nichols & S.S. Humenick (Eds.), *Childbirth education: Practice, research and theory* (pp. 344–361). Philadelphia: W.B. Saunders.

Nicholson, C. (1990). Nursing considerations for the parturient who has received epidural narcotics during labor or delivery. *Journal of Perinatal & Neonatal Nursing, 4,* 14–26.

Rose, A.T., & Hilbers, S.M. (1988). Relaxation: Paced breathing techniques. In F.H. Nichols & S.S. Humenick (Eds.), *Childbirth education: Practice, research and theory* (pp. 216–233). Philadelphia: W.B. Saunders.

Sharts-Engel, N. (1991). Naloxone review and pediatric dosage update. *MCN: American Journal of Maternal-Child Nursing, 16,* 182.

Shrock, P. (1988). The basis of relaxation. In F.H. Nichols & S.S. Humenick (Eds.), *Childbirth education: Practice, research and theory* (pp. 118–132). Philadelphia: W.B. Saunders.

Steffes, S.A. (1988). Relaxation: Imagery. In F.H. Nichols & S.S. Humenick (Eds.), *Childbirth education: Practice, research and theory* (pp. 184–200). Philadelphia: W.B. Saunders.

Steiner, S.H., & Steiner, J.F. (1988). Pharmaceutical pain management strategies. In F.H. Nichols & S.S. Humenick (Eds.), *Childbirth education: Practice, research and theory* (pp. 291–302). Philadelphia: W.B. Saunders.

Taylor, T. (1993). Epidural anesthesia in the maternity patient. *MCN: American Journal of Maternal-Child Nursing, 18,* 86–93.

Wild, L., & Coyne, C. The basics and beyond: Epidural analgesia. *American Journal of Nursing, 92,* 26–34.

Wisenberg, M., & Caspi, Z. (1989). Cultural and educational influences on pain of childbirth. *Journal of Pain and Symptom Management, 4,* 13–19.

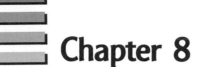

## Chapter 8

# Nursing Care of Women with Complications During Labor and Birth

## OBJECTIVES

*On completion and mastery of Chapter 8, the student will be able to*

- Define each vocabulary term listed.
- Describe each obstetric procedure discussed in this chapter.
- Explain the nurse's role in each obstetric procedure.
- Describe factors that contribute to an abnormal labor.
- Explain each intrapartum complication discussed in this chapter.
- Explain the nurse's role in each intrapartum complication.

Childbirth is a normal, natural event in the life of most women and their families. When the many factors that affect the birth process function in harmony, complications are unlikely. However, some women experience complications during childbirth that threaten their well-being or that of the baby.

## Obstetric Procedures

Nurses assist with several obstetric procedures during birth; they also care for women after the procedures. Some are done in otherwise uncomplicated births. Others are needed for women who have complications during birth.

### AMNIOTOMY

Amniotomy, abbreviated AROM, is artificial rupture of the membranes (amniotic sac, or "bag of waters") by using a sterile sharp instrument. It is performed by a physician or nurse-midwife. Amniotomy is not a nursing function of either the registered or practical nurse. The nurse assists with amniotomy and cares for the woman and fetus afterward.

Amniotomy is done to stimulate contractions. It may provide enough stimulation to start labor before it begins naturally, but it is more often done to enhance contractions that have already begun. It may also be done to permit internal fetal monitoring (see p. 141).

### Technique

To determine if amniotomy is safe and indicated, the physician or nurse-midwife does a vaginal examination to assess the cervical effacement and dilation and the station of the fetus (see pp. 123 and 131). A disposable plastic hook is passed through the cervix, and the amniotic sac is snagged to create a hole and release the amniotic fluid (Fig. 8–1).

### Complications

The three complications associated with amniotomy may also occur if a woman's membranes rupture spontaneously (abbreviated SROM, for spontaneous rupture of membranes). These are prolapse of the umbilical cord, infection, and abruptio placentae.

**Prolapse of the Umbilical Cord.** Prolapse may occur if the cord slips downward with a gush of fluid (see p. 209).

**Infection.** Infection may occur because the membranes no longer block vaginal organisms from entering the uterus. An amniotomy essentially "commits" the woman to delivery. The physician or nurse-midwife delays amniotomy until reasonably certain that birth will occur before the risk of infection markedly increases.

**Abruptio Placentae.** Abruptio placentae (separation of the placenta before birth) is more likely to occur if the uterus is overdistended with amniotic fluid (hydramnios) when the membranes rupture. The uterus becomes smaller with discharge of amniotic fluid, but the placenta stays the same size and no longer fits its implantation site (see p. 87 for more information about abruptio placentae).

### Nursing Care

The main nursing care after amniotomy is the same as that following spontaneous membrane rupture: identifying complications and promoting the woman's comfort.

## Nursing Brief

Observe for wet underpads and linens after the membranes rupture. Change them as often as needed to keep the woman relatively dry.

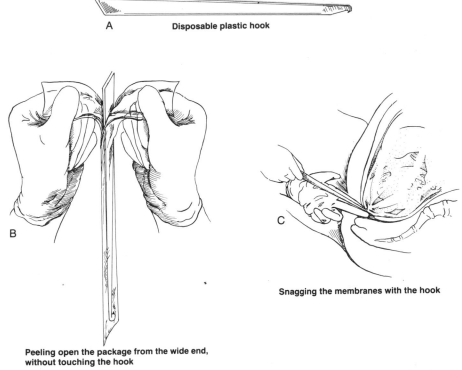

A    **Disposable plastic hook**

B

Peeling open the package from the wide end,
without touching the hook

C

Snagging the membranes with the hook

**Figure 8–1.** Amniotomy. *A*, The Amnihook disposable plastic hook. *B*, Technique to open the Amnihook package for the physician or nurse-midwife. *C*, Method of rupturing the membranes.

**Identifying Complications.** The fetal heart rate is recorded for at least 1 minute after amniotomy. Rates outside the normal range of 110–160 beats/min for a term fetus suggest a prolapsed umbilical cord. A large quantity of fluid increases the risk for prolapsed cord, especially if the fetus is above a 0 station.

The color, odor, amount, and character of amniotic fluid are recorded. The fluid should be clear, possibly with flecks of vernix (newborn skin coating), and should not have a bad odor. Cloudy, yellow, or malodorous fluid suggests infection.

The woman's temperature is taken every 2 hours after her membranes rupture. A maternal temperature of 38°C (100.4°F) or higher suggests infection. An increase in the fetal heart rate, especially if above 160 beats/min, may precede the woman's temperature increase.

Green fluid means that the fetus passed the first stool (meconium) into the fluid before birth. Meconium-stained amniotic fluid is more common if the gestation is post term (more than 42 weeks) or if the placenta is not func-

tioning well. The fluid may range from barely green-tinged and watery, to thick with meconium and scant ("pea soup"). Meconium-stained amniotic fluid, especially if thick, is associated with fetal compromise during labor and infant respiratory distress after birth (see p. 329).

**Promoting Comfort.** When amniotomy is anticipated, several disposable underpads are placed under the woman's hips to absorb the fluid, extending from about her mid-back to her knees. Amniotic fluid continues to leak from the woman's vagina during labor. Disposable underpads are changed often enough to keep her reasonably dry and to reduce the moist, warm environment that favors growth of microorganisms.

## INDUCTION OR AUGMENTATION OF LABOR

*Induction* of labor is the initiation of labor before it begins naturally. *Augmentation* is the stimulation of contractions after they have begun naturally.

## Indications

Labor is induced if continuing the pregnancy is more hazardous for the woman and fetus than shortening it by artificial means. Examples of hazardous conditions are

- Pregnancy-induced hypertension (see p. 88)
- Ruptured membranes without spontaneous onset of labor (see p. 206)
- Infection within the uterus
- Medical problems in the woman that worsen during pregnancy, such as diabetes, kidney disease, or pulmonary disease
- Fetal problems, such as slowed growth, prolonged pregnancy (see p. 208), or incompatibility between fetal and maternal blood types (see p. 98)
- Fetal death

Convenience for the physician or family is not an indication for induction of labor. However, the woman who has a history of rapid labors and lives a long distance from the birth facility may have her labor induced because she has a risk of giving birth en route if she awaits spontaneous labor.

## Contraindications

Labor is not induced if spontaneous labor should not occur, such as in these conditions:

- Placenta previa (see p. 86)
- Umbilical cord prolapse (see p. 209)
- Abnormal fetal presentation
- High station of the fetus, which suggests a preterm fetus or a small maternal pelvis
- Active herpes infection in the birth canal, which the baby can acquire during birth (see p. 108)
- Abnormal size or structure of the mother's pelvis
- Previous classic (vertical) cesarean incision (see p. 197)

The physician may attempt labor induction in a preterm pregnancy if continuing the pregnancy is more harmful to the woman and/or fetus than the hazards of prematurity would be to the infant.

## Technique

Amniotomy may be the only method used to initiate labor, but it is more likely to be used in addition to oxytocin to stimulate contractions.

Induction and augmentation of labor may employ drug and nondrug methods.

**Cervical Ripening.** Induction of labor is easier if the woman's cervix is soft, partially effaced, and beginning to dilate. These prelabor cervical changes occur naturally in most women. Methods to produce the changes, or "ripen" the cervix, ease labor induction.

Prostaglandin gel (Prepidil) softens the cervix when applied before labor induction. It is given in the hospital, and the woman is observed in the labor area for a short time after application. Oxytocin induction is begun 6–12 hours after application of the prostaglandin gel. Some women who receive the gel begin labor without oxytocin stimulation.

An alternative to prostaglandin gel for cervical ripening is insertion of one or more laminaria into the cervix. A laminaria is a narrow cone of a substance that absorbs water. The laminaria swells inside the cervix, thus beginning cervical dilation. Oxytocin induction follows, usually on the next day.

**Oxytocin Induction and Augmentation of Labor.** Initiation or stimulation of contractions with oxytocin (Pitocin) is the most common method of labor induction and augmentation in hospital births. Oxytocin is administered by registered nurses with additional training in induction of labor and electronic fetal monitoring. Augmentation of labor with oxytocin follows a similar procedure.

Oxytocin for induction or augmentation of labor is diluted in an intravenous solution. The oxytocin solution is a secondary (piggyback) infusion that is inserted into the primary (nonmedicated) intravenous solution line so that it can be stopped quickly while an open intravenous line is maintained.

Infusion of oxytocin solution is regulated with an infusion pump. Administration begins at a very low rate and is adjusted upward or downward according to how the fetus responds to labor and to the woman's contractions. There is no standard dose. Augmentation of labor usually requires less total oxytocin than induction of labor, because the uterus is more sensitive to the drug.

Continuous electronic fetal monitoring is the usual method to assess and record fetal and maternal responses to oxytocin. Many physicians prefer internal methods of fetal monitoring when oxytocin is used, because these are more accurate than external methods, although they require that the membranes be ruptured.

**Nondrug Methods to Stimulate Contractions.** The nurse has several nondrug options to help the woman whose contractions have become less effective.

*Walking.* Many women benefit from a change in activity if their labor slows. Walking stimulates contractions, eases pressure of the fetus on the mother's back, and adds gravity to the downward force of contractions. If she does not feel like walking, other upright positions often improve the effectiveness of each contraction. She cannot walk if an epidural block is in effect.

*Nipple Stimulation of Labor.* Stimulating the nipples causes the woman's posterior pituitary gland to secrete natural oxytocin. This improves the quality of contractions that have slowed or weakened, just as synthetic intravenous oxytocin does. She can stimulate her nipples by

- Pulling or rolling them, one at a time
- Gently brushing them with a dry washcloth
- Using water in a whirlpool tub or a shower
- Applying suction with a breast pump (see p. 240)

If contractions become too strong with these techniques, the woman stops them.

## Complications of Oxytocin Induction and Augmentation of Labor

The most common complications, related to overstimulation of contractions, are fetal compromise and uterine rupture. Fetal compromise can occur because blood flow to the placenta is reduced if contractions are excessive. See page 210 for discussion of uterine rupture.

Water intoxication sometimes occurs because oxytocin inhibits excretion of urine and promotes fluid retention. Water intoxication is not common with the small amounts of oxytocin and fluids given intravenously during labor, but it is more likely to occur if large doses of oxytocin and fluids are given intravenously after birth.

Oxytocin is discontinued, or its rate reduced, if signs of fetal compromise or excessive uterine contractions occur. Fetal heart rates outside the normal range of 110–160 beats/min, late decelerations, and loss of variability (see p. 142) are the most common signs of fetal compromise. Excessive uterine contractions are most often evidenced by frequency less than every 2 minutes, durations longer than 90 seconds, or resting intervals shorter than 60 seconds. The resting tone of the uterus (muscle tension when it is not contracting) is often higher than normal.

Internal uterine activity monitoring allows determination, in millimeters of mercury (mmHg), of peak uterine pressures and uterine resting tone.

In addition to stopping the oxytocin infusion, the registered nurse chooses one or more of these measures to correct adverse maternal or fetal reactions:

- Increasing the nonmedicated intravenous solution
- Keeping the woman on her side or repositioning her
- Giving oxygen by face mask

The physician is notified after corrective measures are taken. A tocolytic (drug that reduces uterine contractions) may be ordered if contractions do not quickly decrease after oxytocin is stopped.

### Nursing Care

Nursing care in labor induction and augmentation is directed by the registered nurse and by hospital policies. Baseline maternal vital signs are assessed and a fetal monitor tracing is done to identify contraindications to induction or augmentation.

During induction or augmentation, the principal nursing observations are the fetal heart rate and character of uterine contractions. If abnormalities are noted in either, the nurse stops the oxytocin and begins measures listed to reduce contractions and increase placental blood flow.

The woman's blood pressure, pulse, and respirations are taken every 30–60 minutes. Her temperature is taken every 4 hours (every 2 hours after her membranes rupture). Recording her intake and output identifies water intoxication.

### VERSION

Version is a method of changing the fetal presentation, usually from breech to cephalic.

## Nursing Brief

Women who have oxytocin stimulation of labor may find their contractions are difficult to manage. Help them stay focused on breathing and relaxation techniques with each contraction.

There are two methods, external and internal. External version is the more common one. A successful version reduces the likelihood that the woman will need cesarean delivery.

### Risks and Contraindications

There are few maternal and fetal risks associated with version, especially external version. Version is not indicated if there is any maternal or fetal reason why vaginal birth should not occur, since that is its goal. Examples of maternal conditions that are contraindications for version are

- Abnormal uterine or pelvic size or shape
- Most cases of previous cesarean birth
- Abnormal placental placement

The main risk to the fetus is that it will become entangled in the umbilical cord, thus compressing the cord. This is more likely to happen if there is not adequate room to turn the fetus, such as in multifetal gestation (e.g., twins) or when the amount of amniotic fluid is small. Version is not done if there are signs that the placenta is not functioning normally.

### Technique

External version is done after 37 weeks of gestation. The procedure begins with a non-stress test or biophysical profile (see Table 5–5, p. 93) to determine if the fetus is in good condition and if there is adequate amniotic fluid to perform the version. The woman receives a tocolytic drug to "quiet" her uterus during the version.

Using ultrasound to guide the procedure, the physician pushes the fetal buttocks upward out of the pelvis while pushing the fetal head downward toward the pelvis (Fig. 8–2). After the external version is completed (or the effort abandoned), the tocolytic drug is stopped. Rh-negative women receive a dose of Rh immune globulin (RhoGAM).

Internal version is an emergency procedure. The physician performs internal version during vaginal birth of twins to change the fetal presentation of the second twin. An external version may be done for the same purpose.

### Nursing Care

Nursing care of the woman having external version includes assisting with the procedure

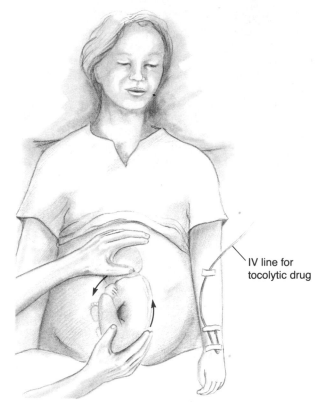

**Figure 8–2.** External version. After the uterus is relaxed by a tocolytic drug, the physician pushes the breech of the fetus upward out of the pelvis while at the same time pushing the head downward toward the pelvis.

IV line for tocolytic drug

and observing the mother and fetus afterward for about 1 or 2 hours. Baseline maternal vital signs and a fetal monitor strip (part of the non-stress test or biophysical profile) are taken. The mother's vital signs and the fetal heart rates are observed to ensure return to normal levels after the version.

Vaginal leaking of amniotic fluid suggests that manipulating the fetus caused a tear in the membranes, and is reported. Uterine contractions usually decrease or stop shortly after the version. The physician is notified if they do not. The nurse reviews signs of labor with the woman because version occurs near term, when spontaneous labor is expected.

### EPISIOTOMY AND LACERATIONS

Episiotomy is the surgical enlargement of the vagina during birth. Either the physician or a nurse-midwife performs and repairs an episiotomy.

# Nursing Brief

Pay special attention to a woman's diet and fluids if she had a third- or fourth-degree laceration. Roughage in the diet and adequate fluids help prevent constipation that might break down the area where the laceration was sutured.

Lacerations of the perineum and episiotomy incisions are treated similarly. Lacerations are classified according to how far they extend from the vagina toward the anus. First- and second-degree lacerations are usually uncomplicated because they do not affect the rectal sphincter. A third-degree laceration extends into the rectal sphincter; the fourth-degree laceration extends completely through the rectal sphincter. Women with third- and fourth-degree lacerations may have more difficulty if they are constipated after birth.

## Indications

Fetal indications are similar to those for forceps or vacuum extraction (see p. 194). Additional maternal indications include

- Better control over the direction and amount that the vaginal opening is enlarged
- An opening with a clean edge, rather than the ragged opening of a tear (controversial)

Routine episiotomy has been challenged by several recent studies that do not support many of its supposed benefits. Nevertheless, it is so common that the nurse can expect to give postpartum care to many women with episiotomies.

## Risks

As in other incisions, infection is the primary risk in an episiotomy or laceration. An additional risk is extension of the episiotomy with a laceration into or through the rectal sphincter (third- or fourth-degree).

## Technique

The episiotomy is done with blunt-tipped scissors just before birth. One of two directions is chosen (Fig. 8–3):

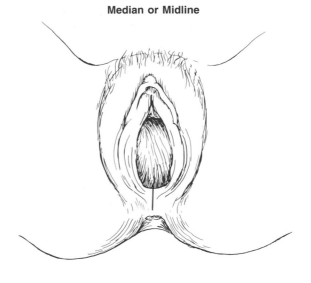

**Median or Midline**

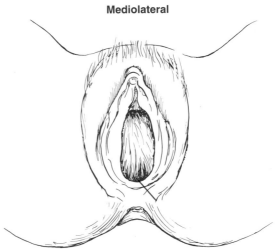

**Mediolateral**

**Figure 8–3.** Episiotomies. The median and a left mediolateral episiotomy is shown here.

- *Median (also called midline)*, extending directly from the lower vaginal border toward the anus
- *Mediolateral*, extending from the lower vaginal border toward the mother's right or left

The median episiotomy is easier to repair and heals neatly, but it does not enlarge the opening as much as the mediolateral incision. The mediolateral incision provides more room, but greater scarring during healing may cause painful sexual intercourse. A laceration that extends a median episiotomy is much more likely to go into the rectal sphincter than one that extends the mediolateral episiotomy.

## Nursing Care

Nursing care for an episiotomy or laceration begins during the fourth stage of labor. Cold packs reduce pain, bruising, and edema during the first 12–24 hours. After this time, warm applications increase blood circulation, enhancing comfort and healing. Mild oral analgesics are usually sufficient for pain management. (See p. 224 for postpartum nursing care of the woman with an episiotomy or laceration.)

## FORCEPS AND VACUUM EXTRACTION BIRTHS

These two procedures are done by the physician to aid the woman's pushing efforts at the end of labor. Forceps are instruments with curved blades that fit around the fetal head without unduly compressing it (Fig. 8–4). Several styles are used to assist the birth of the fetal head in a cephalic presentation. Forceps may also help the physician extract the fetal head through the incision during cesarean birth. Piper forceps are a special type used to deliver the head during vaginal birth of the fetus in a breech presentation.

A vacuum extractor uses suction applied to the fetal head so that the physician can assist

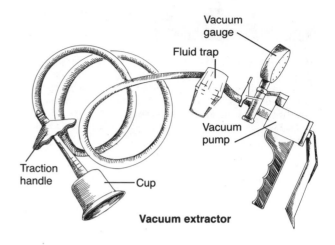

**Vacuum extractor**

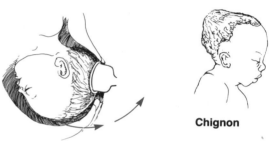

**Vacuum extractor applied,** showing direction of traction

**Chignon**

**Figure 8–5.** The vacuum extractor cup with its attachments to regulate suction. The chignon is scalp edema where the cup was applied.

the mother's expulsive efforts (Fig. 8–5). The vacuum extractor can be used to assist birth of the head during cesarean birth. It cannot be used to deliver the aftercoming head of a fetus in breech presentation. One advantage of the vacuum extractor is that it does not take up room in the mother's pelvis, as forceps do.

## Indications

Forceps or vacuum extraction may be used to end the second stage of labor if it is in the best interests of the mother and/or fetus. The mother may be exhausted, or she may be unable to push effectively because of a regional block. Women with cardiac or pulmonary disorders often have forceps or vacuum extraction births, because prolonged pushing can worsen these conditions. Fetal indications include conditions in which there is evidence of an increased risk to the fetus near the end of labor.

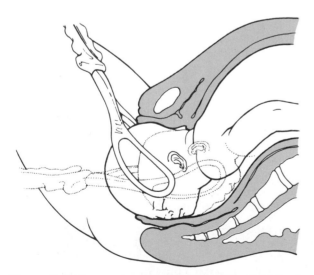

**Figure 8–4.** Forceps to assist the birth of the fetal head. After applying the forceps to each side of the fetal head and locking the two blades, the physician pulls, following the pelvic curve.

These may include minor degrees of placental disruption or questionable fetal heart rate patterns.

## Contraindications

Forceps or vacuum extraction cannot substitute for cesarean birth if the maternal or fetal condition requires a quicker delivery. These techniques are not done if they would be more traumatic than cesarean birth, for example, when the fetus is high in the pelvis or too large for the pelvis.

## Risks

Trauma to maternal and/or fetal tissues is the main risk when forceps or vacuum extraction is used. The mother may have a laceration or hematoma (collection of blood in the tissues) in her vagina. The infant may have bruising, facial or scalp lacerations or abrasions, cephalohematoma (see p. 299), or intracranial hemorrhage. The vacuum extractor causes a harmless area of circular edema on the infant's scalp (chignon) where it was applied.

## Technique

If the woman has not urinated recently, the physician catheterizes her to prevent trauma to her bladder and to make more room in her pelvis. After the forceps are applied, the physician pulls in line with the pelvic curve. An episiotomy is usually done. After the fetal head is brought under the mother's symphysis, the rest of the birth occurs in the conventional way.

Birth assisted with the vacuum extractor follows a similar sequence. The physician applies the cup over the fetal occiput, and suction is created with a machine to hold it there. Traction is applied by pulling on the handle of the extractor cup.

## Nursing Care

If use of forceps or vacuum extraction is anticipated, the nurse places the sterile equipment on the delivery instrument table. A catheter is added to empty the woman's bladder.

After birth, care is similar to that for episiotomy and perineal lacerations. Ice is applied to the perineum to reduce bruising and edema.

## Nursing Brief

Many parents are concerned about the marks made by forceps. Reassure them that they are temporary and usually resolve without treatment.

---

The physician is notified if the woman has signs of vaginal hematoma, which include severe and poorly relieved pelvic or rectal pain.

The infant's head is examined for lacerations, abrasions, or bruising. Mild facial reddening and molding (alteration in shape) of the head are common and require no treatment. Antibiotic ointment is sometimes ordered for skin breaks. Cold treatments are not used on neonates because they disrupt temperature regulation.

Pressure from forceps may injure the infant's facial nerve. It is evidenced by facial asymmetry (different appearance of right and left sides), which is most obvious when the infant cries. Facial nerve injury usually resolves without treatment.

## CESAREAN BIRTH

Cesarean delivery is the surgical birth of the fetus through incisions in the mother's abdomen and uterus. Of all births in the United States, 20–25% are by cesarean delivery.

## Indications

Several conditions may require cesarean delivery:

- Abnormal labor
- Inability of the fetus to pass through the mother's pelvis (cephalopelvic disproportion, also called fetopelvic disproportion)
- Maternal conditions such as pregnancy-induced hypertension, or diabetes
- Active maternal herpes, which may cause serious or fatal infant infection
- Previous surgery on the uterus, including some types of cesarean incisions
- Fetal compromise, including prolapsed umbilical cord and abnormal presentations
- Placenta previa or abruptio placentae

### Contraindications

There are few contraindications to cesarean birth, but it is not usually done if the fetus is dead or too premature to survive, or if the mother has abnormal blood clotting.

### Risks

Cesarean birth carries risks to both mother and baby. Maternal risks are similar to those of other types of surgery and include

- Risks related to anesthesia (see Chap. 7)
- Infection
- Hemorrhage
- Injury to the urinary tract
- Blood clots
- Delayed intestinal peristalsis (paralytic ileus)

Risks to the newborn may include

- Unforeseen preterm birth
- Respiratory problems because of excessive lung fluid remaining in the infant's lungs
- Injury, such as laceration or bruising

Unintentional birth of a premature fetus is the greatest risk. The physician often performs amniocentesis before a planned cesarean birth to determine if the fetal lungs are mature (see Table 5–5, p. 93) and avoid this complication.

### Technique

Cesarean birth may occur under planned, unplanned, or emergency conditions. Although the sequence is similar for each, preparations are severely abbreviated for cesarean birth under emergency conditions.

#### PREPARATIONS FOR CESAREAN BIRTH

As in other surgery, several laboratory studies are done to identify anemia or blood clotting abnormalities. Complete blood count, coagulation studies, and blood typing and screening are common. One or more units of blood may be typed and crossmatched if the woman is likely to need a transfusion.

The woman does not usually receive premedication, as is commonly done in other surgeries, because the drugs can affect the infant's adaptation after birth. She receives a drug to reduce gastric acidity, such as sodium citrate with citric acid (Bicitra), in case general anesthesia is required. Most physicians order prophylactic antibiotics to prevent infection. Sterile antibiotic solution may be flushed into the abdomen before the incision is closed.

The woman's abdomen is shaved from just above her umbilicus to her mons pubis, where her thighs come together. If a Pfannenstiel (transverse, or "bikini") skin incision is planned, the upper border of the shave is about 3 inches above her pubic hairline.

An indwelling Foley catheter is inserted to keep the bladder empty during birth and prevent trauma to it. The circulating nurse will scrub the abdomen by using a circular motion that goes outward from the incisional area.

#### TYPES OF INCISIONS

There are two incisions in cesarean birth: a skin incision and a uterine incision. The directions of these incisions are not necessarily the same.

**Skin Incisions.** The skin incision is done in either a vertical or a transverse direction. The vertical incision allows more room if a large fetus is being delivered, and it is usually needed for an obese woman. In an emergency, the vertical incision can be done more quickly. The transverse, or Pfannenstiel, incision is nearly invisible when healed but cannot always be used in the obese woman or with a large baby.

**Uterine Incisions.** The more important of the two incisions is the one that cuts into the uterus. There are three types of uterine incisions (Fig. 8–6): low transverse, low vertical, and classic.

*Low Transverse.* This uterine incision is preferred because it is not likely to rupture during another birth, has less blood loss, and is easier to repair. It may not be an option if the fetus is large or if there is a placenta previa in the area where the incision would be made. This type of incision makes vaginal birth after cesarean (VBAC) possible for subsequent births.

*Low Vertical.* This uterine incision produces minimal blood loss and allows delivery of a larger fetus. However, it is more likely to rupture during another birth, although less so than the classic incision.

*Classic.* This uterine incision is rarely used, because it involves more blood loss and is the most likely of the three types to rupture during another pregnancy. However, it may be the only choice if the fetus is in a transverse lie or if there is scarring or a placenta previa in the lower anterior uterus.

Low transverse incision

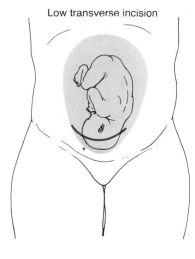

Low vertical incision

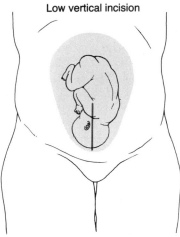

Classic incision

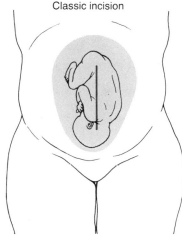

**Figure 8–6.** Three types of uterine incisions for cesarean birth. The low transverse incision is preferred, because it is not likely to rupture during a subsequent birth, allowing vaginal birth after a cesarean birth. The low vertical and classic incisions must occasionally be used.

## SEQUENCE OF EVENTS IN CESAREAN BIRTH

When the woman is anesthetized, scrubbed, and draped, the physician makes the skin incision. After making the uterine incision, the physician ruptures the membranes (unless they are already ruptured) with a sharp instrument, such as a clamp with teeth. The amniotic fluid is suctioned from the operative area, and its amount, color, and odor are noted.

The physician reaches into the uterus to lift out the fetal head or buttocks. Forceps or vacuum extraction may be used to assist birth of the head. The infant's mouth and nose are quickly suctioned to remove secretions, and the cord is clamped. The physician hands the infant to the nurse, who receives the infant into sterile blankets or drapes. Care of the infant is essentially the same as that during vaginal birth.

After birth of the baby, the physician scoops out the placenta and examines it for intactness. The uterine cavity is sponged to remove blood clots and other debris. The uterine and skin incisions are then sutured in layers.

### Nursing Care

The registered nurse assumes most of the preoperative and postoperative care of the woman. This includes obtaining the required laboratory studies, administering medications, preoperative teaching, and preparing for surgery.

Women who have cesarean birth usually need greater emotional support than those having vaginal births. They are usually happy and excited about the newborn but may also feel grief, guilt, or anger because the expected birth did not occur. These feelings may linger and resurface during another pregnancy.

Women who plan VBAC but need a repeat cesarean delivery often experience diverse feelings. A woman may feel positive in spite of needing another cesarean, because she did her best to give vaginal birth a chance. Another woman may have feelings of failure, especially if she strongly wanted a vaginal birth. The nurse avoids using phrases such as "failed VBAC," which a woman may interpret as a personal failure.

Anxiety is normal in confronting a new or unexpected experience. Childbirth, including cesarean childbirth, may be a woman's first hospital experience. Procedures and equipment that are familiar to health-care personnel seem overwhelming when first experienced. Explaining procedures and the role of all persons in the operating room helps reduce her anxiety. A calm voice and quiet environment promote relaxation.

Emotional care of the partner and family is essential; they are included in explanations of the surgery as much as the woman wishes. The partner may be terrified when an emergency cesarean is needed but may not express these feelings because the woman needs so much support. The partner may be almost as exhausted as the woman, if cesarean birth is done after hours of labor. The thoughtful nurse includes the partner and promotes his or her emotional and physical well-being.

A support person is present for most cesarean births. The nurse informs the partner of when he or she may enter the operating room, because 1/2 hour or more may be needed for administration of regional anesthesia and for surgical preparations. During this wait, the partner dons surgical attire.

After birth, the mother, infant, and partner are not separated if possible. The woman and her partner are encouraged to talk about the cesarean birth so that they can integrate the experience. The nurse answers questions about events surrounding the birth. The focus is the *birth*, rather than the surgical, aspects of cesarean delivery.

Nursing assessments after cesarean birth are similar to those after vaginal birth, including assessment of the uterine fundus. Assessments are done every 15 minutes for the first 1 or 2 hours, according to hospital policy. Recovery room assessments after cesarean birth include

- Vital signs to identify hemorrhage or shock; a pulse-oximeter is often used to identify depressed respiratory function
- Intravenous site and rate of solution flow
- Fundus for firmness, height, and midline position
- Dressing for drainage
- Lochia for quantity, color, and presence of clots
- Amounts of urine output from the indwelling catheter

The fundus is checked as gently as possible. The woman flexes her knees slightly and takes slow, deep breaths to minimize the pain of fundal assessments. The fingers are "walked" from the side of the uterus toward the midline. Massage is not needed if the fundus is already firm.

The woman is told to take deep breaths at each assessment and to cough to move secre-

## Nursing Brief

Although assessing the uterus after cesarean birth causes discomfort, it is important to do so regularly. The woman can have a relaxed uterus that causes excessive blood loss, regardless of the type of delivery she had.

tions from her airways. Changing her position every hour or two helps expand her lungs and also makes her more comfortable.

Pain relief after cesarean birth may be by patient-controlled analgesia (PCA) pump or by intermittent injections of narcotic analgesics. Epidural narcotics provide long-lasting pain relief but are associated with delayed respiratory depression and itching (see p. 176). After about the first 24 hours, the woman is changed to oral analgesics. Nursing Care Plan 8–1 details interventions for selected nursing diagnoses that pertain to the woman with an unplanned cesarean birth.

## Abnormal Labor

The "four Ps" of labor (see p. 122) interact constantly throughout the birth. Abnormalities in the powers, passenger, passage, or the psyche may result in abnormal labor. Additionally, the length of labor may be abnormally short or long. Labor abnormalities may require forceps or cesarean delivery, or they may result in injury to the mother and baby.

### PROBLEMS WITH POWERS OF LABOR

A woman may have abnormal contractions that are hypotonic or hypertonic. She may not have adequate pushing efforts to bring about fetal descent. Some women have a lax abdominal wall that impedes normal fetal descent.

### Hypotonic Labor Dysfunction

A woman has hypotonic labor if her contractions are too weak to be effective. Hypotonic labor usually occurs during active labor. The woman begins labor normally, but contractions diminish during the active phase (after 4 cm of cervical dilation). Hypotonic labor is more likely to occur if her uterus is overdistended, such as with twins or excess amniotic fluid. Women who

| NURSING CARE PLAN 8–1 | | |
|---|---|---|
| **Selected Nursing Diagnoses for the Woman with an Unplanned Cesarean Birth** | | |
| Goals | Interventions | Rationale |

**Nursing Diagnosis:** Anxiety related to development of complications.

| | | |
|---|---|---|
| Woman and her partner will express decreased anxiety after explanations about the planned surgery | 1. Reinforce all explanations given by physician, expressing them in simpler terms, if needed | 1. Anxiety tends to narrow attention; although physician may have explained need for surgery, woman and her partner may not have comprehended everything they were told |
| | 2. Encourage woman to continue using breathing and relaxation techniques she learned in prepared childbirth classes; tell her the techniques may help with pain control after birth | 2. Learned pain management techniques increase woman's sense of control; control over a situation reduces feelings of helplessness and decreases anxiety |
| | 3. Tell woman what operating room looks like and who will be present; explain basic equipment such as catheter, narrow table, monitors for her heart and blood pressure, anesthesia machine, and large overhead lights; explain that all personnel will wear masks, gowns, gloves, hats, and shoe covers; personnel at operating table will also have eye protection, such as goggles or face shield | 3. Commonplace equipment and attire in an operating room can be intimidating for someone who has not seen them before; unfamiliarity increases anxiety; preparation reduces anxiety and fear of the unknown |
| | 4. Describe usual postoperative care—assessment of the vital signs, fundus, vaginal bleeding, dressing, and catheter; tell her she will be asked to take deep breaths and change position regularly | 4. If woman understands common postoperative care, she is more likely to cooperate with it, even if assessments are uncomfortable |
| | 5. Encourage her partner to be with her during surgery and do not separate family afterward, if possible | 5. Companionship of familiar persons helps reduce anxiety; keeping new family together promotes bonding |

**Nursing Diagnosis:** Pain related to effects of surgery (incisional, slowed gastric peristalsis).

| | | |
|---|---|---|
| Woman will state that pain is manageable with the pharmacologic and nonpharmacologic methods used | 1. Assess nature of pain: location, quality, intensity, duration, and factors that increase or decrease it | 1. Proper assessment allows nurse to choose most appropriate interventions, such as repositioning or medication |
| | 2. Provide analgesics as ordered, usually intramuscular or patient-controlled analgesia (PCA) pump for the first 24 hr and oral analgesics after this time; do not allow pain to become too intense before medicating woman | 2. Analgesics inhibit brain's ability to interpret pain; early and frequent use of measures to relieve pain allows optimal control and facilitates healing |
| | 3. Assess bowel sounds each shift or more frequently if they are diminished; ask woman to report when she begins passing flatus (gas) rectally | 3. Cesarean birth may delay the return of bowel function; accumulation of intestinal gas will cause abdominal distention and cramping; passing flatus indicates return of bowel function |
| | 4. Encourage woman to get out of bed about 24 hr after surgery, as ordered; progressively increase her ambulation | 4. Activity stimulates intestinal peristalsis, which reduces accumulation of gas and limits discomfort from this source |

*Continued*

**NURSING CARE PLAN 8–1 *Continued***

**Selected Nursing Diagnoses for the Woman with an Unplanned Cesarean Birth**

| Goals | Interventions | Rationale |
|---|---|---|
| **Nursing Diagnosis:** Pain related to effects of surgery (incisional, slowed gastric peristalsis). | | |
| | 5. Discourage woman from drinking carbonated drinks or drinking through a straw | 5. These activities tend to increase swallowed gas and can increase gastric discomfort |
| **Nursing Diagnosis:** High risk for ineffective airway clearance related to reduced breathing efforts secondary to incisional pain. | | |
| Woman will have a normal respiratory rate of 12–24 breaths/min, clear lung sounds | 1. Assess vital signs and lung sounds according to length of time since surgery (usually every 15 min in the recovery area, then every 4 hr after stabilized) | 1. Tachypnea or congested lung sounds suggest that woman is not moving secretions from her airways; temperature elevation over 38°C (100.4°F) suggests infection, which could have several sources, including respiratory |
| | 2. Have woman take deep breaths and cough every 2 hr; teach her to press a pillow or folded blanket over her incision area to splint it | 2. Deep breathing and coughing help move secretions from airways; splinting incision reduces strain on it and reduces pain so woman can cough more effectively |
| | 3. Encourage changing position every 2 hr before ambulating, turning side to side | 3. Helps move secretions from airways and prevents congestion, which is a favorable environment for growth of infectious organisms |
| **Nursing Diagnosis:** High risk for altered tissue perfusion related to bleeding secondary to uterine atony. | | |
| Woman will have adequate tissue perfusion as evidenced by saturation of no more than one pad per hour during recovery period. | 1. Assess vital signs every 15 during recovery area, then according to hospital policy | 1. Rising pulse and falling blood pressure suggest shock, which is most often dur to hemorrhage |
| | 2. Assess uterine fundus for firmness, height, and position (midline or deviated) with vital signs; massage fundus until it is firm if necessary; explain reason for this assessment, and have woman bend her knees and breathe slowly and deeply while you assess fundus. | 2. Firm fundus compresses bleeding blood vessels at placenta site; this procedure is often painful if woman had a cesarean birth, especially with a vertical skin incision; if she understands its importance and takes measures to minimize discomfort, she is more likely to accept needed assessment |
| | 3. Assess lochia for amount, color, and odor when uterine fundus is assessed; report over one pad per hour saturated during recovery period or persistent clots | 3. Signs of excessive blood loss require prompt medical and nursing intervention to avoid altering tissue perfusion. |
| | 4. Assess catheter for patency and for amount of urine output with vital signs and fundal and lochia checks; assess voided output until woman is urinating adequate amounts (over 100 ml) regularly. | 4. A full bladder inhibits uterine contraction and can lead to hemorrhage; adequate urine output verifies patency of catheter and reflects and adequate circulating blood volume. |
| | 5. Check dressing and incision with each fundal check | 5. Bloody drainage on dressing suggests breakdown in incision line; gapping of incision (after dressing is removed) suggests infection and can lead to hemorrhage (see Chap. 9 for more information about postpartum infection) |

have had many babies (grand multiparas) are more likely to have hypotonic labor, because they have poorer uterine muscle tone.

**Medical Treatment.** The physician usually does an amniotomy if the membranes are intact. Augmentation of labor with oxytocin or by nipple stimulation increases the strength of contractions. Intravenous or oral fluids may improve the quality of contractions if the woman is dehydrated.

**Nursing Care.** The woman is usually comfortable, but frustrated because her labor is not progressing. In addition to providing care related to amniotomy and labor augmentation, the nurse gives emotional support to the woman and her partner. She is allowed to express her frustrations. The nurse tells her when she makes progress, to encourage continuing her efforts.

Position changes may help relieve discomfort and enhance progress. Contractions are usually stronger and more effective when the woman lies on her side, although they may be less frequent. Walking or nipple stimulation may intensify contractions. Nursing Care Plan 8–2 details interventions for selected nursing diagnoses that pertain to the woman with hypotonic labor dysfunction.

### Hypertonic Labor Dysfunction

Hypertonic dysfunction is characterized by contractions that are frequent, cramplike, and poorly coordinated. They are painful and nonproductive. The uterus is tense, even between contractions, which reduces blood flow to the placenta.

Hypertonic labor dysfunction usually occurs during the latent phase of labor (before 4 cm of cervical dilation). It is less common than hypotonic dysfunction. Box 8–1 summarizes differences between hypotonic and hypertonic labor dysfunction.

**Medical Treatment.** Medical treatment may include mild sedation to allow the woman to rest. Tocolytic drugs (see p. 927), such as terbutaline (Brethine), may be ordered to reduce the high uterine resting tone (resting muscle tension).

**Nursing Care.** Women with hypertonic dysfunction are uncomfortable and frustrated. Anxiety about the lack of progress impairs their ability to tolerate pain. They may lose confidence in their ability to give birth.

The nurse should accept the woman's frustration and that of her partner. Both may be exhausted from the near-constant discomfort. It is important not to equate the amount of pain a woman reports with how much she "should" feel at that point in labor. The nurse provides general comfort measures that promote rest and relaxation.

### Ineffective Maternal Pushing

The woman may not push effectively during the second stage of labor because she does not understand which techniques to use or she fears tearing her perineal tissues. Epidural or subarachnoid blocks (see p. 174) may depress or eliminate the natural urge to push. An exhausted woman may be unable to gather her resources to push out her baby.

**Nursing Care.** Nursing care focuses on coaching the woman about the most effective techniques for pushing. If she cannot feel her contractions because of regional anesthesia, the nurse tells her when to push, as each contraction reaches its peak.

The exhausted woman may benefit from pushing only when she feels a strong urge or perhaps with every other contraction. The fearful woman may benefit from explanations that sensations of tearing or splitting often accompany fetal descent but that her body is designed to accommodate to the baby. Pushing every two or three contractions allows her tissues to adjust to the distention caused by fetal descent.

### Weak Abdominal Wall

Some women have weak abdominal muscles that allow the uterus to rotate sharply forward with each contraction or push. This action keeps the fetus from aligning with the pelvic canal. An abdominal binder contains the uterus so that each contraction or pushing effort directs the fetus into the pelvis. Upright positions also improve alignment of the fetus with the pelvis and make use of gravity.

### PROBLEMS WITH THE FETUS

Several fetal conditions can contribute to abnormal labor, including fetal size, presentation, or position. Multifetal pregnancies are associated with difficult labor. Some birth defects alter the fetal body in such a way as to impede birth.

### Fetal Size

A large fetus (macrosomia) is generally considered to be one weighing over 4000 gm (8.8

| NURSING CARE PLAN 8–2 | | |
|---|---|---|
| **Selected Nursing Diagnoses for the Woman with Hypotonic Labor Dysfunction** | | |
| **Goals** | **Interventions** | **Rationale** |

**Nursing Diagnosis:** High risk for infection related to loss of barrier (ruptured membranes).

| | | |
|---|---|---|
| Woman's temperature will remain under 38°C (100.4°F), and the amniotic fluid will remain clear with a mild odor | 1. Take woman's temperature every 2 hr; at same time, assess the amniotic fluid drainage for color, clarity, and odor | 1. Elevated temperature is a sign of infection; cloudy, yellow, or foul-odored fluid suggests infection; meconium (green) staining suggests fetal compromise but is also seen with prolonged pregnancy |
| | 2. Monitor fetal heart rates (see p. 141) | 2. Fetal tachycardia (rate > 160/min) may be the first sign of infection; poor fetal oxygenation also may occur, especially with abnormal labor |
| | 3. After birth, continue to assess woman's temperature every 4 hr until she is stable; assess the lochia (postbirth vaginal drainage) for a foul odor or brown color | 3. Woman may not show these signs of infection until after birth |
| | 4. Observe neonate for a temperature below 36.2°C (97°F) or over 37.8°C (100°F); observe for poor feeding, lethargy, irritability, or "not looking right" | 4. Neonate may become infected in utero and display these signs of infection after birth; neonatal sepsis may occur with prolonged rupture of membranes and is a potentially fatal infection |

**Nursing Diagnosis:** Ineffective individual coping related to frustration with slow labor and delayed birth.

| | | |
|---|---|---|
| Woman will use breathing and relaxation techniques that she and her partner learned in prepared childbirth class | 1. If there is no contraindication, such as epidural block, encourage woman to walk or to sit upright in bed or chair; walking may not be wise if membranes are ruptured and fetus is high | 1. Upright positions enhance fetal descent; walking strengthens labor contractions; walking when membranes are ruptured and fetal station is high could lead to umbilical cord prolapse |
| | 2. Help woman use natural methods to stimulate contractions, such as nipple stimulation; encourage a shower or whirlpool if available and not contraindicated | 2. Nipple stimulation causes woman's posterior pituitary gland to secrete natural oxytocin, which strengthens contractions; water may help woman relax, which improves labor; all nondrug methods to stimulate labor enhance her sense of control |
| | 3. Assist registered nurse with oxytocin augmentation if it is ordered; observe contractions for excessive frequency (more frequent than every 2 min), duration (over 90 sec), or inadequate rest interval (under 60 sec); observe fetal heart rate for rates outside normal 110–160 beats/min | 3. Primary risks of oxytocin augmentation or induction of labor relate to overstimulating the uterus; excessive contractions can reduce fetal oxygen supply; these are signs of potential uterine overstimulation |
| | 4. Explain to woman how each method is expected to help her labor advance; tell her any time she makes progress, either in improved contractions or increasing cervical dilation | 4. If woman understands reason for any interventions, she will more likely cooperate with them and feel more in control; knowing that her efforts are having desired effect encourages her to continue with her learned coping methods |
| | 5. Help woman relax and use breathing techniques she learned in prepared childbirth class; praise and support her when she uses them | 5. Relaxation promotes normal labor; woman with a long labor may feel that there is no use in continuing relaxation and breathing if she is not making progress; praise encourages her to continue |

| BOX 8-1 | Differences Between Hypotonic Labor and Hypertonic Labor Dysfunction |
|---|---|

**Hypotonic Labor**

Contractions weak and ineffective

More common than hypertonic labor dysfunction

Occurs during active phase, after 4 cm cervical dilation

More likely if uterus is overdistended or if woman has had many other births

Medical management includes amniotomy, oxytocin augmentation, and hydration

Nondrug stimulation methods include walking, upright positions, and nipple stimulation

Other nursing interventions include position changes and encouragement

**Hypertonic Labor**

Contractions poorly coordinated, frequent, and painful

Uterine resting tone between contractions is tense

Less common than hypotonic labor dysfunction

More likely to occur during latent labor, before 4 cm of cervical dilation

Medical management includes mild sedation and tocolytic drugs

Nursing interventions include acceptance of the woman's discomfort and frustration and provision of comfort measures

pounds) at birth. The large baby may not fit through the woman's pelvis. A very large fetus distends the uterus and can contribute to hypotonic labor dysfunction.

Shoulder dystocia sometimes occurs, usually when the fetus is large. The fetal head is born, but the shoulders become impacted above the mother's symphysis pubis. A shoulder dystocia is an emergency, because the fetus needs to breathe. The physician may request that the nurse apply firm downward pressure just above the symphysis, to push the shoulders toward the pelvic canal. Squatting or sharp flexion of the thighs against the abdomen may also loosen the shoulders.

**Nursing Care.** If the woman successfully delivers a large infant, observe mother and child for injuries after birth. The woman may have a large episiotomy or laceration. The large infant is more likely to have a fracture of one or both clavicles (collarbones). The infant's clavicles are felt for crepitus (creaking sensation) or defor-

mity of the bones, and the arms are observed for equal movement.

### Abnormal Fetal Presentation or Position

Labor is most efficient if the fetus is in a flexed, cephalic presentation and in one of the occiput anterior positions (see p. 129). Abnormalities of fetal presentation and position prevent birth from being most efficient.

**Abnormal Presentations.** The fetus in an abnormal presentation, such as the breech or face presentation, does not pass easily through the woman's pelvis. Abnormal presentations, such as the brow presentation, may also increase the size of the presenting part (see Fig. 6–6, p. 127). Abnormal presentations prevent smooth dilation of the cervix and interfere with the mechanisms of labor (p. 130).

In the United States, most fetuses in the breech presentation are born by cesarean delivery. During vaginal birth in this presentation, the trunk and extremities are born before the head. After the fetal body delivers, the umbilical cord can be compressed between the fetus and the mother's pelvis. The head, which is the single largest part of the fetus, must be quickly delivered so that the infant can breathe. Delay in birth of the head could cause brain damage or death.

External version is being used to avoid some cesarean deliveries for a breech presentation. However, external version cannot always be done, and the fetus sometimes returns to the abnormal presentation.

**Abnormal Positions.** A common cause of abnormal labor is the fetus's remaining in a persistent occiput posterior position (left [LOP] or right [ROP]). The fetal occiput occupies either the left or right posterior quadrant of the mother's pelvis. In most women, the fetal head rotates in a clockwise or counterclockwise direction until the occiput is in one of the anterior quadrants of the pelvis (left [LOA] or right [ROA]).

Rotation does not occur in every woman. Labor is likely to be longer when the fetus remains in this position. Intense back and leg pain that is poorly relieved characterizes labor when the fetus is in the occiput posterior position. Most women with an average-size pelvis cannot deliver their infants in an occiput posterior position. The physician may use forceps to rotate the fetal head into an occiput anterior position. If forceps rotation is not successful, cesarean delivery is usual.

*Nursing Care.* During labor, the nurse should encourage the woman to assume positions that favor fetal rotation and descent. These positions also reduce some of the back pain. Good positions for back labor include

- Sitting or kneeling, leaning forward on a support
- Hands and knees (Fig. 8–7)
- Side-lying
- Squatting

See Chapter 6 for further information about labor positions.

After birth, mother and infant are observed for signs of birth trauma. The mother is more likely to have a hematoma of her vaginal wall (see p. 254) if the fetus remained in the occiput posterior position for a long time. The infant may have excessive molding (alteration in shape) of the head, caput succedaneum (scalp edema), and possibly injury from forceps or the vacuum extractor.

## Multifetal Pregnancy

If the woman has more than one fetus, dysfunctional labor is likely for two reasons:

- Uterine overdistention contributes to poor contraction quality.
- Abnormal presentation or position of one or all fetuses interferes with normal labor mechanisms.

Because of the difficulties inherent in multifetal deliveries, cesarean birth is common. Birth is almost always cesarean if three or more fetuses are involved.

*Nursing Care.* When the woman has a multifetal pregnancy, each fetus is monitored separately during labor. The woman should avoid lying on her back. A side-lying position with the head slightly elevated to facilitate breathing is usually most comfortable. Labor care is similar to that for single pregnancies, with observations for hypotonic labor.

The nursery and intrapartum staffs prepare duplicate equipment and medications for every infant expected. An anesthesiologist is often present at birth because of the potential for maternal and/or neonatal problems. One nurse is available for each infant, and one or more pediatricians are usually present. Another nurse focuses on the mother's needs.

### Fetal Anomalies

Some birth defects distort the fetal body so that birth is difficult. Hydrocephalus (collection of fluid within the brain) causes the fetal head to be large. The large fetal head usually keeps the fetus from assuming the normal head-down presentation, and it may not fit through the pelvis. Excessive amniotic fluid often occurs with fetal hydrocephalus and may result in uterine overdistention with hypotonic labor. Hydrocephalus is discussed more fully on page 337.

## PROBLEMS WITH PELVIS AND SOFT TISSUES

The woman's pelvic size or shape and the characteristics of her soft tissues can either facilitate or impede birth.

### Bony Pelvis

Some women have a pelvis that is small or abnormally shaped, thus impeding the normal mechanisms of labor. There are four basic pelvic shapes: gynecoid, which is the most favorable for vaginal birth; anthropoid; android; and platypelloid, which is unfavorable for vaginal birth (see Fig. 2–7). Most women do not have a pure shape, but have a mixture of different pelvic types.

Absolute pelvic measurements are rarely helpful to determine whether a woman's pelvis is adequate for birth. A woman with a "small" pelvis may still deliver vaginally if other factors are favorable. If her fetus is not too large, the head is well flexed, contractions are good, and her soft tissues yield easily to the forces of labor, she often delivers vaginally.

In contrast, some women have vaginally delivered several infants well over 9 pounds but

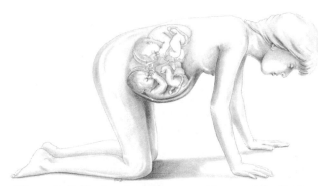

**Figure 8–7.** The hands-and-knees position can help the fetus rotate from an occiput posterior to an occiput anterior position. Gravity causes the fetus to float downward toward the pool of amniotic fluid.

cannot deliver one weighing 10 pounds. Obviously, the pelvis of each was "adequate," or even "large," according to standard measurements. However, the pelvis was not large enough for the largest infant. The ultimate test of a woman's pelvic size is whether her baby fits through it at birth.

### Soft Tissue Obstructions

The most common soft tissue obstruction during labor is a full bladder. The woman is encouraged to urinate every 1 or 2 hours. Catheterization may be needed if she cannot urinate, especially if regional anesthesia and/or large quantities of intravenous fluids were given.

Less common soft tissue obstructions include pelvic tumors, such as benign (noncancerous) fibroids. Some women have a cervix that is scarred from previous infections or surgery. The scar tissue may not efface or dilate normally.

### PSYCHOLOGICAL PROBLEMS

Labor is stressful. However, women with adequate social and professional support usually adapt to this stress and can labor and deliver normally. If their stress is too high, however, they perceive more pain and often have inadequate contractions. Their body responds to stress with a "fight-or-flight" reaction that impedes normal labor. For example, the fight-or-flight reaction

- Uses glucose the uterus needs for energy
- Causes secretion of hormones that inhibit uterine contractions
- Diverts blood from the uterus
- Increases tension of pelvic muscles, which impedes fetal descent
- Increases perception of pain, creating greater anxiety and stress, and worsening the cycle

**Nursing Care.** Promoting relaxation and helping the woman conserve her resources for the work of childbirth are the principal nursing goals. The nurse uses every opportunity to spare her energy and promote her comfort. See Chapter 7 for more information about promoting comfort.

### ABNORMAL DURATION OF LABOR

Labor that is either longer or shorter than normal can cause problems in the mother or in her fetus or infant.

## Nursing Brief

In any abnormal labor, observe the fetus for compromised oxygen supply. Observe the woman and newborn for signs of injury or infection.

### Prolonged Labor

Any of the previously discussed factors may be associated with a long or difficult labor (dystocia). The average rate of cervical dilation during the active phase of labor is about 1.2 cm/hr for the woman having her first baby and about 1.5 cm/hr if she had a baby before. A *Friedman curve* (Fig. 8–8) is often used to graph the progress of cervical dilation and fetal descent.

Prolonged labor can result in several problems:

- Maternal or newborn infection, especially if the membranes have been ruptured for a long time (usually about 24 hours)
- Maternal exhaustion
- Postpartum hemorrhage (see p. 252)

Additionally, mothers who have difficult and long labors are more likely to be anxious and fearful about their next labor.

**Nursing Care.** Nursing care focuses on helping the woman conserve her strength and encouraging her as she copes with the long labor. Observe for signs of infection during or after birth in both the mother and newborn:

- Mother: temperature 38°C (100.4°F) or higher; foul-odored, cloudy, or yellowish am-

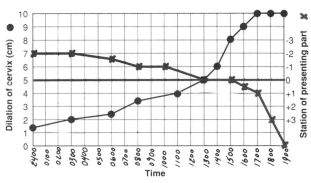

**Figure 8–8.** A Friedman graph is a record of the woman's labor progress. Dots indicate cervical dilatin; "X's" indicate fetal station.

## Nursing Brief

A woman who had a difficult labor and birth must recover physically before she has much interest in caring for her newborn.

---

niotic fluid; foul-odored vaginal drainage after birth
- Infant: axillary temperature under 36.2°C (97.0°F) or over 37.8°C (100°F); lethargy or irritability; poor feeding; not "looking right"

See page 256 for further information about postpartum infection and page 358 for discussion of neonatal infection.

### Precipitate Labor

Precipitate labor is completed in less than 3 hours. Labor often begins abruptly and intensifies quickly, rather than having a more subtle onset and gradual progression. Contractions may be frequent and intense.

Precipitate labor is not the same as precipitate birth. A precipitate birth is one that occurs unexpectedly, with no trained birth attendant present. Precipitate birth may occur after a labor of any duration.

If the mother's pelvis is adequate for the size of her baby and her soft tissues yield easily during fetal descent, neither she nor her baby usually has problems. However, if her tissues do not yield easily, she may have uterine rupture (see p. 210), cervical lacerations, or hematoma.

Fetal oxygenation can be compromised by intense contractions, because the placenta is resupplied with oxygenated blood between contractions. In precipitate labor, this interval may be very short. Birth injury from rapid passage through the birth canal may become evident in the infant after birth. These injuries can include intracranial hemorrhage or nerve damage.

**Nursing Care.** Care for the woman in precipitate labor includes methods to promote fetal oxygenation and cope with discomfort. A side-lying position and supplemental oxygen improve fetal oxygenation. A tocolytic drug may be ordered to reduce intense contractions.

Pain control is difficult in precipitate labor. Regional anesthetics may not be effective soon enough to be useful. Narcotics should not be given near the time of birth (usually within 1 hour), to avoid depressing the newborn's respirations. The nurse must rely heavily on the nonpharmacologic techniques discussed in Chapter 7. The nurse stays with the woman and breathes with her to help her focus on coping with each contraction.

After birth, the nurse observes the mother and infant for signs of injury. Excessive pain or bruising of the woman's vulva is reported. Cold applications limit pain, bruising, and edema. Abnormal findings on the newborn's assessment (see p. 296) are reported to the physician.

## Premature Rupture of Membranes

Premature rupture of the membranes (PROM) is rupture of the membranes at term (38 or more weeks' gestation) before labor contractions begin. A related term, *preterm premature rupture of the membranes* (PPROM), is rupture of the membranes before term (before 38 weeks' gestation), with or without uterine contractions. Medical management of each condition depends on the gestation and whether other complications accompany the ruptured membranes.

Infection of the amniotic sac, called chorioamnionitis, may cause prematurely ruptured membranes; or it may be a consequence of rupture because the barrier to the uterine cavity is broken. After the rupture, the risk for infection increases as time elapses. There is no exact time of infection, but the risk is known to increase greatly after 24 hours.

Umbilical cord compression may occur because the amniotic fluid cushion is lost. The newborn may have infection and may also have respiratory distress and other problems of immaturity (see p. 317) if born prematurely.

**Medical Treatment.** Medical therapy depends on the gestation (term or preterm) and on whether there is evidence of infection, umbilical cord compression, or other complication. If the fetus is immature, the physician carefully weighs the benefits of continued maturation against the risk of infection or other complications. If there are no signs of infection, the woman is usually kept on bed rest at home or in the hospital.

If the fetus is at or near term (about 36 weeks' gestation), the physician usually induces labor with oxytocin if it does not begin spontaneously. Oxytocin induction is rarely successful far from term, because the uterus is not sensitive to the drug.

**Nursing Care.** The woman is observed for signs of infection, as discussed previously. If sent home, she usually remains on bed rest, except to go to the bathroom. The nurse must emphasize that too much activity can precipitate preterm labor. The woman should take her temperature as prescribed, and observe for uterine contractions (see discussion of preterm labor). Sexual intercourse is avoided because it can trigger labor and increases the risk for infection.

## Preterm Labor

Preterm labor occurs after 20 and before 38 weeks of gestation. The main risks are the problems of immaturity in the newborn.

Just as it is not known exactly why labor begins at term, it is not known why some women begin labor early. However, a large number of factors are associated with preterm labor (Box 8–2).

Early prenatal care can identify many women at risk early in pregnancy. It may be possible for the woman to reduce or eliminate some risk factors. The woman can be taught to observe for signs of preterm labor so that it can be interrupted before a baby is born prematurely.

Preterm labor often has vague symptoms at its onset. The symptoms vary considerably, but they include

- Contractions that may be either uncomfortable or painless
- Feeling that the baby is "balling up" frequently
- Menstrual-like cramps
- Constant backache
- Pelvic pressure, or a feeling that the baby is pushing down
- A change in the vaginal discharge
- Abdominal cramps, with or without diarrhea
- Thigh pain
- "Just feeling bad" or "coming down with something"

### Medical Treatment

Medical care involves quickly identifying and halting preterm labor. If birth of an immature infant is likely despite interventions to stop preterm labor, the physician may order drugs to speed maturation of the fetal lungs.

**Identifying Preterm Labor Early.** A key ele-

| BOX 8–2 | Some Risk Factors for Preterm Labor |
|---|---|

Exposure to diethylstilbestrol (DES)
Being underweight
Illness such as diabetes or hypertension
Previous preterm labor or birth
Previous pregnancy losses
Uterine or cervical abnormalities
Uterine distention
Abdominal surgery during pregnancy
Infection (especially urinary tract)
Anemia
Premature rupture of the membranes
Inadequate prenatal care
Poor nutrition
Age under 15 or over 35
Low education level
Poverty
Smoking
Substance abuse
Chronic stress
Non-Caucasian

ment of both medical and nursing care is to teach women, especially those at higher risk, about the symptoms of preterm labor. The physician may order home uterine activity monitoring for women at risk for preterm labor. The monitor assesses contractions only; it does not assess fetal heart rates. The monitor is designed for effectively detecting contractions when the uterus is small. The uterine activity is recorded for a specific period, then transmitted by telephone to a central office where a nurse interprets it and counsels the woman. There is no paper strip or screen on the monitoring machine in the home.

**Stopping Preterm Labor.** The initial measures to stop preterm labor include bed rest and hydration. Even minor degrees of dehydration can increase the irritability of the uterus and increase contractions. Urinary tract infections increase the risk for preterm labor and birth, so urinalysis is done to identify them.

Tocolytic drugs may be given to inhibit uterine contractions before a preterm birth occurs. Ritodrine (Yutopar) is the only drug that the United States Food and Drug Administration has approved as a tocolytic. Ritodrine has several serious side effects, such as maternal and fetal tachycardia, maternal hypoglycemia and elevated potassium, and maternal hypotension and other blood pressure alterations. Pulmonary edema is an infrequent, but critical, side effect. These side effects are more pronounced with intravenous administration than with oral administration.

Because of these side effects, other drugs may be given to stop preterm labor. These drugs are well-established for other uses, but their use as a tocolytic is investigational. They are given for their secondary effect of inhibiting contractions. These drugs include

- Terbutaline (Brethine)
- Magnesium sulfate
- Indomethacin (Indocin)
- Nifedipine (Procardia)

The woman on home care may take terbutaline, either orally, or by means of a continuous subcutaneous infusion pump. Side effects of terbutaline are similar to those of ritodrine, although less powerful. Interventions for magnesium sulfate are the same as those for the drug when given to prevent seizures in pregnancy-induced hypertension (see p. 91).

**Speeding Fetal Lung Maturation.** If it appears that preterm birth is inevitable, the physician may give the woman steroid drugs to increase fetal lung maturity. Dexamethasone and betamethasone are two drugs for this purpose. Steroids may be repeated in 1 week if delivery has not occurred.

### Nursing Care

Nurses should be aware of the symptoms of preterm labor because they may occur in any pregnant woman, with or without risk factors. Symptoms are taught and regularly reinforced for women who have risk factors.

Lengthy activity restrictions are often needed to prevent preterm birth. A critical nursing function is to help the woman maintain bed rest and reduce complications of prolonged inactivity.

If the woman remains at home, the nurse reinforces the exact level of activity the physician prescribed. For example, the physician may order bed rest except for going to the bathroom, showering, and eating meals. After a few days, most women begin to think, "It probably won't hurt if I just empty the dishwasher or wash clothes." The nurse should anticipate these temptations and emphasize that maintaining rest as prescribed is the most important work she is doing for her

baby right now. If she departs from the physician's recommendations and has recurrent preterm labor, the nurse should not make her feel guiltier about it than she already does.

To reduce boredom, the woman can set up two places to rest, such as her living room and bedroom. This provides a change of scenery and helps her feel more involved in family activities. A telephone should be nearby in both locations. A picnic cooler packed with drinks and snacks limits walking.

Women with other children have the greatest difficulty in maintaining bed rest. The nurse helps them identify who can assist in child care and transportation to school and other activities.

The nurse helps the woman identify enjoyable activities that can be done in bed. Television, videos, video games, puzzles, reading, letter writing, and hand needlework are some options.

## Prolonged Pregnancy

Prolonged pregnancy lasts longer than 42 weeks. Other terms for prolonged pregnancy include *postmature*, *postdate*, or *postterm*. Many pregnancies seem to be prolonged, yet are really only term, or even preterm. The woman may have had irregular menstrual periods or may have forgotten the date of her last menstrual period. Clarification of uncertain gestation is much more difficult if the woman has not had regular prenatal care.

**Risks.** The greatest risks of prolonged pregnancy are to the fetus. As the placenta ages, it delivers oxygen and nutrients to the fetus less efficiently. The fetus may lose weight, and the skin may begin to peel. Meconium may be expelled into the amniotic fluid, which can cause severe respiratory problems at birth. Low blood sugar is a likely complication after birth.

The fetus with placental insufficiency does not tolerate labor well. Because the fetus has less reserve than needed, the normal interruption in blood flow during contractions may cause excessive stress on the baby.

If the placenta continues functioning well, the fetus continues growing. This can lead to a large fetus and the problems accompanying macrosomia.

There is little physical risk to the mother, other than laboring with a large baby. Psychologically, however, she often feels that pregnancy will never end. She becomes more anxious about when labor will begin and when her physician or nurse-midwife will "do something."

**Medical Treatment.** The physician or nurse-midwife will evaluate whether pregnancy is truly prolonged or if the gestation has been miscalculated. If the woman's pregnancy has truly reached 42 weeks, labor is usually induced by oxytocin. Prostaglandin gel makes induction more likely to be successful if her cervix is not ripe.

**Nursing Care.** Nursing care involves careful observation of the fetus during labor to identify signs associated with poor placental blood flow, such as late decelerations (see p. 144). After birth, the newborn is observed for respiratory difficulties and hypoglycemia.

# Emergencies During Childbirth

Several intrapartum conditions can endanger the life or well-being of the woman or her fetus. Although these problems do not occur often, they require prompt nursing and medical action to reduce the likelihood of damage. Nursing and medical management often overlap in such emergencies.

## PROLAPSED UMBILICAL CORD

The umbilical cord prolapses if it slips downward in the pelvis after the membranes rupture. In this position, it can be compressed between the fetal body and the woman's pelvis, interrupting blood supply to and from the placenta. It may slip down immediately after the membranes rupture, or the prolapse may occur much later.

A prolapsed cord can be classified in one of three ways (Fig. 8–9):

- *Complete:* the cord is visible at the vaginal opening
- *Palpated:* the cord cannot be seen, but it can be felt as a pulsating structure when a vaginal examination is done
- *Occult:* the prolapse is hidden and cannot be seen or felt; it is suspected on the basis of abnormal fetal heart rates

**Risk Factors.** Prolapse of the umbilical cord is more likely if the fetus does not completely fill the space in the pelvis or if fluid pressure is great when the membranes rupture. These conditions are more likely in the following situations:

- Fetus high in the pelvis when the membranes rupture
- Very small fetus, as in prematurity
- Abnormal presentations, such as footling breech or transverse lie
- Hydramnios (excess amniotic fluid)

**Medical Treatment.** The main risk of a prolapsed cord is to the fetus. When prolapsed cord occurs, the first action is to displace the fetus upward to stop compression against the pelvis. Positions such as the knee-chest or Trendelenburg (head-down) accomplish this displacement. The experienced nurse or physician may push the fetus upward from the vagina. Oxygen and a tocolytic drug, such as terbutaline, may be given. The primary focus is to deliver the fetus by the quickest means possible, usually cesarean delivery.

**Nursing Care.** In addition to assisting with emergency procedures, the nurse should remain calm to limit the woman's anxiety. Prolapsed cord is a sudden development; anxiety and fear are inevitable reactions. Calm, quick actions on the part of nurses help the woman and her family feel that she is in competent hands.

After birth, the nurse helps the woman understand the experience. She may need several explanations of what happened and why.

## UTERINE RUPTURE

A tear in the uterine wall occurs if the muscle cannot withstand the pressure inside the organ (Fig. 8–10). There are three variations of uterine rupture:

- *Complete rupture:* there is a hole through the entire uterus, from the uterine cavity to the abdominal cavity
- *Incomplete rupture:* the uterus tears into a nearby structure, such as a ligament, but not all the way into the abdominal cavity
- *Dehiscence:* an old uterine scar, usually from a previous cesarean birth, separates; the separation may be bloodless (a "bloodless window")

Dehiscence is a relatively common occurrence, and the woman may have no signs or symptoms. It may be found during a subsequent cesarean or other abdominal surgery.

**Risk Factors.** Uterine rupture is more likely if the woman had previous surgery on her uterus, usually a previous cesarean delivery. The low-transverse uterine incision (see p. 196) is least likely to rupture. Because the classic uterine incision is prone to rupture, vaginal birth after this type incision is not recommended.

Uterine rupture may occur in the unscarred uterus if a woman

- Had many other births (grand multiparity)
- Has intense labor contractions, such as with oxytocin stimulation
- Had blunt abdominal trauma, such as from a vehicle accident or battering

**Characteristics.** The woman may have no symptoms, or she may have sudden onset of severe signs and symptoms:

- Shock due to bleeding into the abdomen (vaginal bleeding may be minimal)
- Abdominal pain
- Pain in the chest, between the scapulae (shoulder blades), or with inspiration
- Cessation of contractions
- Abnormal or absent fetal heart rates
- Palpation of the fetus outside the uterus, because the fetus is pushed through the torn area

**Medical Treatment.** If the fetus is living when the rupture is detected and/or if blood loss is excessive, the physician performs surgery to deliver the fetus and stops the bleeding. Hysterectomy (removal of the uterus) is likely for an extensive tear. Smaller tears may be repaired if the woman wants more children.

**Nursing Care.** Oxytocin is carefully administered during labor, and the woman observed for excessive contractions. If signs or symptoms of uterine rupture occur, the physician is promptly notified. The nurse incorporates measures to allay the woman's anxiety before and after birth, as discussed with prolapsed umbilical cord.

Uterine rupture is sometimes not discovered until after birth. In these cases, the woman does not have dramatic symptoms of blood loss. However, she may have continuous bleeding that is brighter red than the normal postbirth bleeding. A rising pulse and falling blood pressure suggest shock, which may occur if blood loss is excessive.

## UTERINE INVERSION

Uterine inversion occurs if the uterus turns inside out after the baby is born. There are

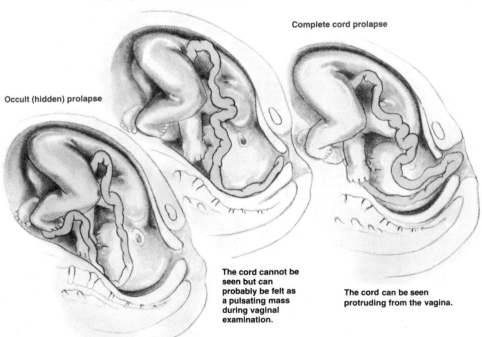

Cord prolapsed in front of the fetal head

Complete cord prolapse

Occult (hidden) prolapse

The cord cannot be seen but can probably be felt as a pulsating mass during vaginal examination.

The cord can be seen protruding from the vagina.

The cord is compressed between the fetal presenting part and pelvis but cannot be seen or felt during vaginal examination.

**Figure 8–9.** Three different degrees of prolapsed umbilical cord.

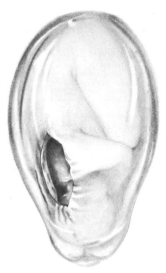

**Figure 8–10.** Uterine rupture.

varying degrees of uterine inversion. The physician may note a minor depression in the top of the uterus or may discover that the uterus is not in the abdomen and protrudes from the vagina with its inner surface showing. Rapid onset of shock is common.

Uterine inversion is more likely to occur if the uterus is not firmly contracted, especially if the birth attendant pulls on the umbilical cord to deliver the placenta. It can also occur during recovery if the uterus is pushed downward toward the pelvis when it is not firm.

**Medical Treatment.** The physician will try to replace the inverted uterus while the woman is under general anesthesia. The anesthetic agent is chosen to cause uterine relaxation; tocolytic drugs also may be used. After the uterus is replaced, oxytocin is given to contract the uterus and control bleeding. If replacement of the uterus is not successful, the woman needs a hysterectomy.

**Nursing Care.** Nursing care during the emergency supplements medical management. Two intravenous lines are usually established to administer fluids and combat shock.

During the recovery period, the woman's uterus is assessed every 15 minutes for firmness, height, and deviation from the midline. Her vital signs and the amount of vaginal bleeding are assessed at the same time. An indwelling catheter may be used to keep her bladder empty so that the uterus can contract well. The catheter is assessed for patency and

the output recorded; output may fall to less than 30 ml/hr with shock. She takes nothing orally until stable and the physician orders oral intake.

After birth, the nurse provides explanations and emotional support to the woman and her partner. The birth may have been completely normal until the uterine inversion occurred. Suddenly, the woman was surrounded by people who inserted additional intravenous lines in her arm and was quickly anesthetized. Her partner was probably sent from the room to sit, terrified, in the waiting room. Both will need explanations about what happened and why the actions were taken to correct the problem. The explanations may need to be reinforced several times before they can integrate the experience.

## AMNIOTIC FLUID EMBOLISM

This uncommon embolism occurs when amniotic fluid, with its particles such as vernix, fetal hair, and sometimes meconium, enters the woman's circulation and obstructs small blood vessels in her lungs. It is more likely to occur during a very strong labor because the fluid is "pushed" into small blood vessels that rupture as the cervix dilates.

The woman has abrupt and severe respiratory distress and circulatory collapse. Coagulation abnormalities may occur because amniotic fluid is rich in factors that promote blood clotting. Immediate cardiac and pulmonary support are begun. Clotting defects are corrected with appropriate blood factors.

The likelihood of death from amniotic fluid embolism is high, especially if meconium was in the fluid. The embolism may occur before or after the infant is born.

## TRAUMA

The pregnant trauma victim may be encountered anywhere, from an accident scene, to the hospital emergency department. The priority is management of the woman's life-threatening injuries. Once the woman is stabilized, the fetus can be considered. As the woman's injuries are treated, a small wedge is placed under one hip to displace her uterus from her large blood vessels. This action helps stabilize her blood pressure and improves blood flow to the placenta. The staff should remain alert to signs and symptoms that suggest abruptio placentae (see p. 88) and uterine rupture, which are more likely to occur with trauma to the pregnant woman's abdomen.

## KEY POINTS

- The nurse observes the character of the amniotic fluid and the fetal heart rate when the membranes are ruptured.
- The nurse observes the fetal condition and character of contractions if any methods to stimulate labor are used. These may include amniotomy, oxytocin, walking, or nipple stimulation.
- After version, the nurse observes for persistent contractions that may indicate labor has begun and leaking amniotic fluid. Before discharge, signs of labor are reviewed with the woman.
- Nursing care after episiotomy or perineal lacerations includes comfort measures, such as cold applications and analgesics.
- Nursing care after cesarean birth is similar to that after vaginal birth, with these additions: surgical dressing, indwelling catheter patency, and intravenous flow. The woman and her partner may need extra emotional support after cesarean birth.
- Nursing measures such as encouraging position changes, aiding relaxation, and reminding the woman to empty her bladder can promote a more normal labor.
- Nursing care after births involving instruments (forceps or vacuum extraction) and after abnormal labor and birth includes observations for maternal and newborn injuries or infections.
- Infection is the most common hazard after membranes rupture prematurely, especially if there is a long interval before delivery.
- Nurses should be aware of the subtle symptoms a woman may have at the beginning of preterm labor and encourage her to seek care at the hospital promptly.
- After any kind of emergency, the woman and her family need emotional support, explanations of what happened, and patience with their repeated questions.

# Study Questions

1. A woman has been in labor for 14 hours, and her membranes have been ruptured for 16 hours. What signs suggest that she is developing an infection?
2. What nursing measures can improve the quality of contractions and facilitate progress if a woman is having a slow labor?
3. A baby is born with assistance of the vacuum extractor. The parents want to know why the baby has "that funny lump" on his head. What should the nurse tell them?
4. A friend had a cesarean birth for her first baby and is pregnant again. Her physician is encouraging her to try for a vaginal birth this time. She asks you, "I thought if you had one cesarean, all your babies had to be born by cesarean. Isn't labor dangerous for me?" What is the best answer?
5. Why is it important to address the woman's psychological needs during labor as well as her physical needs?
6. One of your friends who is 7 months pregnant calls you and says, "I don't really hurt, but I'm sure having a lot of pressure down low." What should you suggest?

# Multiple Choice Review Questions

*Choose the most appropriate answer.*

1. Green amniotic fluid indicates
   a. that the baby is probably premature
   b. passage of the first bowel contents into the fluid

c. that the mother and infant are at risk for infection

d. a normal assessment during labor

3. Contractions during oxytocin induction of labor are every 2 minutes, they last 95 seconds, and the uterus remains tense between contractions. What action is expected based on these assessments?

   a. no action expected; the contractions are normal
   b. rate of oxytocin will be increased slightly
   c. pain medication or an epidural block will be offered
   d. infusion of oxytocin will be stopped

4. Select the appropriate nursing intervention during the early recovery period to increase the woman's comfort if she had forceps-assisted birth and a median episiotomy.

   a. application of a cold pack to her perineal area
   b. encouragement of perineal stretching exercises
   c. application of warm, moist heat to the perineum
   d. administration of stool softeners as ordered

5. It is especially important to observe for respiratory distress in the infant born by cesarean birth because

   a. infants pass meconium in their amniotic fluid before birth
   b. a cool operating room depresses the infant's reflexes to breathe
   c. fluid remains in the airways longer than after vaginal birth
   d. the cesarean-born infant is more likely to be preterm

6. A woman has an emergency cesarean delivery after having a prolapsed umbilical cord. She repeatedly asks similar questions about what happened at birth. The nurse's interpretation of her behavior is that she

   a. cannot accept that she did not have the kind of delivery she planned
   b. is trying to understand her experience and move on with postpartum adaptation
   c. thinks the staff is not telling

her the truth about what happened at birth

   d. is confused about events because general anesthesia effects are persisting

7. What nursing intervention during labor can increase space in the woman's pelvis?

   a. promote adequate fluid intake
   b. position on the left side
   c. assist her to take a shower
   d. encourage regular urination

8. A woman having her fourth baby comes into labor at 8 cm of cervical dilation. The most appropriate way to help her with pain management is to

   a. breathe along with her during each contraction
   b. give her a narcotic drug, such as butorphanol (Stadol) or meperidine (Demerol)
   c. notify the anesthesiologist to administer an epidural block
   d. explain that she should not be in labor much longer

9. A woman is being cared for in the antepartum unit because her membranes ruptured at 30 weeks' gestation. While giving morning care, the nursing student notices that the fluid draining has a strong odor. The most appropriate action to take at this time is to

   a. continue morning care, but caution the woman to remain in bed until her physician visits
   b. ask the woman if she is having any more contractions than usual
   c. take the temperature; report it and the fluid odor to the registered nurse
   d. prepare the woman for an immediate cesarean delivery

10. If the cord prolapses, the woman's hips are elevated higher than her head to

   a. promote rotation of the fetal head within the pelvis
   b. increase blood flow through the umbilical cord
   c. delay an excessively rapid birth
   d. decrease intensity of labor contractions

11. While in the emergency department, a nursing student is helping to care for a woman, 8 months pregnant, who was in a car accident. She has no obvious injuries. The woman complains that her upper middle back hurts more than anything else. The student should
   a. reassure the woman that she will probably have lots of aches and pains for the next few days
   b. turn the woman on her left side and have her take several slow, deep breaths
   c. palpate her abdomen to determine if she is having any uterine contractions
   d. report the woman's complaints to the registered nurse who is supervising her care

## BIBLIOGRAPHY

AWHONN (Association of Women's Health, Obstetric, and Neonatal Nurses). (1993). *Cervical ripening and induction and augmentation of labor.* Washington, DC: Author.

Biancuzzo, M. (1993). How to recognize and rotate an occiput posterior fetus. *American Journal of Nursing, 93,* 38–41.

Bowes, W.A. (1989). Clinical aspects of normal and abnormal labor. In R.K. Creasy & R. Resnik (Eds.), *Maternal-fetal medicine: Principles and practice* (pp. 510–546). Philadelphia: W.B. Saunders.

Brouillard-Pierce, C. (1993). Indications for induction of labor. *MCN: Journal of Maternal-Child Nursing, 18*(Suppl.), 14–22.

Canadian Preterm Labor Investigators' Group. (1992). Treatment of preterm labor with the beta-adrenergic agonist ritodrine. *New England Journal of Medicine, 327,* 308–312.

Clay, L.S., Criss, K., & Jackson, U.C. (1993). External cephalic version. *Journal of Nurse-Midwifery, 38*(Suppl.), 72S–79S.

Cowan, M. (1993). Home care of the pregnant woman using terbutaline. *MCN: American Journal of Maternal Child Nursing, 18,* 99–105.

Dineen, K., Rossi, M., Lia-Hoagberg, B., & Keller, L.O. (1992). Antepartum care services for high-risk women. *JOGNN: Journal of Obstetric, Gynecologic, and Neonatal Nursing, 21,* 121–125.

Gorrie, T.M., McKinney, E.S., & Murray, S.M. (1994). *Foundations of maternal-newborn nursing.* Philadelphia: W.B. Saunders.

Graham, A.D.M. (1992). Preterm labor and premature rupture of membranes. In N.F. Hacker & J.G. Moore (Eds.), *Essentials of obstetrics and gynecology* (2nd ed., pp. 270–280). Philadelphia: W.B. Saunders.

Griese, M.E., & Prickett, S.A. (1993). Nursing management of umbilical cord prolapse. *JOGNN: Journal of Obstetric, Gynecologic, and Neonatal Nursing, 22,* 311–315.

Keppy, K.A., McTigue, M., & Guzman, E.R. (1993). Premature rupture of the membranes. In R.A. Knuppel & J.E. Drukker (Eds.), *High-risk pregnancy: A team approach* (pp. 378–395). Philadelphia: W.B. Saunders.

Knuppel, R.A. & Drukker, J.E. (1993). Twins and other multiple gestations. In R.A. Knuppel & J.E. Drukker (Eds.), *High-risk pregnancy: A team approach* (pp. 433–467). Philadelphia: W.B. Saunders.

Lipshitz, J., Pierce, P.M., & Arntz, M. (1993). Preterm labor. In R.A. Knuppel & J.E. Drukker (Eds.), *High-risk pregnancy: A team approach* (pp. 396–421). Philadelphia: W.B. Saunders.

Lynam, L.E., & Miller, M.A. (1992). Mothers' and nurses' perceptions of the needs of women experiencing preterm labor. *JOGNN: Journal of Obstetric, Gynecologic, and Neonatal Nursing, 21,* 126–136.

Maloni, J.A. (1993). Bed rest during pregnancy: Implications for nursing. *JOGNN: Journal of Obstetric, Gynecologic, and Neonatal Nursing, 22,* 422–426.

Maloni, J.A., Chance, B., Zhang, C., Cohen, A.W., Betts, D., & Gange, S.J. (1993). Physical and psychosocial side effects of antepartum hospital bed rest. *Nursing Research, 42,* 197–203.

Mayberry, L.J., Smith, M., & Gill, P. (1992). Effect of exercise on uterine activity in the patient in preterm labor. *Journal of Perinatology, 12,* 354–358.

Miller, A.M., & Lorkovic, M. (1993). Prostaglandin E$_2$ for cervical ripening. *MCN: American Journal of Maternal Child Nursing, 18*(Suppl.), 23–30.

Newnham, J.P., & Hobel, C.J. (1992). Operative delivery. In N.F. Hacker & J.G. Moore (Eds.), *Essentials of obstetrics & gynecology* (2nd ed., 308–315). Philadelphia: W.B. Saunders.

Papke, K.R. (1993). Management of preterm labor and prevention of premature delivery. *Advances in Clinical Nursing Research, 28,* 279–288.

Penney, D.S., & Perlis, D.W. (1992). Shoulder dystocia: When to use suprapubic pressure. *MCN: American Journal of Maternal Child Nursing, 17,* 34–36.

Petrie, R.H., & Williams, A.M. (1993). Induction of labor. In R.A. Knuppel & J.E. Drukker (Eds.), *High-risk pregnancy: A team approach* (pp. 303–315). Philadelphia: W.B. Saunders.

Phelan, J.P., Bendell, A., & Colburn, V.G. (1993). Cesarean birth. In R.A. Knuppel & J.E. Drukker (Eds.), *High-risk pregnancy: A team approach* (pp. 337–361). Philadelphia: W.B. Saunders.

Reichert, J.A., Baron, M., & Fawcett, J. (1993). Changes in attitudes toward cesarean birth. *JOGNN: Journal of Obstetric, Gynecologic, and Neonatal Nursing, 22,* 159–167.

Resick, L.K., & Erlen, J.A. (1990). Vaginal birth after cesarean: Issues and implications. *Journal of the American Academy of Nurse Practitioners, 2,* 100–106.

Resnik, R. (1989). Post-term pregnancy. In R.K. Creasy & R. Resnik (Eds.), *Maternal-fetal medicine: Principles & practice* (pp. 505–509). Philadelphia: W.B. Saunders.

Sala, D.J., Moise, K.J. (1990). The treatment of preterm labor using a portable subcutaneous terbutaline pump. *JOGNN: Journal of Obstetric, Gynecologic, and Neonatal Nursing, 19*, 108–115.

Tighe, D., & Sweezy, S.R. (1990). The perioperative experience of cesarean birth: Preparation, considerations, and complications. *Journal of Perinatal & Neonatal Nursing, 3*, 14–30.

U.S. Preventive Services Task Force. (1993). Home uterine activity monitoring for preterm labor. *JAMA: Journal of the American Medical Association, 270*, 371–376.

Wilcox, L.S., Stobino, D.M., Baruffi, G., & Dellinger, W.S. (1989). Episiotomy and its role in the incidence of perineal lacerations in a maternity center and a tertiary hospital obstetric service. *American Journal of Obstetrics and Gynecology, 160*, 1047–1052.

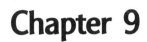

## Chapter 9

# The Family Following Birth

Immediate Postpartum Period: Fourth Stage
System Changes in the Mother: Nursing Care
   Reproductive System
   Cardiovascular System
   Urinary System
   Gastrointestinal System
   Integumentary System
   Musculoskeletal System
   Immune System
   Changes After Cesarean Birth
   Emotional Changes
**Care of the Newborn**
   Airway
   Breathing
   Providing Warmth
   Umbilical Cord
   Blood Coagulation, Anemia, and Hypoglycemia
   Preventing Infection
   Identification
   Meconium Aspiration Syndrome
   Gestational Age Assessment
   Screening Tests
   Reactivity
   Bonding and Attachment
   Rooming-in
   Tender, Loving Care
   Daily Care
**Breast Feeding**
   Beginning Breast Feeding
   Hygiene
   Position
   Procedure
   Milk Supply
   Burping
   Relieving Breast Engorgement

Relieving Sore Nipples
Breast Feeding after Complicated Births
Maternal Nutrition
Weaning
Suppression of Lactation
**Bottle Feeding**
**Discharge Planning**
Postpartum Instructions
Follow-up Care

# OBJECTIVES

*On completion and mastery of Chapter 9, the student will be able to*

■ Define each vocabulary term listed.
■ Define the fourth stage of labor.
■ Name two reasons why the nurse should try to make her interventions culture-specific.
■ Describe how to check the fundus properly.
■ List the main cause of morbidity and mortality during the puerperium.
■ Describe the nursing care of a new mother in the hospital during the postpartum period.
■ Describe the process of lactation.
■ Identify advantages and disadvantages of breast feeding.
■ List the four forms of prepared formulas for newborns.
■ Describe how to bottle feed a baby.

This chapter covers the first few hours after delivery, the postpartum period, and discharge. The postpartum period or *puerperium* (*puer*, "child," and *parere*, "to bring forth") is defined as the 6 weeks following childbirth. This period is also referred to as the "4th trimester" of pregnancy.

During the postpartum period, the new mother undergoes dramatic physical and psychological changes as her body returns to the prepregnant state. The father, siblings, and grandparents also experience role changes. Their participation in the postpartum period depends on their past history, personal security, and acceptance of the pregnancy and outcome.

In the ideal situation, when the delivery has gone well, family members share joy and relief. Even though they may have mixed feelings and new responsibilities, the family remains cohesive. For others there are disappointment and

alienation. One mother who had a cesarean delivery noted that she felt she had "missed the parade." For a few, the much-awaited event ends in apprehension and grieving as the precious baby is admitted to the neonatal intensive care unit or transferred to another institution for care.

**Adaptations for Specific Populations and Cultures.** During the puerperium, the nurse continues to assess the woman's progress carefully and identifies deviations from normal. Families are instructed at their level of understanding. Interventions are adapted to circumstances, such as those of the single or adolescent parent, the poor, those who are physically or mentally challenged, and those with language barriers.

Various ethnic groups have a number of rituals and traditions concerning the postpartum mother. They are often aimed at restoring universal balance between the equal and opposite forces of hot and cold. For many Mexican Americans and Asian Americans, cold is avoided after birth. This may include cold in their environment, water, and diet. The mother must be kept warm and given warm beverages. Bathing is restricted in many cultures.

Nourishment can be a problem. Some women cannot read hospital menus. Others may find the food selection inconsistent with their beliefs. In such instances, family members are encouraged to bring in more traditional meals to entice the mother to eat.

Most Southeast Asians restrict activity after childbirth for 1 or 2 months. Elders take care of the mother. Often the grandmother cooks, cleans, and cares for the baby. It is appropriate that others wait on the mother. The unknowing nurse may see the mother as "lazy" or unwilling to cooperate.

Nurses must be open to incorporating practices different from their own, whenever feasible. This not only provides a more inviting environment for the woman but, one hopes, inspires her to continue contact with health-care professionals following discharge.

## Immediate Postpartum Period: Fourth Stage

The process of labor and delivery is divided into four stages (see Table 6–2).

During the fourth stage, the immediate postpartum period, the new mother is closely monitored for signs of *hypovolemic shock* and *hemor-*

*rhage.* She may be observed in the recovery area or the delivery room, in the birthing room, or in the assigned postpartum room. Once the danger of bleeding is past, the primary concern is *preventing infection.*

In a general hospital setting, once the mother's condition stabilizes, she may be transferred from the recovery area in the delivery suite to her room on the postpartum unit. This transfer may not be necessary when labor, delivery, and postpartum procedures are completed in the same room. In the alternative birthing unit, the mother and baby may go home within hours of delivery.

The receiving nurse is given a full report of the mother's progress and the details of her delivery. This includes vital signs, the level and consistency of her fundus (upper part of uterus), the amount of vaginal discharge, and the existence and/or type of episiotomy. If the mother has voided, the time and amount of urine are reported and documented. Any unusual circumstances at the time of delivery, or afterward, are made known.

The woman who has had a cesarean delivery is not only a postpartum but also a postsurgical patient. Appropriate additional information is added to the chart when she is transferred back to the maternity unit. The condition, weight, sex, and location of the newborn are important for the staff to know.

*Postpartum hemorrhage,* a major threat during the fourth stage, is the leading cause of maternal morbidity and mortality. The nurse closely observes the new mother following delivery of the placenta (afterbirth) for *bleeding* and for *hypovolemic shock* (see p. 250). Particular attention is paid to the fundus and the episiotomy site. Observations at this time serve as baseline data for comparison, should difficulties arise. The color and amount of vaginal bleeding are noted, as is the appearance of the perineum. The perineal pad is changed, and the area beneath the buttocks is carefully checked for excessive or accumulated blood. A fresh gown and a warm blanket provide comfort during bonding.

## Nursing Brief

Painless, bright red vaginal bleeding is immediately reported.

## System Changes in the Mother: Nursing Care

Box 9–1 summarizes the standard nursing assessments for the postpartal woman. Refer to Nursing Care Plan 9–1 to find interventions for selected diagnoses in the postpartum woman.

### REPRODUCTIVE SYSTEM

**Involution of Uterus.** Following childbirth, the uterus undergoes a rapid reduction in size and weight. The rate of decrease in weight varies with the weight of the newborn and the number of previous pregnancies. *Involution* is the term used for the decrease in size of the uterus and a return to its normal condition and position. *Oxytocin* is the hormone responsible for uterine involution and for initiation of the let-down of milk for breast feeding. Nursing stimulates the production of oxytocin, which causes the uterus to contract and hastens involution. The placental site heals by *exfoliation,* or the scaling off of dead tissue. This leaves the uterine lining smooth. By the 10th postpartum day, the fundus of the uterus can no longer be palpated through the abdominal wall.

Barring complications, the uterus returns to the nonpregnant size by 5–6 weeks. The nurse observes the location and consistency (firmness) of the fundus to avoid *uterine atony,* a lack of tone (see p. 252). This condition can lead to increased bleeding. Multiparity, multiple births, prolonged labor, a full bladder, and incomplete expulsion of afterbirth may increase the risk of uterine atony and postpartum hemorrhage.

After delivery, the fundus is at about the level of the umbilicus or slightly lower. On palpation, it should be firm and about the size of a grapefruit. The nurse feels the fundus through the abdominal wall, noting its consistency and

## Nursing Brief

The nurse assesses the progress of involution by palpating the fundus and recording its descent. It descends one fingerbreadth daily. Any changes in consistency are immediately remedied by massage.

## BOX 9–1 Summary of Nursing Assessments of the Postpartum Woman

*General appearance*: Observe patient from head to toe (color and warmth of skin, respiratory status, state of exhaustion); assess the responsiveness of patient (level of consciousness, dizziness, orthostatic hypotension)

*Pulse and blood pressure*: Take and record vital signs as per protocol; blood pressure, pulse, and respiration are generally taken every 15 min for 1 hr or until stable and then every 4 hr; bradycardia is normal in the 1st week post partum (50–70 beats/min)

*Temperature*: It is taken orally to avoid vaginal contamination; a rise in temperature above 38°C (100.4°F) after the 1st 24 hr is suspicious for postpartal infection

*Fundus*: Evaluate the consistency, location, and height of the fundus

*Breasts*: Assess the condition of breasts, such as general appearance, soreness, engorgement, lactation, and discharge from nipples

*Lochia*: Determine the character, color, and amount of lochia, including odor, presence of clots

*Voiding*: Because diuresis begins shortly after delivery, the bladder becomes filled quickly; determine first voiding, frequency, and signs and symptoms of bladder distention

*Perineum*: Observe perineum for edema, bruising, or hematoma

*Episiotomy*: Observe episiotomy site for redness, edema, ecchymosis, discharge, edges well approximated (REEDA)

*Cesarean incision*: Evaluate incision site of cesarean section for (REEDA)

*Hemorrhoids*: Note number and size

*Extremities*: Assess for thrombophlebitis (Homans' sign), edema, tenderness

*Pain*: Observe for pain and discomfort; woman may experience afterpains; woman who had cesarean delivery may experience incisional pain

*Bowels*: Assess amount of time since last defecation, observe bowel sounds: auscultate all four quadrants, especially post cesarean delivery

*Hydration*: Assess hydration and nutritional status (PO intake, intravenous lines, nausea, vomiting, hunger)

*Emotional health*: Evaluate psychological status (weepiness, depression, interaction with family and nurse)

*Attachment*: Observe for attachment to newborn

*Cultural variations*: Assess cultural needs

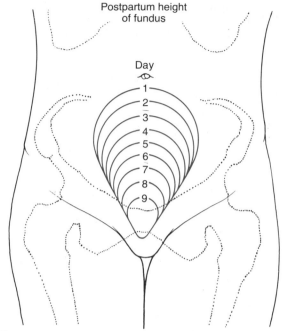

**Figure 9–1.** Uterine involution showing changes in the height of the fundus.

height (i.e., at or below the umbilicus) (Fig. 9–1).

If the consistency of the uterus is boggy (soft, spongy and difficult to feel), the fundus is immediately massaged until the uterus is again contracted. This is accomplished by placing one hand over the fundus and the other just above the pubic bone and massaging in a circular motion (Fig. 9–2). This technique contracts the uterus and prevents it from becoming inverted. This contraction is important in sealing off the large vessels that fed the placenta before it detached at delivery. Generally, tightening of the uterine muscles can be immediately felt under the nurse's hand.

The fundal area is sensitive after labor and delivery. The nurse explains to the woman that she may feel some discomfort during massage. The woman is also instructed to palpate and massage her own fundus. After the uterus is massaged until firm, the blood that has accumulated in the uterine cavity and vagina may be expressed. This is accomplished by gently pressing down on the fundus, forward and outward.

If uterine atony continues, the physician may order the administration of oxytocic drugs. Oxytocin (Pitocin) is often routinely ordered in

> ### NURSING CARE PLAN 9–1
>
> ### Selected Nursing Diagnoses for the Woman Following Childbirth
>
> | Goals | Nursing Interventions | Rationale |
> |---|---|---|
> | **Nursing Diagnosis:** High risk for altered tissue perfusion related to blood loss during delivery and atony of uterus. | | |
> | Woman will maintain adequate tissue perfusion as evidenced by normal vital signs, firm fundus, and saturation of no more than one pad per hour | 1. Assess vital signs every 15 min during initial period, then according to hospital procedure<br>2. Assess uterine fundus by daily evaluating height, position, and firmness; massage if boggy, until well contracted<br>3. Observe lochia for amount, color, consistency, odor, and persistent clots | 1. Rising pulse and falling blood pressure may be signs of shock from excessive bleeding<br>2. A firm fundus compresses bleeding vessels at placental site<br>3. These measures help determine whether there is excessive blood loss; continued bright red lochia signifies possible retained placental fragments; a foul odor indicates infection |
> | **Nursing Diagnosis:** High risk for alterations in urination, retention related to trauma of labor and delivery. | | |
> | Woman will empty bladder completely at regular intervals<br>Fundus will be firm and at appropriate level | 1. Evaluate bladder for distention and measure urinary output<br><br><br><br><br>2. Pour warm water over perineum; run water faucet<br>3. Encourage fluid intake<br><br>4. Woman may require catheterization if other measures fail | 1. A full bladder pressing on the uterus interferes with contraction and involution; urethra may be traumatized because of delivery; less than 150 mL voided may be overflow from a distended bladder<br>2. Warm water may relax urinary sphincter<br>3. Increased fluids may precipitate voiding<br>4. A full bladder may lead to hemorrhage by inhibiting uterine contraction; stasis of urine in bladder can lead to infection |

the postpartum period, to be administered intravenously or intramuscularly. Occasionally, methylergonovine maleate (Methergine) may be ordered.

**Lochia.** Vaginal discharge after delivery is called *lochia rubra*. It is composed of endometrial tissue, blood, and lymph. Lochia is assessed for quantity, type, and characteristics. During the immediate postpartum period, it is red and moderate to heavy. The nurse estimates the amount of flow on the menstrual pad in 1 hour as follows:

- Scant: less than 2.5 cm (1 inch)
- Light: less than 10 cm (4 inches)
- Moderate: less than 15 cm (6 inches)
- Heavy: saturated menstrual pad
- Excessive: menstrual pad saturated in 15 minutes

If a mother experiences flow problems, have her apply a clean pad and check it within 15–20 minutes. The nurse and mother can also count the number of peripads applied during a given time period or weigh them to help determine the amount of vaginal discharge.

Lochia is heavier when the mother ambulates. This increase results from the release of pooled lochia. A few small clots may be seen at this time. These may be alarming to the new mother if she is not prepared for them. Large clots should not be present. Lochia increases with strenuous exercise and initial stair climbing. Women who have had a cesarean delivery have less lochia during the first 24 hours because the uterine cavity was evacuated at delivery. Breast-feeding mothers have less lochia because of the release of oxytocin during nursing. All women have some lochia, and the *absence* may indicate postpartum infection.

When the amount of lochia is assessed as heavy (more than one pad saturated within 1 hour), the fundus is massaged to improve the

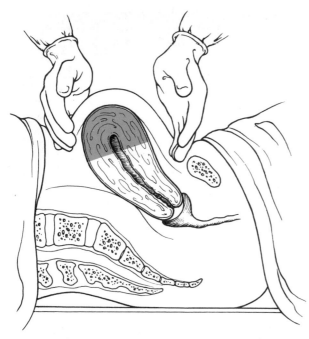

**Figure 9–2.** When massaging the fundus, the nurse keeps one hand firmly on the lower uterus, just above the symphysis pubis. The uterus is massaged in a firm, circular motion. After the uterus becomes firm, the nurse pushes downward, toward the outlet, to expel accumulated blood.

## PROCEDURE FOR ASSESSING AND MASSAGING THE UTERINE FUNDUS

### Materials

Unsterile gloves are worn. Offer perineal care and provide a clean pad. Explain the procedure before beginning.

### Method

1. Identify the need for fundal massage. In most cases, the uterus will be soft and higher than the umbilicus.
2. Have the woman empty her bladder, because a distended bladder raises and displaces the uterus.
3. Place the woman in a supine position with the knees slightly flexed. Lower the perineal pad to observe lochia as the fundus is palpated.
4. Place the outer edge of nondominant hand just above the symphysis pubis, and press downward slightly to anchor the lower uterus.
5. Locate and massage the uterine fundus with the flat portion of the fingers of the dominant hand in a firm circular motion.
6. When the uterus is firm, gently push downward on the fundus, toward the vaginal outlet, to expel blood and clots that have accumulated inside the uterus. *Keep the other hand on the lower uterus to avoid inverting the organ.*
7. Measure the number of fingerbreaths at which the fundus is felt either above or below the umbilicus.
8. Document the consistency and location of the fundus. For example, "FF 2 ↓ U" means the fundus is firm and two fingerbreaths below the umbilicus.
9. Notify registered nurse if the uterus does not become firm or if the fundus becomes boggy when massage has stopped.

muscle tone of the uterus. The nurse reports the passage of large clots or tissue, which may be a sign of retained secundines or afterbirth fragments. The tissue is saved for the physician to observe, to determine if medical or surgical intervention is needed.

Lochia gradually changes from red to pinkish-brown to creamy white. This is a result of the healing process taking place at the placental implantation site. The stages are medically termed *lochia rubra* (red), *lochia serosa*, and *lochia alba* (white). The types and characteristics of lochia are described in Table 9–1.

The nurse prepares the mother in advance for these changes. The process may last 3–6 weeks and varies from woman to woman. Lochia may have a menstrual odor, but it is *never* foul. The nurse emphasizes to the new mother the need to report immediately a foul odor of the lochia. This may indicate an infection of the uterus, which can be serious. Also instruct mothers to report a *return* to lochia rubra, which may indicate a late postpartal hemorrhage. Because some women are being discharged as early as 4 hours following delivery,

the educational component of care becomes increasingly important.

**Afterpains.** Afterpains, most common in multiparas, are painful, intermittent uterine contractions (similar to menstrual cramps) following delivery. They are not usually experienced after the birth of the first child, as the tone of uterus of the primipara is generally good. In the multipara or in women whose uterus has been very distended, such as those with multiple births, afterpains can be severe, particularly

**Table 9–1.** TYPES AND CHARACTERISTICS OF LOCHIA

| Types | Characteristics |
|---|---|
| Lochia rubra | Red, duration 1–3 days; composed of blood, fragments of decidua, mucus, blood cells; menstrual-like odor; foul odor, saturation of pads, and large clots indicate infection |
| Lochia serosa | Pinkish-brown, duration 3–10 days, serosanguineous; no foul odor, not excessive |
| Lochia alba | White, duration 10–14 days or longer, mostly mucus; no foul odor, no change of color back to pink or red; cessation indicates that cervix is closed, less chance of infection from vagina to uterus |

during breast feeding. An analgesic, such as ibuprofen (Motrin), acetaminophen (Tylenol), propoxyphene (Darvon), or oxcodone (Percocet), is administered as ordered to provide relief (Table 9–2). Heat is *not* applied to the abdomen because it may increase bleeding.

**Cervix.** The cervix regains its muscle tone but never closes as tightly as during the prepregnant state. Some edema persists for a few weeks after delivery. Heavy bleeding indicates a cervical or vaginal laceration.

**Vagina.** The vaginal orifice undergoes a great deal of stretching during childbirth. The *rugae*, or vaginal folds, disappear, and the walls of the vagina become smooth and spacious. The rugae reappear 3–4 weeks post partum. The introitus is swollen and erythematous for several weeks of the postpartum period.

**Perineum.** The perineum is tender, even without an episiotomy, because of the tremendous amount of stretching. The episiotomy heals in 5–6 weeks if infection or hematoma does not occur. If no episiotomy is present, the perineum regains its muscle tone in 2–3 weeks.

The patient with an episiotomy or laceration repair is carefully watched for signs of bleeding, infection, and development of a hematoma. Some discomfort of the episiotomy site is anticipated, but intense pain may indicate formation of a hematoma under the episiotomy repair. Large or expanding hematomas may require surgical excision.

An ice pack may be applied following the episiotomy to reduce swelling and increase comfort. Later, an ice pack may be used for its analgesic effect for up to 24 hours. Commercial cold packs combined with perineal pads are available. A disposable rubber glove filled with ice chips and taped at the wrist may also be useful. The patient is instructed to cover the glove to avoid ice burn to the perineum.

**Teaching Self-Care.** Following vaginal delivery, if all has gone well and her condition is stable, the mother may take a sponge bath or shower. She generally needs some assistance. The nurse instructs the mother in the use of the call button and remains close by. This is an excellent opportunity to observe and instruct the mother. The areas of her body at greatest risk for infection are the breasts and the perineum. After a cesarean birth, the abdominal incision is also of concern.

The mother is instructed to use clear water on her breasts and to cleanse in a circular mo-

**Table 9–2.** COMMONLY USED POSTPARTUM SYSTEMIC ANALGESICS

| Trade Name | Generic Name | Dosage | Comments |
|---|---|---|---|
| Darvon | Propoxyphene | 65-mg capsules given PO every 4–6 hr or as ordered | Narcotic analgesic used for mild to moderate pain; alters perception of pain by multiple actions in central nervous system; taking capsule with one-half to one glass of water speeds onset of analgesia |
| Perococet | 5 mg oxycodone, 325 mg acetaminophen | 1–2 tablets PO every 4–6 hr or as ordered | Semisynthetic narcotic analgesic used for relief of moderate to moderately severe pain; rapid onset of analgesia 10–15 min; causes decrease in alertness |
| Motrin | Ibuprofen | 400 mg PO every 4–6 hr | Assess for GI upset |
| Tylenol | Acetaminophen | 325–650 mg PO every 4–6 hr | Side effects are rare |
| Vicodin | Hydrocodone bitartrate | 5–10 mg every 4–6 hr | Effect of medication is reduced if full pain recurs before next dose |

tion from the nipple outward. After drying her breasts with a towel, the nursing mother may air-dry her nipples for 15 minutes.

The mother is also instructed in perineal self-care. This relieves episiotomy discomfort, promotes adequate healing, and most important, prevents infection. Nursing care and teaching self-care of the episiotomy site are detailed in Nursing Care Plan 9–2.

Perineal care is done each time the woman voids or defecates. Soft cloths and a peribottle are used for external cleansing. The mother is instructed to cleanse gently from front to back —that is, from the vulva to the rectum. This method is essential to preventing contamination.

The mother is also taught the proper application and removal of the peripad. It should be placed over the vulva and then over the anus and secured so that it does not slip. When she removes the pad, it should be moved downward, toward the anus, and disposed of properly. The use of cold and heat are described in Nursing Care Plan 9–2. The setup for a sitz bath is shown in Fig. 9–3.

**Topical Anesthetics.** Topical anesthetics are applied to relieve discomfort of the perineal area. These include benzocaine (Americaine or Dermoplast) sprays. Anesthetic pads (Tucks) or ointments may be applied to the rectal area to provide relief from hemorrhoids. The side-lying position is recommended.

---

| NURSING CARE PLAN 9–2 |
|:---:|
| **Selected Nursing Diagnoses for the Woman with an Episiotomy** |

| Goals | Nursing Interventions | Rationale |
|---|---|---|
| **Nursing Diagnosis:** Knowledge deficit related to self-care measures to promote comfort and healing of episiotomy. | | |
| Woman will verbalize feelings of increased perineal comfort<br>Woman will demonstrate self-care measures for comfort before discharge | 1. Explain importance of cleansing episiotomy site to promote healing | 1. Moist heat increases circulation and relaxes the tissue to provide comfort and reduce edema and/or infection |
| | 2. Check perineal area every 8 hr; have mother lie on side with upper leg forward to inspect (Sims' position) | 2. The perineum is assessed for signs of infection, unusual swelling, discoloration, and sharp pain, which may indicate hematoma; Sims' position allows a good view of the inspection area |
| | 3. Instruct in use of peribottle | 3. Peribottles filled with warm water are used for cleansing after each voiding or defecation; perineal pad is applied from front to back to avoid contamination with feces |
| | 4. Use an ice pack for pain relief for 1st 24 hr | 4. This numbs tissues and reduces swelling; woman should cover the ice pack to prevent ice burn |
| | 5. Use a perineal warm pack after 24 hr | 5. Chemically treated pads provide heat to the area; they are gradually replacing heat lamps, which can be a source of cross-contamination |
| | 6. Instruct mother in sitz bath procedure | 6. A sitz bath is a portable basin that circulates warm water; it fits over toilet seat; water flows over perineum to reduce edema associated with episiotomy or hemorrhoids; is used for 20 min as often as woman desires (usually 3 or 4 times daily) |
| | 7. Discuss use of analgesics and topical anesthetics | 7. A mild analgesic such as acetaminophen (Tylenol) and topical anesthetics such as benzocaine (Dermoplast) spray or dibucaine (Nupercainal) ointment are commonly used to relieve discomfort |

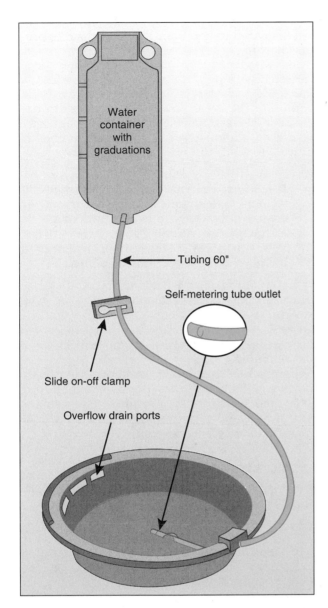

**Figure 9–3.** The sitz bath is a portable basin that fits on the toilet seat. Cool or warm swirling water cleanses and promotes healing of the perineum. (Courtesy of Baxter Health Care Corporation, McGaw Park, IL. Redrawn with permission.)

The mother increases her fluid intake, if an increase is not contraindicated. A stool softener may also be helpful. She is instructed to apply ointments after the sitz bath, to avoid burning the tender tissue. Perineal pads that incorporate a chemical hot pack are gradually replacing heat lamp treatments (Nursing Care Plan 9–2).

**Lactation.** Lactation refers to the production of milk, which begins in pregnancy under the influence of estrogen and progesterone. Following delivery the levels of these and other hormones fall and the level of *prolactin* increases. This phenomenon leads to lactation and resumption of a woman's periods. The anatomy and physiology of the breasts are depicted on page 25.

Late in pregnancy and during the first few days after delivery, *colostrum* is secreted by the breasts. This yellowish fluid is rich in protective antibodies and is the breast-fed infant's first food. It provides protein, vitamins A and E, essential minerals, and nitrogen. It is also said to have a laxative effect, which aids in eliminating *meconium*, a sticky substance that fills the gastrointestinal tract of the newborn.

By the 3rd day, transitional milk becomes noticeable. The breasts become distended and engorged because of the accumulation of milk and increased blood flow to the area. The infant's sucking stimulates the release of *oxytocin* from the posterior pituitary gland. Oxytocin is the hormone responsible for the milk *let-down* reflex. The mother may notice a tingling sensation in both breasts at the time of let-down. Leaking from the opposite breast while feeding is also evidence that the let-down reflex is taking place.

Milk is maintained by the sucking of the newborn. The breasts of women who do not breast feed return to their prepregnant size in about 1–2 weeks.

**Return of Ovulation and Menstruation.** The production of *placental* estrogen and progesterone ceases when the placenta is delivered. This change causes a rise in the production of follicle-stimulating hormone and the return of ovulation. Ovulation, which resumes in approximately 12–18 weeks, also depends on increasing prolactin levels. Menstrual cycles in the nonnursing mother begin in about 6–12 weeks. Most lactating women resume menstruation within 12 weeks, although some may not resume their periods until they discontinue nursing. A woman may ovulate without menstruating. *The absence of menstrual flow does not mean that the woman cannot get pregnant.*

## CARDIOVASCULAR SYSTEM

Following delivery, the heart returns to its normal position because of a shift in the diaphragm and abdominal contents. Cardiac out-

## Nursing Brief

Diagnostic studies commonly ordered during the puerperium include hemoglobin and hematocrit (Hgb/HCT) and possibly urinalysis (UA).

put increases during the first and second stages of labor and declines rapidly thereafter. The additional blood volume seen during pregnancy is decreased by diuresis and blood loss at delivery. The blood loss is approximately 200–500 ml for a vaginal birth and 700–1000 ml with cesarean birth. Hemoglobin and hematocrit levels may fluctuate. These are generally tested in the postpartum period to detect anemia from blood loss or from the pregnancy.

**Chills.** Many mothers complain of being chilled after the delivery. They may visibly shake and tremble uncontrollably. Postpartum chills are believed to be caused by a nervous response or vasomotor changes in the body. This is frightening to the new mothers and their families. The nurse reassures the family and mother (preferably in advance) that this is normal. A blanket is provided. Chills accompanied by fever after the first 24 hours indicate infection.

### URINARY SYSTEM

In the early postpartum period, *diuresis* (increased urine production) occurs as the body rids itself of the excess fluid retained during the pregnancy. Output is measured for the first 24 hours after delivery. The patient's bladder is checked for distention. A full bladder can displace the uterus and prevent proper contraction and involution of the uterus (see p. 253). Signs of this condition are a boggy uterus that is above the level of the umbilicus

## Nursing Brief

The patient who voids frequent, small amounts of urine may be experiencing residual urine. Residual urine in the bladder may cause hemorrhage and is an excellent medium for bacterial growth, which can lead to cystitis.

and displaced to one side. This may lead to profuse bleeding.

Following delivery, the mother may lose the sensitivity and ability to void. This loss is due to decreased muscle tone, to unavoidable trauma to the area during delivery, and to the effects of certain types of anesthesia that may have been administered. If the mother finds it difficult to void, the nurse may try these measures:

1. If it is not contraindicated, encourage the woman to ambulate to the bathroom, or ensure her privacy in using the bedpan.
2. Run water in faucets of sink.
3. Pour warm water over her perineal area to aid in relaxing the urethral sphincter.

Catheterization may be necessary if all other measures fail. Because the perineum may be swollen, it is often difficult to visualize the urinary meatus. Care must be taken not to invade the vagina, as the delicate womb may become contaminated.

Often, when the bladder is emptied and with the aid of massage, the uterus becomes firm again and bleeding is controlled. The urinary system recovers its normal functioning within 6 weeks if no infections develop.

### GASTROINTESTINAL SYSTEM

The gastrointestinal system resumes activity shortly after delivery. Generally, the mother is hungry because during labor she had little, if any, solid food. A light meal is usually provided unless she is nauseated. Complaints of thirst are common because of restricted fluids and excessive perspiration.

The mother may be unable to move her bowels for 2 or 3 days after delivery. Constipation may persist as a problem during the postpartum period for the following reasons:

1. Anesthesia may slow peristalsis.
2. Stretched abdominal muscles lack tone.
3. The perineum may be sore from the episiotomy or hemorrhoids.
4. Anal sensation may be reduced or lost because of tremendous pressure experienced during birth.

A stool softener is commonly ordered. The mother is encouraged to drink lots of fluids, to include roughage in her diet, and to ambulate. These measures are generally sufficient to correct the problem.

The mother who has experienced a cesarean delivery will generally receive intravenous fluids for the first 24 hours or until bowel sounds are heard. Then, clear fluids and a regular diet are offered. The woman may be uncomfortable from flatus. Simethecone (Mylicon), 40–80 mg after each meal and at bedtime, may be prescribed to decrease flatulence and abdominal distention. Stool softeners are useful, as for the mother who has delivered vaginally. Early ambulation assists in relieving these discomforts.

## INTEGUMENTARY SYSTEM

Hyperpigmentation of the skin, seen in the pregnant woman, usually disappears. *Striae* (stretch marks) fade, from reddish-purple to silver.

Postpartum *diaphoresis* (excessive perspiration) is the body's mechanism of reducing the retained fluids associated with pregnancy. The new mother may experience profuse sweating during the day and at night. The nurse prepares the mother for this process and suggests personal hygiene measures, such as a daily shower and frequent change of clothing. She is also encouraged to increase her fluid intake. This process aids in weight loss.

With the delivery of the uterine contents, there is a weight loss of approximately 12–13 pounds. Between the 2nd and 5th days, about 2 liters of body fluid is eliminated by diuresis and diaphoresis. This elimination results in a further loss of approximately 5 pounds. By the 6th to the 8th week, weight has stabilized. Dieting is not recommended until after the 6-week checkup, when the mother's body has returned to its prepregnant state.

## MUSCULOSKELETAL SYSTEM

The abdominal musculature has been greatly stretched during pregnancy. It may now have a "doughy" appearance. Abdominal wall weakness may remain for 6–8 weeks and may contribute to constipation. After a brief recuperative period, all mothers may begin exercising to regain their figures and abdominal muscle tone. The woman who has experienced a cesarean delivery consults her health-care provider to determine when to begin exercising.

During the early postpartum period, the mother is physically exhausted. She should not place any strenuous demands on herself, but she may begin some simple exercises as early as the 1st day after delivery. The main areas of concern are the perineum and abdominal areas. Kegel exercises, which the mother has done during the prenatal period, may be resumed immediately after delivery. These promote circulation and healing of the area. The mother is instructed to tighten the muscles of the perineal area, as if to stop the flow of urine, and then relax them. She should inhale, tighten for a count of 10, exhale, and relax. She may do the exercise five times each hour for the first few days. Then she may increase the number of repetitions.

Another exercise that can be done early in the postpartum period is abdominal tightening. Abdominal isometrics may be done in the supine or erect position. The woman is instructed to inhale by taking a long, slow breath; exhale slowly while contracting the abdominal muscles; count to 10; and then relax. She should begin slowly with three repetitions, and increase the number to five, then ten. This may be done three times and then five times daily, up to 10 times each day.

The head lift may be done on the 2nd postpartum day. The woman lies flat on her bed without a pillow and inhales. While exhaling, she lifts her head, chin to chest, and looks forward at her feet. She holds this position to a count of three, then relaxes. This is repeated several times. After the 3rd week, or when the physician permits, the head lift may progress to include the head and shoulders. This may be done five to 10 times daily.

The pelvic tilt may also be done at this time. While the woman lies supine, knees bent and feet flat, she inhales and exhales, flattening the small of her lower back to the bed or exercise surface and contracting her abdominal muscles. She holds the position to a count of three. She begins with five repetitions and works up to 10 repetitions daily.

## IMMUNE SYSTEM

**Prevention of Rh Sensitivity.** Early in pregnancy, blood typing and Rh factor are ascertained by the physician as an important part of prenatal care. The patient who is Rh-negative undergoes further antibody titering throughout the course of her pregnancy (see discussion of Rh sensitization on p. 98).

The Rh-negative mother, within 72 hours after the delivery of an Rh-positive baby, should be given a vaccine called $Rh_o(D)$ immune globulin (RhoGAM). The physician orders RhoGAM, which is obtained through the blood bank. A sample of the mother's blood is mixed with a sample of RhoGAM to ensure compatibility. The registered nurse may obtain the RhoGAM at the blood bank, or the vaccine may be delivered directly to the unit.

The procedure and protocol used for giving any blood derivative are followed for giving RhoGAM. Two nurses check the label, name, and numbers on the vial and on the laboratory slips before administration. The patient's consent is obtained and witnessed. RhoGAM is given by deep intramuscular injection, most often into the buttocks. Side effects are rare. The patient receives an identification card stating that she is Rh-negative and has received RhoGAM on that particular date. The RhoGAM vial is returned to the blood bank, and appropriate slips are attached to the patient's chart.

RhoGAM should also be given to the Rh-negative patient who aborts or has an ectopic pregnancy or amniocentesis. If abortion or ectopic pregnancy occurs in the 1st trimester, a smaller (50-$\mu$g) dose of $Rh_o$ immune globulin (MICRhoGAM or Mini-Gamulin Rh) is used (Olds, 1992).

**Rubella (German Measles) Vaccination.** Rubella titers are done early in the pregnancy as part of the prenatal work-up. A titer of 1:8 or greater indicates immunity to the rubella virus. The mother who is not immune is vaccinated in the immediate postpartum period. This is the best time to administer the vaccine to a woman, because there is no danger of her being pregnant. Mothers must read the material about the vaccine and sign their name to indicate that this was done. The vaccination protects the mother from acquiring the rubella virus during subsequent pregnancies and causing fetal infection that could lead to congenital rubella syndrome. Some of the birth defects associated with this syndrome are deafness, mental and motor retardation, cataracts, cardiac defects, and retarded interuterine growth.

The rubella virus vaccine (Meruvax II) is supplied in a single-dose vial, and it must be kept in the refrigerator until administered. The total volume of the vial of vaccine is given subcutaneously, usually in the outer aspect of the upper arm. Adverse reactions are uncommon, but the patient may complain of pain or burning at the injection site. She may experience some mild symptoms of rubella, such as rash, malaise, sore throat, headache, joint pain, and slight fever. The nurse advises the patient that these symptoms are transient. The nurse also explains that the woman should not get pregnant for the next 3 months, as the vaccine uses a live virus that could cause birth defects in the fetus. Do not administer the vaccine if the patient is sensitive to Neomycin or if she has had a transfusion within the last 3 months.

## CHANGES AFTER CESAREAN BIRTH

The woman is treated as a postoperative patient (see Nursing Care Plan 8–1). Blood pressure, pulse, and respiration are closely monitored. Hemorrhage is a particular threat, because the patient may have a boggy uterus and bleed from the vagina or from internal blood vessels not securely tied. This is most prevalent during the 1st hour of recovery and remains a threat for 24 hours. The dressing and vaginal pad are frequently observed. Lochia is generally lighter than in women who have delivered vaginally.

The fundus may be gently palpated from the side of the abdomen to avoid placing pressure on a vertical incision. It should remain firm, in the midline, and below the umbilicus. Intravenous oxytocin (Pitocin) may be ordered to stimulate uterine contractions and prevent hemorrhage.

If the patient has received a spinal or epidural anesthetic, the nurse checks sensation of the extremities until feeling returns. An indwelling urinary catheter is generally removed in 24–48 hours. Urine is observed for blood, which may indicate surgical trauma to the bladder. Intake and output are measured. Bowel signs are assessed.

Pain control is important for the comfort of the patient and to prevent surgical complications such as thrombophlebitis or pneumonia from inactivity. The nurse assesses the patient to determine the amount, frequency, and location of discomfort. Patients are instructed to support the incision when moving about.

Patient-controlled analgesics (PCAs) have gained popularity. This technique allows moth-

## Nursing Brief

Women who have had a cesarean delivery are both postpartum and postsurgical patients.

ers to administer their own analgesics with an intravenous pump. A preset safety lock prevents overadministration. Among other benefits, PCAs give the mother a greater sense of control and avoids repeated intramuscular medication. If the woman has had an epidural block, an epidural injection of a narcotic is often given to provide sustained comfort.

## EMOTIONAL CHANGES

**Mothers.** The transition to motherhood brings many hormonal changes, changes in body image, and intrapsychic reorganization. Rubin's psychological changes of the puerperium (Rubin, 1977) are depicted in Box 9–2. During phase 1, the "taking in" phase, the nurse listens and encourages the mother to talk about her experience. Phase 2, "taking hold," is an excellent time for teaching and reassurance. In phase 3, the mother redefines her new role. This phase continues after discharge.

It is normal for a mother to experience conflicting feelings. When they develop after delivery, they are sometimes referred to as "postpartum blues." The mother may feel let down, but overall she finds pleasure in life. The symptoms are self-limiting. When mild depression occurs, the mother may cry for no apparent reason. She may be irritable, nervous, anorexic, and at times unable to sleep (see p. 264). The nurse explains that this experience is not unusual. The mother needs reassurance that, in time, these feelings will pass. Sometimes a shoulder to cry on and a kind ear are all a mother needs. Support groups are available in some areas. *Postpartum depression*

---

**BOX 9–2** **Rubin's Psychological Changes of the Puerperium**

*Phase 1—taking in*: Mother exhausted from birth is passive; conversation centers on labor and delivery, wonder of this beautiful baby

*Phase 2—taking hold*: Mother begins to initiate action; may begin self-care, may walk to nursery, becomes interested in caring for baby; this may occur within a matter of hours if birth is uncomplicated

*Phase 3—letting go*: Woman redefines her new role of mother and continues to move forward; this involves some grief work and is ongoing

---

is more serious than the "blues" and is discussed on page 264.

Less well recognized is that some women experience depression *during* pregnancy. The onset of motherhood may activate unresolved issues of childhood, conflict pertaining to the pregnancy itself, or crises in self-confidence related to upcoming responsibilities. Other issues, including poverty, unemployment, and lack of family support, can intensify anxieties. Women at risk can be identified by a thorough assessment so that early interventions may be instituted.

*Postpartum psychosis* is less common than depression, but more serious. Women experiencing this disorder have an impaired sense of reality. Symptoms include agitation, restlessness, suicidal ideation, irrational behavior, hallucinations, and more extreme fluctuations in mood. (See also page 265.)

If there is a history of psychiatric problems or if prenatal stressors have been high (poor partner relationship, death of a loved one, or difficult pregnancy), postpartum psychosis can occur. Of particular concern are thoughts of harm to herself or the newborn. In such situations, a referral to the psychiatric nurse clinician, social services, or psychiatrist is essential for prompt intervention. The nurse waits with the mother until a resource person arrives and does not leave her alone with the newborn. Possible nursing diagnoses useful in caring for patients experiencing emotional stress include the following: ineffective individual coping, altered bonding, powerlessness, fear, altered family processes, parental role conflict, and high risk for violence to self or others.

**Fathers.** Childbirth may be a maturational crisis for fathers as well as mothers. Although most literature speaks of this time as a happy one, problems may arise, particularly if earlier developmental issues have not been resolved. The increased responsibility and financial demands, reemergence of childhood anger toward parents or siblings, and frustration about spousal attention may surface. Stuart and Sundeen (1991) relate that approximately 2% of hospitalized patients with a diagnosis of paranoid psychosis developed symptoms in relation to fatherhood.

**Grieving Parents.** Although nurses generally think of the maternity unit as being essentially a place of happiness, the potential for grief is ever-present. Even a healthy baby may deviate from the parents' expectations of sex or appearance. Women who suffer miscarriage or choose abortion may experience regret, remorse, and sorrow. This can be one of the most difficult kinds of grief. Anniversaries of these events are painful, and these feelings may last for many years, if not forever ("We have one child, but we almost had two").

If the condition of a newborn is poor, the parents may wish to have a baptism performed. The minister or priest is notified. In an emergency, the nurse may perform the baptism by pouring water on the baby's forehead while saying, "I baptize thee in the name of the Father, and of the Son, and of the Holy Spirit." If there is any doubt as to whether the baby is alive, the baptism is given conditionally: "If you are capable of receiving baptism, I baptize you in the name of the Father, and of the Son, and of the Holy Spirit."

Nursing interventions for these families include listening, correcting misconceptions, encouraging ventilation of feelings (e.g., tears, anger, jealousy of mothers with healthy babies). Occasionally, parents pin small medals to the baby's blankets or clothing. The nurse must be extremely careful not to lose these, because they are of great sentimental value to the parents, particularly if the baby dies. If there are local bereavement groups, such as a hospice or Compassionate Friends, a referral may be advised. Further information on death of a child is presented in Chapter 34.

**Parenthood.** Whether the parents have one or several children, becoming a parent requires learning new roles and making adjustments (Fig. 9–4). Parents having their first child find themselves in a triangular relationship (the "we" has become an "us"). Many parents say that parenthood, not marriage, made the greatest change in their lives. Adjustments are even greater for women who have professions or who are in the work force, because the changes are more extensive.

The demands of parenthood affect communication between the partners, and there is little doubt that at times children detract from the relationship. It is not unusual for one member to feel left out. The division of responsibility can be a source of conflict, particularly when both parents work. Parents often feel inept, which may cause lower self-esteem, depression, and anger. These feelings can be overwhelming.

Fatigue often precipitates irritability. Even in the ideal situation, waking up two or three times every night is wearing. For the new

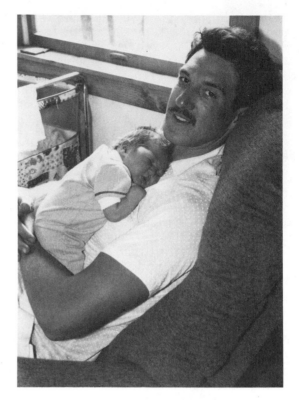

**Figure 9–4.** It is important for the father to take an active role in the care of the newborn.

mother, physiologic changes continue to play a part in her emotional lability. Both parents are concerned with increased economic responsibilities. Loss of freedom and a decrease in socialization may play a part in isolation and loneliness; however, usually this is not as intense with the first-born.

Preparing new parents for the lifestyle changes that occur with a new baby is important. Parenting courses, group discussions, and means of support from relatives or friends can be explored. Social service agencies, public health nurses, and other professional resources should be suggested, as appropriate. Encouraging parents to share their concerns and worries with one another and to keep communication lines open is paramount. Reestablishing a relationship into which the newborn fits with a minimum of disruption can be accomplished when the parents identify their own needs, set priorities, maintain their sense of humor, and relax their standards.

These tools can make the transition to parenthood, although sometimes difficult, a rewarding experience—one in which the stable family can grow and become stronger. Parents who find themselves at an impasse should seek early intervention with a professional counselor.

# Care of the Newborn

### AIRWAY

Regardless of the site of delivery (home, birthing room, taxicab), clearing the newborn's airway is an immediate concern. At delivery this procedure is carried out by the physician or certified nurse-midwife (CNM). The infant is usually held in a slightly head-dependent position to allow secretions to drain from the airways. A rubber bulb syringe may be used to remove exudate from the nose and mouth. This provides very gentle suction, which protects the delicate tissues. When feasible, the parents are taught how to use the bulb syringe (see p. 302).

### BREATHING

Breathing should begin within a few seconds. If it does not, resuscitative measures are begun. The nurse observes the baby for cyanosis (blue color), grunting respirations, retractions of the abdomen under the ribs, flaring of the nostrils, and a sustained respiratory rate higher than 60 breaths/min.

The need for resuscitation can often be anticipated by the history of the mother's pregnancy, abnormal progression of labor, size of the newborn, and difficulty of delivery. Well-trained personnel and properly functioning equipment are imperative. Periodic review of techniques is also required.

Resuscitation methods are directed toward clearing the airway, inflating the lungs, and maintaining circulation. The administration of appropriate drugs, such as sodium bicarbonate, epinephrine, dextrose, or calcium gluconate, may also be warranted. Naxolone hydrochloride (Narcan) is used to reverse respiratory depression in newborns of addicted mothers.

Procedures progress from the simple to the more complex. Measures such as tactile stimulation (rubbing the newborn's back), assisted ventilation by bag and mask or endotracheal tube, intermittent positive-pressure breathing, and external cardiac massage may be necessary. The infant is transferred to the nursery in a prewarmed transport unit. Assisted ventilation via a mechanical respirator may be required in the nursery.

A system for recording the condition of the newborn and the immediate need for resuscitation was devised by Dr. Virginia Apgar, an anesthesiologist. It is called the *Apgar score* and is widely used. The first assessment is made 1 minute after delivery. This is generally the lower score. A second evaluation is made 5 minutes after delivery. Criteria include heart rate, respiratory status, muscle tone, reflexes, and color. The Apgar scoring system is shown in Table 9–3. A score of 8–10 indicates that the newborn is in good condition.

When there are no complications, the new-

**Table 9–3.** APGAR SCORING SYSTEM

| Sign | 0 | 1 | 2 |
|---|---|---|---|
| Heart rate: strong and steady? | Not detectable | Slow (less than 100 beats/min) | Above 100 beats/min |
| Respiratory effort: breathing frequently and regularly? | Absent | Slow, irregular | Good; crying |
| Muscle tone: kicking feet and making fists? | Flaccid | Some flexion of extremities | Active motion |
| Reflex irritability: lusty cry elicited if catheter is pushed up one nostril or soles of feet are prodded? | No response | Grimace, cry; cough or sneeze | |
| Color: pink all over, or hands and feet bluish? | Blue, pale | Body pink, extremities bluish | Completely pink |
| Total | | | |

The Apgar scoring system provides a quick and accurate way of evaluating the baby's physical status right at birth, regardless of what combination of weaknesses or debilities he or she may have. The physician or nurse observes the five vital signs and records the score for each. Each sign is evaluated according to the degree to which it is present: 0 (poor), 1 (fair), or 2 (good). The five scores are then added together; Apgar scores range from 0 to 10. A score of 10 means the baby is in the best possible condition. A score of 9, 8, or 7 indicates good condition; 6, 5, or 4 indicates fair condition. A score of 3, 2, 1, or 0 indicates poor condition and the need for prompt diagnosis and treatment of specific disorders.

born is placed on a warming table. Slight Trendelenburg position may be used initially to drain secretions. Following this, the newborn is positioned on the side with the head slightly elevated to facilitate breathing. The infant is gently dried. Alert mothers are given the baby to hold and inspect.

## PROVIDING WARMTH

Newborns lose heat quickly after birth because fluid evaporates from their body, drafts move heat away, and they are sometimes placed on cold surfaces (Table 9–4). Neonatal hypothermia may ultimately lead to respiratory distress as the baby tries to increase its metabolic rate to generate heat. An increased metabolism requires more oxygen, and the infant is limited in ability to increase oxygenation.

Preheated warming tables are available in most delivery rooms. The newborn is thoroughly dried (especially the hair) and placed, uncovered, under a radiant warmer. In the warmer, a skin probe is applied to the right or left abdomen. The skin probe acts as a thermostat, causing the warmer to increase or decrease the heat output to maintain the infant's temperature within a set range. By placing the infant on the mother's chest, skin-to-skin contact is maintained. A portable radiant warmer can keep both mother and baby warm during the get-acquainted period. The nurse remains with the mother and child to ensure their safety and monitor progress.

**Table 9–4.** NURSING INTERVENTIONS FOR HEAT LOSS IN NEWBORNS

| Type of Heat Loss | Mechanism | Conditions Contributing to Heat Loss | Nursing Interventions |
|---|---|---|---|
| Conduction | Conduction to surfaces that touch skin | Cool temperature of contact surfaces<br>Thermal conductivity of material of contact surfaces | Avoid placing infant on cold surfaces (e.g., scales, x-ray plates, circumcision board); pad with a warm diaper or blanket; warm hands and stethoscope before touching baby |
| Evaporation | Insensible evaporation from skin | Insensible evaporation accounts for 25% of heat loss | Maintain relative humidity of 50–80% |
| | Evaporation of moisture on skin (e.g., amniotic fluid, bath water) | Increased skin permeability leads to insensible water loss and thus evaporative heat loss | Keep skin dry; do not bathe baby unless temperature is stable |
| | Evaporation from mucosa of respiratory tract | Tachypnea increases rate of heat loss from respiratory tract | Bathe and dry only small area at a time; warm any soaks or solutions applied to skin; keep warm; change wet diapers promptly |
| Convection | Air moving over the skin | Exposure to currents of air, including oxygen that has not been warmed and humidified | Avoid drafts from open doors, air conditioning, people moving around |
| | Warm air expired during respiration; convection of heat to skin surface | Thermal sensors on face and forehead are sensitive to cold, even when rest of body is warm | Warm and humidify oxygen; when infant must leave nursery (e.g., for surgery), transport in prewarmed unit |
| Radiation | Transfer from infant's skin to surrounding environment | Difference between skin temperature and environment (e.g., walls of single-walled incubator) | Raise isolette air temperature to 36°C; clothe infant when possible; keep infant's bed away from outside walls and out of drafts |
| | | Total radiating surface of infant— the smaller the infant, the greater the surface area in relation to weight and thus the greater the loss; large surface area of infant's head exacerbates loss | Use a warming unit; swaddle infant; put cap or bonnet on baby (when out of radiant warmer) |

Adapted from Moore, M.L. (1981). *Newborn, family and nurse* (2nd ed.). Philadelphia: W. B. Saunders

A newborn's head is a major site of heat loss. A hat is kept on the head when the infant is outside the radiant warmer. The cap is not worn in the warmer, because it would block heat to the baby. The head must be dried before the cap is applied, or the hat will become damp and accelerate heat loss rather than retain it.

The infant is wrapped in two or more blankets when out of the warmer. The blankets and other clothing or bedding are changed if they become damp, because damp cloth can increase evaporative heat loss. In an out-of-hospital delivery, the newborn and mother can be wrapped together in a sleeping bag.

## UMBILICAL CORD

The umbilical cord, which is attached to the placenta at birth, is cut by the attending physician. Before the clamp is applied, the cord is inspected to determine that two arteries and one vein are present. A single umbilical artery is often indicative of genitourinary anomalies. The findings are recorded.

Cord blood analysis is performed to determine the health status of the baby. Blood gases and fetal tissue pH are helpful to determine respiratory status and other complications, especially when abnormal fetal heart rate patterns have occurred. The nurse observes the cord for *bleeding*, particularly during the first 24 hours.

The cord stump gradually shrinks, discolors, and finally falls off. The blood, vessels of the cord, and their extension into the abdomen are a potential portal of entry for disease organisms until the umbilical wound completely heals. In the nursery, antibiotic ointments, triple dye, povidone-iodine (Betadine), or other preparations may be ordered to promote drying and decrease infection. Because infection may develop after discharge from the hospital, the mother is taught to keep the navel dry. Some recommend swabbing with 70% alcohol daily. Others suggest doing nothing to it. The mother is instructed to report to her physician any redness, odor, or discharge from the baby's umbilicus.

## BLOOD COAGULATION, ANEMIA, AND HYPOGLYCEMIA

Vitamin K is frequently given to promote blood clotting and prevent hemorrhage in the newborn. A mild vitamin K deficiency is not unusual in newborns and is common in preterms. Oozing of blood from the umbilicus, ecchymosis, and bloody stools may be signs of vitamin K deficiency. The intestinal flora of newborns is sterile at birth. The baby is unable to synthesize vitamin K, which is necessary for the formation of several blood factors (VII, IX, X). Normal intestinal flora is established after birth. Vitamin K (AquaMEPHYTON) is administered intramuscularly via the lateral anterior aspect of the thigh.

In the past, infants in the nursery were placed prone with the foot of the bassinet raised to facilitate the drainage of mucus. This practice is no longer recommended because it might increase the likelihood of cerebral pressure and intracranial bleed. The prone position has also been implicated as a possible cause of sudden infant death syndrome.

A hematocrit to determine *anemia* and *polycythemia* (an excess of red blood cells) is generally performed by heel stick. Anemia can be caused by bleeding either externally or internally and by other causes. Polycythemia is often caused by an excess flow of blood into the infant from the umbilical cord. It increases the risk of jaundice and damage to other organs due to blood stasis. A normal hematocrit value in the newborn ranges from 45–65%.

A glucose recording may be performed on stressed babies of diabetic mothers, those small for gestational age, those large for gestational age, and others. Hypoglycemia is common in newborns, as cold and other stressors increase the rate at which glucose is metabolized. A blood glucose level of 35–40 mg/dl or less in the first 72 hours for the term infant is considered to indicate hypoglycemia (see discussion of hypoglycemia in the preterm, p. 320). Oral dextrose in water is given to the newborn to correct this. Follow-up consists of testing blood from the infant's heel and reading it by Destrostix or Chemstrip and Accu-Check II. Hypoglycemia is treated quickly to prevent depletion of glucose in the brain and possible brain damage.

## PREVENTING INFECTION

*Handwashing by all persons involved in the delivery room and nursery is imperative.* Clean gloves, covergowns, or scrubs are worn. The umbilical cord is clamped by using aseptic technique. Keeping the cord dry reduces moistness in the environment that favors growth of organisms. The prevention of infection in newborns is discussed in detail on page 308.

# Nursing Brief

Advise parents to limit the newborn's exposure to crowds during the early weeks of life, as infants have difficulty forming antibodies against infection until about 2 months of age.

---

An agent such as erythromycin (Ilotycin), tetracycline 1%, silver nitrate 1% solution, or penicillin is instilled into the newborn's eyes to prevent *ophthalmia neonatorum*. This condition causes blindness if the newborn becomes exposed to gonococcal infection during the birth process. A chemical conjunctivitis from the use of silver nitrate is common and generally disappears after 24–36 hours. This condition is explained to the parents. Silver nitrate is not effective against *Chlamydia* ophthalmia. Treatment of mothers with the infection remains of utmost importance (see p. 110).

## IDENTIFICATION

Proper identification of the newborn is of utmost importance for safety, security, and parental well-being. It is also imperative legally. The American Academy of Pediatrics recommends that two identical identification bands be placed on the infant while still in the delivery room. Bracelets are placed on both wrists or both ankles, or on one of each (Fig. 9–5). The neonate loses weight after birth, so bracelets must be snug. Information on the bracelet includes the mother's hospital number, the mother's full name, and the sex, date, and time of the baby's birth. Fingerprinting the mother and newborn and footprinting the baby are alternatives (Fig. 9–6). The value of footprinting is controversial at this writing. If required, the footprint is kept with the newborn's chart.

Identification is reaffirmed with the mother's bracelet number each time the baby is brought to her, moved to and from a crib, or moved elsewhere. Some hospitals also place bracelets on fathers or significant others. Identification is reaffirmed on admission to the nursery and before transferring the newborn to a regional care center. Many hospitals are instituting stringent security methods to protect newborns from abduction. This may include security cameras, doors that open with special identification

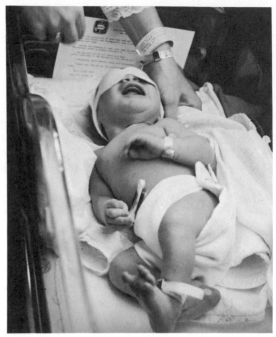

**Figure 9–5.** Identification. Note double identification bands on mother and 2-day-old baby. The eye mask is for protection during phototherapy.

cards, identification badges for employees, and educational programs for parents. A picture of the family may be requested as yet another means of protecting the newborn. *Always be certain of the identity of anyone to whom you give a baby.*

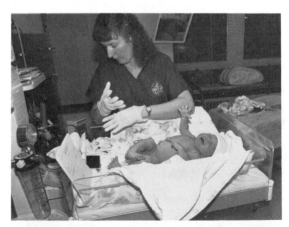

**Figure 9–6.** The nurse takes footprints of a newborn in the delivery room before transfer to the nursery. Note the gloves on the nurse and the certificate near the baby's feet.

## MECONIUM ASPIRATION SYNDROME

Aspiration of stained amniotic fluid is sometimes seen in the term or postterm newborn. If the fetus had been in distress while in utero, hypoxia may occur. This causes the anal sphincter to relax, and meconium is passed. Aspiration of meconium may occur with the first breath. This results in small airway obstruction manifested by tachypnea, retractions, grunting respirations, and cyanosis. Respiratory distress may be immediate or delayed, and pneumothorax may result. If the course is mild, improvement may occur within 48 hours. Immediate suctioning of the nasopharynx by the birth attendant is indicated. A chest x-ray study may show coarse, patchy densities.

Atelectasis sometimes occurs. Resuscitated newborns are transferred to the intensive care nursery for close observation and support of respiratory function.

## GESTATIONAL AGE ASSESSMENT

The Dubowitz scoring system, which is used to determine gestational age, is presented in Chapter 13 (see p. 320). The gestational age of the newborn refers to the number of complete weeks of fetal development, calculated from the 1st day of the mother's last normal menstrual period.

The components of the Dubowitz scoring system consist of evaluation of physical characteristics and neuromuscular tone. This examination is carried out in the nursery, usually within 24 hours of birth.

## SCREENING TESTS

Parents are informed of all normal screening tests done on the newborn. These tests detect conditions that could prove fatal or that could cause mental retardation or physical handicaps. At this writing, tests that can be identified from heel-prick blood include phenylketonuria (PKU), galactosemia, sickle cell disease, maple syrup urine disease, homocystinuria, and hypothyroidism. In order for the PKU level to be accurate, the newborn must have ingested protein for at least 48 hours. If the mother's stay is long enough, PKU and tri-iodothyronine ($T_3$) may be done before discharge and then again in approximately 7–14 days. Retesting is advised to prevent a false-positive result. Further information on PKU and sickle cell disease is found on pages 349–351 and 724–727, respectively. Parents are given written appointments for returning to the clinic to obtain or complete screening tests.

## REACTIVITY

After delivery, the vigorous newborn exhibits a characteristic pattern of activity. These patterns are termed the 1st and 2nd periods of reactivity. During the 1st period, which lasts for about 30 minutes after birth, the newborn is awake and active. The heart and respiratory rates are rapid, and grimacing and sucking movements and random motor activity occur. As eye contact is important to the bonding process, the instillation of eye medication may be postponed until the parents have become acquainted with the baby. A check list for procedures ensures that the medication is not overlooked. This activity is followed by a period of rest, which lasts 2–4 hours. The resting newborn is disinterested in sucking and stimulation.

The 2nd period of reactivity occurs on awakening. This lasts 4–6 hours. The newborn's responsiveness returns. Periods of apnea may be seen, and mucus production increases. The color of the newborn may vary between mildly mottled and cyanotic. Bowel sounds become audible, and meconium stools are passed.

## BONDING AND ATTACHMENT

The term *bonding* refers to the connection that forms soon after birth between parents and the newborn (Fig. 9–7). The term *attachment* generally refers to the infant's connection to the parent, which occurs gradually over time. Frequently the terms are used interchangeably. Bonding begins within the 1st hour after delivery, if it is not contraindicated for mother or infant. Identification of the baby as their own is important at this time.

Both father and mother should view, hold, and most important, *touch* the baby. The parents are allowed to unwrap the baby. In the past, infants were rushed to the nursery as soon as possible for fear of their being chilled. It is true that a newborn's temperature-regulating mechanism is erratic after delivery, so one has to use discretion. However, there is little harm in looking at the unclothed infant for a few minutes. Most parents want to see whether it is a boy or a girl and whether all the fingers and toes are there.

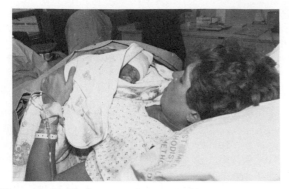

**Figure 9-7.** Mother spends time bonding with her newborn. Note the intravenous infusion being given to the mother and the warm cap and blankets on the baby.

Mothers are praised for their efforts and cooperation. Fathers are praised for their support. If the father was not present during the delivery, he is reunited with his family as soon as possible. Both parents are encouraged to admire and touch the baby. Significant others are included in the bonding process in nontraditional families. The nurse can point out various behaviors of the newborn, encourage eye contact, and provide periods of privacy for the couple. Siblings are encouraged to participate, as appropriate.

Parents often spend the bonding time pointing out familial characteristics of the newborn (Fig. 9-8). This is a common and integral part

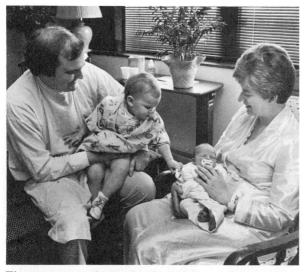

**Figure 9-8.** A family bonding with its new member. (Courtesy of Blank Memorial Hospital for Children, Des Moines, IA.)

## Nursing Brief

To evaluate the attachment process, the nurse observes parents and the reciprocal interaction of the baby during feeding, bathing, and soothing periods.

of accepting and claiming the new family member. The mother may wish to breast feed at this time. This provides closeness and comforting skin-to-skin contact for the newborn. This early identification with the newborn helps the couple to establish the beginnings of parental behavior and love.

For some, parental feelings do not come naturally. These parents are assured that with time and caring for the newborn, parental behavior can be learned and acquired. When there is difficulty in bonding or when rejection or indifference is seen in one or both parents, this observation is recorded and a consultation arranged with social services. Parenting classes may be helpful.

Although early bonding is believed to be beneficial, the evidence from studies is inconclusive. Guilt and apprehension may arise in adoptive parents who have not had this opportunity. For them, it is wise to emphasize that the process of bonding and attachment is complex and that initial contact is one of many factors that affect it.

### ROOMING-IN

*Rooming-in* or *mother-baby units* refers to a concept in which mother and baby reside in the same room. In some hospitals, one nurse cares for both the mother and baby. This practice works easily when labor, delivery, recovery, and postpartum care are confined to one room. In other facilities, mother is cared for by the postpartum staff, and the newborn is supervised by the nursery personnel. This arrangement affords the mother an opportunity to care for the infant, except when the baby is in the nursery. Flexibility in this policy is important because the new mother may be exhausted and uncomfortable. She is permitted to return the baby to the nursery as necessary. Another arrangement is to return the baby to the nursery at night.

Rooming-in enables new parents to become acquainted with their baby and to learn parenting skills. Feeding, diapering, and bathing demonstrations are given by experienced personnel. With the assistance of trained staff, parents gain knowledge and confidence in caring for their infant. They are informed of parenting classes.

Nursing assessment includes observation of specific parenting behaviors, such as amount of affection and interest shown to the baby. The amount of physical contact, stimulation, eye-to-eye contact, and time spent interacting with the baby are significant. The extent to which the parents encourage involvement of siblings and grandparents with the newborn's arrival is also noteworthy. This information provides a basis for nursing interventions that may encourage bonding and foster positive family relationships.

The nurse who calls the baby by name, encourages holding en face, discusses particular behavior patterns, and points out unique characteristics helps to enhance the bonding process. This is especially important if the parents' "fantasy child" differs from the "real" child in sex, physical attributes, or health.

### TENDER, LOVING CARE

The love an infant receives is just as important as physical care. Gentleness in caring for the child is an expression of love and makes physical care, such as bathing and feeding, a pleasure. This expression helps the baby to develop trust. Each infant is an individual. Just as no two look alike, so each is different in disposition, activity, and response to people and surroundings. A baby soon learns that crying brings comforting help. Because mother usually answers the plea, she is preferred over others. The infant who is secure in the care mother provides will accept similar care from others. Love, affection, security, and feeling wanted are necessary for a healthy personality and physical growth.

The nurse relaxes, handles the newborn gently, and speaks in a soft voice. The nurse who keeps the baby warm, dry, and comfortably positioned makes the baby feel secure. After painful procedures, the nurse holds the baby for a few minutes so that the infant does not associate only discomfort with his or her care. Tactile stimulation and establishment of routines based on the needs of the newborn are also important. One hospital has developed a "cuddler program," which enlists volunteer senior citizens to rock and cuddle babies in the intensive care nursery.

### DAILY CARE

The newborn in the hospital needs to wear only a shirt and a diaper and to be covered with a light blanket. A shirt that ties or snaps on in a double-breasted fashion simplifies dressing and gives added warmth to the chest. Many hospitals use disposable diapers, but the nurse should be familiar with the use of cloth diapers, because ecology is becoming a major worldwide consideration.

The cloth diaper may be folded in a triangle or rectangle and pinned at the hips. If the diaper is secured with pins, the nurse emphasizes to parents that the points should be directed toward the side of the baby's abdomen. The nurse should slip two fingers of one hand between the infant's body and the pin in order to prevent injury. The baby girl needs the thickness of the diaper low under her buttocks when lying on her back and in front when lying on her stomach. The baby boy needs padding over the penis. Tabs are used by most manufacturers to keep disposable diapers in place. See Chapter 12 on the term newborn for more information on care of the newborn after the initial period of birth.

# Breast Feeding

An important function of the nurse is to assist and teach new mothers feeding techniques. Nutrition is extremely important in the first few months of life because the brain grows rapidly then. Energy maintenance is high because of the newborn's immature systems. A more in-depth discussion of the nutritional needs of the infant is found on pages 432–440. The mother may choose to nurse her baby or bottle feed. The nurse educates and supports the mother in either decision.

Breast feeding has many advantages for the newborn. These include the following:

- Breast milk is the ideal food for the newborn because it contains a full range of nutrients.
- No commercial formula has the exact nutritional value of breast milk.

# Nursing Brief

Anticipatory guidance concerning problems associated with breast feeding helps the mother to see them as common occurrences and not as complications.

- Breast milk contains the ideal electrolyte and mineral composition.
- Breast milk is easily digested by the baby's developing digestive system.
- It provides "natural immunity"—the mother transfers antibodies through the milk.
- Breast milk has several antiinfection properties.
- The motion provides for good teeth and jaw development.
- It is economical and convenient.
- The milk is readily available at the correct temperature.
- It hastens uterine involution.
- Milk production utilizes maternal fat stores.
- It enhances a warm, close mother-child relationship.

There are some disadvantages and/or contraindications to breast feeding:

- There is a potential for most medications to enter breast milk.
- The mother may be in poor physical health. Women who have active tuberculosis, have advanced cancer, are positive for human immunodeficiency virus, or have cytomegalovirus are counseled to avoid breast feeding.
- The mother's mental health status may be poor.
- Neonatal jaundice may occasionally result from breast milk.
- Working mothers may have little flexibility in their working environment schedule.

## BEGINNING BREAST FEEDING

During a hospital stay, the newly breast-feeding mother relies on the guidance and assistance of the professional staff. The nurse should have knowledge of the lactation process, breast-feeding techniques, and problems that may arise. Some hospitals have a certified lac-

tation nurse as a resource. The baby is put to breast as soon after delivery as possible. There are generally 8–12 feedings in a 24-hour period. The nurse assesses both the mother and newborn during breast feeding.

## HYGIENE

The mother washes her hands before feeding the baby. The breasts and nipples should be cleansed with warm tap water. Soap is used sparingly because it removes the natural oils provided by the body. The nursing mother should wear a supportive nursing bra late in pregnancy and 24 hours a day after delivery. When leaking occurs, soft cotton pads made from handkerchiefs, diapers, or gauze pads are recommended.

## POSITION

The mother is seated comfortably in a chair, with her back and arm supported (Fig. 9–9). The baby's head may rest in the crook of the mother's arm, and the baby's lower arm may be

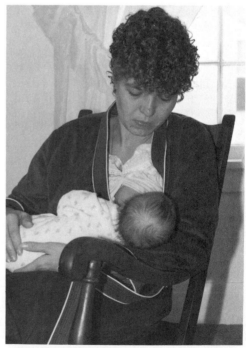

**Figure 9–9.** When nursing, the mother is seated comfortably with her arm supported. The baby's entire body is turned toward the breast.

tucked around the mother's waist. The entire body of the newborn is turned toward the mother's breast. For night feedings, the mother may be on her side with the baby facing her and use a rolled towel or blanket to support the baby's back. Providing for maximum relaxation during breast feeding enhances the let-down reflex and ensures a rewarding experience for both mother and baby.

## PROCEDURE

The baby is brought to the breast to avoid strain on the mother's back. The mother is instructed to hold the breast behind the areola with the thumb on top and the rest of the fingers underneath for support. Brushing the baby's cheek with the nipple elicits the rooting reflex. The baby's head instinctively turns toward the breast; the mouth is open, searching for the nipple. A little milk may be expressed into the baby's mouth to give encouragement, if necessary. The nipple and areola are gently guided into the baby's mouth (Fig. 9–10). The baby should not suck on the nipple only, since this causes soreness and cracking. In the early months of life, the baby is a nose breather. The mother lifts the breast to ensure that it does not block the nose.

The length of feeding varies somewhat from baby to baby but is generally about 10–30 minutes. Some newborns nurse briefly, then fall asleep. This behavior generally decreases as the digestive system matures. The baby can be moved about, burped, and otherwise gently stimulated to awaken. It is helpful to remind concerned mothers that most of the milk is taken by the baby in the first 5 minutes of feeding. The longer sucking time provides for complete satisfaction of the baby's need for sucking. Alternating the breasts increases milk production, particularly *hind milk*, which has a higher protein and fat content. Breast-fed babies are fed on demand. During the first days and weeks, feeding is generally done every 2–3 hours and once during the night. To remove the baby from the breast, the mother gently inserts her finger into the corner of the baby's mouth and breaks the suction, so that the baby releases the nipple. Pulling the baby from the breast without breaking the seal is painful and may lead to sore, cracked nipples. Table 9–5 provides a summary of breast-feeding instructions for the new mother.

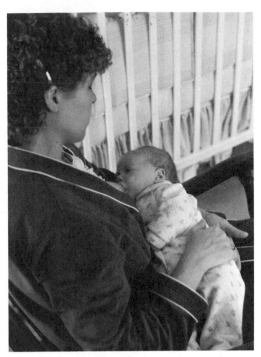

**Figure 9–10.** It is important that the newborn grasp the areola fully in order to compress the milk ducts below.

## MILK SUPPLY

The mother's milk supply is increased as the baby sucks longer at the breast. A smooth sucking and swallowing pattern with pauses in between may be heard. A common worry of breast-feeding mothers is that the baby may not be getting enough milk. If the baby appears comfortable at the breast, is satisfied after feeding, is sleeping well, has six to eight wet diapers per day, has one or more stools a day, and is gaining weight, the baby is getting enough milk. The mother will also notice that her firm breasts become softer as they are emptied during feedings. The nurse encourages the new mother and answers all her questions in order to prevent anxiety, which can cause a decrease in milk supply.

## BURPING

Burping helps remove any swallowed air that may become trapped in the baby's stomach. The baby is burped when the mother changes the feeding from one breast to the other. Three positions for burping are as follows:

**Table 9–5.** SUMMARY OF BREAST-FEEDING INSTRUCTIONS FOR THE NEW MOTHER

| Instruction | Rationale |
| --- | --- |
| Wash hands before proceeding; wash nipples with warm water, no soap | Prevents infection of the newborn and breast |
| Position<br>  Comfortably seated in chair with back and arm support<br>  Side-lying with pillow beneath head, arm above head<br>  Mother needs to experiment initially to find most comfortable positions for her<br>  Entire body of infant turned to mother's breast | Alternating positions facilitates breast emptying and prevents sore nipples |
| Stroke baby's cheek with nipple | Utilizes rooting reflex; baby will turn toward nipple |
| Baby's mouth should cover entire areola | Compresses ducts, lessens tension on nipples |
| After 3rd day, empty first breast completely before changing to second breast (attach safety pin to bra as reminder of where to start) | Alternating breasts increases milk production |
| Lift baby or breast slightly if breast tissue blocks nose | Baby will release nipple if unable to breathe |
| Break suction by placing finger in corner of baby's mouth | Removing baby in this way prevents irritation to nipples |
| The newborn is nursed shortly after birth and approximately every 2–3 hr thereafter | Initial feedings provide colostrum; establishing a pattern helps baby develop own schedule |
| Burp baby halfway through and following feeding | Rids stomach of air bubbles, reduces regurgitation |

- Hold the baby upright, over one shoulder, and gently pat the baby's back.
- Lay the baby across the lap—face down—and gently pat the back.
- Sit the baby up, supporting the chest and head, and gently rub or pat the back.

### RELIEVING BREAST ENGORGEMENT

About 3–4 days after delivery, milk comes into the breasts under the influence of prolactin. The breasts may become distended, engorged, and shiny. They are hard and sensitive to touch. At first this is due to venous congestion, but later the condition is intensified by the accumulating milk. Nurses can help prevent engorgement by encouraging early and frequent breast feeding. The mother may complain of pain and have a slight temperature. Warm compresses provide some relief and enhance the letdown reflex when the baby is put to breast. Ice packs may be utilized between feedings to constrict the circulation and decrease edema and pain. Massage of the breasts causes release of oxytocin and increases the release of milk. Analgesics that are safe for use during breast feeding may be prescribed by the doctor.

A breast pump may be needed to relieve engorgement. Hand or electric pumps are available. Most hospitals use an electric pump. Caution must be taken not to apply a great deal of suction as this could traumatize the tender breast. Several different hand pumps are available at pharmacies. Some are battery operated. Specific directions for their use are provided. Pumping is not done in nonnursing mothers because it stimulates milk production.

Manual expression of milk may relieve occasional engorgement or provide for milk when the mother may be away for a short time. The procedure becomes simple with practice. One hand is placed around the areola to express the milk while the other holds the sterile container to collect it. First, the hand is pressed in toward the chest. Second, the thumb and fingers are tightened together. Pressure on the reservoirs forces out a stream of milk. The position of the hand is changed in a clockwise direction as the sinuses are emptied. Rhythmically repeating this procedure simulates the action of the infant's nursing.

### RELIEVING SORE NIPPLES

Shortly after breast feeding begins, some mothers have pain from cracked or sore nipples. Fissures are a potential portal of entry for bacteria and require treatment. A small amount of expressed breast milk applied to the nipple and areola helps keep the area soft and pliable and has been shown to be successful in treating cracked nipples (Olds, 1992). Lanolin and breast creams are controversial; some feel they may cause allergic reactions, may cause irritation, and/or may be contaminated.

The mother is instructed to change the baby's

position frequently and to start the baby's feeding on the less tender breast, as the most vigorous sucking occurs on the first breast offered. Proper positioning of the infant limits soreness. The mother should air-dry her nipples after each feeding and change nursing pads when they are damp. The nurse assesses the condition of the mother's breasts after each feeding for degree of engorgement, skin integrity, or areas of redness, lumps, or tenderness. Breast feeding that is continued with sore breasts or cracked nipples may lead to an abscess that may require surgical intervention.

The obstetrician, CNMs, lactation specialists, and La Leche League will provide and recommend literature and guidance for breast-feeding mothers both during pregnancy and after the baby is born. Many excellent video tapes are also available. La Leche League is an international organization of breast-feeding mothers who provide assistance and support to new breast-feeding mothers. Because many breast-feeding problems arise after discharge, mothers should receive anticipatory guidance and resource numbers before they leave the hospital.

## BREAST FEEDING AFTER COMPLICATED BIRTHS

**Cesarean Birth.** The mother delivered by cesarean section needs extra assurance from the nursing staff that she can breast feed while recuperating. The nurse stays with the mother during the entire feeding in order to provide assistance in positioning the baby, especially when there is an intravenous infusion. The side-lying position may be appropriate. The football hold is helpful in that it avoids pressure on the incision (see pp. 196 and 197). If the mother needs extra rest, her breasts may be pumped to stimulate and provide milk, and the baby can be fed in the nursery by the staff.

**Multiple Births.** Twins may be fed one at a time or simultaneously. The mother's body adjusts the milk supply to the greater demand. Supplemental feedings may be required and allow father to help with feedings.

**Premature Birth.** Breast feeding is often recommended for a premature baby. Colostrum and breast milk are beneficial to the baby. Most premature babies have a weak sucking reflex, so the mother is instructed to pump her breasts and the nurse feeds the breast milk by gavage. The mother must pump her breasts on a regular schedule in order to maintain the lactation cycle and to prepare her breasts for the time when her baby is strong enough to nurse.

## MATERNAL NUTRITION

As discussed in Chapter 4, a nursing mother must maintain a balanced nutritional regimen to provide optimal nutrition for her baby (see Table 4–4). An increase of 500 cal/day is needed, as is a balanced selection of foods from the basic food groups: (1) meat, fish, poultry, eggs, beans, and nuts; (2) milk and various dairy products; (3) vegetables and fruits; and (4) breads and cereals. A fluid intake of at least six to eight glasses of liquids per day is essential. Milk or other dairy products high in calcium promote bone and teeth development during the infant's early growth. Women with lactose intolerance may use such substitutes as tofu, soy milk, and canned salmon with bones. Usually the birth attendant continues to prescribe prenatal vitamins for the mother during the breast-feeding period.

The nurse informs the mother that whatever she eats directly affects her breast milk. Her food may change the taste of the milk or cause the baby to have gas. A food is tasted in breast milk about 6 hours, and up to 24 hours, after consumption. The infant lets the mother know which foods are tolerated and which should be avoided. Gassy foods, such as cabbage, beans, and broccoli, may be eaten in small quantities. If certain foods are found to cause colic in the infant, they should be completely eliminated from the mother's diet.

Cigarette smoking exposes the infant to nicotine and may reduce milk production. Alcohol may have an adverse effect on the let-down reflex, making successful nursing of the baby difficult. Any medication, including all over-the-counter drugs, may seriously harm a newborn and should be avoided, unless specifically ordered by the doctor. When medications are required by the mother or if a mother has a drug abuse problem, breast feeding is discontinued in order to prevent harm

## Nursing Brief

The nurse reassures the patient that the process of lactation may assist her in losing weight, as fat stores are drawn on to produce milk.

to the newborn (see Appendix C for drugs harmful to the newborn).

### WEANING

Mothers usually wean their babies from 1–6 months or longer. They do so gradually, because abrupt weaning can lead to breast engorgement for the mother and an upset baby. Weaning is not attempted when the baby is ill. Complementary or relief bottles may be used throughout the period of nursing or only occasionally; the mother should consult her health-care provider for specific questions. Decreasing fluid consumption and feedings helps dry up the mother's milk. If the mother becomes pregnant, she discontinues breast feeding, which would be an added strain.

### SUPPRESSION OF LACTATION

When the mother does not wish to breast feed, lactation is suppressed. In the past, bromocriptine (Parlodel) was widely used; however, it is no longer recommended for this purpose. Currently, nonpharmaceutical methods are preferred. A snug bra should be worn around the clock (except to shower) to help alleviate the mother's discomfort. The mother stands with her back to the shower spray to avoid stimulating the nipples. A breast binder may be used if the woman's bra is not suitable. Ice packs are applied over the axillary area of each breast several times a day. Analgesics are ordered for pain. The nurse reassures the mother that in a few days the engorgement will subside.

## Bottle Feeding

When a mother chooses to bottle feed, a commercially prepared formula is ordered by the pediatrician. Most formulas try to duplicate the nutritional components of breast milk. Bottle feeding is rewarding and can enhance the mother-child bonding process when the baby is held.

Formula is available in four forms: (1) ready-to-feed in cans, (2) ready-to-use in disposal bottles, (3) concentrated liquid, which must be diluted with equal amounts of water, and (4) powdered form, which must be diluted according to package directions. In general, products requiring no or little preparation are more ex-

## Nursing Brief

Instruct mothers who are preparing formula made from concentrate (either powder or liquid) to read and follow the directions carefully.

pensive than those requiring mixing. The ready-to-use formula in 4-oz bottles is used today in most hospitals. It is given at room temperature.

For products that require the addition of water, tap water may be used if it comes from an uncontaminated source. If there is doubt, as during traveling, the water is boiled for 5 minutes, then allowed to cool.

The nurse stresses to all new bottle-feeding mothers the importance of *reading the dilution directions* on the formula can. Newborns have become ill, and in severe cases have died, when parents did not understand the need for following these guidelines. This issue is of special concern if there are language barriers. Parents are instructed *not* to save formula from one feeding to the next, because bacteria form quickly in milk that is left open to the air and/or is warm for an extended time. These multiplying microorganisms can cause stomach upset in the baby. Mothers are taught to estimate how much the baby will eat, to feed the baby immediately, and discard the remaining milk.

Some infants with allergies or special needs may need a meat- or soybean-based formula. Allergies are generally not determined until the baby has been bottle fed for a period of time. Cow's milk (whole or skim) is not given before 1 year of age because the curd is not easily digested.

Most mothers prefer to warm the formula somewhat, although studies have shown that babies fed cold milk from the refrigerator do very well. A glass bottle may be heated in a pan of water on the stove (it should be watched carefully—if the water evaporates the bottle will burst).

Microwave heating of infant formula is a common practice despite concerns of oral cavity and esophageal burns. Because of the uneven heating of microwave ovens, the center of the formula becomes very hot and may burn the baby. The baby food industry has designed specific protocols for safe microwave heating of *refrigerated* infant formula (Grant et al, 1992). They suggest that if a bottle is heated in a mi-

They suggest that if a bottle is heated in a microwave, it should be stood up and left uncovered to allow heat to escape. Heat only 4 oz or more. At full power, 4-oz bottles may be heated for 30 seconds, 8-oz bottles for 45 seconds. The nipple is replaced and the bottle inverted 10 times. Formula should be cool to the touch. *Always* test formula before administering.

The nurse instructs the new mother to wash her hands before each feeding. The mother assumes a comfortable position in bed or in a chair. The mother holds the baby's head in the crook of her arm and rests the baby's body in her lap (Fig. 9–11). She should be relaxed with her back supported. Propping the bottle for feedings is discouraged.

The nurse instructs the mother to avoid handling the nipple. The nipple is placed in the baby's mouth over the tongue. The bottle is tilted so that the nipple is filled with formula. This prevents the baby from swallowing large amounts of air. The nipple is tested before each feeding in order to ensure proper flow. A clogged or small hole prevents adequate flow, and most infants respond by fussing and crying. They may gag or choke if the nipple allows a too-fast flow.

The baby is burped after every ½–1 ounce consumed. Two ounces is usually enough to satiate a newborn. Most infants fall asleep when they are full and have had enough. Unused portions of formula are discarded. After feeding, the baby is propped on the right side to facilitate drainage from the stomach and prevent aspiration if regurgitation should occur. The amount of formula taken and retained is reported to the nursery staff after each feeding.

Fathers or significant others are encouraged to assist with feedings. In the beginning, they may need a lot of encouragement and guidance. The nurse instructs them in the proper way to bottle feed and burp the baby. The nurse's presence during feedings is often comforting to new parents.

The following points are observed by the nurse when feeding the baby by bottle:

1. Wear a covergown.
2. The baby wears a bib. Change diaper as needed. Wash hands afterward.
3. Hold the baby unless contraindicated. If a baby cannot be removed from the crib, sit by the crib and elevate the head and shoulders.
4. Observe the kind and amount of formula in the bottle.
5. Let a few drops of formula fall on the inner aspect of your wrist to test
    a. Temperature: the formula may be cold, or room temperature, but not hot.
    b. Size of nipple hole: formula should drop but not flow in a steady stream. If the holes are too small, the weak newborn will tire and fail to finish the feeding. If they are too large, the newborn may choke or miss the satisfaction of sucking.
6. Hold the bottle so that the nipple is full of formula. This prevents the baby from swallowing air.
7. Burp the baby halfway through the feeding and at the end of feeding.
    a. Place a diaper or small towel over your shoulder to protect your gown. Place the baby firmly against your shoulder and pat the back.
    b. Place the baby in a sitting position. Put a towel beneath the chin. Support the chest and head with one hand. Gently rub the back with the other.

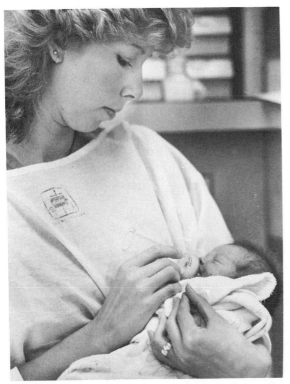

**Figure 9–11.** Position for bottle feeding the newborn. (Courtesy of Blank Memorial Hospital for Children, Des Moines, IA.)

## Nursing Brief

If a pacifier is used to provide extra sucking, instruct parents to obtain a one-piece type to prevent choking. They should use an alligator clip to secure the pacifier to the baby's clothing. If use of the pacifier is continued after 5–6 months, it is likely to become a transitional object, which may become more difficult to give up.

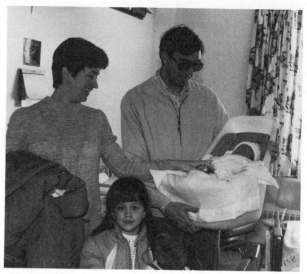

**Figure 9–12.** One happy family prepares to leave the hospital. (Courtesy of St. Joseph Hospital, Nashua, NH.)

8. The feeding should take 15–20 minutes. Do not hurry or force the baby to eat too much.
9. Leave the baby clean and dry. Prop on right side to promote digestion and prevent aspiration of regurgitated milk or vomitus.
10. Chart the amount of formula offered, the amount taken and retained, regurgitation or vomiting, how the formula was taken, and whether or not the baby appeared satisfied following the feeding. (Note that regurgitation is an overflow of milk that occurs shortly after feeding. Vomiting means bringing up a more substantial amount of partially digested milk.)

The majority of babies are fed every 3 or 4 hours. In the hospital or home, the baby who is fed when hungry ("demand feedings") will soon adopt a flexible schedule. Prompt fulfillment of babies' needs assures them that the world is a good place in which to live.

## Discharge Planning

Discharge planning ideally begins on admission. This is of primary concern today when mother and newborn may be discharged after only 1 day (Fig. 9–12). The nurse continually educates parents by role modeling and by direct demonstrations. A review of the patient's admission history suggests areas to target. Follow-up appointments with both the pediatrician and obstetrician are made. The social worker is involved if there is economic need, to ensure that the newborn will receive ongoing care, and that families at risk are directed to an agency sensitive to their needs. This is of particular importance with teenage parents.

The nurse reminds parents of the importance of using infant car seats (Fig. 9–13). The baby is placed in the back seat (never in the front), facing the rear until he or she is old enough and large enough to face forward (at 20 pounds or age 1). The harness is always snugly fastened. Air bags can prevent serious injuries. However, the American Academy of Pediatrics (1993) warns that if a car has a passenger-side air bag, and if the baby is in the front seat facing backward, the opening air bag can seriously injure the baby's head (Fig. 9–14).

Alert parents to the fact that the hospital nursery is open 24 hours a day and that the nurses are available to provide guidance by telephone during the first weeks of the newborn's life. In one hospital a new program titled Training Wheels has been established. Nurses from the maternal-child department provide home visits to educate and assess parental needs. Areas of instruction in baby care include feeding, bathing, safety, cord care, immunizations, methods of soothing the baby, bowel movements, newborn jaundice, and more, as individual circumstances warrant. Topics related to mother include bonding, fatigue, depression, perineal care, formula preparation, breast feeding, and her need for family support and socialization. This program not only is helpful for parents but provides personal feedback for the nurse who has played an important role in the newborn's existence.

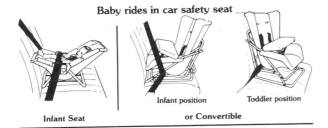

Baby rides in car safety seat

Infant Seat    Infant position    Toddler position
or Convertible

Never carry baby in your arms

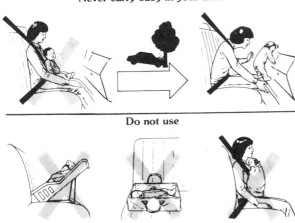

Do not use

Household carrier    Travel bed    Cloth carrier

**Figure 9–13.** The baby must always ride in a car safety seat placed on the back seat of the car; household carriers and travel beds are *not* to be used. The infant faces the rear; the toddler, who is older and larger, can face forward. The infant is never carried in one's arms. The infant's clothing should be comfortable and have legs for a snug fit of the harness. The back should be flat against the car seat, and the head and body should be supported with rolled diapers or blankets. (Adapted courtesy of Evenflow Juvenile Furniture Company, Los Angeles, CA.)

## POSTPARTUM INSTRUCTIONS

The nurse is responsible for reviewing the instructions and ensuring that the mother understands the directions.

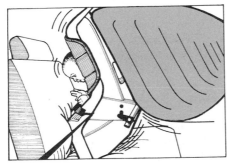

**Figure 9–14.** A passenger air bag could strike the back of the safety seat, and the impact could seriously injure a baby's head. To prevent this injury, always place the baby in the back seat. (From *Safe Ride News*. [Spring, 1993]. American Academy of Pediatrics, Elk Grove Village, IL)

**Rest.** The mother is instructed to avoid strenuous activity and do no heavy lifting or climbing of stairs. Naps, when the baby is napping, are recommended.

**Hygiene.** A daily shower or bath is recommended. Perineal care is continued at home for as long as lochia discharge persists. Douches and tampons should be avoided until after the 6-week checkup.

**Sexual Intercourse.** Coitus should be avoided until the episiotomy is fully healed and the lochia flow has stopped. Having sexual relations before that time can lead to infection and trauma.

The mother's vagina may initially be dry because of hormonal imbalance. Lubrication with K-Y jelly is recommended. Other methods of intimacy, such as kissing, cuddling, and the expression of feelings, are encouraged. Contraception or control of future pregnancies is discussed. The mother's financial income can affect compliance; the nurse should ascertain whether it is a factor.

**Exercises.** Simple abdominal and perineal exercises may be done. Other exercises should be postponed until after the 6-week checkup.

**Diet.** Usually a regular diet that is well balanced is encouraged. Breast-feeding mothers are reminded of the necessity for extra nutrition and fluids.

**Danger Signs.** Heavy bleeding or foul-smelling discharge from the vagina is promptly reported to the physician or CNM. Other symptoms that should be reported are breast pain, elevated temperature, dragging backache, calf pain, and persistent abdominal or pelvic pain.

A follow-up appointment is also made for the newborn's first checkup, which is usually at 2 weeks of age. All infants should remain under medical care by a family physician, pediatrician, or persons in charge of a local child health clinic.

The location of the nearest health clinic may be determined by calling the health department or the Visiting Nurse Association. Its main purpose is to provide health supervision for infants and children who would not otherwise receive these services. Here, under the supervision of competent physicians and public health nurses, healthy infants are weighed, examined, and immunized. Mothers are given guidance in promoting the physical and emotional health of their child. Nurses should become acquainted with the health and welfare facilities in their town or city. The classified section of the telephone book is a good place to begin investigations. Many agencies are listed under "Social Service."

## FOLLOW-UP CARE

At the 6-week appointment, the mother's general health and recuperation are assessed. She is weighed, her vital signs are taken, and she is prepared by the nurse for vaginal examination. The physician or CNM examines the uterus to ensure that adequate involution has taken place. The episiotomy site is examined to see if healing has occurred. The breasts are carefully examined for any signs of problems.

Occasionally a complete blood count is done, and vitamins or iron supplements, or both, are ordered.

Contraception is readdressed, and the mother is educated about the various methods available (see Chap. 11). She is reminded about breast examination and the importance of regularly obtaining a Papanicolaou smear.

The woman has the opportunity to discuss any problems she may be having, whether physical or psychological. The physician and the nurse usually inquire how she is adapting to motherhood. Is she getting enough rest? How is breast feeding coming along? Does she have help at home? How is the father adapting to his new role?

The woman should leave the health care provider's office feeling that all her questions have been answered. It is essential that both the physician and the nurse maintain a link with the family. Maintaining contact increases the parents' feelings of security, and compliance with future visits is more likely.

## KEY POINTS

- During the first 24 hours following delivery, the mother is closely supervised for hypovolemic shock and hemorrhage. After the danger of bleeding has passed, infection is also a concern.
- The nurse observes the new mother for signs of bleeding, height and consistency of the fundus, condition of the perineum, and wound healing if an episiotomy was performed.
- Lochia is the vaginal discharge seen following delivery. It progresses from rubra to serous to alba. The nurse observes it for type, amount, and characteristics.
- Common discomforts of the postpartum mother include swelling of the perineum, hemorrhoids, afterpains, engorged breasts, episiotomy tenderness, and alterations in urination.
- A full bladder may displace the uterus and lead to bleeding.
- The breasts of the new mother are examined for size, shape, reddened areas, tenderness, and condition of the nipples. Education and support of breast-feeding mothers by the nurse will facilitate a positive experience.
- Immediate care of the newborn includes assessment of breathing, provision of warmth, proper identification, and prevention of infection.
- The Apgar score is a means of evaluating the newborn at 1 minute and 5 minutes after delivery. The highest possible score is 10.
- Mother-baby units or rooming-in provides opportunities for the family to interact with the newborn and to learn parenting skills.
- Because of the trend toward early discharge, teaching the new mother self-care and baby care begins soon after delivery. Written information is supplied, and telephone calls to the unit are encouraged. Follow-up supervision is carefully arranged.

# Study Questions

1. Bleeding during the fourth stage of labor may be excessive for several reasons. Identify two of them and the nursing interventions required to resolve the bleeding.
2. What are the names of two medications that may be given to a new mother after delivery to control postpartum bleeding?
3. How does involution of the uterus take place? Describe complications that may occur.
4. Describe what a nurse teaches a new mother about perineal care.
5. Describe the three types of lochia and what to assess.
6. During the fourth stage, how does the nursing care of the mother who had a cesarean delivery differ from that of the woman who had a vaginal delivery?
7. What care is given to the umbilicus of the newborn? Why is this care important?
8. List and compare the advantages and disadvantages of breast feeding and bottle feeding.
9. How may the nurse reassure the breast-feeding mother that her baby is getting enough milk?
10. What special nutritional considerations should a breast-feeding mother be made aware of by the nurse?
11. How can the nurse on the busy maternity unit satisfy the needs of the baby for tender, loving care?
12. Describe three positions for burping the baby.
13. What are the instructions a nurse reviews with a new mother before her discharge from the hospital?

# Multiple Choice
# Review Questions

*Choose the most appropriate answer.*

1. The puerperium, or the postpartum period, is best defined as the
   a. 3–5 days of hospitalization following delivery
   b. first 24 hours after delivery, during which the woman's body returns to the prepregnant state
   c. 6–week period after delivery, during which the woman's body returns to the prepregnant state
   d. time just before delivery
2. On palpation during the postpartum period, the uterus should be
   a. firm and below the umbilicus
   b. soft and boggy
   c. above the umbilicus and firm
   d. at the umbilicus and boggy
3. An *immediate* priority after delivery is for the parents to
   a. notify the relatives
   b. discuss contraception
   c. bond with the newborn
   d. visit with the siblings
4. The term *involution* refers to
   a. the process by which the uterus shrinks to its prepregnant state
   b. a sloughing of the endometrium
   c. the discharge of the ovum from the graafian follicle
   d. firming of the uterine muscle
5. To prevent edema and reduce pain at the site of the episiotomy during the first 24 hours post partum, the nurse provides
   a. a heat lamp
   b. warm compresses
   c. an analgesic spray
   d. an ice pack

6. The hormone that is secreted by the pituitary gland after delivery and stimulates milk production is called
   a. oxytocin
   b. prolactin
   c. estrogen
   d. colostrum
7. A new mother who breast feeds her baby
   a. will gain weight because of increased caloric intake needed to provide the milk
   b. will be more tired than a non-nursing mother because of the frequent breast feedings
   c. will be able to lose weight despite the additional caloric intake because milk production uses energy from the fat reserves
   d. must have 1000 extra calories and at least an extra 4 hours of sleep each day
8. Lochia that has a foul odor should cause the nurse to
   a. consider this normal during the first few days after delivery
   b. discontinue the use of perineal pads for a few days
   c. suggest perineal cleansing in order to reduce odor and provide comfort for the new mother
   d. identify this as an indication of infection and report it immediately
9. Diaphoresis in the early postpartum period is
   a. an indication of infection
   b. retention of body fluids
   c. an elimination of excess body fluids
   d. an elimination of urine
10. Afterpains are caused by
    a. uterine contractions after delivery
    b. constipation after delivery
    c. trauma during delivery
    d. a prolapsed uterus after delivery

## BIBLIOGRAPHY

American Academy of Pediatrics. (1993, Spring). *Safe Ride News.* Elk Grove Village, Ill.

Bernard-Bonnin, A., et al. (1989). Hospital practices and breastfeeding duration: A meta-analysis of controlled trials. *Birth,* 2:64–66.

Blackburn, S.T., & Loper, D.L. (1992). *Maternal, fetal, and neonatal physiology: A clinical perspective.* Philadelphia: W.B. Saunders.

Bond, L. (1993). Physiological changes. In S. Mattson & J.E. Smith (Eds.), *Core curriculum for maternal-newborn nursing* (pp. 315–323). Philadelphia: W.B. Saunders.

D'Avanzo, C.E. (1992). Bridging the cultural gap with Southeast Asians. *MCN: American Journal of Maternal Child Nursing, 18,* 38–43.

Flaskerud, J.H., & Ungvarski, P.J. (1992). *HIV/AIDS: A guide to nursing care* (2nd ed.). Philadelphia: W.B. Saunders.

Glenn, L. (1993). Adaptation to extrauterine life. In S. Mattson & J.E. Smith (Eds.), *Core curriculum for maternal-newborn nursing* (pp. 367–372). Philadelphia: W.B. Saunders.

Grant, M., Bush, G., & Ramaswamy, A. (1992). Microwave heating of infant formula: A dilemma resolved. *Pediatrics, 90,* no. 3.

Hacker, N.F., & Moore, J.G. (1992). *Essentials of obstetrics and gynecology* (2nd ed.). Philadelphia: W.B. Saunders.

Ladewig, P.W., London, M.L., & Olds, S.B. (1994). *Essentials of maternal-newborn nursing* (3rd ed.). Redwood City, CA: Addison-Wesley.

Levine M., Carey, W., Crocker A., Gross, R. (1992). *Developmental-behavioral pediatrics.* Philadelphia: W.B. Saunders.

Olds S.B., London M., & Ladewig, B. (1992). *Maternal-newborn nursing 4.* Reading, MA: Addison-Wesley.

Pillitteri A. (1992). *Maternal and child health nursing.* Philadelphia: J.B. Lippincott.

Rubin, R. (1977). Bonding in the postpartum period. *Maternal Child Nursing Journal, 6,* 67.

Stuart, G., & Sundeen, S. (1991). *Principles and practice of psychiatric nursing 4.* St. Louis: C.V. Mosby.

Whaley, L., & Wong, D. (1991). *Nursing care of infants and children 4.* St. Louis: C.V. Mosby.

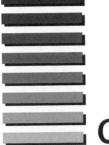

# Chapter 10

# Nursing Care of Women with Complications Following Birth

# OBJECTIVES

*On completion and mastery of Chapter 10, the student will be able to*

- Define each vocabulary term listed.
- Describe signs and symptoms for each postpartum complication.
- Identify factors that increase a woman's risk for developing each complication.
- Explain nursing measures that reduce a woman's risk for developing specific postpartum complications.
- Describe additional problems that may result from the original postpartum complication.
- Describe medical management of postpartum complications.
- Explain general and specific nursing care for each complication.

Most women who have a baby recover from pregnancy and childbirth uneventfully. However, some have complications after birth that slow their recovery. Most childbearing women fully recover from these complications, but the problems interfere with their ability to assume their new role.

A woman can have any medical problem after birth, but most complications fall into one of five categories:

- Hemorrhage
- Thromboembolic disorders
- Infections
- Subinvolution of the uterus
- Mood disorders

Of these classifications, hemorrhage and infection are the two most commonly encountered. Thromboembolic disorders may occur either during pregnancy or after birth.

# Hemorrhage

Postpartum hemorrhage is defined as blood loss greater than 500 ml after vaginal birth, or 1000 ml after cesarean birth. Postpartum blood losses that exceed 500 ml are fairly common, but losses exceeding 1000 ml are unusual.

Most cases of hemorrhage occur immediately after birth, but some are delayed up to several weeks. *Early postpartum hemorrhage* occurs within 24 hours of delivery; *late postpartum he-* *morrhage* occurs later than 24 hours after birth.

## OVERVIEW

The major risk of hemorrhage is hypovolemic (low-volume) shock, which interrupts blood flow to body cells. This prevents normal oxygenation, nutrient delivery, and waste removal at the cell level. Although a less dramatic problem, anemia is likely to occur after hemorrhage, and may require some time to correct.

**Hypovolemic Shock.** Hypovolemic shock occurs when the volume of blood is depleted and cannot fill the circulatory system. The woman will die if blood loss does not stop and if shock is not corrected.

The body initially responds to reduced blood volume with increased heart and respiratory rates. These reactions increase the oxygen content of each erythrocyte (red blood cell) and more quickly circulate the remaining blood. *Tachycardia (rapid heart rate) is usually the first sign of inadequate blood volume.*

The first blood pressure change is a narrow pulse pressure (a falling systolic pressure and rising diastolic pressure). The blood pressure continues falling, and eventually cannot be detected.

Blood flow to nonessential organs gradually stops so that more is available for vital organs, specifically the heart and brain. This change causes the woman's skin and mucous membranes to become pale, cold, and clammy (moist). As blood loss continues, flow to the brain falls, resulting in mental changes, such as anxiety, confusion, restlessness, and lethargy. As blood flow to the kidneys decreases, they respond by conserving fluid. Urine output decreases and eventually stops.

Medical management of hypovolemic shock resulting from hemorrhage may include the following:

- Stopping the blood loss
- Giving intravenous fluids to maintain circulating volume and replace fluids
- Giving blood transfusions to replace lost erythrocytes
- Giving oxygen to increase saturation of remaining blood cells
- Placing an indwelling (Foley) catheter to assess urine output, which reflects kidney circulation

Intensive care may be required to allow inva-

| NURSING CARE PLAN 10–1 |
|---|

## Selected Nursing Diagnoses for the Woman with Postpartum Hemorrhage

| Goals | Interventions | Rationale |
|---|---|---|

**Nursing Diagnosis:** High risk for altered tissue perfusion related to excessive blood loss secondary to uterine atony or birth injury.

| Goals | Interventions | Rationale |
|---|---|---|
| Woman's blood pressure and pulse will be within 10% of her values when she was admitted<br>Woman will not have signs or symptoms of hypovolemic shock | 1. Identify whether woman has added risk factors for postpartum hemorrhage<br><br>2. According to facility protocol, or more often if risk factors are present, assess woman's<br>  ■ Fundus for height, firmness, and position<br>  ■ Lochia for color, quantity, and clots; count pads and degree of saturation (weigh pads for greatest accuracy)<br>  ■ Blood pressure, pulse and respiratory rates<br><br>3. Observe for less obvious signs of bleeding:<br>  ■ Constant trickle of brighter red blood with a firm fundus<br>  ■ Severe, poorly relieved pain, especially if accompanied by changes in the vital signs or shock signs and symptoms<br>4. Observe for other signs and symptoms of hypovolemic shock<br>5. If signs of hemorrhage are noted, take appropriate actions, according to probable cause for hemorrhage:<br>  ■ Uterine atony: massage uterus until firm—do not overmassage; expel blood from uterine cavity when uterus is firm; have breast-feeding woman nurse baby; notify registered nurse and/or physician or nurse-midwife for orders and medication if uterus does not become firm and stay firm<br>  ■ Lacerations: notify registered nurse and/or physician/nurse-midwife to examine woman<br>  ■ Hematoma: notify registered nurse and/or physician or nurse-midwife to examine woman; apply cold pack to small hematomas on the vulva | 1. Women who have risk factors should be assessed more frequently than those who do not; usual protocols may not be frequent enough for woman at increased risk for hemorrhage<br>2. The fundus must be firm to compress bleeding vessels at the placenta site; bladder distention interferes with uterine contraction and causes the fundus to be high and displaced to one side; rising pulse rate is often first sign of inadequate blood volume; rising pulse and falling blood pressure also occur; most blood lost after birth is visible rather than concealed—observing lochia provides an estimate of actual blood loss<br>3. Most postpartum hemorrhage is caused by uterine atony, which has dramatic blood loss; however, blood loss from a laceration or hematoma can be significant, even though it is less obvious<br><br>4. Excessive blood loss can result in hypovolemic shock<br>5. Hemorrhage can cause death of a new mother if not promptly corrected; most minor episodes of uterine atony are easily corrected with fundal massage and infant suckling; if the uterus does not remain firm, physician or nurse-midwife examines woman to identify and correct cause of bleeding; oxytocin (Pitocin) infusions are often ordered to contract uterus—other drugs, such as methylergonovine (Methergine) or prostaglandin, may be needed; overmassage of uterus can tire it, possibly resulting in inability to contract<br>  Trauma such as laceration or hematoma may require repair by physician or nurse-midwife; small hematomas on vulva can be limited by cold applications because they reduce blood flow to area; cold applications also numb area and make woman more comfortable |

*Continued*

| NURSING CARE PLAN 10–1 *Continued* | | |
| --- | --- | --- |
| **Selected Nursing Diagnoses for the Woman with Postpartum Hemorrhage** | | |
| Goals | Interventions | Rationale |

**Nursing Diagnosis:** High risk for injury (falls) related to anemia secondary to blood loss.

| | | |
| --- | --- | --- |
| Woman will not fall or have other injury while in birth facility | 1. Caution woman not to get out of bed without help until her condition has stabilized | 1. While lying in bed, woman may not realize that she is likely to be dizzy or lightheaded when she ambulates |
| | 2. When helping woman out of bed, partially elevate head of bed, then help her slowly rise to a sitting position on the side of the bed | 2. Blood loss reduces amount of circulating blood volume; woman may not have enough volume to maintain circulation to all parts of her body if she changes position quickly |
| | 3. Before she stands or walks, have her sit on side of bed for a few minutes; have her rotate her feet and ankles and move her legs as she sits on bed | 3. Gradual changes of position reduce risk that she will fall because her circulatory system adapts to the change; moving her feet and legs prevents blood from pooling in her lower extremities |
| | 4. Remain with woman when she walks; after she is stable and has been up several times, a family member can walk with her | 4. Someone accompanying woman can prevent her from falling if she becomes dizzy or faint |
| | 5. If woman feels faint, have her sit down immediately; if she faints, gently lower her to floor | 5. Prevents injury due to a fall if woman does faint |

sive hemodynamic monitoring of the woman's circulatory status.

Nursing Care Plan 10–1 specifies interventions for the woman at high risk for altered tissue perfusion related to hemorrhage.

**Anemia.** Anemia occurs after hemorrhage because of the lost erythrocytes. Anemia resulting from blood loss occurs suddenly, and the woman may be dizzy, lightheaded, and likely to faint. These symptoms are more likely to occur if she changes position quickly, particularly from a lying position to an upright one.

Until her hemoglobin and hematocrit return to near-normal values, she will probably be exhausted and have difficulty meeting her needs and those of her infant. She is more likely to develop an infection while her body defenses are down.

Medical management of anemia is usually iron supplements to provide adequate amounts of this mineral for manufacture of more erythrocytes. Some physicians and nurse-midwives have the woman continue taking the remainder of her prenatal vitamins, which usually provide enough iron to correct anemia.

See Nursing Care Plan 10–1 for interventions for the woman at high risk for injury related to anemia.

## EARLY POSTPARTUM HEMORRHAGE

Early postpartum hemorrhage is due to one of three causes:

- Uterine atony
- Lacerations (tears) of the reproductive tract
- Hematomas in the reproductive tract

Of these three, uterine atony is the most common. Table 10–1 summarizes care for these causes of hemorrhage.

### Uterine Atony

Atony describes a lack of normal muscle tone. The uterus is a large, hollow organ having three layers of muscle. One layer has interlacing "figure-eight" fibers. The uterine blood supply must pass through this network of muscle fibers. Contraction of the uterine muscle after birth is essential to limit blood loss.

Blood clotting is not adequate to control blood loss after birth of the placenta; blood flows from open uterine vessels too rapidly to allow clotting. After the placenta detaches, the uterus contracts and the muscle fibers compress bleeding vessels. If the uterus is atonic, these muscle fibers are flaccid and do not compress the ves-

**Table 10–1.** TYPES OF EARLY POSTPARTUM HEMORRHAGE

|  | Uterine Atony | Lacerations | Hematoma |
|---|---|---|---|
| Characteristics | Soft, high uterine fundus that is difficult to feel through the woman's abdominal wall<br>Heavy lochia, often with large clots<br>Bladder distention that causes uterus to be high and usually displaces it to one side<br>Possible signs of hypovolemic shock | Continuous trickle of blood that is brighter than normal lochia<br>Fundus that is usually firm<br>Onset of hypovolemic shock that may be gradual and easily overlooked | If visible, blue or purplish mass on the vulva<br>Severe and poorly relieved pain and/or pressure in vulva, pelvis, or rectum<br>Large amount of blood lost into tissues, which causes signs and symptoms of hypovolemic shock<br>Lochia that is normal in amount and color |
| Contributing factors | Bladder distention<br>Abnormal or prolonged labor<br>Overdistended uterus<br>Multiparity, especially over 5 births<br>Use of oxytocin during labor<br>Medications that relax uterus<br>Retained placenta | Rapid labor<br>Use of instruments, such as forceps or vacuum extractor, during birth | Prolonged or rapid labor<br>Large infant<br>Use of forceps or vacuum extractor |

sels. Uterine atony allows the blood vessels at the placenta site to bleed freely and usually massively.

**Normal Postpartum Findings.** After birth, the uterus should easily be felt through the abdominal wall as a firm mass about the size of a grapefruit. The fundus (top) should be about the level of the umbilicus or slightly lower.

Lochia rubra (bloody drainage after birth) should be dark red. The amount of lochia during the first few hours should be no more than one saturated perineal pad within 1 hour. (Perineal pads containing cold packs absorb less than regular perineal pads.) A few small clots may appear in the drainage, but large clots are not normal.

**Characteristics of Uterine Atony.** When uterine atony occurs, the woman's uterus is difficult to feel, and when found, it is boggy (soft). The fundal height is high, often above the umbilicus. If the bladder is full, the uterus is higher and pushed to one side rather than being in the midline of the abdomen (Fig. 10–1). The uterus may or may not be soft if the bladder is full. However, a full bladder interferes with the ability of the uterus to contract and if not corrected, eventually leads to uterine atony.

Lochia is increased, and may contain large clots. The nurse must remember that some lochia will be retained in the relaxed uterus because the cavity is enlarged. Thus, the true amount of blood loss may not be immediately apparent. Collection of blood within the uterus

# Nursing Brief

To determine blood loss most accurately, weigh perineal pads before applying them and after removal. One gram of weight equals about 1 ml of blood lost.

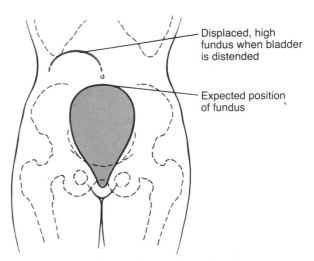

- Displaced, high fundus when bladder is distended

- Expected position of fundus

**Figure 10–1.** A distended bladder pushes the uterus upward and usually to one side of the abdomen. The fundus may be boggy or firm. If not emptied, a distended bladder can result in uterine atony and hemorrhage, because it interferes with normal contraction of the uterus.

interferes with contraction and increases the severity of atony and postpartum hemorrhage.

**Risk Factors.** Uterine atony can occur in women who have no added risk factors, but it should be anticipated in some women. Uterine atony is more common in these situations:

- Urinary bladder distention
- Abnormal labor (see p. 198)
- Uterine overdistention from any cause, such as a multifetal pregnancy, large infant, or excessive amniotic fluid (hydramnios)
- Multiparity, especially over five births
- Stimulation of labor with oxytocin
- Medications that relax the uterus, such as magnesium sulfate or tocolytic drugs (see p. 207)
- Retention of a large piece of the placenta

If a woman has risk factors, more frequent postpartum assessments of the uterus and lochia are needed.

**Medical and Nursing Treatment.** Care of the woman with uterine atony combines nursing and medical measures. When the uterus is boggy, the nurse should immediately massage it until it is firm. One nurse institutes emergency measures, such as fundal massage, while another notifies the physician or nurse-midwife.

The uterus should not be overmassaged. Because it is a muscle, excessive stimulation to contract the uterus will tire it and can actually worsen uterine atony. If the uterus is firmly contracted, it is left alone.

Bladder distention is an easily corrected cause of uterine atony. If the woman cannot urinate in the bathroom or on a bedpan, she must be catheterized. Most physicians and nurse-midwives include an order for catheterization, if needed, to avoid delaying this corrective measure. First, the uterus should be massaged to firmness, then the bladder emptied to keep the uterus firm.

Infant suckling at the breast stimulates the woman's posterior pituitary gland to secrete oxytocin, which causes uterine contraction. Dilute oxytocin (Pitocin) infusion is the most common drug ordered to control uterine atony. Other drugs to increase uterine tone include methylergonovine (Methergine) or prostaglandin $F_{2\alpha}$. Methylergonovine increases blood pressure and should not be given to a woman with hypertension.

The physician may examine the woman in

## Nursing Brief

The woman who develops a hemorrhagic complication should be kept NPO until the physician or nurse-midwife evaluates her in case she needs general anesthesia for correction of the problem.

the delivery or operating room to determine the source of her bleeding and correct it. The physician may perform bimanual compression, a technique to compress the uterus between one hand in her vagina and the other on her abdomen. Rarely, hysterectomy is required to remove the bleeding uterus that does not respond to other measures. The woman should have nothing by mouth until her bleeding is controlled.

### Lacerations of the Reproductive Tract

Lacerations of the perineum, vagina, cervix, or area around the urethra (periurethral lacerations) can cause postpartum bleeding. They are more likely to occur if the woman has a rapid labor or if instruments, such as forceps or a vacuum extractor, are needed to assist the birth.

Blood lost in lacerations is usually a brighter red than lochia and flows in a continuous trickle. Typically, the uterus is firm. *A continuous trickle of blood can result in as much, or more, blood loss than the dramatic bleeding associated with uterine atony.*

**Treatment.** If the woman has signs of a laceration, bleeding with a firmly contracted uterus, the physician or nurse-midwife should be notified. Expect the injury to be sutured in the delivery or operating room. The woman is given nothing by mouth until further orders are received because she may need a general anesthetic for repair of the laceration.

### Hematomas

A hematoma is a collection of blood within the tissues. Hematomas resulting from birth trauma are usually on the vulva or inside the vagina. They may be easily seen as a bulging, bluish or purplish mass (Fig. 10–2). Hematomas deep within the vagina are not visible from the outside.

A particularly serious hematoma is a broad-ligament hematoma. The broad ligament is a

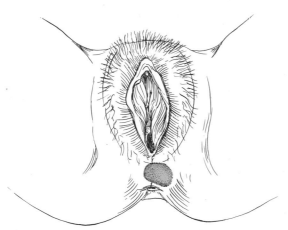

**Figure 10-2.** A hematoma on the vulva is a collection of blood within the soft tissues. It is a blue or purple mass. Cold applications may limit the hematoma.

wide sheet of tissue extending from the side of the uterus to the side walls of the pelvis (see p. 22). Several large arteries and veins are in the broad ligament. Thus, a hematoma in this area can result in massive concealed blood loss.

Discomfort after childbirth is normally minimal and easily relieved with mild analgesics. The woman with a hematoma usually has severe, unrelenting pain that analgesics do not relieve. Depending on the amount of blood in the tissues, she also may describe pressure in the vulva, pelvis, or rectum.

The woman does not have unusual amounts of lochia, but she may develop signs of concealed blood loss. Her pulse and respiratory rates rise, and her blood pressure falls. She may develop other signs of hypovolemic shock if blood loss into the tissues is substantial.

Risk factors for development of a hematoma include

- Prolonged or rapid labor
- Large baby
- Use of forceps or vacuum extractor

**Treatment.** Small hematomas usually resolve without treatment. Larger ones may require incision and drainage of the clots. The bleeding vessel is ligated or the area packed with a hemostatic material to stop bleeding.

Nursing care involves being aware of women who have increased risk for hematoma formation and observing for the typical symptom: excessive, poorly relieved pain. Cold packs to the vulva can limit hematoma formation by causing blood vessel constriction. The physician is promptly notified if the woman has symptoms of a hematoma, even if none can be seen on the outside. She is given nothing by mouth until the physician examines her and other orders are received.

## LATE POSTPARTUM HEMORRHAGE

Late postpartum hemorrhage (later than 24 hours after birth) usually occurs because small fragments of the placenta are retained within the uterus. It may also occur if the "scab" that forms over the placental site is disrupted. Late postpartum hemorrhage usually occurs after discharge. It begins without warning and may be profuse.

Late postpartum hemorrhage is more likely to occur if the placenta does not separate cleanly from its implantation site after birth. This may occur if the placenta is manually removed (removed by hand, rather than being pushed away from the uterine wall spontaneously as the uterus contracts). It is also more likely to occur if the placenta grows more deeply into the uterine muscle than is normal.

**Treatment.** Treatment consists of drugs, such as oxytocin (Pitocin) or methylergonovine (Methergine), to contract the uterus. If bleeding continues, curettage (scraping or vacuuming the inner surface of the uterus) is done to remove small blood clots and placental fragments. Antibiotics are usually prescribed to prevent infection.

The nurse should teach each postpartum woman what to expect about changes in the lochia (see p. 223). She should be taught to report signs of late postpartum hemorrhage to her physician or nurse-midwife:

- Persistent red bleeding
- Return of red bleeding after it has changed to pinkish or white

If a late postpartum hemorrhage occurs, the nurse assists in implementing drug and surgical treatment.

## Nursing Brief

Because postpartum women often have a slow pulse, suspect hypovolemic shock or infection if it is higher than 100 beats/min.

# Thromboembolic Disorders

Venous thrombosis is more likely to occur when three conditions exist:

- Presence of increased clotting factors
- Venous stasis
- Injury to the inner surface (intima) of the vein

In normal pregnancy, two of these conditions exist: increased clotting factors and venous stasis caused by pressure of the growing uterus on veins that return blood to the heart. Injury to the inner vein surface is unlikely to occur unless the woman has a pelvic infection or cesarean delivery.

**Manifestations.** Signs and symptoms depend on whether the disorder is a superficial vein thrombosis or deep vein thrombosis. Superficial vein thrombosis is characterized by a painful, hard, reddened, warm vein that is easily seen. Deep vein thrombosis is characterized by pain, calf tenderness, leg edema, color changes, and pain when the foot is dorsiflexed (Homans' sign). The primary risk of deep vein thrombosis is that a clot will break off (embolize) and lodge in the blood vessels of the lungs (pulmonary embolism).

Pulmonary embolism may have dramatic signs and symptoms, such as sudden chest pain, cough, dyspnea (difficulty breathing), depressed consciousness, and signs of heart failure. A small pulmonary embolism may have nonspecific signs and symptoms, such as shortness of breath, palpitations, hemoptysis (bloody sputum), faintness, and low-grade fever. Table 10–2 compares the manifestations and likelihood of pulmonary embolism of superficial vein thrombosis with those of deep vein thrombosis.

**Table 10–2.** ASSESSMENT OF VENOUS THROMBOSIS

| Location | Manifestations | Pulmonary Embolism |
|----------|----------------|--------------------|
| Superficial vein | Tender, painful hard, reddened area along warm vein; easily visible | Rare |
| Deep vein | Increased pain and calf tenderness, leg edema, color changes, pain when foot is dorsiflexed (Homans' sign), occasional fever rarely over 101°F (38.3°C) | Possible |

**Treatment.** Superficial vein thrombosis is treated with analgesics, local application of heat, and elevation of the legs to promote venous drainage. Deep vein thrombosis is treated similarly, with the addition of heparin anticoagulation. Anticoagulant therapy is continued with heparin or warfarin (Coumadin) for 6 weeks after birth to minimize the risk of embolism. See a medical-surgical nursing text for treatment of pulmonary embolism.

**Nursing Care.** The nurse observes for signs and symptoms that suggest venous thrombosis before and after birth. Dyspnea, coughing, and chest pain suggest pulmonary embolism and are reported immediately.

Pregnant women should not cross their legs, which impedes venous blood flow. When the legs are elevated, there should not be sharp flexion at the groin or pressure in the popliteal space behind the knee, which would restrict venous flow. Measures to promote venous flow should be continued during and after birth, because levels of clotting factors remain high for several weeks.

The woman on anticoagulant therapy is taught to give herself the drug and is taught about signs of excess anticoagulation, as one would discuss with a patient with heart disease. Home nursing visits are often prescribed to obtain blood for laboratory clotting studies and to help the woman cope with therapy.

# Infection

New mothers may acquire a variety of infections after birth. Many of these have their origins during pregnancy or labor but may not become apparent until after birth. The most likely sites for postpartum infection are

- Wounds such as from an episiotomy, laceration, or surgical incision
- Uterus
- Urinary tract
- Breast

Table 10–3 lists characteristics, medical treatment, and nursing care for these infections.

## OVERVIEW

Regardless of their location or the causative organism, postpartum infections have several common features.

**Table 10–3.** POSTPARTUM INFECTIONS

| | Wound Infections | Endometritis (Uterus) | Urinary Tract | Mastitis (Breast) |
|---|---|---|---|---|
| Characteristics | Signs of inflammation (redness, edema, heat, pain)<br>Separation of suture line<br>Purulent drainage | Tender, enlarged uterus<br>Prolonged, severe cramping<br>Foul-smelling lochia<br>Fever and other systemic signs of infection | *Cystitis (bladder)*<br>Low temperature elevation<br>Burning, urgency, and frequency of urination<br>*Pyelonephritis (kidneys)*<br>High fever with a pattern of spikes<br>Chills<br>Pain in the costovertebral angle or flank<br>Nausea and vomiting | Reddened, tender, hot area of the breast<br>Edema and a feeling of heaviness in the breast<br>Purulent drainage, which may occur if an abscess forms |
| Medical treatment | Culture and sensitivity of wound exudate<br>Antibiotics | Culture and sensitivity of uterine cavity<br>Antibiotics, by intravenous (IV) route initially | Clean-catch or catheterized urine specimen for culture and sensitivity testing<br>Antibiotics (initially by IV route for pyelonephritis) | Antibiotics (usually oral, although may be IV initially if woman has an abscess)<br>Incision and drainage of abscess |
| Nursing care | Aseptic/sterile technique for all wound care, as indicated<br>Teaching of proper perineal hygiene to reduce fecal contamination<br>Sitz baths for perineal wound infections | Teaching woman usual progression of lochia, since infection often occurs after discharge<br>Fowler's position to facilitate drainage of infected lochia<br>Analgesics<br>Observation for absent bowel sounds, abdominal distention, and nausea or vomiting, which suggest spread of infection | Teaching perineal hygiene<br>Encouraging fluid intake of 3 L/day<br>Teaching which foods increase acidity of urine, such as apricots, cranberry juice, plums, and prunes | Teaching effective breast-feeding techniques (see p. 237)<br>Moist heat applications with a warm pack<br>Warm shower before nursing to start milk flow<br>Massage of affected area to reduce congestion<br>Regular and frequent nursing or pumping to keep breasts empty |

**Manifestations.** Puerperal (postpartum) morbidity (illness) is defined as a temperature of 38°C (100.4°F) or higher after the first 24 hours, and occurring on at least 2 days during the first 10 days after birth. Slight temperature elevations, with no other signs of infection, often occur during the first 24 hours because of dehydration. The nurse should look for other signs of infection if the woman's temperature is elevated, regardless of the time since birth.

Other signs and symptoms of infection may be localized (in a small area of the body) or systemic (throughout the body). Redness, edema, and pain are examples of localized signs and symptoms. Fever, malaise, achiness, and loss of appetite are examples of systemic signs and symptoms of infection.

White blood cells (leukocytes) are normally elevated during the early postpartum period to about 20,000–30,000/dl, which limits the usefulness of the blood count to identify infection. Leukocyte counts in the upper limits are more likely to be associated with infection than lower counts, however.

**Risk Factors.** Childbirth involves some amount of trauma, providing a portal of entry for microorganisms that naturally inhabit the vaginal and rectal area. Breast feeding can result in small cracks in the nipples. The warm, dark, moist environment of the uterus provides a good growth medium for bacteria. Additionally, the vagina is less acidic than usual after birth, which fosters growth of microorganisms.

The organs of the reproductive tract are especially vulnerable to infection because they are interconnected. During pregnancy and for a time after birth, the reproductive organs are richly supplied with blood. These two characteristics make it easy for an infection in one organ to spread to another or to enter the circulation and infect a distant part of the body.

Some women have added risk for infection. Conditions that increase a woman's risk for developing infection include

- Cesarean birth
- Use of forceps or a vacuum extractor
- Long labor
- Prolonged rupture of membranes, especially for longer than 24 hours
- Urinary catheterization
- Repeated vaginal examinations during labor
- Retained fragments of placenta

- Anemia
- Poor nutritional state

These risk factors are often linked to one another. For example, the woman who has a long labor often has prolonged ruptured membranes, many vaginal examinations, and a forceps or cesarean birth.

**General Medical Treatment.** The goals of medical treatment are to

- Limit the spread of infection to other organs
- Eliminate the infection

A culture and sensitivity of the site of the suspected infection is done to determine what antibiotics are effective. A culture and sensitivity requires 2 or 3 days to complete. In the meantime, antibiotics that are effective against typical organisms that cause the infection are administered to limit the spread of infection to nearby structures.

**General Nursing Care.** Nursing care objectives focus on preventing infection and if one occurs, on facilitating medical treatment. To achieve these goals, the nurse should

- Use and teach hygienic measures to reduce the number of organisms that can cause infection, such as handwashing and perineal care
- Promote adequate rest and nutrition for healing
- Observe for signs of infection
- Teach signs of infection that the woman should report after she is discharged
- Teach the woman to take all of the antibiotics prescribed rather than stopping them after her symptoms go away

Women should be taught to wash their hands before and after doing self-care that may involve contact with secretions. The nurse should explore ways to help the woman get enough rest. Nursing Care Plan 10–2 details interventions for the woman at high risk for infection.

Ultimately, a woman's own body must over-

## Nursing Brief

Proper handwashing is the primary method to avoid spread of infectious organisms. Gloves should be worn when contacting any body secretion.

| NURSING CARE PLAN 10–2 | | |
| --- | --- | --- |
| **Selected Nursing Diagnoses for the Woman with Postpartum Infection** | | |
| **Goals** | **Interventions** | **Rationale** |

**Nursing Diagnosis:** High risk for infection related to loss of skin integrity (cesarean incision) and increased risk factors (prolonged labor).

| | | |
| --- | --- | --- |
| Woman will not have signs of infection, as evidenced by oral temperature below 38°C (100.4°F) and normal progression of lochia that does not have a foul odor | 1. Use handwashing when providing care; teach woman personal hygiene measures, such as handwashing, perineal care, regular changes of perineal pads | 1. Limits transfer of infectious organisms between clients and from one area of the body to another; regular pad changes also reduce amount of time organisms have to multiply in its warm, dark, and moist environment |
| | 2. Assess vital signs every 4 hr, or more frequently if signs of infection are present | 2. An elevated temperature and rising pulse are signs of infection; if they occur, woman should be assessed for other signs and symptoms of infection |
| | 3. Assess lochia for amount, color, and odor with vital signs | 3. Endometritis is more common if a woman has a cesarean birth and is evidenced by foul-smelling lochia that may be increased or decreased; it is sometimes brown |
| | 4. Assess uterus for height, firmness, and descent | 4. Endometritis is characterized by an enlarged, tender uterus |
| | 5. Assess for cramping or other pain | 5. Prolonged cramping may occur with endometritis; a wound infection may be painful |
| | 6. Assess the wound each shift for redness, edema, discharge, and intactness | 6. A wound infection is characterized by signs of inflammation; suture line may separate if there is infection in the area |
| | 7. Assess for signs and symptoms of urinary tract infection (see p. 262). Encourage high fluid intake (3 liters/day) | 7. Identifies possible presence of urinary tract infection so that it can be reported to the physician; high fluid intake regularly flushes microorganisms from bladder and reduces chance that they will infect urinary tract |

**Nursing Diagnosis:** High risk for altered nutrition, less than body requirements, related to increased demand for nutrients secondary to infection.

| | | |
| --- | --- | --- |
| After teaching, woman will verbalize foods that provide nutrients she needs for healing | 1. Determine foods woman usually eats | 1. Identifies her preferences and areas of nutrient adequacy or inadequacy; nurse can build on her preferences and dislikes |
| | 2. Teach sources of foods high in protein, vitamin C, and iron:<br>■ Protein: eggs, meats, cheeses, milk, legumes, combinations of grain foods<br>■ Vitamin C: citrus fruits and juices, strawberries, cantaloupe, tomatoes, broccoli, peppers, cabbage<br>■ Iron: meats, enriched cereals and breads, dark-green leafy vegetables, dried beans and fruits | 2. Protein and vitamin C are necessary for healing; anemia, which is usually related to iron deficiency, can be corrected by high-iron foods; vitamin C also improves body's ability to use iron |

*Continued*

| | | |
|---|---|---|
| **NURSING CARE PLAN 10–2 Continued** | | |
| **Selected Nursing Diagnoses for the Woman with Postpartum Infection** | | |
| Goals | Interventions | Rationale |

**Nursing Diagnosis:** High risk for altered nutrition, less than body requirements, related to increased demand for nutrients secondary to infection.

| Goals | Interventions | Rationale |
|---|---|---|
| | 3. Reinforce physician's orders about vitamin supplements | 3. Many physicians have woman take remainder of her prenatal vitamins to be certain she has adequate nutrients |
| | 4. If woman is breast feeding, incorporate diet recommendations for nursing mother into teaching (see p. 241) | 4. Nursing mother requires added nutrients to meet her own needs for healing and restoration, plus enough to make breast milk |
| | 5. Have woman restate appropriate foods to meet her nutritional needs after teaching her | 5. Identifies if she learned and identifies need for further teaching |
| | 6. Refer to social services for financial assistance, such as the Women, Infants, and Children (WIC) program for food supplementation | 6. Helps overcome financial barriers to obtaining adequate food |

come infection and heal any wound. Nutrition is an essential component of her body defenses. She is taught about foods that are high in protein (meats, cheese, milk, legumes) and vitamin C (citrus fruits and juices, strawberries, cantaloupe) because these nutrients are especially important for healing. Foods high in iron to correct anemia include meats, enriched cereals and breads, and dark green, leafy vegetables. Refer to Nursing Care Plan 10–2 for interventions for the woman at high risk for altered nutrition related to infection.

## WOUND INFECTION

Wound infections can occur in a surgical incision, episiotomy, or lacerations. The signs and symptoms are typical of localized infection anywhere in the body:

- Redness
- Warmth
- Edema
- Pain and localized tenderness
- Purulent (pus-containing) drainage, which may have a foul odor
- Separation of the suture line

The woman also may experience systemic signs and symptoms, such as fever and malaise.

**Medical Treatment.** The physician or nurse-midwife usually obtains a sample of the wound's exudate for a culture and sensitivity. Antibiotics are prescribed, usually by the oral route unless the infection is severe. The wound may be opened to allow drainage of the purulent exudate. Analgesics are usually prescribed.

**Nursing Care.** Nursing care begins with regular assessment of wounds for the signs of infection. If they are found, they should be reported to the physician.

Cleanliness is promoted by using and teaching a good handwashing technique. The woman should do perineal care after each time she urinates or has a bowel movement. To reduce the risk of carrying fecal organisms from the rectum to the vagina, she should be taught to use a front-to-back motion when she

- Performs perineal care
- Applies a perineal pad
- Wipes the perineal area after toileting

The nurse observes for signs of infection and teaches the woman to report fever or increasing pain from any wound to her physician or nurse-midwife. Normally, pain after birth decreases steadily. Persistent or increasing pain is often associated with infection. Any drainage should be reported as well.

Sitz baths several times each day may increase comfort and speed healing of infections located in the perineal area. Sitz baths may be done with a disposable unit or in a bathtub. At home, the woman should run warm water in her tub to a depth of about 6 inches, just enough to immerse the affected area. She should remain in the tub about 20 minutes. Staying longer in the sitz bath will not harm her, but it has no added benefit.

## UTERINE INFECTION

Endometritis is an infection of the uterine lining, often at the site of the placenta. The woman has systemic signs and symptoms of infection and looks sick. Specific signs and symptoms of endometritis include

- Uterine tenderness
- Enlarged uterus
- Prolonged and severe cramping
- Foul-smelling lochia that may be increased or decreased in amount

**Complications.** The major risk of endometritis is that it may spread: the organisms may infect nearby organs or enter the circulation (Fig. 10–3). Infection from the uterus may spread to the

- Fallopian tubes (salpingitis)
- Ovaries (oophoritis)
- Connective tissues and ligaments (parametritis)
- Lining of the abdomen and pelvis (peritonitis)

The spreading infection also may contribute to pelvic thrombophlebitis.

**Medical Treatment.** Therapy includes culture and sensitivity studies, followed by immediate initiation of antibiotic treatment. Common antibiotics are ampicillin and cephalosporins. The antibiotics are usually begun by the intravenous route and may be continued by the oral route after the acute phase of the infection. Analgesics for pain are ordered.

The breast-feeding mother may have to stop nursing to conserve her energy for healing if she is quite ill. A few antibiotics cannot be taken during breast feeding. If the mother wants to resume nursing after the infection, she may pump her breasts to maintain lactation.

**Nursing Care.** The woman is placed in a Fowler's (semisitting) position to promote drainage of the infected lochia. Regular perineal care and pad changes to make the woman more comfortable are encouraged. Perineal hygiene reduces the number of infectious organisms that may spread to the reproductive organs, an episiotomy incision or laceration, or the urinary tract.

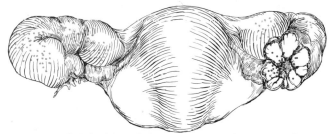

A    **Salpingitis:** Infection in fallopian tubes causes them to become enlarged, hyperemic, and tender

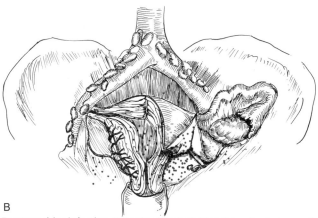

B
**Parametritis:** Infection spreads via lymphatics through uterine wall to connective tissue of broad ligament or entire pelvis

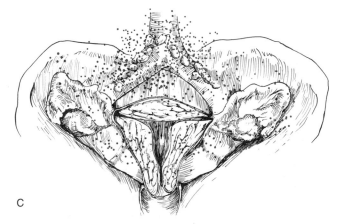

C

**Peritonitis:** Infection spreads via lymphatics to peritoneum; formation of a pelvic abscess may occur

**Figure 10–3.** *A to C,* Endometritis can spread to nearby organs if it is not eradicated promptly.

Antibiotics and analgesics are given as ordered. The woman is observed for signs of improvement or worsening of her condition. Her fever and discomfort should decline. Persistent or worsening discomfort, absence of bowel sounds, abdominal distention, or nausea and vomiting suggest that the infection has spread beyond the uterus.

## URINARY TRACT INFECTION

Infections of the bladder or kidneys are common after birth. Trauma during delivery and incomplete emptying of the bladder increase the risk for infection. Many women are catheterized during labor, sometimes several times, which can carry organisms from the lower urethra into the bladder.

Infection may occur in the bladder (cystitis) or the kidneys (pyelonephritis). Cystitis is characterized by

- Low fever
- Burning pain during urination
- Urgency to urinate
- Increased frequency of urination, with small amounts voided each time

Pyelonephritis has more severe signs and symptoms:

- High fever with a spiking (abrupt up-and-down) pattern
- Chills
- Pain in the back, about the waistline, when the area is tapped (costovertebral angle [CVA] tenderness)
- Flank pain
- Nausea and vomiting

**Medical Treatment.** Oral antibiotics, such as ampicillin, are prescribed for cystitis. Intravenous antibiotics and supplemental fluids are ordered for pyelonephritis.

**Nursing Care.** The nurse maintains the prescribed antibiotic therapy to help eliminate the infection. The woman usually continues antibiotic therapy after discharge and should be taught how to take the prescribed drug.

Most microorganisms in the urinary tract are flushed out with each voiding. The woman needs to drink large quantities (about 3 liters) of liquid each day to promote the self-cleaning action of the urinary tract. Acidic urine inhibits growth of infectious organisms. Foods that increase urine acidity include apricots, cranberry juice, plums, and prunes.

Many women are prone to recurrent episodes of urinary tract infection, usually cystitis. The postpartum period is a good time to teach preventive measures, such as adequate fluid intake and foods to acidify the urine. Urination immediately after sexual intercourse flushes out organisms that may have entered the urethra.

## BREAST INFECTION

Mastitis is an infection of the breast. It usually occurs about 2 or 3 weeks after birth (Fig. 10–4). Mastitis occurs when organisms from the skin or the infant's mouth enter small cracks in the nipples or areola. These cracks may be microscopic. Breast engorgement (congestion) and inadequate emptying of milk are associated with mastitis.

Signs and symptoms of mastitis include

- Redness and heat in the breast
- Tenderness
- Edema and a heaviness in the breast
- Purulent drainage (may or may not be present)

The woman usually has fever, chills, and other systemic signs and symptoms. If not treated, the infected area becomes walled off, and pus collects in a pocket (abscess). The infection is usually outside the ducts of the breast, and the milk is not contaminated. If an abscess develops, it may rupture into the ducts and contaminate the milk.

**Medical Treatment.** Oral antibiotics are usually sufficient to treat mastitis. Mild analgesics make the woman more comfortable. If an abscess forms, the woman may require an incision and drainage of the infected material. Intravenous antibiotics are usually given to begin treatment for a breast abscess.

The mother can usually continue to breast feed unless an abscess forms. If she should not nurse her infant, she can pump her breasts and discard the milk. The mother should not wean her baby when she has mastitis, because weaning leads to engorgement and stasis of milk, which worsens the condition.

**Nursing Care.** Heat promotes blood flow to the area, comfort, and complete emptying of the breast. Moist heat can be applied with chemical packs. An inexpensive warm pack can be made by wetting a disposable diaper with hot water and applying it to the breasts. A warm shower

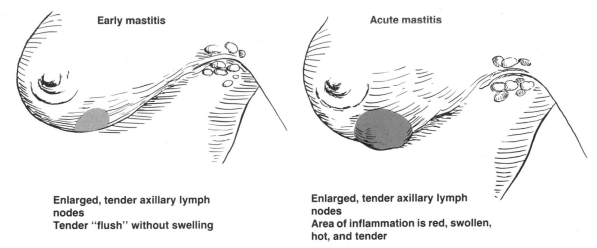

**Early mastitis**

Enlarged, tender axillary lymph nodes
Tender "flush" without swelling

**Acute mastitis**

Enlarged, tender axillary lymph nodes
Area of inflammation is red, swollen, hot, and tender

**Figure 10–4.** Mastitis is a breast infection. It typically occurs several weeks after birth in the woman who is breast feeding. Bacteria usually enter the breast through small cracks in the nipples. Breast engorgement and milk stasis increase the risk for mastitis.

provides warmth and stimulates the flow of milk if done just before nursing.

Both breasts should be emptied regularly (every 1½–2 hours) to reduce milk stasis, which increases the risk for abscess formation. If the affected breast is too painful for the mother to nurse, she can use a pump to empty it. She can massage the area of inflammation to improve milk flow and reduce stasis. Nursing first on the unaffected side starts the milk flow in both breasts and can improve emptying.

Other nursing measures include

- Encouraging fluid intake, about 3 liters/day
- Wearing a good support bra to support the breasts and limit movement of the painful breast
- Supporting the woman emotionally and reassuring her that she can continue to breast feed

## Subinvolution of the Uterus

Involution is the return of the uterus, after birth, to its nonpregnant condition. Subinvolution is a slower-than-expected return of the uterus to its nonpregnant condition. Infection and retained fragments of the placenta are the most common causes of uterine subinvolution.

The uterus normally descends about one fingerwidth each day after birth. By 10 days, it is usually small enough that it cannot be felt through the abdomen. Lochia progresses in a predictable sequence of lochia rubra, lochia serosa, and lochia alba. See Chapter 9 for more information about the normal maternal changes after birth.

These expected changes in the uterine size and progression of lochia do not occur at the normal pace in subinvolution of the uterus. Two typical signs of subinvolution are

- Fundal height greater than expected for the amount of time since birth
- Persistence of lochia rubra or a slowed progression through the three phases

Other signs and symptoms are similar to those of endometritis, and the two conditions often occur together. The other signs and symptoms are

- Pelvic and back pain
- Tenderness of the uterus
- Fatigue and general malaise

The woman often has fever and other signs that accompany infection.

**Medical Treatment.** Medical treatment is selected to correct the cause of the subinvolution. It may include any or all of these measures:

- Methylergonovine (Methergine) to maintain firm uterine contraction
- Antibiotics for infection
- Dilation of the cervix and curettage to re-

move fragments of the placenta from the uterine wall

**Nursing Care.** The mother has almost always been discharged when subinvolution of the uterus occurs. Nursing care focuses on teaching all new mothers about the normal changes to expect so that they can recognize a departure from the normal pattern. Women should report fever, persistent pain, persistent red lochia (or return of bleeding after it has changed), or foul-smelling vaginal discharge.

The woman may be admitted to the hospital on the gynecology unit. Nursing care involves assisting with medical therapy and providing analgesics and other comfort measures. Specific nursing care depends on whether the subinvolution is due to infection or another cause.

## Disorders of Mood

"Postpartum blues," or "baby blues," are common after birth. The woman has periods when she feels let down, but overall, she finds pleasure in life and in her new role as mother. Her roller-coaster emotions are self-limiting as she adapts to the changes in her life.

A mood is a pervasive and sustained emotion that can color one's view of life. A psychosis involves serious impairment of one's perception of reality. Postpartum depression and postpartum psychosis are disorders of mood. They are more serious than the "blues."

### POSTPARTUM DEPRESSION

The woman with postpartum depression persistently exhibits characteristics such as these:

- Lack of enjoyment in life
- Disinterest in others; loss of normal give-and-take in relationships
- Feelings of inadequacy and inability to cope
- Loss of mental concentration
- Disturbed sleep
- Constant fatigue and feelings of ill health

## Nursing Brief

If a postpartum woman seems depressed, the nurse should not assume that she has the common "baby blues" or that she will "snap out of it."

The woman who has postpartum depression has impaired function because she is listless and withdrawn most of the time. However, she remains in touch with reality. Nevertheless, postpartum depression can seriously disrupt her life and that of her family. It may persist for months before it finally lifts.

No specific cause of postpartum depression is identified. Factors associated with the disorder include

- Complications of pregnancy or birth
- Complications in the newborn
- History of depression, mental illness, or alcoholism in the woman or her family
- Immature personality
- Low self-esteem
- Isolation from sources of support
- Financial worries
- Rapid changes in hormone levels after birth

As in many other complications, one of these factors often leads to another. For example, complications during pregnancy may result in the birth of an infant who is ill.

**Nursing Care.** The nurse is more likely to encounter the woman with postpartum depression in the physician's office or a pediatric clinic. The nurse may help the mother by being a sympathetic listener. Women may be reluctant to express dissatisfaction with their new role, especially if they have waited a long time for a baby.

The nurse should elicit the new mother's feelings about motherhood and her infant. The nurse also observes for complaints of sleeplessness or chronic fatigue. The mother's expressions of feeling are pursued, including feeling like a failure or feeling hopeless, lonely, or isolated.

Isolation can be both a cause and a result of depression. The new mother is helped to identify sources of emotional support among her family and friends. Many of her friends may have stopped including her because she has withdrawn from them. She may not have the emotional energy to reach out to them again.

The woman who is physically depleted often has an exaggerated feeling of let-down and depression. The nurse determines if she is getting enough exercise, sleep, and proper nutrition to improve her physical health and sense of well-being. She is helped to identify ways to meet her own needs and reassured that she is not being selfish.

A new mother may feel guilty because she is not happy all the time. The nurse explains that her feelings are not right or wrong; feelings simply exist. She is referred to support groups if these are available in the area. Discussing her feelings with others who have similar difficulties can help her realize that she is not alone.

## POSTPARTUM PSYCHOSIS

Women having a postpartum psychosis have an impaired sense of reality. Psychosis is much less common than postpartum depression. A woman may have any psychiatric disorder. Those more often encountered are

- *Bipolar disorder:* a disorder characterized by episodes of mania (hyperactivity, excitability, euphoria, and a feeling of being invulnerable) and depression

- *Major depression:* a disorder characterized by deep feelings of worthlessness, guilt, serious sleep and appetite disturbance, and sometimes delusions about the infant's being dead

Postpartum psychosis may be fatal for both mother and infant. The mother may endanger herself and her baby during manic episodes because she uses poor judgment and has a sense of being invulnerable. Suicide and infanticide are possible, especially during depressive episodes.

Care of the woman with postpartum psychosis requires psychiatric professionals and is beyond the scope of maternity nursing. She is usually treated in the same way as other people with similar disorders.

## KEY POINTS

- The nurse must be aware of women who are at higher risk for postpartum hemorrhage and assess them more often.
- A constant small trickle of blood can result in significant blood loss, as can a larger one-time hemorrhage.
- Persistent and more severe pain is characteristic of a hematoma in the reproductive tract.
- It is essential to identify and limit an infection before it spreads to adjacent organs or through the blood stream to a distant site.
- The woman who has a difficult labor or birth is more likely to have postpartum hemorrhage or infection.
- The nurse should teach new mothers about normal postpartum changes and indications of problems they should report.
- Careful listening and observation can help the nurse identify a new mother who is suffering from postpartum depression.
- Postpartum psychoses are serious disorders that are potentially life-threatening to the woman and others, including her infant.

# Study Questions

1. If a woman has excessive bleeding 1 hour after a vaginal birth, what should the nurse do first? What is the most likely reason for the excessive bleeding?

2. How do these postpartum bleeding complications differ from one another?

   - Uterine atony
   - Vaginal or cervical laceration
   - Hematoma

3. How can breast feeding her baby limit a woman's blood loss after birth?

4. A woman complains of continued pain 2 hours after a forceps-assisted vaginal birth, despite having received an analgesic 45 minutes ago. What is the most likely reason for her symptoms? What is the best nursing action?

5. What should the new mother be taught about complications that develop after she goes home, such as late hemorrhage or infection?

6. A woman has a temperature of 38.3°C (101°F) 12 hours after a cesarean birth for failure to progress in labor. What are possible causes of her temperature elevation? What should the nurse do?

7. What are some measures to prevent reproductive and urinary tract infections that can be taught to every postpartum woman?

8. What nursing measures promote comfort and resolution of the infection when the woman has mastitis? Explain the rationale for each.

9. A woman returns to her nurse-midwife for a checkup 2 weeks after an uncomplicated vaginal birth. The CNM notes that her uterus is about 2 cm above the symphysis and that the lochia is dark brown-red. Are these assessments normal? If not, what is the most likely complication?

10. How does postpartum depression or psychosis differ from the common "baby blues"?

# Multiple Choice Review Questions

*Choose the most appropriate answer.*

1. The earliest finding in hypovolemic shock is usually
   a. low blood pressure
   b. fast pulse
   c. pale skin color
   d. soft uterus

2. A woman has her fifth baby, a 9-pound (4082-gm) infant. What complication should the nurse particularly observe her for?
   a. subinvolution of the uterus
   b. mastitis
   c. endometritis
   d. uterine atony

3. The proper hand position for doing uterine massage is
   a. both hands at the top of the uterus
   b. one hand on the fundus and one just above the symphysis
   c. one hand in the vagina and the other on the abdomen
   d. both hands on the symphysis

4. A bleeding laceration typically exhibits
   a. a soft uterus that is difficult to locate
   b. low pulse and blood pressure
   c. bright red bleeding and a firm uterus
   d. profuse dark red bleeding and large clots

5. The white blood cell (leukocyte) count is normally_____during the postpartum period.
   a. higher
   b. lower
   c. unchanged

6. The best position for a woman who has endometritis is
   a. lying on her left side
   b. in a slightly head-down position
   c. with the head of the bed elevated
   d. with a pillow to elevate her hips

7. Select the food that is highest in iron.
   a. orange
   b. enriched oatmeal
   c. cranberry juice
   d. cheese

8. How does high fluid intake help resolve urinary tract infection?
   a. reduces fever
   b. decreases bladder muscle tone
   c. increases urine acidity
   d. removes microorganisms

9. If a woman has mastitis, the nurse should expect to
   a. explain methods to empty the milk from the breast
   b. teach exercises to increase blood flow to the area

c. help her wean her infant from the breast immediately

d. avoid clothes or support garments for the breasts

10. A woman is having her checkup with her nurse-midwife 6 weeks after birth. She seems disinterested in others, including her baby. She tells the nurse she does not think she is a very good mother. The nurse should

a. reassure her that almost all new mothers feel let down after birth

b. ask her how her partner feels about the new baby

c. explore her feelings with sensitive questioning

d. refer her to a psychiatrist

## BIBLIOGRAPHY

Cunningham, F.G., MacDonald, P.C., & Gant, N.F. (1989). *Williams Obstetrics* (18th ed.). Norwalk, CT: Appleton & Lange.

Gibbs, R.S., & Sweet, R.L. (1989). Maternal and fetal infections: Clinical disorders. In R.K. Creasy & R. Resnik (Eds.), *Maternal-fetal medicine: Principles and practice* (2nd ed., pp. 656–725). Philadelphia: W.B. Saunders.

Hayashi, R.H. (1992). Postpartum hemorrhage and puerperal sepsis. In N.F. Hacker & J.G. Moore (Eds.), *Essentials of obstetrics & gynecology* (2nd ed., pp. 289–298). Philadelphia: W.B. Saunders.

Hayashi, R.H., & Castillo, M.S. (1993). Bleeding in pregnancy. In R.A. Knuppel & J.E. Drukker (Eds.), *High-risk pregnancy: A team approach* (pp. 539–560). Philadelphia: W.B. Saunders.

Hibbard, L. (1990). Postpartum pelvic hematomas. In E.J. Quilligan & F.P. Zuspan (Eds.), *Current therapy in obstetrics and gynecology 3* (pp. 232–233). Philadelphia: W.B. Saunders.

Higgins, P. (1993). Postpartum complications. In S. Mattson & J.E. Smith (Eds.), *Core curriculum for maternal-newborn nursing* (pp. 639–656). Philadelphia: W.B. Saunders.

Martell, L.K. (1990). Postpartum depression as a family problem. *MCN: Journal of Maternal-Child Nursing, 15,* 90–93.

McCormac, M. (1990). Managing hemorrhagic shock. *American Journal of Nursing, 90,* 22–29.

Quilligan, E.J. (1990). Postpartum hemorrhage. In E.J. Quilligan & F.P. Zuspan (Eds.), *Current therapy in obstetrics and gynecology 3* (pp. 233–235). Philadelphia: W.B. Saunders.

Ross, M.G., & Hobel, C.J. (1993). Normal labor, delivery, & the puerperium. In N.F. Hacker & J.G. Moore (Eds.), *Essentials of obstetrics and gynecology* (2nd ed., pp. 119–133). Philadelphia: W.B. Saunders.

Stuart, G.W., & Sundeen, S.J. (1991). *Principles & practice of psychiatric nursing.* St. Louis: Mosby.

Varcarolis, E.M. (1994). *Foundations of psychiatric mental health nursing.* Philadelphia: W.B. Saunders.

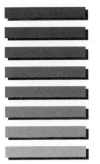

# Chapter 11

# The Nurse's Role in Reproductive Health

## VOCABULARY

basal body temperature (279)
climacteric (287)
coitus interruptus (280)
dyspareunia (288)
implant (272)
osteoporosis (288)
perimenopause (287)
spermicide (276)
sterilization (280)
symptothermal (277)

Family Planning (Contraception)
   Abstinence
   Oral Contraceptives (the Pill)
   Norplant
   Morning-After Pill
   Contraceptive Injection (Depo-Provera)
   Intrauterine Device
   Diaphragm and Cervical Cap
   Contraceptive Sponge
   Spermicides
   Male Condom
   Female Condom
   Natural Family Planning and Fertility Awareness
   Coitus Interruptus
   Voluntary Sterilization
Toxic Shock Syndrome
Fertility Counseling
   Cultural Considerations
   Male-Related Factors and Tests
   Female-Related Factors and Tests
   Medical and Psychological Considerations
Menopause
   Cultural Variations
   Symptoms
   Cardiovascular Changes
   Bone Density Changes (Osteoporosis)
   Hormone Replacement Therapy

## OBJECTIVES

*On completion and mastery of Chapter 11, the student will be able to*

- Define each vocabulary term listed.
- Describe the various methods of birth control.
- List the side effects and contraindications of each method.
- Discuss contraceptives suitable for the postpartum woman.
- List three methods of natural family planning.
- Describe four vasomotor symptoms seen in the perimenopausal period.
- Discuss the nurse's role in contraceptive education.
- List two tests performed to determine a woman's fertility.

# Family Planning (Contraception)

Family planning (birth control) is an individual matter. It is personal and difficult for couples to discuss with health professionals. The physician, nurse practitioner, or nurse-midwife is often the person who provides information about contraceptive methods. The environment should be private and the client assured of confidentiality.

Information about family planning is widely available in nonprofessional periodicals and the news media. Sometimes this information is misleading or erroneous. Nurses must be familiar with the various types of birth control and their effectiveness in order to dispel myths and impart accurate information to the public.

Many factors influence the choice of a contraceptive. Some of these are age, health status, religion, culture, personality, career ambitions, and even the national economy. Other key considerations include the method's effectiveness, frequency of intercourse, convenience, expense, degree of spontaneity desired, and degree of comfort the partners have with touching their bodies.

The number of sex partners and whether the individual has a history of sexually transmitted disease is also important, particularly because of the acquired immunodeficiency syndrome (AIDS) epidemic. Some methods involve the partner more than do others (e.g., male condoms versus diaphragms). This may be a consideration for the individual. A couple's choice of contraception may change according to its practicality. For example, a woman who has been on the pill and does not want any more children may decide on sterilization. A person who was once married and is currently dating also might change her method of contraception. Figure 11–1 is a graph showing the percentage of women accidentally becoming pregnant in their 1st year of continuously using various contraceptives. The following is a description of the various methods of birth control that the client needs to understand in order to make an informed choice.

## ABSTINENCE

Abstinence means not having vaginal intercourse. The woman cannot become pregnant if sperm do not enter the vagina. It is 100% effective in preventing pregnancy and sexually transmitted diseases (STDs). Many religious groups support abstinence among unmarried people.

## ORAL CONTRACEPTIVES (THE PILL)

The pill is one of the most popular, effective, and reversible methods of birth control available to women in this country. It is obtained by prescription. Oral contraceptives contain combined hormones (estrogen and progesterone) or progesterone alone (minipill). Combination pills prevent ovulation. Minipills, not used as commonly today, can also prevent ovulation, but they usually work by thickening the cervical mucus. This prevents the sperm from joining with the egg. Minipills may also prevent the ovum from implantation in the womb. Minipills are useful for the woman who cannot take estrogen. There is evidence that the use of the pill decreases the risk of ovarian and endometrial cancer and causes no greater risk for breast cancer.

To obtain oral contraceptives, the woman must first visit a private doctor or family planning clinic, where a complete history is taken. She also must have a thorough physical examination. A pelvic examination and Papanicolaou (Pap) smear are performed. The woman must have this examination at least once a year in order to renew her prescription. The clinician may initially recommend a follow-up visit in 3 months.

The pills are taken as directed and are shown in Figure 11–2. In contrast to past practice,

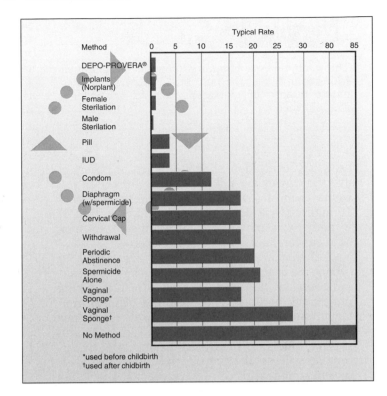

**Figure 11-1.** Percentage of women experiencing an accidental pregnancy in the first year of continuous use of various contraceptives. (Adapted by UpJohn Co. from Trussell et al. [1990]. *Obstetrics and Gynecology, 76,* 558.)

women taking the pill no longer need periodic breaks from it. The pill is also being used more by older women and may even be prescribed into the perimenopausal years. This requires *reeducation* of women who may have preconceptions about how the pill needs to be taken. Because the pill does not protect the woman from sexually transmitted disease, it should be used with the condom.

**Side Effects and Contraindications.** Unpleasant side effects, such as nausea, vomiting, weight gain, spotting between periods, depression, and breast tenderness, may occur in some females. These effects generally disappear within a few months and are less frequently seen when low-dose estrogen is used. Women taking oral contraceptives tend to have more regular and comfortable periods and lighter menstrual flow. Oral contraceptives are thought to decrease the incidence of iron-deficiency anemia, ectopic (tubal) pregnancy, and pelvic inflammatory disease.

Certain risk factors contraindicate oral contraceptives. Women who have a history of thromboembolic disorders (blood clots), cere-

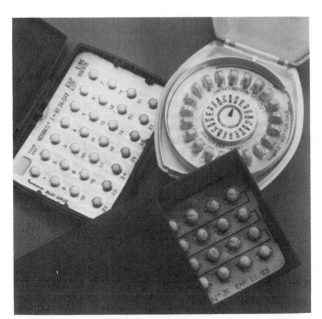

**Figure 11-2.** Birth control pills. (Courtesy of Planned Parenthood Federation of America, Inc., New York, NY.)

## Nursing Brief

Smoking greatly increases the chance of experiencing pill-related complications.

# Nursing Brief

The woman who is planning to become pregnant refrains from taking the pill. She should use an alternative method of contraception until ovulation is reestablished.

brovascular accident, heart disease, or breast or uterine cancer are not candidates for the pill. A woman who is over 35 and smokes more than 15 cigarettes a day should not take the pill. A woman with malignant melanoma, a form of skin cancer, is also not a candidate.

Oral contraceptives are rarely prescribed for breast-feeding mothers because they decrease milk supply. They are contraindicated during pregnancy because of the danger of fetal malformations. Women with medical conditions such as diabetes, liver disease, undiagnosed vaginal bleeding, sickle cell disease, and hypertension will require further individualized evaluation and testing to determine whether they should be placed on the pill. *Patients are taught always to inform the physician or practitioner of any preexisting health condition.* More detailed information about the risks of oral contraceptives is included in package inserts. Figure 11–3 illustrates complications for which the woman taking oral contraceptives should contact her health-care provider.

Certain medications should not be taken with oral contraceptives. These include anti-epileptics, some antibiotics, and certain drugs used in treatment for tuberculosis. The woman needs to make a list of medications that she is taking and inform health-care personnel about them. She also reports to her health-care provider any change in medication or physical health.

## NORPLANT

Norplant is a newer, reversible method of birth control. Six matchstick-sized progestin-releasing capsules are surgically implanted under the skin of the underside of the upper arm, midway between the elbow and armpit (Fig. 11–4). A local anesthetic is used to numb the area. Levonorgestrel, the synthetic progestin, is released slowly and in small amounts. It prevents ovulation and lasts for 5 years. The effectiveness is considered to be close to 100%. Its advantages are that it does

not need to be taken daily and it does not need to be insert-ed before intercourse. It can be removed at any time but is generally replaced after 5 years.

**Side Effects and Contraindications.** Contraindications to Norplant include acute liver disease, jaundice, unexplained vaginal bleeding, thromboembolic disorders, pregnancy, and known or suspected breast cancer (King, 1992). Again, the woman is advised to inform the health-care provider of *any* preexisting health condition. It is still inconclusive whether

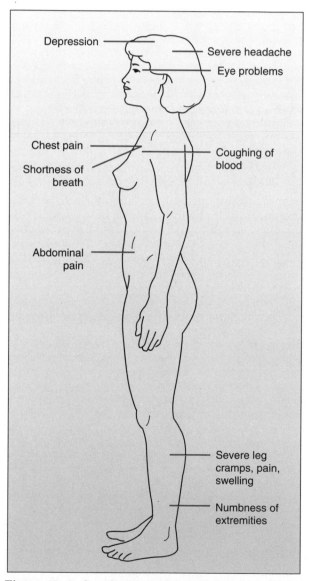

**Figure 11–3.** Complications of the pill for which the female should contact her health-care provider.

women using Norplant are at a slightly increased risk for heart attack or stroke and how smoking interacts with Norplant. Currently, women using Norplant are advised to stop smoking.

A common side effect of Norplant is menstrual irregularity. Symptoms of complications include heavy vaginal bleeding, arm pain, abdominal pain, amenorrhea, pain, pus, or bleeding at implant site, or implant disruption. The cost, including medical examination, implants, and insertion, is between $500 and $600. This amounts to about $100 a year over 5 years (Planned Parenthood, 1992).

## MORNING-AFTER PILL

The morning-after pill is used to prevent pregnancy in cases of unprotected intercourse. More specifically, it is administered to women who have been raped. It contains a high level of estrogen, which prohibits implantation of the egg. This pill is not used routinely in the United States and is prescribed with caution because it can cause malformations of the fetus if the pregnancy is not terminated.

## CONTRACEPTIVE INJECTION (DEPO-PROVERA)

Depo-Provera is a reversible, injectable form of contraception. The injection is given intramuscularly in the buttock or upper arm once every 12 weeks. The first injection is given within the first 5 days after the beginning of menses, within 5 days after childbirth for non–breast-feeding women, or within 6 weeks after childbirth for breast-feeding women. It contains medroxyprogesterone acetate, a synthetic form of progesterone. It does not contain estrogen. It does not prevent lactation.

Depo-Provera acts by preventing ovulation. It also changes the lining of the uterus, making it less likely that a pregnancy will occur. It is con-

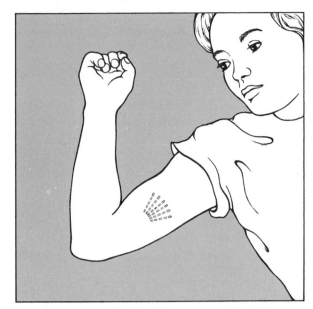

**Figure 11–4.** The Norplant contraceptive system.

sidered to be 99% effective (UpJohn Company, 1993). This is a prescription medication, and the woman must see her health-care provider for a physical examination before using it.

**Side Effects and Contraindications.** Side effects of Depo-Provera include weight gain, *irregular menses*, amenorrhea, headache, nervousness, stomach pain or cramps, dizziness, fatigue, and decreased sex drive. These effects generally diminish over time. A decrease in bone mineral stored in the body may increase the risk of bone fractures. These changes are greatest when the woman begins taking the medication. Because certain blood tests are altered by the hormones, the woman must inform her physician before the tests are administered. Some anticancer drugs may significantly decrease the effectiveness of Depo-Provera (UpJohn Company, 1993).

Depo-Provera is contraindicated during pregnancy and in women who have breast cancer, stroke, thromboembolic disease, liver disease, or allergies to Depo-Provera. It is also contraindicated in women who have vaginal bleeding from unknown causes.

The woman should tell her health-care provider about any preexisting condition, such as family history of breast cancer, abnormal mammograms, fibrocystic disease, breast nodules, bleeding from the nipples, kidney disease, irregular or scanty menstrual periods, high

## Nursing Brief

Because more young teenagers are becoming pregnant each year, they must be educated about contraception, reproductive health, and the dangers of unprotected sex.

blood pressure, migraine headaches, asthma, epilepsy, diabetes, or history of depression.

## INTRAUTERINE DEVICE

Intrauterine devices (IUDs) are a reversible prescription method of birth control. Two types are currently approved for use in the United States: ParaGard (380A) and Proges-tasert (Fig. 11–5A). ParaGard is a small T-shaped plastic device containing copper. It can be left in place for 6–8 years. Progestasert is also T-shaped and contains progesterone in the stem. The progesterone in this type of device must be replenished yearly. Neither method changes the hormone levels in the body.

IUDs work because the presence of a foreign body apparently prevents implantation of the egg, although the exact mechanism is still unclear. In the time of early Christianity, the nomads used a similar practice, placing a stone in the womb of each female camel. This kept the camels from getting pregnant on long journeys.

One of the most serious complications of the IUD is pelvic inflammatory disease. This can cause scarring of the fallopian tubes and result in infertility. For this reason it is not recommended for persons with multiple sex partners, whose risk of contracting an STD is high (King, 1992).

**Insertion of Intrauterine Device.** The woman must first see her health-care provider for a physical and pelvic examination. A test for STDs and a Pap smear are also performed. The IUD is inserted by a physician or nurse practitioner during menstruation, when the cervical canal os is slightly dilated. It may also be implanted during the 4–6-week postpartum checkup. More recently it has been inserted immediately after the placenta is delivered (Olds, London, & Ladewig, 1992). A consent form must be read and signed to ensure the woman's understanding of the process and possible complications.

The IUD is inserted with the T portion collapsed. A string protrudes through the cervix into the vagina (Fig. 11–5B). The woman is instructed to feel for the string periodically, especially following her period. Some women may expel the IUD within the first 24 hours. Replacement depends on the clinical judgment of the health-care provider and the woman's willingness. Antibiotics may be given to reduce the chance of infection. Cramping and pain are generally experienced initially. There may be spotting for 2 or 3 weeks.

**Side Effects and Contraindications.** The woman is instructed to report to her physician the following signs of complications: inability to feel the string; missed, late, or light periods; severe cramping or an increase in pain in the lower abdomen; pain or bleeding during intercourse; fever and chills; or foul-smelling vaginal discharge. Contraindications include history of pelvic infection, ectopic pregnancy, uterine anomaly, and cancer of the uterus. IUDs are not recommended for women with no previous pregnancies.

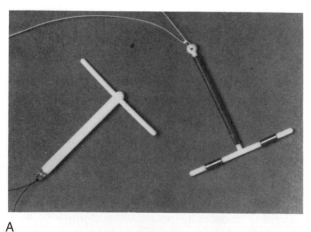

A

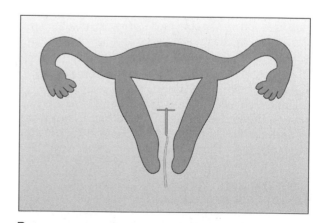

B

**Figure 11–5.** *A and B,* The intrauterine device. (*A,* Courtesy of Planned Parenthood Federation of America, Inc., New York, NY.)

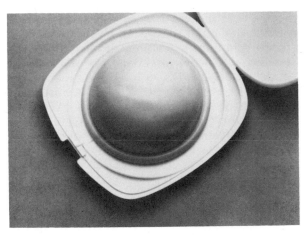

**Figure 11–6.** The diaphragm. (Courtesy of Planned Parenthood Federation of America, Inc., New York, NY.)

## DIAPHRAGM AND CERVICAL CAP

Diaphragms and cervical caps are reversible barrier methods of birth control (Figs. 11–6 and 11–7). They are called barriers because they block semen from entering the woman's cervix. This prevents sperm from entering the uterus and fallopian tubes. These flexible rubber devices fit securely over the cervix. They are used in conjunction with spermicidal creams or jellies, which kill sperm that might pass the mechanical barrier. Jelly also provides some protection against STDs.

The diaphragm and cervical cap are prescribed and initially fitted by a health-care worker. They cost about $13 to $15 plus the cost of the spermicidal jelly. The diaphragm may be inserted up to 6 hours before intercourse and can be left in place for 24 hours. The cervical cap may be left in place for up to 48 hours. These devices must be in place each time the woman has intercourse and need to be left in place for at least 6 hours afterward. If sex is repeated within 6 hours, the diaphragm does not have to be removed, but more cream or jelly must be inserted into the vagina. Using additional spermicide with the cap is optional (Planned Parenthood, 1992).

Before each instance of intercourse, the woman needs to check that the device covers the cervix. The diaphragm or cervical cap needs to be observed routinely for weak spots or pinholes. This can be accomplished by holding the device up to the light. Women should not

## Nursing Brief

The nurse advises the woman that she needs to have her diaphragm refitted if she loses 10–20 pounds or more, after a full-term pregnancy, after a miscarriage of a fetus older than 3 months, and after pelvic surgery.

douche with these barriers in place. The cap is considered somewhat more difficult to insert and remove. Women who are uncomfortable touching their bodies may prefer other forms of contraception. When used as directed, they are considered safe, effective methods of birth control. They are particularly valuable for mothers who are nursing their babies and for women who cannot take the pill or use the IUD.

**Side Effects and Contraindications.** Women who have an allergy to rubber or spermicides are not good candidates for the diaphragm or cervical cap. These devices are not recommended for women who have a history of toxic shock syndrome (see p. 284), because the diaphragm or cap must remain in the body for a period of time. Certain anomalies of the uterus preclude their use. Some women tend to de-

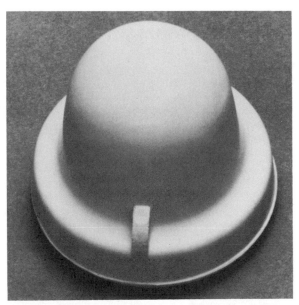

**Figure 11–7.** The cervical cap. (Courtesy of Planned Parenthood Federation of America, Inc., New York, NY.)

velop bladder infections because pressure from the device on the urethra may interfere with complete emptying of the bladder. They are not worn during menstruation or in cases of vaginal bleeding. A woman should contact her health-care provider if she notices discomfort, difficulty in keeping the device in place, vaginal irritation, or a foul odor or discharge.

## CONTRACEPTIVE SPONGE

The contraceptive sponge is soft, round, and about 2 inches in diameter (Fig. 11–8). Each sponge has a nylon loop attached to it for easy removal. It fits snugly over the cervix and acts as a barrier. It prevents pregnancy by releasing the spermicide nonoxynol-9. It is moistened with water and inserted into the vagina before intercourse. One size fits all. The contraceptive sponge may be worn for up to 24 hours after insertion. It must remain in place for at least 6 hours after intercourse. The sponge is an over-the-counter product. Manufacturer's directions should be carefully followed. The spermicides in the sponge offer some protection against certain STDs, including AIDS.

**Side Effects and Contraindications.** The sponge has few side effects or complications. Women who have uterine anomalies, those who are allergic to polyurethane or irritated by sper-

micides, and those with a history of toxic shock syndrome should refrain from its use. Some women complain of vaginal dryness with continued use. It is not intended to be worn during menstruation or if a woman is experiencing vaginal bleeding from other causes. It is not used after childbirth, miscarriage, or abortion until a health-care provider approves its use. Effectiveness rates are seen in Figure 11–1.

## SPERMICIDES

Spermicidal foam, cream, jelly, and suppository capsules are nonprescription over-the-counter contraceptives. An applicator is supplied by the manufacturer. They are inserted into the vagina at least 10 minutes (some suggest 1 hour) before intercourse. They neutralize vaginal secretions, destroy sperm, and block entrance to the uterus. Detailed instructions accompany the product. They need to be read and closely followed. Women should not douche for 8 hours following intercourse. A spermicide is more effective when used with a condom.

**Side Effects and Contraindications.** Spermicides have a low rate of toxicity and are popular because they are readily available. They can irritate the vagina and therefore should not be used by women with inflammation of the cervix. Spermicides can also irritate the penis. Couples may need to try several brands before they find one that is best for them. Some women complain that spermicides are messy and leak. Many adolescents use this type of contraceptive because it is inexpensive and easy to obtain. They must be cautioned that these methods are not as effective in preventing pregnancy as other methods (see Fig. 11–1). Teenagers must also understand that products labeled "for personal hygiene use" are not intended as methods of birth control but are for cleansing purposes (Pillitteri, 1992).

## MALE CONDOM

Male condoms are sheaths of thin rubber or animal tissue (skin condoms) worn on the penis during intercourse (Fig. 11–9). Condoms collect semen before, during, and after ejaculation. They come in various styles, such as ribbed, lubricated, and colored, and they come with or without spermicide. Plain condoms cost as little as 25 or 30 cents. They are nonprescription items and are widely available from vending

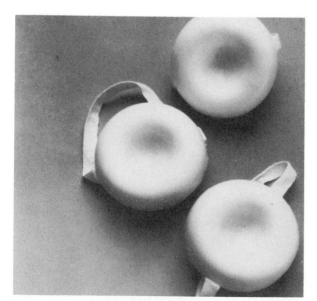

**Figure 11–8.** The contraceptive sponge. (Courtesy of Planned Parenthood Federation of America, Inc., New York, NY.)

machines, drugstores, and family planning clinics. They provide very good protection, although not complete protection, from STDs, including human immunodeficiency virus (HIV).

**Side Effects and Contraindications.** Side effects and contraindications are rare. Some men are allergic to latex. Water-soluble lubricants such as K-Y jelly are advocated if the condom or vagina is dry. These do not damage the latex or cause breakage. The penis is withdrawn immediately if the man feels that the condom is breaking or becoming dislodged. The condom is removed and replaced (a spare should be carried).

Condoms are not reused, because even a pinhole can lead to pregnancy or permit the entry of viruses, including HIV. The condom is applied before *any* contact with the opening of the vagina, including foreplay. Animal skin condoms do not shield the person from STDs as the latex types do. Condoms with the spermicide nonoxynol-9 are advocated in addition to other methods of birth control, unless both partners are certain that they have no STDs, including HIV, and both have no other sex partners. Box 11–1 explains how to apply a condom.

## FEMALE CONDOM

Female condoms are new on the market. They are essentially used for the same purpose as male condoms, to prevent pregnancy and to protect the woman from HIV and other STDs. Marketed in the United States under the name Reality, the condom consists of two rings, one that fits into the vagina and one that remains outside.

Female condoms are connected by a loose-fitting sheath. Because the outer rim protects the labia and the base of the penis, it more effectively shields the reproductive organs than does the male condom, thus it may offer more protection (Fig. 11–10). It comes prelubricated, does not have to be fitted by a health-care professional, and does not need to be placed precisely over the cervix (Anastasi, 1993).

The method of inserting the female condom is much like that for a diaphragm. The condom can be inserted up to 8 hours before intercourse, although most women insert it shortly before coitus. It is meant for one-time use. It is stronger than male latex condoms and less likely to break or tear. In contrast to the male condom, it allows vaginal penetration before a complete erection. Following intercourse, the

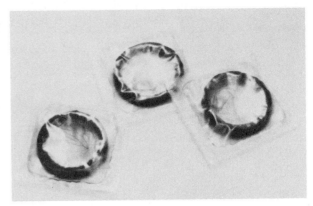

**Figure 11–9.** The male condom. (Courtesy of Planned Parenthood Federation of America, Inc., New York, NY.)

outer ring is squeezed and sealed to keep sperm inside (see package directions). It is removed and discarded. The nurse may find that initially, clients find it unattractive. The nurse emphasizes its usefulness in giving the woman control and in preventing the spread of HIV.

**Side Effects and Contraindications.** No significant allergic reactions to the female condom have been reported. The rate of breaks and tears is less than 1% (Anastasi, 1993). Women who are allergic to latex can use it. It costs about $2.50.

## NATURAL FAMILY PLANNING AND FERTILITY AWARENESS

Natural family planning includes menstrual cycle charting and abstinence during days of fertility. The woman is taught how to predict ovulation and to be aware of her fertile periods. She needs to be aware that the ovum may be fertilized 18–24 hours after ovulation and that sperm are viable for 48–72 hours. There are several ways for a woman to predict when she is fertile. These include taking and recording basal body temperature, observing cervical mucus, and using the calendar, or rhythm, method. It is best to combine basal body temperature, cervical mucus, and calendar methods; this is called the *symptothermal* method. In addition, the woman observes for bloating, breast changes, and other symptoms. The term *fertility awareness methods* refers to the woman who determines her fertility period and uses a barrier contraceptive during "unsafe" days.

| BOX 11–1 | How to Use a Male Condom Safely |
| --- | --- |

1. Squeeze the air from the tip. Leave a half inch of space at the tip to allow sperm to collect and to prevent breakage.

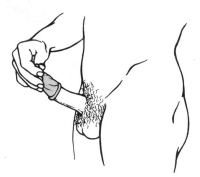

2. Hold the tip while you unroll the condom completely

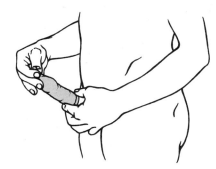

3. Do not use petroleum jelly, grease, or oil because they can cause the condom to burst. Instead, use K-Y jelly or some other water-based lubricant.

4. To remove the condom, hold onto it at the base of the penis, and withdraw it while the penis is still hard.

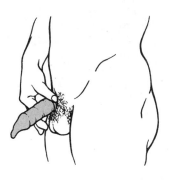

5. Remove the condom. Be sure that no semen spills from it.

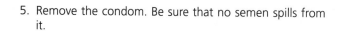

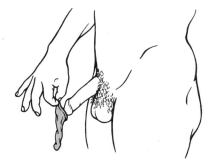

6. Place the condom in the trash or in some safe disposal. Use a new condom each time. Check the expiration date on packages, as condoms may deteriorate over time.

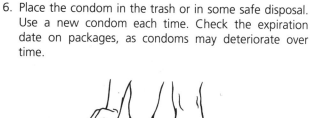

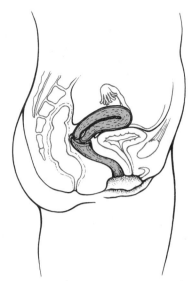

**Figure 11–10.** The female condom can protect the woman from sexually transmitted disease and offer her a sense of control over her own body.

**Basal Body Temperature.** The woman is instructed to take her temperature with a basal thermometer every morning before arising and record it on a graph (Fig. 11–11). This is her basal body temperature (BBT). A basal thermometer calibrated in tenths of a degree is used. It may be purchased in a drugstore. Shortly after ovulation her temperature will increase between 0.4°F and 0.8°F. This increase is due to the influence of progesterone. The temperature remains at this level until menstrua-

tion. The woman maintains abstinence from this point until 3 full days later (the life of ova and sperm). Because the temperature does not rise until after ovulation occurs, some couples prefer to abstain for a few days before the rise as well.

**Cervical Mucus.** This method is also referred to as the Billings, ferning, or ovulation method. The amount and character of cervical mucus change during the menstrual cycle. This change is the result of estrogen and progesterone influences on the mucus-secreting glands of the cervix.

The woman must observe for changes in mucus all through the first part of her menstrual cycle. At first the mucus is cloudy and tacky. However, within a few days of ovulation, it becomes slippery and clear. It will stretch between the fingers. This stretching is referred to as *spinnbarkeit* (Fig. 11–12). It is greatest at the time of ovulation. Spinnbarkeit enhances the mobility of the sperm.

*Ferning* refers to the fernlike pattern of cervical mucus seen during fertile days. It is due to increased estrogen levels around the time of ovulation that decrease near menstruation. The woman must abstain from vaginal intercourse immediately before ovulation, during ovulation, and for 3 days afterward to avoid conception. She must refrain from douching until the fertile period is over because she may not be able to observe the mucus. Assessing the character of secretions following intercourse is unreliable, because the woman may not be able to differentiate seminal fluid from ovulatory mucus.

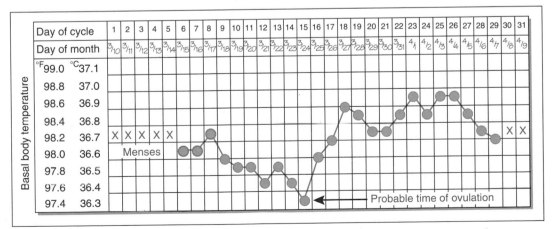

**Figure 11–11.** Basal body temperature chart. By taking and recording her temperature, the woman can determine the probable time of ovulation.

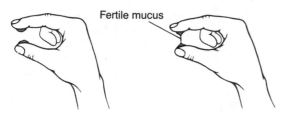

Fertile mucus

**Figure 11–12.** Spinnbarkeit. The woman tests the ability of her cervical mucus to stretch. This helps determine the time of ovulation.

**Calendar, or Rhythm, Method.** The woman charts her menstrual cycles on a calendar for several months. If they are regular, she may be able to predict ovulation. The rhythm method is based on the assumption that ovulation generally takes place approximately halfway through the 28-day menstrual cycle, counting from the 1st day. Intercourse is avoided from 4 days before ovulation to 3 days afterward. In a 28-day cycle, the couple would abstain from day 10 through day 17.

**Side Effects and Contraindications.** There are no medical or hormonal side effects of these methods. They are accepted by most religious groups, and they are inexpensive. Women who are in good health, who are monogamous, and who have the cooperation of their partners have the most success with these natural methods. Vaginal infections or personal hygiene products may alter cervical mucus. Illness may alter temperature readings. Some women have irregular periods that make calculations difficult. Careful instructions are required. These are available from family health, family planning, and church-affiliated programs.

## COITUS INTERRUPTUS

Coitus interruptus, or penis withdrawal before ejaculation, is one of the oldest and least reliable methods of birth control. It is least reliable because it demands great self-control on the part of the male and because preejaculatory secretions often contain sperm. When explaining this to clients the term "come" may be bet-

## Nursing Brief

A woman can become pregnant while breast feeding.

ter understood (e.g., explain that it means withdrawing the penis before the man "comes"). Douching after intercourse is not a form of birth control and may actually transport sperm farther into the birth canal.

## VOLUNTARY STERILIZATION

Voluntary sterilization is a permanent method of birth control. It can be accomplished surgically in either a man or a woman. Although at times the procedure may be reversed, this is expensive and not always successful. Therefore, clients should carefully think about this decision. It is not recommended for adolescents because the desire for children may change as one matures. Instead, the young person is directed to less permanent methods of contraception.

Persons who may use sterilization are those who have all the children they desire, those who have a hereditary disease, women whose health would be in jeopardy, and those who are sure they have no desire for children (Planned Parenthood, 1992).

**Male Sterilization.** Male sterilization, termed *vasectomy*, is performed by making a cut in each side of the scrotum. The vas deferens, the

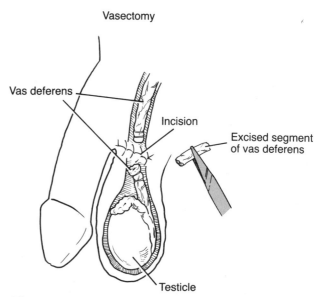

Vasectomy

Vas deferens

Incision

Excised segment of vas deferens

Testicle

**Figure 11–13.** Vasectomy. (From Black, J.M., & Matassarin-Jacobs, E. [1993]. *Luckmann and Sorensen's medical-surgical nursing: A psychophysiologic approach* [4th ed.]. Philadelphia: W.B. Saunders.)

tubes through which the sperm travel, are blocked (Fig. 11–13). This is generally accomplished by ligation; however, the use of a silicone plug is under investigation. This would make the procedure more reversible.

Men need information about the anatomy and physiology of their sex organs. They need reassurance that they will still have erections and ejaculations and that intercourse will remain pleasurable. They also need emotional support because this procedure is usually very anxiety-producing.

The surgery takes about 20 minutes and is performed on an outpatient basis under local anesthesia. There is some pain, bruising, and swelling after the surgery. Occasional infection can result. Rest, a mild analgesic, and the application of an ice pack provide an increase in comfort. Because some sperm remain in the system following surgery, pregnancy can occur. Other methods of birth control are recommended until laboratory tests show that there are no more sperm. Intercourse can generally be resumed in about 1 week.

**Female Sterilization.** Female sterilization, called *tubal ligation*, involves blocking or ligating the fallopian tubes. It can be accomplished by using electrocautery or clips. The most common operation, called a *laparoscopy*, is usually performed in same-day surgery under local or general anesthesia (Fig. 11–14). The *minilaparotomy* is similar to a laparotomy but uses a suprapubic incision. It is sometimes used following childbirth or abortion.

The laparoscopy is done on an inpatient or outpatient basis. It is nicknamed "Band Aid" surgery by the general public. A small incision is made near the navel. Carbon dioxide gas is infused, by means of a needle, into the abdominal cavity. The gas pushes the intestine away from the uterus and fallopian tubes. A lighted *laparoscope* allows the surgeon to see within. An electric current is passed through the instrument to coagulate and seal the tube.

There is a certain amount of discomfort following laparoscopy. Some women experience nausea from the anesthesia. Abdominal pain and bloating from the gas are also reported. Even though this is not considered major surgery, the woman must plan a minimum of 1 or 2 days to recuperate. Potential complications, although unusual, include coagulation

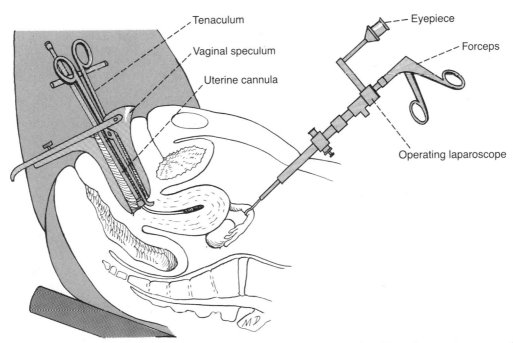

**Figure 11–14.** Laparoscopy. (From Black, J.M., & Matassarin-Jacobs, E. [1993] *Luckmann and Sorensen's medical-surgical nursing: A psychophysiologic approach* [4th ed.]. Philadelphia: W.B. Saunders.)

**Table 11–1.** METHODS OF CONTRACEPTION

| Method | Failure Rate: Accidental Pregnancy Rate (Typical Use: First Year) (%) | Postpartum Use | Risks and Disadvantages | Benefits |
|---|---|---|---|---|
| Abstinence | 0 | Is the method of choice for first 4–6 wk, especially for operative deliveries, complications, and lacerations | May be unacceptable to woman or partner; may cause relationship problems when there is disagreement | Promotes healing and involution |
| Oral contraceptives (two types) 1. Regular pill: combined estrogen plus progestin 2. Minipill: progestin only | 3 | May interfere with lactation by decreasing milk supply; if lactating, use minipill or wait until lactation is well established | Minor side effects are breast tenderness, nausea, irregular bleeding (especially with minipill); major risks are rare in women age 36 and younger who do not smoke; blood clots, liver tumor, cerebrovascular accident, myocardial infarction, gallbladder disease; requires regular monitoring by health-care provider | May be acceptable for healthy women aged 36–50 yr who do not smoke; menses are lighter and shorter, and there are fewer cramps; may protect against breast, ovarian, and uterine disease |
| Norplant | 0.04 | No studies are available of use during first 6 wk; lactating concerns same as those for the birth control pill | Requires insertion and removal of implants in arm by trained health-care provider; change in bleeding pattern common; risks similar to minipill; expensive | Contains progestin only; circulating hormone level less than that with minipill; lasts 5 yr; little monitoring required after insertion |
| Depo-Provera | 0.04 | Not recommended first 6 wk; does not prevent lactation; can be passed to infant via breast milk; no known harmful effects on newborn | Must be given by health-care provider; irregular menses common; risks similar to those of minipill | Injected intramuscularly every 12 wk; lasts for 3 mo |
| Intrauterine device (IUD) | 3 | Is not recommended during postpartum period | Must be inserted by a health-care provider during menses; has an increased risk of pelvic infection; may increase menstrual flow and cramps | Once in place, requires little monitoring by woman; for suitable candidate, may be inserted during first menses after childbirth |
| Diaphragm with spermicide | 18 | Is not recommended; decreased levels of estrogen make the vagina thinner and drier than normal and insertion difficult; must be refitted after a pregnancy; proper fitting is not possible until involution is complete | Causes irritation, allergic reactions, bladder irritation, must be inserted before intercourse and left in place for 6 hr; some positions may dislodge | Not appropriate during the early postpartum period |

| | | | | |
|---|---|---|---|---|
| Cervical cap with spermicide | 18 | Same as diaphragm | Are same as for diaphragm, except may leave in place longer; may increase risk of cervical neoplasia; few health-care providers fit caps | Not recommended during the postpartum period |
| Sponge | 28 | May cause irritation related to decreased levels of estrogen; may increase risk of pelvic infection | Is difficult to remove; causes irritation and allergic reactions; linked to toxic shock syndrome | Is available over the counter; may be left in place longer than diaphragm; is disposable |
| Spermicide alone | 21 | May cause irritation because of decreased levels of estrogen | May cause allergic reactions; is messy; insert just before intercourse | Available over the counter, affords some protection against sexually transmitted diseases |
| Foams with condoms, used together | 3 | Has no contraindications | Irritation and allergic reactions are rare; must be inserted/put on just before intercourse; is messy; may decrease sensation | As effective as the pill when used together; foam is lubricant; available over the counter; protect against sexually transmitted diseases |
| Condoms alone | 12 | Have no contraindications | Irritation and allergic reactions are rare; may break or leak; may decrease sensation; must use correctly | Available over the counter; affords protection against sexually transmitted diseases |
| Natural family planning, fertility awareness, periodic abstinence | 20 | Are not recommended; requires signs and symptoms of hormone fluctuation during normal cycling; this cycling does not occur during the postpartum period, especially during lactation | No risks; require practice and education from trained professional; require self-monitoring and record keeping as well as varying periods of abstinence | Require no devices or chemicals; may be acceptable for couples who do not wish to use other methods because of religious or other reasons |
| Withdrawal | 18 | Has no contraindications | Requires interruption of sexual response cycle; fluid with sperm is often released before ejaculation | Requires no devices or chemicals |
| Vasectomy or male sterilization | 0.15 | Has no contraindications | Is permanent; requires minor surgery | No further monitoring required after verification that all sperm in system have been ejaculated |
| Bilateral tubal ligation or female sterilization | 0.4 | May be performed during cesarean delivery; may be performed soon after vaginal delivery | Is permanent; may present surgical complications | Requires no further monitoring |

Adapted from Mattson, S. & Smith, J.E. (1993). *Care curriculum for maternal-newborn nursing.* Philadelphia: W.B. Saunders.

burns of the bowels, infection, hemorrhage, and adverse effects of anesthesia. Surgical sterilization is extremely effective. In addition, sexual relationships may be enhanced because the fear of childbearing is removed.

Table 11–1 lists methods of contraception and their failure rates, postpartum use, risks, and benefits.

## Toxic Shock Syndrome

Toxic shock syndrome (TSS) is a disease of women in their childbearing years. Its incidence is higher in younger women. It is caused by *Staphylococcus aureus*, which produces a specific toxin that enters the blood stream. This is what causes the shocklike symptoms. High-absorbency tampons are closely linked to this condition; however, leaving a diaphragm, cervical cap, or sponge in place beyond the specified time may also increase the risk of TSS. Infection can also be carried along the IUD string to the uterus. Postpartum women should not use tampons for at least 6–8 weeks (Nursing Care Plan 11–1).

Any menstruating woman who develops a fever along with diarrhea and vomiting needs to be assessed for TSS, which can be fatal (Table 11–2). A careful vaginal examination with removal of any particles of tampons is essential. Cervical and vaginal cultures for *S. aureus* are taken. Women are usually hospitalized and given intravenous fluids, medication to maintain blood pressure, and antibiotics. The incidence of TSS has fallen with increasing knowledge of the correct use of tampons and birth control devices.

---

### NURSING CARE PLAN 11–1

#### Selected Nursing Diagnoses: Education of Woman about Toxic Shock Syndrome

| Goals | Nursing Interventions | Rationales |
|---|---|---|
| **Nursing Diagnosis:** Knowledge deficit related to tampon use. | | |
| The client will verbalize seven common practices for safe tampon use | 1. Teach woman to wash hands thoroughly before inserting barrier contraceptives or tampons | 1. Handwashing is single most effective mechanism for preventing the spread of infection |
| | 2. Emphasize the need to change tampons every 3–4 hr | 2. Blood-soaked tampons are an ideal medium for bacteria to thrive in |
| | 3. Instruct woman not to leave barrier contraceptives in body for more than the time recommended by manufacturer | 3. Use of the diaphragm, cervical cap, and contraceptive sponge has been linked to toxic shock syndrome |
| | 4. Suggest alternately using tampons with perineal pads (use perineal pads during night) | 4. Prolonged tampon use may cause chronic vaginal ulcerations through which *Staphylococcus aureus* is absorbed |
| | 5. Teach woman to avoid deodorant and superabsorbency tampons | 5. Superabsorbent tampons containing cellulose may present problems; bacteria can break down cellulose, providing a ripe environment for organism growth; may cause vaginal dryness, particularly at end of period when flow diminishes; women tend to leave them in longer; deodorant tampons may cause irritation or allergic response |
| | 6. Advise postpartum woman not to use tampons for 6–8 wk | 6. The healing cervix is subject to trauma and infection |
| | 7. Instruct woman to contact her health-care provider if fever, vomiting, and diarrhea occur during menstrual cycle | 7. Symptoms are often mistaken for influenza; tampons are not recommended for women with prior history of toxic shock syndrome |

## Nursing Brief

When assessing sexual needs of a couple, the nurse uses the word "partner" until the couple indicates that they prefer an alternative term.

## Fertility Counseling

*Infertility* is the inability or diminished ability to produce offspring. Couples who have unprotected, unlimited sex for 1 year without a pregnancy are considered infertile. Infertility is termed *primary* when conception has never occurred and *secondary* when there have been one or more pregnancies before the infertility.

This condition is on the increase. Although statistics vary, it is estimated that one of every six married couples in the United States suffers from primary infertility. A variety of reasons account for this upsurge. Many couples are delaying childbearing well into their thirties, making conception more difficult. There is an increase in STDs, which are known to affect fertility. Also, more couples are seeking medical help for infertility (Saulsbery & Pohlhaus, 1992).

When a couple is seen in the fertility clinic, a complete history is obtained. They are given thorough physical examinations, including blood work and urinalysis. A Venereal Disease Research Laboratory (VDRL) test and an Rh-factor test are done for both partners. A Pap smear is obtained from the woman, and prostate and urethral cultures from the man. Protocols go from less intrusive procedures to more complex ones.

### CULTURAL CONSIDERATIONS

In many areas of the world, fertility is considered a female function. It may be closely linked to the woman's social status. The stigma of infertility can lead to divorce and rejection from family and society. To be treated for infertility may involve the couple's going against societal norms.

Acquiring cultural information is often difficult because clients may be reluctant to discuss their feelings and beliefs. In addition, many ethnic groups are not exposed to routine physical examinations, pelvic examinations, and requests for specimens. Latin, Indian, Pakistani,

and subcontinental women may cover their faces during vaginal examinations, particularly if the physician is a man (Blenner, 1991). Many men from various cultures have difficulty masturbating to produce semen specimens.

The lack of cultural sensitivity by the health-care provider may lead to labeling of the patient as uncooperative or difficult. An awareness of cultural differences can lead to greater understanding and compliance. This promotes a higher level of satisfaction for both client and health-care professional.

### MALE-RELATED FACTORS AND TESTS

Congenital abnormalities such as undescended testes, trauma, endocrine imbalance, obstruction, autoimmunity, illness, age, impotence, drug or alcohol abuse, irradiation, anabolic steroids, and occupational and environmental hazards can affect the production of sperm. Mumps with orchitis, tuberculosis, and STDs are also causative factors. A *varicocele*, an enlargement of the veins of the testicles, has been implicated in male infertility. The venous congestion is believed to raise the temperature in the scrotum, thus destroying sperm. Premature ejaculation due to physical or psychological problems may reduce fertility.

A *semen analysis* (often more than one) is obtained from the man early on. This determines such factors as the amount, concentration, and mobility of the sperm. An infertility diagnosis in the male may be one of reduced sperm concentration, reduced sperm count, or reduced motility, or a combination of any of these factors. The exact sperm count necessary for fertilization is controversial. A specimen that has less than 20 million sperm per milliter of seminal fluid is considered infertile. A low or absent sperm count can be caused by increased scrotal

**Table 11–2.** CLINICAL MANIFESTATIONS OF TOXIC SHOCK SYNDROME

| | |
|---|---|
| Fever over 38.9°C (102°F) | Inflamed mucous membranes |
| Sunburn-like rash | Disorientation |
| Vomiting, diarrhea | Impaired renal function |
| Dizziness, headache | Peeling of skin |
| Aching muscles | Impaired liver function |
| Hypotension, shock | Decrease in platelets |
| (Blood pressure below 90 mmHg systolic) | |

heat from hot tubs or saunas. Wearing tight underwear has also been cited. Usually the diagnosis of male infertility is not anticipated, and this can have a devastating impact on the couple (Cant, 1993).

## FEMALE-RELATED FACTORS AND TESTS

Female factors that may cause infertility include absence of ovulation, obstruction of the fallopian tubes, infections or growths in the uterus, and cervical and vaginal changes. The health-care provider obtains a detailed menstrual history, which includes all contraceptives and medications used in the past. It is determined if the woman ever used or was exposed to diethylstilbestrol, a drug known to cause uterine anomalies and cervical changes. Initial laboratory studies for women include hormonal assays for estrogen, prolactin, progesterone, luteinizing hormone (LH), and follicle-stimulating hormone (FSH). Thyroid function tests may also be indicated because endocrine conditions can also contribute to infertility.

*Anovulation* is the most serious problem for the female. This may be caused by below-normal hormone levels. Methods of determining ovulation include BBT readings and testing of cervical mucus. The woman is also asked to test her urine to determine the increase in LH that occurs just before ovulation. Instructions are included in the kit.

Medical therapies (fertility drugs) may be chosen to induce ovulation if other methods fail. These drugs include clomiphene citrate (Clomid), human chorionic gonadotropin (hCG), Menotropin (Pergonal), and urofollitropin (Metrodin). Often they produce multiple births. Women undergoing ovulation induction are monitored carefully.

Another condition causing infertility in women is obstruction of the fallopian tubes. Obstruction may be due to infections, congenital defects, adhesions, or scarring from surgery. Tubal patency is usually assessed by *hysterogram*. This technique involves injecting a radioactive dye into the uterus and viewing its passage through the tubes by fluoroscopy. A *culdoscopy* may also be scheduled. In this test, the pelvic cavity is examined through the vagina by an endoscope. Laparoscopy is another procedure that affords direct examination of the pelvic organs. A small incision is made in the area of the umbilicus, and inspection is made by means of a thin, hollow, lighted tube.

Congenital abnormalities of the uterus may be present. Fibromas or malignant growths may interfere with implantation and block the tubes. There may be a history of pelvic inflammatory disease. The endometrium may be inadequate because of inadequate secretions of progesterone, making it impossible for the fertilized ovum to be implanted. *Endometriosis*, a condition in which endometrial tissue appears outside the uterus, is known to affect fertility by blocking tubes, ovaries, and other areas of the reproductive tract. An endometrial biopsy may be considered if the woman does not have an active infection. Endometriosis and adhesions may be treated by cautery or laser in some cases.

Cervical and vaginal changes can interfere with pregnancy. Erosions of the cervix, infection, trauma from past abortion, dilation and curettage, and cervical conization may cause scarring or other damage to the reproductive tract. An incompetent cervix (a dilated internal cervical os) may prevent pregnancy.

Cervical mucus is examined for infection and the estrogen effects of ferning and spinnbarkeit (see p. 279). Another procedure less frequently used is the *postcoital* test. This evaluates midcycle cervical mucus–spermatozoa interaction. The couple has intercourse 1–3 hours before the office visit. A pelvic examination is performed on the woman, and a sample of mucus is obtained from the cervix for examination.

## MEDICAL AND PSYCHOLOGICAL CONSIDERATIONS

Fertility protocols are time-consuming and expensive (not always covered by insurance), and the procedures are sometimes uncomfortable. When a cause (e.g., an infection) is discovered, it is treated. Anovulation may be treated with fertility drugs if the couple decides to choose that option. Premature ejaculation is sometimes treated with microsurgery if there is an obstruction. In some cases, the tests themselves will open a passageway and correct the condition.

Couples who are unable to conceive with more conventional therapies may decide to try

## Nursing Brief

Childlessness due to infertility can alter the aspects of personal and social identity that are linked to parenthood.

*assisted reproductive therapies (ARTs)*. A summary of ARTs is provided in Table 11–3. The educational and counseling components of an ART program are of particular relevance for compliance. There are legal and ethical consid-

**Table 11–3.** SUMMARY OF ASSISTED REPRODUCTIVE THERAPIES (ARTs)

| Therapy | Description |
| --- | --- |
| Artificial insemination | Donor sperm are instilled into the uterus; sperm may be husband's artificial insemination (AIH) or donor's artificial insemination (AID) |
| In vitro fertilization (IVF) | The woman's eggs are recovered from her ovaries by laparoscopy or transvaginal aspiration under sonography; they are then fertilized with sperm in the laboratory and transferred to her uterus after a day or two, when normal embryonic development has begun |
| Gamete intrafallopian transfer (GIFT) | The transfer of oocytes and sperm into the distal end of the fallopian tube. Fertilization occurs in the tube (in vivo) rather than in the laboratory (in vitro) |
| Direct intraperitoneal insemination (DIPI) | Sperm are directly instilled through the posterior wall of the vagina into cul-de-sac of Douglas; done by ultrasonography |
| Donor oocyte (eggs) | Process by which the eggs are donated by IVF, inseminated, and then transferred into the prepared uterus of the infertile woman |
| Embryo transfer (ET) | As above, only embryo is transferred to the uterus of the infertile female when it reaches the four- to six-cell stage |
| Surrogate mother | The woman agrees to have her eggs impregnated by the man's sperm via artificial insemination; biological mother agrees to relinquish the child after birth |
| Gestational carrier | Process in which the couple undergoes IVF and the embryo(s) is transferred to another woman's uterus (the carrier); unlike the surrogate mother, the carrier has no genetic investment in the baby |

erations of enormous complexity. The Human Fertilization and Embryology Act 1990 provides guidelines for these treatments.

For most couples, diagnosis and treatment are emotionally difficult. They necessitate intrusion into their private sexual behaviors, which creates anxiety and embarrassment. Their lives revolve around trying to conceive. It is difficult to plan ahead because of the unpredictability of the process. Intercourse "on cue" often lacks spontaneity and can lead to anger, guilt, and marital stress. Menstruation becomes the monthly reminder of failure. Depression and grief are common.

Health-care providers should avoid statements that the couple may view as blaming either partner. Instead, infertility needs to be presented as a complex and sometimes baffling condition with multitudinous variables. In many cases, it is not possible to determine the cause of the infertility, which makes the diagnosis difficult to accept. A national support group called Resolve is an important resource for these couples. A collaborative effort by health professionals is essential to ensuring a positive outcome. For some couples, this may mean the decision to discontinue therapy and try other avenues.

## Menopause

When a woman's menstrual periods have ceased for a period of 1 year she is termed "menopausal." Menopause signals the end of her reproductive cycle. This is a normal and natural process that may present few or many symptoms. The *climacteric* is the time in a woman's life surrounding this event, when many physical and psychological changes occur. It is also referred to as the *perimenopausal period*.

This transition is a gradual process. Most women have their first period at about 13 years of age and begin the perimenopausal transition ("the change") around age 48. Perimenopausal symptoms have been known to occur as early as age 35.

Education and treatment of menopausal women is usually a collaborative process. The physician or nurse practitioner generally provides the initial education and course of treatment. The nurse plays an important role in assessing the woman's understanding of what she has been told, reaffirming important information, and acting as a liaison between the woman and health-care provider.

The final menstrual period is generally experienced between 52 and 55 years if the woman has not had a hysterectomy. Any spontaneous bleeding after 12 consecutive months of no periods needs to be investigated. Menopause may be induced at any age by hysterectomy, pelvic irradiation, or extreme stress. When menopause does not occur before the late fifties or early sixties, it is considered delayed and requires investigation.

Perimenopausal symptoms are due to a decrease in ovarian function and changes in hormone production. There is an increase in the FSH. The ovaries stop producing progesterone and estrogen. Ovulation gradually ceases. Certain vasomotor changes accompany these fluctuations. Blood tests are available to determine hormone levels. Elevation of FSH and LH in the presence of minimal estrogen is indicative of the process.

Because cells in the reproductive organs are estrogen-dependent, noticeable physical changes occur. The uterus shrinks because of a decrease in myometrium. The ovaries atrophy. The sacral ligaments relax and pelvic muscles weaken. The cervix becomes pale and shrinks. The vagina becomes shorter, narrower, and less elastic. There is less lubrication. Some women notice a change in *libido* (sexual desire) at this time.

## CULTURAL VARIATIONS

Women from different cultures have different experiences of menopause. How the society views aging, the role of the female, and femininity itself has a bearing. In countries in which age is revered, menopause is practically a "non-event." In the United States, with its emphasis on youth, sex appeal, and physical beauty, menopause can threaten the female's feelings of health and self-worth.

A positive aspect of menopause is that it is also a time of liberation from monthly cramps and the fear of unwanted pregnancy. It is the beginning of postreproductive life. Gail Sheehy calls this stage a coalescence—the mirror image of adolescence, a time in which women can tap into the new vitality that Margaret Mead called "postmenopausal zest" (Sheehy, 1992).

## SYMPTOMS

Perimenopausal symptoms related to *vasomotor* changes include hot flashes, mild to drenching sweats, chills, occasional palpitations, dizziness, and tingling sensation of the skin, particularly in the extremities. In addition, periods may become irregular and lighter or heavier.

Vaginal dryness, burning, and itching may cause *dyspareunia* (painful sex). There may be an increase in vaginitis. The uterus may prolapse. The urethra may atrophy, causing an increase in bladder problems. Pubic hair thins and may change to gray or white. Eventually the breasts lose their firmness. Insomnia is common because of night sweats and disturbances in rapid-eye-movement sleep. Concentration difficulties may arise.

## CARDIOVASCULAR CHANGES

It has long been thought that estrogen produced until menopause protected women from coronary artery disease. It seems that menopausal women have an increased incidence of atherosclerotic changes in their bodies. The addition of estrogen causes vessels to dilate, cardiac palpitations to diminish, and peripheral blood flow to improve. It is believed that these and other factors protect the woman from myocardial infarction and ischemic heart disease. However, progesterone may have a countereffect, in which case the benefit of estrogen may be lost.

Other cardiac risk factors must also be considered. More women are smoking, which is a major cause of coronary artery disease. Obesity, lack of exercise, and stress are known contributors. In one seminar taught to mid-life women who had experienced coronary bypass surgery, six of eight believed that they were type A personalities. The type-A personality is noted for being impatient, perfectionistic, extremely competitive, and often irritable and angry. These characteristics, plus financial and family difficulties, cause symptoms that sometimes exacerbate or are difficult to differentiate from menopausal symptoms (e.g., insomnia and anxiety).

## BONE DENSITY CHANGES (OSTEOPOROSIS)

A reduction in bone mass is termed *osteoporosis*. Skin, bone, and joints all contain cells that respond to estrogen by producing better-quality collagen. Estrogen is also necessary for the metabolism of calcium in the bones. A decrease or absence of estrogen may lead to osteoporosis.

About 250,000 women suffer from fractured hips each year in the United States. Compression fractures of the spine and lower forearm fractures are also common in postmenopausal women. Calcium and vitamin D supplements, exercise, and limiting or avoiding cigarettes and alcohol help to avert this condition.

Foods rich in calcium include milk, dairy products, and green leafy vegetables. The effectiveness of increased calcium in reducing osteoporosis and the proper dosage is subject to controversy. The National Institutes of Health Consensus Conference on Osteoporosis recommends that premenopausal women consume 1000 mg of calcium per day and postmenopausal women consume 1500 mg calcium daily (Mahan & Arlin, 1992). The U.S. recommended daily allowance for vitamin D is 400 IU.

A woman should consult her medical care provider about the advisability and dosage of calcium supplements because they vary and may differ in absorption. They are contraindicated in certain disease conditions. A high calcium intake does not substitute for hormone replacement therapy (HRT). Other therapeutic modalities to prevent osteoporosis may include calcitonin and sodium fluoride.

## HORMONE REPLACEMENT THERAPY

HRT may be provided to relieve the discomforts of the climacteric. In the 1970s, estrogen replacement therapy (ERT) alone was linked to endometrial hyperplasia, a possible forerunner of uterine cancer. For this reason, unopposed estrogen is not recommended for women who have an intact uterus.

A variety of types of estrogen are used in ERT. These include Premarin, Estrace, and Estraderm. Estrogen comes in tablets, transdermal skin patches, vaginal creams, injections, and pellets. The goal of therapy has a bearing on dosage and form prescribed (e.g., whether for temporary relief of hot flashes or for osteoporosis.) Vaginal changes can be treated locally with vaginal creams or systemically, or both ways. Estrogen should not be discontinued abruptly.

Currently, estrogen is given with progesterone. This mimics the normal menstrual cycle and protects against cancer of the uterus. Treatment routines vary and are still controversial. One commonly prescribed dosage is 0.625 mg estrogen with 2.5 mg Provera taken daily.

## Nursing Brief

When completing laboratory slips, indicate whether the woman is on hormone replacement therapy.

The advantage of continuous combined therapy is that withdrawal bleeding generally stops in about 6 months. Some think that replacement therapy should be continued throughout the life span.

**Side Effects and Contraindications.** Side effects are usually related to progesterone. These include depression, weight gain, premenstrual tension, and breast tenderness. For these reasons and because progesterone may unfavorably alter cholesterol ratios of high-density lipoprotein and low-density lipoprotein, unopposed estrogen is recommended for women who have undergone a hysterectomy (Black & Matassarin-Jacobs, 1993).

Certain conditions contraindicate ERT. These include pregnancy, history of endometrial or breast cancer within the last 5 years, thromboembolic disorder, acute liver disease, gallbladder or pancreatic disease, poorly controlled hypertension, and undiagnosed genital bleeding. Fibrocystic breast disease, diabetes, or obesity may require extra caution (Kee & Hayes, 1993).

Suspected breast cancer must be ruled out before hormone therapy begins. First, a physical examination and Pap smear are necessary. The woman should also see a health-care provider every year for a pelvic and breast examination and a blood pressure check. The woman is taught to examine her breasts monthly (Fig. 11–15) and to obtain mammograms regularly.

**Nursing Care.** The nurse needs to assess the woman's knowledge of the climacteric and menopause. Both pharmacologic and nonpharmacologic treatments are reviewed. In particular, the nurse ascertains the woman's understanding of the risks and benefits of HRT. Current educational materials are provided in the health-care setting.

The woman is instructed to stop treatment and contact her primary-care provider if she has headaches, visual disturbances, signs of thrombophlebitis, heaviness in her legs, chest pain, or breast lumps. If she desires to stop replacement therapy, she should do so with the physician's supervision.

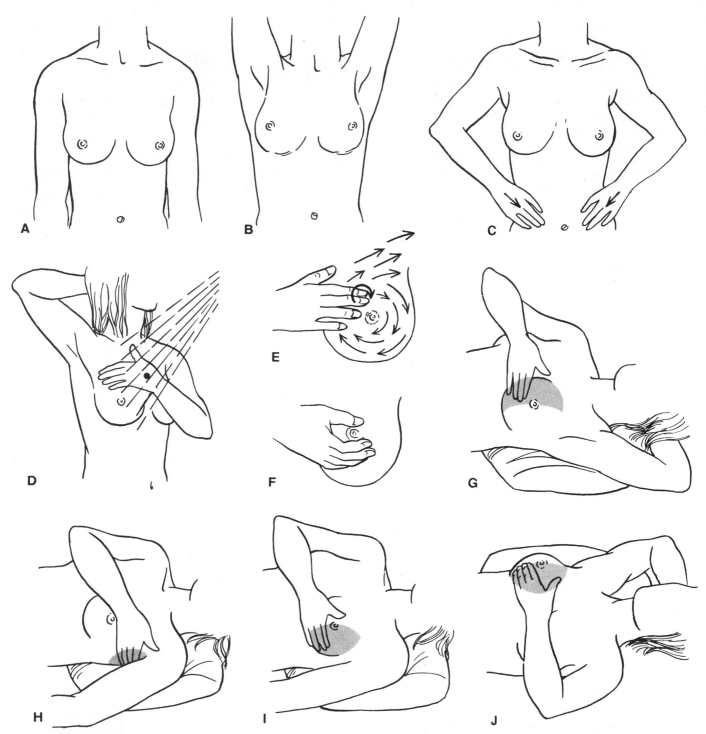

**Figure 11–15.** *A to J*, Self-examination of female breasts and axillae, accomplished by observation and palpation. Various positions are assumed while standing in front of a mirror. *A*, Relax the arms at the sides. Lean forward. *B*, Raise the arms high overhead. Press the arms behind the head. *C*, Place the hands on the hips and firmly press inward to flex the chest muscles. *D*, In the shower, examine the breast contours. *E*, Method of palpating the breast. Use the fingers to press gently in small circular motions around an imaginary clock face (begin at 12 o'clock). Move outward, an inch at a time. *F*, Finally, squeeze the nipple gently between thumb and index finger. *G to I*, Palpate the breast while lying down: *G*, Position to palpate inner breast. *H*, Position to examine the axilla. *I*, Position to examine the outer breast. *J*, Repeat the entire process for opposite breast and axilla. (From Black, J.M., & Matassarin-Jacobs, E. [1993]. *Luckmann and Sorensen's medical-surgical nursing: A psychophysiologic approach* [4th ed.]. Philadelphia: W.B. Saunders.)

| NURSING CARE PLAN 11–2 | | |
|---|---|---|
| **Selected Nursing Diagnoses: The Woman Experiencing Perimenopausal Symptoms** | | |
| **Goals** | **Nursing Interventions** | **Rationales** |

**Nursing Diagnosis:** Knowledge deficit related to vasomotor symptoms (hot flashes).

| | | |
|---|---|---|
| Woman will verbalize four measures to increase her comfort during vasomotor symptoms | 1. Suggest that she wear layered cotton clothes | 1. This allows the woman to take off or put on clothes during hot flashes or chills |
| | 2. Advise her to avoid caffeine (coffee, tea, colas, chocolate) | 2. Hot flashes often occur at night; caffeine is a stimulant and will contribute to insomnia and perspiration |
| | 3. Suggest she consult her physician about the use of vitamin E | 3. Vitamin E, a mild prostaglandin inhibitor, improves circulation; although practice is not fully substantiated, many women report a relief in vasomotor symptoms with use of vitamin E supplements |
| | 4. Explain that stress exacerbates the condition; therefore, she needs to maintain a healthful lifestyle | 4. Stress affects virtually every system of the body, including endocrine and cardiovascular systems |
| | 5. Suggest she discuss hormone replacement therapy (HRT) with her physician | 5. Each woman should have the choice of whether to participate in HRT; both HRT and estrogen therapy (ET) relieve vasomotor symptoms |

**Nursing Diagnosis:** Altered sexuality related to dyspareunia.

| | | |
|---|---|---|
| Woman will express no discomfort with coitus | 1. Instruct woman to use K-Y jelly before intercourse | 1. Thinning of vaginal walls and drying of secretions can lead to discomfort during intercourse unless additional lubrication is used; water-soluble lubricants do not dry mucosa as do petroleum products (Vaseline) |
| | 2. Explain that commercial over-the-counter products, such as Replens, are available for use as indicated on package | 2. These products help lubricate vagina and increase sexual comfort; come with own applicator |
| | 3. Advise woman that physicians sometimes prescribe a topical application of estrogen; it is inserted at bedtime for best absorption | 3. Topical applications of estrogen, such as Estraguard, may alleviate signs and symptoms of vaginal atrophy |
| | 4. Explain that overuse of feminine hygiene products may contribute to dryness and irritation of vagina | 4. These products can destroy the natural flora and secretions of vaginal walls |
| | 5. Suggest she discuss HRT with her health-care provider | 5. HRT promotes a return of vaginal secretions and may increase libido |

Relief from vasomotor symptoms can be promoted by suggesting measures depicted in Nursing Care Plan 11–2. Applying the nursing process to matters of sexual health requires openness and a willingness to approach the subject. It is wise to start with issues less highly charged. For instance, nurses may begin with questions about the woman's periods or known disorders of the reproductive organs. Phrases such as "some women experience" can be helpful and helps lessen the client's anxiety about being "different."

## KEY POINTS

- Contraception is an individual choice. The nurse must be aware of her own biases when assisting in the education of clients.
- The nurse provides women with clear information about feminine hygiene.
- Periodic abstinence and fertility awareness methods prevent pregnancy by determining the time of ovulation. This is accomplished mainly by taking body temperature readings, observing cervical mucus, and using the rhythm method.
- The pill, Norplant, intrauterine device, periodic abstinence, fertility awareness methods, and withdrawal offer no protection against sexually transmitted diseases.
- Menopause refers to the cessation of periods for 12 months.
- Perimenopause and the climacteric refer to the period of about 3–5 years leading up to menopause.
- Common menopausal symptoms include "hot flashes," chills, night sweats, palpitations, dyspareunia, and dizziness. These stem from the cessation of ovulation and decrease in hormonal activity, particularly that of estrogen and progesterone.
- Infertility can be either primary or secondary.
- The process by which a woman's eggs are collected from her ovaries, fertilized in the laboratory with sperm, and transferred to her uterus is called in vitro fertilization.
- The nurse helps couples deal with the grief that they often experience when seeking fertility treatments.

# Study Questions

1. List four factors that might influence a woman's choice of contraception.
2. What two hormones does the pill contain?
3. Why is it important that the health-care provider know of a woman's pre-existing health conditions?
4. List the complications for which a woman taking birth control pills should contact her health-care provider.
5. What types of contraceptives are suitable for the postpartum woman?
6. What types of contraceptives are suitable for the nursing mother?
7. List three methods of natural family planning.
8. Name two support resources for infertile couples.
9. List five vasomotor symptoms commonly seen in the premenopausal period.
10. What is the connection between menopause and osteoporosis?

# Multiple Choice Review Questions

*Choose the most appropriate answer.*

1. Which of the following contraceptives are most effective in preventing pregnancy?
   a. coitus interruptus, sterilization, intrauterine device (IUD)
   b. diaphragm, cervical cap, Depo-Provera
   c. sterilization, the pill, subdermal implants
   d. female condom, fertility awareness, spermicidal foam

2. Juanita is nursing her newborn. She plans to have more children. Which contraceptives would be her best option in the first 4–6 weeks?
   a. Norplant, cervical cap
   b. the pill, Depo-Provera
   c. abstinence or male condoms
   d. IUD, abstinence
3. Which risk is associated with the IUD?
   a. Pelvic inflammatory disease
   b. cervical dysplasia
   c. inflamed leg veins
   d. migraine headaches

4. The term used when a woman's periods have ceased for 1 year is
   a. climacteric
   b. perimenopausal
   c. menopause
   d. dyspareunia
5. This condition is a result of tampon misuse.
   a. amenorrhea
   b. toxic shock
   c. menarche
   d. mittelschmerz

## BIBLIOGRAPHY

Anastasi, J. (1993). AIDS update. What to tell patients about the female condom. *Nursing, 23,* 71–73.

Assessing contraceptive needs during the menopause. (1993). *Professional Nurse, 8,* 258.

Black, J.M., & Matassarin-Jacobs, E. (1993). *Luckmann and Sorensen's medical-surgical nursing: A psychophysiologic approach* (4th ed.). Philadelphia: W.B. Saunders.

Blenner, J. (1991). Health care providers' treatment approaches to culturally diverse infertile clients. *Journal of Transcultural Nursing, 2*(2).

Braverman, A., & English, M. (1992). Creating brave new families with advanced reproductive technologies. *NAACOG's Clinical Issues in Perinatal and Women's Health Nursing, 3*(2), 353–363.

Bullough, B., & Bullough, V. (1991). Contraceptives for teenagers. *Journal of Pediatric Health Care, 5:*277–284.

Cant, S. (1993). Infertility: Causes and treatment. *Nursing Standard, 7,* 28–30.

Harper, D.C. (1990). Perimenopause and aging. In R. Lichtman & S. Papers (Eds.), *Gynecology: Well woman care.* (pp. 405–425). East Norwalk, CT: Appleton & Lange.

Kee, J.L., & Hayes, E. (1993). *Pharmacology: A nursing process approach.* Philadelphia: W.B. Saunders.

King, J. (1992). Helping patients choose an appropriate

method of birth control. *MCN: American Journal of Maternal Child Nursing, 17,* 91–95.

Lewis, J., Reame, N., & English, M. (1992). *NAACOG's clinical issues in perinatal and women's health nursing.* Philadelphia: J.B. Lippincott.

Lichtman, R.C. (1991). Perimenopausal hormone replacement therapy: Review of the literature. *Journal of Nurse Midwifery, 36,* 30–48.

Mahan, L.K., & Arlin, M.T. (1992). *Krause's food, nutrition & diet therapy* (8th ed.). Philadelphia: W.B. Saunders.

Olds, S., London, M., & Ladewig, P. (1992). *Maternal newborn nursing* (4th ed.). Reading, MA: Addison-Wesley.

Pearson, L. (1992). The stigma of infertility. *Nursing Times, 87,* 21.

Pillitteri, A. (1992). *Maternal and child health nursing.* Philadelphia: J.B. Lippincott.

Planned Parenthood. (1992, October). *Facts about birth control.* New York: Author.

Saulsbery, S., & Pohlhaus, M. (1992). Assessment and initial management of infertility. *Journal of the American Academy of Nurse Practitioners, 4,* 53–57.

Sheehy, G. (1992). *The silent passage: Menopause.* New York: Random House.

Sotile, W. (1992). *Heart illness and intimacy.* Baltimore: Johns Hopkins University Press.

UpJohn Company. (1993, April). *Depo-Provera contraceptive injection.* Kalamazoo, Michigan: Author.

# Part 4 The Newborn

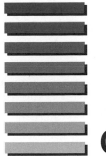

## Chapter 12

# The Term Newborn

## OBJECTIVES

*On completion and mastery of Chapter 12, the student will be able to*

- Define each vocabulary term listed.
- Briefly describe three normal reflexes of the neonate, including the approximate age of their disappearance.
- List four types of heat loss in the newborn.
- List two symptoms of physiologic jaundice in the newborn.
- Define the following skin manifestations in the newborn: lanugo, vernix caseosa, mongolian spots, milia, acrocyanosis, desquamation.
- List the clinical signs of infection in the newborn.
- Describe home phototherapy.

The arrival of the newborn, or neonate, begins a highly vulnerable period during which many psychological and physiologic adjustments to life outside the uterus must be made. In the United States, approximately three-quarters of the deaths in the 1st year of life occur in the first 28 days (Whaley & Wong, 1991). The fetus that remains in the uterus until maturity has reached a major goal. The baby's genetic background, the health of the recent uterine environment, a safe delivery, and the care during the 1st month of life contribute to this adjustment.

The *infant mortality rate* is the ratio between the number of deaths of infants younger than 1 year of age during any given year and the number of live births occurring in the same year. The rate is usually expressed as the number of deaths per thousand live births. The infant death rate is highest in the first month and is referred to as the *neonatal mortality rate*. The first 24 hours of life are the most dangerous ones. The infant mortality rate is considered to be one of the best means of determining the health of a country. In order to obtain accurate figures, all births and deaths must be registered. In the United States, this registration is required by law. Each birth certificate is permanently filed with the state Bureau of Vital Statistics.

*Morbidity* (*morbidus*, "sick") refers to the state of being diseased or sick. Morbidity rates show the incidence of disease in a specific population during a certain time frame. *Perinatology* is the study and support of the fetus and neonate. The term *perinatal mortality* designates fetal and neonatal deaths related to prenatal conditions and delivery circumstances.

## Adjustment to Extrauterine Life

When a baby is born, an orderly, continuous adaptation from fetal life to extrauterine life takes place. All the body systems undergo some change. Respirations are stimulated by chemical changes within the blood and by chilling. Sensory and physical stimuli also appear to play a role in respiratory function. The first breath opens the alveoli. The baby then enters the world of air exchange, at which time an independent existence begins. This process also instigates cardiopulmonary interdependence. The newborn's ability to metabolize food is hampered by the immaturity of the digestive system, particularly deficiencies in enzymes from the pancreas and liver. The kidneys are structurally developed, but their ability to concentrate urine and maintain fluid balance is limited because of a decreased rate of glomerular flow and limited renal tubular reabsorption. Most neurologic functions are primitive (see discussion of the individual body systems later in this chapter).

## Physical Characteristics and Nursing Assessment

This discussion covers the physical characteristics and nursing assessment of the newborn, by body system. Refer to Chapter 9 for postpartum care of the newborn.

### NERVOUS SYSTEM

**Reflexes.** The nervous system directs most of the body's activity. Newborns can move their arms and legs vigorously but cannot control them. The reflexes full-term babies are born with, such as winking, sneezing, gagging, sucking, and grasping (Fig. 12–1), help keep them alive. They can cry, swallow, and lift their heads slightly when lying on their stomach. If the crib is jarred, they draw their legs up and fold their arms across the chest in an embrace position. This is normal and is called the *Moro reflex* (Fig. 12–2). Its absence may indicate abnor-

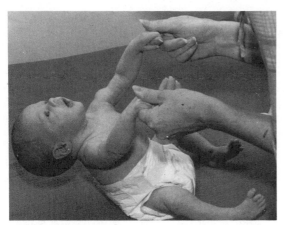

**Figure 12–1.** Grasp reflex and head lag help to determine the maturity of the newborn. (From Marlow, D.R., & Redding, B.A. [1988]. *Textbook of pediatric nursing* [6th ed.]. Philadelphia: W.B. Saunders, p. 369.)

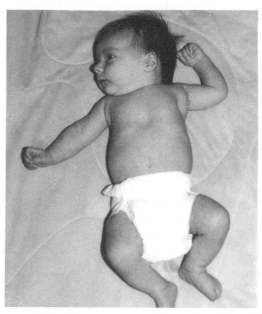

**Figure 12–3.** Spontaneous tonic neck reflex. (From Marlow, D.R., & Redding, B.A. [1988]. *Textbook of pediatric nursing* [6th ed.]. Philadelphia: W.B. Saunders, p. 369.)

malities of the nervous system. The *rooting reflex* causes the infant's head to turn in the direction of anything that touches the cheek, in anticipation of food. The nurse utilizes this when helping a mother to breast feed her infant. A breast touching the cheek causes the infant to turn toward it to find the nipple.

The *tonic neck reflex* is a postural reflex that is sometimes assumed by sleeping babies. The head is turned to one side, and the arm and leg are extended on the same side, while the opposite arm and leg are flexed in a "fencing" position. This reflex disappears about the 20th week of life (Fig. 12–3). Prancing movements of the legs, seen when a baby is held upright on

the examining table, are termed the *dancing reflex*. Table 12–1 lists ages at which the neurologic signs of infancy appear and disappear.

**Head.** The newborn's head is large in comparison with the rest of the body, for the brain grows rapidly before birth. The normal limits of head circumference range from 13.2 to 14.8 inches (Fig. 12–4*A*). The head may be out of shape from *molding* (the shaping of the fetal head to conform to the size and shape of the

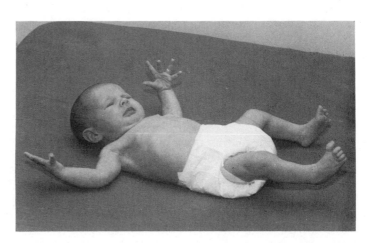

**Figure 12–2.** Moro reflex. Sudden jarring causes extension and abduction of the extremities and spreading of the fingers. (From Marlow, D.R., & Redding, B.A. [1988]. *Textbook of pediatric nursing*. [6th ed.]. Philadelphia: WB. Saunders, p. 369.)

**Table 12–1.** AGES OF APPEARANCE AND
DISAPPEARANCE OF NEUROLOGIC
SIGNS PECULIAR TO INFANCY

| Response | Age at Time of Appearance | Age at Time of Disappearance |
|---|---|---|
| *Reflexes of Position and Movement* | | |
| Moro reflex | Birth | 1–3 mo |
| Tonic neck reflex (unsustained)* | Birth | 5–6 mo (partial up to 2–4 yr) |
| Palmar grasp reflex | Birth | 4 mo |
| Babinski response | Birth | Variable† |
| *Responses to Sound* | | |
| Blinking response | Birth | |
| Turning response | Birth | |
| *Reflexes of Vision* | | |
| Blinking to threat | 6–7 mo | |
| Horizontal following | 4–6 wk | |
| Vertical following | 2–3 mo | |
| Postrotational nystagmus | Birth | |
| *Food Reflexes* | | |
| Rooting response awake | Birth | 3–4 mo |
| Rooting rsponse asleep | Birth | 7–8 mo |
| Sucking response | Birth | 12 mo |
| *Other Signs* | | |
| Handedness | 2–3 yr | |
| Spontaneous stepping | Birth | |
| Straight line walking | 5–6 yr | |

*Arm and leg posturing can be broken by child despite continued neck stimulus.
†Usually of no diagnostic significance until after age 2 yr.
Adapted from *Children are different*. Columbus, OH, Ross Laboratories, © 1986.

birth canal) (Fig. 12–4*B*). There may also be swelling of the soft tissues of the scalp, which is termed *caput succedaneum* (Fig. 12–4*C*). It gradually subsides without treatment. Occasionally, a *cephalohematoma* (*cephal*, "head," and *hemato*, "blood" + *oma*, "tumor") protrudes from beneath the scalp (Fig. 12–4*D*). This condition is caused by a collection of blood beneath the cranial bone. It may be seen on one or both sides of the head but does not cross the suture line. This condition usually recedes within a few weeks. Some newborns have much hair, which eventually is replaced by new hair. It is washed daily when the baby is bathed and is brushed into place.

The *fontanels* are unossified spaces or soft spots on the cranium of a young infant. They protect the head during delivery by the process of molding and allow for further brain growth during the next 1½ years. The *anterior fontanel* is diamond-shaped and located at the junction of the two parietal and two frontal bones. It usually closes by 12–18 months of age. The *posterior fontanel* is triangular and located between the occipital and parietal bones. It is smaller than the anterior fontanel and is usually ossified by the end of the 2nd month. The nurse can see the pulsating of the anterior fontanel. These areas are covered by a tough membrane, and there is little chance of their being injured during ordinary care.

The features of the newborn's face are small. The mouth and lips are well developed, as they are necessary to obtain food. The newborn can both taste and smell. In fact, the newborn can recognize the scent of the mother's breastpad.

**Visual Stimuli and Sensory Overload.** The healthy newborn can see and can fixate on points of contrast. The newborn shows preference for observing a human face and follows moving objects. Visual stimulation is thus an important ingredient in care of the newborn. Toys that make sounds and have contrasting colors attract the newborn. *Sensory overload* can occur if there is too much detrimental stimulation. This overload can happen in the hospital environment, where lights are bright and voices carry. The nurse can help to modify this situation by responding quickly to alarms and by speaking quietly when working near the baby.

**Hearing.** The ears are well developed at birth but are small. Hearing is thought to be keener than was once believed. Increased responses to vocal stimulation, particularly higher-pitched female voices, have been documented. DeCasper and Fifer (1980) note that the ability to discriminate between the mother's voice and others' voices occurs as early as 3 days of age. Hearing is important to speech. The nurse observes and records how the newborn reacts to sound, such as a rattle or the voice of the caretaker. One test used to measure infant hearing is a Crib-O-Gram. It analyzes hearing by comparing the movement of the newborn before and after a sound. The sensor is placed beneath the isolette mattress, and a read-out is generated by a microprocessor (Whaley & Wong, 1991).

The ears and nose need no special attention, except for cleansing with a soft cloth during the bath. Occasionally, they may be *externally* cleansed with a cotton ball moistened slightly

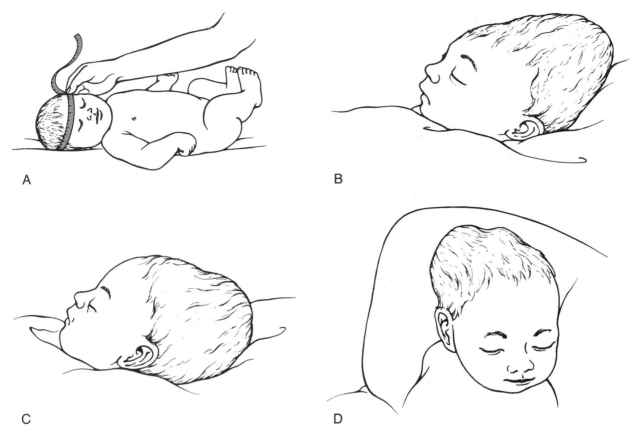

A
B
C
D

**Figure 12–4.** *A*, The circumference of the head is measured during a routine physical examination. *B*, Molding of the head occurs as a result of overriding of the parietal bones as the head passes through the birth canal. The head appears to be longer than normal. This condition disappears without treatment within a few weeks. *C*, Caput succedaneum is a collection of fluid under the scalp. *D*, Cephalohematoma. Blood vessels rupture, and blood collects between the surface of the cranial bone and periosteal membrane.

with water. *Do not* use toothpicks or wooden applicators. They may cause serious injury to the tympanic membrane if inserted too far into the ear canals, or if the baby moves suddenly.

**Sleep.** The baby sleeps approximately 15–20 hours a day. There is a gradual change in the quantity and quality of sleep as the newborn matures. Differentiation between active and quiet sleep is based primarily on whether rapid eye movement (REM) occurs. The sleep of the newborn consists of approximately 50% REM sleep, as opposed to sleep of the 5-year-old, which is only 20% REM. During REM sleep, respirations are rapid and more irregular, movements of the eye are evident beneath the eyelid, and movements of the limbs and mouth may be seen. Preterm infants have an even higher proportion of REM sleep than do babies

born at term. Investigators theorize that REM sleep stimulates the growth of the nervous system. The pattern of sleep gradually develops into one in which the newborn is awake during the day and asleep during the night.

**Pain.** In the past, it was believed that newborns did not experience pain because of immaturity of the nerve pathways to the brain. Pain in newborns was discredited also because it was believed that newborns did not possess a memory. It was thought that anesthesia was risky, and suitable types of anesthesia had not yet been developed. These impressions are being questioned by several studies (Anand & Hickey, 1987; Porter, 1989; and Shapiro, 1989).

It is now thought that fibers that conduct pain stimuli to the spinal cord are in place early in fetal life. These are called *nociceptors*

## Nursing Brief

Advise parents that even the youngest of babies can roll off a changing table or bed when left unattended.

(*noci*, "pain," and *ceptus*, "to receive"). It is also being discovered that the newborn produces catecholamines and cortisol in response to stress. Heart rate and respiratory rates change. Blood pressure increases and blood glucose levels rise. These findings raise concern about the fact that newborns often are not medicated for pain, even when discomfort is anticipated. In addition, the assessment of pain in newborns is difficult. Medications to control pain, particularly narcotics, carry the potential for overdose and/or withdrawal symptoms. These problems present challenges in how to assess and manage pain appropriately in the newborn.

**Conditioned Responses.** A conditioned response or reflex is one that is learned over time. It is an unconscious response to an external stimulus. An example is the hungry baby who stops crying merely at the sound of the caregiver's footsteps, even though food is not yet available. Emotions are particularly subject to this type of conditioning. As an infant matures, the mere sight of an object that once caused pain can precipitate fear. Learning mechanisms such as these are of particular interest to behavior theorists, who hold that the proper focus of psychology is the study of behavior alone.

**Neonatal Behavioral Assessment Scale.** The Neonatal Behavioral Assessment Scale, developed by T. B. Brazelton, has increased our understanding of the newborn's capabilities. Among other areas of assessment, the scale measures the inherent neurologic capacities of the newborn and responses to selected stimuli. Areas tested include alertness, response to visual and auditory stimuli, motor coordination, level of excitement, and organizational process in response to stress.

### RESPIRATORY SYSTEM

The unborn fetus is completely dependent on its mother for all vital functions. The fetus needs oxygen and nourishment in order to grow. These nutrients are supplied through the blood stream of the pregnant woman by way of the placenta and umbilical cord. The fetus is relieved of the waste products of metabolism by the same route. The lungs are not inflated and are almost completely inactive. The circulatory system is adapted only to life within the uterus. Little blood flows through the pulmonary artery because of natural openings within the heart and vessels that close at birth or shortly thereafter. When the umbilical cord is clamped and cut, the lungs take on the function of breathing oxygen and removing carbon dioxide. The first breath helps to expand the collapsed lungs, although full expansion does not take place for several days. The physician assists the first respiration by holding the newborn's head down and removing mucus from the passages to the lungs. The baby's cry should be strong and healthy. The most critical period for the newborn is the 1st hour of life, when the drastic change from life within the uterus to life outside the uterus takes place.

**Apgar Score.** The Apgar score is a standardized method of evaluating the newborn's condition immediately after delivery. Five objective signs are measured: heart rate, respiration, muscle tone, reflexes, and color. The score is obtained at 1 and 5 minutes (see Table 9–3). On admission of the newborn to the nursery, the Apgar score is reviewed to determine any particular difficulties encountered during the birth process. The physician's orders are noted. The nurse must observe the newborn *very closely*. Respiratory distress may be shown by the rate and character of respirations (Fig. 12–5), color (watch for cyanosis), and general behavior. Sternal retractions are reported immediately (Fig. 12–6). Mucus may be seen draining from the nose or mouth. It is wiped away with a sterile gauze square. Gently clearing mucus with a bulb syringe may also be indicated. The bulb is depressed, and the tip is inserted into the nose or mouth. The depression is slowly released, creating the necessary suction (Fig.

## Nursing Brief

The nurse must adhere to universal precautions while working in the delivery room and/or nursery. These guidelines are of particular importance during the initial care of the newborn, when exposure to secretions, blood, and amniotic fluid is high.

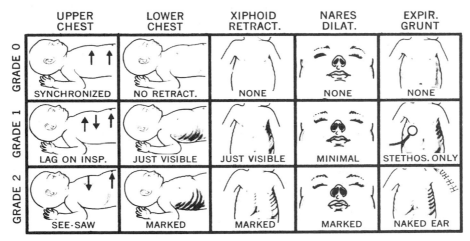

|  | UPPER CHEST | LOWER CHEST | XIPHOID RETRACT. | NARES DILAT. | EXPIR. GRUNT |
|---|---|---|---|---|---|
| GRADE 0 | SYNCHRONIZED | NO RETRACT. | NONE | NONE | NONE |
| GRADE 1 | LAG ON INSP. | JUST VISIBLE | JUST VISIBLE | MINIMAL | STETHOS. ONLY |
| GRADE 2 | SEE-SAW | MARKED | MARKED | MARKED | NAKED EAR |

**Figure 12–5.** Criteria of respiratory distress. Grade 0 for each criterion indicates no respiratory distress; grade 2 for each criterion indicates severe distress. (dilat., dilation; expir., expiratory; insp., inspiration; retract, retraction; and stethos, stethoscope.) (Courtesy of Mead Johnson, Evansville, IN. Modified from Silverman, W., & Andersen, D. [1956]. Controlled clinical trial of effects of water mist on obstructive respiratory signs, death rate, and necropsy findings among premature babies. Reproduced by permission of *Pediatrics*, *17*, 1, copyright 1956.)

12–7). When this procedure is done orally, the tip is inserted into the side of the mouth to avoid stimulating the gag reflex. Parents are instructed in the use of the bulb syringe and to keep one next to the newborn during the early weeks. The DeLee-type catheter attached to low suction is also used in the hospital to remove mucus from the stomach.

## CIRCULATORY SYSTEM

The mother's blood has brought essential oxygen to each cell of the fetus in the uterus. The obstetrician cuts off this supply by severing the umbilical cord. Thereafter, the newborn has not only a systemic circulation but also a pulmonary circulation. (There is some pulmonary circulation prior to birth, although it is less than after the lungs have expanded.)

The circulation of the fetus differs from that of the newborn in that most of the fetal blood bypasses the lungs (see Fig. 3–6). Some of the blood goes from the right atrium to the left atrium of the heart through an opening (the foramen ovale) in the septum. Some goes from the pulmonary artery to the thoracic aorta by way of the ductus arteriosus. These normal openings close soon after birth. If they fail to close or if there are congenitally abnormal openings, the baby may be cyanotic, because part of the blood continues to bypass the lungs and does not pick up oxygen.

Murmurs are caused by blood leaking through openings that have not yet closed. Murmurs may be thought of as functional (innocent) or organic (due to improper heart formation). Functional murmurs are due to the

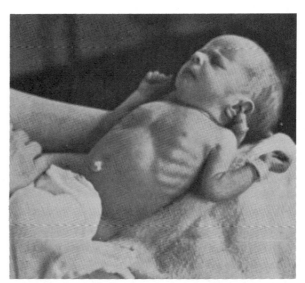

**Figure 12–6.** Sternal retractions. Note the triangular indentation over the area of the chest, which indicates marked retraction during inspiration. Intercostal retractions are also evident. The infant is inactive. All of his energy is being used to breathe. (From Kalafatich, A. [1966]. *Pediatric nursing.* New York: G.P. Putnam's Sons. Copyright 1966, The Putnam Publishing Group.)

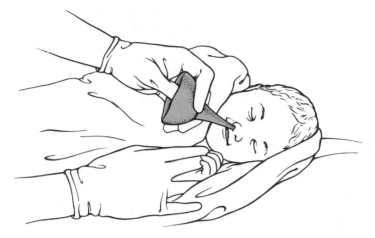

**Figure 12–7.** Nasal and oral suctioning. The bulb is compressed before it is inserted into the nose or mouth; then the bulb is released. If the bulb is depressed after being inserted, mucus will be forced farther into the respiratory passages.

sound of blood passing through normal valves. Organic murmurs are due to blood passing through abnormal openings or normal openings that have not yet closed. The majority of heart murmurs are not serious. However, they should be checked periodically in order to rule out other possibilities.

**Providing Warmth.** The newborn has an unstable heat-regulating system. Body temperature falls immediately after birth to about 96°F. Within a few hours, it climbs slowly to a range of 98–99°F (36.6–37.2°C). The body temperature is influenced by that of the room and the number of blankets covering the baby. The temperature of the nursery, or the mother's room in the case of rooming-in, is kept at 68–75°F. The humidity should be 45–55%. The air in the room must be fresh, but there should be no drafts. A good way to determine whether a baby is warm or cool is to observe facial color. If it is flushed, the baby is too warm; if it is pale or bluish, the baby is too cold. The hands and feet are not used as a guide because the baby's extremities are cooler than the rest of the body. *Acrocyanosis* (*acro* "extremity," and *cyanosis*, "blue color") is also evident. The newborn cannot adapt to changes in temperature. The nurse wraps the baby in a blanket whenever the baby leaves the nursery. Because the baby's heat perception is poor, the nurse must be careful when applying any form of external heat.

**Obtaining Temperature, Pulse, and Respirations.** Some birth facilities recommend that the initial temperature of the newborn be taken by rectum to determine that it is patent. When the temperature is taken rectally, the nurse must be gentle to avoid injuring the rectal mucosa. Daily routine temperatures are taken by axilla. To obtain the axillary temperature, the glass thermometer is held firmly in the center of the axilla for 5 minutes. During this time, the arm is held against the baby's side. Digital thermometers are read when the indicator sounds. Tympanic membrane thermometers (ear thermometers) provide a reading in about 1 second).

The newborn's pulse and respirations are counted before the temperature is taken, because the baby is apt to cry when disturbed, especially when the thermometer is inserted into the rectum. Figure 12–8 illustrates the apical pulse being obtained from a newborn infant. The newborn's pulse is irregular and rapid, varying from 110 to 160 beats/min. Blood pressure is low and may vary with the size of the cuff used. The average blood pressure at birth is 80/46. The respirations are approximately 35–50 breaths/min. The nurse always reports the following changes:

- Temperature elevated to 100°F or below 97°F
- Pulse elevated to 160 beats/min or below 110 beats/min
- Respirations elevated to 60 breaths/min or below 30 breaths/min

## MUSCULOSKELETAL SYSTEM

**Movements, Eye Coordination, and Tremors.** The bones of the newborn are soft because they are chiefly made up of cartilage, in which there is only a small amount of calcium. The skeleton is flexible. The joints are elastic in order to accommodate the passage through the birth canal. Because the bones of the child are easily molded by pressure, position must be changed frequently. If the baby lies constantly in one position, the bones of the head can become flattened.

The movements of the newborn are random and uncoordinated. The newborn lacks the muscular control to hold the head steady. The development of muscular control proceeds from head to foot and from the center of the body to the periphery (see discussion of cephalocaudal and proximodistal control, p. 386). Therefore, the baby holds the head up before sitting erect. In fact, the head and neck muscles are the first ones under control. The legs are small and short and may appear bowed. There should be no limitation of movement. Fingers clenched in a fist should be separated and observed.

An examination of the newborn for maturity includes checking for the *Scarf sign* (Fig. 12–9). This refers to the full-term infant's resistance to attempts to bring one elbow farther than the midline of the chest. No resistance would be observed in the preterm infant.

Most newborns appear cross-eyed because their eye muscle coordination is not fully developed. At first, the eyes appear to be blue or gray; however, the permanent coloring becomes

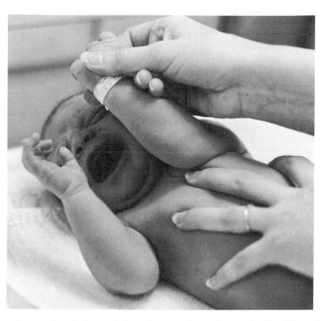

**Figure 12–9.** Examining the newborn for maturity. The full-term newborn's elbow resists attempts to bring it beyond the midline of the chest. Little or no resistance is seen in the preterm infant. This is called the Scarf sign.

fixed between 6 and 12 months. The eyelids are closed most of the time. Tears do not appear until approximately 1–3 months because of the immaturity of the lacrimal gland ducts.

The baby needs freedom of movement. The infant stretches, sucks, and makes faces, and vigorously moves the whole body when crying. Tremors of the lips and extremities during crying are normal. Constant tremors during sleep may be pathologic. These are often accompanied by eye movements and are not related to particular stimuli. The morning bath provides excellent opportunities for the newborn to exercise and the nurse to inspect and assess the baby's condition. When handled, the infant should not feel limp. General body proportions are noted. Bathing is also an excellent means of stimulation for the newborn.

**Length and Weight.** The length of the average newborn is 19–21½ inches (46–56 cm). The weight varies from 6 to 9 pounds (2700–4000 gm) (Fig. 12–10). Girls generally weigh a little less than boys. African-American, Asian-American, and Native-American babies may be somewhat smaller. In the first 3–4 days after birth, the baby loses about 5–10% of the birth weight. The loss may be as high as 15% for preterm infants. This may be due to with-

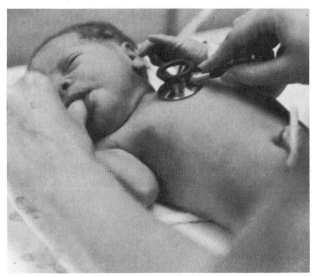

**Figure 12–8.** Apical pulse. An apical pulse is obtained from newborns and infants.

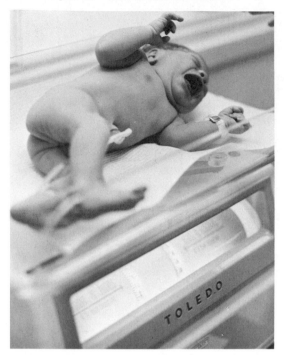

**Figure 12–10.** The newborn weighs 2700–4000 gm (6 to 9 pounds). Weight loss of about 10% occurs within the first 2 days because of fluid shifts.

drawal from maternal hormones, fluid shifts, and the loss of feces and urine. Mothers are prepared for this and reassured that weight will normalize after 3 or 4 days. Newborns are weighed at the same time each day, when morning care is given. (Instructions for measuring and weighing the baby are provided on pp. 572 and 574.)

## GENITOURINARY SYSTEM

The kidneys function normally at birth but are not fully developed. The glomeruli are small. Renal blood flow is only about one-third that of the adult. The ability to handle a water load is reduced, as is the excretion of drugs. The renal tubules are short and have a limited capacity for reabsorbing important substances such as glucose, amino acids, phosphate, and bicarbonate. There is a decrease in the ability to concentrate urine and to cope with fluid imbalances. It is important to note the first voiding of the newborn. This may occur in the delivery room or may not occur for several hours. If voiding does not occur within the first 8 hours, the physician is notified. The nurse must keep an accurate record of the frequency of urina-

tion. Anuria, changes in color, and any unusual findings are brought to the attention of the physician.

**Male Genitalia.** The genitals of the male are developed at birth, although their maturation varies. The testes of the male descend into the scrotum before birth. Occasionally, they remain in the abdomen or inguinal canal. This condition is called *cryptorchidism*, or undescended testes, and is described on pages 800–801. With proper surgical treatment, the prognosis is good.

Routine retraction of the foreskin of the newborn for cleansing is no longer recommended. Lund (1990) states that nonretractability is normal in newborns. The foreskin and glans penis gradually separate, beginning in the prenatal period. This process is generally completed between 3 and 5 years (Olds et al., 1992). Parents are instructed to test occasionally for retraction during the daily bath. If it has occurred, gentle washing of the glans is begun. The foreskin is then returned to its unretracted position.

*Circumcision.* Circumcision is the surgical removal of the foreskin. The procedure is subject to much controversy. The position of the American Academy of Pediatrics has been that there are no valid medical indications for circumcision. In 1989 the AAP modified this, suggesting that circumcision had both advantages and disadvantages (AAP, 1989). The disadvantages include infection and hemorrhage. Infants with congenital anomalies of the penis, such as hypospadias (the opening of the urethra on the undersurface of the penis), should not be circumcised because the skin may be needed for surgery. Studies linking cancer and the absence of circumcision are considered by some to be incomplete. There appears to be an increased incidence of HIV in uncircumcised males (Gelbaum, 1992). A discussion of the pros and cons of this procedure is included as part of prenatal and postpartum education. Regardless of whether the male is circumcised, at an appropriate age he is taught daily hygiene of the genitals. This includes special attention to skin folds, retraction of the foreskin, cleansing of the penis, and examination for lumps or swelling.

The baby should be at least 12 hours old before circumcision. This allows a period of time for the newborn to become stabilized. This stress should be avoided immediately following delivery, when it may also interfere with bonding. The newborn is restrained on a circumcision board (Fig. 12–11). The Gomco clamp and the Plastibell clamp are two devices commonly used for performing circumcisions. If the Gomco clamp is used, a thin layer of petroleum jelly (Vaseline) or petroleum jelly–impregnated gauze may be applied to the end of the penis to protect it from moisture and from sticking to the diaper. The area is observed for bleeding, infection, and irritation. Voidings are recorded.

When a Plastibell is used, the foreskin is tied over a fitted plastic ring and the excess prepuce cut away. The rim usually drops off 5–8 days after circumcision. Parents are instructed not to remove it prematurely. No special dressing is required, and the baby is bathed and diapered as usual. A dark brown or black ring encircling the plastic rim is natural. This disappears when the rim drops off. Parents are instructed to consult their physician if there are any questions, if there is increased swelling, if the ring has not fallen off within 8 days, or immediately if the ring has slipped onto the shaft of the penis.

The Jewish religious custom of circumcision, comparable to baptism in the Christian faith, is performed on the 8th day after birth if the newborn's condition permits. The baby receives his Hebrew name at that time.

The nurse's role in circumcision includes assessing parental knowledge, checking to see that the surgical consent has been signed, and preparing the newborn. The baby is not fed for 1–2 hours prior to the procedure to prevent possible vomiting and aspiration. A bulb syringe is kept handy in case suctioning is required. A light blanket is placed under the infant on the "circ" board, and the diaper is removed. A heat lamp is positioned to avoid cold stress.

The physician may administer a local anesthetic to minimize pain during the procedure and to prevent irritability and sleep disturbances following it (Lund, 1990). Additional comfort measures include holding and soothing the baby and using a pacifier. If bleeding occurs, gentle pressure is applied to the site with a sterile gauze pad, and the physician is notified. The amount and characteristics of the urinary stream are recorded, as edema could cause an obstruction.

**Female Genitalia.** The female genitals may be slightly swollen. Blood-tinged mucus (pseudomenstruation) may be discharged from the vagina. This discharge is due to hormonal withdrawal from the mother at birth. The nurse cleanses the vulva from the *urethra to the anus*, using a clean cotton ball or different sections of a wash cloth for each stroke in order to prevent fecal matter from infecting the urinary tract. The importance of this is stressed to parents.

## INTEGUMENTARY SYSTEM

**Skin.** The skin of newborn Caucasian babies is red to dark pink. The skin of African-American babies is reddish-brown. Infants of Latin descent may appear to have an olive or yellowish tint. The body is usually covered with fine hair called lanugo, which tends to disappear during the 1st week of life. This is more evident in premature infants. *Vernix caseosa*, a cheeselike substance that covers the skin of the newborn, is made of cells and glandular secretions; it is thought to protect the skin from irritation and the effects of a watery environment. White pinpoint pimples caused by obstruction of sebaceous glands may be seen on the nose and chin. These are called *milia* and disappear within a few weeks. *Stork bites* (telangiectatic nevi) are flat, red areas seen on the nape of the neck and on the eyelids. They result from the dilation of small vessels (see Color Figure 1).

*Mongolian spots*, bluish discolorations of the skin, are common in babies of African-American parents, Native-American parents, and parents of Mediterranean races. They are usually found over the sacral and gluteal areas (see Color Figure 2). They disappear spontaneously during the early years of life. Acrocyanosis, or peripheral blueness of the hands and feet, is normal. Pallor is not normal and should be reported, because it may indicate neonatal anemia or another more serious condition.

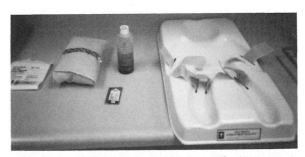

**Figure 12–11.** Circumcision board, sterile instruments, surgical blade, antiseptic, and gloves. (Courtesy of Columbia/HCA Portsmouth Regional Hospital, Portsmouth, NH.)

Many hospitals identify newborns by footprints. The skin is constructed with ridges and grooves so that each person has a unique pattern that never changes, except to grow larger. That is why fingerprints or footprints positively identify a person.

Tissue turgor refers to the hydration or dehydration of the skin. To test tissue turgor (elasticity), the nurse gently grasps and releases the skin. It should spring back to place immediately. When the skin remains distorted, tissue turgor is considered poor. Figure 12–12 illustrates the method of testing tissue turgor.

Desquamation, or peeling of the skin, occurs during the early weeks of life. Skin in areas such as the nose, knees, elbows, and toes may break down because of friction from rubbing against the sheets. The involved area is kept dry, and the baby's position is changed frequently. The buttocks need special attention. A wet diaper should be changed immediately to prevent chafing. The buttocks are washed and dried well.

Physiologic jaundice, also called icterus neonatorum, is characterized by a yellow tinge of the skin. It is caused by the rapid destruction of excess red blood cells, which the baby does not need now, being in an atmosphere that contains more oxygen than was available during prenatal life. Plasma levels of bilirubin rise from a normal 1 mg/dl to an average of 5–6 mg/dl between the 2nd and 4th days. Physiologic jaundice becomes evident between the 2nd and the 3rd days of life and lasts for about 1 week. This is a normal process and is not harmful to the baby. However, genetic and ethnic factors may affect its severity, resulting in pathologic hyperbilirubinemia. Evidence of jaundice is reported and charted, and the newborn is frequently evaluated to ensure safety.

**Bathing the Baby.** The bath is an excellent time to observe the naked newborn. Special attention must be given to areas of the skin that

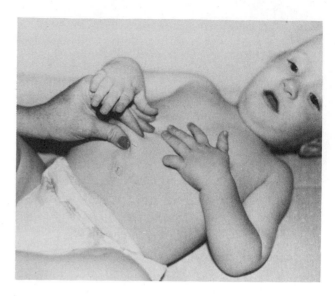

**Figure 12–12.** Testing tissue turgor. *Turgor* refers to the elasticity of the skin, which is affected by the extent of hydration. The nurse tests turgor by gently grasping the skin. When the skin is released, it should instantly spring back into place; if it does not, tissue turgor is considered poor. (From Thompson, E.D., & Ashwill, J.W. [1992]. *Pediatric nursing: An introductory text* [6th ed.]. Philadelphia: W.B. Saunders, p. 92.)

come in contact with each other, because chafing may occur there. These areas are found in the neck, behind the ears, in the axillae, and in the groin. They should be dried well. Powder is seldom used in the hospital, because it can irritate the respiratory tract. Parents are educated about this fact. The use of lotions and oil and the type of soap vary with each institution. The baby is bathed when his or her temperature is stable; the bath removes blood and vernix. The nurse adheres to universal precautions during the procedure.

The following method for giving a sponge bath may be used in the nursery or pediatric unit and in the home until the cord has healed. The nurse has to adapt it to the patient's condition and the routine of the hospital. The newborn's parents are involved in this procedure as much as possible.

### GASTROINTESTINAL SYSTEM

**Stools.** The intestinal tract functions as an outlet for amniotic fluid as early as the 5th month of fetal life. The normal functions of the gastrointestinal tract begin after birth: Food is prepared for absorption into the blood and is

## Nursing Brief

Emphasize flexibility in the time of the bath. Stress the need to gather all materials beforehand in order to avoid leaving the newborn unattended or chilled. The nurse attempts to help parents relax by emphasizing that there is nothing baffling about bathing a baby.

## PROCEDURE FOR GIVING A SPONGE BATH

### Equipment

Linen
  Bath towel
  Wash cloth
  Shirt
  Diaper
  Quilted pad
  Crib sheet
  Receiving blanket
Bath tray
  Cotton balls
  Mild soap
  Baby oil or lotion
  Comb
Paper bag
Wash basin
Gown, mask, gloves as needed for universal precautions (in hospital)

### Method

1. Temperature of room 75–80°F. Temperature of water 100–105°F (test with elbow or bath thermometer). Wash hands. Don clean covergown and gloves.
2. Wash baby's face with plain water and dry.
3. Clean outer nostrils as needed. Use a separate cotton ball moistened with water for each side of the nose.
4. Wrap wash cloth around one finger and cleanse outer ear.
5. Squeeze cheeks gently to examine mouth. Gums should be pink and clean, breath should be sweet.
6. Wash scalp by making a lather of soap on the hands. Wash the scalp thoroughly. Observe fontanels.
7. Using football position, hold head over tub, and rinse off soap with a wet wash cloth. (If there is a scaly crust [cradle cap], apply oil at night and the scale will come off more readily with the next morning's shampoo.) Dry gently with a soft towel.
8. Remove diaper and cleanse diaper area with a cotton ball dipped in water. Wash from front to back, using a separate cotton ball for each stroke.
9. Remove baby's shirt, soap hands, and go over the entire body, front and back. Rinse with wash cloth. Pay special attention to creases, folds, and genitals.
10. Pat dry and re-dress. Comb hair.

### Method

11. Apply clean crib sheet and quilted pad to crib. Cover baby with clean receiving blanket. Tidy unit.

absorbed, and waste products are eliminated. *Meconium*, the first stool, is a mixture of amniotic fluid and secretions of the intestinal glands. It is dark green, thick, and sticky and is passed 8–24 hours following birth. The stools gradually change during the 1st week. They become loose and are greenish-yellow with mucus. These are called *transitional* stools.

The stools of a breast-fed baby are bright yellow, soft, and pasty. There may be three to six stools a day. With age the number of stools decreases. The bowel movements of a bottle-fed baby are more solid than those of the breast-fed baby. They vary from yellow to brown and are generally fewer in number. There may be one to four a day at first, but this gradually decreases to one or two a day. The stools are darker when a baby is receiving iron and green when a baby is under the bilirubin lamp. Small, putty-like stools and diarrhea and bloody stools are abnormal. When there is a question, the nurse saves the stool specimen for the physician to observe. The nursery nurse keeps an accurate record of the number and character of stools each newborn passes daily.

**Constipation.** Constipation refers to the passage of hard, dry stools. Newborns differ in regularity. Some pass a soft stool every other day. This is not constipation. The nurse explains to parents that straining in the newborn period is due to undeveloped abdominal musculature. This is normal and no treatment is required. As the baby grows older and if a formula change is made, constipation is sometimes seen. Increasing water intake may be all that is necessary to remedy this constipation. If the baby is on solid foods, an increase in intake of fruits, vegetables, and whole-grain cereals is usually sufficient. The nurse encourages mothers to telephone their physician's office when questions arise and ask to speak to the nurse. This is particularly emphasized to new mothers, who may be afraid of appearing "ignorant." Very often there is a simple solution that can relieve hours of anxiety.

**Hiccups.** Hiccups appear frequently in newborns and are normal. Most disappear spontaneously. Burping the baby and offering warm water may help.

**Digestion.** Breast-fed babies may be put to breast on the delivery table to help stimulate milk production and for psychological benefits. Bottle feedings are begun in about 5 hours. A baby's hunger is evidenced by crying, restlessness, fist sucking, and the rooting reflex. The capacity of the stomach is about 90 ml. Emptying time is 2–3 hours, and peristalsis is rapid. Deficiency of pancreatic lipase limits fat absorption. The liver is immature, especially in its ability to conjugate bilirubin, regulate blood sugar, and coagulate blood.

**Vitamins.** Babies need extra vitamins C and D. Breast milk contains sufficient vitamin C if the mother's diet is rich in citrus fruits and certain vegetables. Vitamin D may be added to milk, which is labeled "vitamin D milk." Commercial concentrated preparations may also be prescribed. The fluid is drawn up in the dropper to the prescribed amount (0.3 or 0.6 ml) and is placed directly in the baby's mouth. This is done each morning at approximately the same time to avoid forgetting the vitamins.

# Preventing Infection

Infections that are relatively harmless to an adult may be fatal to the newborn. Symptoms are often subtle in the early stages, and their recognition can be crucial. The nurse caring for the newborn reviews the ways in which germs enter and leave a person's body. Briefly, the portals of entry are the respiratory tract, the gastrointestinal tract, the genitourinary tract, and breaks in the skin. The portals of exit are the same as those just mentioned, and the germs are in the excretions from the various systems: sneezes, sputum, vomitus, feces, saliva, urine, and discharges from the skin and mucous membranes.

Nursery standards are developed and enforced by various professional agencies, such as the American Academy of Pediatrics, hospital accreditation boards, and local health agencies. The infection control nurse in each hospital also provides education and surveillance. Provisions governing space, control of temperature and humidity, lighting, and safety from fire and other hazards are considered.

Each newborn has an individual crib, bath equipment, and linen supply. Any communal equipment is sterilized following each use.

Protective precautions may be employed for patients in pediatric units, especially preterm babies, newborns, and infants. The meaning of protective precautions is implied by the name; they protect the patient from microorganisms. Children with burns or leukemia and persons receiving certain therapeutic regimens, such as body irradiation or steroids, may also be on protective precautions. Handwashing is the most reliable procedure available. The nursery nurse washes her hands between handling different babies. Alcohol foam may be used for brief encounters. A private room is also suggested when appropriate. The nurse stresses to parents the need for proper handwashing in the home.

## HANDWASHING TECHNIQUE

As just mentioned, one of the most effective procedures employed in the prevention of infections is *proper handwashing*. The nurse must conscientiously wash and rinse the hands and forearms before handling each baby and before and after handling equipment. Although most organisms are transmitted by direct contact, some are capable of remaining alive for a time outside the body and may be transferred indirectly by articles. Personnel entering the newborn nursery scrub their hands and forearms with an antiseptic. In other areas of the hospital, hands are washed with soap under running water. Parents and relatives are taught the importance of this simple but highly effective procedure.

## OTHER MEANS OF PROTECTION

Nursery personnel wear clean scrub gowns while in the nursery and wear covergowns if they leave the nursery for any reason. The use of caps and masks varies with each institution. Physicians, technicians, and nonnursery personnel wear a covergown, cap, and mask, as appropriate, when on duty in the nursery. Universal precautions are adhered to for the protection of personnel.

Health examination of personnel before employment and annually minimizes the spread of infection from unhealthy persons. Many hospitals require throat cultures and stool examina-

## PROCEDURE FOR HANDWASHING

**Equipment**

Running water
Soap
Paper towels

**Method**

1. Keep the hands lowered over the basin throughout the procedure.
2. Wet the hands.
3. Soap the hands well, working up a lather.
4. Rinse the bar of soap, leaving it clean for the next use. (Soap dispensers are used in many institutions.)
5. Use friction; rub well between the fingers and around the nails; wash the hands, wrists, and forearms thoroughly; rinse well.
6. Repeat steps 2, 3, 4, and 5 three times.
7. Dry the hands well.
8. If there is no foot pedal, turn off the faucet with a paper towel.

tions for personnel assigned to specific areas, such as the nursery, although the value of this practice is questionable. The nurse who has signs of a cold, earache, skin infection, or intestinal upset should not work in the nursery or care for ill children. Visitors are instructed not to come to the hospital or be around hospital patients if they are not feeling well.

The signs and symptoms of infection in the newborn are presented in Table 12–2.

# Discharge Planning

Discharge teaching ideally begins with the admission of the woman to the hospital or birthing center. Many hospitals have flow sheets, which are helpful in ensuring that all topics have been addressed and that patients understand what has been explained to them. Areas of concern include

1. Basic care of the baby, including bathing, cord care, feeding, and elimination
2. Safety measures
3. Immunizations
4. Support groups, such as La Leche League

5. Return appointments
6. Nursery number (note 24-hour availability)
7. Signs and symptoms of problems and who to contact; for example, temperature above 38.4°C (101°F) rectally or 38°C (100.4°F) by axilla, refusal of two feedings in a row, two green watery stools, frequent or forceful vomiting, lack of voiding or stooling.

Nursing Care Plan 12–1 specifies nursing interventions for assisting the mother, parents, or other caregivers in caring for the infant after discharge from the hospital.

**Table 12–2.** CLINICAL PRESENTATION OF INFECTION BY SITE OF INFECTION

| System Involved | Signs and Symptoms |
|---|---|
| Central nervous system | Lethargy or irritability |
| | Jitteriness or hyporeflexia |
| | Tremors or seizures |
| | Coma |
| | Full fontanel |
| | Abnormal eye movements |
| | Hypotonia or increased tone |
| Respiratory system | Cyanosis |
| | Grunting |
| | Irregular respirations |
| | Tachypnea or apnea |
| | Retractions |
| Gastrointestinal tract | Poor feeding |
| | Vomiting (may be bile-stained) |
| | Diarrhea or decreased stools |
| | Abdominal distention |
| | Edema or erythema of abdominal wall |
| | Hepatomegaly |
| Skin | Rashes or erythema |
| | Purpura |
| | Pustules or paronychia |
| | Omphalitis |
| | Sclerema |
| Hematopoietic system | Jaundice |
| | Bleeding |
| | Purpura or ecchymosis |
| | Splenomegaly |
| Circulatory system | Pallor, cyanosis, or mottling |
| | Cold, clammy skin |
| | Tachycardia or arrhythmia |
| | Hypotension |
| | Edema |
| Whole-body system | "Not doing well" |
| | Poor temperature control (fever or hypothermia) |

Adapted from Klaus M.H., & Fanaroff, A.A. (1993). *Care of the high-risk neonate,*(4th ed.). Philadelphia: W.B. Saunders.

| | NURSING CARE PLAN 12–1 | |
|---|---|---|
| | **Selected Nursing Diagnoses for Discharge of the Newborn** | |
| **Goals** | **Nursing Interventions** | **Rationales** |

**Nursing Diagnosis:** Knowledge deficit; parents or single mother, related to inexperience, lack of information, feelings of inadequacy.

| Goals | Nursing Interventions | Rationales |
|---|---|---|
| Parents or single mother will verbalize understanding of instructions and display phone numbers to call for assistance | 1. Role model and demonstrate safe care of newborn during such procedures as bathing, holding, and feeding; provide demonstrations and reinforcement of knowledge as indicated; this is begun immediately after birth and continued throughout hospitalization | 1. New mothers observe and look to nurse for information—actions speak louder than words; return demonstrations provide practice and assist nurse in determining weak areas |
| | 2. Role model and teach healthy interaction with newborn; encourage caretakers to verbalize understanding of bonding and attachment processes; if this is weak, refer to social service or other appropriate agency | 2. Nurse can do much to help caretakers feel comfortable with the newborn and understand the importance of healthy interaction, which promote mutual love and trust |
| | 3. Encourage participation in parenting classes or single-parenting classes, as indicated | 3. Parenting classes provide group discussion of common problems; members receive support from one another; they also provide needed change of environment; single-parenting groups are of particular value for above reasons |
| | 4. Review all areas on flow sheet to assess understanding and to answer questions | 4. Flow sheet provides a means of documentation of teaching; parents may sign sheet to acknowledge their understanding of material presented |
| | 5. Ascertain that mother knows who to call for help | 5. It is extremely important to denote availability to parents, particularly new ones or those whose baby has experienced even a minor problem; some nurseries provide a 24-hour telephone number; birthing units are expanding their care by providing one or two home visits by nurse; parents can call baby clinic or physician |
| | 6. Stress importance of keeping follow-up appointments | 6. Newborn screening can detect such conditions as galactosemia, phenylketonuria, sickle cell disease, and hypothyroidism; immunizations protect the newborn from many diseases; many apprehensions can be lessened during these visits; they also provide continued supervision and education |
| | 7. Ensure that the newborn returns home in an approved car seat | 7. Motor vehicle accidents cause more deaths in all pediatric age groups after age 1 yr than any other disease or injury. Some service clubs and hospitals have loan programs; baby's first ride home in a car seat sets a precedent and stresses importance that medical profession places on this protective measure |

| Goals | Nursing Interventions | Rationale |
|---|---|---|

**Nursing Diagnosis:** Altered family processes related to new member, change in family unit.

| | | |
|---|---|---|
| Family or significant other demonstrates willingness to learn caretaking activities such as holding or diapering; appears interested in newborn | 1. Assess interaction; encourage verbalization of expectations related to new family member; be a good listener<br>2. Ask caregivers about change in general, the family's previous adaptation to change, and what challenges they expect to face at home; discuss coping mechanisms used in the past<br>3. Identify specific behaviors of the newborn, such as sleeping a lot, eating, alert stages, and how they can be incorporated into the family lifestyle<br>4. Have siblings draw and discuss "bringing baby (name) home." | 1. This is an ideal time to pick up many cues for intervention, such as parenting skills or unreal expectations of themselves<br>2. Change is stressful, even when it is a good change and a much-anticipated one; an unwanted pregnancy can place additional strain on a relationship<br>3. This helps establish uniqueness of individual newborn and fosters bonding; also can stimulate parental thinking about home care<br>4. Including siblings makes acceptance of new baby easier; drawing provides an opportunity to express their feelings in a less threatening way than through conversation |

# Home Care

## FURNISHINGS

It helps if the newborn has a separate room. Simple, durable, easy-to-clean furnishings are necessary. A crib with a firm mattress is a suitable place for the infant to sleep for several years. Crib slats should adhere to safety standards. Mattress covers of thin rubber that are large enough to tuck in at the sides may be used. *Plastic bags are never used for this purpose.* Sheeting that has a flannelette backing on both sides stays in place. Contour sheets are convenient. Blankets of lightweight cotton are warm and easy to launder. A knitted shawl stays tucked in and is also a nice wraparound for going places. The newborn does not require a pillow.

Pictures are attached securely to the wall with wall tapes. Thumbtacks may be swallowed by the growing child. A chest of drawers for clothing, an adult chair (preferably a rocker), and a flat-topped table for changing clothes are necessary. The baby needs a separate bathtub, which may be merely a plastic basin. A tray containing frequently used articles saves time and energy. These might include a ther-mometer, hairbrush and comb, baby wipes, and baby oil or lotion. A diaper pail is also necessary.

## CLOTHING

Clothing must be soft, washable, of the proper size, and easy to put on and take off. Instruct parents to launder new clothing and sheets before using them in order to prevent skin irritation. Nightgowns with drawstring necks are avoided because they may lead to strangulation. Buttons need to be sewed on tightly. Snaps or Velcro fasteners are safer. If the mother does not have a clothes dryer, she needs a clothes rack to dry the infant's garments when the weather is inclement.

Disposable diapers are handy and most commonly used in hospitals. They have an outer waterproof layer. Diapers are made of gauze, knitted cotton, or bird's-eye or cotton flannel. Contoured and prefolded types are available and are convenient if a diaper service is used. However, they take longer to dry when laundered at home and are more costly. Diaper liners are specially treated tissues placed within the diaper. When diapers are soiled, the stool is rinsed into the toilet. The diapers are soaked in cold water, washed with a mild soap, rinsed thoroughly, and dried by clothes dryer or outdoors in the sun. Diapers that have been improperly washed and rinsed may aggravate rashes.

Waterproof pants should be loose and cut so that air can circulate through them. They are not used when the skin is irritated. If a rash is present, the buttocks are kept exposed to the air as often as possible. Diapers are changed as soon as they are wet. Disposable diapers are avoided for the time being because the plastic covering prevents evaporation. If a rash becomes increasingly worse, the physician is consulted.

The quantity of items that the mother needs is determined by her washing facilities and the climate of the area in which she lives. It is wise to obtain sufficient amounts of the few articles that have to be changed often, for example, three or four dozen diapers, six shirts and blankets, six nightgowns, and two or three sweater sets. Figure 12–13 illustrates the simplest way to dress the newborn.

### HOME PHOTOTHERAPY

Home phototherapy programs are being suggested for newborns with mild to moderate physiologic (normal) jaundice. These programs are advocated because bilirubin levels generally begin to rise on the 2nd or 3rd day after birth, when the mother and newborn are being discharged. Currently, many women are leaving the hospital within 12–24 hours of birth, and a rise in bilirubin levels necessitates the newborn's return to the hospital and possible separation of mother and baby. Home therapy is less costly. Referral for home care is made by the baby's pediatrician on the basis of the newborn's health, bilirubin levels (generally between 10 and 14 mg/dl), evidence of jaundice,

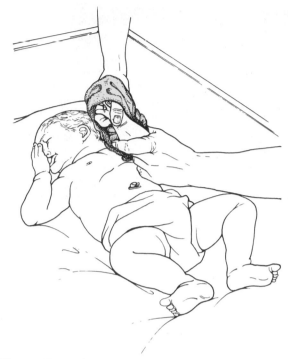

**Figure 12–13.** The simplest way to dress the newborn is to put your hand through the sleeve, grasp the baby's hand, and gently pull it through.

and suitability of the family for complying with the home program.

Lights may be rented from vendors of medical supplies. Fiberoptic phototherapy blankets are also being utilized. They allow for holding the baby and decrease the risk of eye damage. Written instructions are given to the parents. Parents keep a daily record of their baby's temperature, weight, intake and output, stools, and feedings. A nursing care plan for the baby receiving phototherapy appears on page 330.

## KEY POINTS

- The newborn is born with certain reflexes. Three of these are the Moro reflex, the rooting reflex, and the tonic neck reflex.
- The fontanels are soft spots on the baby's head.
- The Apgar score is a standardized method of evaluating the newborn's condition immediately following delivery. Five objective signs are measured. These include heart rate, respiration, muscle tone, reflexes, and color.

- The most critical period for the newborn is the 1st hour of life, when drastic change from life within the uterus to life outside it takes place.
- Physiologic jaundice becomes evident between the 2nd and 3rd day of life and lasts for about 1 week.
- The newborn has an unstable heat-regulating system and must be kept warm.
- Although the kidneys function at birth, they are not fully developed. Likewise, the immune system is not fully activated.
- Cryptorchidism is the medical term for undescended testes.
- Vernix caseosa is a cheeselike substance that covers the skin of the newborn at birth.
- Meconium, the first stool of the newborn, is a mixture of amniotic fluid and secretions of the intestinal glands. They change in color from tarry green, to greenish-yellow (transitional stools), to yellow-gold.

# Study Questions

1. What is the meaning of an Apgar score of 8?
2. Define the following: meconium, vernix caseosa, fontanels, Moro reflex, rooting reflex, and tonic neck reflex.
3. Define circumcision. Describe how you would teach Mrs. Zimmerman how to care for newly circumcised Harold.
4. What measures must the nurse take in order to prevent infection of the newborn in the newborn nursery? On the children's unit? In the home?
5. Baby Rand is crying loudly in her bassinet. List several discomforts that might be the cause of her unhappiness. What can the nurse do to alleviate them? How can you help Mrs. Rand interpret her newborn's crying?
6. Define skin turgor. How does the nurse test for good skin turgor?

# Multiple Choice Review Questions

*Choose the most appropriate answer.*

1. When a baby is born, an orderly series of adaptations from fetal life to extrauterine life takes place. This includes all but
   a. the stimulation of respiration through chilling and chemical changes within the blood
   b. the opening of the alveoli
   c. the beginning of closure of the foramen ovale
   d. the beginning of development of amniocentesis
2. The soft spots on a newborn's head are termed
   a. hematomas
   b. fontanels
   c. sutures
   d. petechiae

3. Infections in the newborn require prompt intervention because
   a. they spread more quickly
   b. infections that are relatively harmless to an adult can be fatal to the newborn
   c. the portals of entry and exit are more numerous
   d. the newborn has no defenses against infection

4. White pinpoint pimples caused by obstruction of sebaceous glands seen on the nose and chin of the newborn are termed
   a. vernix caseosa
   b. acrocyanosis
   c. milia
   d. mongolian spots

5. Which of the following is not a normal finding in the newborn?
   a. heart rate of 60–80 beats/min
   b. acrocyanosis
   c. 97°F temperature
   d. Moro reflex

## BIBLIOGRAPHY

American Academy of Pediatrics (AAP). (1989). Report of the AAP Task Force on Circumcision. *Pediatrics, 84* (4), 388–391.

Anand, P., & Hickey, P. (1987). Pain and its effects in the human neonate and fetus. *New England Journal of Medicine, 317,* 1321.

Behrman, R., & Vaughan V. (1992). *Nelson's textbook of pediatrics* (14th ed.). Philadelphia: W.B. Saunders.

Blackburn, S., & Loper, D. (1992). *Maternal, fetal, and neonatal physiology.* Philadelphia: W.B. Saunders.

Brazelton, T.B. (1973). *The neonatal behavioral assessment scale.* Philadelphia: J.B. Lippincott.

CDC clarifies "Universal Precautions." (1988). *American Journal of Nursing, 88,* 1322.

De Casper, A.M., & Fifer, W.P. (1980). Of human bonding: Newborns prefer their mothers' voices. *Science, 208,* 1174–1176.

Ellis, J. (1985). Home phototherapy for newborn jaundice. *Birth, 12*(Suppl. 3), 15–17.

Gelbaum, I. (1992). Circumcision. *J Nurse Midwifery, 37,* (Suppl. 2):97s.

Graef, J., & Cone, T. (1985). *Manual of pediatric therapeutics.* Boston: Little, Brown.

Green, M., & Haggerty, R. (1990). *Ambulatory pediatrics IV.* Philadelphia: W.B. Saunders.

Kelts, D., & Jones, E. (1985). *Manual of pediatric nutrition.* Boston: Little, Brown.

Levine, M.D., Carey, W.B., & Crocker, A.C. (1992). *Developmental-behavioral pediatrics.* Philadelphia: W.B. Saunders.

Ludwig, M. (1990). Phototherapy in the home setting. *Journal of Pediatric Health, 4,* 304–308.

Lund, M.M. (1990) Perspectives on newborn male circumcision. *Neonatal Network, 9,* 7.

Mott, S., James, S.R., & Sperhac, A.M. (1990). *Nursing care of children and families* (2nd ed.). Reading, MA: Addison-Wesley.

Olds, S.B., London, M., & Ladewig, B. (1992). *Maternal-newborn nursing* (4th ed.). Reading, MA: Addison-Wesley.

Porter, F. (1989). Pain in the newborn. *Clinics in Perinatology, 16,* 549.

Shapiro, C. (1989). Pain in the neonate: Assessment and intervention. *Neonatal Network, 8,* 7.

Slater, L., & Brewe, M. (1984). Home versus hospital phototherapy for term infants with hyperbilirubinemia: A comparative study. *Pediatrics, 73,* 515.

Thompson, E.D., & Ashwill, J.W. (1992). *Pediatric nursing: An introductory text* (5th ed.). Philadelphia: W.B. Saunders.

Whaley, L., & Wong, D. (1991). *Nursing care of infants and children* (4th ed.). St. Louis: C.V. Mosby.

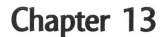

# Chapter 13

# Preterm and Postterm Newborns

# OBJECTIVES

*On completion and mastery of Chapter 13, the student will be able to*

- Define each vocabulary term listed.
- Differentiate between the preterm and the low-birth-weight newborn.
- List three causes of preterm birth.
- Describe the handicaps of preterm birth and the nursing goals associated with each handicap (e.g., "poor control of body temperature—keep warm in isolette.")
- Contrast the techniques for feeding preterm and full-term newborns.
- Discuss two ways to help facilitate maternal-infant bonding for a preterm newborn.
- Devise a nursing care plan for the baby receiving phototherapy.
- List three characteristics of the postterm baby.

## The Preterm Newborn

The preterm (also known as premature) newborn is the most common admission to the intensive care nursery. With increased specialization and sophisticated monitoring techniques, many babies who in the past would have died are now surviving. The nurse's role has become more and more complex, with greater emphasis placed on subtle clinical observations and technology. This chapter acquaints the student with the preterm baby in order to encourage appreciation of this baby's struggle for survival and the intense responsibility placed on those entrusted with this care. The words *preterm* and *premature* are used synonymously, although the former is now considered more accurate.

An interesting historical perspective is provided by Klaus and Kennell (1976). They describe how premature infants were commercially cared for in "child hatcheries" by Martin Cooney, an early neonatologist. Because these babies were not expected to live, they were given to Cooney for exhibition. He settled on Coney Island and successfully cared for more than 5000 premature infants, displaying them in almost all major fairs and expositions from 1902 to 1940. In 1932, at the Chicago World's Fair, the receipts he brought in were "second only to those of Sally Rand the fan dancer" (Fig. 13–1).

When premature infants moved from the fairgrounds to the hospital, most of Cooney's strict practices were adopted, including prohibiting mothers from entering the nursery. The advent of antibiotics and more recent findings on the importance of maternal-infant bonding, however, have changed the tide to favor liberalizing nursery and hospital practices.

Any newborn whose life or quality of existence is threatened is considered to be in a high-risk category and requires close supervision by professionals. Preterm newborns con-

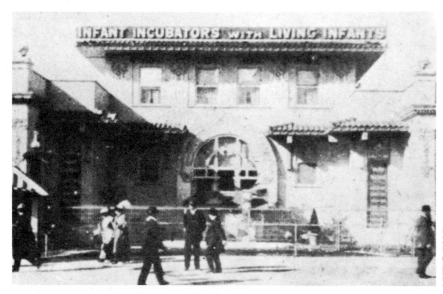

**Figure 13–1.** Outside Cooney's exhibit in San Francisco in 1915. (From Klaus, M.H., & Kennell, J.H. [1976]. *Maternal-infant bonding.* St. Louis: C.V. Mosby.)

stitute a majority of these patients and account for the largest number of admissions to the neonatal intensive care unit. Premature birth is responsible for more deaths during the 1st year of life than any other single factor. Preterm babies also have a higher percentage of birth defects. Prematurity and low birth weight are often concomitant, and both factors are associated with increased neonatal morbidity and mortality. The less a baby weighs at birth, the greater the risks to life during delivery and immediately thereafter.

In the past, a newborn was classified solely by birth weight. Emphasis is now placed on gestational age and level of maturation (Fig. 13–2). Current data also indicate that intrauterine growth rates are not the same for all babies and that individual factors must be considered. *Gestational age* refers to the actual time, from conception to birth, that the fetus remains in the uterus. For the preterm this is less than 38 weeks, for the term baby it is 38–42 weeks, and for the postterm baby it is beyond 42 weeks. One standardized method used to estimate gestational age is the *Dubowitz scoring system*, based on the baby's external characteristics and neurologic development (Figs. 13–3 and 13–4).

*Level of maturation* refers to how well developed the baby is at birth and the ability of the organs to function outside the uterus. The physician can determine much about the maturity of the newborn by careful physical examination, observation of behavior, and family history. A baby who is born at 34 weeks' gestation, weighs 3½ pounds at birth, has not been damaged by multifactorial birth defects, and has had a good placenta may be healthier than a full-term, "small for date" baby whose placenta was insufficient for any of a number of reasons. It is also probably in better condition than the heavy but immature baby of a diabetic mother. Each child has different, distinct needs.

## CAUSES

The predisposing causes of prematurity are numerous; in many instances the cause is unknown. Prematurity may be caused by multiple births, illness of the mother (e.g., malnutrition, heart disease, diabetes mellitus, or infectious conditions), or the hazards of pregnancy itself, such as PiH, placental abnormalities that may result in premature rupture of the membranes,

placenta previa (the placenta lies over the cervix instead of higher in the uterus), and premature separation of the placenta.

Studies also indicate relationships between prematurity and poverty, smoking, alcohol consumption, and cocaine and other drug abuses. Adequate prenatal care to prevent preterm birth is extremely important. Following delivery, early parental interaction with the baby is recognized as essential to the bonding (attachment) process. The presence of parents in special care nurseries is commonplace. Some preterm babies are born into families with numerous other problems. The parents may not be prepared to handle the additional financial and emotional strain imposed by a preterm infant. Parent aides and other types of home support and assistance are vital, particularly because current studies indicate a correlation between high-risk births and child abuse and neglect.

## PHYSICAL CHARACTERISTICS

Preterm birth deprives the newborn of the complete benefits of intrauterine life. The baby whom the nurse sees in the isolette may resemble a fetus of 7 months' gestation. The skin is transparent and loose. Superficial veins may be seen beneath the abdomen and scalp. There is a lack of subcutaneous fat, and fine hair (lanugo) covers the forehead, shoulders, and arms. The cheeselike vernix caseosa is abundant. The extremities appear short. The soles of the feet have few creases, and the abdomen protrudes. The nails are short. The genitals are small. In girls, the labia majora may be open.

## RELATED HANDICAPS

Figure 13–5 graphs various types of neonatal morbidity as a function of weight and gestational age.

**Inadequate Respiratory Function.** Important structural changes occur in fetal lungs during the second half of the pregnancy. The alveoli, or air sacs, enlarge, which brings them closer to the capillaries in the lungs. The failure of this phenomenon leads to many deaths attributed to previability (*pre*, "before," and *vita*, "life"). In addition, the muscles that move the chest are not fully developed; the abdomen is distended, causing pressure on the diaphragm; the stimu-

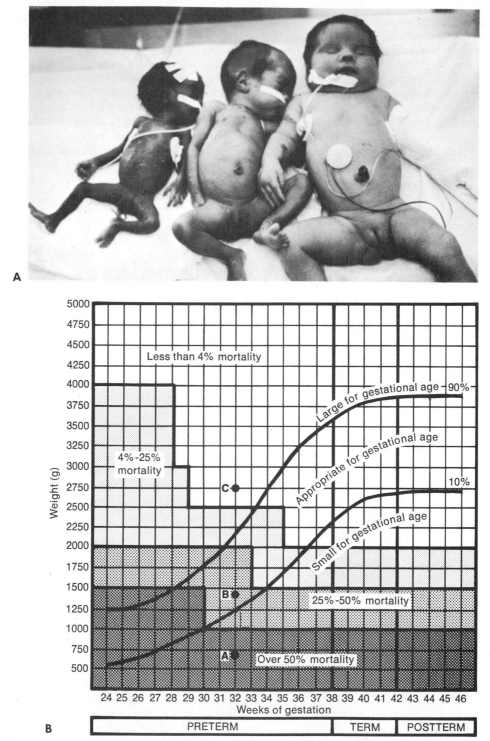

**Figure 13-2.** *A*, Three babies of the same gestational age (32 weeks) weighing 600, 1400, and 2750 gm, respectively, from left to right. (From Korones, S.B. [1986]. *High risk newborn infants: The basis of intensive nursing care* [4th ed.]. St. Louis: C.V. Mosby.) *B*, Classification of the newborn as indicated by relationship of weight to gestational age. The status of the babies in *A* plotted at 32 weeks (dots A, B, and C). (From Battaglia, F.C., & Lubchenco, L.O. [1967]. A practical classification of newborn infants by weight and gestational ages. *Journal of Pediatrics, 71,* 59.)

lation of the respiratory center in the brain is immature; and the gag and cough reflexes are weak because of inadequate nerve supply.

**Respiratory Distress Syndrome.** Respiratory distress syndrome (RDS), also called hyaline membrane disease, is a result of immaturity of the lungs, which leads to decreased gas exchange. An estimated 50% of all neonatal deaths result from RDS or its complications (Behrman, 1992). In this disease, there is a deficient synthesis or release of *surfactant*, a chemical in the lungs. Surfactant is high in lecithin, a fatty protein necessary for absorption of oxygen by the lungs. A test to determine the amount of surfactant in amniotic fluid is the lecithin/sphingomyelin (L/S) ratio. Areas of *atelectasis*, or collapse, also occur, and the functional residual capacity (FRC) of the lungs fails to develop.

*Manifestations.* The symptoms of respiratory distress are generally apparent after delivery, although they may not be manifested for several hours. Respirations increase to 60 or more breaths/min. Rapid respirations (tachypnea) are accompanied by gruntlike sounds, nasal flaring, cyanosis, and intercostal and sternal retractions. As the condition becomes more severe, edema, lassitude, and apnea occur. Mechanical ventilation may be necessary. The treatment of these babies is ideally carried out in the neonatal intensive care unit.

*Treatment.* If insufficient amounts of surfactant are detected through amniocentesis, it is possible to increase its production by giving the mother injections of corticosteroids, such as betamethasone. Administration 1 or 2 days before delivery may reduce the chances of RDS. Surfactant replacement, a new treatment modality, shows some promise. It is administered into the trachea of the preterm via endotracheal tube immediately after birth or within 24 hours. It appears to improve pulmonary function, but its ability to reduce further complications and/or death is yet to be proved.

Continuous positive airway pressure through an intubated airway or an oxygen hood has proved beneficial in preventing postnatal collapse of the alveoli. The lungs begin to produce surfactant generally within 2 or 3 days. Evaluation of the baby's oxygen needs is determined by color and by intermittent arterial blood gas assessment. Behrman (1992) noted that the long-term prognosis of healthy lungs is excellent in newborns surviving this disease.

**Atelectasis.** The lungs are collapsed during fetal life. The lungs must expand somewhat with the first breath, although they do not fully develop until days later. Primary atelectasis, in which the alveoli fail to expand, is common in preterms and infants with damage to the respiratory center of the brain. Secondary atelectasis occurs when the lungs collapse after they have once inflated. This collapse may be caused by pressure from misplaced organs, aspirated mucus, or pulmonary disease. Because this condition is most common among preterm infants, babies born by cesarean delivery, and babies born by difficult labor and delivery, prevention depends on proper prenatal care and delivery.

*Manifestations.* The infant exhibits irregular, rapid respirations. They may be accompanied by a respiratory grunt and flaring of the nostrils. The skin is cyanotic and mottled. Inter-rib and sternal retractions may be noticeable. X-ray films that reveal increased density, sometimes throughout both lungs, confirm the diagnosis. The prognosis depends on the general condition of the baby and the cause of the atelectasis.

**Apnea.** Apnea is defined as the cessation of breathing for 20 seconds or longer. It is not uncommon in the preterm newborn. Apnea may be accompanied by *bradycardia* (fewer than 100 beats/min) and cyanosis. Apnea monitors alert nurses to this complication. Gentle rubbing of the baby's feet, ankles, and back may stimulate breathing following this occurrence. When these measures fail, suctioning of the nose and mouth and raising of the baby's head usually facilitates breathing. If breathing does not begin, an Ambu bag is utilized. Apnea is believed to be related to immaturity of the nervous system.

**Sepsis.** Sepsis is a generalized infection of the blood stream. Preterm newborns are at risk for developing this complication because of the immaturity of many body systems. The liver of the premature infant is immature and forms antibodies poorly. Body enzymes are inefficient. There is little or no immunity received from the mother, and stores of nutrients, vitamins, and iron are deficient. There may be no local signs of infection, which also hinders diagnosis. Table 12–2 outlines the signs and symptoms of sepsis.

The prevention of sepsis or other milder infections is of utmost importance. Merely placing the preterm newborn in an isolette does not en-

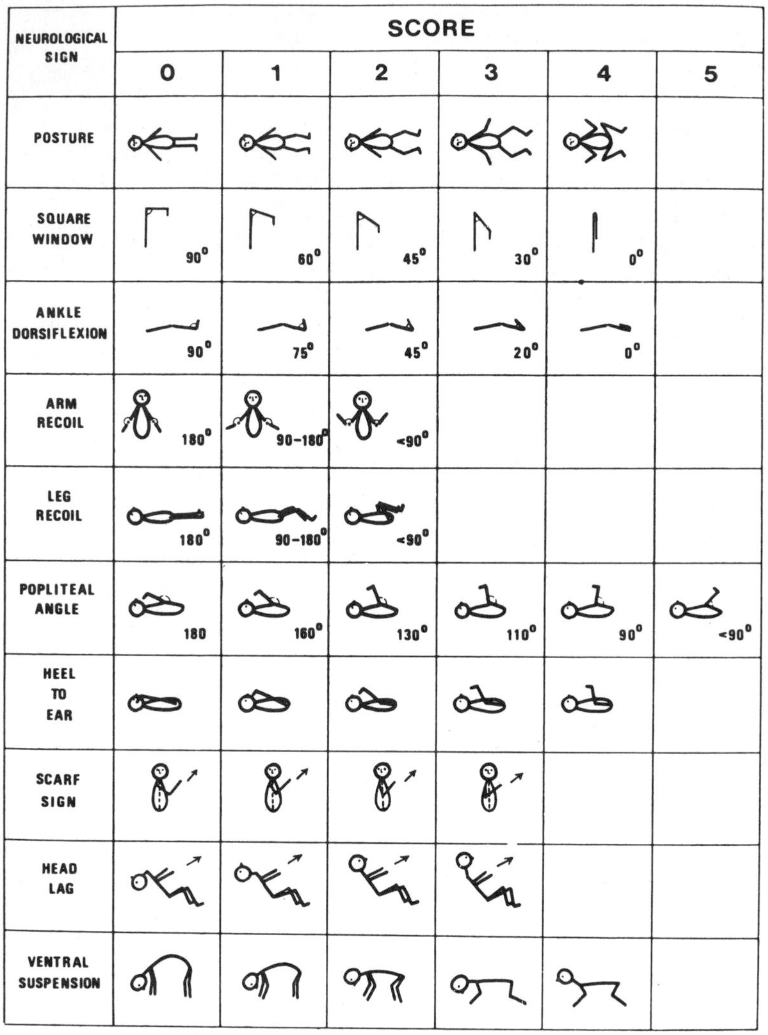

| NEUROLOGICAL SIGN | SCORE | | | | | |
|---|---|---|---|---|---|---|
| | 0 | 1 | 2 | 3 | 4 | 5 |
| POSTURE | | | | | | |
| SQUARE WINDOW | 90° | 60° | 45° | 30° | 0° | |
| ANKLE DORSIFLEXION | 90° | 75° | 45° | 20° | 0° | |
| ARM RECOIL | 180° | 90–180° | <90° | | | |
| LEG RECOIL | 180° | 90–180° | <90° | | | |
| POPLITEAL ANGLE | 180 | 160° | 130° | 110° | 90° | <90° |
| HEEL TO EAR | | | | | | |
| SCARF SIGN | | | | | | |
| HEAD LAG | | | | | | |
| VENTRAL SUSPENSION | | | | | | |

A

**Figure 13–3.** *A,* Dubowitz scoring system for neuromuscular criteria. Add scores for all signs and apply that score to *B.*

sure freedom from infection. The hands must be meticulously washed before and after handling the newborn and between handling different babies. Equipment that is not disposable must be scrupulously cleaned. Each baby should have individual clothing supplies. The baby is handled very gently and as little as possible in order to prevent infection and to conserve energy. The baby is kept warm. If sepsis occurs, the baby is isolated to prevent the infection from spreading throughout the nursery.

**Poor Control of Body Temperature.** Keeping the preterm infant warm is a nursing challenge. Heat loss in the preterm is due to several factors:

1. The preterm infant has a lack of fat, which is the body's insulation.
2. There is excessive heat loss by radiation from a surface area that is large in proportion to body weight. As explained by Olds, London, and Ladewig (1992), this means that the preterm infant's ability to produce heat (body weight) is much smaller than the potential for losing heat (surface area).
3. The heat-regulating center of the brain is immature.
4. The sweat glands are not functioning to capacity.
5. The premature infant is inactive, the mus-

**Score** **Units**

| | 0 | 1 | 2 | 3 | 4 | 5 | 6 | 7 | 8 | 9 |
|---|---|---|---|---|---|---|---|---|---|---|
| 0 | | | | | | 26.0 | 26.0 | 26.5 | 26.5 | 27.0 |
| 10 | 27.0 | 27.5 | 27.5 | 28.0 | 28.0 | 28.5 | 29.0 | 29.0 | 29.5 | 29.5 |
| 20 | 30.0 | 30.0 | 30.5 | 30.5 | 31.0 | 31.0 | 31.5 | 31.5 | 32.0 | 32.0 |
| 30 | 32.5 | 33.0 | 33.0 | 33.5 | 33.5 | 34.0 | 34.0 | 34.5 | 34.5 | 35.0 |
| 40 | 35.0 | 35.5 | 35.5 | 36.0 | 36.0 | 36.5 | 36.5 | 37.0 | 37.5 | 37.5 |
| 50 | 38.0 | 38.0 | 38.5 | 38.5 | 39.0 | 39.0 | 39.5 | 39.5 | 40.0 | 40.0 |
| 60 | 40.5 | 40.5 | 41.0 | 41.0 | 41.5 | 42.0 | 42.0 | 42.5 | 42.5 | 43.0 |
| 70 | 43.0 | | | | | | | | | |

B

**Figure 13–3** *Continued. B*, The way to determine gestational age in weeks is illustrated by the following example: For a score of 44, find 40 in the far left column. Then read across to the column headed by 4. The gestational age is 36.0 weeks. (From Dubowitz, L.M., Dubowitz, V., & Goldberg, C. [1970]. Clinical assessment of gestational age in the newborn infant. *Journal of Pediatrics,77*, 1.)

cles are weak and less resistant to cold, and the baby cannot shiver.

6. The posture of the preterm infant's extremities is one of leg extension. This increases the surface area exposed to the environment and increases heat loss.
7. Metabolism is high, and the preterm infant is prone to low blood glucose (hypoglycemia).

These and other factors make the preterm newborn vulnerable to *cold stress*, which causes an increased need for oxygen and glucose. Early detection can prevent complications.

**Hypoglycemia and Hypocalcemia.** Hypoglycemia (*hypo*, "below," and *glycemia*, "sugar in the blood") is common among preterm babies. They have not remained in the uterus long enough to acquire sufficient stores of glycogen and fat. This condition is aggravated by the need for increased glycogen in the brain, heart, and other tissues as a result of asphyxia, sepsis, RDS, unstable body temperature, and the like. Any condition that increases energy requirements places more stress on these already-deficient stores. Plasma glucose levels of less than 30 mg/dl are indicative of hypoglycemia. Early feeding is one major method of preventing hypoglycemia. Intravenous infusion of glucose is another method.

Hypocalcemia (*hypo*, "below," and *calcemia*, "calcium in the blood") is also seen in preterm and sick newborns. Calcium is transported across the placenta throughout pregnancy, but particularly during the 3rd trimester. Early birth can result in babies with lower serum calcium levels. Other stressors, such as perinatal asphyxia, trauma, or a diabetic mother, may predispose the newborn to hypocalcemia. "Early" neonatal hypocalcemia is seen in the first 2 or 3 days of life. It usually is temporary. "Late" hypocalcemia appears about 1 week after birth. Hypocalcemia may result from decreased activity of the parathyroid glands, especially if the mother is diabetic. This condition is also referred to as "neonatal tetany." Serum calcium levels are monitored for all high-risk newborns. Normal levels range from 8.0 to 10.5 mg/dl. Hypocalcemia is treated by early feedings and calcium supplements when possible.

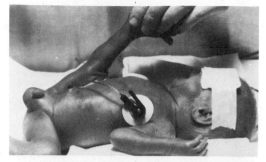

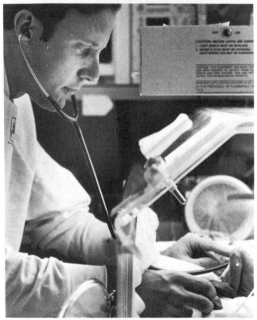

**Figure 13–4.** *A,* The popliteal angle is 180 degrees, rating a score of 0. (From Moore, M.L. [1982]. *Family, newborn, and nurse.* Philadelphia: W.B. Saunders.) *B,* Physical assessment of the preterm infant is an ongoing process. (Courtesy of Blank Memorial Hospital for Children, Des Moines, IA.)

Calcium gluconate may also be given intravenously.

**Increased Tendency to Bleed.** Premature babies are more prone to bleeding than full-term babies because their blood is deficient in prothrombin, a factor of the clotting mechanism. Fragile capillaries of the head are particularly susceptible to injury during delivery, causing intracranial hemorrhage. Ultrasonography is helpful in detecting this problem.

**Retinopathy of Prematurity.** Retinopathy of prematurity (ROP) is a disease that produces separation and fibrosis of the retina, which can lead to blindness (Fig. 13–6). Damage to immature blood vessels is thought to be caused by high oxygen levels of arterial blood. The disease was formerly termed "retrolental fibroplasia," but the term ROP is currently used because it is more precise. It refers to all stages of the disease, from mild to severe—not just end-stage disease. It is the leading cause of blindness in newborns weighing less than 1500 gm. It was believed at first to be caused by oxygen toxicity alone, but now many other factors have been discovered, some of which are not fully understood. The disorder is classified into several stages, and preterm babies who have milder forms of the disorder may have no residual effects or visual disabilities (Behrman, 1992). Prevention of preterm births and the problems that beset preterm infants are the key to resolving ROP. Careful monitoring of arterial blood gases in high-risk infants continues to be a priority in the nursery. Gorrie clarifies further that it is the level of oxygen in the blood, rather than the amount of oxygen received, that is of importance (Gorrie et al., 1994). Consultation with an experienced ophthalmologist is necessary when pathologic signs appear.

**Poor Nutrition.** The stomach capacity of the premature baby is small. The sphincter muscles at both ends of the stomach are immature, contributing to regurgitation and vomiting, particularly after overfeeding. Sucking and swallowing reflexes are immature. The baby's ability to absorb fats is poor (this includes fat-soluble vitamins).

**Necrotizing Enterocolitis.** Necrotizing enterocolitis (NEC) is an acute inflammation of the bowel that leads to bowel *necrosis.* The cause is unknown. Preterm newborns are particularly susceptible to NEC, and the rising incidence of this disease may reflect their improved survival rate (Behrman, 1992). The distal ileum and proximal colon are generally the sites of involvement. Factors implicated in the cause include infectious agents, such as bacteria and rotavirus, and a diminished blood supply to the mucosal cells lining the bowel wall. When the preterm baby is fed, bacteria may multiply. Signs include abdominal distention, bloody stools, diarrhea, and bilious vomitus. Specific nursing attention is directed to observing vital signs, maintaining infection control techniques, carefully resuming oral fluids as ordered, and avoiding taking temperatures

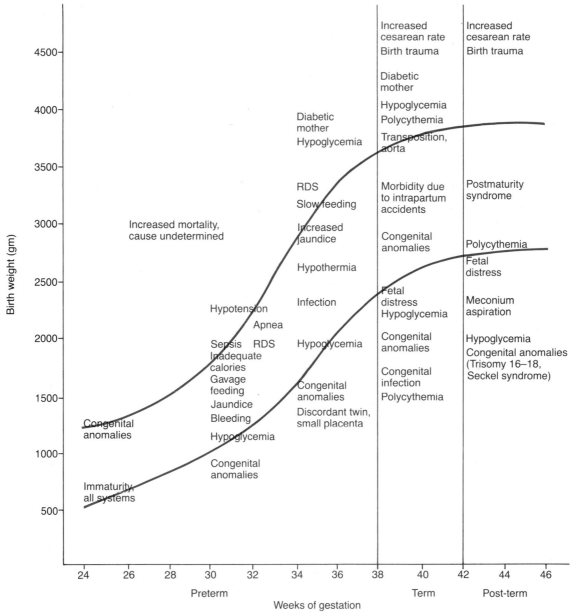

**Figure 13–5.** Neonatal morbidity by birth weight and gestational age. (Modified from Lubchenco, L.O. [1976]. *The high-risk infant*. Philadelphia: W.B. Saunders.)

rectally to prevent bowel perforation. Measuring the abdomen and listening for bowel sounds are also important. Treatment includes antibiotics and the use of parenteral nutrition to rest the bowels. An ostomy may be necessary.

**Immature Kidneys and Skin.** Improper elimination of body wastes contributes to electrolyte imbalance and disturbed acid-base relationships. Dehydration occurs easily. Tolerance to salt is limited, and susceptibility to edema is increased.

**Jaundice (Hyperbilirubinemia).** The liver of the newborn is immature, which contributes to a condition called *icterus* or jaundice (Table 13–1). Jaundice causes the skin and whites of

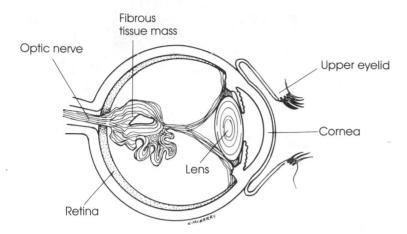

**Figure 13-6.** Advanced retinopathy of prematurity.

the eyes to assume a yellow-orange cast. The liver is unable to clear the blood of bile pigments that result from the normal postnatal destruction of red blood cells. In addition, there may be a deficiency in the enzyme glucuronyl transferase. This enzyme limits the amount of bilirubin that can be conjugated. The amount of bile pigment in the blood serum is expressed as milligrams of bilirubin per deciliter. The higher the bilirubin level, the deeper the jaundice and the greater the risk. An increase of more than 5 mg/dl in 24 hours requires careful investigation. Physiologic jaundice is normal and is discussed on page 306. Pathologic jaundice is more serious. It occurs within 24 hours of birth and is secondary to an abnormal condition such as ABO-Rh incompatibility.

The preterm baby's level of bilirubin increases more rapidly than that of the full-term newborn. Early detection is more difficult because the preterm lacks subcutaneous fat. Race is a factor in this condition. There is a lower incidence among African-American babies, and it is more prevalent among Native Americans, Eskimos, and Asian-Americans. The reason for

this finding is not clear. There is more evidence of jaundice in babies who are breast-fed. Breast-milk jaundice begins to be seen about the 4th day, when the mother's milk supply develops. The newborn does well but is carefully monitored to rule out more serious disease. Breast feeding may be temporarily discontinued.

The aims of treatment for hyperbilirubinemia are to prevent *kernicterus,* a serious neurologic complication that can cause brain damage, and to reverse the hemolytic process caused by blood incompatibilities such as erythroblastosis fetalis (see pp. 355–357). Nursing care and treatment for hyperbilirubinemia consist of phototherapy and other treatments, as designated by the seriousness of the newborn's condition.

## SPECIAL NEEDS

The doctor appraises the physical status of the preterm newborn at delivery. The immediate needs are to clear the baby's airway and to provide warmth. The baby is given care for the umbilical cord and eye care and is then properly identified. Weighing is sometimes omitted until later if the baby's condition is poor. It is placed naked in an isolette and taken to the nursery. The nurse in charge is given a report on the general condition of the newborn, the type of delivery, and any complications that have occurred. Today, many hospitals transfer their preterm infants to special centers geared to care for them. The transport team is briefed by the neonatologist and is dispatched to the referring hospital. A life-support infant-transport

**Table 13-1.** NEONATAL JAUNDICE

| Type | Appears | Peak Bilirubin Concentration | Duration |
|---|---|---|---|
| Physiologic | | | |
| Full-term | 2–3 days | 10–12 mg/dl | 4–5 days |
| Preterm | 3–4 days | 15 mg/dl | 7–9 days |
| Pathologic | 1st day | Unlimited | Varies |
| Breast milk | 4–7 days | 15–20 mg/dl | 16 weeks |

incubator that can be carried by ambulance, and sometimes helicopter, is utilized. Box 13–1 lists some nursing goals for care of the preterm newborn.

### Thermoregulation (Warmth)

*The Isolette.* The preterm newborn is placed in an isolette in order to maintain environmental conditions similar to those of the uterus. The isolette is designed to provide proper heat, humidity, oxygen, and mist; isolation; and protection from infection. The top of the isolette is transparent to enable personnel to view the newborn clearly at all times. Models include alarms to indicate overheating or lack of circulating air, facilities for positioning, and a scale to weigh the baby without removal from the warm environment. Nurses must understand how to use the isolettes available in the nurseries to which they are assigned. They should request assistance if needed. The temperature of the isolette is generally kept at 85–95°F. The nurse records the temperature every 4 hours. The temperature of the baby is stabilized by monitoring with a heat-sensitive probe, which is taped to the abdomen or back. Axillary temperatures are also taken. A relative humidity of 60% or higher is desirable. Overheating should be avoided because it increases the baby's oxygen and calorie requirements.

*Radiant heat.* Radiant heat cribs that supply overhead heat have the advantage of pro-

**BOX 13–1 Nursing Goals for the Preterm Newborn**

The nursing goals in caring for the preterm newborn are to

- Improve respiration
- Maintain body heat (keep the "premie" warm)
- Conserve energy
- Prevent infection
- Provide proper nutrition and hydration
- Give good skin care
- Observe the baby carefully and record observations
- Support and encourage the parents

viding easier access to the patient while maintaining a neutral environment (Fig. 13–7). Refer to Nursing Care Plan 13–1 to find nursing interventions for selected nursing diagnoses pertinent to care of the preterm newborn.

*Kangaroo Care.* Kangaroo care is a new method of care for preterm infants that uses skin-to-skin contact. It is becoming popular in the United States. This method of holding the baby is similar to the way a kangaroo keeps its offspring warm in its pouch (Fig. 13–8). The practice began in 1979 in Bogota, Colombia, in response to a shortage of isolettes and staff.

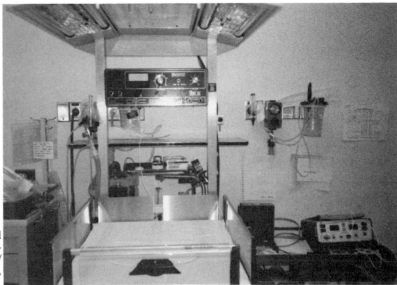

**Figure 13–7.** The radiant warmer is used to conserve the baby's body heat. Note phototherapy lights. (Courtesy of Columbia/HCA Portsmouth Regional Hospital, Portsmouth, NH.)

| NURSING CARE PLAN 13–1 |
| :---: |
| **Selected Nursing Diagnoses for the Preterm Newborn** |

| Goals | Nursing Interventions | Rationales |
| --- | --- | --- |

**Nursing Diagnosis:** High risk for hypothermia related to decreased subcutaneous tissue, immature body temperature control.

| Goals | Nursing Interventions | Rationales |
| --- | --- | --- |
| Baby's temperature will remain at 97.6° F with Servocontrol | 1. Monitor temperature with skin probe or by axillary method | 1. These methods provide best indication of infant's core temperature and are less invasive |
| | 2. Adjust isolette or radiant warmer to maintain skin temperature | 2. A neutral thermal environment permits baby to maintain a normal core temperature with minimum oxygen consumption and caloric expenditure |
| | 3. Observe for signs of cold stress, such as decreased temperature, pallor, and lethargy | 3. Preterm babies have little or no muscular activity; they remain in an extended posture because of lack of muscle tone; they cannot shiver |
| | 4. Use discretion in bathing | 4. Temperature of a wet baby drops quickly as a result of evaporation |
| | 5. Avoid cold surfaces | 5. Conductive heat loss occurs when a baby is weighed on a cold scale; prewarm surfaces or use receiving blanket for protection |

**Nursing Diagnosis:** High risk for impaired skin integrity related to immature skin, poor nutrition, and immobility.

| Goals | Nursing Interventions | Rationales |
| --- | --- | --- |
| Skin will remain intact | 1. Change position regularly | 1. This prevents pressure sores and aids respiration and circulation |
| | 2. Be gentle when removing dressings, tape, and electrodes | 2. The preterm's skin is fragile and bruises easily; use as little tape as possible |
| | 3. Cleanse skin with clear water or approved cleansers | 3. Avoid hexachlorophene cleaners because of their toxic effect; all products need to be carefully assessed before use because permeability of preterm's skin fosters absorption of ingredients |
| | 4. Observe skin for signs of infection while recognizing that there may be no local inflammatory response, only vague signs and symptoms | 4. Heel pricks and other invasive procedures are often necessary; preterm baby's immune system is immature and healing becomes difficult |

The baby, wearing only a diaper and small cap, rests at the mother or father's naked breast. The skin warms and calms the child and promotes bonding. Anderson (1991) describes several research studies that indicate that the babies were warm enough; had adequate oxygenation; had fewer episodes of periodic breathing, apnea, and bradycardia; and had no increase in infection. Protocols for use are being established in several U.S. hospitals. Long-term outcomes have not yet been determined.

**Nutrition.** Feeding of the preterm newborn varies with gestational age and health status. There is currently controversy about the type and timing of feedings. One reason for this con-troversy is that the optimal growth rate is unclear. In the past, the preterm newborn was given nothing by mouth for the first 24–72 hours. Today, early feedings of sterile water or glucose solution are given to prevent dehydration, hyperbilirubinemia (*hyper*, "excessive," *bilirubin*, "bile," and *emia*, "blood"), and hypoglycemia (low blood sugar). The preterm newborn is at risk because early birth has denied the baby time to store needed nutrients, such as glycogen and fat. In addition, water and caloric requirements are higher.

Human milk is ideal because its fat is absorbed readily. Breast milk is sometimes supplemented with a glucose solution, such as

Polycose, to increase caloric intake. The use of milk obtained from milk banks or donors is no longer popular because of many factors, including the risk of human immunodeficiency virus and cytomegalovirus infections. A number of commercial formulas for the preterm infant are available.

The preterm may be fed orally, by gavage (tube feeding), or parenterally. Oral feedings are ordered in milliliters; as little as 2–4 ml may initially be given. Special nipples that are small and soft are used. Often the infant is fed while still in the isolette warming bed. Fluids may be administered intravenously by a catheter passed into the umbilical vein. Again, only very small amounts of fluid are given, sometimes as little as 5 ml/hr. Because the preterm infant's suckling may be weak and swallowing reflexes are immature, gavage feedings may be necessary. Supplemental vitamins (C, D, and E) may be prescribed.

The technique of formula feeding is similar to that for the term newborn, with adjustments for the preterm infant's smaller stomach capacity, lower gastric acidity, and poor absorption of fats. The feeding should take no longer than 15–20 minutes to avoid the expenditure of necessary calories. Overfeeding is dangerous. The hazards of aspiration are increased because gag and cough reflexes are weak, which makes airway clearance more difficult. Careful burping is necessary. Following the feeding, the preterm is placed on the right side with the head slightly raised unless the position is contraindicated by other conditions.

The nurse reports the number of voidings and color of the patient's urine, periodically measures specific gravity, and watches for signs of edema. The hydration needs of the patient are reviewed daily on the basis of intake, output, weight, blood chemistries, and general appearance. *Hyperalimentation*, that is, total parenteral nutrition, provides fluid, calories, electrolytes, and vitamins to sustain growth. It may be lifesaving for an infant whose birth weight is very low.

**Close Observation.** The doctor examines the preterm newborn when the patient's condition permits and writes specific orders for treatment and nursing care. When the doctor leaves the nursery, the nurse is responsible for reporting any significant changes in the baby's condition. The experienced nurse in the preterm nursery observes and charts care and treatment in great detail (Fig. 13–9). For example, a chapter

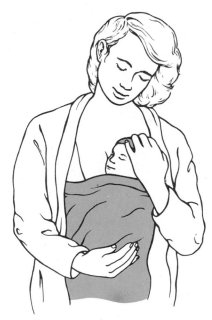

**Figure 13–8.** Kangaroo care (nature's incubator).

could be spent on observations of the preterm infant's behavior during feedings. Table 13–2 lists *general* observations to guide care of the preterm newborn. Sudden changes are immediately reported.

**Positioning, Skin Care, and Phototherapy.** The preterm newborn is positioned on the back with the head of the mattress slightly elevated unless contraindicated. In this position the abdominal contents do not press against the diaphragm and impede breathing. The baby should not be left in one position for long periods because it is uncomfortable and may harm the lungs. Changing the position also prevents breakdown from pressure on the infant's delicate skin. If such a breakdown should occur, the area is exposed to the air, and a suitable ointment is applied as prescribed by the doctor (see p. 305 for a more extended discussion on the skin of the newborn).

As mentioned earlier, jaundice is caused by too much bilirubin in the tissues of the body. It can be detected by observing the color of the skin and the whites of the eyes, both of which assume a yellowish cast. Another sign is the presence of bilirubin by-products in the urine. Pale stools in the presence of jaundice indicate an obstruction in the bile duct system. Although jaundice is common, particularly in

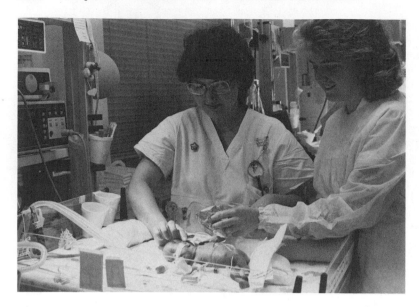

**Figure 13–9.** Although sophisticated monitoring devices are now available, the nurse's astute observation of the patient remains crucial. (Courtesy of Mercy Hospital Medical Center, Des Moines, IA.)

preterm newborns, all cases should be reported so that the possibility of a more serious underlying condition can be ruled out. Because bilirubin breaks down faster in the presence of light, phototherapy is used to manage jaundice. Nursing Care Plan 13–2 outlines care for newborns receiving phototherapy.

**Table 13–2.** NURSING OBSERVATIONS IN CARE OF THE PRETERM BABY

| Observation | Signs to Look for |
|---|---|
| Color | Paleness, cyanosis, jaundice |
| Respirations | Regularity, apnea, sternal retractions, labored breathing |
| Pulse | Rate and regularity |
| Abdomen | Distention |
| Stools | Frequency, color, consistency |
| Skin | Rashes, irritations, pustules, edema |
| Cord | Discharge |
| Eyes | Discharge |
| Feeding | Sucking ability, vomiting or regurgitation, degree of satisfaction |
| Mucous membranes | Dryness of lips and mouth, signs of thrush |
| Voiding | Initial, frequency |
| Fontanels | Sunkenness or bulging |
| General activity | Increase or decrease in movements, lethargy, twitching, frequency and quality of cry, hyperactivity |

## PROGNOSIS

In the absence of severe birth defects and complications, the growth rate of the preterm newborn nears that of the term baby by about the 2nd year. Very-low-birth-weight infants may not catch up, especially if there has been chronic illness, insufficient nutritional intake, or inadequate caretaking (Behrman, 1992). Additional studies are needed in order to determine the effects of these factors at various age levels. Parents need to be prepared for relatives' comments on the baby's small size and slower development. In general, growth and development of the preterm infant is based on current age minus the number of weeks before term the infant was born; for example, if born at 36 weeks' gestation, a 1-month-old infant would be at a newborn's achievement level. This calculation ensures that no one has unrealistic expectations for the infant.

## FAMILY REACTION

Parents need guidance throughout the infant's hospitalization to help prepare them for this new experience. They may be disheartened by the unattractive appearance of the preterm newborn. They may believe that they are to blame for the baby's condition. They may fear that the baby will die but may be unable to express their feelings. They need time to look at

## Nursing Brief

Encourage parents to talk about their feelings and fears concerning the preterm baby. Answer questions about home care.

and touch the baby, and to begin to see the child as uniquely their own. This touch and immediate human contact are vital for the infant as well. The mother is usually concerned with her ability to care for such a small and helpless creature. When she feels ready, she may assist the nurse in diapering, bathing, feeding, and so on. During these times, other aspects of baby care are also stressed.

Often a mother is discharged without her baby. This is difficult for the entire family and makes attachment and bonding more complicated. The nurse encourages the family to keep in touch by telephone and by visits. Parents can help siblings accept the infant by addressing the child by name, sharing news of progress, taking pictures of the infant, and encouraging communication by drawings and cards. Listening to what siblings are saying provides information for discussion.

Discharge planning begins at birth. The parents will require demonstration and practice in routine and/or specialized care. Visits by the nurse to assess home care and provide additional support are valuable. Continued medical supervision is important. The nurse stresses the importance of well-baby examinations, immunizations, and prevention of infection. Good prenatal care for subsequent pregnancies is emphasized because this mother is at high risk for future preterm births.

## The Postterm Newborn

The newborn is considered *postterm* if a pregnancy goes beyond 42 weeks. *Postmaturity* refers to the infant's showing characteristics of the postmature syndrome. Identification of babies who are not tolerating the extra time in the uterus is the major goal of treatment. Death is uncommon today because of early detection and intervention. What causes postma-

turity is not yet clear; however, it is known that the placenta does not function adequately as it ages, which could result in fetal distress. The *mortality* rate of late babies is higher than that of newborns delivered at term. *Morbidity* rates are also higher. Once the baby makes it through delivery, the risks are fewer.

The late birth is a psychological strain on the mother, father, and other members of the family, who are eagerly awaiting the arrival of the baby. The nurse encourages parents to verbalize their feelings and concerns about the delay. Very large newborns, such as those of diabetic mothers, are not necessarily postmature but are larger than normal because of rapid abnormal growth before delivery. The following problems are associated with postmaturity:

- Asphyxia due to chronic hypoxia in the uterus from a deteriorated placenta
- Meconium aspiration; hypoxia and distress may cause relaxation of the anal sphincter; meconium can be aspirated into the fetal lungs
- Poor nutritional status; depleted glycogen reserves cause hypoglycemia
- Increase in red blood cell production (polycythemia) due to hypoxia
- Difficult delivery due to increased size of baby
- Birth defects
- Seizures as a result of the hypoxic state

### PHYSICAL CHARACTERISTICS AND CARE

The postterm infant is long and thin and looks as though weight has been lost. The skin is loose, especially about the thighs and buttocks. There is little lanugo (downy hair) or vernix caseosa. Loss of the cheeselike vernix caseosa leaves the skin dry; it cracks, peels, and is almost like parchment in texture. The nails are long and may be stained with meconium. The baby has a good head of hair and looks alert. Many postterm babies suffer few adverse effects from the delay, but they still require careful observation in the nursery.

The management of postmaturity may include a nonstress test and a contraction stress test. Cesarean deliveries are now commonly performed if the pregnancy is determined, by testing, to be past 42 weeks or if there are signs of fetal distress or maternal risk.

| NURSING CARE PLAN 13–2 | | |
|---|---|---|
| **Selected Nursing Diagnoses for the Baby Receiving Phototherapy** | | |
| **Goals** | **Nursing Interventions** | **Rationale** |

**Nursing Diagnosis:** High risk for injury to eyes and gonads related to phototherapy.

| Baby does not have eye drainage or irritation<br>Genitals are protected | 1. Apply eye patches over infant's closed eyes before placing infant under lights<br>2. Remove patches at least once per shift to assess eyes for conjunctivitis<br>3. Remove patches to allow eye contact during feeding<br>4. Cover ovaries or testes with diaper | 1. Closing eyes prevents corneal abrasion, protects retina from damage by high-intensity light<br>2. Facilitates early detection of inflammation and jaundice (sclera may yellow)<br>3. Provides for visual stimulation and bonding<br>4. Protects gonads from damage by heat |

**Nursing Diagnosis:** Altered skin integrity related to immature structure and function, immobility.

| Skin remains intact as evidenced by absence of skin rash, excoriation, or redness | 1. Observe for maculopapular rash<br><br>2. Cleanse rectal area gently, as stools are often green and liquid<br><br>3. Reposition at least every 2 hr<br><br>4. Assess for jaundice or bronzing (note: serum bilirubin may be high even though baby may not appear jaundiced under lights)<br><br>5. Observe for pressure areas | 1. Rashes and burns have been known to occur as a result of phototherapy<br>2. Frequent stools may cause breakdown of skin; loose stools are result of increased bilirubin excretion<br>3. Repositioning provides exposure of all skin areas<br>4. Observation of jaundice may be initial sign of hyperbilirubinemia. Bronze baby syndrome appears in preterms who do not excrete the photooxidation products adequately.<br>5. Early intervention prevents skin breakdown |

**Nursing Diagnosis:** High risk for fluid volume deficit related to increased water loss through skin and loose stools.

| Baby does not become dehydrated, as evidenced by good skin turgor, normal fontanels, and moist tongue and mucous membranes<br>Weight maintenance, urine output satisfactory | 1. Monitor intravenous fluids<br><br><br>2. Check skin turgor<br><br>3. Observe for depressed fontanel<br>4. Anticipate the need for additional water between feedings<br><br>5. Daily weights unless contraindicated | 1. IV fluids are sometimes used to prevent dehydration or in anticipation of exchange transfusion<br>2. Helps determine extent of dehydration<br>3. Sign of dehydration<br>4. Adequate hydration facilitates elimination and excretion of bilirubin<br>5. Assess progress; helps determine extent of dehydration |

**Nursing Diagnosis:** High risk for hyperthermia or hypothermia.

| Baby does not become overheated or chilled; temperature will be maintained between 36.3 and 37.4°C (97.4 and 99.4°F) | 1. Monitor baby's temperature<br><br><br>2. Adjust isolette to maintain neutral thermal environment | 1. Hyperthermia and hypothermia are common complications of phototherapy<br>2. Avoid overheating isolette or warming unit |

| NURSING CARE PLAN 13–2 *Continued* | | |
|---|---|---|
| **Selected Nursing Diagnoses for the Baby Receiving Phototherapy** | | |
| Goals | Nursing Interventions | Rationale |

**Nursing Diagnosis:** High risk for neurologic injury related to nature of hyperbilirubinemia.

| Goals | Nursing Interventions | Rationale |
|---|---|---|
| Baby will show no signs of neurologic involvement (lethargy, twitching) | 1. Anticipate daily bilirubin blood levels | 1. Phototherapy success determined by frequently measuring serum bilirubin levels |
| | 2. Turn off phototherapy lights when blood is being drawn in order to avoid false readings | 2. Promotes accuracy of blood test |
| | 3. Observe parameters for neurologic deficit (e.g., twitching, lethargy) | 3. Kernicterus (brain damage) is rare but is evidenced by neurologic sequelae such as hypotonia, diminished reflexes, twitching, lethargy |

**Nursing Diagnosis:** Nutrition alterations: less than body requirements.

| Goals | Nursing Interventions | Rationale |
|---|---|---|
| Baby receives adequate nutrients as evidenced by stabilization of weight, laboratory reports | 1. Provide feedings as ordered | 1. Early feedings within 4–6 hr following delivery tend to decrease high bilirubin levels as well as to provide nourishment |
| | 2. Assist mother to reestablish breast feeding if temporarily halted | 2. Encourage mother, help her to feel more in control, promotes bonding; opinions of physicians vary as to discontinuance of breast feeding, as the cause of breast milk jaundice is not known |

**Nursing Diagnosis:** High risk for injury related to immobility, electrical apparatus.

| Goals | Nursing Interventions | Rationale |
|---|---|---|
| Baby will show no signs of burns or other breaks in skin integrity. | 1. Ascertain that all electrical outlets are grounded | 1–3. Safety is an important consideration in all procedures involving patients and equipment |
| | 2. Record number of hours lights have been in use, change as necessary | |
| | 3. Use plexiglass cover or shield to protect baby in case of lamp breakage | |

**Nursing Diagnosis:** Parental anxiety related to knowledge deficit, crisis of having a baby with jaundice.

| Goals | Nursing Interventions | Rationale |
|---|---|---|
| Parents express fears concerning baby's welfare | 1. Explain procedures and treatment | 1. Information decreases parental stress |
| | 2. Provide reassurance | 2. Parents are in need of support persons |
| | 3. Provide follow-up | 3. Follow-up care is reassuring to parents and medical personnel that family is progressing nicely without complications |

# Transporting the High-Risk Newborn

Transportation of the high-risk newborn to a regional neonatal center requires organization and the expertise of a special team. A nurse and sometimes a doctor accompany the baby unless specialists (e.g., life-flight helicopter personnel) are part of the transport team. Stabilization of the baby before discharge is important. Baseline data, such as vital signs and blood work (blood gases and glucose levels), are obtained. The baby is weighed if this is not contraindicated. Copies of all records are made. This includes the baby's record, the mother's prenatal history and delivery, and pertinent admission data. A transport incubator is provided for warmth. Batteries are kept fully charged.

The mother is shown the newborn before departure. If the mother is unable to hold the baby because of its condition, the isolette is wheeled to the bedside for her observation. A picture is taken and given to the parents. On occasion, a mother is unable to see her baby because of her own unstable condition. Such situations require special empathy from nursing personnel. Once the baby has safely reached its destination, the parents are contacted by telephone. It is also thoughtful if the receiving hospital personnel provide feedback to the transport team so that they may enjoy the results of their efforts.

## KEY POINTS

- Early identification of the high-risk fetus facilitates treatment and nursing care.
- Studies indicate that there is a relationship between prematurity and poverty, smoking, alcohol consumption, and narcotics use.
- The preterm newborn is observed very carefully, and a detailed record of progress is maintained by the nurse.
- Respiratory distress syndrome has a high mortality rate, and it may precipitate long-term effects.
- Problems associated with prematurity include asphyxia, meconium aspiration, hypoglycemia, hypocalcemia, hemorrhage from fragile vessels, poor resistance to infection, and inadequate nutrition.
- Heat or thermoregulation is essential for the preterm newborn's survival. Cold stress is to be avoided.
- Nursing goals in caring for the preterm newborn are to improve respirations, maintain body heat, conserve baby's energy, prevent infection, provide nutrition and hydration, give good skin care, and support and encourage the parents.
- Oxygen is administered very carefully to preterm newborns to help prevent eye complications, such as retinopathy of prematurity.
- Phototherapy is used to treat jaundice.
- The postterm newborn is born after 42 weeks of gestation and shows certain characteristics that place the baby at risk.

# Study Questions

1. List the handicaps associated with the preterm baby.
2. What is an isolette? A radiant warmer? Kangaroo care?
3. How does the nursing care of the premature baby differ from that of the full-term newborn?
4. Define the following: preterm, sternal retractions, oxygen analyzer, phototherapy.
5. What is retinopathy of prematurity?
6. Close observation is extremely important in the care of the preterm newborn. List several significant changes that should be reported to the nurse in charge.
7. What problems confront the parents of the preterm newborn? In what ways might the nurse facilitate maternal-infant bonding?

# Multiple Choice Review Questions

*Choose the most appropriate answer.*

1. A standardized method of determining gestational age based on appearance and neuromuscular criteria is the
   a. Gesell graph
   b. Dubowitz score
   c. Washington guide
   d. Friedman curve

2. Some preterm babies are fed by gavage because of
   a. poor digestion
   b. overdeveloped gag and cough reflexes
   c. refusal of formula
   d. weak sucking and swallowing reflexes

3. Phototherapy is used to correct
   a. hypoglycemia
   b. jaundice
   c. macrosomia
   d. glycosuria

4. The actual time that the fetus remains in the uterus is termed
   a. gestational age
   b. interuterine growth rate
   c. neurologic age
   d. level of maturation

5. Excessive arterial oxygen in a preterm may cause
   a. hyaline membrane disease
   b. cyanosis
   c. retinopathy of prematurity
   d. primary atelectasis

## BIBLIOGRAPHY

Affonso, D., Bosque, E., Wahlberg, V., & Brady, J.P. (1993). Reconciliation and healing for mothers through skin to skin contact provided in an American tertiary level intensive care nursery. *Neonatal Network, 12,* 25–32.

Anderson, G. (1991). Current knowledge about skin-to-skin (kangaroo) care for preterm infants. *Journal of Perinatology, 11.*

Behrman, R. (1992). *Nelson textbook of pediatrics* (14th ed.). Philadelphia: W.B. Saunders.

Betz, C., Hunsberger, M., & Wright, S. (1994). *Family-centered nursing care of children.* Philadelphia: W.B. Saunders.

Blackburn, S., & Loper, D. (1992). *Maternal, fetal, and neonatal physiology.* Philadelphia: W.B. Saunders.

Creasy, R., & Resnik, R. (1992). *Maternal-fetal medicine.* Philadelphia: W.B. Saunders.

Gorrie, T., McKinney, E., & Murray, S. (1994). *Foundations of maternal newborn nursing.* Philadelphia: W.B. Saunders.

Graef, J., & Cane, T. (1988). *Manual of pediatric therapeutics.* Boston: Little, Brown.

Klaus, M.H., & Fanaroff, A.A. (1993). *Care of the high-risk neonate* (4th ed.). Philadelphia: W.B. Saunders.

Klaus, M.H., & Kennell, J. (1976). *Maternal-infant bonding.* St. Louis: C.V. Mosby.

Mott, S., James, S.R., & Sperhac, A.M. (1990). *Nursing care of children and families* (2nd ed.). Redwood City, CA: Addison-Wesley.

Nelson, L. (1984). *Pediatric ophthalmology.* Philadelphia: W.B. Saunders.

Olds, S.B., London, M., & Ladewig, P. (1992). *Maternal-newborn nursing* (4th ed.). Reading, MA: Addison-Wesley.

Thompson, E.D., & Ashwill, J.W. (1992). *Pediatric nursing: An introductory text.* Philadelphia: W.B. Saunders.

Whaley, L., & Wong, D. (1988). *Essentials of pediatric nursing* (3rd ed.). St. Louis: C.V. Mosby.

Whaley, L., & Wong, D. (1991). *Nursing care of infants and children* (4th ed.). St. Louis: C.V. Mosby.

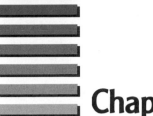

# Chapter 14

---

# The Newborn with Special Needs

# OBJECTIVES

*On completion and mastery of Chapter 14, the student will be able to*

- Define each vocabulary term listed.
- List and define the more common disorders of the newborn period.
- Describe five classifications of birth defects.
- Outline the nursing care for the infant with hydrocephalus.
- Outline the preoperative and postoperative nursing care of a newborn with spina bifida cystica.
- Describe the symptoms of increased intracranial pressure.
- Differentiate between cleft lip and cleft palate.
- Discuss the early signs of dislocation of the hip.
- Discuss the care of the newborn with Down syndrome.
- Outline the causes and treatment of hemolytic disease of the newborn (erythroblastosis fetalis).
- List four infectious diseases seen in the newborn period.
- Formulate a nursing care plan for the patient with acquired immunodeficiency syndrome (AIDS).

| BOX 14–1 | Classification of Birth Defects |
|---|---|

**Malformations Present at Birth**

Structural defects, such as hydrocephalus, spina bifida, congenital heart malformations, cleft lip and palate, clubfoot, and congenital hip dysplasia

**Metabolic Defects (Body Chemistry)**

Cystic fibrosis, phenylketonuria, Tay-Sachs disease, family hypercholesterolemia—high cholesterol that often causes early heart attack, and others

**Blood Disorders**

Sickle cell anemia, hemophilia, thalassemia, defects of white blood cells and immune defense, and others

**Chromosomal Abnormalities**

Down syndrome, Klinefelter's syndrome, Turner's syndrome, trisomies 13 and 18, and many others; most involve some combination of mental retardation and physical malformations ranging from mild to fatal in severity

**Perinatal Damage**

Infections, drugs, maternal disorders, abnormalities unique to pregnancy (Rh disease, difficult labor or delivery, premature birth)

Data from *Birth defects* (1992). White Plains, NY: March of Dimes Birth Defects Foundation.

Birth defects affect more than 250,000 infants in the United States each year. According to the March of Dimes Birth Defects Foundation (Birth Defects, 1992), they occur in 1 of every 14 births, affecting millions of families. An abnormality of structure, function, or metabolism may result in a physical or mental handicap, may shorten life, or may be fatal. Box 14–1 shows the system of classification of birth defects. Because these disorders include so many conditions, it has been necessary to limit the number discussed in this chapter and to place others in relevant areas of the text (see Index for specific conditions).

*Defects present at birth* often involve the skeletal system; limbs may be missing, malformed, or duplicated. Some abnormalities, such as congenital hip dysplasia, are more subtle, and the nurse must be alert to detect them. *Inborn errors of metabolism* include a number of inherited diseases that affect body chemistry. There may be an absence or a deficiency of a substance necessary for cell metabolism. The deficient substance is usually an enzyme. Almost any organ of the body may be damaged. Examples of inborn errors of metabolism include cystic fibrosis and phenylketonuria (PKU). In *disorders of the blood*, there is a reduced or missing blood component or an inability of a component to function adequately. Sickle cell anemia, thalassemia, and hemophilia fall into this category. *Chromosomal abnormalities* number in the hundreds. Most involve some type of mental retardation, and some are incompatible with life. The newborn with Turner's syndrome or Klinefelter's syndrome may be retarded in physical growth and sexual development. *Perinatal damage* has many causes and is seen in a variety of forms, the most common of which is premature birth.

"Few birth defects can be attributed to a single cause. The majority are thought to result from an interplay between environment and

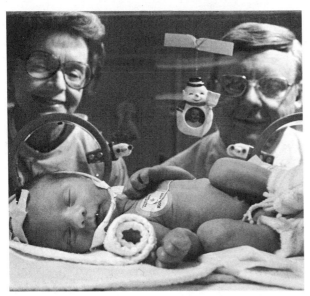

**Figure 14–1.** Visits from relatives are encouraged in the neonatal unit when a newborn is detained for an extended period of time. (Courtesy of Blank Memorial Hospital for Children, Des Moines, IA.)

heredity, depending on inhcrited susceptibility, stage of pregnancy, and degree of environmental hazard" (Birth Defects, 1992). Newborns with birth defects may have to remain in the neonatal unit for an extended period (Fig. 14–1).

# Malformations Present at Birth

This discussion covers *congenital* malformations, or those present at birth, according to body systems.

### NERVOUS SYSTEM

### Hydrocephalus

**Description.** Hydrocephalus (*hydro*, "water," and *cephalo*, "head") is a condition characterized by an increase of cerebrospinal fluid (CSF) in the ventricles of the brain, which causes an increase in head size and pressure changes in the brain. It results from an imbalance between production and absorption of CSF. Hydrocephalus may be congenital or acquired. It is most commonly caused by an obstruction, such as a tumor, or by improper formation of the ventricles. It may occur with a meningomyelocele or as a sequela of infections (including congenital TORCH* infections, encephalitis, or meningitis) or perinatal hemorrhage. The symptoms depend on the site of obstruction and the age at which it develops.

Hydrocephalus is classified as noncommunicating (obstructive) or communicating. *Noncommunicating hydrocephalus* results from obstruction of CSF flow from the ventricles of the brain to the subarachnoid space. Communicating hydrocephalus results when CSF flow is not obstructed in the ventricles but is inadequately reabsorbed in the subarachnoid space. Hydrocephalus may proceed slowly or rapidly. Two forms of hydrocephalus are the Arnold-Chiari malformation and the Dandy-Walker syndrome.

The nurse recalls that the brain and spinal cord are surrounded by fluid, membranes, and bone. The three membranes, called *meninges*, are the dura mater, the arachnoid, and the pia mater. The arachnoid, or middle membrane, resembles a cobweb with fluid-filled spaces. CSF is also found in spaces of the brain called *ventricles*. The primary site of formation is believed to be the *choroid plexus*.

**Manifestations.** The signs and symptoms of hydrocephalus depend on time of onset and severity of the imbalance. The classic sign is an increase in head size. The direction of skull expansion depends on the site of the obstruction. Transillumination (*trans*, "across," and *illuminare*, "to enlighten"), the inspection of a cavity or organ by passing a light through its walls, is a simple diagnostic procedure useful in visualizing fluid. A flashlight with a sponge-rubber collar is held tightly against the infant's head in a dark room. The examiner observes for areas of increased luminosity. A small ring of light is normal; a large halo effect is not (Fig. 14–2).

A bulging anterior fontanel and separation of the cranial sutures are other signs of this condition. The scalp is shiny, and the veins are dilated. In advanced cases, the pupil of the eyes may appear to be looking downward, while the sclera may be seen above the pupil, much like the look of a setting sun (Fig. 14–3). The infant is helpless and lethargic. The body becomes

---

*TORCH stands for *t*oxoplasmosis, *r*ubella, *c*ytomegalovirus, and *h*erpes simplex (see p. 108).

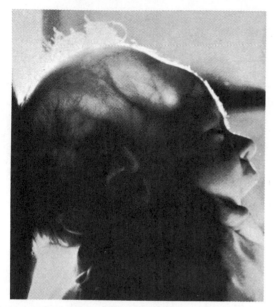

**Figure 14-2.** A halo of light through the skull indicates a loss or thinning of cerebral cortex. (From Jarvis, C. [1992]. *Physical examination and health assessment.* Philadelphia: W.B. Saunders.)

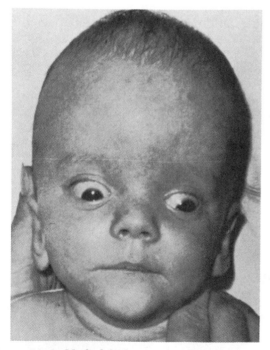

**Figure 14-3.** Marked hydrocephalus with "setting sun" sign and divergence of the eyes. (From Youmans, J.R. [1982]. *Neurological surgery* [2nd ed.]. Philadelphia: W.B. Saunders.)

thin, and the muscle tone of the extremities is often poor. The cry is shrill and high-pitched. Irritability, vomiting, and anorexia are present, and convulsions may occur.

**Diagnosis.** The child's head is measured daily. Echoencephalography, computed tomography (CT) scan, and magnetic resonance imaging (MRI) are tests used to visualize the enlarged ventricles and identify the area of obstruction. A ventricular tap or puncture may be performed in the treatment room using sterile technique. The equipment needed is the same as that for a lumbar puncture. A specimen is labeled and sent to the laboratory for analysis.

**Treatment.** After careful evaluation of preoperative test results, the decision of whether to operate is made. The surgeon attempts to bypass or *shunt* the point of obstruction. The CSF may thus be carried to another area of the body, where it is absorbed and finally excreted. This is accomplished by inserting special tubing, which is replaced at intervals as the child grows. Two widely used procedures are the ventriculoatrial shunt and the ventriculoperitoneal shunt (Fig. 14-4).

The prognosis for the child with this condition has improved with modern drugs and surgical techniques. If the brain is not seriously damaged before the operation, mental function may be preserved. Motor development is sometimes slower if the child cannot lift the head normally. Complications of shunts are usually mechanical (kinking or plugging of tubing) or infection. The shunt acts as a focal spot for infection and may need to be removed if infection persists.

**Nursing Care.** The general nursing care of an infant with hydrocephalus who has not undergone surgery presents several problems. The child may be barely able to raise the head. Mental development is delayed. Lack of appetite, a tendency to vomit easily, and poor resistance to infections present challenging problems.

The position of the patient must be changed frequently in order to prevent hypostatic pneumonia and pressure sores. Hypostatic pneumonia occurs when the circulation of the blood in the lungs is poor and the patient remains in one position too long. It is particularly prevalent in patients who are poorly nourished or weak, or who have a debilitating disease. When the nurse turns the patient with hydrocephalus, the head must always be supported.

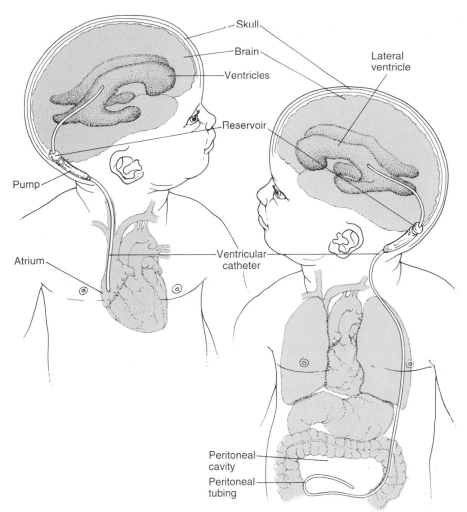

**Figure 14–4.** Shunting procedure for hydrocephalus, in which a catheter drains the ventricular system into either the right atrium or the peritoneal cavity.

To turn the patient in bed, the weight of the head is borne in the palm of one hand, and the head and body are rotated together to prevent a strain on the neck. When the patient is lifted from the crib, the head must be supported by the nurse's arm and chest.

Pressure sores may occur if the patient's position is not changed at least every 2 hours. The tissues of the head and ears as well as the bony prominences have a tendency to break down. A pad of lamb's wool or sponge rubber placed under the head may help prevent these lesions. If the skin becomes broken, it is given immediate attention to prevent infection. The patient must be kept dry, especially around the creases of the neck, where perspiration may collect.

In most cases the nurse may hold the infant for feedings. The nurse sits with the arm supported because the baby's head is heavy. A calm, unhurried manner is necessary. The room should be as quiet as possible. After the feeding, the infant is placed on the side. The patient is not disturbed once settled, since vomiting occurs easily. The nurse must organize daily care so that it does not interfere with meals.

Observations to be made include type and amounts of food taken, vomiting, condition of skin, motor abilities, restlessness, irritability, and changes in vital signs. Fontanels are inspected for size and signs of bulging. Symptoms of increased pressure within the head are an increase in blood pressure and a decrease in pulse and respiration. Signs of a cold or other infection are immediately reported to the nurse in charge and are recorded.

Postoperative nursing care is complex. Often students assist or are coassigned with a graduate. In addition to routine postoperative care and observations, the nurse observes the patient for signs of increased intracranial pressure (ICP) and of infection at the operative site or along the shunt line.

Bacterial infection is a life-threatening complication that sometimes necessitates removing the shunt. Signs of infection include an increase in vital signs, poor feeding, vomiting, pupil dilation, decreased levels of consciousness, and seizures. The operative area is observed for signs of inflammation. A flushing device may be used to determine the functioning of the tube and ensure patency, particularly when increased ICP is suspected. The physician may order the pump to be routinely depressed a certain number of times each day to facilitate drainage. This is accomplished by compressing the antechamber or reservoir.

Positioning of the patient depends on several factors and may vary with the patient's progress. If the fontanels are sunken, the infant is kept flat because too-rapid reduction of fluid may lead to seizures or cortical bleeding. If the fontanels are bulging, the patient is usually placed in the semi-Fowler position to promote drainage of the ventricles through the shunt. The patient is always positioned so as to avoid pressure on the operative site. The surgeon leaves orders for the patient's position and activity.

Assessment of skin remains a priority. Head and chest measurements are recorded; in patients with peritoneal shunts, the abdomen is measured or observed to detect malabsorption of fluid.

As the patient's condition improves, parents are instructed in care of the shunt. The management of hydrocephalus is ongoing for the family, and they require careful instructions and support. The National Hydrocephalus Foundation (NHF) is an important resource.

### Myelodysplasia and Spina Bifida

Myelodysplasia refers to a group of central nervous system disorders characterized by malformation of the spinal cord, one of which is spina bifida.

**Description.** Spina bifida (divided spine) is a congenital embryonic neural tube defect in which there is an imperfect closure of the spinal vertebrae. There are two forms, occulta (hidden) and cystica (sac or cyst).

*Spina bifida occulta* is a relatively minor variation of the disorder in which the opening is small and there is no associated protrusion of structures. It is often undetected and occurs most commonly at L5 and S1 levels. There may be a tuft of hair, a dimple, a lipoma, or a portwine birthmark at the site. Generally, treatment is not necessary unless neuromuscular symptoms appear. These symptoms consist of progressive disturbances of gait, footdrop, or disturbances of bowel and bladder sphincter function.

*Spina bifida cystica* consists of the development of a cystic mass in the midline of the spine (Fig. 14–5). Meningocele and meningomyelocele are two types of spina bifida cystica. A *meningocele* (*meningo*, "membrane," and *cele*, "tumor") contains portions of the membranes and CSF. The size varies from that of a walnut to that of a newborn's head.

More serious is a protrusion of the *membranes* and *spinal cord* through this opening, or a *meningomyelocele*. Although it resembles a meningocele, there may be associated paralysis

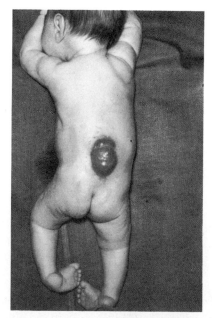

**Figure 14–5.** Newborn with spina bifida and bilateral clubfoot. (From Moore, K.L., & Persaud, T.V.N. [1993]. *The developing human: Clinically oriented embryology* [5th ed.]. Philadelphia: W.B. Saunders, p. 397.)

of the legs and poor control of bowel and bladder functions. Hydrocephalus is common. Prenatal detection is possible by ultrasonography and by testing for increased alpha$_1$-fetoprotein (AFP) in the amniotic fluid of the mother.

**Treatment.** The treatment for spina bifida is surgical closure. The prognosis for patients with these conditions depends on the extent of involvement. In a meningocele patient with no weakness of the legs or sphincter involvement, surgical correction is performed with excellent results. Surgery is also indicated in a meningomyelocele patient for cosmetic purposes and to help prevent infection. In some cases, surgery may diminish neurologic symptoms. A multidisciplinary approach is necessary because, depending on the extent of the defect, the child may have difficulties with hydrocephalus, orthopedics, and urinary function.

Habilitation is necessary after the operation because the legs remain paralyzed and the patient is incontinent of urine and feces. Habilitation, rather than rehabilitation, is the term used to describe this treatment because the patient is handicapped from birth and therefore is learning, not relearning. The aim of habilitation is to minimize the child's disability and put to constructive use the unaffected parts of the body. Every effort is made to help the child develop a healthy personality so that a happy and useful life may be experienced. Eventually, the child can be taught to use a wheelchair and possibly to walk with braces and crutches. The child may also be able to maintain some control over fecal and bladder incontinence.

**Nursing Care.** The student nurse needs demonstrations and careful explanations when assisting with the care of these infants in the hospital. The main objectives of the extensive nursing care required include prevention of infection of or injury to the sac; correct position to prevent pressure on the sac and deformities; good skin care, particularly if the baby is incontinent of urine and feces; adequate nutrition; tender, loving care; accurate observations and charting; education of the parents; continued medical supervision; and habilitation.

Immediate care of the sac is essentially the same regardless of whether the cord is involved. On delivery the newborn is placed in an isolette. Moist, sterile dressings of saline or an antibiotic solution may be ordered to prevent drying of the sac. Some method of protecting the mass is necessary if surgery is to be de-

layed. Pertinent nursing observations include a description of the newborn, the size and area of the sac, and any tears or leakage. The extremities are observed for deformities and movement. There may be spasticity or paralysis of the limbs, or they may be normal, depending on the type and location of the cyst. The head is measured to determine the possibility of associated hydrocephalus. Fontanels are observed to provide baseline data. Lack of anal sphincter control and dribbling of urine are significant in the differential diagnosis. In general, the higher the defect is on the spine, the greater the neurologic deficit. Data are recorded along with the routine observations made for every newborn.

Positioning of the patient is of importance. The goal is to avoid pressure on the sac and to prevent postural deformities. When positioning patients with multiple deformities, the nurse must try to guard against aggravating existing problems. The infant is usually placed prone with a pad between the legs to maintain abduction and counteract hip subluxation. A small roll is placed under the ankles to maintain foot position. Some patients may be supported in a side-lying posture to provide periods of relief. The disadvantage of this position is that it reduces movement of the arms and flexes the hips. The physical therapy staff may provide a helpful consultation. Fortunately, surgery is generally done early.

Postoperative nursing care involves neurologic assessment and prevention of infection. The status of the fontanels and any signs of increased ICP, such as irritability or vomiting, are significant. Sometimes a shunt is performed along with closure of the spine. Complications that can be life-threatening include meningitis, pneumonia, and urinary tract infection.

Urologic monitoring is essential, since many of these patients have urinary incontinence. Medication to prevent urinary tract infections is routinely given. In infants, the Credé method of bladder emptying may be employed. Older children may be taught intermittent, clean self-catheterization. This technique can be per-

## Nursing Brief

The Spina Bifida Association of America provides services for families of children with spinal lesions.

formed by parents and learned by children. Implanted artificial sphincters are another avenue.

Skin care is a challenge. Diapering is generally contraindicated. Constant dribbling of feces and urine irritates the perineal area and can infect the sac or the incision. Meticulous cleanliness is necessary. Bedding must be dry and wrinkle-free. Frequent cleansing, application of a prescribed ointment or lotion, and light massage help maintain skin integrity. If range-of-motion exercises are ordered, they are performed gently.

Feeding of the patient is facilitated by early closure of the defect. In delayed cases, gavage may be used. To bottle feed the patient, one nurse may hold the infant over her shoulder while another administers the formula. Nipple holes should be large enough to prevent exhausting the infant by making suckling difficult. A side-lying position in or out of the crib (on the nurse's lap) is effective with some babies.

These patients need cuddling and sensory stimulation. If the infant cannot be held, the nurse soothes him by touch. The nurse talks to the baby and, when possible, provides face-to-face (en-face) communication. Mobiles are placed appropriately. Periodically moving the isolette or crib provides diversity of view. Soft music is also soothing.

Special consideration must be given to the establishment of parent-infant relationships. This problem is complicated if the infant is transferred to a large medical center. Understanding and support are given to the parents, who may be overwhelmed. It is not unusual for them to be repulsed by the cyst. Most experience a sense of loss for what was to have been their "perfect baby." Steps of the grieving process may be recognized by the astute nurse. If the malformation is complex and incompatible with life, a decision must be made about the feasibility of surgical intervention. This is a crisis situation for the most mature of people and an area in which guidelines are not clearly defined. Information and education about this disorder can be obtained from the Spina Bifida Association of America.

A crucial factor for the nurse is recognition of personal feelings about these patients, which often include sorrow, anger, frustration, guilt, and fear of incompetence. Group discussions that provide a safe, nonthreatening environment in which nurses can express their feelings are healthy. Physical outlets, such as exercise, active sports, and screaming rooms, prevent illness and displacement of repressed feelings on innocent parties. These resources are essential if emotional burnout is to be avoided (see discussion of facing death, pp. 889–891).

## GASTROINTESTINAL SYSTEM

### Cleft Lip (Harelip)

**Description.** A cleft lip is characterized by a fissure or opening in the upper lip (Fig. 14–6). It is a result of the failure of the embryonic structures of the face to unite. In many cases, it seems to be caused by hereditary predisposition coupled with a minor deviation of the intrauterine environment. This disorder appears more frequently in boys than in girls and may occur on one or both sides of the lip. The extent of the defect may vary from slight to severe. Sometimes it is accompanied by a cleft palate, a fissure in the midline of the roof of the mouth. Cleft lip and palate are common congenital anomalies, occurring in about 1 in 600 to 1250 births. Transculturally, they occur more often in Asian Americans and Native Americans and less commonly in African Americans (Jarvis, 1992).

**Treatment and Nursing Care.** The initial treatment for cleft lip is surgical repair. The

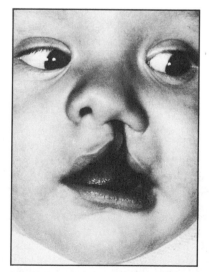

**Figure 14–6.** Cleft lip. (From Behrman, R.E., & Kliegman, R.M. [1992]. *Nelson textbook of pediatrics* [14th ed.]. Philadelphia: W.B. Saunders.)

cleft lip is repaired first, because it interferes with the infant's ability to eat. The baby cannot create a vacuum in the mouth and is unable to suck. Surgery not only improves the infant's sucking but also greatly improves appearance. Indirectly, this influences the amount of affection the baby receives, because some refrain from cuddling a baby who is obviously disfigured. Currently, the operation is performed any time after birth if the infant is in good general health and free from infection.

Before surgery, a complete physical examination is done and blood tests are ordered. Photographs may also be taken. Any signs of infection, such as a cold, are reported to the nurse manager. The doctor may order restraints to prevent the patient from scratching the lip and to acquaint the baby with them because they are necessary postoperatively. An Asepto syringe with a rubber tip or a Haberman feeder is used to feed the baby before and after surgery, since sucking motions must be avoided to decrease tension on the suture line (Fig. 14–7). Sometimes a cleft-lip nipple is used before surgery.

The procedure for feeding babies with both cleft lip and cleft palate is described on page 344. The nurse needs to allow more time than the usual 20 minutes required for bottle feedings.

Postoperative nursing goals for this patient include (1) preventing the baby from sucking and crying, which could cause tension on the suture line, (2) careful positioning (never on the abdomen) to avoid injury to the operative site, (3) cleansing of the suture line to prevent crusts from forming that could cause scarring, (4) applying restraints to prevent injury to the opera-

tive site and use of a Logan bow, and (5) cuddling and other forms of affection to provide for the infant's emotional needs, which are of particular importance because the baby cannot obtain the usual satisfactions from sucking.

The infant receives feedings by dropper until the wound is completely healed (1–2 weeks). The mother who has fed her baby preoperatively and has been allowed to assist with feedings during hospitalization will feel more confident after discharge. The immediate improvement as a result of surgery is encouraging to the parents, particularly if the child must have further surgery for cleft palate repair.

### Cleft Palate

**Description.** A cleft palate is more serious than a cleft lip. It forms a passageway between the nasopharynx and the nose, which not only complicates feeding but also easily leads to infections of the respiratory tract and middle ear. It is generally responsible for speech difficulties that occur in later life. Unlike cleft lip, cleft palate is more common in females than in males.

**Treatment.** The best time for surgery is a subject of controversy, although some surgeons prefer to operate before 18 months of age, if at all possible, so that speech patterns are not affected. To facilitate communication, a dental speech appliance may be used if surgery has been deferred or has been contraindicated because of extensive malformation. This appliance must be changed periodically as the child grows.

Treatment of the child with a cleft lip and

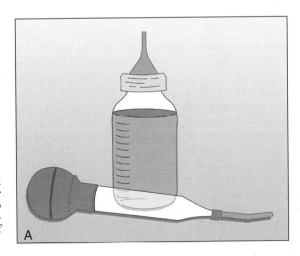
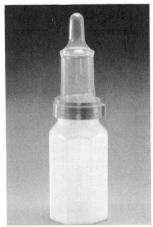

**Figure 14–7.** Equipment to feed the infant with a cleft lip or palate. *A,* Gravity feeder, cleft-lip nipple. *B* shows the new Haberman feeder. (*B,* Courtesy of Medela, Inc., McHenry, IL.)

## PROCEDURE FOR FEEDING NEWBORNS WITH A CLEFT LIP OR CLEFT PALATE, OR BOTH

### Equipment

Sterile medicine dropper with rubber tip *or*
Asepto syringe with rubber tip
Formula
Covergown for nurse
Bib

### Method

1. Check to see that the baby is dry and warm. Change the diaper as needed. Wash your hands following this. Leave restraints on during feeding.
2. Hold the baby in a sitting position. Draw the formula into an Asepto syringe or medicine dropper.
3. Place the rubber tip of the feeder just inside the lips, on the opposite side of the mouth from the cleft or repaired area.
4. Exert gentle pressure on the bulb of the feeder, allowing a small amount of fluid to drop into the mouth.
5. Allow the baby to swallow before giving more. Prevent sucking motions as much as possible.
6. Bubble frequently. Sit the baby up and gently pat the back with one hand while supporting the chest with the other. *Note:* The doctor may wish to have the formula followed by a small amount of sterile water to cleanse the mouth.
7. Following the feeding, return the baby to the crib. Place on right side. Support the back with a rolled blanket or small pillow.
8. Chart: Time of feeding, method, amount offered, amount taken and retained, and untoward results (vomiting).

palate requires expert teamwork over a long period. Emotional problems that sometimes occur with this condition require more extensive attention than does the repair itself. A child born with a facial deformity encounters many problems. Feedings are difficult and are not relaxed in the initial period. As the child grows, irregular tooth eruptions, drooling, delayed speech, and the need for intermittent hospitalization and frequent clinic appointments can be frustrating. It is difficult not to be attractive when society places such emphasis on good looks.

A mother's first reaction to a disfigured newborn is one of shock, hurt, disappointment, and guilt. Some parents regard the deformity as a result of their inadequacies. They may desire to hide the child from relatives and friends. The developing child senses the parents' feelings and acquires either a positive or a negative self-image. The patient and family need understanding, a concrete basis for hope, and practical advice.

In large cities, special cleft palate clinics are available in which several specialists can work together in convenient consultation. The parents are instructed about the resources available in the state in which they live. Financial assistance is usually indicated because of the length of treatment required.

### Postoperative Treatment and Nursing Care

*Nutrition.* Fluids are taken by a cup, although a gravity feeder may be desirable in some cases. The method varies with the plastic surgeon. The diet is progressive. At first it consists of clear fluids and then full fluids. By the time of discharge, a soft diet can generally be taken. Hot foods and liquids are avoided to prevent injury to the operative site. The patient must not suck on a straw. When feeding with a spoon, place only its side into the mouth. The spoon must not touch the roof of the mouth. The nurse teaches parents that objects such as the child's thumb, tongue blades, toast, cookies, forks, and pacifiers are kept out of the mouth. The child is prevented from placing fingers or objects in the mouth. The tongue should be kept away from the sore part of the mouth. The diet is advanced only on consultation with the physician.

*Oral Hygiene.* The mouth is kept clean at all times. Feedings are followed by a little water. The doctor may prescribe a mild antiseptic mouthwash.

*Restraints.* Elbow restraints are generally sufficient. They are removed one at a time and periodically, to prevent constriction of circulation and to allow normal movement. In the home, they may be made of rolled cardboard tied with string.

*Speech.* It is helpful to speak slowly and distinctly to the child. The child is encouraged to pronounce words correctly. Children who have had extensive repairs or have associated deafness need the help of a speech therapist. The speech therapist evaluates the child and assists the parents in specific activities that will facilitate speech development.

*Diversion.* Crying is to be avoided as much as possible. Play should be quiet, particularly in the immediate postoperative period. The nurse reads, draws, or colors with the child.

*Complications.* Earaches and dental decay may accompany this condition. Parents are instructed to take the child to the doctor at the first signs of earache. Regular visits to the dentist are scheduled.

## MUSCULOSKELETAL SYSTEM

### Clubfoot

**Description.** Clubfoot, one of the most common deformities of the skeletal system, is a congenital anomaly characterized by a foot that has been twisted inward or outward. The incidence is about 1 in 700–1000 live births. Many mild forms are due to improper position in the uterus, and these clear up with little or no treatment when the extremity is allowed unrestricted activity. In contrast, true clubfoot does not respond to simple exercise. Many believe that this is because of an abnormal degree of compression and molding of the infant's feet in the uterus. Several types are recognized. Talipes (*talus*, "heel," and *pes*, "foot") equinovarus (*equinus*, "extension," and *varus*, "bent inward") is seen in 95% of patients. The feet are turned inward, and the child walks on the toes and the outer borders of the feet. It generally involves both feet. Boys are affected twice as often as girls.

**Treatment and Nursing Care.** The treatment of clubfoot is started as early as possible; otherwise the bones and muscles continue to develop abnormally. During infancy, conservative treatment, consisting of manipulation and casting to hold the foot in the right position, is carried out (Fig. 14–8). A Denis Browne splint may also be used, usually for children under 1 year of age. It is made of two footplates attached to a crossbar. When it is fitted to the shoes, the feet may be put in various positions of angulation by sets of screws. When the infant kicks, the feet are automatically forced into the correct position. Passive stretching exercises may also be recommended. If these methods are not effective, surgery is indicated. The infant with a clubfoot is under medical supervision for a long time. Parents need to be instructed in developmental behaviors of the infant as well as the clinical aspects of care. Ongoing support is paramount.

**Cast Care.** Casts are made of plaster or synthetic materials such as fiberglass or polyurethane. The plastic cast consists of crinoline that has powdered plastic in its meshwork. It is placed in warm water before being applied over cotton wadding or stockinette. The wet plaster of Paris hardens as it dries. This type of cast dries from the inside out and takes 24–48 hours to dry.

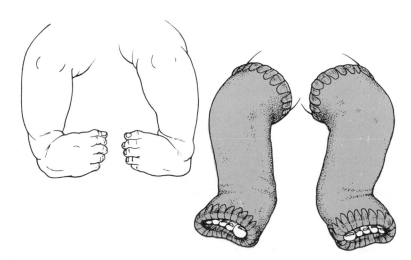

**Figure 14–8.** Bilateral talipes equinovarus (clubfoot) before and after application of plaster casts. Adhesive "petals" have been placed around the ends of the casts in order to prevent plaster from irritating the skin.

# Nursing Brief

In the long-term care of orthopedic patients, educating the parents about orthopedic devices, cast care, exercise, hygiene, and treatment goals is necessary. The nurse explains the importance of frequent clinic visits, reinforces doctor information, and clarifies directions as necessary.

---

If the patient returns to the unit before the cast is dry, the cast must be left uncovered and protected from pressures that could cause a depression in it. If the doctor orders that the leg and foot be elevated on pillows to prevent swelling, the nurse who assists must use the palms of the hands, not the fingers, to hold the cast. Indentations made in a wet cast by fingers can press on the underlying skin and cause damage. This precaution is also explained to parents. Lighter synthetic casts dry in less than 30 minutes; however, they are less strong and more expensive.

The toes are left exposed for observation. The nurse checks them for signs of poor circulation, pallor, cyanosis, swelling, coldness, numbness, pain, or burning. If circulation is impaired, the doctor may split the cast in order to relieve the pressure, or the cast may need to be removed and reapplied. The nurse also reports irritation of the skin around the edges of the cast and lack of movement of the toes. Adhesive petals may be placed around the edges of the cast in order to prevent skin irritation.

It is difficult to keep a child's cast free of food particles, which cause skin irritation. Careful supervision during mealtime is necessary in order to prevent the child from placing bits of food under the edges of the cast. Powder and oil are not used following the bath because they may cause irritation.

If surgery on tendons and bones has been performed, the nurse also observes the cast for evidence of bleeding. If a discolored area appears on the cast, it is circled and the time is recorded. Further bleeding can then be estimated. If bleeding is noted, the patient's vital signs are also checked and compared with preoperative readings. After surgery, the cast is changed about every 3 weeks in order to bring the foot gradually into position. When the cast is removed for the final time, exercise and special shoes may be indicated.

**Emotional Support.** The nurse is an important figure in the care of the long-term patient with clubfoot. Nurses review the normal growth and development of children in the patient's age range in order to anticipate problems and to educate caretakers in parenting.

In general, children of up to 4 years of age suffer the most severely from being separated from their parents. They cry loudly when visiting hours end and need the nurse to console them. They may be slow in developing certain motor abilities, and many regress to more babyish behavior. This is particularly true of bowel and bladder control. The nurse does not shame a child if an "accident" occurs.

The parents can give much helpful information about their child. The nurse must be a good listener. Parents are encouraged to participate in the care of their hospitalized child because it brings them satisfaction and a sense of control and reassures the child.

The financial burdens of hospitalization, surgery, special shoes, and continued medical supervision pose a serious problem. If the nurse suspects that the parents need financial help, a social-service referral is made.

## Congenital Hip Dysplasia

**Description.** Congenital hip dysplasia is a common orthopedic deformity. The incidence is about 1 in 1000 births. The term *hip dysplasia* is a broad description applied to various degrees of deformity: subluxation or dislocation, either partial or complete. The head of the femur is partly or completely displaced from a shallow hip socket (acetabulum). Hereditary and environmental factors appear to be causal factors. Hip malformation, joint laxity, breech position, and race may all contribute. Congenital hip dysplasia is seven times more common in girls than in boys. Newborn infants seldom have complete dislocation. However, the baby beginning to walk exerts pressure on the hip, which can cause complete dislocation. Therefore, early detection and treatment are of particular importance.

**Manifestations.** A dislocation of the hip is commonly discovered at the periodic health examination of the baby during the 1st or 2nd month of life. One of the most reliable signs is a limited abduction of the leg on the affected side. When the infant is placed on the back with knees and hips flexed, the doctor can press the femur of the normal hip backward until it almost touches the examining table. This can be

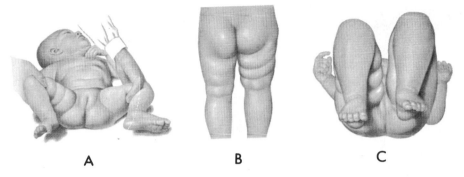

**Figure 14–9.** Early signs of dislocation of right hip. *A*, Limitation of abduction. *B*, Asymmetry of skin folds. *C*, Shortening of femur. (From *Clinical education aid no. 15*. [1986]. Columbus, OH: Ross Laboratories. Reproduced with permission of Ross Laboratories.)

accomplished only partially on the affected side. The knee on the side of the dislocation is lower, and the skin folds of the thigh are deeper and often asymmetric (Fig. 14–9). When the infant is prone, one hip is higher than the other.

In some infants younger than 4 weeks, the doctor can actually feel and hear the femoral head slip into the acetabulum under gentle pressure. This is called Ortolani's sign or Ortolani's click and is considered diagnostic of the disorder. The child who is walking and has had no treatment displays a characteristic limp. Bilateral (*bi*, "two," and *latus*, "side") dislocation may occur; however, unilateral (*uni*, "one," and *latus*, "side") dislocation is more common. X-ray studies confirm the diagnosis.

**Treatment.** Treatment begins immediately on detection of the dislocation. The doctor attempts to form a normal joint by keeping the head of the femur within the hip socket. This constant pressure enlarges and deepens the acetabulum; thus, it corrects the dislocation. The nurse recalls that the bones of small children are fairly pliable because they contain more cartilage than do bones of adults.

There is some controversy over the exact course of treatment; however, some device to maintain abduction of the hips is used. The Pavlik harness is frequently utilized (Fig. 14–10). If the dislocation is severe or is not detected until the child begins to walk, it may be necessary to use traction. This pulls the head of the femur down to the correct position opposite the acetabulum. Casting in a froglike position is then done. This type of cast, known as a *body spica* cast, is shown in Figure 14–11.

The length of time spent in a cast varies according to the patient's progress and growth and the condition of the cast; however, it is usually 5–9 months. During this time, the cast may be changed about every 6 weeks. Sometimes surgery is required. If so, open reduction of the dislocation or repair of the shelf of the hip bone is done. After surgery, a cast is applied to keep the femur in the correct position.

**Nursing Care.** The nursery nurse carefully observes each infant during the morning bath to detect signs of a dislocated hip. When the baby is prone, the nurse observes the buttocks for variation in size. The legs of the infant should be equal in length. The infant should be kicking both legs, not just one leg. There should be no difference in the depth of the skin folds of the baby's upper thighs. In the well-baby clinic, the nurse notes the posture and gait of older children and records observations.

Infants who progress well with the Pavlik harness or Frejka splint, or a similar brace, remain at home. The mother and baby visit the doctor regularly. The parents need assurance that the baby may be held and may sit in a chair. They should be encouraged to ask questions of the clinic nurse and doctor.

The child who is admitted to the hospital with a diagnosis of a congenital dislocated hip is given as much personal attention as possible. The first admission sets the pattern for future hospitalization; therefore, the child must make a satisfactory adjustment. The nurse becomes familiar with the child's habit and care sheet. Every effort is made to provide a homelike environment for patients who are hospitalized for many weeks.

The body spica cast encircles the waist and extends to the ankles or toes. General cast care, discussed on page 345, should be reviewed at

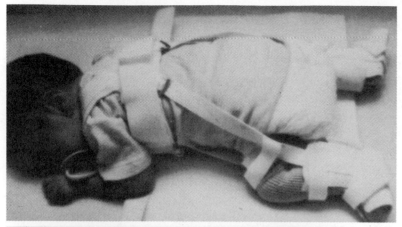
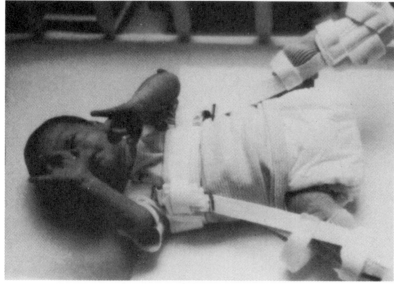

**Figure 14–10. The** Pavlik harness maintains abduction of the hips. (From Behrman, R.E., & Kliegman, R.M. [1992]. *Nelson textbook of pediatrics* [14th ed.]. Philadelphia: W.B. Saunders.)

this point. Nursing Care Plan 14–1 gives selected nursing diagnoses and interventions for the patient with a spica cast.

Firm, plastic-covered pillows are required. These are placed beneath the curvatures of the cast for support. Older children may benefit from an overhead bar and trapeze. The room should be adequately ventilated. A fracture pan should be available in the bedside table.

The head of the patient's bed is slightly elevated so that urine or feces drain away from the body of the cast. One should not elevate the head or shoulders of a child in a body cast by means of pillows, as this thrusts the patient's chest against the cast and causes discomfort or respiratory difficulty. The child who is not toilet-trained may be placed on a Bradford frame to facilitate nursing care. Frequent change of position is important; bed patients need to be turned often. Infants may be held in the nurse's lap after the cast has dried. A ride on a stretcher to the playroom or around the hospital provides changes of position and scenery.

The procedure for changing the position of a child is described on page 349.

Itching is a problem for the patient in a body cast. If at all possible, before applying the cast, a strip of gauze is placed beneath the cast, extending through the opened area required for toilet needs. It is gently moved back and forth to relieve itching. When the strip becomes soiled, a clean one is tied to one end of the soiled gauze and pulled through the cast;

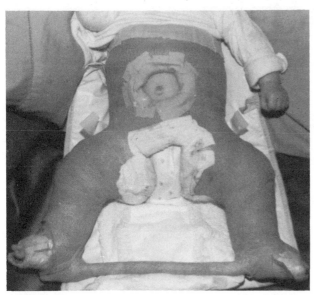

**Figure 14–11.** A spica body cast. This cast maintains the legs in a froglike position and is used to treat congenital dislocations of the hip. Note that the infant is able to move her toes freely. The opening in the center allows for auscultation of bowel sounds.

## PROCEDURE FOR TURNING THE CHILD IN A BODY CAST

### Method

Two people, one on each side of the bed, are needed to turn a child in a body cast.

1. Move the child to the edge of the bed as far as possible, so that the nurse who receives the child is farther away from him or her.
2. The nurse nearer to the child places one hand under the head and back and one hand under the leg part of the cast and turns the child to the midway point on the side.
3. The nurse farther away then accepts the support of the child and cast as the child is turned completely onto the abdomen.

The supporting bar between the legs should not be used as a lever when turning the child. All body curvatures are supported with pillows or sheet rolls. Whenever possible, the older child should be on the abdomen during mealtime to facilitate swallowing and self-feeding. When placing a child in a body cast on a fracture pan, support the upper back and legs with pillows so that body alignment is maintained.

this soiled portion is removed. Other methods that might cause injury to the skin beneath the cast are discouraged because any break in the skin under a cast is difficult to heal.

The child with this long-term disability needs help in meeting everyday needs. This child is growing and developing rapidly. Therefore, frequent adjustments in home and clinic care are necessary. Dressing and clothing are a problem. The child cannot fit into regular furniture and much of the play equipment enjoyed by other children. Transportation is difficult. A special wagon built up with pillows may be used during hospitalization. Home health care is a good resource on discharge.

## Metabolic Defects

### PHENYLKETONURIA

**Description.** Classic phenylketonuria (PKU) is a genetic disorder caused by the faulty metabolism of phenylalanine, an amino acid essential to life and found in all protein foods. The hepatic enzyme phenylalanine hydroxylase, normally needed to convert phenylalanine into tyrosine, is missing. When the baby is fed milk, phenylalanine begins to accumulate in the blood. It can rise to as high as 20 times the normal amount. Its by-product, phenylpyruvic acid, appears in the urine within the first weeks of life. This inborn error of metabolism, which is transmitted by an autosomal recessive gene, is termed "classic PKU" and is associated with phenylalanine levels above 20 mg/dl. It results in severe retardation, evidenced in infancy. Early detection and treatment are paramount. The baby appears normal at birth but begins to show delayed development at about 4–6 months of age. The child may show evidence of failure to thrive, have eczema or other skin conditions, have a peculiar musty odor, or have personality disorders. About one-third of the children have epileptic seizures. PKU occurs mainly in children who are blond and blue-eyed; these features are due to a lack of tyrosine, a necessary component of the pigment melanin. Less severe forms of the disorder are now recognized. They are designated as "atypical PKU" and "mild hyperphenylalaninemia."

**Diagnosis.** The *Guthrie blood test* is widely used and is currently considered the most reliable test. Blood is obtained from a simple heel prick. A few drops of capillary blood are placed

| NURSING CARE PLAN 14–1 | | |
| --- | --- | --- |
| **Selected Nursing Diagnoses for the Neborn/Infant with a Spica Cast** | | |
| Goals | Nursing Interventions | Rationale |

**Nursing Diagnosis:** High risk for altered tissue perfusion due to cast constriction.

| | | |
| --- | --- | --- |
| Tissues and circulation appear adequate as evidenced by pink, warm skin, good capillary refill, and lack of numbness or swelling<br><br>Parents understand signs of inadequate circulation and explain the importance of seeking immediate assistance if these signs appear | 1. Observe exposed extremities and skin distal to the cast every 30 min for the first few hours of a new cast and every 1–4 hr thereafter; watch for signs of pallor, cyanosis, swelling, coldness, numbness, pain, or burning<br>2. Circle any drainage on cast with date and time; monitor and record findings<br>3. Observe nonverbal communication for signs of pain; ask older child if pain is experienced<br><br><br><br><br><br><br><br>4. Educate parents and patient, if old enough, in all of above<br>5. Written instructions are provided | 1. Circulation can be impaired leading to ischemia. Peripheral nerves in contrast to muscles do not degenerate with disuse but loss of *innervation* can take place if nerves are damaged by pressure or if blood supply is disrupted<br>2. An increase in size of circle indicates further bleeding or possibly a draining infection<br>3. Pain, especially after a few days, may indicate *compartment syndrome*; compartment is an area, such as upper and lower extremities, in which a group of muscles and fascia appear; increase in pressure within this closed space may disrupt circulation within space<br>4. Education reduces stress of parents and patient<br>5. Written instructions provide reinforcement and help ensure success of other interventions |

**Nursing Diagnosis:** High risk for injury related to awkwardness and weight of cast.

| | | |
| --- | --- | --- |
| Patient will remain safe and as independent as possible | 1. Restrain patient adequately when on Bradford frame with vests and belts<br>2. Inform older child when turning as to how and when you are going to proceed (e.g., "ready, set, go")<br><br>3. Leave articles and toys within reach<br><br><br><br>4. Some car seats are adapted to accommodate small child in a spica cast | 1. These restraints prevent falls; active children may turn without assistance or move suddenly<br>2. Involving child in procedure as age-appropriate gives patient a sense of control; procedure will go more smoothly<br>3. Child will not need to strain or move awkwardly to reach articles; patient will feel greater mastery if articles can be obtained independently<br>4. These children need protection in car |

on a filter paper and mailed to the laboratory for screening. It is recommended that the blood be obtained after 72 hours of life, preferably after ingestion of proteins, in order to reduce the possibility of false-negative results. Because of early discharge, many states require that the test be done on all newborns before they leave the nursery. A repeat test is performed within 4–6 weeks. The infant can be tested at home by a public health nurse or at the clinic or physician's office. Confirmation of the diagnosis requires quantitative elevations of phenylalanine compound in both blood and urine (Mahan & Arlin, 1992). Screening programs for pregnant women have also been advocated to detect elevated phenylalanine levels that could have an effect on the newborn. Prenatal diagnosis of PKU is possible.

**Treatment.** Treatment consists of close dietary management and frequent evaluation of blood phenylalanine levels. Because phenylalanine is found in all natural protein foods, a syn-

## Nursing Brief

Children with PKU need to avoid the sweetener aspartame (NutraSweet) because it is converted to phenylalanine in the body.

thetic food providing enough protein for growth and tissue repair but little phenylalanine must be substituted. "The most commonly used formulas are Lofenalac for infants and Phenyl-Free for children and adolescents. A dietician may supplement the formula with evaporated milk or regular infant formula during infancy and early childhood to provide high biologic value protein, nonessential amino acids, and sufficient phenylalanine to meet the individualized requirements of the growing child" (Mahan & Arlin, 1992). Solid foods that are low in phenylalanine are added at the same age as are solid foods for infants without PKU. Phenyl-Free is introduced between the ages of 3 and 8 years. Cookbooks and family recipes provide variety. Eventually the child learns to assume full management of the diet.

At the time of this writing (1994), authorities advise continuing the diet indefinitely, as some children taken off the diet at 4–6 years of age showed losses in intellectual performance. Behavioral difficulties, such as poor attention span, have also been cited. Monitoring of blood phenylalanine levels is essential. Formula adjustments are made in order to stabilize serum levels. Researchers hope to be able eventually to supply the missing enzyme that these children fail to produce.

## Blood Disorders

### THALASSEMIA

**Description.** The thalassemias are a group of hereditary blood disorders in which the patient's body cannot produce sufficient adult hemoglobin. The red blood cells are abnormal in size and shape and are rapidly destroyed. This abnormality results in a chronic anemia. The body attempts to compensate by producing large amounts of fetal hemoglobin. These disorders are caused by a deficiency in the normal synthesis of hemoglobin polypeptide chains. They are categorized according to the polypep-

tide chain affected as alpha, beta, gamma, or delta thalassemia.

The most common variety of thalassemia involves impaired production of beta chains and is known as *beta thalassemia*. This variety consists of two forms, thalassemia minor and thalassemia major. Thalassemia major is also called Cooley's anemia. Thalassemia occurs mainly in persons of Mediterranean origin, for example, Greeks, Syrians, Italians, and their descendants elsewhere—the term is derived from the Greek *thalassa*, which means "sea." Thalassemia can also occur from spontaneous mutations.

### Thalassemia Minor

Thalassemia minor, also termed "beta thalassemia trait," occurs by the child's inheriting a thalassemia gene from only one parent, that is, by heterozygous inheritance. It is associated with mild anemia. Hemoglobin concentration averages 2–3 gm/dl, lower than age-related values. These patients are often misdiagnosed as having an iron-deficiency anemia. Symptoms are minimal. The patient is pale, and the spleen may be enlarged. The patient may lead a normal life, with the illness going undetected. This condition is of genetic importance, particularly if both parents are carriers of the trait. Prenatal blood samples can detect thalassemia major in such cases.

### Thalassemia Major (Cooley's Anemia)

When two thalassemia genes are inherited (homozygous inheritance), the child is born with a more serious form of the disease. A progressive, severe anemia becomes evident within the second 6 months of life. It usually occurs when both parents have thalassemia minor; however, one parent may have the trait and the other may carry the trait for sickle cell anemia or another anemia variant.

The patient is pale and hypoxic, has a poor appetite, and may have a fever. Jaundice, which at first is mild, progresses to a muddy bronze color. There is chronic hypoxia. The liver enlarges, and the spleen grows enormously. Abdominal distention is great, which causes pressure on the organs of the chest. Cardiac failure is a constant threat. Bone marrow space enlarges to compensate for hematopoietic (*hema*, "blood," and *poiesis*, "to make") defects,

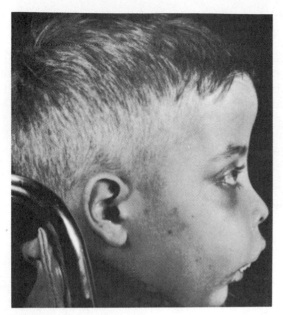

**Figure 14–12.** Appearance of patient with thalassemia major (Cooley's anemia). Note the overgrowth of the upper right jaw bone. (From Behrman, R.E., & Kliegman, R.M. [1992]. *Nelson textbook of pediatrics* [14th ed.]. Philadelphia: W.B. Saunders.)

and weakened bones are subject to fracture. Changes in the facial contour give the child a characteristic appearance (Fig. 14–12). The teeth protrude because of an overgrowth of the upper jaw bone.

The diagnosis is aided by the family history of thalassemia, radiographic bone growth studies, and blood tests. Hemoglobin electrophoresis is helpful in diagnosing the type and severity of the various thalassemias, because it analyzes the quantity and specific hemoglobin variants found in blood (Whaley & Wong, 1991). The prognosis is poor. Death may be due to cardiac failure, severe anemia, or secondary infection.

**Treatment and Nursing Care.** The mainstay of treatment for thalassemia major is frequent blood transfusions to maintain the hemoglobin level above 10 gm/dl. As a result of repeated blood transfusions, excessive deposits of iron may be stored in the tissues. This is termed *hemosiderosis* and is seen especially in the spleen, liver, heart, pancreas, and lymph glands. Deferoxamine mesylate (Desferal Mesylate), an iron-chelating agent, is given to counteract hemosiderosis. Severe splenomegaly may occur in some children. Splenectomy may make the patient more comfortable, increase the abil-

ity to move about, and allow for more normal growth. After surgery these children are given prophylactic antibiotics to prevent infection. Bone marrow transplants are being performed with increasing success.

Nursing measures adhere to the principles of long-term care. The observation of the patient during a blood transfusion is discussed on p. 735. Monitoring of vital signs is necessary to detect irregularities of the heart. Whenever possible, the same nurse cares for the patient during transfusions, blood tests, and other unpleasant procedures in order to provide security. Restricted activity is less needed now than in the past because of frequent transfusions. Instead patients are taught to regulate their activities according to their own tolerance.

The emotional health of the child and parents needs special consideration by the nurse. Every attempt to ease the strain of this prolonged illness must be made. Home care arrangements can be provided through community agencies. Older children need special support to accept changes in their body image and sexual immaturity caused by the disease. Suggestions applicable to the care of the chronically ill child are discussed throughout the text. Care of the dying child is discussed on pp. 890–893.

# Chromosomal Abnormalities

### DOWN SYNDROME

**Description.** Down syndrome is one of the most common chromosomal abnormalities. Its incidence is approximately 1 in 600–800 live births. It is higher among children of mothers 35 years or older. Paternal age is also a factor, particularly when the father is 55 or over. Sometimes, the first baby of a young mother has Down syndrome; however, subsequent children are usually born free of the defect. Children born with this birth defect have mild to severe mental retardation and generally some physical abnormalities. In the past, children with this condition were called "mongoloid" because of the Oriental ("Mongolian") appearance of their faces, but this term is now considered inappropriate.

Three phenotypes (genetic makeups) of Down syndrome are seen. These are trisomy 21, mosaicism, and translocation of a chromosome. The most common type, trisomy 21 syndrome, accounts for 95% of patients. In this instance there are three number 21 chromosomes, rather than the normal two (see Fig. 16–2). It is a result of *nondisjunction*, the failure of a chromosome to follow the normal separation process into daughter cells. The earlier in the embryo's development that this occurs, the greater is the number of cells affected.

When nondisjunction occurs late in development, both normal and abnormal cells are present in the newborn. This condition is *mosaicism*. Patients with this condition tend to be less severely affected in physical appearance and intelligence. The third condition is *translocation*. In translocation, a piece of chromosome in pair 21 breaks away and attaches itself to another chromosome.

What causes these disruptions is unknown. Many hypotheses have been suggested, such as abdominal irradiation prior to conception, autoimmunity (particularly thyroid autoimmunity), and endocrine changes in older women. Although there are many unanswered questions about the etiologic aspects of this disorder, current information points to multiple causality (Levine, Carey, & Crocker, 1992). Down syndrome has been reported to occur in all races.

**Manifestations.** The signs of Down syndrome, which are apparent at birth, are close-set and upward-slanting eyes, small head, round face, flat nose, protruding tongue that interferes with sucking, and mouth breathing (Fig. 14–13*A*). The hands of the baby are short and thick, and the little finger is curved (Fig. 14–13*B*). There is a deep straight line across the palm, which is called the *Simian crease*. There is also a wide space between the first and the second toes. The undeveloped muscles and loose joints enable the child to assume unusual positions. Physical growth and development may be slower than normal (Tables 14–1 and 14–2). The child is limited intellectually. Some children have been found to have IQs in the borderline to low-average range. Congenital heart deformities are also associated with this condition.

These happy-go-lucky children are very lovable. They may be restless and somewhat more difficult to train than the normal youngster. Their resistance to infection is poor, and they are prone to respiratory and ear infections. They are also prone to speech and hearing problems. The life spans of children with Down syndrome has been increased with the widespread use of antibiotics. The incidence of acute leukemia is higher in these children than in the normal population. Plastic surgery to facilitate nose breathing, speaking, and eating is being performed for selected Down syndrome patients.

**Counseling Parents.** The counseling of families of Down syndrome is ongoing. It takes exceptional strength and time to accept this diag-

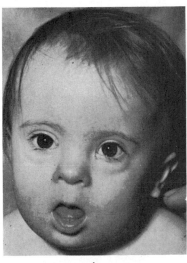
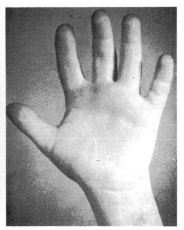

**Figure 14–13.** *A*, Typical facial appearance of an infant with Down syndrome. (From Smith, D.W. [1982]. *Recognizable patterns of human malformation* [3rd ed.]. Philadelphia: W.B. Saunders.) *B*, Typical broad, spadelike hand of a 12-year-old boy with Down syndrome. Note the shortness of all fingers. (From Vaughan, V.C., et al. [1979]. *Nelson textbook of pediatrics* [11th ed.]. Philadelphia: W.B. Saunders.)

A                                    B

**Table 14–1.** TIME OF OCCURRENCE OF DEVELOPMENTAL MILESTONES IN NORMAL CHILDREN AND THOSE WITH DOWN SYNDROME

| Milestone | Children with Down Syndrome | | Normal Children | |
|---|---|---|---|---|
| | *Average (Months)* | *Range (Months)* | *Average (Months)* | *Range (Months)* |
| Smiling | 2 | 1.5–4 | 1 | 0.5–3 |
| Rolling over | 8 | 4–22 | 5 | 2–10 |
| Sitting alone | 10 | 6–28 | 7 | 5–9 |
| Crawling | 12 | 7–21 | 8 | 6–11 |
| Creeping | 15 | 9–27 | 10 | 7–13 |
| Standing | 20 | 11–42 | 11 | 8–16 |
| Walking | 24 | 12–65 | 13 | 8–18 |
| Talking, words | 16 | 9–31 | 10 | 6–14 |
| Talking, sentences | 28 | 18–96 | 21 | 14–32 |

From Levine, M.D., Carey, W.B., & Crocker, A.C. (1992). *Developmental-behavioral pediatrics* (2nd ed.). Philadelphia: W.B. Saunders.

nosis. Maternity nurses need to be aware of their own feelings before they can effectively support parents. They too will feel saddened at the birth of an imperfect child. They may identify with the parents. It is appropriate to express one's feelings of initial helplessness, and it may encourage the parents to verbalize their concerns. The nurse must listen and provide honest, tactful, and compassionate support.

Sometimes parents cannot accept the fact that their baby is retarded and are ashamed to tell anyone of the baby's condition. The nurse can support and encourage the parents' need to cry. Empathy from the nurse is particularly important. Involving parents in the care and planning for the infant from the start facilitates bonding. The need for the staff's warm concern cannot be overestimated. Pampering the baby by putting a little curl in the hair, for example, shows that others care even though the baby is different. Parents watch for evidence of rejection of their child; they are sensitive to such indicators as placement in the nursery.

Siblings of the patient need to be informed and included in discussions about the new baby. Even very young children are aware of parental distress, and their imaginations can be more frightening than the reality. Open communications early on will prevent isolation, avoid misconceptions, and promote an easier transition period. The nurse should connect the family with a Down syndrome support group in their area, if there is one. Other parents with a Down syndrome child are an important resource. The National Association for Down Syndrome is one organization that provides education and sup-

**Table 14–2.** TIME OF OCCURRENCE OF SELF-HELP SKILLS IN NORMAL CHILDREN AND THOSE WITH DOWN SYNDROME

| Milestone | Children with Down Syndrome | | Normal Children | |
|---|---|---|---|---|
| | *Average (Months)* | *Range (Months)* | *Average (Months)* | *Range (Months)* |
| Eating | | | | |
|   Finger feeding | 12 | 8–28 | 8 | 6–16 |
|   Using spoon and fork | 20 | 12–40 | 13 | 8–20 |
| Toilet training | | | | |
|   Bladder | 48 | 20–95 | 32 | 18–60 |
|   Bowel | 42 | 28–90 | 29 | 16–48 |
| Dressing | | | | |
|   Undressing | 40 | 29–72 | 32 | 22–42 |
|   Putting clothes on | 58 | 38–98 | 47 | 34–58 |

From Levine, M.D., Carey, W.B., & Crocker, A.C. (1992). *Developmental-behavioral pediatrics* (2nd ed.). Philadelphia: W.B. Saunders.

port to families. (For further discussion of nursing care of the mentally retarded child, see p. 880.)

# Perinatal Damage

## HEMOLYTIC DISEASE OF THE NEWBORN: ERYTHROBLASTOSIS FETALIS

**Description.** Erythroblastosis fetalis (*erythro*, "red," and *blast*, "a formative cell," and *osis*, "disease condition") is a disorder that becomes apparent in fetal life or soon after birth. It is one of many congenital hemolytic diseases found in the newborn. There is an excessive destruction of the red blood cells of the baby due to maternal antibodies that pass through the placenta (see p. 98). The terms *isoimmunization* and *sensitization* refer to this process. The incidence of erythroblastosis fetalis has greatly decreased as a result of the protective administration of an Rh vaccine (RhoGAM) to women at risk. Incompatibility of ABO factors is now more common and generally less severe than Rh incompatibility (see p. 99).

The process of maternal sensitization is depicted in Figures 14–14 and 14–15. The mother accumulates antibodies with each pregnancy; therefore, the chance that complications may occur increases with each gestation. If large numbers of antibodies are present, the baby may be severely anemic. In the gravest

form, *hydrops fetalis*, the progressive hemolysis causes fetal *hypoxia*, *anasarca* (generalized edema), and heart failure. This is rare today because of early-detection methods.

**Diagnosis and Prevention.** An extensive history is obtained. Of particular interest are previous sensitizations, an ectopic pregnancy, abortion, blood transfusions, or children who developed jaundice or anemia during the neonatal period. The mother's blood titer is carefully monitored. An *indirect Coombs test* on the mother's blood will indicate previous exposure to Rh-positive antigens. Not every Rh-negative woman has erythroblastotic babies. Some women never become sensitized, even though they bear several Rh-positive children.

Diagnosis of the disease in the prenatal period is confirmed by amniocentesis and monitoring of bilirubin levels in the amniotic fluid. Information gained from these tests helps determine early interventions such as induction of labor or intrauterine exchange transfusion. In the latter procedure, a needle is inserted into the abdomen of the fetus. The position of the needle is guided and verified by ultrasonography, and a transfusion is given. Repeated transfusions may be required. Intravascular transfusions are now being performed in utero (Behrman, 1992). These procedures are hazardous; therefore, they are done only in carefully selected cases, and the parents are informed of possible complications. Improved intrauterine diagnosis has led to fewer fetal deaths.

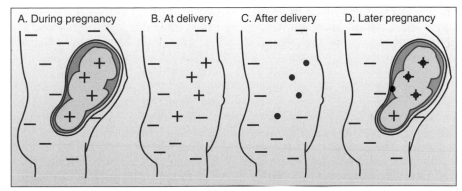

+ Baby's Rh-positive blood cells
− Mother's Rh-negative blood cells
● Mother's Rh antibodies

**Figure 14–14.** *A,* An Rh-negative mother is carrying an Rh-positive baby. *B,* Some of the baby's Rh-positive blood enters the mother's body. *C,* Her body produces antibodies against this factor. *D,* When she carries a subsequent Rh-positive baby, the antibodies cross the placenta and attack the baby's red blood cells.

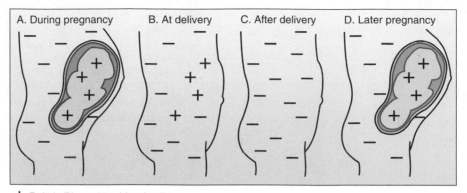

+ Baby's Rh-positive blood cells
− Mother's Rh-negative blood cells

**Figure 14–15.** *A*, After birth, the baby's blood is tested. *B*, If the blood is Rh-positive, RhoGAM is given to the Rh-negative mother within 72 hours after delivery. *C*, It prevents formation of Rh antibodies. *D*, The next Rh-positive fetus is protected. The procedure is repeated with each pregnancy or miscarriage.

Prevention of erythroblastosis by the use of $Rh_o(D)$ immune globulin (RhoGAM) is now routine. An intramuscular injection is given to the mother within 72 hours of delivery of an Rh-positive infant, provided she has not previously been sensitized (Fig. 14–15). RhoGAM may also be given to the pregnant woman at 28 weeks' gestation. This is important in a primigravida who may have unknowingly miscarried or in a multigravida who may not have received her postpartum RhoGAM. It is also administered, when appropriate, following a spontaneous or therapeutic abortion, following amniocentesis, and to women who have bleeding during pregnancy, because fetal blood may leak into the mother's circulation at these times. Mothers who deliver at home and are potential candidates for sensitization must not be overlooked.

**Manifestations.** At the time of delivery, a sample of the baby's cord blood is sent to the laboratory. The *direct Coombs test* detects damaging antibodies. The symptoms of erythroblastosis fetalis vary with the intensity of the disease. Anemia and jaundice are present. The anemia is due to hemolysis of large numbers of erythrocytes. This *pathologic jaundice* differs from *physiologic jaundice* in that it becomes evident within 24 hours following delivery. The liver is unable to handle the massive hemolysis, and bilirubin levels rise rapidly, causing hyperbilirubinemia (*hyper*, "excess," *bilis*, "bile," *rubor*, "red," and *emia*, "blood"). Early jaundice is immediately reported to the physician.

Enlargement of the liver and spleen and extensive edema may develop. The circulating blood usually contains an excess of immature nucleated red blood cells (erythroblasts) caused by the baby's attempts to compensate for the destruction of cells. The oxygen-carrying power of the blood is diminished, as is the blood volume, so shock or heart failure may result. Severe jaundice may cause *kernicterus* (accumulation of bilirubin in the brain tissues). This may cause serious brain damage, may leave the newborn mentally retarded, and frequently results in death.

**Treatment and Nursing Care.** Treatment includes prompt identification, laboratory tests, drug therapy, phototherapy, and exchange transfusion if indicated. Phototherapy may be utilized to reduce serum bilirubin levels in the skin. It may be used alone or in conjunction with an exchange transfusion. It may decrease the need for an exchange transfusion or the number required. The newborn is placed under a bank of fluorescent lights. Specific protocols are carried out. Although this procedure may prevent the rise of bilirubin, it has no effect on the underlying cause of jaundice, and hemolysis may continue to produce anemia (Olds, London, & Ladewig, 1992). The nursing care of the infant receiving phototherapy is presented on pp. 330–331.

During an exchange transfusion, a plastic catheter is inserted into the umbilical vein of the newborn, small amounts of blood (10–20 ml) are withdrawn, and equal amounts of Rh-negative blood are injected. In this way, healthy cells are added to the infant's blood and antibodies are removed. Additional small transfusions may be necessary later. Antibiotics may be given to prevent infection. The nurse is usually responsible for the following: observing the newborn's color and reporting any evidence of jaundice during the 1st and 2nd day; applying wet, sterile compresses to the umbilicus if ordered, until an exchange transfusion is ruled out; stressing to mothers the importance of good prenatal care for subsequent pregnancies; helping to interpret the treatment to parents by giving reassurance as needed; observing and assisting the physician with the exchange transfusion.

Terms helpful in understanding Rh sensitization are listed in Box 14–2. Problems in preventing Rh immunization are listed in Box 14–3.

## INTRACRANIAL HEMORRHAGE

Intracranial hemorrhage, the most common type of birth injury, may result from trauma or anoxia. It occurs more frequently in the preterm infant, whose blood vessels are fragile. Blood vessels within the skull are broken, and

---

> ### BOX 14–2 Terms Helpful in Understanding Rh Sensitization
>
> **Antigen (*anti*, "against," and *gen*, "to produce"):** A substance that induces the formation of antibodies; the antigen-antibody reaction is the basis of immunity
>
> **Coombs test:** Indirectly measures Rh-positive antibodies in *mother's* blood; directly measures antibody-coated Rh-positive red cells in *baby's* blood
>
> **Erythroblastosis fetalis:** The severe form of this disease, which produces anemia in the *fetus* as a result of the incompatibility of the red blood cells of the mother and those of the fetus
>
> **RH$_o$(D) immune globulin (RhoGam):** Immunoglobulin given after delivery of an Rh-positive fetus to an Rh-negative mother, to prevent the maternal Rh immune response
>
> **Sensitization (isoimmunization):** The phenomenon in which the Rh-negative mother develops antibodies against the Rh-positive fetus

---

> ### BOX 14–3 Problems in the Prevention of Rh Immunization
>
> Allergic reactions to Rh$_o$(D) immune globulin (RhoGam)
> Failure to give treatment after delivery of Rh-positive baby
> Failure to give treatment after abortion
> Failure to give treatment after amniocentesis
> Failure of RhoGam to confer protection (because of massive transplacental hemorrhage or inadvertent Rh-positive transfusion)
> Occurrence of Rh immunization late in pregnancy or soon after delivery, before prophylaxis is given
> Occurrence of Rh immunization during infancy ("grandmother theory")
> Very weak Rh antibody in an Rh-negative woman
>
> From Creasy, R., & Resnik, R. (1989). *Maternal-fetal medicine: Principles and practice* (2nd ed.). Philadelphia: W.B. Saunders.

---

bleeding into the brain occurs. When the diagnosis is made, the specific location of the hemorrhage may be noted, that is, subdural, subarachnoid, or intraventricular. This injury may also occur during precipitated delivery or prolonged labor or when the newborn's head is large in comparison with the mother's pelvis.

**Manifestations.** The symptoms of intracranial hemorrhage may occur suddenly or gradually. Some or all symptoms are present, depending on the severity of the hemorrhage. They include inability to move normally, lethargy, poor sucking reflex, irregular respirations, cyanosis, twitching, forceful vomiting, a high-pitched shrill cry, and convulsions. Opisthotonic posturing may be observed. The fontanel may be tense and under pressure, rather than soft and compressible. One pupil of the eye is likely to be small and the other large. If the symptoms are mild, most patients have a good chance of complete recovery. Death results if there is a massive hemorrhage. The infant who survives an extensive hemorrhage may suffer residual defects, such as mental retardation or cerebral palsy. The diagnosis is established by the history of the delivery, computed tomography (CT) scan, magnetic resonance imaging (MRI), evidence of an increase in pressure of the cerebrospinal fluid, and the symptoms and course of the disease.

**Treatment and Nursing Care.** The newborn is placed in an isolette, which allows proper temperature control, ease in administering oxygen, and continuous observation. The baby is handled gently and as little as possible. The head is elevated. The doctor may prescribe vitamin K to control bleeding and phenobarbital if twitching or convulsions are apparent. Prophylactic antibiotics as well as vitamins may be used. The baby is fed carefully because the sucking reflex may be affected. The infant vomits easily. The nurse observes the baby for signs of increased intracranial pressure (see p. 666) and convulsions and assists the doctor with such procedures as lumbar punctures and aspiration of subdural hemorrhage.

If a convulsion occurs, observation of its character by the nurse aids the doctor in diagnosing the exact location of the bleeding. The following are of particular importance: Were the arms, legs, or face involved? Was the right or left side of the body involved? Was the convulsion mild or severe? How long did it last? What was the condition of the infant before and after the seizure? The nurse records observations in the nurses' notes.

## INFECTIONS

### Thrush (Oral Candidiasis)

**Description.** Thrush is an infection of the mucous membranes of the mouth caused by the fungus *Candida*. This organism is normally present in the mother's vagina and is nonpathogenic. However, the altered conditions in the vagina produced by pregnancy may lead to the development of monilial vaginitis. The mucous membranes of the baby's mouth may become infected by direct contact with this infection during delivery, or by contact with the mother's or nurse's contaminated hands. Cross-infection of other newborns may result.

**Manifestations.** White patches that resemble milk curds appear on the tongue, inner lips, gums, and oral mucosa. They are painless but cannot be wiped away. Anorexia may be present. The systemic symptoms are mild if the infection remains in the mouth; however, it can pass along the mucous membranes into the gastrointestinal tract, causing inflammation of the esophagus and stomach. Pneumonitis may also develop. Epstein's pearls, which are small,

## Nursing Brief

In the home, parents are taught to drop nystatin or other medication slowly into the front of the baby's mouth. Medication needs to remain in contact with "patches" as long as possible. Instruct parents to watch for dehydration (e.g., decrease in number of wet diapers due to the baby's refusal to take fluids because of mouth discomfort).

white, epithelial cysts that appear along both sides of the midline of the hard palate, are sometimes mistaken for thrush. These are harmless and gradually disappear.

**Treatment and Nursing Care.** This infection responds well to local application of an antibiotic suspension, such as nystatin (Mycostatin). The mouth is swabbed three or four times a day between feedings with a sterile applicator moistened with the prescribed solution. With proper care, the condition disappears within a few days following its onset.

Newborns suspected of having thrush are isolated. Individual feeding equipment is necessary, and the equipment should be sterile. Disposable bottles or prefilled formula bottles are used. Nipples require scrupulous cleansing because they come in direct contact with the lesions. Disposable nipples, as well as bottles, are preferred. Nurses who care for newborns with infectious conditions do not give daily care to other, healthy babies.

Prevention of this infection begins in the prenatal period. Mothers suspected of having *Candida* infection can then be properly treated. Effective handwashing to prevent reinfection from the mother is necessary. This is particularly true if she is breast feeding her infant. Nurses and other personnel must maintain a high quality of nursing care in order to prevent cross-infection.

### Diarrhea

**Description.** Despite improved care of the newborn, infectious diarrhea continues to be a serious problem in many areas of the world. It is defined as the excessive loss of water and electrolytes in stools, which usually results from disturbed solute transport in the intestine. Infectious diarrhea is highly contagious and may be *fatal*.

Diarrhea may be caused by a variety of

organisms, and often the offender cannot be identified. Viral gastroenteritis is the most widespread type and is self-limiting. Rotavirus is the major etiologic agent during winter (Behrman, 1992). Often it is preceded by respiratory infection. *Escherichia coli* often affects children under 2 years of age. *Shigella*, *Salmonella*, and *Staphylococcus* may also cause diarrhea.

Diarrhea may accompany antibiotic therapy, which sometimes alters the normal flora of the intestinal tract. Food allergies, emotional strain, fatigue, and the unwise use of laxatives can precipitate this disorder in older children. Overfeeding, unbalanced diets containing excessive amounts of sweets, and spoiled foods are additional offenders in the early years.

A carefully obtained medical history yields valuable information. The age of the child is significant in determining etiology. Travel, personal contacts, and history of food allergy are relevant. Diarrhea may last from a few days to several weeks. Functional diarrhea differs from infectious diarrhea in that it is due to organic disease rather than to infection.

**Manifestations.** The symptoms of diarrhea may be mild or extremely severe. The stools are watery and are expelled with force. They may be yellowish-green. The baby becomes listless, refuses to eat, and loses weight. The temperature may be elevated, and the infant may vomit. Dehydration is evidenced by sunken eyes and fontanel and by dry skin, tongue, and mucous membranes. Urination may become less frequent. In severe cases, the excessive loss of bicarbonate from the gastrointestinal tract results in *acidosis*.

**Treatment and Nursing Care.** Constant observation of each newborn in the nursery is of utmost importance. If diarrhea is suspected, it is reported immediately and the baby is isolated. The infection-control nurse is notified. A warm stool specimen is sent to the laboratory for culture. The nurse accurately describes the stools in the nurses' notes as to consistency; frequency; color; odor; presence or absence of blood, mucus, or pus; and force with which the stool is expelled. In older patients, cramping and *tenesmus*, or involuntary straining to empty the bowel, may be observed and should be recorded.

The gastrointestinal tract of the newborn is especially vulnerable to infection. The nurse must constantly protect infants against exposure to pathogenic organisms and must strictly adhere to nursery routines. The preparation of formula requires undivided attention to prevent microorganisms from being carried to the newborn through this medium. Careful feeding techniques are necessary. If a nipple becomes contaminated, a new one must be applied. Proper handwashing is essential. If clothing or blankets fall on the floor, they are sent to the laundry.

The skin of the buttocks receives special care to prevent excoriation. Removing the diaper and exposing the area to the air may be beneficial. A hair dryer on a low setting also helps dry the skin. Daily *accurate weights* are taken to help ascertain the amount of water loss. Careful observation and charting of intravenous fluids are necessary (see pp. 589–593). *Strict intake and output sheets are maintained.*

If the causative organism is identified, specific chemotherapy is instituted. Supportive treatment designed to combat the loss of water and salts is initiated. If vomiting occurs, the baby is given nothing by mouth until the vomiting ceases. Intravenous fluids may be required. As the baby's condition improves, frequent sips of fluid to replace the fluids lost through vomiting and diarrhea are given. Commercial rehydration solutions such as Lytren and Pedialyte are utilized. Breast feeding can generally be continued. The fat and carbohydrate contents of a baby's formula is reduced, and half-strength skimmed milk or skimmed lactic acid milk may be ordered. Parents are taught to consult with their physician or nurse practitioner about how to advance the infant's diet, because this process is individualized according to the baby's age and condition.

Mild diarrhea in older children may be treated at home under a doctor's direction, provided that there is a suitable caregiver. Treatment is essentially the same. The intestine is rested by reducing intake of solid foods. Clear fluids, such as flat ginger ale, gelatin desserts (Jell-O), tea, and Popsicles, are usually well tolerated. High-sodium broths are avoided to prevent electrolyte imbalance. Other foods are added to the diet gradually. A soft diet (sometimes called a BRAT diet, for *b*ananas, *r*ice cereal, *a*pplesauce and *t*oast with jelly) may be resumed when liquids are well tolerated. Creamed soups are avoided. Crackers and pretzels are gradually added. A regular intake is usually resumed within 2–3 days. Milk and butter are cautiously added as the patient's condition improves. Medications such as diphenoxylate hydrochloride and atropine (Lomotil), paregoric, and pectin, which slow intestinal mobility, are generally avoided in the treatment of children because of their narrow margin of safety.

Nursing Care Plan 14–2 provides selected diagnoses and nursing interventions for the infant with diarrhea.

## Acquired Immunodeficiency Syndrome

**Description.** Acquired immunodeficiency syndrome (AIDS) in children was first reported in 1983. By the 1990s, the human immunodeficiency virus (HIV) epidemic was spreading rapidly among infants and children (Fig. 14–16). Today it is among the top 10 causes of death for children 1–4 years old. By 1994, an estimated 7500 children in the United States will have developed AIDS from being infected before or during birth, or from breast feeding after birth. During the next decade, at least 125,000 children will become orphans of the epidemic (U.S. Public Health Service [1993]).

AIDS is caused by a retrovirus known as the human immunodeficiency virus type 1 (HIV-1). HIV attacks lymphocytes (the white blood cells

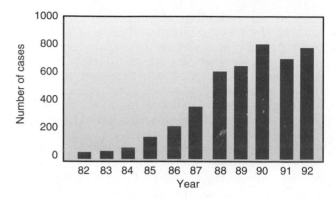

**Figure 14–16.** New cases of acquired immunodeficiency syndrome each year among children 13 years of age and younger in the United States, 1982–1992. (From U.S. Public Health Service, Centers for Disease Control and Prevention [1993].. *Facts about the scope of the HIV/AIDS epidemic in the United States.* National AIDS Clearinghouse.)

that protect one from disease). It appears to cause an imbalance between the helper T cells (CD4+) that support the immune system and the suppressor T cells that shut it down. In a person not infected with HIV, the number of

| NURSING CARE PLAN 14–2 |
| --- |
| **Selected Nursing Diagnoses for the Newborn/Infant with Diarrhea** |

| Goals | Nursing Interventions | Rationale |
| --- | --- | --- |
| **Nursing Diagnosis:** Fluid volume deficit related to active loss of body fluid. | | |
| Bowel movements will be reduced in number by 24 hr<br>Infant's fluid loss will be restored as evidenced by maintenance or increase in weight, skin turgor and other parameters | 1. Weigh infant daily | 1. Daily accurate weights are necessary to ascertain amount of water lost through liquid stools |
| | 2. Obtain warm stool specimen for analysis; wear gloves to handle stool | 2. Warm stool specimen is necessary for culture of pathogenic organisms; gloves protect caregiver from infectious organisms |
| | 3. Record intake and output *accurately* | 3. Accurate intake and output measurement is necessary to determine fluid replacement and kidney function |
| | 4. Offer Pedialyte or other rehydration fluid as ordered | 4. Rehydration fluid decreases mobility of colon, and rests intestinal tract |
| | 5. Observe intravenous fluids if instituted | 5. Fluid depletion occurs very rapidly in babies; infants and small children have different proportions of body water and body fat than adults, and water needs and water losses of baby per unit of body weight are greater (see Fig. 23–23); if hydration status does not improve, intravenous therapy is needed to prevent dehydration, electrolyte imbalance, shock, and death |

*Continued*

| NURSING CARE PLAN 14–2 *Continued* | | |
|---|---|---|
| **Selected Nursing Diagnoses for the Newborn/Infant with Diarrhea** | | |
| Goals | Nursing Interventions | Rationale |

**Nursing Diagnosis:** High risk for altered skin integrity related to frequency of stools.

| | | |
|---|---|---|
| Skin in diaper area is not erythematous and will appear improved within 24 hr | 1. Change diaper frequently; cleanse perianal area with clear water; avoid wipes with alcohol, which will sting | 1. Stools of diarrhea are very irritating to skin |
| | 2. Expose buttocks to air when explosive stools decrease | 2. Air helps dry skin and promotes healing |
| | 3. Apply a soothing ointment such as A and D | 3. This decreases baby's discomfort by soothing irritated skin |

**Nursing Diagnosis:** High risk for transmission of infection related to pathogenic organisms.

| | | |
|---|---|---|
| Organisms will be contained by enteric isolation technique during hospitalization | 1. Institute enteric isolation (gown to enter room, gloves to handle stools) | 1. Many organisms that cause diarrhea are infectious |
| Parents will verbalize their understanding of procedures | 2. Wash hands thoroughly before leaving room | 2. Handwashing is major mode of containing infection |
| | 3. Instruct parents in proper procedures | 3. Parents need to participate safely in infant's care |

**Nursing Diagnosis:** Parental knowledge deficit related to diarrhea in babies.

| | | |
|---|---|---|
| Parents will verbalize understanding of the seriousness of diarrhea in children, compared with in adults | 1. Teach parents that over-the-counter remedies for diarrhea can be harmful to infants and small children | 1. Absorbents such as kaolin and pectin may alter the consistency and appearance of stools and decrease the frequency of evacuation but do not reduce amount of fluid loss and may actually mask significant fluid losses (Whaley & Wong, 1991); labels caution their use in children under 2 yr of age |
| | 2. Explain that dehydration occurs rapidly in infants and that this can be dangerous; because of this, parents need to seek help of a health professional early on so that patient can be assessed and followed | 2. Early detection helps prevent more severe forms of disorder; if infant refuses fluids, if number and consistency of stools increase, and/or if child is vomiting, instruct parents to contact a physician or nurse practitioner |

CD4+ cells remains constant over time. In an HIV-infected person, as months and years go by, the number of CD4+ cells drops.

The CD4+ cell count is a measure of the damage to the immune system caused by HIV and of the body's ability to fight infection (U.S. Public Health Service [1993]). A physician uses the CD4+ cell count to help decide what medical treatments are best for the individual.

A series of terms for this disorder have been developed, but the disease is now classified along a continuum by the Centers for Disease Control. The categories include

1. *Asymptomatic infection.* This refers to a latent period. Individuals in this category have positive antibody tests, indicating exposure to the virus, but are not ill. The current belief is that future critical illness is inevitable.
2. *Symptomatic HIV infection.* Many individuals have this earlier and milder condition (compared with AIDS). This has formerly been referred to as AIDS-related complex, or ARC.
3. *AIDS.* This refers to the most advanced involvement, which includes the finding of HIV antibodies in the patient's blood, the presence of complicating opportunistic infections, and other criteria.

**Transmission.** Only blood, semen, vaginal secretions and human milk have been implicated in the transmission of AIDS. More specifically, AIDS is transmitted by oral, anal, or vaginal sex with someone infected with the virus (either heterosexual or homosexual). It can also be transmitted by sharing drug needles and syringes with an infected person.

Some of the earliest cases of pediatric AIDS resulted from the use of blood products administered to hemophiliacs and from infected blood transfusions. A baby can also become infected through breast milk if the mother is infected. In the United States, if the mother is infected, the baby should be given formula instead (U.S. Public Health Service [1993]).

Children do not get AIDS from casual relationships at schools and medical facilities or through family living. The virus is infectious but not highly contagious, and the circumstances for acquiring it are specific, as indicated. Improved attention to hygiene practices in response to this disease can only be applauded.

Children with AIDS include infants born to mothers with the infection, infants and children who live in households at high risk for AIDS, children sexually abused by intravenous drug users, children with hemophilia, and adolescents who practice unsafe sex. Babies of women infected with the virus may be born with the infection because it can be transmitted from the mother to the baby before or during birth. This *perinatal transmission* is on the rise.

Because passive transmission of antibodies from the mother occurs, babies are born with antibodies that crossed the placenta. Some babies' systems become clear of antibodies in about 15 months, whereas other babies eventually experience the infection. Because of the transference of antibodies, the standard enzyme-linked immunosorbent assay (*ELISA*) and *Western blot* tests used to diagnose HIV infection in older children and adults are less reliable. Antigen tests, and tests to determine the presence of the virus (HIV culture) are currently underway.

Transculturally, the disease is higher among African Americans and Hispanics. "Nearly 84 percent of children with AIDS who were infected before, during, or after birth are black or Hispanic. In New York State, AIDS has been the leading cause of death since 1988 for Hispanic children 1–4 years of age, and the second leading cause of death for black children in the same age group" (U.S. Public Health Service [1993]).

**Manifestations.** Criteria for the disease in children have been outlined by the Centers for Disease Control in Atlanta. The patient becomes subject to overwhelming infection. Oppor-

tunistic infections, such as oral thrush, *Pneumocystis carinii* pneumonia, herpes viruses, and cytomegalovirus take advantage of the body's depressed immune system. Kaposi's sarcoma, a rare type of skin cancer, appears to be less common in children than in adults. Serious bacterial infections, such as meningitis, impetigo, and urinary tract problems, are reported in children. Isolated organisms include *Streptococcus pneumoniae*, *Haemophilus influenzae*, *E. coli*, and *Salmonella*.

The symptoms of HIV infection generally develop more rapidly in infants, and this may be attributed to the infant's immature immune system (Flaskerud & Ungvarski, 1992). Suspicious symptoms in infants include failure to thrive, chronic diarrhea, repeated respiratory tract infections, chronic ear infections, recurrent fever, developmental delays, oral candidiasis, anemia, and enlargement of the liver and spleen. In children as in adults, HIV affects all of the organ systems.

**Treatment and Nursing Care.** Treatment and nursing care are supportive because there is no cure for AIDS at this time. Assessment and care of the child with HIV or AIDS are critically important. Vital signs are taken routinely. Changes in respiratory status are reported. The child's skin is carefully examined for diaper rash, or other breakdown. The inside of the mouth is inspected for lesions. The patient is encouraged to eat high-protein, high-calorie foods to prevent weight loss and maintain tissue growth. Daily weights are obtained, recorded, and compared. Comfort measures are employed. The patient is protected from persons with infection. Health-care workers can reduce the risk of being infected on the job by using universal precautions (see Appendix F). Nursing Care Plan 14–3 provides selected nursing diagnoses and interventions for the patient with AIDS.

Psychological support for these children is paramount. Sensory stimulation and touching are especially important for infants. The effects of isolation and of being ostracized can be physically and emotionally devastating to the developing child. Many babies are abandoned, outlive their mothers, or must live in foster care. Other unique programs such as Children's AIDS Program (CAP) provide homelike respite-care environment and day care ("A place for infants with HIV," 1992). The goal of the program is to help families living with HIV infection stay together.

## Selected Nursing Diagnoses for the Newborn/Infant with AIDS

| Goals | Nursing Interventions | Rationale |
|---|---|---|
| **Nursing Diagnosis:** High risk for infection related to HIV attack on T lymphocytes and the suppression of antibody function. | | |
| Patient remains free from infection as evidenced by intact skin, absence of respiratory distress, and normal laboratory findings | 1. Anticipate opportunistic infections, as patient's immune system is depressed | 1. Opportunistic infections are those that occur due to opportunity afforded by poor health of patient; newborns and preterms have immature immune systems, so are particularly susceptible; once infected, they have few reserves |
| | 2. Monitor respiratory status closely; watch for restlessness, apprehension | 2. Lungs are a target for infection; patients are subject to pneumonia, particularly *P. carinii* |
| | 3. Examine patient regularly for infection (puncture sites, mouth, rectum, pierced ears) | 3. Thrush and herpes simplex are common in children; perianal region is in danger of secondary infection from feces |
| | 4. Reposition frequently | 4. Frequent repositioning reduces pooling of secretions in lungs |
| | 5. Administer antipyretics and antibiotics as prescribed | 5. These will increase patient comfort; may help ward off infection; pneumonia requires aggressive efforts to identify pathogen; fever is common |
| **Nursing Diagnosis:** Nutritional alterations: less than body requirements related to anorexia, anemia, thrush. | | |
| Nutrition maintained as evidenced by normal healing, muscle tone, and body weight | 1. Offer small portions of high-calorie bland foods often | 1. Child has poor appetite; may have mouth sores |
| | 2. Provide oral formula to infants as prescribed | 2. Must have sufficient nutrients to meet growth and development and to maintain body expenditures |
| | 3. Administer nasogastric tube feedings if ordered | 3. Preterms and weakened infants may require nasogastric feedings |
| | 4. Provide hyperalimentation therapy if ordered | 4. Nutritional supplements may be necessary as disease progresses; prognosis is poor, despite aggressive management |
| | 5. Provide for mobility to ensure muscle strength | 5. Immobility contributes to wasted muscles; toddlers need to be up and around as condition permits |
| | 6. Chart intake and output, daily weights | 6. These patients become easily dehydrated. Daily weights will determine nutritional progress |
| **Nursing Diagnosis:** High risk for injury related to changes in central nervous system and from decreased blood components. | | |
| Parents become aware of potential sources of injury; parents recognize signs of bleeding<br>Child will not show signs of injury as evidenced by absence of petechiae | 1. Provide developmentally safe environment | 1. Children are accident prone; normal cuts and abrasions become easily infected; impetigo can be very dangerous for this child |
| | 2. Observe skin for petechiae and bruising, explain to parents | 2. Thrombocytopenia is common; Kaposi's sarcoma, a form of skin cancer, is rare in children, but may be seen in adolescents; looks like bruise in early stages |
| | 3. Monitor laboratory reports (prothrombin times, hematocrit, and so on) | 3. Cultures of blood, urine, throat, and stool may be ordered; child may be unable to generate a white cell response great enough to be detected in laboratories; may also be abnormal response of cells |

*Continued*

## Selected Nursing Diagnoses for the Newborn/Infant with AIDS

| Goals | Nursing Interventions | Rationale |
|---|---|---|
| **Nursing Diagnosis:** Skin integrity: impaired integrity related to immunosuppression. | | |
| Skin remains intact; patient is able to eat without discomfort | 1. Inspect mouth often for lesions (*Candida albicans*)<br>2. Apply nystatin suspension if ordered<br>3. Observe frequently for diaper rash; apply prescribed ointment; maintain skin intactness by thorough, gentle cleansing | 1. Mouth sores may prevent child from eating<br>2. Nystatin may soothe and promote healing<br>3. Skin is subject to breakdown and infection |
| **Nursing Diagnosis:** Infection: high risk for transmission related to disease organism. | | |
| Infection is contained through the use of universal blood and body fluid precautions | 1. Observe isolation technique; use universal precautions for blood and body fluids; maintain enteric and needle precautions similar to those for hepatitis B; wear gloves for diaper change, specimen collections (especially blood); handle secretions and excretions with care; utilize good handwashing techniques | 1. Centers for Disease Control and Prevention regulations request universal precautions to prevent body secretions, especially blood, from infecting caregivers (see Appendix F) |
| **Nursing Diagnosis:** Knowledge deficit of family. | | |
| Family verbalizes understanding of disease process, transmission, and precautions necessary | 1. Clarify misconceptions about the disease<br><br>2. Help prepare parents for possible poor prognosis<br><br><br><br>3. Prepare parents adequately for discharge from hospital<br><br>4. Encourage parents to stay abreast of current, unfolding information<br><br>5. Provide ongoing support services | 1. Misconceptions create anxiety; there are a lot of misconceptions about acquired immunodeficiency syndrome (AIDS)<br>2. Prognosis is generally death; zidovudine (AZT) is showing promise for delaying onset of AIDS if used after positive serologic testing; much controversy about testing exists<br>3. Children should remain with their families and, if possible, be managed out of the hospital with medical and social supports<br>4. Newer developments may change picture of disease; instills some hope in family<br>5. Because of the stigma, possible length, and prognosis of this disease, families require much support |
| **Nursing Diagnosis:** Fear (parents and patient). | | |
| Parents verbalize fears; family develops coping skills that assist them in managing stress related to life-threatening disease | 1. Encourage family to support one another and keep lines of communication open<br>2. Alert parents to self-help groups<br><br><br><br>3. Acquire accurate knowledge about disease<br><br>4. Dispel inordinate fears of general public | 1. Fear is reduced if it can be shared<br><br>2. AIDS support groups, hospice; discuss value of life support measures; families may be faced with such difficult decisions<br>3. There is much inaccurate information about how AIDS is acquired and transmitted<br>4. It is important that pediatric nurses be well informed about the disease |

Since the prognosis for HIV-infected children is poor, the nurse anticipates interventions related to the care of the child with a life-threatening disease. Efforts to support families in crisis are particularly pertinent. Often the extended family must take over. Many families have few financial resources and are exhausted from the child's frequent hospitalizations and physical care. They need to be introduced to such agencies as social service, financial aid, AIDS and grief support groups, home health, nutritional programs such as Women, Infants, and Children (WIC), and hospice services (see discussion of AIDS in pregnancy, p. 111).

The principal medications used for the management of AIDS are zidovudine (AZT: Retrovir), didanosine (ddI: Videx), and zalcitabine (ddC: Hivid). The two latter drugs are used mainly in children who have not responded to zidovudine. The Food and Drug Administration has made the review process faster for AIDS drugs.

Other agents that prevent or manage many of the opportunistic infections include trimetho-methoprim-sulfamethoxazole (Bactrim), isethionate, nystatin (Mycostatin), acyclovir (Zovirax), steroids, and others. Intravenous gamma globulin is used as indicated to provide passive immunity to children.

Research is also being carried out to find ways to strengthen the body's immune system. The major difference in the childhood immunization of affected children is that live poliovirus vaccine is omitted. Instead, inactivated poliovirus vaccine is substituted. Tuberculosis testing is done routinely and as needed. Several antiviral drugs are being tested in children. Early diagnosis and treatment can improve the quality and length of life for many patients.

# Infant of a Diabetic Mother

Diabetes in the mother presents various problems for the newborn infant. These are determined by the severity and duration of the disease in the mother, the degree of control of her condition, and the gestational age of the baby. Diabetes in pregnancy is discussed on page 99.

Many newborn infants of diabetic mothers have serious complications. When the mother is hyperglycemic, large amounts of glucose are transferred to the fetus. This makes the fetus hyperglycemic. In response, the fetal pancreas (islet cells) produces large amounts of fetal insulin, which acts as a growth hormone. Hyperinsulinism, along with excess production of protein and fatty acids, often results in a newborn infant who weighs over 9 pounds. Such a baby is designated large for gestational age (LGA). The condition is termed *macrosomia* (macro—large + soma—body). This infant is prone to injuries at birth because of its size. Following delivery, it often has *low blood sugar* levels because of the abrupt loss of maternal glucose.

The babies have a characteristic *cushingoid* appearance owing to increased subcutaneous fat. The face is round and appears puffy; the babies appear lethargic. The size of these newborn infants makes them appear healthy, but this is deceptive as they often have developmental deficits and may suffer complications of respiratory distress syndrome (RDS) or congenital anomalies. In contrast, an infant born to a mother with severe diabetes may be small for gestational age (SGA) because of poor placental perfusion. These babies suffer from problems of hypoglycemia, hypocalcemia, and hyperbilirubinemia, which are discussed on pp. 320–322 and pp. 323–324.

## KEY POINTS

- Measuring the size of the infant's head is important in babies with hydrocephalus.
- Spina bifida is a congenital embryonic neural tube defect in which there is an imperfect closure of the spinal vertebrae.
- Postoperative nursing care of the baby with a cleft lip includes preventing the baby from sucking and crying, which could impair the suture line.
- The body spica cast encircles the waist and extends to the ankles or toes. It is used in the treatment of congenital dislocations of the hip.
- Down syndrome is a congenital defect of the embryo.
- RhoGAM is given after delivery of an Rh-positive fetus to an Rh-negative mother, to prevent the maternal Rh immune response.

■ In intracranial hemorrhage, blood vessels within the skull are broken and bleeding into the brain occurs.

■ Diarrhea can be life-threatening to newborns and infants because they become dehydrated very quickly.

■ HIV infection and AIDS is a worldwide epidemic that is now known to be caused by a retrovirus.

■ Universal precautions are necessary to protect workers from HIV and AIDS and to contain the disease.

# Study Questions

1. What is the most obvious symptom of hydrocephalus?
2. What complications may arise from neglecting to turn the patient with hydrocephalus?
3. List the symptoms of increased intracranial pressure.
4. What does the term *maternal-infant bonding* mean to you? How can the nurse facilitate this process?
5. Baby Jones has just been admitted to the newborn nursery. His mother has Rh-negative blood. The nurse must observe the baby for what symptoms?
6. What is the most effective procedure carried out by the nurse in preventing the spread of infection?
7. What care is given to the buttocks of the infant with diarrhea? List five characteristics of the baby's stool that the nurse must record.
8. Describe the method of feeding the patient with a cleft lip and palate.
9. What resources are available in your community for speech training of the child with a cleft palate?
10. Define *clubfoot*. Why is it necessary to begin treatment early?
11. Billy, who has congenital clubfoot, had his cast changed in the early morning. List several signs of impaired circulation that might appear.
12. Baby Rico has been admitted with the diagnosis of congenital hip dysplasia. List the signs and symptoms of this orthopedic disorder.
13. How is HIV transmitted?

# Multiple Choice Review Questions

*Choose the most appropriate answer.*

1. The inspection of a cavity by passing a light through its wall to visualize fluid is called
   a. transillumination
   b. phototherapy
   c. hydrotherapy
   d. photosynthesis

2. A congenital defect that results in enlargement of the patient's head and pressure changes within the brain is
   a. hydrocephalus
   b. microcephalus
   c. hydrocele
   d. anencephaly

3. Meningomyelocele is
   a. a protrusion of the meninges through an opening in the spine
   b. primarily a disorder of the muscular tissue of the body
   c. a protrusion of the membranes and cord through an opening in the spine
   d. a tumor in the meningele space
4. A Pavlik harness is sometimes used to correct
   a. clubfoot
   b. juvenile arthritis
   c. congenital hip dysplasia
   d. fractured femur
5. When bathing an infant, the nurse observes the hips for dislocation. One sign of this is
   a. toes turned inward
   b. limitation of abduction
   c. asymmetry of epicanthal folds
   d. shortening of patella

## BIBLIOGRAPHY

A place for infants with HIV. Spotlight (1992). *MCN: American Journal of Maternal-Child Nursing, 17,* 264.

Behrman, R.E. (1992). *Nelson textbook of pediatrics* (14th ed.). Philadelphia: W.B. Saunders.

Bernstein, L., Krieger, B., Novick, et al. (1985). Bacterial infection in the acquired immunodeficiency syndrome of children. *Pediatric Infectious Diseases, 4,* 472.

*Birth defects* (1992). White Plains, NY: March of Dimes Birth Defects Foundation.

Chinn, J. (1990). Current and future dimensions of the HIV/AIDS pandemic in women and children. *Lancet, 336,* 221–224.

Creasy, R.K., & Resnik, R. (1989). *Maternal-fetal medicine: Principles and practice* (2nd ed.). Philadelphia: W.B. Saunders.

Flaskerud, J.H., & Ungvarski, P.J. (1992). *HIV/AIDS: A guide to nursing care* (2nd ed.). Philadelphia: W.B. Saunders.

Jarvis, C. (1992). *Physical examination and health assessment.* Philadelphia: W.B. Saunders.

Klaus, M.H., & Fanaroff, A.A. (1993). *Care of the high-risk neonate* (4th ed.). Philadelphia: W.B. Saunders.

Levine, M.D., Carey, W.B., & Crocker, A.C. (1992). *Developmental-behavioral pediatrics* (2nd ed.). Philadelphia: W.B. Saunders.

Mahan, L.K. & Arlin, M.T. (1992). *Krause's food, nutrition & diet therapy* (8th ed.). Philadelphia: W.B. Saunders.

Mott, S., James, S.R., & Sperhac, A.M. (1990). *Nursing care of children and families.* Reading, MA: Addison-Wesley.

Olds, S., London, M., & Ladewig, P. (1992). *Maternal-newborn nursing* (4th ed.). Reading, MA: Addison-Wesley.

Scott, G.B., Hutto, C., Makuch, R.W., et al. (1989). Survival in children with perinatally acquired human immunodeficiency virus type 1 infection. *New England Journal of Medicine, 221,* 1791–1796.

Selekman, J. (1990). The multiple faces of immunodeficiency in children. *Pediatric Nursing, 16,* 351–355, 361.

U. S. Department of Health and Human Services, Centers for Disease Control and Prevention (1993). *Facts about the scope of the HIV/AIDS epidemic in the United States.* Rockville, MD: National AIDS Clearinghouse.

U. S. Public Health Services, Center for Disease Control and Prevention. (1993). *Surgeon General's report to the American public on HIV infection and AIDS.* Rockville, MD: Health Resources and Services Administration, National Institutes of Health.

Whaley, L. & Wong, D. (1991). *Nursing care of infants and children* (4th ed.). St. Louis: C.V. Mosby.

# Unit 2

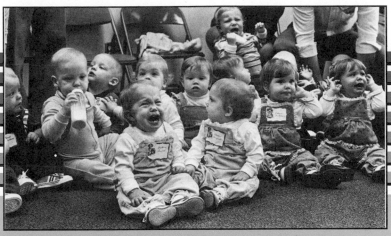

A reunion of twins at a local hospital.

# The Growing Child and Family

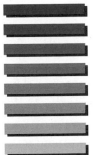

# Chapter 15

# History of Pediatrics

## OBJECTIVES

*On completion and mastery of Chapter 15, the student will be able to*

- Define each vocabulary term listed.
- List four historical developments that have affected the care of children.
- Contrast present-day concepts and attitudes of child care with those of the early 19th century.
- Discuss the contribution to pediatrics made by Lillian Wald.
- Name two international organizations concerned with children.
- List five federal programs that assist mothers and children.
- Discuss the American Nurses' Association Standards for Maternal-Child Health Nursing Practice.
- State the purpose of the Children's Bureau and its location.
- Review and list a minimum of six provisions for children cited by the Children's Charter.

## Pediatrics Then and Now

*Pediatrics* is defined as the branch of medicine that deals with the child's development and care and with the diseases of childhood and their treatment. The word is derived from the Greek *pais*, *paidos*, "child," and *iatreia*, "cure." Abraham Jacobi (1830–1919) is known as the father of pediatrics because of his many contributions to the field. The establishment of pediatric nursing as a specialty paralleled that of departments of pediatrics in medical schools, the founding of children's hospitals, and the development of separate units for children in foundling homes and general hospitals.

In the Middle Ages, the concept of childhood did not exist. Infancy lasted until about the age of 7, at which time the child was assimilated into the adult world. Art of that time depicts the child wearing adult clothes and wigs. Most children did not attend school. Childhood became a separate entity only when large numbers of people entered the middle class and leisure time increased. Because infants were surviving for a longer time, parents were willing to become more invested in them.

Today we no longer consider the child a "miniature adult." Childhood has become a separate phase of life, which in Western society is characterized by schooling. Children's rights are protected by laws and customs. As youths have become free from the labor of farms and factories, adolescence as a separate entity has also emerged.

Children are composed of physical, intellectual, emotional, and spiritual natures, and we should relate to each as a whole person. As the organic causes of death and disability seen in the past are reduced, we turn to improving the quality of care by helping to provide an environment for optimum growth and development. Names of child experts such as Erikson, Bowlby, and Piaget are now well known in the health-care fields.

### CULTURAL INFLUENCES

Methods of child care have varied throughout history. The culture of a society has a strong influence on standards of child care. Many primitive tribes were nomads. Strong children survived, whereas the weak were left to die. This practice of infanticide (French and Latin *infans*, "infant," and *caedere*, "to kill") helped ensure the safety of the group. As tribes became settled, more attention was given to children, but they were still frequently valued for their productivity. Certain peoples, such as the Egyptians and the Greeks, were advanced in their attitudes. The Greek physician Hippocrates (460–370 BC) wrote of illnesses peculiar to children.

Christianity had a considerable impact on child care. In the early 17th century, several children's asylums were founded by Saint Vincent de Paul. Many of these eventually became hospitals, although their original concern was for the abandoned. The first children's hospital was founded in Paris in 1802. In the United States, numerous homeless children were cared for by the Children's Aid Society, founded in New York City in 1853. In 1855 the first pediatric hospital in the United States, The Children's Hospital of Philadelphia, was founded.

## Nursing Brief

Cultural beliefs today, as in the past, affect how a family perceives health and illness. Holistic nursing includes being alert for cultural diversity and incorporating this information into nursing care plans.

## Nursing Brief

Innovative community programs such as foster grandparents, home health or parent aids, and Phone a Friend (a call-in program for children home alone after school) are of particular value to dysfunctional or isolated families.

## ADVANCES

Many advances have been made in medical and surgical techniques through the years. For instance, children with heart problems are now treated by a pediatric cardiologist. Much of the complex surgery needed by the newborn with a congenital defect is provided by the pediatric surgeon. Emotional problems are managed by pediatric psychiatrists. Many hospital laboratories are better equipped to test pediatric specimens. Congenital and heritable defects have increasing importance. Chromosomal studies and biochemical screening have made identification and family counseling more significant than ever. The field of perinatal biology has advanced to the forefront of pediatric medicine.

The medical profession and allied agencies work as a team for the total well-being of the patient. Children with defects previously thought to be incompatible with life are taken to special diagnostic and treatment centers where they receive expert attention. Following discharge, many of these children are being cared for in their homes. Some are dependent on sophisticated hospital equipment such as ventilators and home monitors. The nursing care may require the suctioning of a tracheotomy, central line care, and other highly technical skills. Parents must be carefully educated and continually supported. Although this type of care is cost effective and psychologically sound for the child, respite care is extremely important, because 24-hour-a-day care is extremely taxing for the family, both physically and psychologically.

## The Children's Bureau

Lillian Wald, a nurse who was interested in the welfare of children, is credited with suggesting the establishment of a federal children's bureau. She believed that if a nation could have a bureau dedicated to its farm crops, it should

certainly have one to look after its "child crop" (Bradbury & Oettinger, 1962). She and Florence Kelley, an ardent foe of child labor, were jointly responsible for the far-reaching conception of a children's bureau. The time was 1903. It took several years for the bill to be given the needed support by the first White House Conference on Children and Youth. The act directed the Children's Bureau "to investigate and report upon all matters pertaining to the welfare of children and child life among all classes of people."

Once the Children's Bureau was established in 1912, it focused its attention on the problems of infant mortality. This study was followed by one that dealt with maternal mortality. These investigations gave great impetus to drives for improvement in maternal and child health. Another early effort was made in the area of birth registration. This study eventually led to birth registration in all states.

In the 1930s, the Children's Bureau began to investigate the effects of the economic depression on children. It found that the health and nutrition of children throughout the nation were declining because of the great increase in poverty. As a result of the research done in this area, hot lunch programs were established in many schools.

During the Depression, many adolescents found home life unbearable because of unemployment. Great numbers of young people wandered throughout the country in search of work. Because there was none to be found, they were not welcome in most communities. In 1933 the chief of the Bureau made suggestions that were instrumental in the establishment of the Civilian Conservation Corps. These work camps provided opportunities for training in a wholesome environment, and they proved very successful.

Throughout this period, the Children's Bureau had been observing the conditions under which children were forced to work. The observations were appalling. A description of 13- and 14-year-old children working in coal mines was particularly vivid.

## Nursing Brief

Today the Children's Bureau is administered under the auspices of the Department of Health and Human Services.

Black coal dust is everywhere, covering the windows and filling the air and lungs of the workers. The slate is sharp so that slate pickers often cut or bruise their hands; the coal is carried down the chute in water and this means sore and swollen hands for the pickers. The first few weeks after the boy begins to work his fingers bleed almost continuously, and are called "red tops" by the older boys (Bradbury & Oettinger, 1962).

These studies paved the way for a federal government law that controls child labor. The Fair Labor Standards Act, passed in 1938, established a general minimum working age of 16 (Fig. 15–1) and a minimum working age of 18 for jobs considered hazardous. More important, this act paved the way for the establishment of

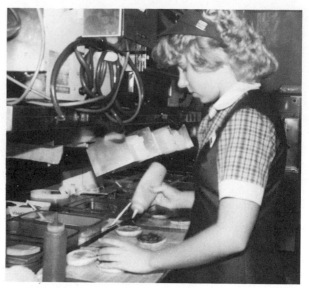

**Figure 15–1.** The Fair Labor Standards Act of 1938 stipulates a minimum working age of 16 years.

# Nursing Brief

Two international organizations concerned with children are the United Nations Children's Fund (UNICEF) and the World Health Organization (WHO).

national minimum standards for child labor and provided a means of enforcement. Table 15–1 provides a summary of federal programs designed to promote the welfare of children and their families.

**Table 15–1.** SUMMARY OF FEDERAL PROGRAMS AFFECTING MATERNAL-CHILD HEALTH

| Program | Year of Inception | Comment |
|---|---|---|
| Social Security Act | 1935 | Provides matching state and federal funds for maternal and child care and for crippled children, supports preventive health programs (immunizations, screenings) |
| Fair Labor Standards Act | 1938 | Establishes minimum working age of 16 |
| Maternal-Child Health Infant Care Project | 1963 | Attempts to decrease infant and maternal mortality |
| Children and Youth Project | 1965 | Targets low-income and less accessible children requiring health care |
| Crippled Children's Service | 1965 | Provides services to disabled children under 21 |
| National School Lunch Act and Child Nutrition Act | 1966 | Provides reduced-cost or free meals to low-income families |
| Head Start | 1969 | Assists disadvantaged preschool children, increases educational skills |
| Medicaid Early and Periodic Screening, Diagnosis and Treatment (EPSDT) | 1972 | Provides EPSDT for poor children (implemented in each state) |
| Women, Infants, and Children (WIC) | 1972 | Provides supplemental food programs for women, infants, and children of low income |
| Child Abuse Prevention and Treatment Act | 1974 | Established National Center on Child Abuse; receives reports, research |
| Education for All Handicapped Children Act | 1975 | PL 94-142, provides free public education to all handicapped children ages 3–21; provides necessary supportive services |
| Administration for Children, Youth and Families (ACYF) | 1977 | Coordinates all children's programs |
| Community Mental Health Centers (CMHCs) | 1982 | Attempts to increase availability of mental health centers to low-income families |
| Missing Children Act | 1982 | Nationwide clearinghouse for missing children (National Crime Information Computer) |

# White House Conferences

The First White House Conference on Children and Youth was called by President Theodore Roosevelt in 1909. It gathered every 10 years.

In the White House Conference on Child Health and Protection (1930), the Children's Charter was drawn up (Box 15–1). This is considered to be one of the most important documents in child care history. It lists 19 statements related to needs of children in the areas of education, health, welfare, and protection. This declaration has been widely distributed throughout the world.

---

**BOX 15–1  The Children's Charter of 1930**

I. For every child spiritual and moral training to help him or her to stand firm under the pressure of life.

II. For every child understanding and the guarding of personality as a most precious right.

III. For every child a home and that love and security which a home provides; and for those children who must receive foster care, the nearest substitute for their own home.

IV. For every child full preparation for the birth, the mother receiving prenatal, natal, and postnatal care; and the establishment of such protective measures as will make child-bearing safer.

V. For every child protection from birth through adolescence, including: periodical health examinations and, where needed, care of specialists and hospital treatment; regular dental examinations and care of the teeth; protective and preventive measures against communicable diseases; the ensuring of pure food, pure milk, and pure water.

VI. For every child from birth through adolescence, promotion of health, including health instruction and health programs, wholesome physical and mental recreation, with teachers and leaders adequately trained.

VII. For every child a dwelling-place safe, sanitary, and wholesome, with reasonable provisions for privacy; free from conditions which tend to thwart development; and a home environment harmonious and enriching.

VIII. For every child a school which is safe from hazards, sanitary, properly equipped, lighted, and ventilated. For younger children nursery schools and kindergartens to supplement home care.

IX. For every child a community which recognizes and plans for needs; protects against physical dangers, moral hazards, and disease; provides safe and wholesome places for play and recreation; and makes provision for cultural and social needs.

X. For every child an education which, through the discovery and development of individual abilities, prepares the child for life and through training and vocational guidance prepares for a living which will yield the maximum of satisfaction.

XI. For every child such teaching and training as will prepare him or her for successful parenthood, home-making, and the rights of citizenship and, for parents, supplementary training to fit them to deal wisely with the problems of parenthood.

XII. For every child education for safety and protection against accidents to which modern conditions subject the child—those to which the child is directly exposed and those which, through loss or maiming of the parents, affect the child directly.

XIII. For every child who is blind, deaf, crippled, or otherwise physically handicapped and for the child who is mentally handicapped, such measures as will early discover and diagnose his handicap, provide care and treatment, and so train the child that the child may become an asset to society rather than a liability. Expenses of these services should be borne publicly where they cannot be privately met.

XIV. For every child who is in conflict with society the right to be dealt with intelligently as society's charge, not society's outcast; with the home, the school, the church, the court, and the institution when needed, shaped to return the child whenever possible to the normal stream of life.

XV. For every child the right to grow up in a family with an adequate standard of living and the security of a stable income as the surest safeguard against social handicaps.

XVI. For every child protection against labor that stunts growth, either physical or mental, that limits education, that deprives children of the right of comradeship, of play, and of joy.

XVII. For every rural child as satisfactory schooling and health services as for the city child, and an extension to rural families of social, recreational, and cultural facilities.

## Nursing Brief

The American Academy of Pediatrics (AAP), made up of pediatricians from across the nation, has established its position of leadership in setting health standards for children.

The 1980 White House Conference on Families focused on involving the states at the grass-roots level. A series of statewide hearings was held to identify the most pressing problems of families in the various localities. A tremendous range of viewpoints on many subjects was shared, and specific recommendations were made. All participants had the common concern of *strengthening and supporting the American family*. Further White House Conferences have been canceled, and at this point, none will be rescheduled until the current president makes a decision about their relevance and funding.

## International Year of the Child

The year 1979 was designated as the International Year of the Child (IYC). Its purpose was to focus attention on the critical needs of the world's 1.5 billion children and to inspire the nations, the organizations, and the individuals of the world to consider how well they are providing for children (U.S. Commission of the International Year of the Child, 1980). At this time the United Nations reaffirmed the Declaration of the Rights of the Child (Box 15–2). Although the United States has some of the finest health-care facilities in the world, the following information, cited in this report, indicates how far children's health in the United States fell short of the ideal:

- Several other countries do a better job than the United States in keeping babies alive in the 1st year of life. In the United States, the death rate for African-American infants is higher than that of Caucasian infants. Death rates for other minorities are also high, but accurate data are not available.
- Nearly 10 million American children have no known regular source of primary health care.

| BOX 15–2 | The United Nations Declaration of the Rights of the Child |
| --- | --- |

The general assembly proclaims that the child is entitled to a happy childhood and that all should recognize these rights and strive for their observance by legislative and other means:

1. All children without exception shall be entitled to these rights regardless of race, color, sex, language, religion, politics, national or social origin, property, birth, or other status.
2. The child should be protected so that he or she may develop physically, mentally, morally, spiritually, and socially in freedom and dignity.
3. The child is entitled at birth to a name and nationality.
4. The child is entitled to healthy development which includes adequate food, housing, recreation, and medical attention. He or she shall receive the benefits of Social Security.
5. The child who is handicapped physically, mentally, or emotionally shall receive treatment, education, and care according to his or her need.
6. The child is entitled to love and a harmonious atmosphere, preferably in the environment of his or her parents. Particular love, care, and concern need to be extended to children without families and to the poor.
7. The child is entitled to a free education and opportunities for play, recreation, and to develop his or her talents.
8. The child shall be the first one protected in times of adversity.
9. The child shall be protected against all forms of neglect, cruelty, and exploitation. He or she should not be employed in hazardous occupations or before the minimum age.
10. The child shall not be subjected to racial or religious discrimination. The environment should be peaceful and friendly.

- Many children who are handicapped receive no services.
- Fully one-half of the children who require vision care do not receive it, whether the care be eye examinations, eyeglasses, vision therapy, or surgery.
- Of children under age 12, 47% have never been to a dentist for treatment.
- More and more of the health problems among children and youths are psychoso-

cial, for example: *Alcohol abuse*—an estimated 3.3 million problem drinkers exist in the 14–17-year-old age bracket, representing 19% of this population. *Adolescent pregnancy*—every year more than 200,000 babies are born to teenage girls between 15 and 17 years of age. An additional 11,000 children are born to mothers under the age of 15. *Physical and sexual abuse*—more than 1 million children in the United States are abused each year. It is estimated that 2000–5000 children die every year as a result of child abuse. An additional 10,000 children are severely battered; 50,000–200,000 children are sexually abused.

- Mental health services are not available to the majority of children who are in need of them. The President's Commission on Mental Health in 1978 declared that mental health care was "inadequate or nonexistent" for children and adolescents.
- Accidents, homicides, and suicides account for about three-fourths of all deaths among teenagers. Accidents are the leading cause of death of all children over the age of 1 year. If no child died in a car accident, total childhood mortality would be reduced by 20%. (U.S. National Commission on the International Year of the Child, 1980.)

At this writing, many of these important issues remain a challenge. There are no plans at present for another IYC.

## Missing Children's Act

In 1982 Congress passed the Missing Children's Act. This act set up a nationwide clearinghouse for missing children. Local law enforcement officials must enter into the Federal Bureau of Investigation's National Crime Information Computer the names of children under 17 years of age who had been missing for 48 hours and who have no history of previously running away. This information is available to police departments across the nation. If this is not done, the parents, legal guardians, or next of kin may enter the name themselves. The act also mandated that information on unidentified bodies be placed on the computer and that this be available to coroners and law enforcement officials nationwide.

Parental kidnapping, which is of equal concern, has been addressed in the Parental Kidnapping Prevention Act. This law requires all states to honor child custody decrees of other states and use the Fugitive Felon Act to help officials locate children abducted by estranged parents.

## Public Health Department

The public health department assumes a great deal of responsibility for the prevention of disease and death during childhood. This is done on national, state, and local levels. The water, milk, and food supplies of communities are inspected. Maintenance of proper sewage and garbage disposal is enforced. Epidemics are investigated, and when necessary, persons capable of transmitting diseases are isolated. The public health department is also concerned with the inspection of housing.

Law requiring the licensing of physicians and pharmacists indirectly affect the health of children and the general public. Protection is also afforded by the Pure Food and Drug Act, which controls medicines, poisons, and purity of foods. Programs for disaster relief, care and rehabilitation of handicapped children, foster child care, family counseling, family day care, protective services for abused or neglected children, and education of the public are maintained and supported by governmental and private agencies. State licensing bureaus control the regulation of motor vehicles. This and the protection of the public by law enforcement agencies are ever more important because automobile accidents rank among the leading causes of injury and death of children.

## The Pediatric Nurse as Advocate

Pediatric nurses are increasingly assuming a role as child advocates. An advocate is a person who intercedes or pleads in behalf of another. Advocacy may be required for both the child's physical and emotional health and may include other family members. Hospitalized children frequently cannot determine or express their needs. When nurses feel that the child's best interests are not being met, they must seek assistance. This usually involves taking the problem through the normal chain of command. Nurses need to document their efforts to seek instruction and direction from their head nurse, supervisors, or the physician.

## The Pediatric Nurse as Teacher

The nurse teaches in a variety of settings. The pediatric nurse may be involved in teaching both the parents and the child. Because of brief hospital stays, teaching must be accomplished in a short time. This calls for the organization of information. In the hospital, most teaching is done informally, using checklists to ensure that nothing is omitted. Teaching is most effective if the learner is involved in the process rather than just being a passive listener. Repetition of skills increases retention and feelings of competence. Cultural influences affect learning. Summarizing important concepts is effective. It is important to allow time for questions concerning the new material.

## Current Challenges

Child health nurses face many challenges in attempting to provide holistic care for children. The American Nurses Association (ANA) develops standards of care that serve as a guide to meet some of these challenges. These standards are used when policies and procedures are established. Also, each state has a nurse practice act that determines the scope of practice for the registered nurse, practical nurse, and certified nurse assistant. These descriptions vary from state to state, so nurses must keep ir̃ormed about the laws in the state where they are employed. Pediatric nurses practice in a variety of settings, some of which are listed in Box 15–3.

Cost containment is a major motivation in health care, especially when health costs rise without decreases in morbidity and mortality. Many hospitals are merging to increase their buying power and reduce duplication of services.

Insurance reimbursement has become an important consideration in health care. The federal government has had to revise its Medicare and Medicaid programs. Among other changes it instituted Diagnosis Related Groupings (DRGs). DRGs refer to a Medicare system that determines payment for a hospital stay based on the patient's diagnosis. This

| BOX 15–3 | Current Pediatric Nursing Settings |
|---|---|

Community nurse
School nurse
Camp nurse
Office nurse
Day care nurse
Home nurse
Hospital nurse
Children's long-term care facility nurse
Hospice nurse

mandate has had a tremendous impact on health care delivery. Patients are being discharged earlier, and more care is being given in skilled nursing facilities and in the home. Some insurance companies are employing nurses in the role of case managers. Nurses remaining in institutions also may be required to assume the role of case managers and to become more flexible through cross training. Nurses are expected to be concerned with keeping hospital costs down while maintaining quality care. Many suggest that the future of nursing may depend on how well nurses can demonstrate their value and cost effectiveness.

Health maintenance organizations (HMOs) and preferred provider organizations (PPOs) have emerged as alternative medical care delivery systems. Insurers and providers of care have united to hold costs down and yet remain competitive. A two-tiered system has evolved: one tier serves the more financially stable people (private insurance, HMOs/PPOs), and the other serves the less financially stable people (Medicare and Medicaid). In addition, a large percentage of persons are uninsured or underinsured. This presents problems in access and quality of health care.

Health promotion continues to assume increased importance. Preventing illness or disability is cost effective; more importantly, it saves the family from stress, disruptions, and financial burden. Healthy children are spending fewer days in the hospital. Many conditions are treated in same-day surgery, ambulatory settings, or emergency rooms. Rather than being distinct, hospital and home care have become interdependent.

Chronically ill children are living into adulthood, creating the need for more support ser-

## Nursing Brief

Expanded nursing roles include the clinical nurse specialist, the pediatric nurse practitioner, the school nurse practitioner, the family practitioner, and the certified nurse-midwife.

vices. Medically fragile and technology-dependent children may change the profile of chronically ill children. The nurse is often the instigator of support services to these patients through education and referral. Ideally these services will assist the child to become as independent as possible, to lead a productive life, and to be integrated into society. In the past, the term *mainstream* was used to describe the process of integration of a physically or mentally challenged child into society. The term *full inclusion*, an expansion of the mainstream policy, is being used more frequently today. Early infant intervention programs for children with developmental disabilities attempt to reduce or minimize the effects of the disability. These services may be provided in a clinic or in the home. The need for in-home family-centered pediatric care will continue to grow with the number of children with chronic illness who survive.

Quality of life is particularly relevant. Organ transplants have saved some children; however, the complications, limited availability, and expense of these transplants create moral and ethical dilemmas. Older children with life-threatening conditions need to be included in planning modified advance directives with their families and the medical team.

These developments, along with the explosion of information, emphasis on individual nurse accountability, new technology, and the use of computers in medicine, make it especially desirable for nurses to maintain their knowledge and skills at a level necessary to provide safe care. Employers often offer continuing education classes for their employees. Most states require proof of continuing education for renewal of nursing licenses.

Professional journals of interest to the pediatric nurse include *Maternal-Child Nursing Journal, Pediatric Nursing, Issues in Comprehensive Pediatric Nursing,* and the *Journal of Pediatric Nursing*. Bimonthly information on current topics may also be found in the *Pediatric Clinics of North America*. Organizations that share information on children and their families include the Society of Pediatric Nurses as well as subspecialty groups such as the Association of Pediatric Oncology Nursing.

## KEY POINTS

- The culture of a society has a strong influence on the family and child care.
- Lillian Wald, a nurse, is credited with suggesting the establishment of the Children's Bureau.
- The Fair Labor Standards Act, passed in 1938, controls child labor.
- The White House Conferences on Children and Youth investigated and reported on matters pertaining to children and their families among all classes of people.
- The physicians' organization that helps set health standards for children is the American Academy of Pediatrics.
- The Children's Charter of 1930 is considered one of the most important documents in child-care history.
- The United Nations Declaration of the Rights of the Child calls for freedom, equality of opportunity, social and emotional benefits, and enhancement of each child's potential.
- The American Nurses' Association (ANA) has written standards of maternal-child health practices.
- Diagnosis-related groups, a form of cost containment, continue to affect nursing practice.
- Nurses must carry on their historical role of focusing on the human aspects of child health care.

# Study Questions

1. Define the following: infanticide, pediatrics, pediatrician, Children's Charter, Fair Labor Standards Act.
2. How often did the White House Conference on Children and Youth meet?
3. Contrast present-day concepts and attitudes of child care with those of the early 19th century.
4. List two organizations concerned with child care.
5. Discuss the purpose of the International Year of the Child.

# Multiple Choice Review Questions

*Choose the most appropriate answer.*

1. The man known as the father of pediatrics is
   a. Benjamin Spock
   b. John Bowlby
   c. Abraham Jacobi
   d. Hippocrates
2. The nurse credited with suggesting the establishment of a Federal Children's Bureau is
   a. Lillian Wald
   b. Florence Nightingale
   c. Eleanor Thompson
   d. Mary Adelaide Nutting
3. An important document drawn up in 1930 that lists the needs of children is
   a. Pledge to Children
   b. Children's Charter
   c. Declaration of the Rights of the Child
   d. Missing Children's Act
4. The constitutional amendment that controls child labor is
   a. Smith Hughes Act
   b. Fair Labor Standards Act
   c. Social Security Act
   d. Hill-Burton Labor Act
5. The leading cause of death in children over the age of 1 year as determined by IYC is
   a. cancer
   b. heart disease
   c. accidents
   d. pneumonia

## BIBLIOGRAPHY

Bradbury, D., & Oettinger, K. (1962). *Five decades of action for children*. Washington, DC: Children's Bureau, Department of Health, Education, and Welfare.

Betz, C., Hunsberger, M., & Wright, S. (1994). *Family-centered nursing care of children* (2nd ed.). Philadelphia: W.B. Saunders.

Brodie, B. (1985). Reflections on the first decade of MCN. *American Journal of Maternal-Child Nursing, 10*, 11–12, 17.

Cone, T. (1980). *History of American pediatrics*. Boston: Little, Brown.

Grad, R. (1989, July/August). National Commission acts on behalf of children. *American Journal of Maternal-Child Nursing*.

Mott, S., James, S., & Sperhac, A. (1990). *Nursing care of children and families* (2nd ed.). Reading, MA: Addison-Wesley.

*Standards of maternal-child nursing practice* (1986). Kansas City: American Nurses' Association.

U. S. National Commission on the International Year of the Child (1980). *Report to the President*. Washington, DC: Government Printing Office.

Velsor-Friedrich, B. (1991). Health goals for children and their families: 1991 and beyond. *Journal of Pediatric Nursing, 6*, 62.

Whaley, L., & Wong, D. (1991). *Nursing care of infants and children* (4th ed.). St. Louis: C.V. Mosby.

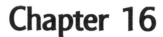

## Chapter 16

# Growth, Development, and Nutrition

*On completion and mastery of Chapter 16, the student will be able to*

■ Define each vocabulary term listed.
■ Differentiate between dominant and recessive genes.
■ Discuss the role of the genetic counselor.
■ Explain the differences among growth, development, and maturation.
■ Recognize and read a growth chart for children.
■ List five factors that influence growth and development.
■ Discuss the nursing implications of growth and development.
■ Discuss the nutritional needs of growing children.
■ Differentiate between the permanent and the deciduous teeth and list the times of their eruption.

## Heredity

Most of us understand that something that is inherited is received from one's ancestors. It may be money or a desired heirloom. It is also possible to inherit physical traits and sometimes even a disorder, such as hemophilia. A person's sex and all the person's inherited characteristics are determined at the moment of conception, when the male sperm cell unites with the female ovum. There are 23 pairs of chromosomes, 22 autosomes (chromosomes common to both sexes), and 1 pair of sex chromosomes (XX in girls and XY in boys). These contain the blueprint, or genetic code, for an individual. Modern cytogenetics (*cyto*, "cell" and *genetic*, "origin") has led to the identification of chromosomes as bearers of genes and deoxyribonucleic acid (DNA) as the key molecule of the gene. Like chromosomes, genes are paired.

Although matching genes in a pair of chromosomes have the same basic function, they do not act with equal power. Some are *dominant*, others *recessive*. If a gene is recessive, its instructions are overpowered if it is matched with a dominant gene. However, if a child inherits two recessive genes (one from each parent), the particular characteristics associated with them will prevail. When any two members of a pair of genes carry the same genetic instructions, the person carrying those genes is said to be *homozygous* for that trait. When the two genes in a pair carry different instructions, the person is *heterozygous* for the trait. One member of a heterozygous pair of genes is the dominant gene.

The concept of dominant and recessive genes is important in studying birth defects because some parents who carry defective genes can have normal children or children who are carriers but are not themselves affected. It also explains how supposedly normal parents can give birth to a defective baby. An individual's particular set of genes is known as a *genotype*. Researchers have localized many genes to specific chromosomes. This is termed *gene mapping*. Such techniques make an *accurate family health history more vital than ever*. Family medical forms are available from The National Foundation/March of Dimes. They provide space for vital information covering three generations. The family history record is called a pedigree chart or *genogram*.

### KARYOTYPES

Geneticists are able to photograph the nuclei of human cells and to enlarge them enough so that one can see the 46 chromosomes. These are cut from the picture, matched in pairs, and grouped from large to small. The result is called a karyogram (*karyo*, "nucleus," and *gram*, "chart"). The karyogram of a normal individual shows 22 pairs of chromosomes called *autosomes*. These chromosomes, which are alike in both girls and boys, direct the development of the individual. An example of an autosomal defect is Down syndrome, also known as trisomy 21 because patients have a third number 21 chromosome in most of the cells in their bodies (Fig. 16–1).

The remaining pair of chromosomes are sex chromosomes. These differ in boys and girls, determining sex and secondary sexual characteristics. The female sex chromosomes appear as XX, the male as XY. Defects in sex chromosomes are more prevalent than those in autosomes and account for a greater variety of abnormal conditions. The Y chromosome is small and apparently carries only the genes for masculinity. The X chromosome is much larger and carries the female genes plus many others essential to life, such as those that direct various aspects of metabolism, blood formation, color blindness, and defense against bacteria.

Omissions and duplications of chromosomes can occur during meiosis (the cell division, seen

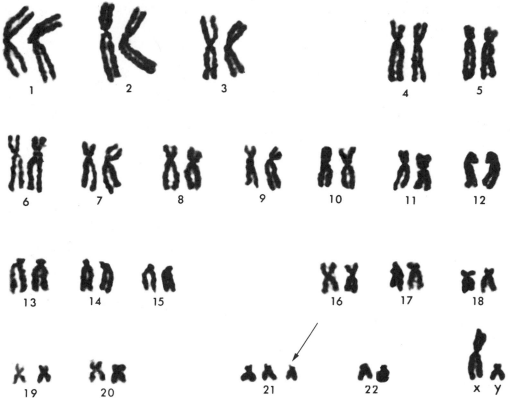

**Figure 16-1.** A karyogram depicting Down syndrome with trisomy 21. (From Robbins, S.L., Angell, M., & Kumar, V. [1981]. *Basic pathology* [3rd ed.]. Philadelphia: W.B. Saunders, p. 169.)

only in sex cells, in which the chromosomes divide in half before the cell divides in two). When a piece of a chromosome, or an entire one, becomes joined to another chromosome, or when broken segments exchange places, the abnormality is termed a *translocation*. When the genes that cause a specific condition are known to be carried on the sex chromosomes, the disorder is termed *sex-linked*.

*Mutations* or mistakes in the DNA of a specific gene are not completely understood. Once a gene becomes abnormal, the defect is repeated whenever the chromosome on which it appears reproduces itself during normal cell division. Radiation in the form of x-rays, radium, atomic energy, and isotopes is known to cause mutations. Because a defect may not appear for generations, the amount of radiation a person can safely be exposed to is difficult to determine. New gene mutations also occur.

A mutation of a gene that directs the production of an enzyme can result in a disruption in the orderly process of metabolism. These bio-chemical disorders are termed *metabolic defects* or *inborn errors of metabolism*. Without proper direction of the enzymes, harmful chemical products accumulate in the system. An example of this is phenylketonuria (PKU), discussed on page 349. Another kind of error results when an essential substance is absent. This occurs in persons with albinism (*albus*, "white," and *ismos*, "condition") a disorder in which there is a total lack of pigment in the skin, hair, and eyes. Some other examples of inherited pathologic conditions discussed in this text are cystic fibrosis, sickle cell anemia, and hemophilia. If a genetic mistake affects only an unimportant link in the metabolism chain or if the body otherwise compensates, no abnormal symptoms may occur even though a gene is defective.

## GENETIC RESEARCH AND COUNSELING

As researchers gather more knowledge about the mysteries of the gene, they are able to discover ways to prevent and treat genetic mishaps. The role of the genetic counselor has broadened and taken on greater importance. Patterns of inheritance are known for hundreds of specific birth defects. Counselors can often predict the percentage of risk a couple with a hereditary disorder may face and can suggest laboratory tests to determine if prospective parents are carriers (Figs. 16-2 and 16-3). Counselors are a good source of information about modern treatment and prevention of birth defects. A list of the locations of genetic counseling services can be obtained from The National Foundation/March of Dimes.

In specific genetic disorders in which a precise enzyme or protein is missing, it is often possible to supply the necessary factor. For example, clotting agents may be given to hemophiliacs and pancreatic enzymes to those afflicted with cystic fibrosis. In other disorders, eliminating the offending substance can correct the problem. This is seen in PKU, in which the elimination of foods high in phenylalanine can prevent brain damage.

Medical researchers are on the threshold of important breakthroughs in this large group of disorders. For example, the gene associated with cystic fibrosis has been identified. The gene that causes fragile X syndrome, an inherited form of mental retardation, has also been found. A gene that causes an inherited form of colon cancer has been identified. As biochemists learn to create some of these vital factors in

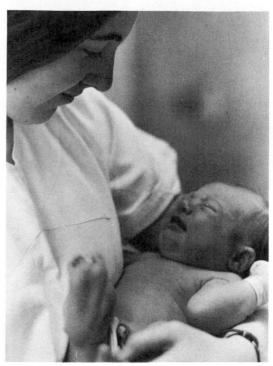

**Figure 16-3.** Not all inherited disorders are present at birth. Awareness of a family disease can alert the physician to the need for early testing of the baby. (Courtesy of Rivier College/St. Joseph Hospital School of Practical Nursing, Nashua, NH.)

laboratories, and as the genetic code is further deciphered, it is hoped that we will learn how to send messages to the nuclei of cells and supply the minute amount of DNA needed to correct the mistake.

Other scientists anticipate the development of long-lasting enzymes that the patient could take perhaps once a year. Tissue and organ transplants are another area of investigation. Although this field is in its infancy, physicians have been able to transplant active cells into the bone marrow of individuals in order to produce missing antibodies. The transplant of insulin-making cells is being carefully investigated.

The role of the nurse in genetic counseling is to identify families at risk, to support and clarify the family's understanding of the specific condition, to provide comfort and support, and to ensure continuity of follow-up care.

## ADVANCES IN FETAL RESEARCH

The quality of the uterine environment is as important to the fetus as the quality of genetic

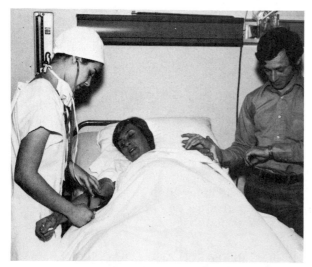

**Figure 16-2.** Preparing for a healthy baby includes genetic counseling, good prenatal care, and family involvement. (Courtesy of Rivier College/St. Joseph Hospital School of Practical Nursing, Nashua, NH.)

## Nursing Brief

The first birth conceived by in vitro fertilization (IVF) took place in Great Britain in 1978. This development raises many questions about the role of biologic parents. Mother surrogates, sperm banks, and embryo transplants with all their ethical and legal problems have transformed conjecture into reality.

makeup. If the fetus inherits a susceptibility to a seemingly harmless drug or minor pathogenic organism, great harm can ensue. Certain chemicals and radiation are known *teratogens* (*terato*, "monster," and *genēs* (born), "to produce"). These substances are hard to pinpoint, as the defect may not be apparent for several months after delivery. The offenders are most harmful during the first weeks after conception, before a mother is aware that she is expecting. In many cases, the culprit is impossible to single out, and it is thought that many disorders are *multifactorial*. Cleft lip or palate, clubfoot, congenital dislocation of the hip, spinal bifida, hydrocephalus, and pyloric stenosis are defects now thought to be multifactorial in origin.

It is possible to directly monitor the fetus in utero. The amount of oxygen concentration in the blood of the unborn child can be determined. The introduction of *ultrasonography* in the 1950s was a major advance in maternity care. Sound beams are sent into the body tissues to determine early pregnancy, multiple fetuses, fetal growth, location, size, presentation, estimation of gestational age, and other parameters. Both transabdominal and endovaginal methods are used. In the latter, a small lightweight instrument is inserted into the woman's vagina. This type of ultrasonography is useful in assessing early embryonic development and fetal heartbeat and in more clearly visualizing structures. Magnetic resonance imaging (MRI) is also being utilized to distinguish between normal and diseased tissue, and between maternal and fetal structures.

Intrauterine diagnosis has also been greatly facilitated through *amniocentesis*—a procedure in which amniotic fluid is withdrawn from the womb for the purpose of examining fetal cells (see page 92). Certain abnormalities that cause retardation, such as Down syndrome and Tay-Sachs disease, can be determined, as can Rh-negative blood problems. Respiratory distress syndrome (hyaline membrane disease) may also

be detected. Amniocentesis also enables the physician to determine the sex of the baby, which is important in detecting sex-linked disorders. It is also possible to diagnose spina bifida (open spine) and anencephaly (absence of the brain) by testing for elevation of a certain fetal protein, alpha$_1$-fetoprotein (AFP). This procedure can be augmented by ultrasonography.

## Growth, Development, and Maturation

The main difference between caring for the adult and caring for the child is that the latter is in a continuous process of growth and development. This process is orderly and proceeds from the simple to the more complex (Fig. 16–4). Although the process is orderly, at times it is uneven. Growth spurts are often followed by plateaus. One of the most noticeable growth spurts is at the time of puberty. The rate of growth varies with the individual child. Each baby has an individual timetable that revolves about established norms. Siblings within a family vary in growth rate. Growth is measurable and can be observed and studied. This is done by comparing height, weight, increase in vocabulary, physical skills, and other parameters. There are variations in growth within the systems and subsystems. Not all parts mature at the same time. Skeletal growth approximates whole-body growth, whereas the brain, lymph, and reproductive tissues follow distinct and individual sequences.

### TERMINOLOGY

The stages of growth and development that are referred to throughout this text are as follows:

**Fetus:** conception to birth
**Newborn:** birth to 4 weeks
**Infant:** 4 weeks to 1 year
**Toddler:** 1 to 3 years
**Preschool:** 3 to 6 years
**School Age:** 6 to 12 years
**Adolescence:** 12 to 18 years

Growth refers to an increase in physical size, measured in inches and pounds. Development refers to a progressive increase in the function of the body. The two are inseparable. Matura-

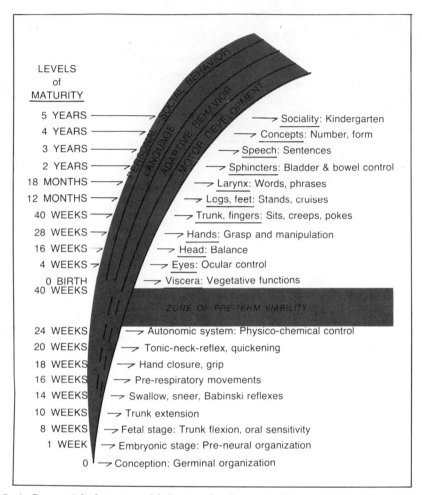

**LEVELS of MATURITY**

| | |
|---|---|
| 5 YEARS | → Sociality: Kindergarten |
| 4 YEARS | → Concepts: Number, form |
| 3 YEARS | → Speech: Sentences |
| 2 YEARS | → Sphincters: Bladder & bowel control |
| 18 MONTHS | → Larynx: Words, phrases |
| 12 MONTHS | → Legs, feet: Stands, cruises |
| 40 WEEKS | → Trunk, fingers: Sits, creeps, pokes |
| 28 WEEKS | → Hands: Grasp and manipulation |
| 16 WEEKS | → Head: Balance |
| 4 WEEKS | → Eyes: Ocular control |
| 0 BIRTH 40 WEEKS | → Viscera: Vegetative functions |

ZONE OF PRE-TERM VIABILITY

| | |
|---|---|
| 24 WEEKS | → Autonomic system: Physico-chemical control |
| 20 WEEKS | → Tonic-neck-reflex, quickening |
| 18 WEEKS | → Hand closure, grip |
| 16 WEEKS | → Pre-respiratory movements |
| 14 WEEKS | → Swallow, sneer, Babinski reflexes |
| 10 WEEKS | → Trunk extension |
| 8 WEEKS | → Fetal stage: Trunk flexion, oral sensitivity |
| 1 WEEK | → Embryonic stage: Pre-neural organization |
| 0 | → Conception: Germinal organization |

**Figure 16–4.** Sequential character of behavior development. The general trends of behavior development are shown from conception to 5 years of age. (From Gesell, A., & Armatruda, C.S. [1969]. *Developmental diagnosis.* New York: Harper & Row.)

tion (*maturus*, "ripe") refers to the total way in which a person grows and develops, as dictated by inheritance (Box 16–1). Although maturation is independent of environment, its timing may be affected by environment.

**Directional Patterns.** Directional patterns are fundamental to all humans. *Cephalocaudal* development proceeds from head to toe. The infant is able to raise the head before being able to sit, and he or she gains control of the trunk before walking. The second pattern is *proximodistal*, or inner to outer. Development proceeds from the center of the body to the periphery (Fig. 16–5). These patterns occur bilaterally. Development also proceeds from the general to the specific. The infant grasps with the hands before pinching with the fingers.

**Height.** At birth the newborn has an average length of about 20 inches (50 cm). Linear growth is caused mainly by skeletal growth. Growth fluctuates throughout life until maturity is reached. Infancy and puberty are both rapid growth periods. Height is generally a

---

**BOX 16–1** | **Key Terms in Child Development**

**growth:** an increase in physical size, measured in feet or meters and pounds or kilograms
**development:** a progressive increase in the function of the body (e.g., baby's increasing ability to digest solids)
**maturation:** the total way in which a person grows and develops, as dictated by inheritance

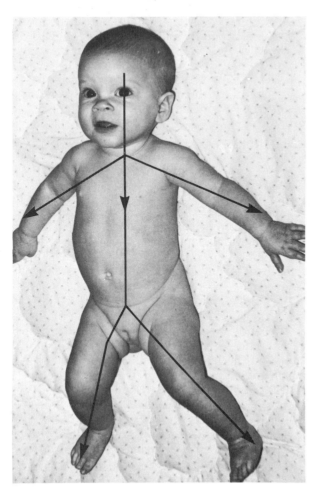

**Figure 16–5.** The development of muscular control proceeds from head to foot (cephalocaudally) and from the center of the body to its periphery (proximodistally). (From Betz, C., Hunsberger, M., & Wright, S. [1994]. *Family-centered nursing care of children* [2nd ed.]. Philadelphia: W.B. Saunders.)

family trait, although there are exceptions. Good nutrition and general good health are instrumental in promoting linear growth. Height is measured during each well-child conference (see p. 574 for procedure).

**Weight.** Weight is another good index of health. The average newborn weighs 6–9 pounds (2.72–4.09 kg). About 5–10% of the birth weight is lost by 3 or 4 days. This is the result of the passage of stools and a limited fluid intake. The quality of the uterine environment has a bearing on weight. Birth weight usually doubles by 5–6 months and triples by 1 year of age. After the 1st year, weight gain levels off to approximately 4–6 pounds (1.81–2.72 kg) per year until the pubertal growth spurt begins. Weight is determined at each office visit. A marked increase or decrease requires further investigation.

**Body Proportions.** Body proportions of the child differ greatly from those of the adult. The head is the fastest-growing portion of the body during fetal life. During infancy the trunk grows rapidly, and during childhood growth of the legs becomes the predominant feature. At adolescence, characteristic male and female proportions develop as childhood fat disappears. Alterations in proportions in the size of head, trunk, and extremities are characteristic of certain disturbances. Routine measurements of head and chest circumference are important indexes of health.

**Metabolic Rate.** The metabolic rate in children is higher than that in adults. Infants require more calories, minerals, vitamins, and fluid, in proportion to weight and height, than do adults. Higher metabolic rates are accompanied by increased production of heat and waste products. The body surface area of young children is far greater in relation to body weight than that of adults. The young child loses relatively more fluid from the pulmonary and integumentary systems.

**Bone Growth.** Bone growth provides one of the best indicators of biologic age. Bone age can be determined by x-ray films. In the fetus, bones begin as connective tissue, which later is converted to cartilage. Through ossification, cartilage is converted to bone. The maturity and rate of bone growth vary within individuals; however, the progression remains the same. Growth of the long bones continues until epiphyseal fusion occurs. Bone is constantly synthesized and reabsorbed. In children, bone synthesis is greater than bone destruction. Calcium reserves are stored in the ends of the long bones. "Vitamin A is necessary for growth and development of skeletal and soft tissue through its effect upon protein synthesis and differentiation of the bone cells" (Mahan & Arlin, 1992).

**Critical Periods.** There appear to be certain periods when environmental events or stimuli have their maximum effect on the child's development. The embryo, for example, is adversely affected during times of rapid cell division. Certain viruses, drugs, and other agents are known to cause congenital anomalies during the first 3 months following conception. It is believed that these sensitive periods also apply to factors such as developing a sense of trust during the 1st year of life (and) learning readiness. Most research in this area has been done with animals, and questions have been raised as to its application in humans.

**Integration of Skills.** As the child learns new skills, they are combined with ones previously mastered. For instance, the child who is learning to walk may sit, pull the body up to a table by grasping it, balance, and take a cautious step. Tomorrow the child may take three steps! Children connect and perfect each skill in preparation for learning a more complex one.

## GROWTH STANDARDS

Growth is measured in dimensions such as height, weight, volume, and thickness of tissues, but measurement alone, without any standard of comparison, limits interpretation of the data. A number of standards have been developed to make it possible (1) to compare the measurement of a child to others of the same age and sex, and ideally race, and (2) to compare that child's present measurements with the former rate of growth and pattern of progress. These standards, available as *growth charts*, are among the tools that have been used to assess the child's overall development (Figs. 16-6 and 16-7).

Length refers to horizontal measurement; it is used before a child can stand. Height is measured with the child standing. Some pointers in reading and interpreting growth charts follow:

■ Children who are in good health tend to follow a consistent pattern of growth.
■ At any age, there are wide individual differences in measured values.
■ Percentile charts are customarily divided into seven percentile levels designated by lines. These lines generally are labeled 97th, 90th, 75th, 50th, 25th, 10th, and 3rd, or 95th, 90th, 75th, 50th, 25th, 10th, and 5th.
■ The median (middle), or 50th percentile, is designated by a solid black line. Percentile levels show the extent to which a child's measurements deviate from the 50th percentile or middle measurement. A child whose weight is at the 75th percentile line is one percentile *above* the median. A child whose height is at the 25th percentile is one percentile *below* the median.

■ A difference of two or more percentile levels between height and weight may suggest an underweight or overweight condition and prompts further investigation.
■ Deviations of two or more percentile levels from an established growth pattern require further evaluation.

## INFLUENCING FACTORS

Growth and development are influenced by many factors, such as heredity, nationality, race, ordinal position in the family, sex, and environment. These factors are closely related and dependent on one another in their effect on growth and development. They make each person unique. If a child is ill, physically or emotionally, the developmental processes may be delayed.

**Hereditary Traits.** Characteristics derived from our ancestors are determined at the time of conception by countless genes within each chromosome. Each gene is made of a chemical substance called deoxyribonucleic acid (DNA), which plays an important part in determining inherited characteristics. Examples of these inherited traits are the color of eyes and hair and physical resemblances within families.

**Nationality and Race.** Many physical differences among people of various nationalities and races, who were formerly distinguished with ease, have become less apparent in our age of common environment and customs. For instance, one thinks of a person of Japanese origin as being of short stature. However, Japanese children living in the United States are comparable in height to other children in this country. Nevertheless, ethnic differences extend into many areas, including speech, food preferences, family structure, religious orientation, and moral code. The nurse should ascertain cultural beliefs and practices when collecting data for nursing assessment.

**Ordinal Position in the Family.** Whether the child is the youngest, middle, or oldest in the family has a bearing on growth and development (Light, Keller, & Calhoun, 1989). The youngest and middle children learn from their older sisters and brothers. The motor development of the youngest may be prolonged because the child may tend to be babied by the others in the family. The only child or the oldest child may excel in language development because conversations are mainly with adults. These children are often subject to greater parental

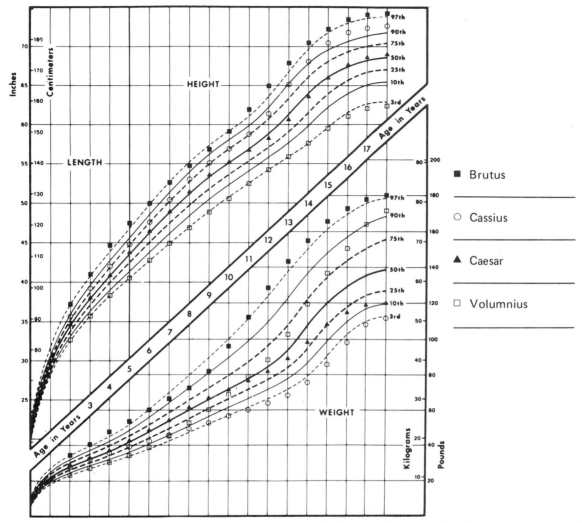

**Figure 16–6.** Sample of a complete growth chart. Note the percentile for length, height, and weight for four boys from birth to age 18 years. (From Valadian, I., & Porter, D. [1977]. *Physical growth and development from conception to maturity.* Boston: Little, Brown.)

expectations. None of these generalizations is an absolute, however, and individual variations abound (Light, Keller, & Calhoun, 1989).

**Sex.** The male infant weighs more and is longer than the female. He grows and develops at a different rate. Parents and relatives treat boys differently from girls by providing sex-appropriate toys and play and by having different expectations of them.

**Environment.** The physical condition of the newborn is influenced by the prenatal environment. The health of the mother at the time of conception and the amount and quality of her diet during pregnancy are important for proper fetal development. Infections or diseases may

lead to malformations of the fetus. A healthy and strong newborn can easily adapt to the surroundings.

The home greatly influences the infant's physical and emotional growth and development. If a family is financially strained by an added member, and the parents are unable to provide nourishing foods and suitable housing, the infant is directly affected. An uneducated mother may not know how to properly cook foods in order to preserve their nutritional value. Immunizations and other medical attention may be neglected. The baby senses tension within the family and is affected by it.

In contrast, when the surroundings are se-

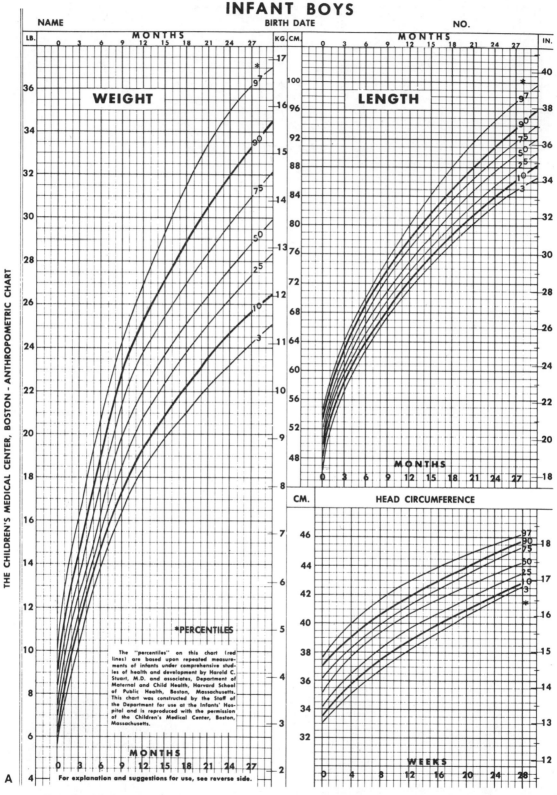

**Figure 16–7.** Growth grids for infant boys (*A*) and girls (*B*). (From Smith, D. [1977]. *Introduction to clinical pediatrics* [2nd ed.]. Philadelphia: W.B. Saunders, pp. 426, 428.)

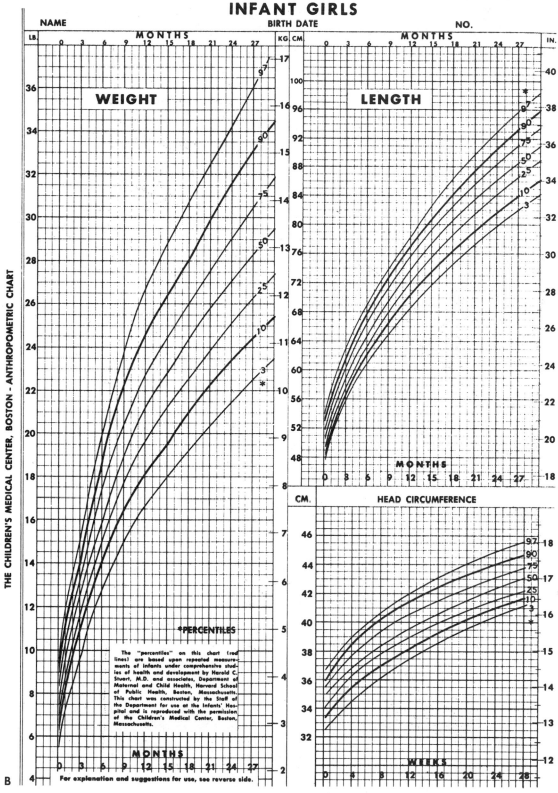

**Figure 16–7.** *Continued*

## Nursing Brief

"Different" does not mean "inferior."

---

cure and stable, and the infant feels secure, wanted, and loved, energies can be directed toward positive development. Most environments are neither completely positive nor completely negative but fall somewhere between the two extremes.

Intelligence plays an important role in social and mental development. Potential intelligence is believed to be inherited but greatly affected by environment.

### THE FAMILY

Raising a child or children can be a most rewarding and satisfying experience. A baby can bring great joy to others. Adults mature around the lives of their children. The role of the father is honored in every Judeo-Christian society. Half of the child's heredity is transmitted through him; the newborn is a continuation of him and the child's mother. A mother's love for her baby is considered to be the strongest emo-

tional tie between two human beings. The family can be a source of strength and security for the child (Figs. 16–8 and 16–9).

Traditionally, the *nuclear*, or biologic, family has been the basic unit of structure in American society (mother, father, siblings). According to recent statistics, nuclear families now constitute only approximately 25% of the household configurations (U.S. Department of Health and Human Services, 1992). This is a highly significant change. Many nuclear families do not share the same household because of single parenthood, divorce, and remarriage. Kinship lines have become blurred and fundamental changes are occurring in the family as it was once perceived. The *extended* family refers to three generations: grandparents, parents, and children. Because of an increasing life span, however, there are a greater number of living grandparents and great-grandparents, and the proportion of them living in the family home may increase. Table 16–1 lists various types of families and a description of each.

Historically in middle-class families, the father was the breadwinner and the mother managed the home and raised the children. This trend has shifted. The fastest-growing group of women in the labor market are moth-

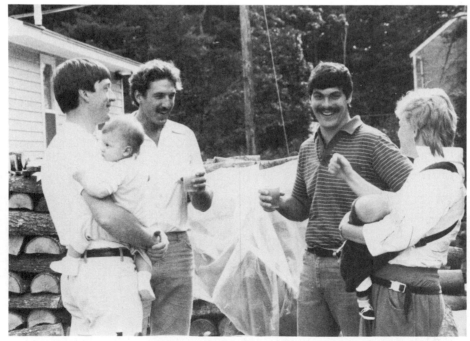

**Figure 16–8.** Caregivers can build on the many strengths of young families.

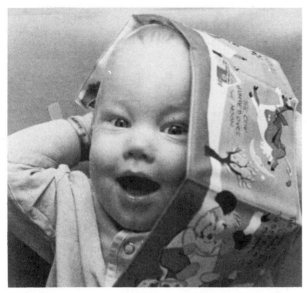

**Figure 16–9.** Infants who are secure and loved can direct their energy toward positive development. (Courtesy of Blank Memorial Hospital for Children, Des Moines, IA.)

ers with infants (Mott, James, & Sperhac, 1991). Because of changing economic conditions, both parents' earnings may be necessary to maintain the family's standard of living. In dual-career families, a father and mother are

often absent for most of the day because of long commutes or the demands of the working environment. Both parents may share child care and domestic chores. The parents may have to transfer to different locations to maintain their careers. This decreases extended family support and makes it necessary for children to change schools frequently.

Divorce, separation, death, and pregnancy outside marriage create many one-parent families (Fig. 16–10). The percentage of children living in single-parent families has more than doubled during the past 20 years, from 11.9% to 24.7%. In 1990 15.9 million children lived in single-parent families (U.S. Department of Health and Human Services, 1992). All single-wage families have an economic disadvantage, but families with women as the single wage earner have considerably lower incomes than those with men. The problem of providing good affordable child care is a serious one for both dual-career families and single parents. Relatives and the noncustodial parent may assist in raising the child. Many single parents remarry, creating the *blended* family. The addition may be merely a stepfather or stepmother, or two families may unite. These family units must make many adjustments. In order to succeed, parents and children have to learn problem-solving techniques, communication skills, and flexibility.

**Table 16–1.** VARIETIES OF FAMILY LIVING

| Type of Family* | Comment |
|---|---|
| Nuclear | Traditional—husband, wife, children (natural or adopted) |
| Extended | Kin, grandparents, parents, children, relatives |
| Single-parent | Women or men establishing separate households through individual preference, divorce, death, illegitimacy, desertion |
| Foster-parent | Parents who care for children who require parenting because of dysfunctional families, no families, or individual problems |
| Alternative | Communal family |
| Dual-career | Both parents work because of desire or need |
| Blended | Remarriage of persons with children |
| Polygamous | More than one spouse |
| Homosexual | Two persons of the same sex who have adopted children or who have had children from a previous marriage |
| Cohabitation | Heterosexual or homosexual couples who live together but remain unmarried |

*May not all be legally sanctioned.

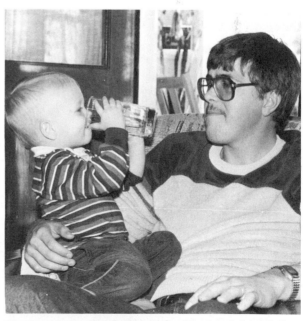

**Figure 16–10.** Single-parent families headed by fathers are no longer uncommon.

**The Family as Part of a Community.** The term *community* is defined in many ways, but here it is used to refer to the immediate geographic area in which the family lives and interacts (e.g., "I come from the south side").

Families are greatly influenced by the communities in which they reside. Nurses must understand the makeup of the community in which they work or to which the patient will return (Table 16–2). Assessment of the community is particularly important in creating discharge plans for families of various cultures. Their lives may be broadened or constricted, depending on the facilities of the community. A few factors to consider are housing, access to public transportation, city services, safety, and health-care delivery. The nurse with her immediate access to the patient becomes an impor-

## Nursing Brief

The family is an important resource for the child and the nurse.

tant liaison between various departments addressing specific needs.

The effect of the family on children will greatly outlast concerns of health-care systems. It is imperative that we take advantage of its strengths while attending to its weaknesses. Nurses are in an excellent position to help the health professions move toward truly contemporary models of family-centered care. The nuclear family of the past is no longer dominant. Pediatric nursing research and care must reflect this phenomenon.

**Table 16–2.** POSSIBLE NURSING DIAGNOSES FOR CHILDREN AND FAMILIES FROM DIVERSE SOCIOCULTURAL BACKGROUNDS

| Functional Health Pattern | Nursing Diagnosis | Related Factors |
|---|---|---|
| Health perception–health management | Altered health maintenance | Lack of communication skills (fluency in language other than English) |
| | | Lack of material resource (unemployed, ineligible for welfare and Medicaid or Medicare) |
| | Noncompliance | Value conflict |
| | | Cultural conflict |
| | | Perceived therapeutic ineffectiveness |
| Activity-exercise | Impaired home-maintenance management | Insufficient finances |
| | | Unfamiliarity with neighborhood resources |
| | | Inadequate support systems |
| | | Homelessness |
| Cognitive-perceptual | Knowledge deficit | Inability to use materials or information resources (cultural and language differences) |
| | | Unfamiliarity with information resources |
| Self-perception–self-concept | Anxiety | Perceived threat to self-concept, health status, role functioning |
| | | Unconscious conflict (essential values, life goals) |
| | Powerlessness | Health-care environment |
| | | Interpersonal interaction (language and cultural) |
| Role-relationship | Social isolation | Inability to engage in satisfying personal relationships (inadequate personal resources) |
| | Impaired social interaction | Communication barriers |
| | | Sociocultural dissonance |
| | | Environmental barriers |
| | Altered family processes | Situational crisis or transition (immigration, legal or illegal, refugee status) |
| | Impaired verbal communication | Cultural difference |
| Coping–stress tolerance | Ineffective individual coping | Situational crises (immigration status, inability to ask for help—language and cultural barriers) |
| Value-belief | Spiritual distress | Separation from religious or cultural ties |

From Mott, S., James, S.R., & Sperhac, A.M. (1990). *Nursing care of children and families* (2nd ed.). Reading, MA: Addison-Wesley. Copyright © 1990 by Addison-Wesley Nursing, a division of the Benjamin/Cummings Publishing Company. Reprinted by permission.

## PERSONALITY DEVELOPMENT

Most people tend to equate personality with social attractiveness: "She has a lot of personality, and he has no personality"; or "There's an example of personality plus." The term is more broadly defined by psychologists. One definition states that personality is a "unique organization of characteristics that determine the individual's typical or recurrent pattern of behavior." No two persons are exactly alike. An individual's personality is the result of interaction between biologic and environmental heritages.

Although no one group of theories can explain all human behavior, each can make a useful contribution to it. Many experts have devoted their lives to understanding why children and families behave as they do. Some, called *systems theorists*, believe that everyone in the family or system is affected by each of its members. This theory focuses on the interrelatedness of the various persons as opposed to an analysis of an individual in the group. Nurses using systems theory focus on caring for the child by caring for the whole family. They see the family as protector, educator, resource, and health provider for the child. In turn, they see the child's health as having an impact on each member of the family as a whole.

Many see human development as a composite of various theories. Abraham Maslow's hierarchy of needs is depicted in Figure 16–11, and the developmental theories of Erik Erikson, Sigmund Freud, Lawrence Kohlberg, Harry Stack Sullivan, and Jean Piaget are presented in Table 16–3. Other theorists are briefly con-

trasted within appropriate chapters devoted to specific age groups. Theories provide a framework for the practitioner; however, humans are not a gathering of isolated parts, even though these parts need to be dissected for investigative purposes (Fig. 16–12).

**Cognitive Development.** Cognition (*cognoscere*, "to know") refers to one's intellectual ability. Children are born with inherited potential, but it must be developed. "It requires opportunities for exploration that are neither too easy nor too hard" (Levine et al., 1992). The development of logical thinking and conceptual understanding is a complex process. One outstanding authority on cognitive development was Piaget, a Swiss psychologist. He proposed that intellectual maturity is attained through four orderly and distinct stages of development, all of which are interrelated. These are sensorimotor (up to 2 years), preoperational (2–7 years), concrete operations (7–11 years), and formal operations (11–16 years). The ages are approximate, and each stage builds on the preceding one.

Piaget believed that intelligence consists of interaction and coping with the environment. Babies begin their interaction by reflex response. As they grow older, their use of symbolism (particularly language) increases. Gradually they acquire a here-and-now orientation (concrete operations) and finally a fully abstract comprehension of the world (formal operations). Current theorists have identified inconsistencies in Piaget's theories; however, he remains one of the foremost authorities in the study of intelligence.

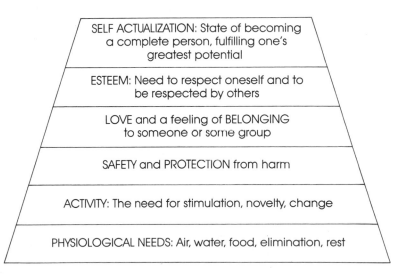

**Figure 16–11.** Maslow's hierarchy of basic needs. The needs at the bottom of the pyramid must be met before one can fulfill needs at the next higher level.

**Table 16–3.** COMPARISON OF THE DEVELOPMENTAL THEORIES OF ERIKSON, FREUD, KOHLBERG, SULLIVAN, AND PIAGET

| Developmental Period | Erikson | Freud | Kohlberg | Sullivan | Piaget |
|---|---|---|---|---|---|
| *Infancy* | Trust/mistrust Getting Tolerating frustration in small doses Recognizing mother as distinct from others and self | Orality—understanding the world by exploration with the mouth | | Security, patterns of emotional response, organization of sensation | Sensorimotor stage (birth to 2 yr)—at birth, responses limited to reflexes; begins to relate to outside events; concerned by sensations and actions that affect self directly |
| *Early childhood* | Autonomy/shame and doubt Trying out own powers of speech Beginning acceptance of reality versus pleasure principle | Anality—learning to give and take | | Mastery of space and objects | Preoperational (2–7 yr)—child is still egocentric; thinks everyone sees world as self does Preconceptual (2–4 yr)—forms general concepts, is not capable of reasoning yet |
| *Late childhood* | Initiative/guilt Questioning Exploring own body and environment Differentiation of sexes | Phallic/oedipal phase—becoming aware of self as sexual being | Preconventional or premoral morality—rules are absolute; breaking rules results in punishment (4–7 yr) | Speech and conscious need for playmates, interpersonal communication | Perceptual (4–7 yr)—capable of some reasoning but can concentrate on only one aspect of a situation at a time |
| *School age* | Industry/inferiority Learning to win recognition by producing things Exploring, collecting Learning to relate to own sex | Latency—focusing on peer relations, learning to live in groups and to achieve | Conventional morality—rules are created for the benefit of all; adhering to rules is the right thing to do (7–11 yr) | Chumship, one-to-one relationship, self-esteem, compassion (homosexuality) | Concrete operations (7–11 yr)—reasoning is logical but limited to own experience; understands cause and effect |
| *Adolescence* | Identity/role diffusion Moving toward heterosexuality Selecting vocation Beginning separation from family Integrating personality (e.g., altruism) | Genitality | Principled morality (autonomous stage) (12 yr on)—acceptance of right or wrong on basis of own perceptions of world and personal conscience | Capacity to love, empathy, partnership (heterosexuality) | Formal operational stage (11–16 yr)—acquires ability to develop abstract concepts for self; oriented to problem-solving |

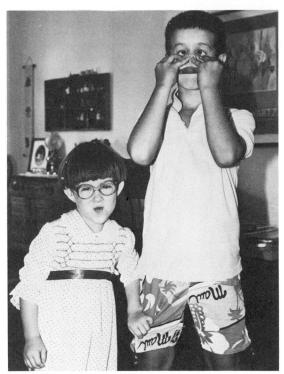

**Figure 16–12.** Each child has a unique personality. The study of how children grow and why they differ attracts researchers in psychology, psychiatry, medicine, and nursing. The most fascinated observers, however, are parents.

In Table 16–4, Piaget's theory is related to feeding and nutrition. It is a good example of how a knowledge of development can help one understand the behavior of a child at a particular time.

**Moral Development.** Lawrence Kohlberg, a childhood theorist, suggests that moral development in children is sequential. His theories on moral development are based on Piaget's cognitive development investigations. He describes three levels with two stages at each level. The three levels are preconventional, conventional, and postconventional. In the preconventional stage (4–7 years), children try to be obedient to their parents for fear of punishment. During the conventional phase (7–11 years), children show conformity and loyalty, and they focus on obeying rules. In the postconventional level (12 years and older), *moral values* are developed to solve complex problems. There is an emphasis on individual conscience within the society. Although rules are still important, changing them to meet the needs of a culture are considered.

## NURSING IMPLICATIONS

An understanding of growth and development, including its predictable nature and individual variation, has value in the nursing process. Such knowledge is the basis of the nurse's anticipatory guidance of parents. For example, the nurse who knows when the infant is likely to crawl can, at the appropriate age, expand teaching on safety precautions. The nurse also incorporates these precautions into nursing care plans in the hospital. Age-appropriate care cannot be administered without an understanding of growth and development.

While explaining various aspects of child care to families, the nurse stresses the importance of individual differences. Parents tend to compare their children's development and behavior with those of other children and with information in popular magazine articles. This may relieve their anxiety or cause them to impose impossible expectations and standards. In addition, many parents had poor role models who influenced their own experiences as children. Lack of knowledge about parenting can be recognized by the nurse and suitable interventions begun.

The nurse who understands that each child is born with an individual temperament and "style of behavior" can help frustrated parents cope with a newborn who has difficulty settling into the new environment. Specific parameters can be used to determine whether an infant is merely on an individual timetable or whether the infant varies from normal.

The nurse must also recognize when to intervene in order to prevent disease and/or accidents. For example, a brief visit with a caretaker may reveal that the child's immunizations are not up-to-date. A review of the characteristics of a 2-year-old with a teenage mother may prevent the ingestion of poisons. Complications of the newborn can be avoided by advising the expectant mother to avoid alcohol and cigarettes. Other threats to health may

## Nursing Brief

Arnold Gesell, founder of the Clinic for Child Development at Yale University, was the first to study children scientifically over a period of time. He coined the term *child development*.

**Table 16–4.** PIAGET'S THEORY OF COGNITIVE DEVELOPMENT IN RELATION TO FEEDING AND NUTRITION

| Developmental Period | Cognitive Characteristics | Relationships to Feeding and Nutrition |
|---|---|---|
| *Sensorimotor (Birth–2 yr)* | Progression from newborn with automatic reflexes to intentional interaction with the environment and the beginning use of symbols | Progression is made from sucking and rooting reflexes to the acquisition of self-feeding skills<br>Food is used primarily to satisfy hunger, as a medium to explore the environment, and to practice fine motor skills |
| *Preoperational (2–7 yr)* | Thought processes become internalized; they are unsystematic and intuitive<br>Use of symbols increases<br>Reasoning is based on appearances and happenstance<br>Approach to classification is functional and unsystematic<br>Child's world is viewed egocentrically | Eating becomes less the center of attention than social, language, and cognitive growth<br>Food is described by color, shape, and quantity, but there is limited ability to classify food into "groups"<br>Foods tend to be classed as "like" and "don't like"<br>Foods can be identified as "good for you," but reasons are unknown or mistaken |
| *Concrete operations (7–11 yr)* | Child can focus on several aspects of a situation simultaneously<br>Cause-effect reasoning becomes more rational and systematic<br>Ability to classify, reclassify, and generalize emerges<br>Decrease in egocentrism permits child to take another's view | Child begins to realize that nutritious food has a positive effect on growth and health but has limited understanding of how or why this occurs<br>Mealtimes take on a social significance<br>Expanding environment increases the opportunities for, and influences on, food selection (peer influence rises) |
| *Formal operations (11–16 yr)* | Hypothetic and abstract thought expand<br>Understanding of scientific and theoretic processes deepens | The concept of nutrients from food functioning at physiologic and biochemical levels can be understood<br>Conflicts in making food choices may be realized (knowledge of nutritious food versus preferences and nonnutritive influences) |

From Mahan, L.K., & Arlin, M.T. (1992). *Krause's food, nutrition & diet therapy* (8th ed.). Philadelphia: W.B. Saunders.

likewise be anticipated. Knowing that specific diseases are prevalent in certain age groups, the nurse maintains a high level of suspicion when interacting with these patients. This approach, based on developmental knowledge, experience, and effective communication, helps ensure a higher level of family care.

Finally, the nurse must understand how to provide nursing care to children of various ages so that their physical, mental, emotional, and spiritual development is enhanced according to their specific needs and comprehension.

# Nutrition

## PREPARING FOR CONCEPTION

Good nutrition ideally begins before conception. Unfortunately, pregnancy is often confirmed well after the critical period of embryonic development has passed. Preparation for conception should especially target women whose nutri-

tional status is sufficient to make them fertile but insufficient for a normal pregnancy. Moderate to high income or educational level does not markedly reduce the incidence of "marginal malnutrition." Underweight women frequently have poor nutritional reserves. Obese women and adolescents are also at risk. Suboptimal maternal nutrition, coupled with alcohol consumption or smoking, often leads to complicated pregnancies and abnormalities of the fetus. Therefore, nutrition counseling cannot begin too early. A well-nourished mother improves her chances for a smooth pregnancy and a healthy baby. Table 16–5 lists and describes various nutrition resources found in the community.

## TEENAGE PREGNANCY

In 1988 the United States had the highest teenage pregnancy rate among developed countries (9.8% of females aged 15–19), and that

**Table 16–5.** NUTRITION RESOURCES WITHIN THE COMMUNITY

| Program | Eligibility | Program Content |
|---|---|---|
| Maternal and Child Health | Pregnant women and children of low-income families | Free or reduced price<br>Improved health-care services for mothers and children at a clinic affiliated with a specific hospital<br>Free vitamins, immunizations |
| Special Supplemental Food Program for Women, Infants, and Children (WIC) | Individuals at nutritional risk:<br>Pregnant women up to 6 mo postpartum<br>Nursing mothers up to 1 yr<br>Infants and children up to age 5 identified as being at nutritional risk<br>Must live in geographically determined low-income area and be eligible for reduced price or free medical care<br>Must be certified by WIC staff member<br>Periodic assessment of risk status | Provision of supplemental foods:<br>>1 yr: iron-fortified formula and infant cereals, fruit juice high in vitamin C<br>Women and children: whole fluid milk or cheese, eggs, iron-fortified hot or cold cereal, fruit or vegetable high in vitamin C<br>Food distribution: directly from participating agency, via voucher system, or home delivery<br>Nutrition education is an integral part of program |
| Program for Children with Special Health Needs (formerly Crippled Children's Services) | Children with developmental disabilities | Under Title V<br>Free nutrition counseling<br>Funds available for equipment or supplies |
| Child Care Food Program (CCFP) | Preschool children in nonprofit facilities, Head Start, day care, afterschool facilities | Year-round program<br>Cash in lieu of commodities available |
| School Breakfast Program | All public and nonprofit private schools<br>Public and licensed nonprofit residential child-care institutions<br>For needy children or those who travel great distances to school | As set by U.S. Dept. of Agriculture<br>Nonprofit breakfasts meeting nutritional standards<br>Served free or at a reduced price to children from low-income families<br>Costs to schools reimbursed by federal funds |
| National School Lunch Program | All public and nonprofit private school pupils of high-school grade or under, some residential institutions and temporary shelters | As set by U.S. Dept. of Agriculture<br>Nonprofit nutritious lunches offered free or at a reduced price to those who cannot pay<br>Lunch follows specified guidelines and meets one-third or more of daily dietary allowance<br>Schools reimbursed by federal and state funds |
| Summer Food Service Programs for children | Public agency–sponsored preschool and school age recreation programs, summer camps | Free lunch to children in summer programs<br>Federal monetary support |
| Special Milk Program<br>Food Distribution (donated foods)<br>Food Stamps | Schools, child care centers, summer camps<br>Supplemental programs for mothers and infants<br>Eligibility based on total income, expenses, number being fed in household<br>Each applicant is considered on an individual basis | Federal reimbursement for all or part of the milk served<br>Distribution of surplus food to eligible persons, schools, institutions<br>Client should apply at local Food Stamp Office within the community, presenting wage slips, sources of income, rent receipts, utility bills<br>Food Stamps are given free of charge, depending on eligibility needs<br>Used like cash to purchase food at authorized food stores (nonfood items and alcoholic beverages not allowed) |

number is rising. Japan has the lowest rate of 1% (Mahan & Arlin, 1992). Whereas the birth rate among married persons has consistently dropped in America in the past 10 years, the birth rate among unmarried adolescents has almost doubled (Burroughs, 1992). In addition, adolescents who become pregnant are likely to have more than one pregnancy. Factors that contribute to this increase include peer pressure, the exploitation of sex by the media, cohabitation, risk taking (sex without protection), and lack of knowledge about contraception (pp. 270–284).

Poverty, the continuing growth of the adolescent, and the growth of the baby make the pregnant teenager a nutritional risk. In addition, teenage mothers are frequently alarmed by weight gain. It is vitally important that the nurse stress the need for the basic food groups and the particular value of enriched flours, cereals, meat, and fruit. Empty caloric foods and cravings for foods that are nonnutritious should be reduced. Exercise appropriate to the pregnant woman is encouraged.

An adequate supply of nutrients during pregnancy also helps ensure good-quality breast milk during lactation. The advantages of breast feeding are now well recognized, and the continued emphasis on its importance has been advocated by the Surgeon General of the United States, the Public Health Service, and the American Academy of Pediatrics. Many young women are successfully breast feeding their babies with guidance and support from family members and health professionals. The mother's dietary habits partly determine the composition of her milk. If her diet is poor in, for example, protein and calcium, her milk continues to provide normal amounts of these nutrients until her stores are depleted. A mother who becomes pregnant at such a time is at nutritional risk.

### THE CHILD'S NUTRITIONAL HERITAGE

After birth, the newborn continues on the nutritional path. The dependent child is fed for many years by adults whose eating habits may be based on misinformation, income level, folklore, fads, or religious, cultural, and ethnic preferences. Table 16–6 describes food patterns of various cultures found in the United States. Many families are poor, others have inadequate knowledge of how to prepare foods, and many rely on convenience foods in order to save time.

## Nursing Brief

Every person who practices conventional or less conventional eating or living habits does not necessarily share all of the practices, beliefs, or values associated with it. Individual habits are assessed in developing care plans.

Some do not consider food a priority in the home. The nurse is in a position to identify children at risk and to help families modify eating habits in order to ensure proper nutrition. *An important resource for the nurse is the nutritionist on the staff of the health agency where the nurse is employed.*

### FAMILY NUTRITION

The United States Departments of Agriculture and Health and Human Services' seven guidelines for good eating are listed in Box 16–2. They are intended to correct misinformation and help Americans make informed decisions about what they eat. *Families who practice such principles are educating their offspring by good example.* A well-balanced diet supplies all the essential nutrients in the amounts that one needs. Food must perform the functions of

---

| BOX 16–2 | Dietary Guidelines for Americans |
|---|---|

Many health problems in middle and old age can be avoided by beginning good nutrition practices in childhood and adolescence:

- Eat a variety of foods
- Choose a diet low in fat, saturated fat, and cholesterol
- Choose a diet with plenty of vegetables, fruits, and grain products
- Maintain a healthy weight
- Use salt and sodium only in moderation
- Use sugars only in moderation
- If you drink alcoholic beverages, do so only in moderation

Data from the U.S. Departments of Agriculture and Health and Human Services, 1990.

**Table 16–6.** CULTURALLY DIVERSE FOOD PATTERNS OF AMERICANS

| Culture | Historical Dietary Pattern* |
|---|---|
| African American | All meats, fish, and chicken; pork often consumed (spareribs, bacon, and sausage); vegetables cooked in salt pork for long periods of time; grits and cornbread muffins; some lactose intolerance. Popular vegetables include collard greens, beet greens, and sweet potatoes |
| Chinese American | Rich in vegetables (bean sprouts, broccoli, bamboo shoots, and mushrooms). Vegetables cooked until crisp; meat consumed in small portions with other food. Soy sauce, tofu, peanut butter; limited milk and cheese; fish baked with native spices; soups with egg, meat, and vegetables. Tea is China's national beverage. Rice is staple of diet |
| Jewish American | Diet varies according to whether family is Orthodox, Reform, or Conservative. For Orthodox family, food must be kosher (clean); meat is soaked in salt water to remove blood; only meat eaten is that of divided hoofed animals that chew a cud; pork and fish without scales (shellfish) are prohibited; milk and meat cannot be combined. Favorites are gefilte fish, lox (smoked salmon), herring, eggs, bagels, cream cheese, and matzo |
| Laotian American | Numerous varieties of freshwater fish and shellfish (eaten fresh, dried, or salted); pork, beef, chicken, rabbit, often mixed with vegetables and spices; eggs, peanuts, black-eyed peas; vegetables eaten raw, as juice, or cooked with meat or fish and preserved by drying or pickling; sticky rice, rice or bean thread noodles, and legumes often used in desserts; soybean drink, sugar cane drink, tea, and coconut juice. Popular seasonings include padek, chilies, curry, tamarind, and red and black pepper |
| Italian American | All meats, fish, and chicken, including cold cuts (salami, mortadella) and Italian pork sausage; pasta (staple of diet), breads, olive oil, wine, cheese, and all varieties of fruits and vegetables |
| Japanese American | Fish and seafood (fresh, smoked, and raw) and beef. Food is cut into small portions. Principal fruit is nasi, which tastes much like a pear. Many vegetables are eaten, such as seaweed, bamboo shoots, onions, beans, and dried mushrooms (shitake); enjoy pickled vegetables. Rice is national staple. Beverages include tea and sake. Little cheese, milk, butter, or cream is consumed. Chief cooking fat is soybean oil or rice oil |
| Mexican American | Chicken, pork chops, wieners, cold cuts, hamburger, eggs (used frequently), beans (eaten mashed or refried with lard), potatoes (basic item, usually fried), chilies, fresh tomatoes, corn (maize—often used as basic grain), tortillas, packaged cereals; little milk because of lactose intolerance |
| Native American Indian | Acorn flour, a staple food made into mush or bread; salmon, fresh or dried; other varieties of fish, deer, duck, geese, and other small game; nuts such as buckeye and hazel; wild berries, seeds, and roots |
| Puerto Rican American | Meat cooked in stews; poultry, pork, fish, dried beans or peas mixed with rice; milk in combination with coffee (cafe con leche), variety of fruits, starchy vegetables (plantains, cassava, sweet potatoes), salad, soft drinks |
| Vietnamese American | Pork—most common meat; meats cut into small pieces and fried, boiled, or steamed; fish—all types of freshwater fish and shellfish, often fried and dipped in fish sauce; eggs, soybeans, legumes, and wide variety of fruits and vegetables; rice often eaten with every meal; seasonings including oyster sauce, soy sauce, monosodium glutamate, ginger, garlic, nuoc mam sauce; tea, coffee, soft drinks, soybean milk |

*More diverse eating patterns occur as future generations of a culture become assimilated.
Data from Mahan, L.K., & Arlin, M.T. (1992). *Krause's food, nutrition & diet therapy* (8th ed.). Philadelphia: W.B. Saunders, and other sources.

providing heat and energy, building and repairing tissues, and regulating body processes. A given food is a mixture of elements, such as minerals (e.g., calcium, phosphorus, sodium, iron), compounds (carbohydrates, fats, proteins, some vitamins), and water. The body needs approximately 50 nutrients, which it absorbs at various sites (Fig. 16–13). Table 16–7 specifies recommended dietary allowances for energy and protein for children.

Children are susceptible to nutritional deficiencies because they are growing and developing. Infants require more calories, protein, minerals, and vitamins in proportion to their weight than do adults. Fluid requirements are also higher for infants. Eating a *variety* of foods selected from the basic food groups ensures good health for children. The *amount* and *size* of portions are important in maintaining a reasonable weight. *There are no known advantages to consuming excessive amounts of any nutrients, and there are risks for overdoses.*

## NUTRITIONAL CARE PLAN

The nutritional care plan can be used in the hospital, home, or outpatient department. Parts

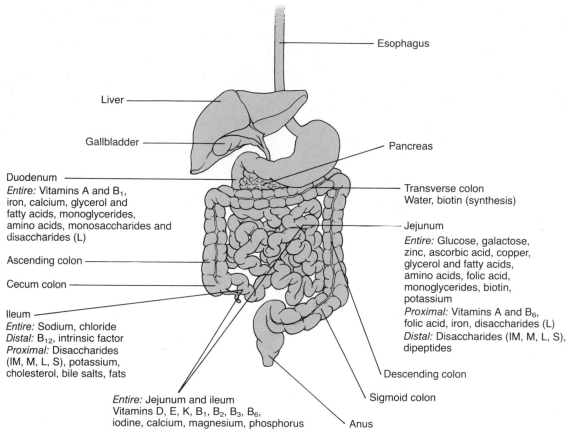

Esophagus

Liver

Gallbladder

Pancreas

Duodenum
*Entire:* Vitamins A and B₁,
iron, calcium, glycerol and
fatty acids, monoglycerides,
amino acids, monosaccharides and
disaccharides (L)

Transverse colon
Water, biotin (synthesis)

Jejunum
*Entire:* Glucose, galactose,
zinc, ascorbic acid, copper,
glycerol and fatty acids,
amino acids, folic acid,
monoglycerides, biotin,
potassium
*Proximal:* Vitamins A and B₆,
folic acid, iron, disaccharides (L)
*Distal:* Disaccharides (IM, M, L, S),
dipeptides

Ascending colon

Cecum colon

Ileum
*Entire:* Sodium, chloride
*Distal:* B₁₂, intrinsic factor
*Proximal:* Disaccharides
(IM, M, L, S), potassium,
cholesterol, bile salts, fats

Descending colon

Sigmoid colon

*Entire:* Jejunum and ileum
Vitamins D, E, K, B₁, B₂, B₃, B₆,
iodine, calcium, magnesium, phosphorus

Anus

**Figure 16–13.** Sites of absorption of major nutrients. The exact absorption sites for manganese, cobalt, selenium, chromium, molybdenum, and cadmium are unknown. (Modified from Kelts, D., & Jones, E. [1985]. *Manual of pediatric nutrition.* Boston: Little, Brown.)

**Table 16–7.** RECOMMENDED DIETARY ALLOWANCES FOR ENERGY AND PROTEIN FOR CHILDREN

| | Kilocalories | | Grams of Protein | | |
| --- | --- | --- | --- | --- | --- |
| **Age** | **Daily** | **Per Kilogram** | **Per Centimeter** | **Daily** | **Per Kilogram** |
| 1–3 | 1300 | 102 | 14.4 | 16 | 1.2 |
| 4–6 | 1800 | 90 | 16.0 | 24 | 1.1 |
| 7–10 | 2000 | 70 | 15.2 | 28 | 1.0 |

Reprinted with permission from *Recommended Dietary Allowances: 10th Edition.* Copyright 1989 by the National Academy of Sciences. Courtesy of the National Academy Press, Washington, D.C.

of the care plan may already have been collected by other professionals, so the nurse should refer to the patient's chart for pertinent data. The care plan provides information and stores it in one place. It can also be put on a computer for ease of retrieval. Figure 16–14 shows a sample form for initial nutritional assessment.

## NUTRITIONAL ADVANCES

In recent years, more has been learned about the nutritional requirements of infants and children. In addition, overnutrition and its possible link to obesity in adults have been explored. The effects of childhood nutrition on adult disease patterns, such as heart disease, are under investigation. Concern is expressed over the level of cholesterol in children. Methods to reduce cholesterol in families are listed in Box 16–3. The National Cholesterol Education Program's recommendations are cited in Box 16–4.

Dietary supplements, formulas, and nutritional support techniques for preterm babies, children with cancer, and those with long-term disorders, such as cystic fibrosis, have become

Name _____ Date of Birth _____ Male/Female

Diet Prescription _____ Diagnosis _____

Activity Level _____ Appetite _____

Medications

<u>Meal Pattern</u>

B          L          S

Food Preferences:                                    Food Intolerances/Dislikes:

_____

<u>Clinical Data:</u> Skin Condition _____ Edema _____

Impairments:   Eyesight _____ Hearing _____ Speech _____ Taste _____

Chewing and Swallowing Ability _____

Present Weight _____ Usual Weight _____ Desired Weight Range _____

Elbow Breadth _____ Midarm Circumference _____ Triceps Skin Fold_____

Height _____

<u>Meal Observation:</u> Percentage of food consumed _____ Fluid intake _____ ml

Type of assistance needed _____

Affective response to food _____

<u>Biochemical Data:</u>

Serum laboratory values: _____

**Figure 16–14.** Sample nutrition assessment and care plan. (From Peckenpaugh, N.J., & Poleman, C.M. [1991]. *Nutrition essentials and diet therapy* [7th ed.]. Philadelphia: W.B. Saunders.)

*Continued*

Urinalysis: ______________________________

Skin Tests: ______________________________

Evaluation and Reommendation:

| Problem/Need | Intervention | By Whom | Goal | Response/Date |
|---|---|---|---|---|
| | | | | |

By: ____________________ Title: __________

Date: ____________________

**Figure 16–14.** *Continued*

**BOX 16–3 Methods to Reduce Cholesterol in School Children**

- Exercise more with your children
- Provide fresh fruit and vegetables rather than empty calories such as found in doughnuts and store-bought pastries
- Decrease trips to fast-food restaurants
- Switch to low-fat foods; use vegetable oil cooking sprays in place of butter; bake or broil foods instead of frying
- If you have a family history of heart disease, have child's as well as adult's levels of cholesterol tested
- Seek advice of nutritionist

sophisticated and are successfully utilized. Total parenteral nutrition allows the physician to choose preparations ranging from amino acids and intravenous fats to complete multivitamins. As technical problems of total parenteral nutrition are resolved, emphasis is placed on short- and long-term goals and particularly on the patient's quality of life.

During the past decade, an oral rehydration solution (ORS) used by Third-World populations for treating acute diarrhea in children has gained acceptance and is now produced and distributed by the World Health Organization. It is composed mainly of sodium, glucose, and water. Health workers are able to teach parents how to save lives of their infants by using this simple solution. Medicine women, the respected leaders of some tribes, are being incorporated into the educational process. A commercial preparation is available in the United States as Hydralyte.

## THE TEETH

**Deciduous Teeth.** The development of the 20 deciduous, or baby, teeth begins at about the 5th month of intrauterine life. The health and

**Nursing Brief**

"Catch-up" growth refers to the process by which a child who has been sick or malnourished and whose growth has slowed or stopped experiences a more rapid period of recovery as the body attempts to compensate.

---

**BOX 16–4**  **NCEP\* Recommendations for Detection and Management of Hypercholesterolemia in Children and Adolescents**

In April, 1991, NCEP made recommendations for management of hypercholesterolemia to be applied to adolescents and children over the age of about 2 yr. This is the first time that there has been consensus among pediatric experts, lipid researchers, and nutrition and health-care communities on this subject.

For the general population of children and adolescents in the United States, NCEP recommended that there be adoption of eating patterns to meet the following criteria:

Nutritionally adequate, varied diet
Adequate energy intake to support growth and development and maintain appropriate body weight
Saturated fat—less than 10% of total calories
Total fat—an average of no more than 30%
Dietary cholesterol—less than 300 mg/day

To implement these patterns means involvement of the entire community—parents, in selection and preparation of food; schools, in modification of school food service; health-care clinics, in health education; government, in improvement of food labeling; and the food industry, in development of low-saturated-fat, low-fat foods appealing to children.

NCEP also aims to identify and treat individual children and adolescents who have hypercholesterolemia

and a family history of premature cardiovascular disease, or whose parents have hypercholesterolemia. For this group, NCEP recommends:

Blood cholesterol screening of children and adolescents whose parents or grandparents, at 55 yr or younger, were found to have coronary atherosclerosis; suffered myocardial infarction, peripheral vascular disease, cerebrovascular disease, or sudden death; or underwent invasive cardiac therapy (balloon angioplasty or coronary artery bypass surgery)
Blood cholesterol screening of offspring of a parent with a blood cholesterol of 240 mg/dl or greater
Appropriate levels for TC and LDL-C (see below)
For children with levels above these, dietary change is recommended

**Levels of Blood Total and LDL-Cholesterol in Children and Adolescents**

| Category | Total Cholesterol | LDL-cholesterol |
|---|---|---|
| Acceptable | <170 mg/dl | <110 mg/dl |
| Borderline | 170–199 mg/dl | 110–129 mg/dl |
| High | ≥200 mg/dl | ≥130 mg/dl |

If after 6 mo to 1 yr of dietary therapy there is insufficient blood lipid lowering, drug therapy can be considered in children over 10 yr of age.

From Mahan, L.K., & Arlin, M.T. (1992). *Krause's food, nutrition, & diet therapy* (8th ed.). Philadelphia: W.B. Saunders.
\*NCEP, National Cholesterol Education Program.

---

diet of the expectant mother affect their soundness. Teeth appear during the first 2½ years of life. It is a normal process and is generally accompanied by little or no discomfort. Wide individual differences in tooth eruption occur in normal, healthy infants. Occasionally a baby is born with teeth (Fig. 16–15). A delay in teething is significant if other forms of immaturity or illness are present. The physician evaluates the process of teething during the baby's regular health checkups.

The first tooth generally appears at about the 7th month. The 1-year-old has about six teeth, four above and two below. The order in which the teeth appear is almost always the same (Fig. 16–16). They are shed in about the same order in which they appear, that is, lower central incisors first, and so forth. Although the Academy of Pediatric Dentistry recommends that the first dental visit occur by 1 year, the majority of children begin seeing the dentist at

about 3 years of age. Tetracycline antibiotics stain developing teeth a yellowish-brown and are to be avoided during pregnancy and in the first 8 years of life.

Parents and nurses must not neglect baby teeth, thinking that they will eventually be lost. A 2-year-old who wants to brush his teeth when Mommy does is encouraged to do so. The deciduous teeth serve not only in the digestive process but also in the development of the jaw. When the deciduous teeth are lost early because of neglect, the permanent teeth become poorly aligned. The nurse checks that all patients 3 years of age and older have toothbrushes. Children sometimes need to be reminded of oral hygiene at bedtime.

**Permanent Teeth.** The 32 permanent teeth develop just before birth and during the 1st year of life. They do not erupt through the gums, however, until the 6th year. Nutrition and general health during the 1st year of life

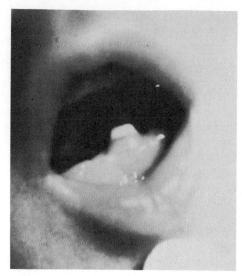

**Figure 16–15.** Neonatal tooth in a newborn. (From Poole, A., & Badwal, D. [1991]. Structural abnormalities of the craniofacial complex and congenital malformations. *Pediatric Clinics of North America, 38,* 1107.)

affect the formation of permanent teeth. This process is not completed until the wisdom teeth appear at about the age of 18–23 years. The first permanent teeth do not replace any of the deciduous teeth but appear behind the deciduous molars. They are important teeth because the whole denture develops around them. Cavities in them are frequently neglected because they are mistaken for baby teeth. The most common site of decay in children is the fissures of the molar teeth. These areas can be protected by the professional application of plastic sealants.

**Oral Hygiene.** Good dental care begins with proper diet to supply adequate nutrients while the teeth are developing in the jaws, especially during the prenatal period and the 1st year. The many essential elements found in milk include calcium, phosphorus, vitamins A and B complex, and protein. Vitamin D, the sunshine vitamin, and vitamin C, found in citrus fruits, are also valuable. Dietary practices influence cavity

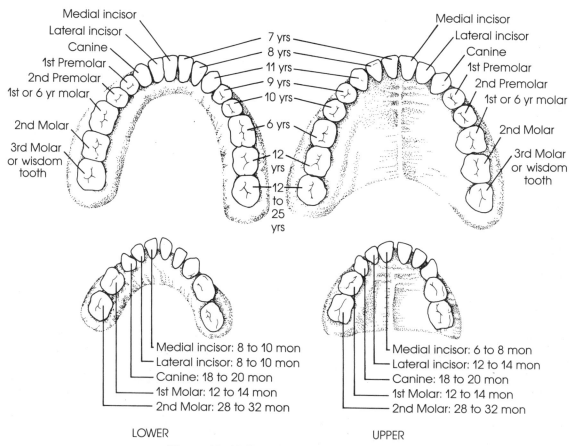

**Figure 16–16.** Permanent and deciduous teeth.

**Table 16–8.** DEVELOPMENTAL DENTAL HYGIENE

| Age | Dental Hygiene Practice |
|-----|-------------------------|
| 1st year of life | A clean wash cloth can be used by parents to wipe the teeth; no toothpaste necessary (baby may not like foaming action or taste). Child is not put to sleep with bottle of milk or juices. If baby must have a bottle, water is used |
| 2–3 yr | Parents introduce soft brush and toothpaste. Only a pea-sized amount of toothpaste is used to minimize fluoride ingestion |
| 3–6 yr | Deciduous teeth erupt, and toward end of this period, baby teeth start to exfoliate (fall out). Parents assist children and remind them to brush. Small, soft toothbrush is used. Bedtime routine of brushing is established, as salivary flow rates slow during sleep, reducing natural protective mechanisms. Parents are advised to brush for the child at least once a day and to clean teeth that are in contact with each other with dental floss. Number of sweets eaten per day is monitored |
| 6–12 yr | First permanent molars appear. The pits and fissures of molars make them primary site for caries. Sealants (plastic coating) professionally applied to molars provide a mechanical barrier against bacteria. Procedure is painless and does not require anesthesia. Parents continue with fluorides, flossing, reducing *frequency* of exposure to carbohydrates. Adolescent gingivitis (*gingi*, "gum," and *itis*, "inflammation of") characterized by redness, swelling, and bleeding is common in children and adolescents and may be aggravated by hormonal changes at puberty. Motivating the adolescent to assume responsibility for dental care may be complicated by rebellion against authority and some incapacity to appreciate long-term consequences. Topical fluorides and fluoride toothpastes are available. Orthodontic treatments place adolescent at high risk for gingivitis and caries around appliances or braces. Discourage use of smokeless tobacco (snuff), which can cause oral cancer and addiction. Mouth protectors should be used to prevent dental injuries from contact sports |

Data from Griffen, A., & Goepferd, S. (1991). Preventive oral health care for the infant, child and adolescent. *Pediatric Clinics of North America, 38.*

rates, and parents are encouraged to limit the *frequency* of sugar intake (Table 16–8).

In the past, total carbohydrate consumption was thought to be the most important dietary consideration for dental health. Today more attention is given to the frequency with which sweets are eaten and how long they stick to the teeth. Sticky retentive foods have more caries (cavity) potential than do sugared drinks that are quickly cleared. Rinsing the mouth after eating sticky foods is recommended. Foods that can be recommended as relatively safe snacks include cheese, peanuts, milk, sugarless gum, and raw vegetables. Items to be avoided include sugared gum, dried fruits, sugared soft drinks, cakes, and candy.

Of most importance in preventing caries is the administration of fluoride by mouth. Ideally, fluorides may be present naturally in the water supply or may be added to it. Systemic fluorides are no longer of benefit after the last permanent tooth erupts at about the age of 13 years (Griffen & Goepferd, 1991). Many fluoride preparations are available, often incorporated with vitamins. These tablets are obtained by prescription and should not be interchanged among children of various ages, as too much fluoride may cause the teeth to become "mottled." Fluoride may also be applied directly to the teeth by the dentist.

Another aspect of tooth care is the prevention of bottle-mouth caries. This occurs when an infant is put to bed with a bottle of milk or sweetened juice. Sugar pools within the oral cavity, causing severe decay. It is seen most often in children between 18 months and 3 years of age. Eliminating the bedtime bottle or substituting water is recommended.

## FEEDING THE HEALTHY CHILD

Table 16–9 specifies nursing interventions that help meet the nutritional needs of children, from infancy to adolescence.

**The Infant.** Infants, in proportion to their weight, require more calories, protein, minerals, and vitamins than adults do. Their fluid requirements are also high. Breast milk is excellent, and a nursing mother may continue this even when her baby is hospitalized. The nurse ensures the mother's privacy by placing a screen around the patient's unit or by posting a "Do not disturb" sign on the door. The nurse stresses that the mother should avoid fatigue because it affects milk production. Breast milk can be manually expressed and refrigerated at the hospital, then given in the mother's absence.

Some babies are unable to tolerate milk be-

**Table 16–9.** NURSING INTERVENTIONS FOR MEETING THE NUTRITIONAL NEEDS OF CHILDREN

| Age | Comment | Nursing Interventions |
|---|---|---|
| *Newborns and infants* | High energy maintenance because of immature systems, e.g., heat loss | Assist mother with breast feeding |
| | | Assist family with bottle feeding |
| | | Teach formula preparation |
| | Immature digestive system | Place infant on right side following feeding |
| | | Burp infant frequently |
| | Nutrient requirements related to body size | Observe infant for tolerance to formula |
| | | Consider vitamin C and D supplementation |
| | | Anticipate iron deficiencies (particularly in preterm newborns) |
| | Need for additional nutrients, satiety | Introduce solids when age-appropriate, at about 6 mo (consider variety, portions, texture) |
| | Danger of choking decreases as swallowing matures | |
| | | Instruct parents not to add salt or sugar to baby foods |
| | | Anticipate allergies |
| | | Explain selection and makeup of soy-based formulas if prescribed |
| | Prevention of dental decay | Encourage use of fluorides |
| | | Encourage weaning as appropriate to prevent bottle-mouth caries |
| | | Rinse infant's mouth after feedings |
| | Continued requirements for basic food groups | Assess educational and financial needs of family |
| | | Utilize supplemental food programs (WIC)* |
| *Toddlers and preschoolers* | Slower rate of growth; although body needs are still high, energy requirements decrease | Emphasize that from a nutritional viewpoint, child can regulate intake if appropriate foods are offered |
| | Picky eater | Provide nutritious snacks |
| | | Respect need for independence; do not force child to eat |
| | | Use colored straws; offer cheese, yogurt† if milk refused; add milk to potatoes |
| | | Offer mild meat in bite-sized portions |
| | | Add fruit to cereal |
| | | Reduce sweets |
| | | Invite playmate to lunch |
| | | Relax at meals |
| | | Promote harmony |
| *Children of school age* | Growth rate that continues to be slow but steady until puberty, some spurts and plateaus | Maintain education in nutrition |
| | | Introduce new foods when eating out |
| | | Assist child in preparing nutritious lunches |
| | | Provide fruits and raw vegetables for snacks when competition exists for meals |
| | | Encourage parents to include children in meal planning, preparation, and food shopping |
| *Adolescent girls* | Girls' caloric requirements less than those of boys | Emphasize that skipping meals can lead to decrease in essential nutrients |
| | Concern with body image may lead to anorexia or bulimia | Encourage physical exercise to maintain body weight |
| | | Educate as to proper nutrients to maintain body weight, e.g., skim milk, fruits |
| | | Avoid high-calorie fast foods |
| | | Consider emotional components related to foods (difficulty with peers, need for love and approval, and so on) |
| | Athletic activities | See interventions for adolescent boys |
| | Oral contraceptives | Explain that oral contraceptives increase requirements for several nutrients (folic acid, vitamin $B_6$, ascorbic acid) |
| | Adolescent pregnancy | Educate client concerning increased nutritional needs to complete growth and nourish fetus |

**Table 16–9.** NURSING INTERVENTIONS FOR MEETING THE NUTRITIONAL NEEDS OF CHILDREN *Continued*

| Age | Comment | Nursing Interventions |
|---|---|---|
| *Adolescent boys* | Concern with body image, bodybuilding | Instruct as to proper nutrition for sports<br>Avoid quack claims<br>Promote proper conditioning, well-balanced diet (increased calories), proper hydration without supplements—salt tablets unnecessary |
| | Overnutrition | Explain that this can lead to adult obesity<br>Instruct clients in order to lose weight:<br>　Eat a variety of foods low in calories and high in nutrients<br>　Eat less fat and fewer fatty foods<br>　Eat less sugar and fewer sweets<br>　Drink less alcohol<br>　Eat more fruits, vegetables, whole grains<br>　Increase physical activity |

*WIC = Women, Infants, and Children.
†Is not fortified with Vitamin D.

cause of intestinal bleeding, allergy, or other negative reactions. Many milk substitutes are available for therapeutic use. Among these are soybean mixtures (such as ProSobee and Isomil) for patients with milk-protein sensitivity. Most products come in dry and liquid forms, and parents need to be made aware of what concentrations the doctor intends.

The nurse needs to be aware of the problems of underfeeding and overfeeding of infants. Underfeeding is suggested by restlessness, crying, and failure to gain weight. Overfeeding is manifested by such symptoms as regurgitation, mild diarrhea, and too-rapid weight gain. Diets high in fat delay gastric emptying and cause abdominal distention. Diets too high in carbohydrates may cause distention, flatus, and excessive weight gain. Constipation may be the result of too much fat or protein, or a deficiency in bulk. Increased amounts of cereals, vegetables, and fruits can often correct this problem.

In general, solids are introduced at about 6 months of age. The infant given large quantities of milk and few solids is a good target for iron-deficiency anemia. This is by far the most common disease of the blood in infants and small children. Because of this, the Nutrition Committee of the American Academy of Pediatrics recommends that all infants who are not breast-fed be on a commercial formula supplemented with iron, until 1 year of age. In the past, it was not common to use such formulas beyond 5–6 months, and there has been an unfortunate reluctance among parents to adopt this suggestion.

Most infants naturally adapt to a schedule of three meals a day by the end of the 1st year. At this time, the appetite fluctuates as the growth rate slows somewhat. The patient may not be interested in eating. Spills are frequent. At 1 year, children cannot manipulate a spoon, but hand-to-mouth coordination is good enough that they enjoy holding a piece of toast while the nurse assists. In the hospital, children in highchairs wear jacket restraints. The nurse remains in constant attendance. Developmental advancements that change food patterns are explained to parents in order to prevent feeding difficulties.

**The Toddler.** By the end of the 2nd year, toddlers can feed themselves. This is important to developing a sense of independence. The toddler may be balky at times, and food may be pushed away or completely refused. Toddlers benefit most from the caretakers' presence at mealtime. Feeding difficulties may result from anxieties of parents and lack of time.

**The Preschool Child.** Preschoolers and toddlers like finger foods. Dawdling is common in this age group, as is regression. Preschoolers in general are more vulnerable to protein-calorie deficiencies; their younger siblings receive priority at home, and older brothers and sisters receive benefits of school lunch programs. The nurse recognizes this problem and offers nourishing snacks, such as dry cereal out of the box, graham crackers, fruit juices, milk, and ice cream.

**The School-Age Child.** School-age children need food from the basic food groups, but in in-

**Table 16–10.** RECOMMENDED ENERGY AND PROTEIN ALLOWANCES*

| Age (years) | Height | | Weight | | | Protein | | | |
|---|---|---|---|---|---|---|---|---|---|
| | Inches | Centimeters | Pounds | Kilograms | Kilocalories per Day | Kilocalories per Kilogram | Kilocalories per Centimeter | Grams per Day | Grams per Centimeter |
| *Females* | | | | | | | | | |
| 11–14 | 62 | 157 | 101 | 46 | 2200 | 47 | 14.0 | 46 | 0.29 |
| 15–18 | 64 | 163 | 120 | 55 | 2200 | 40 | 13.5 | 44 | 0.26 |
| 19–24 | 65 | 164 | 128 | 58 | 2200 | 38 | 13.4 | 46 | 0.28 |
| *Males* | | | | | | | | | |
| 11–14 | 62 | 157 | 99 | 45 | 2500 | 55 | 16.0 | 45 | 0.28 |
| 15–18 | 69 | 176 | 145 | 66 | 3000 | 45 | 17.0 | 59 | 0.33 |
| 19–24 | 70 | 177 | 160 | 72 | 2900 | 40 | 16.4 | 58 | 0.33 |

Reprinted with permission from *Recommended Dietary Allowances: 10th Edition.* Copyright 1989 by the National Academy of Sciences. Courtesy of the National Academy Press, Washington, D.C.

creased quantities in order to meet energy requirements. Their attitudes toward food are unpredictable. Intake of protein, calcium, vitamin A, and ascorbic acid tends to be low. The love of sweets decreases the appetite and provides empty calories.

**The Adolescent.** During the adolescent years, nutrition is particularly important. Teenagers are growing rapidly and expending large amounts of energy. Food needs are great. The nurse attempts to involve the teenager in selecting foods that are nutritious and appetizing. This may be done by reviewing choices made on the daily menu. Sometimes it helps to stress how important good nutrition is to physical appearance and fitness. The need for peer approval is at its height during adolescence, and food fads and skipped meals may result in malnutrition, even in families of means. Fatigue is a common complaint at this age. If it is accompanied by a lack of appetite and irritability, anemia should be suspected.

Table 16–10 lists the recommended energy and protein allowances for adolescents and adults.

## FEEDING THE ILL CHILD

Children in the hospital are in the process of growth. Well-nourished children nearly always show steady gains in weight and height. They are alert; the hair is shiny. They have no fatigue circles beneath the eyes. The skin color is good, the abdomen flat, the posture good, and the muscles well developed. The mucous membranes of the mouth and gums are firm and pink, not swollen or bleeding. There are no lesions in the mouth or on the tongue. The teeth are erupting on schedule. The appetite is generally good, and elimination regular. The child sleeps well at night, the vitality is good, and the child is not irritable. This picture changes somewhat during illness, but the child who is basically well nourished can easily be distinguished from one who is malnourished.

Many hospitalized children have poor appetites. This may be due to age, nature of the illness, type of diet, sudden exposure to strange foods and strange environment, reaction to hospitalization, and degree of satisfaction obtained during mealtimes. The small child may also refuse to eat in an attempt to manipulate the parents, particularly if anorexia was a concern in the past.

The nurse observes the patient's tray to determine if the food is of the right consistency. Does the child have any teeth? Do lesions in the mouth prevent chewing? Can the child use a knife and fork? Children with bandaged limbs or those receiving intravenous fluids require assistance. The size of servings is important. One should serve less than one hopes will be eaten. A tablespoonful of food (not heaping) for each year of age is a good guide to follow. More is given if the patient appears hungry. One item at a time is placed before small children who feed themselves, so that they will not become overwhelmed. The nurse avoids showing personal dislikes be-cause negative attitudes are easily transmitted. The nurse proceeds slowly with unfamiliar children in order to determine their level of mastery. Food is served warm, and sufficient time is allotted. Sweet drinks, Popsicles, and the like should not be served just before meals.

## KEY POINTS

- A person's sex and all the person's inherited characteristics are determined at the moment of conception.
- The concept of dominant and recessive genes is important in studying birth defects.
- Amniocentesis enables the physician to diagnose many genetic diseases in the prenatal period.
- Growth and development are orderly and sequential, although there are plateaus.
- Developmental theories can serve as guides to nursing intervention; however, each child grows and develops at an individual pace.
- Cephalocaudal development proceeds from head to toe.

- Children are susceptible to nutritional deficiencies because they are in the process of growth and development.
- Abraham Maslow depicted human development on the basis of a hierarchy of needs.
- Deciduous teeth are baby teeth. The proper care of the teeth depends on caretaker supervision and the child's physical level of development and mastery.
- Erick Erikson described eight stages of psychosocial development from birth to adulthood.

# Study Questions

1. Describe the differences in the water, nutrient, and metabolism requirements of the child and adult.
2. Define personality. What factors contribute to the formation of a child's personality? Explain.
3. Why is a knowledge of growth and development essential for nurses caring for children and their families?
4. List four characteristics of growth and development and provide an example of each characteristic.
5. Discuss the statement "Development occurs at different rates for various parts of the body." Give examples.
6. Gloria Chinn is 6 years old. Her mother states that she has always been a "picky eater." What advice might be helpful for Mrs. Chinn? Explain your reasons for this advice.
7. Describe four current types of families and their implications for health-care providers.
8. Review Table 16–6, which summarizes culturally diverse food patterns of some Americans. For each culture discussed, state one nutritional concern if the patient adheres to that diet.
9. What is the purpose of a growth chart?
10. You are caring for 20-month-old Perez. What do you know about the growth and development of 20-month-old babies in terms of eating behavior? What foods would you consider appropriate, and which inappropriate? Describe how you would incorporate your knowledge into Perez's nursing care plan.

# Multiple Choice Review Questions

*Choose the most appropriate answer.*

1. A progressive increase in the function of the body is referred to as
   a. maturation
   b. development
   c. growth
   d. metabolism

2. During the 1st week of life, the newborn's weight
   a. increases about 5–10%
   b. decreases about 5–10%
   c. stabilizes
   d. fluctuates widely

3. The first teeth of the newborn are termed
   a. deciduous teeth
   b. indigenous teeth
   c. permanent teeth
   d. preparatory teeth

4. A mistake in the development of a gene is termed a
   a. karyogram
   b. chromosome
   c. genotype
   d. mutation

5. A method of sending sound waves into body tissues in order to detect malformations is called
   a. amniography
   b. ultrasonography
   c. phototherapy
   d. auscultation

## BIBLIOGRAPHY

Behrman, R. (1992). *Nelson textbook of pediatrics* (14th ed.). Philadelphia: W.B. Saunders.

Betz, C. (1992). The "Brady Bunch" approach. *Journal of Pediatric Nursing: Nursing Care of Children and Families, 7,* 303.

Burroughs, A. (1992). *Maternity nursing: An introductory text* (6th ed.). Philadelphia: W.B. Saunders.

Capra, C. (1991). *Shackelton's nutrition: Essentials and diet therapy* (5th ed.). Philadelphia: W.B. Saunders.

Griffen, A., & Goepferd, S. (1991). Preventive oral health care for the infant, child, and adolescent. *Pediatric Clinics of North America, 38,* 1209.

Josell, S. (1991). Pediatric oral health. *Pediatric Clinics of North America, 38.*

Levine, M.D., Carey, W.B., & Crocker, A.C. (1992). *Developmental-behavioral pediatrics* (2nd ed.). Philadelphia: W.B. Saunders.

Light, D., Keller, S., & Calhoun, C. (1989). *Sociology.* New York: Knopf.

Mahan, L.K., & Arlin, M.T. (1992). *Krause's food, nutrition & diet therapy* (8th ed.). Philadelphia: W.B. Saunders.

Mott, S., James, S.R., & Sperhac, A.M. (1991). *Nursing care of children and families* (2nd ed.). Reading, MA: Addison-Wesley.

*Nutrition and your health: Dietary guidelines for Americans* (3rd ed.). (1990). Home and Garden Bulletin No. 232. Hyattsville, MD: U.S. Department of Agriculture, U.S. Department of Health and Human Services.

Olds, S., London, M., & Ladewig, B. (1992). *Maternal-newborn nursing* (4th ed). Reading, MA: Addison-Wesley.

Pillitteri, A. (1992). *Maternal and child health nursing.* Philadelphia: J.B. Lippincott.

Poleman, C.M., & Peckenpaugh, N.J. (1991). *Nutrition essentials and diet therapy.* Philadelphia: W.B. Saunders.

Public Health Service, U.S. Department of Health and Human Services, and NHLBI (1988). National Cholesterol Education Program (NCEP): *Report of the expert panel on detection, evaluation, and treatment of high blood cholesterol in adults* (NIH Publication No. 88-2925). Washington, DC: U.S. Government Printing Office.

Thompson, E.D., & Ashwill, J.W. (1992). *Introduction to pediatric nursing* (6th ed.). Philadelphia: W.B. Saunders.

Thompson, M.W., McInnes, R.R., & Willard, H.F. (1991). *Thompson and Thompson genetics in medicine* (5th ed.). Philadelphia: W.B. Saunders.

U.S. Department of Health and Human Services (1992). *Child health USA '91.* Washington, DC: U.S. Government Printing Office.

Valadian, I., & Porter, D. (1977). *Physical growth and development from conception to maturity.* Boston: Little, Brown.

Whaley, L., & Wong, D. (1991). *Nursing care of infants and children* (4th ed.). St. Louis: C.V. Mosby.

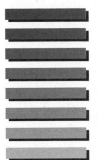

# Chapter 17

# The Infant

## VOCABULARY
colic (431)
extrusion reflex (432)
grasp reflex (416)
immunization (431)
oral stage (416)
parachute reflex (416)
pincer grasp (416)
posterior fontanel (418)
satiety (436)
Washington Guide (430)

General Characteristics
Development and Care
Health Maintenance
   Immunization
   Nutrition Counseling
   Teething

# OBJECTIVES

*On completion and mastery of Chapter 17, the student will be able to*

■ Define each vocabulary term listed.
■ Describe the physical and psychosocial development of infants from 1 to 12 months, listing age-specific events and guidance when appropriate.
■ Discuss the nutritional needs of growing infants.
■ Describe how to select and prepare solid foods for the infant.
■ List four common concerns of parents about the feeding of infants.
■ Discuss the development of feeding skills in the infant.
■ Identify the approximate age for each of the following: posterior fontanel has closed; central incisors appear; birth weight has tripled; child can sit steadily alone; child shows fear of strangers.
■ List the immunizations given during the 1st year using medical terminology, including the approximate age for each, and discussing ways to convince parents of the merits of the type of protection.
■ Discuss teething during infancy.

# General Characteristics

Children, unlike adults, are in the process of growing while they are hospitalized. In order to provide total patient care, the nurse must be able to recognize a patient's needs at various stages of growth and development. The nurse must try to meet them effectively and to administer the specialized nursing care required for the particular patient. *The most common cause for concern about a child is a sudden slowing, not typical for age, of any aspect of development.*

Each baby develops at an individual rate. Although growth is continuous, there are slow and rapid periods. The 1st year of life is a period of rapid growth and development. Brain growth is the most critical organic achievement of infancy. The infant is completely dependent on adults during the first months and gives little in return. Behavior is not consistent.

**Oral Stage.** Sucking brings the infant comfort and relief from tension. This oral stage of personality development is important for the infant's physical and psychological development. The nurse, knowing the importance of sucking to the baby, holds the baby during feedings and allows sufficient time to suck. Infants who are warm and comfortable associate food with love. The baby who is fed intravenous fluids is given added attention and a pacifier to ensure the necessary satisfaction of sucking. When the teeth appear, the infant learns to bite and enjoys objects that can be chewed. Gradually, the baby begins to put the fingers into the mouth. When babies can use their hands more skillfully, they will not suck their fingers as often and will be able to derive pleasure from other sources.

**Motor Development.** The *grasp reflex* is seen when one touches the palms of the infant's hands and flexion occurs. This reflex disappears at about 3 months. *Prehension*, the ability to grasp objects between the fingers and the opposing thumb, occurs slightly later (5–6 months) and follows an orderly sequence of development. By 7–9 months, the *parachute reflex* appears. This is a protective arm extension that occurs when an infant is suddenly thrust downward when prone. By 1 year, the *pincer grasp* coordination of index finger and thumb is well established.

**Emotional Development.** Love and security are vital needs of infants. They require the continuous affection given by parents (Fig. 17–1). If trust is to develop, consistency must be established. Parents are assured that they need not be afraid of spoiling infants by attending promptly to their needs. Loving adults affirm that the world is a good place in which to live. Each day the infant becomes impressed by parental actions and learns to imitate and trust caretakers. A *sense of trust* is vital to the development of a healthy personality. Many consider it to be the foundation of emotional growth. The child who is deprived of this instead learns to mistrust people, which could have a permanently negative effect.

Parents are taught to talk, sing, and touch their babies while providing care. They should not expect too much or too little from them. Babies will easily accomplish various activities if they are not forced before they reach maturity. When an infant shows readiness to learn a task, parents should provide encouragement.

**Need for Constant Care and Guidance.** The constant care of an infant is a strain on the most exemplary parents. The full-time caretaker, in particular, needs and deserves the un-

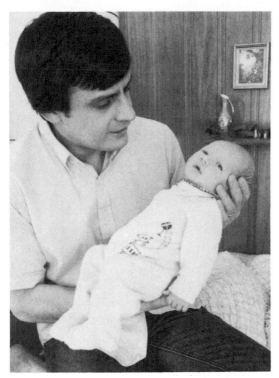

**Figure 17–1.** The role of father, although neglected in the past, is now seen as integral to family-centered nursing.

derstanding of and kind support from relatives at home and from the nurse in the hospital. A short break from pressures provides renewed energy with which to enjoy the baby. A trip to the store or a stroll with the baby in the carriage affords stimulation and a change of environment for the baby and the caretaker. The infant who is constantly left in a crib or playpen and not introduced to a variety of learning experiences may become shy and withdrawn. *Sensory stimulation is essential for development of the baby's thought processes and perceptual abilities.*

If a mother is unable to room-in with her hospitalized infant, personnel should try to imitate her care by promptly fulfilling the infant's physical and emotional needs. In the nursery, the nurse first feeds the baby who appears hungry, rather than delaying feeding to adhere to a specific routine. Wet diapers are changed as soon as possible. The crying child is soothed. The exactness of time or method of bathing or feeding the infant is less important than the care with which it is done. The baby easily rec-

ognizes warmth and affection or the lack of them.

## Development and Care

Table 17–1 is a guide to infant care from the 1st month to the 1st year. The material is arranged under headings and in chronologic order so that the student can easily refer to it. Although convenient, it is merely a summary of data. Some of the aspects of care (e.g., safety measures) are important throughout the entire year.

The nurse explains to parents that physical patterns cannot be separated from social patterns and that abrupt changes do not take place with each new month. Human development cannot be separated into specific areas any more than the body's structure can be separated from its function. *No two infants are just alike at a certain age. This is just a guide!* However, individual variations range about central norms that serve as guidelines in the evaluation of an infant's or child's progress. The addition of the various solid foods to the diet and the time of immunizations vary slightly, depending on the baby's health and the physician's protocol. Nevertheless, the types remain the same.

## Health Maintenance

The prevention of disease during infancy is of the utmost importance and includes all measures that improve the physical health and psychosocial adjustment of the child. The concept of periodic health appraisal is not new. In the late 1800s, "milk stations" were established in various localities throughout the United States to provide safe water and milk for babies in an effort to reduce the number of deaths from infant diarrhea.

Skilled health services today encompass periodic health appraisal, immunizations, assessment of parent-child interaction, counseling in the developmental processes, identification of families at risk (e.g., for child abuse), health education and anticipatory guidance, referrals to various agencies, follow-up services, appropriate record-keeping, and evaluation and audit by peers. They are provided in a variety of health-care facilities. Ideally the infant is seen

**Table 17–1.** PHYSICAL DEVELOPMENT, SOCIAL BEHAVIOR, AND CARE AND
                GUIDANCE OF INFANTS

**1 Month**

*Physical Development*

Weighs approximately 8 lb. Has regained weight lost after birth. Gains about 1 inch in length per month for the first 6 mo

Lifts head slightly when placed on stomach. Pushes with toes. Turns head to side when prone. Head wobbles. Head lags when infant pulled from lying to sitting position. Clenches fists. Stares at surroundings

Vaginal discharge in girls and breast enlargement in boys and girls from maternal hormones received in utero are not unusual and disappear without treatment

*Social Behavior*

Makes small throaty noises. Cries when hungry or uncomfortable

Sleeps 20 of 24 hr. Awakes for 2 AM feeding

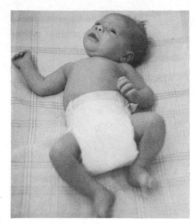

*Joel at 1 month of age.*

**2 Months**

*Physical Development*

Posterior fontanel closes. Tears appear. Can hold head erect in midposition. Follows moving light with eyes. Holds a rattle briefly. Legs are active

*Social Behavior*

Smiles in response to mother's voice. Knows crying brings attention. Awakes for 2 AM feeding

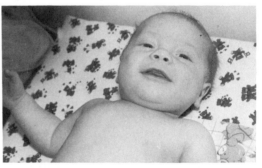

*The 2-month-old's smile delights parents.*

**Table 17—1.** PHYSICAL DEVELOPMENT, SOCIAL BEHAVIOR, AND CARE AND
GUIDANCE OF INFANTS *Continued*

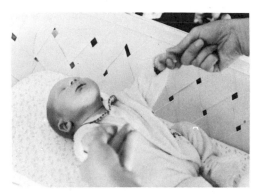

*Note head lag of 1-month-old when pulled from
lying position.*

*Care and Guidance*
   *Sleep.* Back; if side-lying position, support back with
blanket roll. Use a firm, tight-fitting mattress in a crib with
bars properly spaced so that the baby's head cannot be
caught between them. Raise crib rails. Use no pillow
   *Diet.* Breast milk every 2–3 hr or iron-fortified formula
every 4 hr as baby indicates need. Vitamin D (400 IU/day in
dark-skinned infants, breast-fed babies, or infants who are
not regularly exposed to sunlight. Plain, cooled water may
be given between feedings. Bubble baby well
   *Exercise.* Allow freedom from the restraints of clothing
before bath. Provide fresh air and sunshine whenever
possible. Do not leave baby in sun for more than a short
while. Provide protection from insects with netting. Avoid
large crowds until immune system becomes more developed
   Support head and shoulders when holding infant. Attend
promptly to physical needs. Provide colorful hanging toys for
sensory stimulation

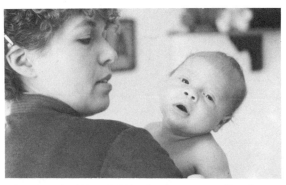

*The 2-month-old can hold his head erect in midline for
brief periods of time.*

*Care and Guidance*
   *Sleep.* Develops own pattern; may sleep from feeding to
feeding
   *Diet.* Breast milk or formula
   *Exercise.* Provide a safe, flat place to kick and be active.
Do not leave baby alone, particularly on any raised surface
   Physical examination by the family doctor, well-baby
clinic, or pediatrician
   *Immunization.* First DTP, an inoculation against
diphtheria, whooping cough, and tetanus. Oral polio vaccine
(OPV), *Haemophilus influenzae* type b (HbCV), and second
HBV vaccine
   Still completely depends on adults for physical care.
Needs a flexible routine throughout infancy and childhood
   *Pacifier.* If used, select for safety. Choose one-piece
construction and loop handle to prevent aspiration
   *Hiccups.* Are normal and subside without treatment. May
offer small amounts of water
   *Colic* (paroxysmal abdominal pain, irritable crying).
Usually disappears after 3 mo. Place baby prone over arms
(Fig. 17–2). Use pacifier. Massage back. Relieve caretaker
periodically

*Continued*

**Table 17–1.** PHYSICAL DEVELOPMENT, SOCIAL BEHAVIOR, AND CARE AND
GUIDANCE OF INFANTS *Continued*

---

**3 Months**

*Physical Development*
  Weighs 12–13 lb. Stares at hands. Reaches for objects but misses them. Carries hand to mouth
  Can follow an object from right to left and up and down when it is placed in front of face. Supports head steadily. Holds rattle

*Social Behavior*
  Cries less. Can wait a few minutes for attention. Enjoys having people talk to him. Takes impromptu naps

---

**4 Months**

*Physical Development*
  Weighs about 13–14 lb
  Drooling indicates appearance of saliva
  Lifts head and shoulders when on abdomen and looks around. Turns from back to side. Sits with support. Begins to reach for objects he sees. Coordination between eye and body movements
  Moves head, arms, and shoulders when excited. Extends legs and partly sustains weight when held upright. Rooting, Moro, extrusion, and tonic neck reflexes are no longer present. Little head lag

*Social Behavior*
  Coos, chuckles, and gurgles. Laughs aloud. Responds to others. Likes an audience. Sleeps through the night. May show preference for certain foods

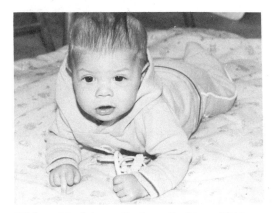

*While on his abdomen the 4-month-old can lift his head and shoulders and look around.*

---

**Table 17–1.** PHYSICAL DEVELOPMENT, SOCIAL BEHAVIOR, AND CARE AND
GUIDANCE OF INFANTS *Continued*

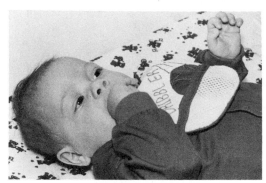

*The 3-month-old carries his hand to his mouth.*

*Care and Guidance*
  *Sleep.* Yawns, stretches, naps in mother's arms
  *Diet.* Mother's milk or formula
  *Exercise.* May have short play period. Enjoys playing with hands

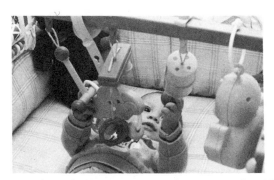

*Visual stimulation is important to the growing infant. The 4-month-old reaches for objects. There is increased coordination between eyes and body movement.*

*Care and Guidance*
  *Sleep.* Stirs about in crib. Sleeps through ordinary household noises—avoid tiptoeing around
  *Diet.* Mother's milk or formula
  *Exercise.* Plays with hand rattles and dangling toys. Start acquainting with a playpen, where baby can roll with safety
  *Immunization.* Second DTP, OPV, and HbCV
  *Elimination.* One or two bowel movements per day. May skip a day

*Continued*

**Table 17–1.** PHYSICAL DEVELOPMENT, SOCIAL BEHAVIOR, AND CARE AND
GUIDANCE OF INFANTS *Continued*

**5 Months**

*Physical Development*
Sits with support. Holds head well. Grasps objects offered.
Puts everything into mouth. Plays with toes

*Social Behavior*
Talks to himself. Seems to know whether persons are
familiar or unfamiliar
May sleep through 10 PM feeding. Tries to hold bottle
at feeding time

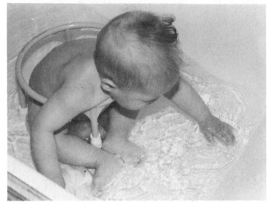

*At 5 months, Joel enjoys water play. Tub safety ring
supports child. Suction cup legs adhere to tub. Baby
can grasp wash cloth and enjoys chewing on it. Do not
leave a baby unattended in tub.*

**6 Months**

*Physical Development*
Doubles birth weight. Gains about 3–5 oz/wk during next
6 mo. Grows about a half inch per month
Sits alone momentarily. Springs up and down when
sitting. Turns completely over. Hitches (moves backward
when sitting). Bangs table with rattle. Pulls to a sitting
position. Chewing more mature. Approximates lips to rim of
cup

*Social Behavior*
Cries loudly when interrupted from play. Increased
interest in world. Babbles and squeals. Sucks food from
spoon. Awakes happy

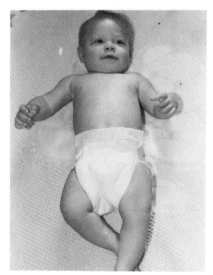

*Joel's weight at 6 months is now 16 pounds, 6 ounces (birth
weight, 8 pounds, 4 ounces).*

**Table 17–1.** PHYSICAL DEVELOPMENT, SOCIAL BEHAVIOR, AND CARE AND
GUIDANCE OF INFANTS *Continued*

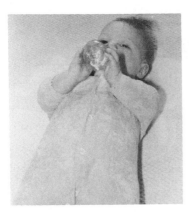

*Joel holds bottle of water.*

*Care and Guidance*
  *Sleep.* Takes two or three naps daily in crib
  *Diet.* Mother's milk or formula
  *Exercise.* Provide space to pivot around. Makes jumping
motions when held upright in lap
  *Safety.* Check toys for loose buttons and rough edges
before placing them in playpen

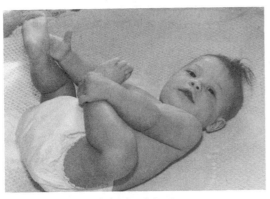

*Joel plays with his feet.*

*Care and Guidance*
  *Sleep.* Needs own room. Should be moved from parents'
room if not previously done. Otherwise, as baby becomes
older, may become unwilling to sleep away from them
  *Diet.* Introduce first solid foods, usually rice cereal fortified
with iron. See Figure 17–6 for progression. Note: The
sequence of supplemental foods varies according to one's
physician. This is not as important as offering a wide variety
of foods during the 1st year
  *Exercise.* Grasps feet and pulls toward mouth
  *Immunization.* DTP, HbCV, and HBV
  *Safety.* Remove toxic plants. Provide a chewable object,
such as a teething ring or face cloth, for enjoyment

*Continued*

**Table 17–1.** PHYSICAL DEVELOPMENT, SOCIAL BEHAVIOR, AND CARE AND
GUIDANCE OF INFANTS *Continued*

### 7 Months

*Physical Development*

Two lower teeth appear. These are the first of the deciduous teeth, the central incisors

Begins to crawl. Moves forward, using chest, head, and arms; legs drag. Can grasp objects more easily. Transfers objects from one hand to the other. Appears interested in standing. Holds an adult's hands and bounces actively while standing. Struggles when being dressed

*Social Behavior*

Shifts moods easily—crying one minute, laughing the next. Shows fear of strangers

Anticipates spoon feeding. Sleeps 11–13 hr at night

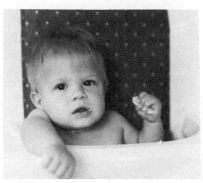

*At 7 months, Joel enjoys finger foods.*

### 8 Months

*Physical Development*

Sits steadily alone. Uses index finger and thumb as pincers. Pokes at object. Enjoys dropping article into a cup and emptying it

*Social Behavior*

Plays pat-a-cake. Enjoys family life. Amuses self longer. Reserved with strangers

Indicates need for sleep by fussing and sucking thumb. Impatient especially when food is being prepared

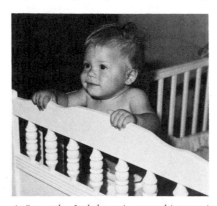

*At 8 months, Joel shows increased interest in standing.*

**Table 17–1.** PHYSICAL DEVELOPMENT, SOCIAL BEHAVIOR, AND CARE AND GUIDANCE OF INFANTS *Continued*

*Care and Guidance*

*Sleep.* Fretfulness due to teething may appear. This is generally evidenced by lack of appetite and wakefulness during the night. In most cases, merely soothing and offering a cup of water are sufficient

*Diet.* Add fruit. Add finger foods, such as toast or zwieback

*Exercise.* Rudimentary locomotion

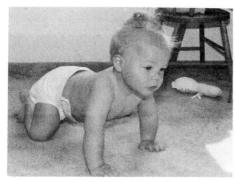

*Joel begins to get around.*

*Care and Guidance*

*Sleep.* Takes two naps a day

*Diet.* Add vegetables. Continue to add new foods slowly

*Exercise.* Enjoys jump chair. Rides in stroller. Stuffed toys or those that squeak or rattle are appropriate

*Safety.* Remain with baby at all times during bath in tub. Protect from chewing paint from window sills or old furniture. Paint containing lead can be poisonous. Close doors to ovens, dishwashers, washing machines, dryers, and refrigerators

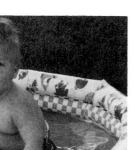

*Joel can sit steadily.*

*Continued*

**Table 17–1.** PHYSICAL DEVELOPMENT, SOCIAL BEHAVIOR, AND CARE AND
GUIDANCE OF INFANTS *Continued*

**9 Months**

*Physical Development*

Shows preference for use of one hand. Can raise self to a sitting position. Holds bottle. Creeps. Carries trunk of body above floor but parallel to it. More advanced than crawling

*Social Behavior*

Tries to imitate sounds, e.g., says "ba-ba" for bye-bye. Cries if scolded

Drops food from highchair at mealtime. May fall asleep after 6 PM feeding

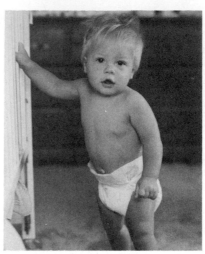

*At 9 months, Joel cruises around holding onto furniture.*

**10 Months**

*Physical Development*

Pulls to a standing position in the playpen. Throws toys to floor for parent to pick up. Cries when they are not returned. Walks around furniture while holding onto it

*Social Behavior*

Knows name. Plays simple games such as peek-a-boo. Feeds himself a cookie. May cry out in sleep without waking

**Table 17–1.** PHYSICAL DEVELOPMENT, SOCIAL BEHAVIOR, AND CARE AND
GUIDANCE OF INFANTS *Continued*

*Care and Guidance*
  *Sleep.* Has generally begun to sleep later in the morning
  *Diet.* Add meat, beans. Introduce chopped and mashed foods. Place newspaper beneath feeding table. Use unbreakable dishes. Allow baby to pick up pieces of food by hand and put them into mouth
  *Safety.* Keep a supply of syrup of ipecac on hand. Know phone number of nearest poison control center. Avoid tablecloths with overhangs baby could reach
  *Exercise.* Is busy most of the day exploring surroundings. Provide sufficient room and materials for safe play
  Help baby to learn. Distract curious child from danger. In this way punishment is limited—avoid excessive spankings and "nos"

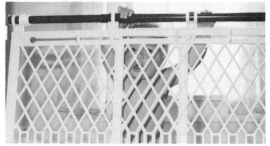

*Stairway gates prevent falls for the infant with increased mobility.*

*Care and Guidance*
  *Sleep.* Avoid strenuous play before bedtime. A night light is convenient for parent and makes baby's surroundings more familiar. Pajamas with feet are warm, as baby becomes uncovered easily
  *Diet.* Takes juice and water from cup. Solid foods in general are taken well
  *Exercise.* Tours around room holding adult's hands. Daytime clothing should be loose so as not to interfere with movement

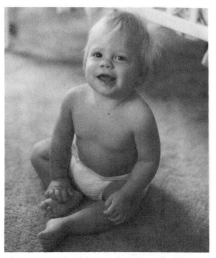

*The 10-month-old. Note lower tooth.*

*Continued*

**Table 17–1.** PHYSICAL DEVELOPMENT, SOCIAL BEHAVIOR, AND CARE AND
GUIDANCE OF INFANTS *Continued*

**11 Months**

*Physical Development*
  Stands upright holding onto adult's hands

*Social Behavior*
  Understands simple directions. Impatient when held.
Enjoys playing with empty dish and spoon following meals

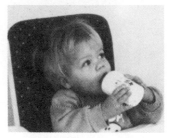

*Drinking from a cup is easy for Joel, who is now 11 months; however, spills still occur.*

**12 Months**

*Physical Development*
  Pulse 100–140 beats/min. Respirations 20–40/min
  Triples birth weight. Height is about 29 inches
  Stands alone for short periods. May walk. Puts arm through sleeve as an aid to being dressed
  Six teeth (four above and two below). Drinks from a cup, eats with a spoon with supervision
  Pincer grasp is well established
  Handedness (the preference for the use of one hand), although not fully established, may be evidenced

*Social Behavior*
  Friendly. Repeats acts that elicit a response
  Recognizes "no-no." Verbalization slows because of concentration on getting about. Enjoys rhythmic music
  Shows emotions such as fear, anger, and jealousy. Reacts to these emotions from adults
  Plays with food, removes it from mouth

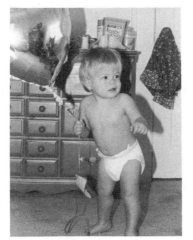

*Happy Birthday, Joel! At 12 months, Joel weighs 21 pounds, 14 ounces, and is 28 ¾ inches tall. He can stand alone for brief periods.*

**Table 17–1.** PHYSICAL DEVELOPMENT, SOCIAL BEHAVIOR, AND CARE AND GUIDANCE OF INFANTS *Continued*

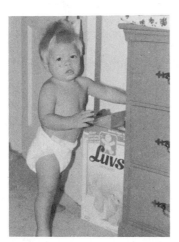

*Directions must be simple for the 11-month-old.*

*Care and Guidance*

*Sleep.* Greets parents in morning with excited jargon

*Diet.* Still spills from cup. Enjoys blowing bubbles

*Exercise.* Plays with toys in tub. Enjoys gross motor activity. Kicks, pulls self up

*Safety.* Cover electrical outlets with tape. Put household cleaners and medicines out of reach if not previously done. Needs to be sat down in playpen at times, since tends to stand until becoming exhausted.

*Care and Guidance*

*Sleep.* May take one long nap daily

*Diet.* Gradually add egg white and fish (baked, steamed, or boiled). Drain oil from tuna or salmon. Add orange juice, if not done earlier. Add well-cooked table foods. Interest in eating dwindles

*Exercise.* Enjoys putting clothespins in a basket and then removing them. Places objects on head

Distraction is an effective way to deal with determination to do what baby wants regardless of outcome

*Skin Test.* Tuberculin

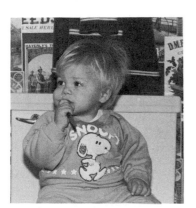

*Joel at 1 year enjoys chewing on his toothbrush.*

at least five times during the 1st year at specific intervals (2 months, 4 months, 6 months, 9 months, and 1 year). The kinds and quality of assistance vary. Private group practice, hospital-based clinics, and neighborhood health centers are examples of medical settings. These visits are as important for parents as they are for the baby. They provide caretaker support and reassurance as well as information and anticipatory guidance for the many developmental changes of the infant's 1st year. Two common concerns, diaper rash and colic, are outlined in Nursing Care Plans 17–1 and 17–2. Figure 17–2 illustrates the "colic carry."

A careful health history is obtained (Fig. 17–3). Growth grids during infancy include measures of weight, length, and head circumference (see pp. 572–574). The reading and recording of growth charts are described on page 388. There are numerous developmental screening tests. The *Denver Developmental Screening Test*, which is widely used, is discussed in Chapter 18 (p. 448). The *Brazelton Neonatal Behavioral Assessment Scale* is of particular value during the newborn period; it helps describe the emerging personality of the baby and includes evaluation of infant reflexes, general activity, alertness, orientation to spoken voice, and response to visual stimuli. Although not a screening test per se, the *Washington Guide to Promoting Development in the Young Child* is also useful in evaluating the child's functional ability in such areas as feeding, sleep, toilet training, play, and motor activity. Expected tasks for each area are listed along with ideas for parental guidance. Although scoring is omitted, it provides a tool for systematic observation of the development of the infant and child from birth through 5 years of age.

The physical examination is adapted to the needs of the infant. Routine assessments of hearing and vision are an integral part of the examination. In the newborn period, loud noises should precipitate the *startle* or *Moro reflex*. Localization of sound during infancy can be roughly ascertained by standing behind the child seated on the mother's lap and ringing a bell or repeating voice sounds. The baby's response is compared with the average for that age level. Vision is mainly assessed by light

---

**NURSING CARE PLAN 17–1**

### Selected Nursing Diagnosis for the Infant with Diaper Rash

| Goal | Nursing Interventions | Rationale |
|---|---|---|
| **Nursing Diagnosis:** High risk for impaired skin integrity, perineal area, related to improper cleansing and infrequent diaper change. | | |
| Skin will remain dry; there will be no signs of redness, irritation, or oozing | 1. Suggest frequent diaper changes | 1. Diaper dermatitis is caused by prolonged and repeated exposure to urine, feces, soaps, detergents, ointments, and friction; changing a wet or soiled diaper promptly eliminates this problem; exposing skin to light and air facilitates drying and healing |
| | 2. Demonstrate how to cleanse the diaper area thoroughly and how to dry between skin folds; have parent return demonstration | 2. After soiling, perineal area is cleansed with plain water and, if needed, a mild soap; disposable wet "wipes" can aggravate a diaper rash if infant is sensitive to an ingredient in product; moisture between skin folds prevents healing |
| | 3. Review changes in diet | 3. Addition of new foods or a change from breast milk to formula may be related to rash |
| | 4. Evaluate finances of family | 4. Socioeconomic factors have a bearing on parent compliance |

| NURSING CARE PLAN 17–2 |
| --- |
| **Selected Nursing Diagnosis for the Infant with Colic** |

| Goals | Nursing Interventions | Rationale |
| --- | --- | --- |
| **Nursing Diagnosis:** Altered family process related to fussiness of infant. | | |
| Parents will demonstrate increased coping behaviors by 1 wk<br>Parents will verbalize feelings of increased confidence in caring for the baby | 1. Educate parents about common manifestations of colic | 1. No one cause has been established for colic; infant appears otherwise healthy but demonstrates cramplike pain, drawing legs to abdomen and demonstrating irritable cry; it is time-limited to about 3 mo |
| | 2. Determine whether other causes have been ruled out by physician | 2. Intestinal obstruction and infection may mimic symptoms of colic; bowel movements are not abnormal with colic |
| | 3. Review caretaker's history and usual day with infant | 3. This helps determine if colic is related to type of feedings, diet of breast-feeding mother, passive smoking, milk allergy, activities of family members while baby is being fed, etc. |
| | 4. Identify soothing measures used by parents and their effectiveness | 4. Environment may be overstimulating infant; parents may not know how to soothe baby |
| | 5. Suggest abdominal massage, wind-up swing, car rides | 5. These measures may help relieve symptoms; burping before and after feedings and placing in an upright position after feedings may also decrease distress |
| | 6. Demonstrate "colic carry" (see Fig. 17–2) | 6. This may comfort infant by applying a little extra pressure on abdomen |
| | 7. Suggest periods of free time for parents | 7. Constant crying by infants produces a great deal of frustration in family members; caution against shaking infant, which can be harmful to the head and neck |
| | 8. Emphasize that colic is not a reflection on their parenting skills | 8. First-time parents may feel anxious and incompetent; nurse provides reassurance and support and builds on their strengths |

perception. The examiner shines a penlight into the eyes and notes blinking, following to midline, and other responses. Laboratory tests include a hemoglobin or hematocrit to detect anemia and a urinalysis. Screening tests for a variety of asymptomatic diseases are assuming greater importance; examples of these are the phenylketonuria (PKU) test, tuberculin test, and sickle cell test.

## IMMUNIZATION

Health personnel must repeatedly stress to parents the importance of immunizations. A crisis in immunization compliance is seen at this writing. A delay can lead to undue risks of serious illness, sometimes with fatal complications. Measles, mumps, and other preventable diseases continue to strike children in the 1990s. A new wave of infant measles is taking place. More than one-quarter of all U.S. measles victims are now under 1 year old. This was almost unheard of in the past. It is believed that vaccinated mothers who are now in their childbearing years are passing on fewer antibodies to their babies than mothers who actually caught the virus and had the disease. This means that their babies become prone to catching measles at an earlier age than their unvaccinated older siblings. In some cities, only about one-half of all 2-year-olds have been vac-

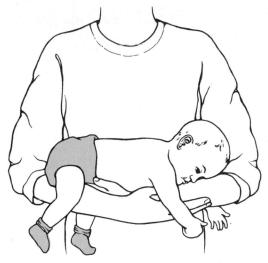

**Figure 17–2.** The colic carry.

cinated. Measles is especially hazardous in infants because of the risk of complications such as diarrhea, ear infections, pneumonia, or encephalitis.

The nurse can stress to working parents that an unprotected child may become sick, making it necessary for them to lose valuable working hours. Immunization also prevents numerous doctor and hospital expenses and is required before school entry. A delay or interruption in a series does not interfere with final immunity. It is not necessary to restart any series, regardless of the length of delay. Accurate records prevent confusion.

*Contraindications* to routine immunizations include acute febrile conditions, some chronic diseases, recent blood transfusion or injection of immune serum globulin, allergy, severe reaction following previous diphtheria, tetanus, and pertussis (DTP) vaccine, malignancy, and steroid therapy. Other stipulations are described in drug circulars. The common cold is not considered sufficient reason for delay. Any questions about these or other maladies should be brought to the attention of the physician *before* immunization. Currently recommended schedules for immunizations are found in Tables 17–2 and 17–3.

**Side Effects.** Parents should be made aware of the possible side effects of the various vaccines. They are usually mild. *The benefits of being protected greatly outweigh the risks.* The physician may recommend prophylactic use of

## Nursing Brief

The Report of the Committee on Infectious Diseases of the American Academy of Pediatrics (the *Redbook*), and the recommendations of the Advisory Committee on Immunization Practices of the Centers for Disease Control, Department of Health and Human Services (*Morbidity and Mortality Weekly Report*) are two authoritative resources that keep the nurse informed about changing immunization schedules.

acetaminophen for fever. Otherwise, no specific treatment is required. Persistent high fever along with other obvious signs of illness is *not* routine and requires further investigation. Possible side effects of DTP vaccine include a mild fever and redness and swelling at the injection site. They last only a day or two. Measles vaccine may produce fever and rash, which occur about 7–12 days following vaccination and last for only a few days. Encephalitis rarely occurs. Mumps vaccine has essentially no side effects other than occasional mild fever. Rubella vaccine may within a few days produce a rash that may last 1 or 2 days. Joint pain and swelling are sometimes seen about 2 weeks following vaccination. One must be aware of the time delay. This side effect is more common in older children. Side effects from polio vaccine are rare.

### NUTRITION COUNSELING

The nutritional needs of infants reflect rates of growth, energy expended in activity, basal metabolic needs, and interaction of nutrients consumed (Mahan & Arlin, 1992). The baby is born with a rooting reflex, which assists in finding the nipple. The suck is rather immature because of the small mouth. There is a forward and backward movement of the tongue. As the infant grows, neuromaturation of the cheeks and tongue enables advancement to a more mature sucking pattern that utilizes negative pressure to obtain milk. This change occurs about the 3rd to 4th month. About this time, the *extrusion reflex* (protrusion), which pushes food out of the mouth in order to prevent intake of inappropriate food, disappears.

I. General Information:

Name _____  Date_____

Age _____  Birth Date _____

Sex _____  Informant _____

Allergies _____  Parents' home and business
                                                                      phones _____

Reason for visit                                          Is child on any
  or admission _____    medication? _____

II. Family Profiles: Health history of:

Mother _____

Father _____

Siblings _____

Paternal grandparents _____

Maternal grandparents _____

Life change events: death; divorce; new baby; moves; illness; separation; other _____

_____

III. Infant Profile:
Newborn status: Did baby come home from hospital with you? _____

Birth defects? _____

Prenatal history: "Tell me about your pregnancy." _____

Developmental history. Age for smile _____ crawl _____ sitting _____ walking _____

speech _____ teeth _____ toilet trained _____ diapers _____ training pants_____

present motor abilities_____

| Immunizations (circle) | DTP 1 2 3 | Booster 1 2 | Measles | HBPV |
| | Polio 1 2 3 | Booster 1 2 | Mumps | |
| | T.B. skin test | | Rubella | |

**Figure 17–3.** Health assessment summary for infants and toddlers.

*Continued*

The digestive system continues to mature. By 6 months, it can handle more complex nutrients and is less susceptible to food allergens. The stomach capacity expands from 10–20 ml at birth to 200 ml by 12 months. This expansion enables the infant to consume more food at less frequent intervals.

Most babies dislike spoon feeding at first. They begin by grasping at the spoon. This response gradually progresses to the point

General Health _____ Previous illness or accident _____

_____

Temperament _____ Behavior problems? _____

How handled? _____

Level of independence _____

Sleep patterns: Crib _____ Bed _____ All night? _____

Naps _____ Security blanket or toy _____ Pacifier _____

Play: Alone _____ With others _____

Patterns of eating and drinking: Bottle _____ Breast _____

Solids _____ Formula _____ Cup _____

Amount of milk consumed daily _____ Vitamins _____

Fluorides _____ Number of stools _____ Character of stools _____

Example of typical foods consumed: Breakfast _____

Lunch _____

Supper _____

IV. Nurse's observations and comments.

General physical description _____

Review of systems _____

_____

Results of screening: Blood _____ Urine _____ DDST _____ Other _____

Individual health education and guidance: _____

Signature of examiner _____

**Figure 17-3.** *Continued*

**Table 17-2.** IMMUNIZATION SCHEDULE

| Immunization Agent | Birth | 2 mo | 4 mo | 6 mo | 15 mo | 4–6 yrs | 4–12 yrs | 14–16 yrs |
|---|---|---|---|---|---|---|---|---|
| Hepatitis B vaccine (HBV) | x | x | | x | | | | |
| Diphtheria, tetanus, pertussis (DTP) | | x | x | x | x | x | | |
| Oral polio vaccine (OPV) | | x | x | | x | x | | |
| *Haemophilus influenzae* type b (HbCV) | | | | | | | | |
| conjugate vaccine | | x | x | x | x | | | |
| Measles, mumps, rubella (MMR) | | | | | x | | x | |
| Tetanus (repeat every 10 yr) | | | | | | | | * |

*Recommended ages for vaccine usage are not absolute. Manufacturer's package insert should be consulted for specific instructions, storage, handling, dosage, and administration.

**Table 17–3.** RECOMMENDED IMMUNIZATION SCHEDULES FOR CHILDREN NOT IMMUNIZED IN THE FIRST YEAR OF LIFE

| Recommended Time/Age | Immunization(s)[a,b] | Comments |
|---|---|---|
| *Younger Than 7 Years* | | |
| First Visit | DTP, Hib, HBV, MMR, OPV | If indicated, tuberculin testing may be done at same visit. |
| | | If child if 5 yr of age or older, Hib is not indicated. |
| Interval after first visit: | | |
| 1 mo | DPT, HBV | OPV may be given if accelerated polio-myelitis vaccination is necessary, such as for travelers to areas where polio is endemic |
| 2 mo | DTP, Hib, OPV | Second dose of Hib is indicated only in children whose first dose was received when younger than 15 mo. |
| ≥8 mo | DPT or DTaP,[c] HBV, OPV | OPV is not given if the third dose was given earlier. |
| 4–6 yr (at or before school entry) | DTP or DTaP,[c] OPV | DTP or DTaP is not necessary if the fourth dose was given after the fourth birthday; OPV is not necessary if the third dose was given after the fourth birthday. |
| 11–12 yr | MMR | At entry to middle school or junior high school. |
| 10 yr later | Td | Repeat every 10 yr throughout life. |
| *7 Years and Older[d,e]* | | |
| First Visit | HBV,[f] OPV, MMR, Td | |
| Interval after first visit: | | |
| 2 mo | HBV,[f] OPV, Td | OPVV may also be given 1 mo after the first visit if accelerated poliomyelitis vaccination is necessary. |
| 8–14 mo | HBV,[f] OPV, Td | OPV is not given if the third dose was given earlier. |
| 11–12 yr | MMR | At entry to middle school or junior high. |
| 10 yr later | Td | Repeat every 10 yr throughout life. |

DTP = diphtheria, tetanus, pertussis, Hib = Haemophilus influenzae type b; HBV = hepatitis B virus; MMR = measles, mumps, rubella; OPB = oral polio vaccine; DTaP = diphtheria tetanus absorbed pediatric; Td = tetanus-diphtheria

[a]If all needed vaccines cannot be administered simultaneously, priority should be given to protecting the child against those diseases that pose the greatest immediate risk. In the US, these diseases for children younger than 2 yr usually are measles and *Haemophilus influenzae* type b infection; for children older than 6 yr, they are measles, mumps, and rubella (MMR).

[b]DTP or DTaP, HBV, Hib, MMR, and OPV can be given simultaneously at separate sites if failure of the patient to return for future immunizations is a concern.

[c]DTaP is not currently licensed for use in children younger than 15 mo of age and is not recommended for primary immunization (ie, first 3 doses) at any age.

[d]If person is 18 yr or older, routine poliovirus vaccination is not indicated in the US.

[e]Minimal interval between doses of MMR is 1 mo.

[f]Priority should be given to hepatitis B immunization of adolescents.

American Academy of Pediatrics. Modified from Peter, G. ed. *1994 Red Book: Report of the Committee on Infectious Diseases* (23rd ed., 1994). Elk Grove Village, IL: American Academy of Pediatrics, 1994: 24.

at which the child scoops a little food but spills most of the contents. As the pincer grasp becomes more developed, the baby can pick up food with tiny fingers and place it in the mouth. By 2 years, the child masters spoon feeding.

**Parental Concerns.** Parents have many concerns about feeding their infant during the 1st year of life. This is a period when readiness to receive nutritional education is usually high; therefore, the nurse looks for opportunities to provide sound information. Assessment of parental knowledge; infant development, behavior, and readiness; parent-child interaction; and cultural and ethnic practices is important. Nutritional care plans based on developmental levels assist parents in recognizing changes in feeding patterns. The components of a nutritional assessment are discussed in Chapter 16 (p. 403).

Mott suggests the following parental guide to determining adequacy of diet: the infant has gained 4–7 oz/wk for the first 6 months, has at least six wet diapers per day, and sleeps peacefully for several hours following feedings (Mott, James, & Sperhac, 1990). Monitoring of weight, height, head circumference, and skin-fold thickness determines if the diet is adequate; therefore, the value of periodic well-baby examinations is stressed. The nurse reassures parents that most children eat enough to grow normally, although intake is seldom constant and varies in quantity and quality. Forced feedings are not appropriate.

**Breast and Bottle Feeding.** Infants, in proportion to their weight, require more calories, pro-

tein, minerals, and vitamins than do adults. Their fluid requirements are also high. Human milk is the best food for infants under 6 months of age. It contains the ideal balance of nutrients in a readily digestible form. Breast feeding soon after birth helps promote bonding and stimulates milk production. It protects the infant from certain bacteria, and allergic reactions are minimal. In addition, it is a safeguard against overfeeding.

Nutritious infant formulas are also available. Many pediatricians recommend iron-fortified ones. A baby who cannot tolerate milk-based formulas may be placed on a soy-based formula. These formulas are nutritionally sound. Whole cow's milk is not recommended for infants, as the tough, hard curd is difficult to digest. This type of milk may also contribute to iron-defi-

**Table 17–4.** INFANT FEEDING BEHAVIORS BY AGE

| Age | Hunger Behavior | Feeding Behavior | Satiety Behavior |
|---|---|---|---|
| Birth to 13 wk (0–3 mo) | Cries; hands fisted; body tense | Rooting reflex; medial lip closure; strong suck reflex; suck-swallow pattern; tongue thrust and retraction; palmomental reflex; gags easily; needs burping | Withdraws head from nipple; falls asleep; hands relaxed; relief of body tension |
| 14–24 wk (4–6 mo) | Eagerly anticipates; grasps and draws bottle to mouth; reaches with open mouth | Aware of hands; generalized reaching; intentional hand-to-mouth movements; tongue elevation; lips purse at corners (pucker); shifts food in mouth (prechewing); tongue protrudes in anticipation of nipple; tongue holds nipple firm; tongue projection strong; suck strength increases; coughs and chokes easily; preference for tastes | Tosses head back; fusses or cries; covers mouth with hands; ejects food; distracted by surroundings |
| 28–36 wk (7–9 mo) | Reacts to food preparation sounds; vocalizes hunger; reaches out | Biting (first teeth); turns palm toward face; draws lower lip with food; thumb-finger grasp and palmar grasp; increased dexterity of hands; lateral tongue movement; mature swallow; chewing begins—vertical jaw protrusion; sucking decreases; holds bottle; handles cup awkwardly | Changes posture; closes mouth; shakes head "no"; plays with and throws utensils |
| 40–52 wk (10–12 mo) | Vocalizes; grasps utensils | Tongue licks food from lower lip; holds and transfers to mouth; drinks from cup with spillage; lateral chewing movement; sticks out tongue; demands to feed self | Shakes head "no"; sputters |

From Mott, S., James, S.R., & Sperhac, A.M. (1991). *Nursing care of children and families* (2nd ed.). Reading, MA: Addison-Wesley. Copyright © 1990 by Addison-Wesley Nursing, a division of The Benjamin/Cummings Publishing Company. Reprinted by permission.

**Table 17–5.** FEEDING, NUTRITION, AND GROWTH IN INFANCY

| Age | Feeding Behaviors | Parental Concerns | Recommended Nutrition | Growth Rate |
|---|---|---|---|---|
| 0–3 mo | Reflexes<br>Rooting<br>Sucking<br>Extrusion | Adequacy of intake<br>Discomfort with breast feeding | 115–130 cal/kg/day<br>Breast milk with 400 IU vitamin D and 0.25 mg fluoride or iron-fortified formula | Weight = 30 gm/day (1 oz/day)<br>Length = 3.5 cm/mo<br>Head circumference = 2 cm/mo |
| 4–6 mo | Reflexes<br>Extrusion and rooting gone<br>Skills<br>Sucking<br>Chewing | Introduction of solids | 100–110 cal/kg/day<br>Breast milk with 400 IU vitamin D and 0.25 mg fluoride or iron-fortified formula | Weight = 20 gm/day (⅔ oz/day)<br>Length = 2 cm/mo<br>Head circumference = 1 cm/mo |
| 6–12 mo | Skills<br>Sucking<br>Chewing<br>Cup drinking (with help)<br>Finger feeding | Messiness<br>Control over feeding | 100–110 cal/kg/day<br>Solids 50% of total calories<br>Limit formula intake to 30 oz/day | Weight = 15 gm/day (½ oz/day)<br>Length = 1.5 cm/mo<br>Head circumference = 0.5 cm/mo |
| 12–24 mo | Skills<br>Spoon<br>Cup drinking<br>Fork | Messiness<br>Selective tastes<br>Decreased appetite | 90–100 cal/kg/day<br>Limit milk to 24 oz/day<br>No foods that can be aspirated | Weight = 220 gm/mo (7 oz/mo)<br>Length = 1 cm/mo<br>Head circumference = 0.27 cm/mo (12–18 mo)<br>Head circumference = 0.15 cm/mo (18–24 mo) |

From Levine, M.D., Carey, W.B., Crocker, A.C., & Gross, R. (1983). *Developmental-behavioral pediatrics*. Philadelphia: W.B. Saunders.

ciency anemia by increasing gastrointestinal blood loss. Formula preparation is discussed on pp. 242–244.

It is suggested that infants remain on human milk or iron-fortified formula for the 1st year of life. Parents are sometimes unsure of when their baby has had enough formula. It is important to explain satiety behavior at the various ages, as depicted in Table 17–4. Coaxing babies to finish the last drop in a bottle is unnecessary.

Table 17–5 describes feeding behaviors, nutrition, and growth rates for different ages throughout infancy. Figure 17–4 illustrates how feeding skills develop in infants and toddlers, and Figure 17–5 shows the effect of the various nutrients on the body systems.

**Addition of Solid Foods.** Parents often wonder when to begin adding solid foods. In the past, recommendations for introduction of solids have varied from 3 days to 4 months. More recently the addition of solid food at about 6 months is recommended. There are a number of commercially prepared brands of baby foods. Parents should be instructed to read the labels on the jars to obtain nutrition informa-

tion. Home-prepared foods may also be utilized.

The sequence in which foods are added is suggested in Figure 17–6. Between 4 and 6 months, sucking becomes more mature, and munching (up-and-down chopping motions) commences. Rice cereal is often recommended as the first solid food because it is less allergenic than others. Three level tablespoonfuls of iron-fortified cereal mixed with liquid provides 7 mg of iron (over half the daily requirement).

Only small amounts are offered at first (1 teaspoonful). Food is placed on the back of the tongue. Cereal may be diluted with formula, water, or juice (if juice has already been introduced). The consistency is thickened and amounts of solid foods are gradually increased as the infant becomes more familiar with them. A spoon with a small bowl and a long, straight handle is suggested. Single-ingredient foods are introduced (green beans rather than mixed vegetables), as it is easier to determine food allergies this way. Only one new food is offered in a 4-day to 1-week period to determine tolerance.

If the baby refuses a certain food, it is temporarily omitted. Mealtime is kept pleasant. The baby is allowed to try new foods, even the

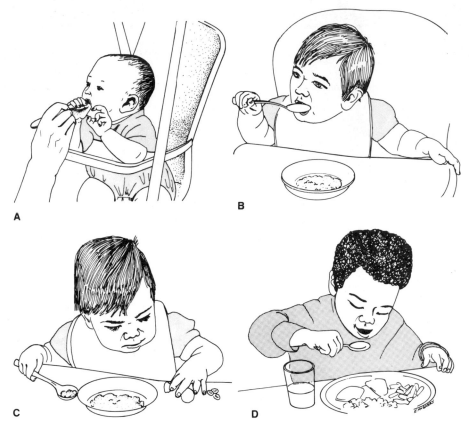

**Figure 17–4.** Development of feeding skills in infants and toddlers. *A,* At 7 months, this child begins to reach for the spoon. *B,* At 9 months, this little girl begins to use her spoon independently, although she is not yet able to keep food on it. *C,* The 9-month-old shows a refined pincer grasp to pick up food. *D,* The 2-year-old is much more skillful at self-feeding, with the ability to both rotate the wrist and elevate the elbow to keep food off the spoon. (Modified from Mahan, L.K., & Arlin, M.T. [1992]. *Krause's food, nutrition & diet therapy* [8th ed.]. Philadelphia: W.B. Saunders, p. 190.)

ones that parents dislike. New foods are not introduced when the baby is ill. The amount of food consumed varies with the child. Fruit juices are generally offered at about 5–6 months of age, when the infant begins to drink from a cup. An exception is the addition of orange juice, which is withheld until the baby is 1 year old, especially when family members have known allergies. Other highly allergenic foods that may be delayed include fish, nuts, strawberries, chocolate, and egg whites.

A spouted plastic cup is helpful at first. The juice is initially diluted. Then the quantity is gradually increased to 3–4 oz/day. The directions for preparing baby food at home are listed in Box 17–1. Baby food can be prepared in a food grinder, electric blender, or food mill or by mashing the food to the desired texture.

The infant's height and weight should increase at approximately the same rate. Variations may be due to illness, improperly prepared formulas (particularly formulas made from powdered concentrates), and other factors. It is important for caregivers to ascertain feeding procedures and practices regularly and to repeat essential information as indicated.

**Buying, Storing, and Serving Foods.** Baby foods stored in jars are vacuum-packed. Parents are taught to check safety seals before purchase. (Directions are generally indicated on the jar, e.g., to reject product if safety button is up.) The expiration date of the product should be checked. Dates are usually found on the caps of jars and on the sides of cereal and bakery items. Unopened jars of baby food and juices are stored in a dry, cool place. Jars are rotated, and those on hand the longest are used first. Baby cereals are kept away from

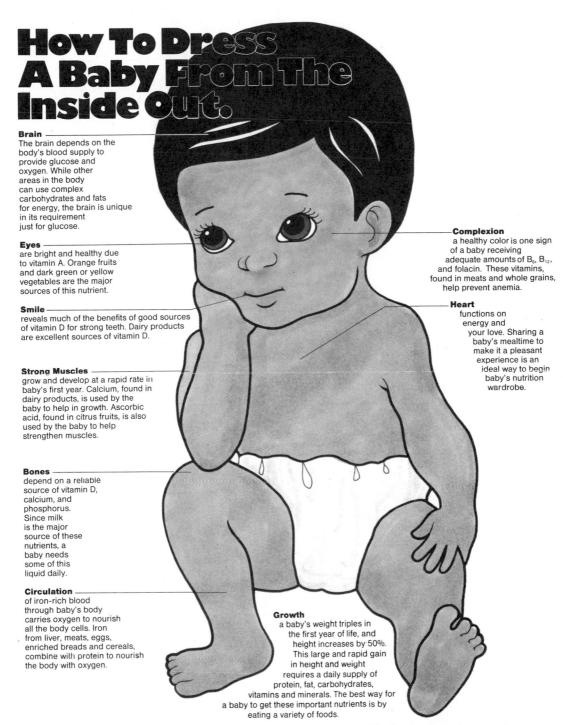

# How To Dress A Baby From The Inside Out.

**Brain**
The brain depends on the body's blood supply to provide glucose and oxygen. While other areas in the body can use complex carbohydrates and fats for energy, the brain is unique in its requirement just for glucose.

**Eyes**
are bright and healthy due to vitamin A. Orange fruits and dark green or yellow vegetables are the major sources of this nutrient.

**Smile**
reveals much of the benefits of good sources of vitamin D for strong teeth. Dairy products are excellent sources of vitamin D.

**Strong Muscles**
grow and develop at a rapid rate in baby's first year. Calcium, found in dairy products, is used by the baby to help in growth. Ascorbic acid, found in citrus fruits, is also used by the baby to help strengthen muscles.

**Bones**
depend on a reliable source of vitamin D, calcium, and phosphorus. Since milk is the major source of these nutrients, a baby needs some of this liquid daily.

**Circulation**
of iron-rich blood through baby's body carries oxygen to nourish all the body cells. Iron from liver, meats, eggs, enriched breads and cereals, combine with protein to nourish the body with oxygen.

**Complexion**
a healthy color is one sign of a baby receiving adequate amounts of $B_6$, $B_{12}$, and folacin. These vitamins, found in meats and whole grains, help prevent anemia.

**Heart**
functions on energy and your love. Sharing a baby's mealtime to make it a pleasant experience is an ideal way to begin baby's nutrition wardrobe.

**Growth**
a baby's weight triples in the first year of life, and height increases by 50%. This large and rapid gain in height and weight requires a daily supply of protein, fat, carbohydrates, vitamins and minerals. The best way for a baby to get these important nutrients is by eating a variety of foods.

**Figure 17–5.** A baby dresses from the inside out. (Courtesy of Gerber Products Company.)

Dietary guidelines handout for parents

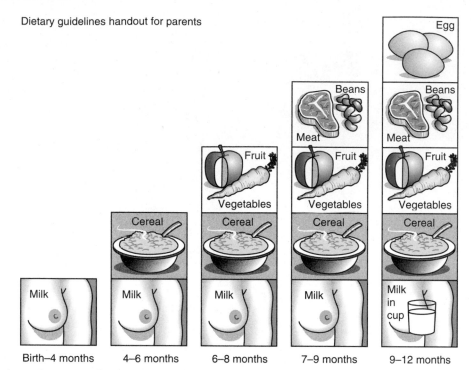

**Figure 17–6.** Approximate ages for introduction of various solid foods. Preparation, consistency, and amount depend on the infant's age and dental development. Note the progressive decrease in reliance on breast milk or formula. (Modified from Kelts, D., & Jones, E. [1985]. *Manual of pediatric nutrition* (p. 101). Boston: Little, Brown.)

## Nursing Brief

Human milk and properly prepared formula supply adequate water for the infant under normal conditions. During illness or hot, humid weather, the infant may require additional water.

other grain products, which may be insect infested.

When a jar is opened, a definite "pop" is heard as the vacuum seal is broken. Food is transferred to a serving dish. One should not feed out of the jar or return leftovers to the jar because saliva may turn certain foods to liquid by digesting them in the jar. Unused portions may be stored in the refrigerator in the original jar. Special precautions are taken when food is heated in the microwave, as sometimes food heats unevenly. All warmed foods are tested. This can be done by tasting or by dropping a portion of a warmed liquid on the hand. Box

17–2 lists a number of concerns parents have about feeding their infants.

### TEETHING

Teething refers to the process in which the crown of the tooth erupts through the periodontal membrane. The gums may be red, swollen, and sensitive. The normal appearance of saliva and drooling at 4 months is frequently attributed to, but rarely due to, teething. The first tooth appears about the 7th month (see p. 406 for a diagram of tooth eruption). The first (deciduous) teeth act as a guide for the proper positioning of the secondary (permanent) teeth.

Teething does not cause infection. However, at this time infants' maternal antibody supplies are low, and infants are more prone to infection. They may be fussy and may wake during the night. Teething is not responsible for respiratory tract infections, rashes, or diarrhea. Cold appears to soothe inflamed gums. A cold wash cloth, a hard-rubber teething ring, or a teething

| BOX 17–1 | Directions for Home Preparation of Infant Foods |
|---|---|

1. Select fresh, high-quality fruits, vegetables, or meats.
2. Be sure all utensils, including cutting boards, grinder, and knives, are thoroughly clean.
3. Wash hands before preparing the food.
4. Clean, wash, and trim the food in as little water as possible.
5. Cook the foods until tender in as little water as possible. Avoid overcooking, which may destroy heat-sensitive nutrients.
6. Do not add salt. Add sugar sparingly. Do not add honey to food for infants less than 1 yr of age.*
7. Add enough water so that the food has a consistency that is easily pureed.
8. Strain or puree the food using an electric blender, food mill, baby food grinder, or kitchen strainer.
9. Pour puree into ice cube tray and freeze.
10. When food is frozen hard, remove the cubes and store in freezer bags.
11. Unfreeze and heat in serving container the amount of food that will be consumed at a single feeding (in water bath or microwave oven).

*Botulism spores have been reported in honey, and young infants do not have the immune capacity to resist this infection.
From Mahan, L.K., & Arlin, M.T. (1992). *Krause's food, nutrition & diet therapy* (8th ed.). Philadelphia: W.B. Saunders.

| BOX 17–2 | Infant Feeding Concerns of Parents |
|---|---|

**Anticipate questions related to**

Demand versus scheduled feedings
How and when to supplement breast feedings
Storing breast milk
Water consumption
Variability in appetite and feeding patterns
Fussiness as a sign of hunger
Spoiling the infant
Sleeping through feedings
Vitamin and fluoride supplements
Introduction of baby foods
Home-prepared foods
Refusal of new foods
Adequacy of feedings
Number of stools
Regurgitation
Teething
Weaning
Colic
Recommended reading

pretzel may bring relief. Acetaminophen is useful when discomfort is clearly related to teeth.

Good oral hygiene during infancy consists of offering water after food and gently wiping the teeth with gauze. Calcium, phosphorus, vitamins C and D, and fluoride help ensure healthy teeth. Bottle-mouth caries are to be avoided (see p. 407). Nursing caries are also being reported in breast-fed babies, particularly in infants who sleep with their mothers and nurse at will throughout the night. To prevent this condition, nocturnal nursing should be discouraged, as should frequent intermittent night feedings after the age of 1 year.

An additional cause of erosion of dental enamel is repeated exposure to gastric acids. This is now being recognized in infants with gastroesophageal reflux who are old enough to have teeth and in teenagers with bulimia. When the effects of gastric acid are recognized early, the teeth can be protected with an acrylic sealant. Parents are taught the cavity-producing (cariogenic) effects of refined sugars, particularly those that are sticky and remain in the mouth for longer periods of time.

## KEY POINTS

- Each infant grows and develops at an individual rate.
- Although growth is continuous, there are periods of slow and rapid growth.
- During infancy all major body systems progressively mature, and there is a corresponding development of fine and gross motor skills.

- The most common cause of concern is a slowing, not typical for age, of any aspect of development.
- A development of a sense of trust begins in infancy and is vital to a healthy personality.
- Breast milk or formula is the most desirable food for the first 6 months of the baby's life, followed by gradual introduction of a variety of solid foods.
- Sensory stimulation is essential for development of the infant's thought processes and perceptual abilities.
- Health maintenance visits are essential during the 1st year to detect variations from normal growth patterns, to provide immunizations, and to educate and support parents.
- The nurse must stress to parents the value of immunizations for infants and children.
- Human milk and properly prepared formula supply adequate water for the infant under normal conditions. During illness or very hot, humid weather, the infant may require additional water.

# Study Questions

1. Why must the pediatric nurse be able to recognize the various stages of growth and development in the infant?
2. Of what value is sucking to the baby?
3. Mrs. Jones tells you that she always props baby Sue's bottle because it saves her so much time. What would you reply?
4. What is the value of attending to the needs of an infant promptly and cheerfully during the 1st year?
5. Mrs. Piper has been bringing Charlene, who is 4 months old, to the well-child clinic since she was 1 month old. What services are provided by a well-child clinic?
6. How does the infant's environment affect physical growth and development? Mental health?
7. What is the primary focus of health maintenance during infancy?
8. List the immunizations given during the 1st year of life and the diseases they prevent.
9. Tommy is 9 months old. Prepare a day's menu for him.
10. Joel is 10 months old. You are giving him green beans for the first time. How would you introduce it to him? List four factors to keep in mind for adding solid foods to a baby's diet.
11. Discuss the needs of the newborn. How do these needs change during the 1st year?
12. Observe a 3-month-old infant on the children's unit. How do physical growth and development compare with those of the healthy 3-month-old infant?
13. Jean, 7 months old, shows a fear of strangers. Discuss various ways in which to handle this problem in the home and in the hospital.

# Multiple Choice
# Review Questions

*Choose the most appropriate answer.*

1. The startle reflex is also known as the
   a. Moro reflex
   b. rooting reflex
   c. pincer reflex
   d. grasp reflex

2. The first diphtheria, tetanus, and pertussis (DTP) vaccine is given at
   a. 6 months
   b. 1 year
   c. 2 months
   d. 4 weeks

3. In order to avoid allergies when feeding new foods,
   a. introduce single-ingredient foods
   b. mix the food with one the infant likes
   c. mix the food with formula
   d. offer two new foods at a time

4. The first tooth appears at about
   a. 2 months
   b. 7 months
   c. 9 months
   d. 12 months

5. The infant can sit alone momentarily about the age of
   a. 4 months
   b. 6 months
   c. 12 months
   d. 15 months

## BIBLIOGRAPHY

American Academy of Pediatrics. (1994). *Report of the Committee of Infectious Disease* (23rd ed.). Elk Grove Village, IL: Author.

American Academy of Pediatrics. (1989). *Measles: Reassessment of the current immunization policy.* Elk Grove Village, IL: Author.

Levine, M.D., Carey, W.B., & Crocker, A.C. (1992). *Developmental-behavioral pediatrics* (2nd ed.). Philadelphia: W.B. Saunders.

Mahan, L.K., & Arlin, M.T. (1992). *Krause's food, nutrition & diet therapy* (8th ed.). Philadelphia: W.B. Saunders.

Mott, S., James, S.R., & Sperhac, A.M. (1990). *Nursing care of children and families* (2nd ed.). Reading, MA: Addison-Wesley.

Phillips, C. (1991). Keeping up with the changing immunization schedule. *Contemporary Pediatrics, 8,* 20–44.

Pillitteri, A. (1992). *Maternal and child health nursing.* Philadelphia: J.B. Lippincott.

Poleman, C.M., & Peckenpaugh, N.J. (1991). *Nutrition essentials and diet therapy* (6th ed.). Philadelphia: W.B. Saunders.

Thompson, E.D., & Ashwill, J.W. (1992). *Pediatric nursing: An introductory text* (6th ed.). Philadelphia: W.B. Saunders.

Whaley, L., & Wong, D. (1991). *Nursing care of infants and children* (4th ed.). St. Louis: C.V. Mosby.

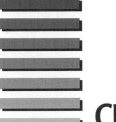

# Chapter 18

# The Toddler

General Characteristics
Guidance
Speech Development
Daily Care
Nutrition Counseling
Dental Health
Toilet Independence
Play
Day Care
Accident Prevention
    Consumer Education
    Toy Safety
    Epidemiologic Framework
    Cardiopulmonary Resuscitation
    Emergency Treatment for Choking

# OBJECTIVES

*On completion and mastery of Chapter 18, the student will be able to*

- Define each vocabulary term listed.
- Describe the physical and psychosocial development of children from 1 to 3 years of age, listing age-specific events and guidance when appropriate.
- List two developmental tasks of the toddler period.
- Describe the Denver II and its uses.
- Discuss speech development in the toddler.
- Discuss how adults can assist small children in combating their fears.
- Identify the principles of toilet training (bowel and bladder) that will assist in guiding parents' efforts to provide toilet independence.
- Describe two aspects of dental health pertinent to the toddler period.
- List two methods of preventing the following: automobile accidents, burns, falls, suffocation and choking, poisoning, drowning, electric shock, and animal bites.
- Describe the Heimlich technique for relief of choking.

## General Characteristics

Children between the ages of 1 and 3 years are referred to as toddlers. They are able to get about by using their own powers and are no longer completely dependent persons. By this time, they have generally tripled their birth weights and gained control of head, hands, and feet. The remarkably rapid growth and development that took place during infancy begins to slow down. The toddler period presents different challenges for the parents and the child. This chapter discusses what toddlers are like as persons and how adults can help them overcome some of the obstacles they must face. Table 18–1 summarizes the toddler's physical development, social behavior, and care at various ages.

Toddlers are curious explorers who get into everything. They gain more control of their bodies as each month passes. Soon they are walking, running, jumping, and climbing. They enjoy repeating these new skills, and with practice they become less clumsy and awkward. Their desire to touch, taste, smell, and smear leads them into difficulties. They quickly discover that much of their conduct is alarming to their parents. Parents no longer accept their actions willingly and without question, as they did when they were infants. Because they cannot understand the need for restrictions, they revolt. Temper tantrums are common and behavior is not consistent. They are negative and unreasonable and say "no" frequently. Ritualism is a characteristic of the toddlers. By making rituals of simple tasks, they increase their sense of security and mastery. Dawdling serves essentially the same purpose. *Egocentric thinking*, in which children refer everything to themselves, predominates.

**Increasing Independence.** The developmental tasks seen during this period are based on a continuum of trust established during infancy. Toddlers are now ready to give up total dependence. They begin to differentiate themselves from others, particularly from mother. They can tolerate brief periods of separation. They learn to delay gratification and to incorporate rudiments of socially acceptable behavior as determined by the limits of their family's culture.

Important self-regulatory functions include toilet independence, eating, sleeping, and perfection of newfound physical skills. The gradual control of these activities provides toddlers with a sense of mastery and contributes to their positive self-concept. According to Erik Erikson, the major task of this period is for the child to acquire a sense of autonomy (self-control) while overcoming shame and doubt.

**Physical Development.** Certain physical changes foster this process. The toddler's body changes proportions (Fig. 18–1). The legs and arms lengthen through ossification and growth in the epiphyseal areas of the long bones. The trunk and head grow more slowly. The rate of brain growth decelerates. The increase in head circumference during infancy is 10 cm (4 inches). During the 2nd year it is only 2.5 cm (1 inch). Chest circumference continues to increase. The size and strength of muscle fibers increase.

Myelination of the spinal cord is practically complete by 2 years, allowing for control of anal and urethral sphincters. Respirations are still mainly abdominal but shift to thoracic as the child approaches school age. The toddler is more capable of maintaining a stable body temperature than is the infant. The shivering process, in which the capillaries constrict or dilate in response to body temperature, has matured.

**Table 18–1.** PHYSICAL DEVELOPMENT, SOCIAL BEHAVIOR, AND CARE AND GUIDANCE OF TODDLERS

| Physical Development | Social Behavior | Care and Guidance |
|---|---|---|
| *1½ yr*<br>Abdomen protrudes<br>Climbs stairs and on furniture<br>Anterior fontanel closes<br>Trunk is long, legs short and bowed<br>Builds a tower of three blocks<br>Takes off shoes and socks<br>Runs clumsily<br>Has sphincter control<br>Turns pages of books | Gets into everything<br>Speaks about 10 words<br>Has rapid shifts of attention<br>Temper tantrums may occur<br>Has egocentric behavior<br>Is aware of ownership<br>Points to common objects when named by adult | *Sleep:* may stay awake in crib after being put to bed<br>*Eating habits:* drinks well from cup; holds and fills spoon, spills contents; likes to play with food<br>*Immunization:* 15 months—Haemophilus b polysaccharide vaccine (HbCV), measles, mumps, rubella (MMR); 15–18 mo—diphtheria, tetanus, pertussis (DTP), oral polio vaccine (OPV)<br>*General:* may begin to signal for potty |

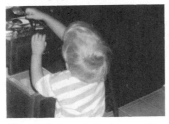

*The toddler's curiosity is unending.*

| | | |
|---|---|---|
| | Talks in short sentences<br>Dawdles<br>Enjoys stories and music<br>Imitative play<br>Has trouble sharing<br>Attention span is increased | If temper tantrum occurs, remove child from focus of attention; keep comments brief; divert child's attention<br>Avoid punishment and giving too much attention<br>Incorporate repetition into routines<br>Identify and repeat names of items and encourage speech |
| *2 yr*<br>Weight 26–28 lb<br>Height about 33 in<br>Pulse 90–120 beats/min<br>Respirations 20–35 breaths/min<br>16 baby teeth<br>Head circumference 49–50 cm (19.6–20 in)<br>Builds a tower of six cubes<br>Runs with a steady gait<br>Visual acuity 20/40 | Is balky—cannot make decisions<br>Is more fearful than before<br>Stuttering is common<br>Speech resembles a monologue<br>Knows first and last names | *Sleep:* has a nighttime ritual; tries to postpone bedtime; may climb out of crib<br>*Eating habits:* feeds self quite well; appetite fluctuates<br>*Exercise:* enjoys outdoor play; needs fenced-in area or constant supervision<br>*General:* setting limits on behavior increases sense of security; praise obedience<br>Encourage self-help in dressing |

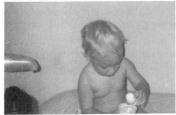

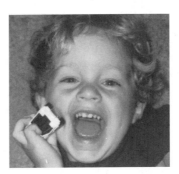

*The 2½-year-old has all of the deciduous teeth.*

*Although 2-year-olds can sit steadily in the tub, parents need to be reminded that it is still not safe to leave them unsupervised. They may slip or turn on hot water and scald themselves.*

*Sleep:* may awaken during night; needs reassurance
*Eating habits:* dawdles at table; easily distracted
*Exercise:* plays actively
Becomes overtired if left to own impulses

*2½ yr*
Has all deciduous teeth
Throws a ball
Builds a tower of eight cubes
Jumps and prances about
May be toilet trained
Walks on tiptoes
Walks up and down stairs, one step at a time
Can jump in place

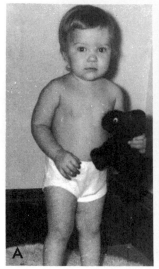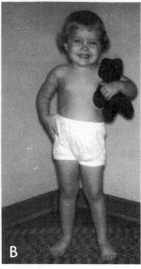

**Figure 18–1.** Compare the growth and development of the child of 20 months (*A*), and the child of 2½ years (*B*).

Developmental screening is a vital component of child health assessment. One widely used tool is the Denver II, a revision of the Denver Developmental Screening Test. This tool assesses the developmental status of children during the first 6 years of life in four categories: personal-social, fine motor–adaptive, language, and gross motor. It is not an intelligence test. Its purpose is to identify children who are unable to perform at a level comparable to their agemates. Failure merely indicates a need for further evaluation. It is designed for use by both professionals and paraprofessionals. Proper administration and interpretation are paramount. Specific instructions for execution and scoring of the results are included in test materials available for purchase from the publisher (Fig. 18–2).

## Guidance

As toddlers struggle for mastery and control of their actions, periods of varying conflict occur. The temperament of children and the temperaments of their caretakers are important factors in these encounters. Cultural and sociologic traditions of raising children also play a role. Some behaviors result from the child's frustration in trying to master a task. Toddlers also show *ambivalence*. They love mother one minute and hate her the next. They cry, kick, and slap when they have decided to play longer outdoors and then turn around and kiss mother for giving them a drink of water. There is no perfect method of managing these behavioral inconsistencies. Ignoring the behavior and distracting the toddler are helpful. At times the child may need to be held until composure is regained.

One of the objectives in the management of toddlers is to help them develop self-control and find socially acceptable outlets for their behavior (Figs. 18–3 and 18–4). Parents who direct all their child's activities cannot expect them to develop confidence in their own abilities. Many activities that are fun, such as writing on the walls, are not acceptable. On the other hand, finger painting in nursery school is just as enjoyable and appropriate.

Toddlers need a certain amount of discipline (guidance). The goal of discipline is not to punish but to teach. The child who is well disciplined is not one who is submissive but rather

The skin becomes tough as the epidermis and dermis bond more tightly, protecting the child from fluid loss, infection, and irritation. The defense mechanisms of the skin and blood, particularly phagocytosis, are working more effectively than they were in infancy. The lymphatic tissues of the adenoids and tonsils enlarge during this period. Eruption of deciduous teeth continues until completion at about 2½ years.

**Sensorimotor and Language Development.** The senses of the toddler do not function independently of one another or of motor abilities. Two-year-old toddlers reach, grasp, inspect, smell, taste, and study objects with their eyes. Their attention becomes centered on characteristics of their surroundings that capture their interest. They can correlate sight with sound, as in the ringing of a bell. Binocular vision is well established by the age of 15 months. By 2 years, visual acuity is about 20/40.

Memory strengthens; toddlers can compare present events with stored knowledge. They assimilate information through trial and error plus repetition. They try alternative methods of accomplishing a goal. Thought processes advance, preparing the way for more complex mental operations. Language development parallels cognitive growth. The increase in the level of comprehension is particularly striking and exceeds verbalization. By 3 years, the child has a rather extensive vocabulary of about 900 words. Speech is more than 90% intelligible.

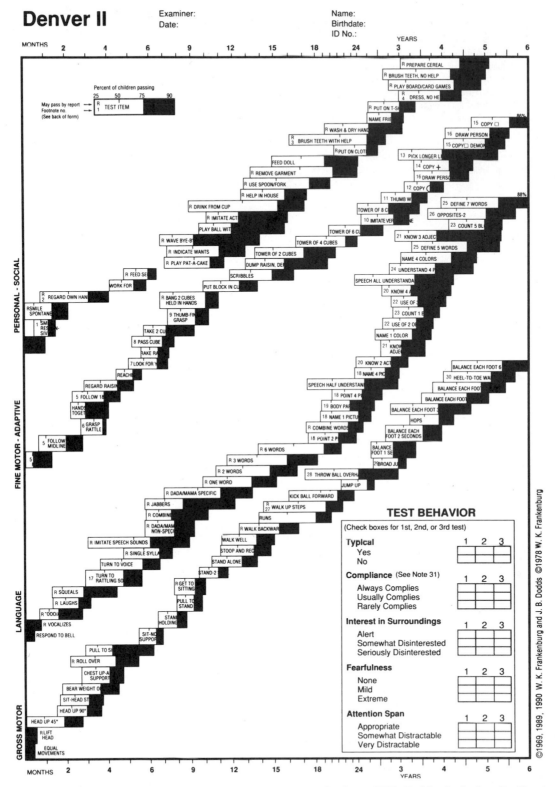

**Figure 18–2.** Denver Developmental Screening Test—II. (From Frankenburg, W.K., Dodds, J., Archer, P., Shapiro, H., & Bresnick, B. (1992). The Denver II: A major revision and restandardization of the Denver Developmental Screening Test. *Pediatrics, 89,* 91.)

*Continued*

# DIRECTIONS FOR ADMINISTRATION

1. Try to get child to smile by smiling, talking or waving.  Do not touch him/her.
2. Child must stare at hand several seconds.
3. Parent may help guide toothbrush and put toothpaste on brush.
4. Child does not have to be able to tie shoes or button/zip in the back.
5. Move yarn slowly in an arc from one side to the other, about 8" above child's face.
6. Pass if child grasps rattle when it is touched to the backs or tips of fingers.
7. Pass if child tries to see where yarn went.  Yarn should be dropped quickly from sight from tester's hand without arm movement.
8. Child must transfer cube from hand to hand without help of body, mouth, or table.
9. Pass if child picks up raisin with any part of thumb and finger.
10. Line can vary only 30 degrees or less from tester's line. |/
11. Make a fist with thumb pointing upward and wiggle only the thumb.  Pass if child imitates and does not move any fingers other than the thumb.

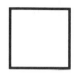

12. Pass any enclosed form.  Fail continuous round motions.

13. Which line is longer? (Not bigger.)  Turn paper upside down and repeat. (pass 3 of 3 or 5 of 6)

14. Pass any lines crossing near midpoint.

15. Have child copy first.  If failed, demonstrate.

When giving items 12, 14, and 15, do not name the forms.  Do not demonstrate 12 and 14.

16. When scoring, each pair (2 arms, 2 legs, etc.) counts as one part.
17. Place one cube in cup and shake gently near child's ear, but out of sight.  Repeat for other ear.
18. Point to picture and have child name it.  (No credit is given for sounds only.)
    If less than 4 pictures are named correctly, have child point to picture as each is named by tester.

 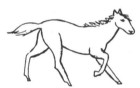 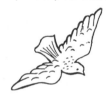 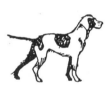 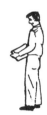

19. Using doll, tell child:  Show me the nose, eyes, ears, mouth, hands, feet, tummy, hair.  Pass 6 of 8.
20. Using pictures, ask child: Which one flies?... says meow?... talks?... barks?... gallops? Pass 2 of 5, 4 of 5.
21. Ask child: What do you do when you are cold?... tired?... hungry?   Pass 2 of 3, 3 of 3.
22. Ask child:  What do you do with a cup?  What is a chair used for?  What is a pencil used for?
    Action words must be included in answers.
23. Pass if child correctly places <u>and</u> says how many blocks are on paper. (1, 5).
24. Tell child: Put block **on** table; **under** table; **in front of** me, **behind** me.  Pass 4 of 4.
    (Do not help child by pointing, moving head or eyes.)
25. Ask child: What is a ball?... lake?... desk?... house?... banana?... curtain?... fence?... ceiling?  Pass if defined in terms of use, shape, what it is made of, or general category (such as banana is fruit, not just yellow).  Pass 5 of 8, 7 of 8.
26. Ask child: If a horse is big, a mouse is __?  If fire is hot, ice is __?  If the sun shines during the day, the moon shines during the __? Pass 2 of 3.
27. Child may use wall or rail only, not person.  May not crawl.
28. Child must throw ball overhand 3 feet to within arm's reach of tester.
29. Child must perform standing broad jump over width of test sheet (8 1/2 inches).
30. Tell child to walk forward, ⚭⚭⚭⚭➡ heel within 1 inch of toe.  Tester may demonstrate.
    Child must walk 4 consecutive steps.
31. In the second year, half of normal children are non-compliant.

**OBSERVATIONS:**

**Figure 18–2.** *Continued*

one who exhibits self-control and positive self-esteem (Levine, Carey, & Crocker, 1992). Expectations need to be commensurate with the child's physical and cognitive abilities. Toddlers get into many situations over their heads. When adults make firm decisions, the problem is resolved, at least for the time being. The child feels secure. An occasional light spanking on the seat of the pants may be helpful, although this debate continues. If, however, parents are constantly punishing a child, further exploration is necessary.

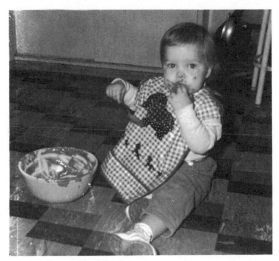

**Figure 18-3.** Adults need to help the toddler find socially acceptable outlets for behavior.

Breaking a child's will must *not* become the focus. In general, successful limit setting includes consistency and selectivity. Battles need to be chosen carefully and issues that are not important overlooked. Frequent renegotiation

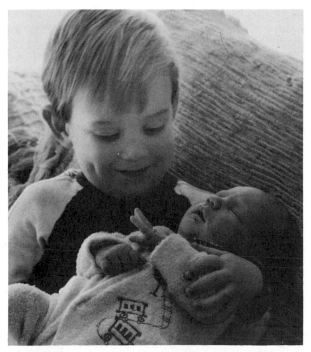

**Figure 18-4.** Note the pride on this toddler's face as he holds his new sister.

is necessary as the child's level of development changes. Limit setting should include praise for desired behavior as well as disapproval for undesired behavior. A 5-minute time-out period in a safe place helps the child to develop self-regulation. Timing should not begin until the child has settled down. The child is praised once calm.

Children, like adults, seek approval. It is effective and helps to increase their self-confidence. The positive approach should be taken as often as possible. One assumes that the toddler is going to be good rather than bad. "Thank you, Johnny, for giving me the matches" will make them arrive in your hand more quickly than "Give me those matches right now," said in a threatening tone.

Fear is a valuable emotion to the child if it does not become too intense. Unfortunately, most children fear many situations that are not in themselves dangerous, and this sometimes deprives them of activities that otherwise would be enjoyable. The physical and mental health of the child at the time of a fear-provoking experience affects the extent of the reaction. Also, if the child is alone, fear may be greater than if someone such as mother or nurse is present. Once a fear has been learned, it is more difficult to eliminate. Favorite possessions and repetitive rituals are *self-consoling behaviors* for the toddler, particularly at bedtime and during separation from parents.

Stress increases fear of separation. Adults should attempt to control their own fears in the presence of young children. Respect and understanding should always be accorded to children who are afraid. Making fun of the fear or shaming the child in front of others is detrimental.

Communicating love and respect to the child can be done as follows:

1. Label the act, not the child. Use "I" messages to relate your thoughts or feelings about the impact of the child's behavior. Example: "I feel frustrated when I can't hear the television because there is so much noise" versus "You are so loud." ("You" messages assign blame and convey criticism; they are a verbal attack.)
2. Do not label the child as "bad," "stupid," or "stubborn." This is demoralizing and suggests a permanent condition with no room for improvement.
3. Provide individual time for child, and give your undivided attention—if only briefly.

## Nursing Brief

Caregivers need to provide safe areas for the toddler to explore. They need to watch carefully before saying "no."

Purposeful conversation suggests that you are trying to understand what the other is feeling and means. Keep exchanges friendly as often as you can.

4. Keep feedback specific, and avoid generalizations such as, "You *never* pick up your toys when I ask." This suggests that the undesirable behavior is a character trait. An "I" message such as "I feel angry when your toys are all over the floor and I cannot vacuum" is more specific. It role models expression of feelings, and is not an attack.
5. Acknowledge positive behaviors, for example, "Thank you for helping to pick up the room, it makes me feel that you want to be helpful."
6. Effective communication involves both listening and talking. Reflect that you understand the child's feelings. "I can see that you are sad [upset, afraid, etc.]."
7. Show faith and confidence in the child.

Behavior problems that can occur during early childhood are detailed in Table 18–2.

## Speech Development

At about the end of the 1st year, the baby begins to make noises that sound like "bye-bye," "ma-ma," and "da-da." When toddlers see the happy response to these sounds, they repeat them. This is true throughout the toddler period. In order for small children to want to learn to talk they must have an appreciative audience.

At first, children refer to animals by the sounds the animals make. For example, before saying "dog," the toddler repeats "bow-bow." Soon the child can say short phrases such as "Daddy gone car." Toddlers also respond to tone of voice and facial expression. If an adult sounds threatening, the toddler may answer "no" and then again in a louder voice.

Toddlers who talk remarkably well and understand more than they say still cannot comprehend much of adult conversation. Sometimes adults forget this, and they scold the child merely for being too young to understand what is requested. Imagine yourself being punished in a foreign country because you could not speak or comprehend the language well enough to defend yourself. Adults who show empathy to the small child can help minimize their frustrations.

Toddlers who have just learned to walk may practically give up repeating words because they are so overjoyed at being able to move about independently. As soon as the initial fascination becomes less pronounced, they take up speech again. Delayed speech does not necessarily indicate that the child is mentally slow. The temperament and personality of the child and the family play an important role. No two toddlers have the same vocabulary at the same age.

If parents are concerned about the child's delayed speech, they can discuss it with their doctor during one of the child's routine physical examinations so that it can be evaluated in the light of total physical growth and development. Many late talkers are perfectly normal children who prefer listening over active participation.

## Daily Care

Adults must simplify their everyday conversation with small children. Offering too many choices confuses them. When talking to the toddler, the adult should be at eye level with the child. In this way, the adult seems less overwhelming. This is of particular importance when the child is in a fear-provoking environment, such as the hospital.

By the time the child becomes a toddler, parents have usually found it easier to give the bath every evening rather than at midmorning. A flexible schedule organized about the needs of the entire household is best. The toddler needs a consistent routine, but it can differ during the summer months, when outdoor water play may make a tub bath optional.

The clothing of toddlers should be simple and easy for them to put on and take off. Slacks with elastic waists are convenient for them to pull down when they go to the toilet. All clothing must be fairly loose to provide freedom of movement for jumping and other strenuous activities. In the summer months, light-skinned children may sunburn quickly and should be protected by clothing and sunscreen to prevent

**Table 18–2.** BEHAVIOR PROBLEMS DURING EARLY CHILDHOOD, NORMAL EXPECTATIONS, AND FACTORS THAT CONTRIBUTE TO PROBLEM BEHAVIOR

| Behavior | Normal Expectations | Factors That Contribute to Problem Behavior | |
|---|---|---|---|
| | | Child Factors | Parent/Home Environment Factors |
| Sleep disorders | Occasional nightmares beginning at about 36 mo Ritual bedtime routine; attempt to delay sleep peaks between 2 and 3 yr Head banging and rocking between 1 and 4 yr provide release of tension Waking between 1 and 5 AM occurs frequently after 6 mo of age (less than once a week) Fearful of darkness between 2 and 5 yr; will settle down with use of rituals, such as having a favorite toy or a night-light | Excessive napping during the day Insufficient adult interaction during the day, leading to use of bedtime as opportunity to gain adult attention Unusual fears related to darkness, being left alone; rituals and night-light do not suffice Illness Development of nighttime bowel and bladder control | Anxiety for child's safety results in frequent checking on child, disturbing sleep Inability to set and maintain limits on delaying tactics Unrealistic expectations; cannot tolerate bedtime rituals Environment noisy, not conducive to sleep Excessive stimulation before bedtime Frightening TV shows before bedtime Environmental stress, such as new sibling or moving |
| Temper tantrums | Tantrums peak at 2 yr of age, decreasing in frequency and intensity until they rarely occur by about 4 yr of age Usually occur in response to frustrated desires of a child, such as wanting a toy that cannot be purchased | Used as a manipulative device to gain control of parental behavior Insufficient positive interaction with adults, leading to use of tantrums to gain attention | Inability to set and maintain limits; parents allow themselves to be manipulated Insufficient positive approaches to child in response to desired behavior Unrealistic expectations; cannot tolerate any tantrum behavior |
| Toilet training and bedwetting | Has full physiologic capacity for day control by 3 yr, night control by 4 yr Daytime and nighttime "accidents" occur throughout early childhood, decreasing in frequency by 4–5 yr Regression occurs with environmental or social changes, such as arrival of sibling, moving, divorce | Fears and anxiety in response to negative means of toilet training inhibit ability to gain control Used as an attention-getting device if positive means of gaining attention are lacking Excessive fluid intake before bedtime | Punishment and other negative approaches to toilet training Unrealistic expectations for control; expect normal control before physiologic ability is present or expect the child to be accident-free Inconsistent recognition of child's signals of needing to use the toilet Inadequate provisions for child's toileting needs, such as small commode Clothing is too difficult for child to manipulate independently Irregular eating patterns |
| Aggressive or quarrelsome behavior; sibling rivalry | Ability to play cooperatively begins to emerge at 4–5 yr Before this age, is seldom able to share toys; often wants toys that another child has Predominant use of physical hitting, shoving to express displeasure; verbal abilities begin to emerge during 5th yr | Insufficient positive adult attention leads to deliberate use of aggression to gain adult attention Aggression may arise from actual or perceived adult preference for sibling or playmate | Insufficient positive interaction in response to desired behavior Unrealistic expectations for cooperative and sharing behavior Actual preferential attention given to sibling or playmate |

*Continued*

**Table 18–2.** BEHAVIOR PROBLEMS DURING EARLY CHILDHOOD, NORMAL EXPECTATIONS, AND FACTORS THAT CONTRIBUTE TO PROBLEM BEHAVIOR *Continued*

| Behavior | Normal Expectations | Factors That Contribute to Problem Behavior | |
| --- | --- | --- | --- |
| | | Child Factors | Parent/Home Environment Factors |
| Inability to separate; excessive shyness | Can separate easily by 3 yr if surroundings are consistent, predictable, positive<br>Continues to protest separation if environment changes or if confronted by total strangers<br>Shy in new and strange surroundings, relaxed and spontaneous in familiar surroundings | Inadequate establishment of self-concept, leading to lack of confidence even in familiar surroundings<br>Uses protest of separation as a manipulative control device<br>Fear of being abandoned | Parental anxiety and guilt over separation<br>Inability to set limits, to leave child after brief, direct explanation<br>Lack of preparation for an anticipated separation, leading to an unpredicted, fearful experience for the child<br>Inconsistent messages and actions, such as telling child parent will stay and then sneaking out, or not returning at a predicted time |

Courtesy of P. Chinn, Denver, CO.
From Chinn, P., & Leitch, C. (1979). *Child health maintenance* (2nd ed.). St. Louis: Mosby–Year Book.

future skin damage. In the winter months, children need outdoor clothing that will protect them from stormy weather. Outdoor garments must be changed when they become wet with snow (Fig. 18–5).

The toddler wears shoes mainly for protection. They should fit the shape of the foot and be ½ inch longer and ¼ inch wider than the foot. The heels must fit securely. Children should

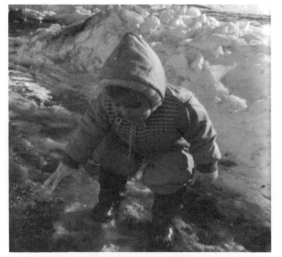

**Figure 18–5.** Tina needs security, but she also needs opportunities to explore her world. She must be dressed suitably for the weather.

wear their usual shoes at their periodic checkups because these show how the shoes have been worn, which indicates to the doctor how the children are using their bodies. Whenever safe and possible, the toddler may go barefoot, since this strengthens the foot muscles. Socks must be large enough that they do not flex the toes. Children are taught to pull socks free from the toes before putting on shoes.

Good posture is the result of proper nutrition, plenty of fresh air and exercise, and sufficient rest. The toddler's mattress must be firm. The chair and play table are adapted to size. In some cases, this can be easily accomplished by placing a few magazines in the seat of the chair. A sturdy small stool placed in the bathroom will bring the child to the proper height for brushing the teeth. As in all areas of learning, the child's posture is greatly influenced by that of other members of the family. The toddler who is happy and is allowed gradually increasing independence develops a sense of security, which is reflected in the posture. Slouching is sometimes seen in children who are insecure and lack self-confidence.

## Nutrition Counseling

The toddler's need for food is not as great as that of the infant, because the toddler does not grow as rapidly, although the activity level increases. Caloric requirements per unit of body weight decline from 120 cal/kg during infancy to 100 cal/kg. Children need an adequate protein intake to cover maintenance needs and to provide for optimum growth. These are mainly provided by milk and other dairy products, meat, and eggs. Milk should be limited to 24 oz/day. Too few solid foods can lead to dietary deficiencies of iron. Children between the ages of 1 and 3 years are high-risk candidates for anemia. "This risk is due to the rapid growth period of infancy with its increase in hemoglobin mass and the continued need to maintain hemoglobin concentration as well as increase total iron mass during growth" (Mahan & Arlin, 1992).

The toddler who is well nourished shows steady proportional gains on height and weight charts and has good bone and tooth develop-

ment. The diet history is adequate. Laboratory values such as blood urea nitrogen, albumin, hemoglobin, hematocrit, lymphocyte count, red and white blood cell counts, cholesterol, sodium, potassium, and glucose are within normal ranges. Excessive calories and large amounts of vitamins are avoided.

The toddler is noted for having a fluctuating appetite with strong food preferences. The nurse reminds parents that any nutritious food can be eaten at any meal; for example, soup for breakfast and cereal for supper. Serving size is important (Table 18–3). Too-large servings are discouraged because they may overwhelm the child and can lead to overeating problems. One tablespoon of solid food per year of age serves as a measurement guide. A quiet time before meals provides an opportunity for the child to

**Table 18–3.** RECOMMENDED FOOD INTAKE FOR GOOD NUTRITION ACCORDING TO FOOD GROUPS AND DAILY DIETARY ALLOWANCES (TODDLERS, 1–3 YR)

| Food Groups | Servings per Day | Serving Size 1 yr | Serving Size 2–3 yr |
|---|---|---|---|
| Bread Group | At least 4 | | |
| • Bread | | ½ slice | 1 slice |
| • Cereal | | ½ oz | ¾ oz |
| • Rice and pasta | | ¼ C | ⅓ C |
| Vegetable Group | At least 3 total | | |
| • Green-yellow vegetables (vitamin A source) | 1 or more | 2 tbsp | 3 tbsp |
| • Other vegetables | 2 | ⅓ C | ½ C |
| Fruit Groups | At least 3 total | | |
| • Citrus fruits, berries, tomato, cabbage, cantaloupe (vitamin C source) | 1 or more (twice as much tomato as citrus) | ⅓ C | ½ C |
| • Other fruits (apple, banana) | 2 | ¼ C | ⅓ C |
| Milk Group | 3 | | |
| • Milk/yogurt | | ½ C | ½–¾ C |
| • Cheese | | 1½ oz cheese = 1 C milk | |
| Meat Group | 2 (6 oz total) | | |
| • Cooked lean meat, poultry, fish | | 2 tbsp | 2 tbsp |
| • Dry beans | | 2 tbsp | 3 tbsp |
| • Egg | | 1 | 1 |
| • Peanut butter | | | 1 tbsp |
| Fats, oils, sweets—USE SPARINGLY | | | |

**Recommended Daily Dietary Allowances**

| Protein | Fat-Soluble | Vitamins | Water-Soluble | Vitamins | Minerals | | Energy Needs |
|---|---|---|---|---|---|---|---|
| 16 g | Vitamin A | 400 μg RE | Vitamin C | 40 mg | Calcium | 800 mg | 1300 kcal |
| | Vitamin D | 10 μg | Thiamine | 0.7 mg | Phosphorus | 800 mg | |
| | Vitamin E | 6 mg α—TE | Riboflavin | 0.8 mg | Magnesium | 80 mg | |
| | Vitamin K | 15 μg | Niacin | 9 mg NE | Iron | 10 mg | |
| | | | Vitamin $B_6$ | 1.0 mg | Zinc | 10 mg | |
| | | | Folate | 50 μg | Iodine | 70 μg | |
| | | | Vitamin $B_{12}$ | 0.7 μg | Selenium | 20 μg | |

From Betz, C., Hunsberger, M., & Wright, S. (1994). *Family-centered nursing care of children* (2nd ed.). Philadelphia: W.B. Saunders.
Adapted with permission from *Recommended Dietary Allowances*: 10th Edition. Copyright 1989 by the National Academy of Sciences. Published by the National Academy Press, Washington, D.C.; and US Department of Agriculture, Human Nutrition Information Service. (1992). *Food guide pyramid*. (Leaflet No. 572). Washington, D.C.
*Key:* RE, retinol equivalent; TE, tocopherol equivalent; NE, niacin equivalent.

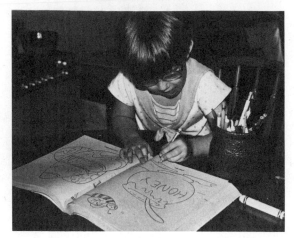

**Figure 18–6.** A quiet time before meals helps the toddler unwind.

"wind down" (Fig. 18–6). The toddler's refusal to eat may be due to fatigue or not being particularly hungry. The child may eat one food with vigor one week and refuse it the next. A flexible schedule designed to meet the needs of the toddler and the rest of the family must be worked out by the individual family. Forcing toddlers to eat only creates further difficulties. They are quick to sense parents' frustration and may use mealtime to obtain attention by behaving poorly and refusing to eat. Discipline and arguments during mealtime only upset everyone's digestion.

Toddlers are fond of ritual. This is frequently seen at mealtime. They want a particular dish, glass, and bib. It is best to go along with the wishes, as long as they do not become too pronounced. It gives them a sense of security and, in the long run, saves time and energy for the adult.

Toddlers have a brief span of attention. They may try to stand in the highchair or wander away from the table. If they have eaten a fair amount of the meal, they may be excused; otherwise distraction of some type is necessary. Toddlers who regularly feed themselves may enjoy being helped by Mommy or Daddy. Some restaurants that cater to families provide a pencil and special placemat to keep the small child occupied until adults finish their dinners. In the hospital, the toddler who is fed in a highchair wears a jacket restraint, and the nurse remains with the patient while in the chair.

The toddler's food is chopped into fine pieces. The portions should be small and separated. A variety of foods are offered, and one should try to plan contrast of colors and textures. A 2-year-old likes finger foods, such as carrot sticks or a lettuce wedge. Foods are served at moderate temperatures. Candy, cake, and soda between meals are to be avoided. Nutritious foods include (1) milk, milk products, eggs, and butter or fortified margarine; (2) vegetables and fruits; (3) meat, fish, and poultry; and (4) enriched breads and cereals.

Children like colorful dishes, which must be made of an unbreakable substance. Washable plastic bibs and placemats are convenient. The floor around the highchair can be protected with newspapers. Silverware should be small enough that it can be handled easily. Seating equipment should be adjusted so that the child is comfortable and maintains good posture. Figure 18–7 illustrates the self-feeding skills of the toddler of 18 months.

## Dental Health

Good dental health is essential to the growing child. Attractive, healthy teeth promote self-esteem and contribute to physical well-being. Today, techniques are available to prevent dental problems in the majority of children. Unfortunately, many poor children seldom visit the dentist's office. Insurance reimbursement may be nonexistent when a parent is out of work. Government allocations for the poor have decreased during the past several years.

Nurses must realize that although most middle-class children see their dentist regularly, tooth decay is still rampant among the poor. They can play an important role in detection, nutrition education, and teaching oral hygiene. They can also direct parents to dental clinics serving low-income clientele.

Prevention of dental problems consists of good nutrition (a diet high in calcium, phosphorus, appropriate vitamins), proper brushing and flossing of the teeth, fluoridation of drinking water or fluoride supplements (not both), and regular dental care. In the past, dental care has been advocated at about the age of 2 years. Recent trends in the field of oral health suggest caring for the teeth as soon as they start to develop. A clinic in one university setting begins preventive care at the age of 1 year. The office visit includes an examination of teeth, gum tissue, and bone structure. It also

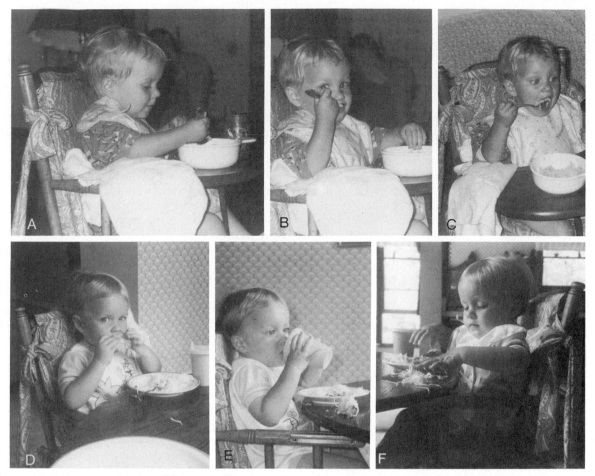

**Figure 18–7.** At 18 months the toddler can hold a spoon *(A)*, can bring food to the mouth *(B)*, does not yet have the ability to rotate the wrist and elevate the elbow to keep food on the spoon *(C)*, manages finger foods *(D)*, drinks well from a cup *(E)*, and enjoys playing with food *(F)*.

includes educating parents about proper nutrition, feeding patterns, tooth cleaning procedures, and fluoride treatments.

Above all, the nurse teaches parents to avoid using the bottle as a daytime or nighttime pacifier. Constant access to a bottle of milk or juice exposes the tiny teeth to hours of sugary acids that can cause severe damage. Low-cariogenic snack foods are also important. Sucking on lollipops and chewing sugary gum are to be discouraged, as their sugar remains longer in the mouth. Parents are instructed to read cereal and other product labels for sugar content. In particular, they should watch for the "ose" ending, which generally refers to sugar (e.g., sucrose, glucose, fructose, lactose).

When brushing is not practical, the child is taught to rinse the mouth several times. The 2-year-old enjoys putting toothpaste on a brush.

Plenty of time is allowed in order to avoid frustration. Technique improves with practice. Parents may need to assist the child to ensure effectiveness.

## Toilet Independence

There are many approaches to toilet training. Much depends on the temperament of both the individual child and the person guiding the child. Readiness is important. Voluntary control of anal and urethral sphincters occurs at about 18–24 months. The child's waking up dry in the morning or from naptime is an indication of maturity. Children must be able to communicate in some fashion that they are wet or need to urinate or defecate. They must be willing to sit on the potty for at least 5–10 minutes.

Toddlers seek approval and like to imitate the actions of parents. They wander into the bathroom and are curious about what is taking place there. If a parent feels that the child will respond to training at this time, the child might first be put in training pants or pull-up diapers. These can be removed quickly and easily, and the child becomes more aware of being wet.

The use of a child's pot chair or a device that attaches to an adult seat is a matter of personal preference. A pot chair may make the toddler feel more secure, for it is small (Fig. 18–8). It should support the back and arms of the child. The feet should touch the floor. The toilet seat type must have a belt to strap the toddler in as a safety measure. The child needs time to become accustomed to this new piece of equipment. Toddlers may want to climb in and out of it and drag it about before they actually try to use it. If a potty seat is not available, the child is placed on the standard-size toilet, facing the toilet tank. This method may increase feelings of security.

Bowel training is generally attempted first;

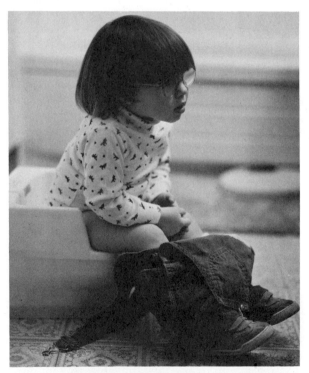

**Figure 18–8.** Toilet training should be a nonstressful experience for the toddler. The nurse assesses the parents' expectations, family and cultural pressures, and developmental readiness of the child before instruction begins.

however, some toddlers become bladder trained during the day because they enjoy listening to the "tinkle" in the potty. If toddlers have bowel movements at the same time each day, they may progress fairly rapidly. They should not be left on the pot chair for more than a few minutes at a time.

If the child's bowel movements are not regular, it might be well to delay training for a while because the toddler will resent being constantly interrupted from play and taken to the bathroom. Toddlers generally enjoy having a parent remain with them during the procedure. Most parents find some phase of toilet training discouraging. Perhaps it is because they work at it too hard, thinking it an obstacle that they must hurdle rather than a normal process that the toddler will easily master when ready. Spankings and threats do more damage than good. Life is smoother for all if the parent remains patient and keeps this new adventure pleasant. Training should not be undertaken when the family or child is under stress, such as during illness or a move to a new location.

Bladder training is begun when the toddler stays dry for about 2 hours at a time. One morning a parent may discover that the toddler has gone the entire night without wetting. It is then logical to put the child on the pot chair and to praise success. Bladder training varies widely, particularly during the night. Restricting fluids before bedtime may help. Placing the half-asleep child on the pot chair accomplishes little.

Most children continue to have occasional accidents until the age of 4–5 years. If the toddler has a mishap, parents should accept it matter-of-factly and merely change the clothes. When adults show continuous affection to their children and accept both bad and good days, they surely benefit from it.

The word that toddlers use to signal defecation or urination should be one that is recognized by others besides the immediate family. Sometimes, a parent may forget to inform the baby-sitter or nursery school teacher of the word that the child uses. This causes the children unnecessary frustration because those about them

## Nursing Brief

Nurses can help parents identify readiness for toilet independence.

cannot understand what they are trying to say.

Toddlers who are toilet trained at home should continue to use the potty in the hospital setting. They may be acutely embarrassed by wetting the crib. Nurses regularly consult children's nursing care plans in order to make the patients feel more at home. Attentive nurses respond quickly to the toddler's plea and ask themselves, "Does this child need to urinate?" Although regression of bowel and bladder training is common during hospitalization, personnel often contribute to it by not taking time to investigate the child's needs.

## Play

Toddlers spend much of the day playing. In this way they develop coordination, which contributes to physical well-being. Play also contributes to mental health by relieving emotional tension. At first the toddler enjoys *parallel play*, that is, play near other children but not with them. This is the beginning of socialization. Gradually, as toddlers learn to communicate more easily and become more skilled in handling toys, cooperative play takes place (Fig. 18–9). They learn to give and take and begin to sense moral values of right and wrong. Play is also of educational value. Learning is continuous as they explore and delight in many new play experiences.

It takes time for small children to learn to share. They clutch toys, shouting, "Mine!" Once in a while they voluntarily offer a toy to a playmate. Parents should not force the toddler to share possessions. This comes at a later stage of development. If toddlers are constantly corrected for hoarding, they may eventually give up their toys when they are supervised, but they seldom share when left to their own designs.

Toddlers need adult supervision during play, especially when other children are involved. The oldest in the group must be distracted from pushing and hugging and from directing the play of others. The youngest child needs protection from being bullied. Toddlers feel secure when they know they will be rescued from alarming experiences. It is unfair to expect them to handle situations beyond their capabilities.

The type of toy the toddler selects for play depends on age. The 15-month-old is content with pots and pans from mother's kitchen and enjoys

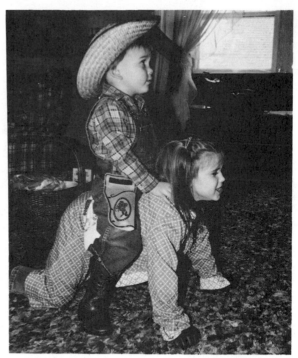

**Figure 18–9.** Siblings help promote socialization.

repeating acts such as removing clothespins from a bucket and replacing them. The toddler likes certain books and looks at the same pictures over and over again (Fig. 18–10). Some children become attached to a certain stuffed toy or blanket. Two year-olds like to unlace and remove their shoes frequently. They are fond of water play and may resent being re-

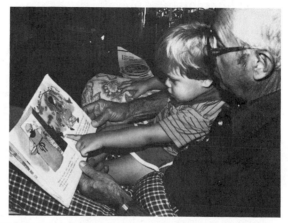

**Figure 18–10.** Active and involved grandparents benefit all three generations.

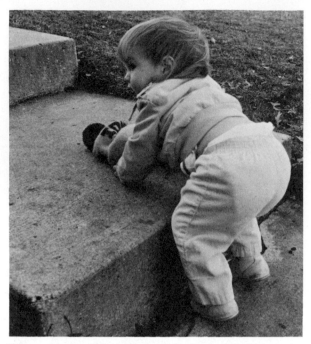

**Figure 18–11.** The toddler usually begins climbing stairs on all fours.

moved from the tub. They enjoy playing in a sand box, scribbling with a crayon and paper, and prancing to rhythmic music.

It is not long before toddlers discover the stairs. Most small children start climbing them on all fours (Fig. 18–11). As children become more accomplished in walking upright, they shift to the method of placing one foot on the stairs and drawing the other foot up to it, supporting themselves by the handrail. Eventually, they can climb the stairs by using their feet alternately, as in walking.

Toys that can be pedaled, such as a tricycle, are adapted to the size of the child. As a rule, wind-up toys cannot be fully enjoyed by the toddlers because they cannot manipulate them alone. Objects that can be pushed or pulled delight the small child. Toys with small, removable parts are dangerous because of possible aspiration.

## Day Care

Family life has changed dramatically since the 1950s. At that time, only 12% of mothers with children under 6 years of age were in the labor force. By 1992 the fastest-growing group of persons in the labor force were women with infants. Not only are more mothers working, but they are also returning to the work force sooner after the child is born. It is clear that alternative methods of child care are necessary. These arrangements must meet families' personal preferences, cultural perspectives, and financial and special needs. Parents must take an active role in ensuring high-quality care (Fig. 18–12). Nurses need to be resource persons and family advocates because finding adequate day care can be stressful.

There are a variety of types of child care. Most children today are cared for by relatives, friends, neighbors, or those who have advertised such services. However, there is little research on these types of home arrangements, and few standards of quality control. Most licensed day-care centers are private businesses run for profit. They are subject to state regula-

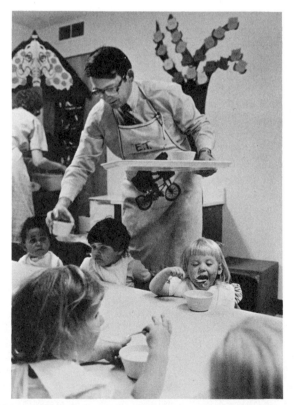

**Figure 18–12.** Parents must take an active role in ensuring high-quality day care. An indication of a good program is the child's degree of happiness while attending the day-care center. (Courtesy of Blank Memorial Hospital for Children, Des Moines, IA.)

tions about physical makeup, number of children per caretaker, education of personnel, and so on. Parents have to plan ahead for times when the child is sick and unable to attend. A few innovative programs for in-home care of sick children are being developed. Employer-supported child care is a rapidly growing area. These programs are very diverse. Some companies provide family day care (care of the child in the provider's home) as well. Other employers assist parents through reimbursement, referral programs, or support of existing child-care programs in the community.

For low-income and some middle-income families, the cost of child care is difficult, if not impossible, to maintain. Some form of continued or expanded government assistance or private funding is necessary. Inspection and monitoring of child-care facilities to ensure compliance with health (physical and mental) and safety standards are paramount. Ideally, all day-care programs would include comprehensive health services and health education programs. Criteria for selecting a day-care center are similar to those discussed for nursery schools (see p. 487).

## Accident Prevention

Accidents kill and cripple more children than any disease known and are the *leading* cause of death in childhood. Unfortunately, we do not have a preventive for this, but we do have a defensive weapon. This weapon is knowledge. If parents understand their child's activities at certain ages, they can prevent many serious injuries by taking necessary precautions. Likewise, when statistics indicate that poisonings or burns are particularly prevalent at a specific age, parents can guard against them (Tables 18–4 and 18–5).

The majority of accidents occur in or near the home (Figs. 18–13 to 18–16). Toddlers are especially vulnerable because they have a natural curiosity for investigating their environment. Parents must allow toddlers some natural experiences, which teach them to look out for their own safety. They should also strive to teach toddlers what is safe and what is not.

Nurses demonstrate safety measures to their patients and their families. This is most effectively done by good example. Measures pertinent to the pediatric unit are discussed on page 560). Nurses in the community can often contribute indirectly to the welfare of others by the example set and by being aware of emergency medical facilities available in the community.

## CONSUMER EDUCATION

The federal government and concerned private agencies have attempted to regulate some of the variables that cause accidents. A few examples are ensuring the use of nonflammable material for children's sleepwear, child-proofing caps on medicine bottles and certain household products, and establishing maximum temperatures for home hot-water heaters. Smoke detectors in homes and public places are commonplace. In 1974, the United States Consumer Product Safety Commission established regulations for crib slats, locks, and latches and mattress size and thickness. Safety warnings on the crib's carton advise buyers to use a snug mattress only.

Laws have been passed in virtually all states that require infants and small children to be restrained while riding in automobiles (Fig. 18–17). These restraints must follow standards established by the Federal Motor Vehicle Safety Department. Rental cars also loan child seat restraints. Many parents still do not understand the importance of safety seats and neglect to use them. This is an essential area of patient teaching, beginning with the first ride home from the hospital.

New homes are required to have smoke detectors. Consumers who live in older homes and apartment complexes are also encouraged to install them. Various other safety codes are mandatory for public buildings, with additional measures required for buildings specifically for the handicapped. The problems of surveillance and upkeep nevertheless are considerable. Many children live in substandard housing with little supervision. The education of parents is of monumental importance in decreasing death and disability.

## TOY SAFETY

In 1970 the Child Protection and Toy Safety Act was passed in an effort to halt the distribution of unsafe toys. In addition, parents must be taught to inspect toys purchased and to buy toys suitable for the age, skills, and abilities of the individual child. Some labels now give

**Table 18–4.** HOW TO PREVENT HAZARDS CAUSED BY THE BEHAVIORAL CHARACTERISTICS OF TODDLERS

| Behavioral Characteristics | Hazard and Prevention Strategies |
|---|---|
| | *Automobile* |
| Impulsive, unable to delay gratification, increased mobility, egocentric | Teach child to look both ways before crossing street |
| | Teach child the meaning of red, yellow, and green traffic lights |
| | Caution children not to run from behind parked cars or snowbanks |
| | Use car-seat restraints |
| | Hold toddler's hand when crossing the street |
| | Supervise tricycle riding |
| | Do not allow children to play in the car or leave them alone in it |
| | Do not allow chldren to ride in the back of open trucks |
| | Drivers must look carefully in front and behind vehicles before accelerating |
| | Teach children what areas are safe for sliding and the like |
| | Watch child under 3 yr at all times or fence in yard |
| | *Burns* |
| Children are fascinated by fire | Teach the child the meaning of "hot" (one mother taught this by allowing the child to touch beach sand warmed by the sun) |
| Toddler can reach articles inaccessible to the infant | Put matches and cigarettes out of reach and sight |
| | Turn handles of cooking utensils toward the back of the stove |
| | Avoid scaldings; do not leave the bathroom when hot water is being drawn or after the tub is filled |
| | Beware of hot coffee; avoid tablecloths with overhang |
| | Keep appliances such as coffee pots, electric frying pans, and food processors out of reach |
| | Test food and fluids heated in microwave ovens to ensure that center is not too hot |
| | Beware of hot charcoal grills |
| | Use snug fireplace screens |
| | Mark children's rooms to alert fire fighters in emergency |
| | Keep a pressure-type fire extinguisher available, and teach all family members who are old enough how to use it |
| | Practice what to do in case of fire in your home |
| | Install smoke detectors |
| | Teach children the danger of smoke inhalation and how to avoid it |
| | *Falls* |
| Toddlers like to explore different parts of the house. They can open doors and lean out open windows. Their depth perception is immature. *Their capabilities change quickly.* Although they may seem quite grown up at times, they still require constant supervision at home and on the playground | Teach children how to go up and come down stairs when they show a readiness for this task |
| | Fasten crib sides securely and leave them up when child is in the crib |
| | Use side rails on a large bed when child graduates from crib |
| | Lock basement doors or use gates at top and bottom of stairs |
| | Mop spilled water from floor immediately |
| | Use window guards |
| | Use car-seat restraints |
| | Keep scissors and other pointed objects away from the toddler's reach |
| | *Suffocation and Choking* |
| Explores with senses, likes to bite on and taste things | Do not allow small chldren to play with deflated balloons, as these can be sucked into windpipe |
| Eats on the run | Inspect toys for loose parts |
| | Remove small objects such as coins, buttons, pins from reach |
| | Avoid popcorn, nuts, small hard candies, chewing gum |
| | Debone fish, chicken |
| | Learn Heimlich maneuver |
| | Inspect width of crib and playpen slats |
| | Keep plastic bags away from small children; do not use as mattress cover |
| | Do not lift child from crib if vomiting; turn on side |
| | Avoid nightclothes with drawstring necks |
| | Discard old refrigerators |

**Table 18–4.** HOW TO PREVENT HAZARDS CAUSED BY THE BEHAVIORAL CHARACTERISTICS OF TODDLERS *Continued*

| Behavioral Characteristics | Hazard and Prevention Strategies |
| --- | --- |
| | *Poisoning* |
| Ingenuity increases, can open most containers | Store household detergents and cleaning supplies out of reach |
| Increased mobility provides child access to cupboards, medicine cabinets, bedside stands, interior of closets | Lock cabinet if toddler is particularly fascinated by items |
| Looks at and touches everything | Do not put chemicals or other potentially harmful substances into food or beverage containers; store in separate cabinets |
| Learns by trial and error | Keep medicines in a locked cabinet; put them away immediately after using them |
| | Use child-resistant caps and packaging |
| | Flush old medicine down toilet |
| | Follow physician's directions when administering medication |
| | Do not allow one child to give another medicine |
| | Do not refer to pills as "candy" |
| | Keep mouthwash away from small children in order to avoid potential alcohol poisoning |
| | Educate parents as to when and how to use ipecac |
| | Explain poison symbols to child (Mr. Yuk stickers and so on) and to parents not fluent in English |
| | Keep telephone number of poison control center available |
| | When painting, use paint marked "for indoor use" or one that conforms to standards for use on surfaces that may be chewed by children |
| | Wash fruits and vegetables before eating |
| | Obtain and record name of any new plant purchased |
| | Alert family of location of poisonous plants on or around property |
| | *Drowning* |
| Lacks depth perception | Watch child continuously while at beach or near a pool |
| Does not realize danger | Empty wading pools when child has finished playing |
| Loves water play | Cover wells securely |
| | Wear recommended life jackets in boats |
| | Begin teaching water safety early |
| | Lock fences surrounding swimming pools |
| | Supervise tub baths; be aware that a young child can drown in a very small amount of water (one 17-month-old toddler drowned in a cleaning pail of bleach water) |
| | *Electric Shock* |
| Pokes and probes with fingers | Cover electrical outlets |
| | Cap unused sockets with safety plugs |
| | Water conducts electricity; teach child not to touch electrical appliances when wet; keep appliances out of reach |
| | *Animal Bites* |
| Immature judgment | Teach child to avoid stray animals |
| | Do not allow toddler to abuse household pets |
| | Supervise closely |

*Keep first aid chart and emergency numbers handy*
*Know location of and how to get to nearest emergency facility*

safety information and intended age. Parents are also taught to inspect toys routinely for breakage.

Notification of recall of a specific toy is generally published in newspapers and consumer journals. Toy boxes and toy chests are also a potential hazard. The most serious injuries caused by a box or chest are the result of the lid's falling on a child or a child's being trapped inside. A parent can report a product hazard by

**Table 18–5.** HOW TO PREVENT HAZARDS IN THE HOME

| Room/Object | Hazard | Prevention Strategies |
|---|---|---|

*Kitchen*

| Room/Object | Hazard | Prevention Strategies |
|---|---|---|
| A—Lower cabinets and drawers | Poisonous and corrosive substances in cabinets or on counters, including spices and extracts used in cooking | Remove and place out of reach in locked cabinet |
| | Alcohol or liquor in lower cabinets | Place in upper cabinet with cabinet lock |
| | Sharp knives, scissors, or other dangerous articles in drawers | Place in upper cabinet with cabinet lock, or use drawer lock |
| | Breakable bowls or pie plates in lower cabinets | Remove or use cabinet lock |
| B—Kitchen table | Pills or medicine on kitchen table or window sills | Lock up with other dangerous substances; use child-proof caps |
| C—Stove | Stove dials easily accessible | Remove until needed |
| | Cookies or other attractive food over stove | Remove to another location; have fire extinguisher available |
| | Stove turned on when not in use | Make sure burners are off and gas pilot is working properly; keep matches in metal container covered and out of reach |
| D—Countertop | Food processor on counter | Remove blades to make them inaccessible; keep processor unplugged to prevent accidental activation |
| | Other electrical appliances on counter-tops—toaster, coffee pot, and so on | Keep unplugged; use short cord, or wind and secure cord |
| E—Sink | Accessible disposal | Keep covered to prevent child from inserting hand in |
| F—Floor | Wastebasket | Have a covered wastebasket to reduce curiosity; keep in closet or cabinet or out of reach |
| | Accessible stepstool might be used for climbing | Keep in kitchen closet; use plastic door handle covers to prevent entry |
| G—Dishwasher | Knives within reach | Keep door closed and locked |
| H—Door | Outside access available to children | Use simple door lock out of child's reach |

*Dining Room*

| Room/Object | Hazard | Prevention Strategies |
|---|---|---|
| A—Table | Tablecloth hanging within reach | Remove cloth or use shorter cloth, particularly when lighted candles are on table |
| B—Buffet with hutch | Breakable item on buffet | Remove |
| | Glass and china items accessible in china cabinet | Use cabinet locks to prevent access |
| | Chafing dishes and hot trays | Keep unplugged until just before use |
| | Accessible wine rack | Move to higher location; keep bottles out of reach |

**Table 18–5.** HOW TO PREVENT HAZARDS IN THE HOME *Continued*

| Room/Object | Hazard | Prevention Strategies |
|---|---|---|
| *Living Room* | Poisonous plants | Identify plants that are poisonous and remove or place out of child's reach |
| A—End table | Lighting fixtures | Make certain table lamps are not easily displaced |
| B—Fireplace | Fireplace or wood stove | Use fireplace screen; place gate around wood stove; dangerous fire-stoking equipment should be out of reach; do not heat water on wood stove; never cook with charcoal in fireplace; keep chimney damper open |
| C—Coffee table and couch | Furniture edges | Sharp-edged furniture should be removed or padded |
|  | Ashtrays | Keep ashtrays empty; dispose of cigarettes properly; keep matches and lighters out of reach |
| D—Window | Curtains and draperies | Short draperies recommended with small children; if using long drapes, make sure drapery rod is securely fastened to wall |
| E—Piano | Pianos and piano benches | Keep cover over keys when not in use |
| F—Book shelves | Stereo equipment | Stereo cabinet with locked doors recommended |
|  | Games | Games with small pieces must be kept out of reach or in locked cabinets |
|  | Books | Check that books cannot be pulled off shelves easily |
| G—Desk | Desk accessories | Remove sharp objects, pencils, pens, paper clips, and so on from desk top; lock drawers if possible |
| H—Dehumidifiers and fans | Blades and motors | Check consumer magazines to purchase child-safe appliance; grates should be too narrow for little fingers |
| *Hallways and Stairs* |  |  |
| A—Carpets | Slippery rugs | Use nonslip rug pad under rugs |
| B—Closets | Attractive playing area | Use plastic door knob covers for all closets containing hazardous items |
| *Bathroom* |  |  |
| A—Tub | Slippery surface, hot water | Apply decorative nonskid strips to bottom; use flexible plastic faucet cover; keep hot water heater turned down; keep shampoo, soap, and razors out of reach |
| B—Medicine cabinet | Dangerous substances | All medicines need child-proof caps and should be in a locked cabinet |
|  |  | Remove any cosmetics, hair dyes, nail polish, and the like and keep in a locked bathroom closet |
| C—Vanity and sink | Dangerous substances | Remove perfumes and powders from vanity top; electric shavers and toothbrushes should not be near water source; use outlet fillers for exposed outlets; use cabinet locks on vanity cabinets; store bathroom cleaners in locked bathroom closet; hair dryers, curling irons, and wastebaskets should be out of reach |
| D—Linen closet | Dangerous substances | Closet should have bolt lock or door handle cover to prevent entry; storage place for dangerous items |

*Continued*

**Table 18–5.** HOW TO PREVENT HAZARDS IN THE HOME *Continued*

| Room/Object | Hazard | Prevention Strategies |
|---|---|---|
| E—Floor | Space heaters | Floor coil heaters should not be available for child's use |
| | Rugs | All bathroom rugs should have nonslip backing |
| | Clothes hamper | Hampers with covers are recommended |
| F—Toilet | Water and dangerous chemicals | Keep toilet cover closed; avoid continuous toilet cleaners |
| *Bedrooms* | | |
| A—Bureaus | Dangerous substances and small objects | Remove cosmetics and small pieces of jewelry from bureau top; put loose change away and out of reach; keep jewelry box locked; drawers should not be easily removable |
| | Fans | Keep fans and air conditioners unplugged; use only when parent is around and never in children's rooms; do not place fans on floor; keep all electrical outlets filled |
| B—Night tables | Breakable objects | Remove breakables; telephones, radios, and so on, should be situated in middle to prevent being pulled off; keep flashlight here for emergencies |
| C—Sewing table | Electrical appliances; small, sharp objects | Keep machine unplugged until needed; keep bobbins, needles, and pins in inaccessible locations |
| D—Closets | Dangerous substances, plastic bags | Remove any mothballs or other insecticides; do not use plastic cleaner bags to store clothing in closets that are unlocked; keep clothes hangers off floors |
| E—Beds | | Do not use too much bedding or pillows for young children; keep children in sleepers if concerned about cold; discourage children from playing on bunk beds or bunk ladders; see information about crib safety |

*Note:* Be alert for dangerous items in the home. Use a common-sense approach to safety.
From Mott, S., James, S., & Sperhac, A. (1990). *Nursing care of children and families* (2nd ed.). Reading, MA: Addison-Wesley. Copyright © 1990, Addison-Wesley Nursing, a division of The Benjamin/Cummings Publishing Company. Reprinted by permission.

writing the United States Consumer Product Safety Commission, Washington DC 20207.

## EPIDEMIOLOGIC FRAMEWORK

An epidemiologic framework for accident prevention is a means of providing a systematic method of evaluation. It consists of three parts: the characteristics of the host (the child), the agent (the direct cause—for example, poisonous plants), and the environment.

**Host and Agent.** The individual characteristics of the child must be assessed by the nurse.

Particular attention is paid to the parents' description of the child. Some children are much more active, independent, and inquisitive than others. The nurse carefully evaluates children who are aggressive or stubborn or show low frustration tolerance. Children who appear accident-prone may be calling attention to themselves in an attempt to reconcile parents (parents usually communicate when the child has an accident) and for many other reasons. Children are less receptive to parental advice when they are tired and hungry.

The child's age and developmental stage

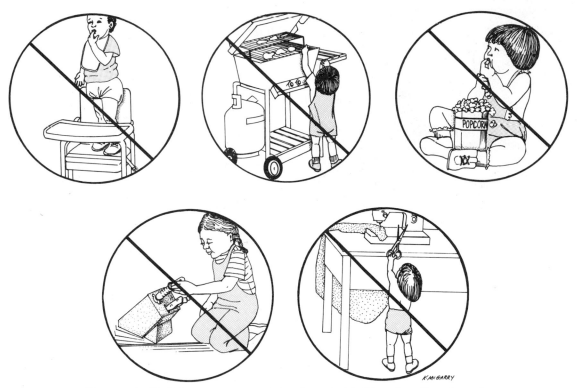

**Figure 18–13.** Safety measures are taken to protect toddlers from these hazards.

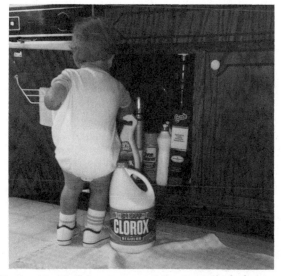

**Figure 18–14.** Poisoning prevention is particularly important for toddlers between the ages of 1 and 4 years.

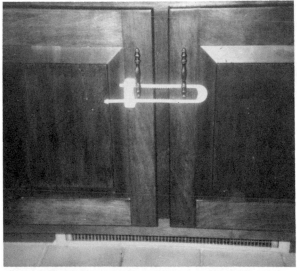

**Figure 18–15.** Inexpensive safety devices, such as these plastic door handle devices, limit access to materials that are dangerous to the inquisitive toddler.

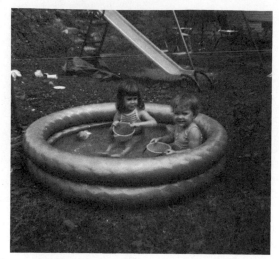

**Figure 18–16.** Pam and Tina enjoy water play. Two-year-olds need continuous supervision for this type of activity.

influence the types of accidents that occur. Toddlers and children under 5 years of age are often injured at home by factors listed in Table 18–5. School children are exposed to other hazards, such as motorized two- and three-wheel bicycles, guns, and fireworks, and participate in sports that predispose them to injuries. Providing anticipatory guidance is important.

Nurses must closely assess children with spe-

cial needs for safety precautions. Children with handicaps such as visual, motor, or intellectual impairments; convulsive disorders; or diabetes require extended instruction according to the child's particular needs. Immobile children need to be protected from sunburn and inclement weather. Adults must also guard these children from mosquitoes and other vectors. Control of the agent of injury involves some of the methods mentioned in the discussion of consumer education (e.g., child-proof caps on medication containers and regulations for children's furniture).

**Environment.** The physical, economic, and social environments of the child are also important in accident prevention. Families may be poor, overcrowded, fatigued, and dysfunctional. Children reared in households burdened by significant stress appear to be at greater risk for accidents. A new parent (or baby-sitter) may underestimate the developmental capabilities of the child. The reverse may occur when a new baby arrives and older children are given tasks beyond their abilities. Some suggest that the time of day has a bearing on accidents. Morning rush hour, after school (particularly for latchkey children), and evening have been cited. Family nationality and lifestyle are also considerations. Vacations and relocations, which place small children in strange environments, are potentially dangerous.

The nurse is often the person in close contact with families and can help them identify specific environmental hazards. A room-by-room survey of the home with the parents can be highly informative. A discussion of the neighborhood environment, for example, playgrounds, school yard, street lights, may also be relevant. The nurse explains the necessity for proper "modeling" of safety precautions because children absorb parental attitudes and behaviors. Community resources such as the library, fire department, and police are used. Problem-solving should be prioritized, information repeated, and effectiveness evaluated (Fig. 18–18).

## CARDIOPULMONARY RESUSCITATION

It is stressful to be faced with a life-threatening emergency. This is true for even the most experienced persons. Except in the newborn period, the number of children who require resuscitation is small; therefore, periodically reviewing and updating skills are essential to prevent

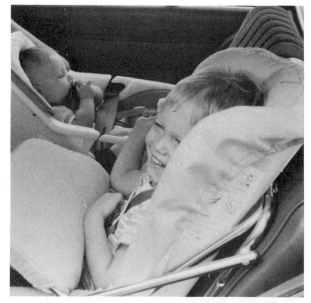

**Figure 18–17.** Automobile restraints save lives.

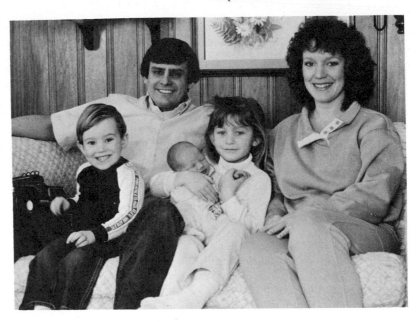

**Figure 18–18.** Family assessment is an integral part of the nursing process.

one from forgetting techniques because of lack of use. Basic life support is the phase of emergency care that (1) prevents respiratory and circulatory arrest through prompt recognition and intervention or (2) supports or provides ventilation and, if necessary, circulation to a victim, without the use of adjuncts. The following information is based on the Standards for Cardiopulmonary Resuscitation (CPR) and Emergency Cardiac Care (ECC), published by the American Medical Association (1992).

## Assessment ABCs

**Airway.** Assessment of the victim and the circumstances is done immediately in all cases. Quickly tap or gently shake the shoulder of the victim, then ask, "Are you O.K.?" (Omit question if not age-appropriate, i.e., for infants.) Then call out, "Help!" Next, position the victim. If the patient is lying face down, turn him or her as a unit with support to the head and neck. Place the patient supine on a firm sur-

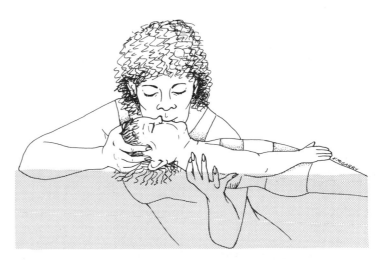

**Figure 18–19.** Drowning. Begin mouth-to-mouth resuscitation immediately, while the victim is still in the water. (From Thompson, E., & Ashwill, J. [1992]. *Pediatric nursing. An introductory text* [6th ed.]. Philadelphia: W.B. Saunders.)

face. In the unconscious patient, the tongue relaxes and falls back, obstructing the airway. Open the airway, by using head-tilt/chin-lift maneuver, to a sniffing or neutral position. One should not overextend the head. If the child is the victim of drowning, mouth-to-mouth resuscitation should be started immediately, while still in the water (Fig. 18–19).

**Breathing.** Determine if the victim is breathing by placing your ear over the victim's mouth and listening for exhaled air. Can you feel the exhaled air? Is the chest rising and falling? This should take only seconds. If the victim is not breathing, ventilate twice at 1–1.5 seconds of inspiration. This is accomplished by placing your mouth over the mouth and nostrils of an infant or small child; older children are ventilated by pinching the nostrils shut while breathing through the mouth. In both cases, make a tight seal. Observe the rise and fall of the chest. If pulse is present, continue rescue breathing at approximately 20 times/min for infants, or 15 times/min for older children, until the victim begins to breathe spontaneously.

**Circulation.** After the initial two breaths, determine if the victim has a pulse. Feel for the carotid pulse on the near side of the victim for 5–10 seconds. In infants with short, fat necks, this may be difficult to palpate. An alternative is to use the brachial pulse on the inner side of the upper arm, midway between the elbow and the shoulder. Maintain head tilt with your other hand.

If you are unable to find a pulse, begin chest compressions in order to maintain the circulation of the blood to the vital organs of the body. They are always accompanied by ventilation of the lungs. In the infant, an imaginary line between nipples is located over the breastbone; the compression site is one fingerbreadth below the intersection of the sternum and the imaginary line. Using two or three fingers, compress $\frac{1}{2}$–1 inch in infants at a rate of at least 100 times/min (five in 3 seconds or less). There is a short pause for ventilation after every fifth compression.

In older children (1–8 years), compressions are applied to the lower sternum, two fingerbreadths above the sternal notch. Pressure is applied with the heel of one hand. The depth of compression is 1–1$\frac{1}{2}$ inches, at a rate of 80–100 times/min (five in 3–4 seconds). Children over 8 years old are generally treated as adults. Compression and ventilations are continued by the mouth-to-mouth method at a ratio of five compressions per one breath (5:1)

until there are signs of recovery as evidenced by a return of pulse, improvement in color, and normal pupil size. In the infant and child, the 5:1 compression-to-ventilation ratio is maintained for both one and two rescuers. Reassessment is performed after about 1 minute and every few minutes thereafter. Figure 18–20 illustrates the procedures for cardiopulmonary resuscitation.

## EMERGENCY TREATMENT FOR CHOKING

An attempt at clearing the airway is desired with children in whom aspiration is witnessed or strongly suspected and in unconscious, non-breathing children whose airways remain obstructed despite the usual maneuvers to open them. The emergency treatment is known as the *Heimlich maneuver*. There remains controversy over the best methods for removing foreign bodies from the airways in children. At this writing, the following approaches are recommended.

**Older Child Standing or Sitting.** Stand behind the standing or sitting victim and wrap your arms around the victim's waist, with one hand made into a fist (Fig. 18–21). The thumb side rests against the victim's abdomen, slightly above the navel and well below the tip of the sternum. Grasp the fist with the other hand and press into the victim's abdomen with a quick upward thrust. Six to ten thrusts may be necessary to dislodge the object. Each thrust should be a separate and distinct movement.

**Older Child Lying Down (Conscious or Unconscious).** Position the child on his back. Kneel at the child's feet if the child is on the floor or stand at the child's feet if on a table. Place the heel of one hand on the child's abdomen in the midline, slightly above the navel and well below the rib cage. Grasp the fist with the other hand and press into the victim's abdomen with a quick upward thrust. Repeat six to ten thrusts as needed. Direct thrusts upward into the midline and not to either side of the abdomen. The smaller the child, the more gentle the procedure should be.

**Infant.** Determine airway obstruction. If the object is visualized, remove it, trying not to push the object deeper into the throat. If this approach is unsuccessful, position the child prone with the head lower than the trunk. (Support head and neck with one hand and straddle the infant face down over your forearm supported on your thigh, as shown in Figure 18–21.) Resting

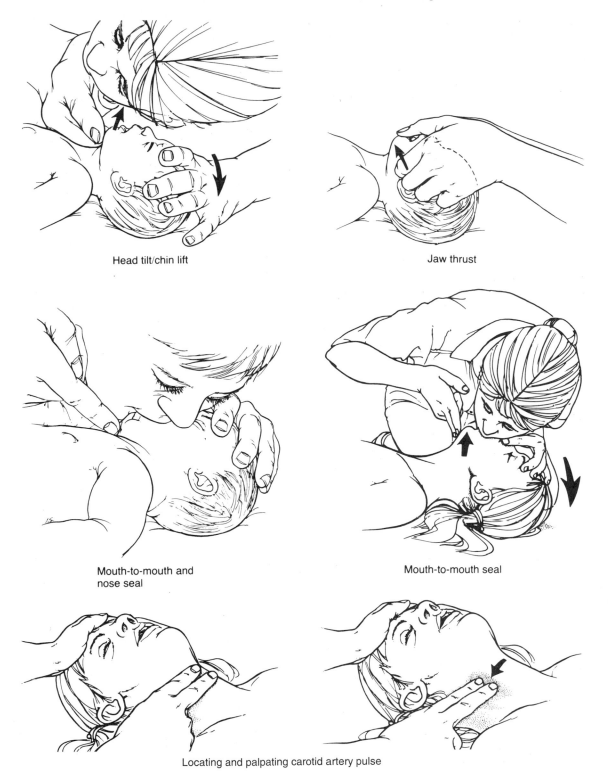

Head tilt/chin lift

Jaw thrust

Mouth-to-mouth and
nose seal

Mouth-to-mouth seal

Locating and palpating carotid artery pulse

**Figure 18–20.** Procedures for pediatric basic life support. (From Guidelines for cardiopulmonary resuscitation and emergency cardiac care [1992]. *JAMA: Journal of the American Medical Association, 268*:2171–2302. Copyright 1992, American Medical Association.)

*Continued*

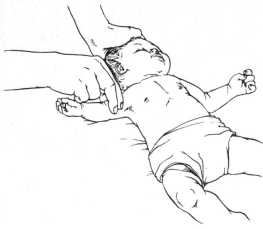

Locating and palpating
brachial pulse

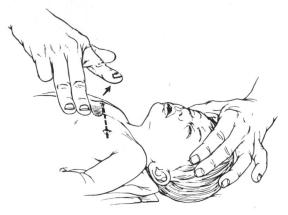

Locating finger position
for chest compressions
in infant

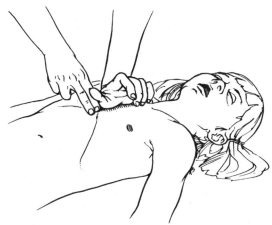

Locating hand position for chest
compressions in child

**Figure 18–20.** *Continued*

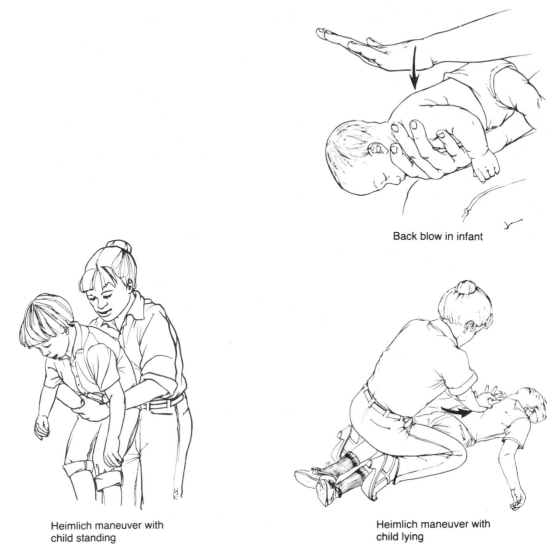

Back blow in infant

Heimlich maneuver with
child standing

Heimlich maneuver with
child lying

**Figure 18–21.** Procedures for clearing an airway obstruction. (From Guidelines for cardiopulmonary resuscitation and emergency cardiac care [1992]. *JAMA: Journal of the American Medical Association*, *268*:2171–2302. Copyright 1992, American Medical Association.)

the infant on the thigh, perform four forceful back blows between the shoulder blades with the heel of the hand. After delivering the back blows, place the free hand on the infant's back, so that the victim is sandwiched between the two hands, and turn the infant on his or her back, with the head still lower than the trunk. Deliver four thrusts in the mid-sternal region in the same manner as for external chest compressions, but at a slower rate (3–5 seconds). Repeat until the foreign body is expelled.

## Nursing Brief

If help arrives, have someone call the emergency medical system. The caller relates information including location of victim, telephone number from which the call is being made, circumstances, and condition of victim. The caller must remain on the telephone until all important information (particularly directions) is obtained by the dispatcher.

## KEY POINTS

- Egocentric (*ego*, "I," and *centric*, "centered") thinking predominates ("I want what I want, when I want it"). Toddlers believe everyone sees the world the way they do.
- Physical changes include the acquisition of fine and gross motor skills, including increased mobility and increased eye-hand coordination.
- Erickson refers to this stage as one in which the child's task is to acquire a sense of autonomy (self-control) while overcoming shame and doubt.
- The most evident cognitive achievements are language and comprehension.
- Some important self-regulatory functions include toilet independence, eating, sleeping, tolerating delayed gratification, separating from parents, and perfecting newfound physical skills and speech.
- The toddler is noted for having a fluctuating appetite and strong food preferences.
- Some methods of dealing with the inconsistencies of the toddler include distraction, ignoring minor infractions, reward and praise, and "time out" in a safe place.
- Use "I" messages as a method of communicating with the child.
- Accident prevention is extremely important during this period because the toddler is very inquisitive and explores everything.
- Good dental health consists of scheduling regular examinations, teaching the toddler how to brush, using fluoride supplements, and avoiding sticky, sugary foods.

# Study Questions

1. How can adults meet the emotional needs of the toddler during the "negative" stage?
2. Prepare a day's menu for the toddler. Include between-meal snacks.
3. List several situations that frighten you. What can you do to keep from transmitting these fears to others?
4. Define "parallel play." Of what value is play to the child?
5. What is the adult's role in the child's speech development?
6. Steve, age 3, recently had his appendix removed. The doctor has written on his chart that Steve has had a regression in bowel and bladder control. What does this mean?
7. Mrs. Jones, your neighbor, is discouraged because 2-year-old Billy signals that he needs to go to the toilet *after* he has soiled his pants. Discuss various ways to cope with this common problem.
8. What factors must be considered in selecting shoes and socks for toddlers?
9. List several factors that contribute to good communication with children.
10. Review your newspaper for 1 week. Bring to class accounts of various accidents that have occurred to children during that week. Be prepared to discuss how they might have been prevented.
11. Make a list of household substances that are potentially poisonous to small children. In what cases would you want to induce vomiting? When would you not want to make a child vomit?
12. Describe mouth-to-mouth resuscitation.

# Multiple Choice
# Review Questions

*Choose the most appropriate answer.*

1. The term used to denote the toddler's concentration on self is
   a. ritualism
   b. negativism
   c. egocentric thinking
   d. egomania
2. By 2 years, visual acuity is about
   a. 20/20
   b. 20/40
   c. 20/60
   d. 20/80
3. All the deciduous teeth are generally present by
   a. 1½ years
   b. 1 year
   c. 2 years
   d. 2 ½ years

4. Nutritionally, the toddler is at high risk for
   a. diabetes
   b. vitamin deficiencies
   c. anemia
   d. failure to thrive
5. One of the developmental tasks of the toddler that is most hazardous to safety is
   a. brief attention span
   b. need for ritual
   c. fluctuating appetite
   d. need to explore

## BIBLIOGRAPHY

Bchrman, R. (1992). *Nelson textbook of pediatrics* (14th ed.). Philadelphia: W.B. Saunders.

Howard, B. (1991). Discipline in early childhood. *Pediatric Clinics of North America, 38.*

Levine, M.D., Carey, W.B., & Crocker, A.C. (1992). *Developmental-behavioral pediatrics* (2nd ed.). Philadelphia: W.B. Saunders.

Mahan, L.K., & Arlin, M.T. (1992). *Krause's food, nutrition & diet therapy* (8th ed.). Philadelphia: W.B. Saunders.

Mott, S., James, S.R., & Sperhac, A.M. (1991). *Nursing care of children and families* (2nd ed.). Reading, MA: Addison-Wesley.

Pillitteri, A. (1992). *Maternal and child health nursing.* Philadelphia: J.B. Lippincott.

Poleman, C.M., & Peckenpaugh, N.J. (1991). *Nutrition essentials and diet therapy* (6th ed.). Philadelphia: W.B. Saunders.

Thompson, E.D., & Ashwill, J.W. (1992). *Introduction to pediatric nursing* (6th ed.). Philadelphia: W.B. Saunders.

Whaley, L., & Wong, D. (1991). *Nursing care of infants and children* (4th ed.). St. Louis: C.V. Mosby.

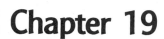

# Chapter 19

## The Preschool Child

# OBJECTIVES

*On completion and mastery of Chapter 19, the student will be able to*

- Define each vocabulary term listed.
- Describe the physical and psychosocial development of children from 3 to 6 years of age, listing age-specific events and guidance when appropriate.
- Discuss the characteristics of a good nursery school.
- Discuss the value of play in the life of a child.
- Designate two toys suitable for the preschool child, and provide the rationale for each choice.
- Describe the speech patterns of the 3-year-old.
- Discuss the value of the following: time-out periods, consistency, role modeling, rewards.
- Describe the developmental characteristics that predispose the preschool child to certain accidents, and suggest methods of prevention for each type of accident.

## General Characteristics

The child from 3 to 6 is often referred to as the *preschool child*. This period is marked by a slowing down of the growth process.

**Physical Development.** The infant who tripled birth weight at 1 year has only doubled the 1-year weight by age 6. For instance, the baby who weighs 20 pounds on the first birthday will probably weigh about 40 pounds by the sixth. The child between ages 3 and 6 grows taller and loses the chubbiness seen during the toddler period. Appetite fluctuates widely. The normal pulse rate is 90–110 beats/min. The rate of respirations during relaxation is about 20/min. The systolic blood pressure is about 85–90 mmHg; the diastolic is about 60 mmHg. Preschool children have good control of their muscles and participate in vigorous play; they become more adept at using old skills as each year passes. They can swing and jump higher. Their gait resembles that of an adult. They are quicker and have more self-confidence than they did as toddlers. Although physical development of the preschool child may seem slower and steadier, certain difficulties stem from increased independence, life in a social world, and increased cognitive ability.

**Cognitive Development.** The thinking of the preschool child is unique. Piaget calls this period the *preoperational phase*. It comprises the ages of 2–7 years and is divided into two

stages, the *preconceptual stage*, age 2–4 years, and the *intuitive thought stage*, age 4–7 years. Of importance in the preconceptual stage is the increasing development of language and symbolic functioning. Symbolic functioning is seen in the play of children who pretend that an empty box is a fort; they create a mental image to stand for something that is not there.

Another characteristic of this period is *egocentrism*, a type of thinking in which children have difficulty seeing any point of view other than their own. Because children's knowledge and understanding are restricted to their own limited experiences, misconceptions arise. One misconception is *animism*. This is a tendency to attribute life to inanimate objects. Another is *artificialism*, the idea that the world and everything in it are created by people. Table 19–1 lists examples of all three characteristics of thought at this age.

The intuitive stage is one of prelogical thinking. Experience and logic are based on outside appearance (the child does not understand that a wide glass and a tall glass can both contain four ounces of juice).

A distinctive characteristic of intuitive thinking is *centering*, the tendency to concentrate on a single outstanding characteristic of an object while excluding its other features.

With time and experience, more mature conceptual awareness is established. The process is highly complex, and the implications for practical application are numerous. Interested students are encouraged to explore these concepts through further study. Box 19–1 summarizes some major theories of personality development for the preschooler.

## Physical, Mental, Emotional, and Social Development

### THE 3-YEAR-OLD

Three-year-olds are a delight to their parents. They are helpful and can assist in simple household chores. They obtain articles when directed and return them to the proper place. Three-year-olds come very close to the ideal picture that parents have in mind of their child. They are living proof that their parents' guidance during the trying 2-year-old period has been rewarded. Temper tantrums are less frequent, and in general the 3-year-old is less erratic. Of course, they are still individuals, but they seem to be able to direct their primitive in-

**Table 19–1.** THE NATURE OF EARLY CHILDHOOD THOUGHT

|  | Sample Questions | Typical Answers |
|---|---|---|
| *Egocentrism* | | |
| | Why does the sun shine? | To keep me warm. |
| | Why is there snow? | For me to play in. |
| | Why is grass green? | Because that's my favorite color. |
| | What are TV sets for? | To watch my favorite shows and cartoons. |
| *Animism* | | |
| | Why do trees have leaves? | To keep them warm. |
| | Why do stars twinkle? | Because they're happy and cheerful. |
| | Why does the sun move in the sky? | To follow children and hear what they say. |
| | Where do boats go at night? | They sleep like we do. |
| *Artificialism* | | |
| | What causes rain? | Someone emptying a watering can. |
| | Why is the sky blue? | It has been painted. |
| | What is the wind? | A man blowing. |
| | What causes thunder? | A man grumbling. |

From Helms, D., & Turner, J. (1978). *Exploring child behavior: Basic principles* (p. 447). Philadelphia: W.B. Saunders

stincts better than previously. They can help dress and undress themselves (Fig. 19–1), use the toilet, and wash their hands. They eat independently, and their table manners have improved.

The 3-year-old talks in longer sentences and can express thoughts: "What are you doing?" "Where is Daddy?" (Box 19–2). They are more company to their parents and other adults because they can talk about their experiences

---

| BOX 19–1 | **Features of Major Theories of Development During Early Childhood** |
|---|---|

**Sigmund Freud**

- Critical period for socialization
- Sensual pleasure centers on genitals
- Child's wishes to satisfy desires lead to conflict with opposite-sex parent
- Child identifies with same-sex parent: conflict is resolved and foundation of appropriate sex role is established
- Response of opposite-sex parent (e.g., degree of warmth and affection) influences child's personality development
- Same-sex parent is model for child's acquisition of adult values

**Erik Erikson**

- Parental and peer responses have major effect on child's socialization
- Child identifies with same-sex parent and adopts that parent's behavior to develop personal identity
- Positive self-image and strong personal identity depend on peer and parental support during child's first efforts toward appropriate sex-role behavior.

**Lawrence Kohlberg**

- Child first understands appropriate sex role, and then identifies with same-sex parent
- Child begins to think and behave as others of that sex, and thus to identify with that sex
- Child's understanding of competent, acceptable behavior is of greatest importance in socialization

**Jean Piaget**

- Sensorimotor development is basis of cognitive development
- Child changes from having limited, reflex responses to the outer world to relating more actively with outside events
- Child is egocentric (thinks everyone sees the same world as self)
- Child can form general concepts but cannot reason

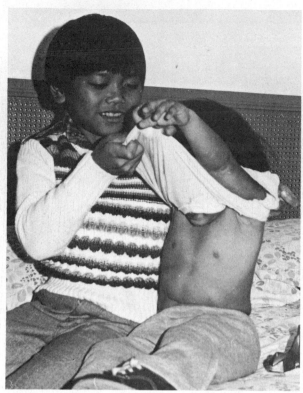

**Figure 19–1.** The preschooler gets an assist from his older brother. (From Tackett, J.J., & Hunsberger, M. [1981]. *Family-centered care of children and adolescents* [p. 389]. Philadelphia: W.B. Saunders.)

(Fig. 19–2). They are imaginative, talk to their toys, and imitate what they see about them. Soon they begin to make friends outside the immediate family. The type of play typical of this period is both *parallel* and *associative*. Children play in loosely associated groups. Their play is often similar. Because they can now converse with playmates, they find satisfaction in joining their activities. Three-year-olds do not play cooperatively for long periods of time, but at least it is a start. Much of their play still consists of watching others, but now they can offer verbal

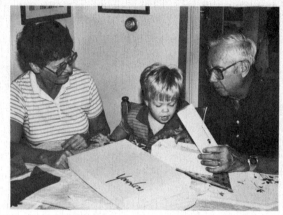

**Figure 19–2.** Happy birthday, Grandpa! The preschool child's world begins to extend outward.

| BOX 19–2 | Linguistic Abilities of the 2-Year-Old and the 3-Year-Old |
| --- | --- |

In language, what a difference a year makes. These lists contain the verbatim comments of two small girls, both of whom were playing with toys in the presence of their mothers and other adults. Note the much greater language skill of the 3-year-old, including her ability to ask questions.

| 2-Year-Old Girl | 3-Year-Old Girl |
| --- | --- |
| The rug | Hey, I found Captain Kangaroo |
| The pretty rug | Mummy? |
| Table | Can I have this? |
| Dish | What shall I fix with this? |
| Doggy tired | What did you found? |
| The book fall down | Won't it be fun to play with these? |
| Want hankie | I show you how to play animals |
| Other side | Hey, this is my dollie |
| Oh, other side | And then now I will line all mine up like this |

From Kagan, J. & Havemann, E. (1968). *Psychology: An introduction.* New York: Harcourt, Brace & World; and Shirley, M.M. (1933). *The first two years.* Institute of Child Welfare Monograph No. 7. Minneapolis: University of Minnesota Press. Copyright 1933 by University of Minnesota.

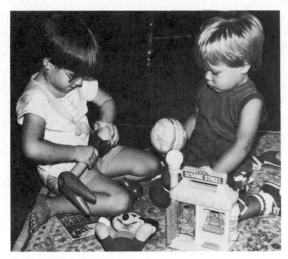

**Figure 19–3.** Preschoolers enjoy both parallel and associative play.

advice, should they feel the need. They can ask others to "come out and play." If 3-year-olds are placed in a strange situation with children they do not know, they commonly revert to "parallel play" because it is more comfortable (Fig. 19–3).

At this time, there is a change in the relationship of the children and parents. They begin to find enjoyment away from Mom and Dad, although they want them nearby when needed. They begin to lose some of their interest in their mother, who up to this time has been more or less their total world. The father's prestige begins to increase. Romantic attachment to the parent of the opposite sex is seen during this period. Mary wants "to marry Daddy" when she grows up. Children also begin to identify themselves with the parent of the same sex.

Preschool children have more fears than the infant or the older child. Some of the many causes of this are increased intelligence, which enables them to recognize potential dangers; development of memory; and graded independence, which brings them into contact with many new situations. Toddlers are not afraid of walking in the street, because they do not understand its danger. Preschool children realize that trucks can injure, and they worry about crossing the street. This fear is well founded, but many others are not.

The fear of bodily harm, particularly the loss of body parts, is peculiar to this stage. The little boy who discovers that baby sister is made dif-

ferently may worry that she has been injured. He wonders if this will happen to him. Masturbation is common during this stage as children attempt to reassure themselves that they are all right (see p. 485). Other common fears include fear of animals, fear of the dark, and fear of strangers. Night wandering is typical of this age group (see Box 18–1).

Preschool children become angry when others attempt to take their possessions. They grab, slap, and hang on to them for dear life. They become very distraught if toys do not work the way they should. They resent being disturbed from play. They are sensitive, and their feelings are easily hurt. Much of the unpleasant social behavior seen during this time is normal and necessary to the child's total pattern of development.

## THE 4-YEAR-OLD

Four is a stormy age. Children are not as eager to please and willing as they were at 3 years. They are more aggressive and like to show off. They are eager to let others know they are superior, and they are prone to pick on playmates, often taking sides and making life difficult for the child who does not measure up to their standards. Four-year-olds are boisterous, tattle on others, and may begin to swear if they are around children or adults who use profanity. They recount personal family activities with amazing recall but forget where their tricycle has been left. At this age, children become interested in how old they are and want to know the exact age of each playmate. It bolsters their ego to know that they are older than someone else in the group. They also become interested in the relationship of one person to another. Timmy is a brother, but also Daddy's son.

Four-year-olds can use scissors with success. They can lace their shoes. Vocabulary has increased to about 1500 words. They run simple errands and can play with others for longer periods of time. Many feats are done for a purpose. For instance, they no longer run just for the sake of running. Instead, they run to get someplace or see something. They are imaginative and like to pretend they are doctors or fire fighters. They begin to prefer playing with friends of the same sex.

The preschool child enjoys simple toys and common objects (Fig. 19–4). Raw materials are more appealing than toys that are ready-made and complete in themselves. An old cardboard

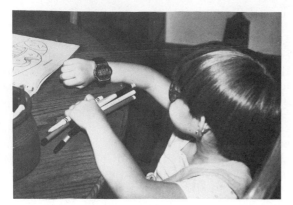

**Figure 19–4.** A watch enthralls this preschooler.

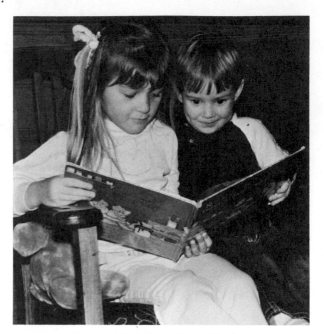

**Figure 19–6.** Story time with sister.

box that can be moved about and climbed into is more fun than a doll house with tiny furniture (Fig. 19–5). A box of sand or colored pebbles can be made into roads and mountains. Parents should avoid showering their children with ready-made toys. Instead, they can select materials that are absorbing and that stimulate the child's imagination.

Stories that interest young children depict their daily experiences (Fig. 19–6). If the story has a simple plot, it must be related to what they understand in order to hold their interest. They also enjoy music; they like records they can march around to, music videos, and simple instruments they can shake or bang. (Make up a song about their daily life, and watch their reaction.)

Children's curiosity about sex continues to heighten. If the parents have answered questions simply, they should not be alarmed to find their children checking up on them. It is common for children of this age to take down their panties in front of friends of the opposite sex. They discuss their differences with their friends. Older children who are more sensitive about their bodies should be told that this is a natural curiosity seen in small children. This may rid them of guilt feelings that they might harbor, particularly if they participated in similar activities during the preschool period. Children are as matter-of-fact about these investigations as they would be about any other learning experience and are easily distracted to other interests.

Between 3 and 4, children begin to wonder about death and dying. They may be the hero who shoots the intruder dead, or they may witness a situation in which an animal is killed. Their questions are direct. "What is 'dead'? Will I die?" There are no specific answers to these

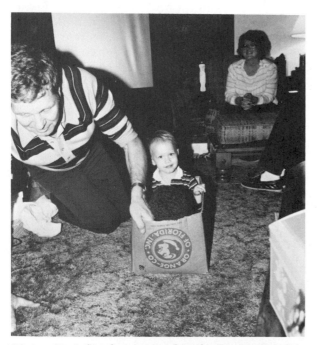

**Figure 19–5.** Simple toys stimulate the imagination of the preschool child.

inquiries. The worldview of the family is important to the interpretation of this complex phenomenon.

Perhaps children can become acquainted with death through objects not of particular significance to them. For instance, the flower dies at the end of the summer. It does not bloom anymore. It no longer needs sunshine or water, for it is not alive. Usually young children realize that others die, but they do not relate death to themselves. If they continue to pursue the question of whether or not they will die, parents should be casual and reassure them that people do not generally die until they have lived a long and happy life. Of course, as they grow older they will discover that sometimes children do die. The underlying idea, nevertheless, is to encourage questions as they appear and gradually help them accept the truth without undue fear. There are many excellent books for children about death. Two that are appropriate for the preschool child are *Geranium Mornings* by S. Powell, and *My Grandpa Died Today* by J. Fassler.

### THE 5-YEAR-OLD

Five is a comfortable age. Children are more responsible, enjoy doing what is expected of them, have more patience, and like to finish what they have started. Five-year-olds are serious about what they can and cannot do. They talk constantly and are inquisitive about their environment. They want to do things correctly and seek answers to their questions from those who they consider to "know" the answers. Five-year-old children can play games governed by rules. They are less fearful because they feel their environment is controlled by authorities. Their worries are less profound than at an earlier age.

The physical growth of 5-year-olds is not outstanding. Their height may increase 2–3 inches, and they may gain 3–6 pounds. The variations in height and weight of a group of 5-year-olds are remarkable. They may begin to lose their deciduous teeth at this time. They can run and play games simultaneously, jump three or four steps at once, and tell a penny from a nickel or a dime. They can name the days of the week and understand what a week-long vacation is. They usually can print their first name.

Five-year-olds can ride a tricycle around the playground with speed and dexterity. They can

use a hammer to pound nails. Adults should encourage them to develop motor skills and not be continually reminding them to "be careful." The practice children experience will enable them to compete with others during the school-age period and will increase confidence in their own abilities. As at any age, children should not be scorned for failure to meet adult standards. Overdirection by solicitous adults is damaging. Children must learn to do tasks themselves in order for the experience to be satisfying.

The number and type of TV programs that parents allow the preschool child to watch is a topic for discussion. Although children enjoyed TV at 3 or 4 years of age, it was usually for short periods of time. They could not understand much of what was going on. The 5-year-old has better comprehension and may spend a great deal of time watching TV. The plan of management differs with each family. Whatever is decided needs to be discussed with the child. TV should not be allowed to interfere with good health habits, for example, sleep, meals, and physical activity. Most parents find that children do not insist on watching TV if there is something better to do (see p. 50).

# Guidance

### DISCIPLINE, SETTING LIMITS

Much has been written on the subject of discipline, which has changed considerably over time. Today, authorities place much importance on the development of a continuous, warm relationship between children and their parents. They believe this helps prevent many problems. The following is a brief discussion that may help the nurse in guiding parents.

Children need limits for their behavior. Setting limits makes them feel secure, protects them from danger, and relieves them from making decisions that they may be too young to formulate. Children who are taught acceptable behavior have more friends and feel better about themselves. They live more enjoyably within the neighborhood and society. The manner in which discipline or setting limits is carried out varies from culture to culture. It also varies among different socioeconomic groups. Individual differences occur among families and between parents and vary according to the characteristics of each child.

The purpose of discipline is to teach and to

gradually shift control from parents to the child, that is, self-discipline. Positive reinforcement for appropriate behavior has been cited as more effective than punishment for poor behavior (Levine, Carey, & Crocker, 1992). Expectations must be appropriate to the age and understanding of the child. The nurse encourages parents to try to be consistent because "mixed messages" are confusing for the learner.

**Timing and Time Out.** Most researchers agree that to be effective, discipline must be given at the time the incident occurs. It should also be adapted to the seriousness of the infraction. The child's self-worth must always be considered. Warning the preschool child who appears to be getting into trouble may be helpful. Too many warnings without follow-up, however, lead to ineffectiveness. Spankings, for the most part, are not productive. The child associates the fury of the parents with the pain rather than with the wrong deed, because anger is the predominant factor in the situation. Thus, the real value of the spanking is lost. Beatings administered by parents as a release for their own pent-up emotions are totally inappropriate and can lead to child-abuse charges. In addition, the parent serves as a role model of aggression. Whether a parent is affectionate, warm, or cold (uncaring) also plays a role in the effectiveness of child rearing. Time-out periods, such as sitting for 5 minutes in a chair or corner, are one alternative to inappropriate punishment. Parents need to be taught to resist using power and authority for their own sake. As the child understands more clearly, privileges can be withheld. The reasons for such actions are carefully explained.

**Reward.** Rewarding the child for good behavior is a positive and effective method of discipline. This can be done with hugs, smiles, tone of voice, and praise. Praise can always be tied with the act: "Thank you, Suzy, for picking up your toys." "I appreciate your standing quietly like that." The encouragement of positive behavior eliminates many of the undesirable effects of punishment.

**Consistency and Modeling.** Being consistent is difficult for parents. Realistically, it is only an ideal to strive for—no parent is consistent all the time. Consistency must exist *between* parents as well as within each parent. It is suggested that parents establish a general style for what, when, how, and to what degree punishment is appropriate to misconduct. Parents who are lax or erratic in discipline and who alter-

nate it with punishment have children who experience increased behavioral difficulties.

The influence of modeling or good example has been widely explored. Studies show that adult models significantly influence children's education. Children identify and imitate adult behavior, verbal and nonverbal. Parents who are aggressive and repeatedly lose control demonstrate the power of action over words. Those who communicate, show respect and encouragement, and set appropriate limits are more positive role models. Finally, parents need assistance in reviewing parental discipline during their own childhood in order to recognize destructive patterns that they may be repeating.

## BAD LANGUAGE

Parents express astonishment at the words that flow from the mouths of their sweet little children during the preschool period. Bad language is inevitable. Caretakers should suppress the desire to shout their disapproval. The small child delights in attention, and it does not matter, unfortunately, whether the attention is good or bad. Swearing at this age is not particularly meaningful because children are merely imitating what they hear—the words have no real significance to them. They use swearing as a way to identify themselves with the older children in the neighborhood and to shock adults. One mother dealt with this problem by saying, "Chad, Mommy doesn't mind if you hear or know what that word means, but we don't use it in our home any more than you would think of going outdoors without your clothes on." Chad felt free to discuss what he heard with his mother, and shortly thereafter his interest was taken up by other subjects.

## JEALOUSY

Jealousy is a normal response to actual, supposed, or threatened loss of affection. Children or adults may feel insecure in their relationship with the person they love. The closer children are to their parents, the greater is their fear of losing them. Children envy the new baby. They love the sibling but resent its presence. They cannot understand the turmoil within themselves (Fig. 19–7). Jealousy of a new baby is strongest in children under 5 years of age and is shown in various ways. Children may be aggressive and may bite or pinch, or they may be rather discreet and may hug and kiss the baby

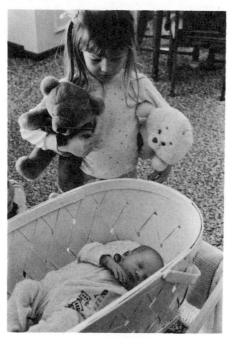

**Figure 19–7.** An additional family member creates a lot of new feelings for the preschool child.

with a determined look on their face. Another common situation is children's attempt to identify with the baby. They revert to wetting the bed or want to be powdered after they urinate. Some 4-year-olds even try the bottle, but it is usually a big disappointment to them.

Preschool children may be jealous of the attention that their mother gives to their father. They may also envy the children they play with if they have bigger and better toys. School-age children are more often jealous of those who are more athletic or popular. There is less jealousy in an only child, who is the center of attention and has a minimum number of rivals. Siblings of varied ages are apt to feel that the younger ones are "pets" or that the older ones have more special privileges.

Parents can help reduce jealousy by the early management of individual occurrences. Preparing the young children for the arrival of the new baby minimizes the blow. They should not be made to think that they are being crowded. If the new baby is going to occupy their crib, it is best to settle the older child happily in a large bed before the baby is born. Children should feel that they are helping with care of the infant. Parents can inflate their ego from time to time by reminding them of the many activities they can do that the new baby cannot.

If it is convenient, the new baby is given a bath or a feeding while the older child is asleep. In this way, the older sibling avoids one occasion in which the mother shows the newborn affection for a relatively long time. Some persons think that giving the child a pet to care for helps. Many hospitals offer sibling courses that assist parents in helping the child to overcome jealousy.

If the child intends to hit the baby or another child, both children must be separated, but the one who has caused or is about to cause the injury needs as much attention as the victim, if not more. Similar aggressiveness is seen when the child is made to share toys. It is even more difficult to learn to share Mother, so the child must be given time to adjust to new situations. Children are assured that they are loved but told that they cannot injure others.

## THUMB-SUCKING

From 1914 to 1921, the United States Children's Bureau pamphlet entitled *Infant Care* cautioned mothers that thumb-sucking would deform the mouth and cause drooling. It also suggested that the thumb or fingers be consistently removed from the mouth while the baby's attention is diverted (Levine, Carey, & Crocker, 1992). Today we recognize that thumb-sucking is an instinctual behavioral pattern that is considered normal. It is seen by sonogram about the 29th week of embryonic life. Although the cause is not fully understood, it satisfies and comforts the infant.

Finger- or thumb-sucking will not have a detrimental effect on the teeth as long as the habit is discontinued before the second teeth erupt. Most children give up the habit by the time they reach school age, although they may regress during periods of stress or fatigue. Management includes education and support of the parents in order to relieve their anxiety and prevent secondary emotional problems in their children. The child who is trying to stop thumb-sucking is given praise and encouragement.

## MASTURBATION

Masturbation is common in both sexes during the preschool years. The child experiences pleasurable sensations, which lead to repetition of the behavior. It is beneficial to rule out other causes of this activity, such as rashes or penile or vaginal irritation. Masturbation is also exhibited in the child who feels emotionally isolated or anxious. A variety of interpretations of masturbation have been postulated; however, many questions about the significance of this behavior for the child remain unanswered. Masturbation at this age is considered harmless if the child is outgoing, sociable, and not preoccupied with the activity. One common fear that could be explored in boys is that of castration.

Education of the parents consists of assuring them that this behavior is normal and not harmful to the child, who is merely curious about sexuality. The cultural and moral background of the family must be considered in assessing the degree of discomfort about this experience. A history of the time and place of masturbation and the parental response is helpful. Punitive reactions are discouraged, as these can potentially harm the child. Parents are advised to ignore the behavior and distract the child with some other activity. The child needs to know that masturbation is not acceptable in public; however, this must be explained in a nonthreatening manner. Children who masturbate excessively and who have experienced a great deal of disruption in their lives benefit from ongoing counseling.

## ENURESIS

**Description.** The term *enuresis* is derived from the Greek word *enourein*, "to void urine." Bedwetting has existed for generations and affects many cultures. There are two types: primary and secondary. Primary enuresis refers to bedwetting in the child who has never been dry. Secondary enuresis refers to a recurrence in a child who has been dry for a period of 1 year or more. *Diurnal*, or daytime, wetting is less common than *nocturnal*, or nighttime, episodes. It is more common in boys than in girls; there is a higher incidence among the poor; and there appears to be a genetic influence. In many children, a specific cause is never determined. By the age of 5 years, about 92% of children achieve daytime dryness. By 12–14 years of age, approximately 98% of children remain dry during the night (Rappaport, 1992).

Some organic causes of nocturnal enuresis are urinary tract infections, diabetes mellitus, diabetes insipidus, seizure disorders, obstructive uropathy, abnormalities of the urinary tract, and sleep disorders. Sudden onset may be due to psychological stress, such as a death in the family or divorce. Giggling may precipitate wetting. Maturational delay of the nervous system and small bladder capacity have also been suggested as causes.

**Treatment and Nursing Care.** A detailed history is obtained. Such factors as the pattern of wetting, number of times per night or week, number of daytime voidings, type of stream, dysuria, amount of fluid taken between dinner and bedtime, family history, stress, and reactions of parents and child are documented. The nurse also determines any medications that the child may be taking and the extent to which social life is inhibited by the problem, for example, inability to spend the night away from home. Developmental landmarks, including toilet training, are reviewed. If there appears to be an organic cause, appropriate blood and urine studies are undertaken. In most cases, physical findings are negative.

Education of the family is extremely crucial to preventing secondary emotional problems. Parents are reassured that many children experience enuresis and that it is self-limited in nature. Power struggles, shame, and guilt are fruitless and destructive. Reassurance and support by the nurse are of great help.

Therapies for bedwetting are subject to controversy. Some modalities include counseling, hypnosis, behavior modification, and pharmacotherapy. Moisture-activated conditioning devices are also commercially available (an alarm rings when the child wets). These have had limited success. Bladder-training exercises, in which the child is asked to withhold the urine for as long as possible, may stretch the bladder and increase its size. The child's bedroom should be as close to the bathroom as possible, and a night-light employed. Limiting fluids at bedtime and awakening the child during the night have not been highly successful. A spontaneous cure may occur with little or no intervention or after other types of treatment have failed.

The nurse prepares the parents for relapses, which are common. The response to various therapies is highly individual. Overzealous treatment is to be avoided. A nonpunitive, matter-of-fact attitude appears prudent. Children are involved in any routine that is adopted and allowed to care for themselves as much as possible. Imipramine hydrochloride (Tofranil) has been found to decrease enuresis in controlled studies. It is administered before bedtime and is used only on a short-term basis. Imipramine has a variety of side effects, including mood and sleep disturbances and gastrointestinal upsets. Overdose can lead to cardiac arrhythmias, which may be life-threatening. Dosage and administration should be closely supervised. It is not recommended for children under age 6. Desmopressin (DDAVP), an antidiuretic hormone, has been used with limited success.

## Nursery School

The change from home to nursery school is a big step toward independence. At this age, children are adjusting to the outside world as well as to the family. Some children have the complicating factor of a new baby in the house. The child also finds that parents are beginning to expect more neatness and more cooperative play with others. This transition period is troublesome.

A good nursery school provides the child with opportunities to release pent-up emotions (Fig. 19–8). There is plenty of room to run and shout. The toys are sturdy, and children can manipulate them because they are the appropriate size. Because the toys are not their own,

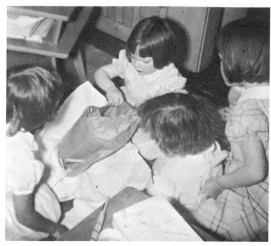

**Figure 19–9.** Socialization is an important phase of the preschool period. Children begin to understand friendship.

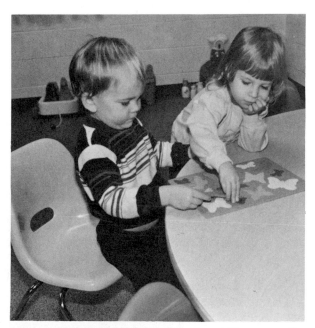

**Figure 19–8.** Although home is cozier, children soon discover that nursery school is fun.

they find them easier to share. Children are not as emotionally involved with their teacher as with their parents. They feel more able to express their negative and positive feelings, and the teacher can be more objective about them. Rules and regulations are kept to a minimum. The teacher expects the children to choose their play materials and playmates. Children take responsibility for their own belongings.

Children are accepted into nursery schools between the ages of 2 and 5 years. Most sessions last about 3 hours. A good nursery school challenges children's imagination, acquaints children with a social world, introduces children to various cultures, and does this so that it adds to their security and increases their independence (Fig. 19–9).

Parents who are considering nursery school for their child should evaluate the following factors: How many teachers are there? What is their educational background? Are the physical facilities adequate? How many children are there per teacher? What is the cost? Is the child ready for nursery school? Parents will also want to visit the school and talk with the person in charge. They may also wish to talk with parents whose children are attending the program.

The student nurse may have the opportunity to visit a nursery school during studies of the well child. This can be a rewarding experience if nurses use their powers of observation. When observing an individual child, they should compare the child with *others* in their age group

| BOX 19–3 | Behavioral Characteristics of the Preschool Child |
|---|---|

Watch for and evaluate the following in terms of a child's security and independence.

**Physical Development**

Ability to walk, run, jump, use play equipment
General health: easily fatigued, etc.

**Emotional Development**

Easily excited
Whines, cries frequently
Evidence of temper tantrums
Persistence in a task
Aggressive
Shy
Reaction to failure

**Social Development**

Talkative
Quiet
Plays with others
Plays near others
Special friends
Tends to lead
Tends to follow
Friendly toward other children and adults
Ability to share
Ability to take turns
Behavior when child desires an object or attention of the teacher

**Degree of Independence**

Removes coat, hat, boots; puts them away
Attends to toilet needs
Gets a drink
Amount of time going from one activity to another
Dependence on adult suggestions and help

**Relaxation**

Relaxes during rest periods
Sits and listens to stories
Is restless, in constant motion

**Specific Routines**

*Music period:* sings, plays games
*Snacks:* Eats lunch, takes other children's food, wanders about, disturbs those nearby, plays with food
*Free play period:* toys preferred, amount of skill using hands, span of interest, evidence of destructive play, plays with others or alone, has imaginary friend

and not merely with one other child. The types of behavior to be observed are outlined in Box 19–3.

## Daily Care

The child between 3 and 6 years of age does not require the extensive physical care given to a baby but still needs a bath each day (more than ever) and a shampoo at least once a week. It is best to keep hairstyles simple. A little girl fares the worst in this area, particularly if her mother expects her to sit still for an elaborate coiffure.

**Teeth.** The child needs to visit a dentist regularly, at least every 6 months. The deciduous teeth are important for the proper formation of the permanent teeth and should not be neglected. The first visit may be merely for an examination. In this way, the child becomes acquainted with the dentist and the appearance of the office. When calling for the appointment, the mother should tell the receptionist that this is Susie's first visit. It also helps to tell Susie a little in advance that she is going and that the dentist will look into her mouth. Too much detail may frighten the imaginative preschool child. The child's diet should continue to emphasize milk, vegetables, and fruits (Table 19–2). Excess sweets, which contribute to dental decay, are restricted. Children are reminded to brush their teeth regularly.

**Need for Independence.** Preschool children like to do things for themselves. Simple clothes make it easy for them to dress. A hook nailed to the door within reach is helpful. These children should dress and undress themselves as much as they can. Mother or Father can assist but not take over. They must be reminded to use the toilet from time to time. Some 3-year-olds may still need assistance to get up onto the seat. There is occasional soiling of garments that embarrasses the preschool child. A stool kept next to the bathroom sink enables children to wash their hands.

**Table 19–2.** RECOMMENDED FOOD INTAKE FOR GOOD NUTRITION ACCORDING TO FOOD GROUPS AND DAILY DIETARY ALLOWANCES: PRESCHOOL (4 TO 6 YEARS)

| Food Groups | Servings per Day | Serving Size | |
|---|---|---|---|
| | | 4–5 yrs | 6 yrs |
| Bread Group | 4–6 | | |
| • Bread | | 1½ slice | 1–2 slices |
| • Cereal | | 1 oz | 1 oz |
| • Rice and pasta | | ⅓ C | ½ C |
| Vegetable Group | 3–5 total | | |
| • Green-yellow vegetables (vitamin A source) | 1 or more | 4 tbsp | 4 tbsp |
| • Other vegetables | 2 or more | 4 tbsp | ⅓ C |
| Fruit Group | At least 3 total | | |
| • Citrus fruits, berries, tomato, cabbage, cantaloupe (vitamin C source) | 1 or more | ½ C | 1 medium |
| • Other fruits (apple, banana) | 2 | ¼ C | ⅓ C |
| Milk Group | 2–3 | | |
| • Milk/yogurt | | ½–¾ C | ½–1 C |
| • Cheese | | (1.5 oz cheese = 1 C milk) | |
| Meat Group | 2 | | |
| • Cooked lean meat, poultry, fish | | 4 tbsp | 4–6 tbsp |
| • Dry beans | | ½ C | ½ C |
| • Egg | | 1 | 1 |
| • Peanut butter | | 2 tbsp | 2–3 tbsp |

Fats, oils, and sweets—USE SPARINGLY

**Recommended Daily Dietary Allowances**

| Protein | Fat-Soluble | Vitamins | Water-Soluble | Vitamins | Minerals | | Energy Needs |
|---|---|---|---|---|---|---|---|
| 24 g | Vitamin A | 500 μg RE | Vitamin C | 45 mg | Calcium | 800 mg | 1800 kcal |
| | Vitamin D | 10 μg | Thiamine | 0.9 mg | Phosphorus | 800 mg | |
| | Vitamin E | 7 mg α—TE | Riboflavin | 1.1 mg | Magnesium | 120 mg | |
| | Vitamin K | 20 μg | Niacin | 12 mg NE | Iron | 10 mg | |
| | | | Vitamin $B_6$ | 1.1 mg | Zinc | 10 mg | |
| | | | Folate | 75 μg | Iodine | 90 μg | |
| | | | Vitamin $B_{12}$ | 1.0 μg | Selenium | 20 μg | |

From Betz, C., et al. (1994). *Family-centered nursing care of children* (2nd ed.). Philadelphia: W. B. Saunders.
Data reprinted with permission from *Recommended dietary allowances: 10th Edition.* Copyright 1989 by the National Academy of Sciences. Published by the National Academy Press, Washington, D.C.; and U.S. Department of Agriculture, Human Nutrition Information Service. (1992). *Food guide pyramid* (Leaflet No. 572). Washington, DC.
*Key:* RE, retinol equivalent; TE, tocopherol equivalent; NE, niacin equivalent.

**Meals.** Preschool children need simple, nourishing meals. Their appetites fluctuate, and they should not be bribed, scolded, or coaxed. Mealtimes should be happy. Parents who use good table manners set an example for children. The milk glass must be unbreakable and not filled completely. A waterproof tablecloth is useful. Children are included in the conversations but not allowed to take over. A nourishing dessert, such as a pudding or fruit, erases the apprehension about what has been left on the child's plate.

**Play.** Preschool children need periods of active play both indoors and outdoors. Their clothes should be loose enough to prevent restriction of movement. Parents who see that their children are having a particularly good time should ask themselves whether it is necessary to interrupt them right at that moment. When children have verbal arguments, parents should avoid rushing in to defend their child. Growth can be painful, but children need to experience it at their own rate.

**Sleep.** Sleep habits vary at this time. Toward the end of the preschool years, children may balk at taking a nap. Instead of insisting that they sleep, parents should see that they engage in something interesting but restful, such as

## Nursing Brief

Imaginary playmates are common and normal during the preschool period and serve many purposes, such as relief from loneliness, mastery of feats, and scapegoat.

reading a story together or playing with a simple puzzle. They need an opportunity to relax.

Prolonging bedtime through ritual routines is still common. Preschool children may awaken frightened during the night. Parents should attend to their needs and reassure them that they are safe and that the parents are close by. A night-light and transitional object, such as a blanket, may help settle the child. If the child persists in awakening and is unusually frightened, professional counseling may be helpful to assess the problem. Usually a few sessions are all that is necessary to provide the child with a sense of control and reassurance.

Children of this age should have a complete physical examination each year. Booster injections of the various immunizations are given when required.

**Accident Prevention.** Accidents are still a major threat during the years from 3 to 5. At this age, children may suffer injuries from a bad fall. Preschool children hurry up and down stairs. They climb trees and stand up on swings. They play hard with their toys, particularly those that they can mount. Stairways must be kept free of clutter. Shoes should have rubber soles, and new ones are bought when the tread becomes smooth. When buying toys, parents must be sure they are sturdy and can take a beating. Preschool children should not be asked to do anything that is potentially dangerous, for example, to carry a glass container or sharp knife to the kitchen sink.

Automobiles continue to be a threat. Children are taught where they can safely ride their tricycle and where they can play ball, and

## Nursing Brief

One mother used color-coded laundry baskets for each of her small children. She placed the clean, folded clothes in the baskets. The children were responsible for taking them to their rooms and putting them away. (Note: The clothes were not always put away, but it is a start!)

they should not be allowed to use sleds on streets that are not blocked off for this purpose. They must not play in or around the car or be left alone in the car. The use of *seatbelt restraints* continues to be important.

Burns that occur at this age are frequently due to the child's experimentation with matches. Children are also intrigued by fancy cigarette lighters. Hot coffee burns are also common. These items are common hazards for this age group; they should be kept well out of reach and their dangers explained to the child.

Poisoning is still a danger. Children try to imitate adults and are apt to sample pills, especially if they smell good. Their increased freedom brings them into contact with many interesting containers in the garage or basement.

Preschool children are also taught the dangers of talking to or accepting rides from strangers. If they are stopped by a driver, they should run to the house of people they know. Parents should make it clear to children in nursery school that they will never send a stranger to call for them. Children must know the dangers of playing in lonely places and of accepting gifts from strangers. Children should always know where to go if Mother or Father or baby-sitter cannot be found. Preschool children still require a good deal of indirect supervision to protect them from dangers that arise from their immature judgment or social environment.

## Play in Health and Illness

### VALUE OF PLAY

It has often been said that play is the business of children. Investigations stress the importance of play to both well and sick children's physical, mental, emotional, and social development. Children climbing on a jungle gym develop coordination of their muscles and exercise all parts of their bodies. They use energy and develop self-confidence. Their imagination may take them to the jungle, where they swing from limb to limb. They face imagined fears and solve problems that would be much more trying, if not impossible, in reality. They communicate with other children and take a further step in developing moral values, that is, taking one's turn and considering others. Other types of play help children learn colors, shapes, sizes, and textures and can teach creativity. This natural and readily available outlet must be tapped by institutional personnel. Children may be unfamiliar with every facet of the hospital, but they know how to play, and playing is a good way for the nurse to establish rapport with them.

## THE NURSE'S ROLE

Some hospitals have well-established programs supervised by play therapists. Play experience may be included in the nurse's educa-

tion. It is not necessary to be an expert in manual dexterity, art, or music; rather one must understand the needs of the child. Play is not just the responsibility of those assigned to it, nor is it confined to certain times or shifts.

Many factors are involved in providing suitable play for children of various ages in the hospital (Table 19–3). The patient's state of health has to be considered. This determines the amount of activity in which they can participate. The nurse can provide many activities

**Table 19–3.** HOW TO CHOOSE AGE-APPROPRIATE TOYS

| Age | Toys | General Considerations |
|---|---|---|
| Infancy | Soft, stuffed animals and dolls<br>Cradle gym<br>Soft balls<br>Bath toys<br>Rattles<br>Pots and pans | Baby likes to pat and hug. Toys should be brightly colored, of different textures, washable; be large enough that they cannot be aspirated; have smooth edges. Infant's attention span is short. Infants look at, reach, grab, chew |
| Toddlerhood | Nest of blocks<br>Push-pull toys<br>Dolls<br>Telephone<br>Rocking horse or chair<br>Wooden pegs and hammer<br>Cloth books<br>Pots and pans<br>Ball | May have favorite toy; enjoys exploring drawers and closets; likes to place things in containers and dump them out; engages in parallel play; may injure others |
| Preschool age | Crayons<br>Simple puzzles<br>Paints with large brushes<br>Finger paints<br>Dolls<br>Dishes, housekeeping equipment<br>Sand box, playground equipment<br>Floating boats for water play<br>Trucks<br>Horns, drums, simple musical instruments<br>Books about familiar circumstances<br>Records, videotapes | Shifts from solitary to parallel to beginning cooperative play; exchanges ideas with others. Engages in active play—climbs, runs, and hammers; imitative play—fire fighter, teacher; imaginative play—let's pretend; creative and dramatic play. Uses toys that do not require fine hand coordination. Plays games that teach safety in everyday life |
| School age | Dolls<br>Doll house<br>Toy housewares<br>Handicrafts<br>Jump rope<br>Skates<br>Construction sets<br>Trains<br>Dress-up materials<br>Table games<br>Books for self-reading<br>Bicycles<br>Puppets<br>Music | Attention span increases; play is more organized, more competitive; child is interested in hobbies or collections of things |

*Continued*

**Table 19–3.** HOW TO CHOOSE AGE-APPROPRIATE TOYS *Continued*

| Age | Toys | General Considerations |
|---|---|---|
| The convalescent child | Ball on string that can be dropped from bed and returned<br>Telephone<br>Easy puzzles<br>Large beads to string<br>Radio<br>Goldfish bowl<br>Miniature autos, trains, dolls, farm animals<br>Stick'ems, paper dolls<br>Hand puppets<br>Lap blackboard<br>Alphabet boards<br>Cutouts<br>(Many toys previously listed are also applicable) | Play should not require a great expenditure of energy; offer a wide variety because the child's interest span is decreased; consider bed limitation; toys should not require long continuous focusing of eyes; consider toys that will be a little easier than those liked when well; pay attention to special interests of individual child |

that relieve stress and provide enjoyment for the patient on bed rest. Overstimulation, nevertheless, would be hazardous for some severely ill children. Nurses are always on guard for signs of fatigue in patients and use their judgment accordingly.

Toys should be safe, durable, and suited to the child's developmental level (Fig. 19–10). Toys should not be sharp or have parts that are easily removed and swallowed. Too many toys at one time are confusing to the child. Complicated toys are frustrating and disappointing. Well-selected toys, such as balls, blocks, and

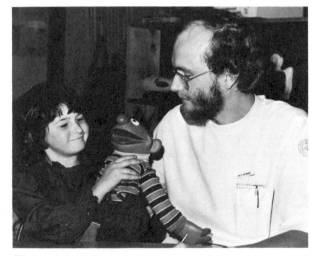

**Figure 19–11.** Puppets are a universal means of communicating with children. (Courtesy of New Hampshire Vocational-Technical College, Claremont, NH.)

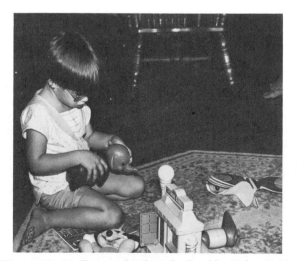

**Figure 19–10.** Toys need to be safe, durable, and suited to the child's developmental needs.

dolls, are useful throughout the years. Each child needs sufficient time to complete the activity. In general, quiet play should precede meals and bedtime for both well and sick children. Investigations have shown that the toys enjoyed by boys and those enjoyed by girls are more similar than dissimilar.

During routine procedures, the nurse can entertain the child with nursery rhymes, stories, nonsense games, songs, finger play, or puppets (Fig. 19–11). Often the other children on the unit can be included for "I'm thinking of something blue, red, and green," and so forth. Simple crafts are fun. The nurse may find various instructions from children's magazines or the local public library. Scrapbooks are entertaining. Children may even enjoy making a storybook about their hospital experience. The nurse involved in enrichment programs for children can make a definite contribution. A student may have helped out at a summer camp, baby-sat, or assisted at Sunday school. Surprise boxes in which a gift is opened every day provide anticipation for the patient. Collections of scraps containing bright ribbons, bits of string, pipe cleaners, paper bags, newspapers, or bits of cotton can be started. Because the turnover of patients is rapid, many projects can simply be repeated with different children.

Music is provided by radio, recorders, and piano. Older children enjoy sending messages to friends via a tape deck. Special children's recordings and videotapes are available. The services of a music therapist are available in some institutions. Drawing materials, finger paints, and modeling clay foster expression and creativity. They require merely a flat surface, such as the overbed table, and a particular medium. The bedridden child can participate in messy projects, too. The bed is simply protected with newspapers or plastic. Children in cribs need adequate back support for such projects. This is done by elevating the mattress or using pillows.

### STORING TOYS

The playroom usually houses most of the toys. Toys should be available for all shifts and should not be locked up at the end of the day. Children may have a durable, washable bag tied to the bed for their possessions. Closets, open shelves, toy chests, cupboards, and bins on rollers may be utilized in the hospital or at home. Pegboards for hanging frequently used items are effective. Sturdy boxes, ice-cream containers, and laundry baskets are other suggestions for housing articles of various sizes and shapes. Children need to be taught how to care for toys following play. If children are to open and close drawers, they should use the handles so that their fingers are not pinched.

### PLAYMATES

Children need playmates to promote social development (Fig. 19–12). The 1-year-old plays

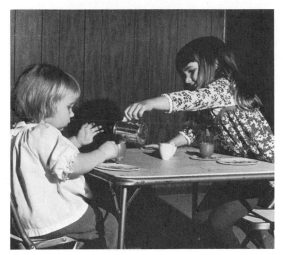

**Figure 19–12.** Playmates promote social development.

near other children. The 2-year-old grabs and pushes and cannot share, but in an individual way acknowledges other children. The older preschool child shows a beginning readiness for cooperative play. The ability to play with others increases during the school years, and in late elementary years girls prefer to play with girls and boys prefer to play with boys. This preference changes during adolescence.

Playmates can be provided in the hospital playroom or on the unit. Children who are ambulatory can visit and play table games with bedridden patients. Of course, the type of illness that each child has must be considered for everyone's protection. If the advisability of a type of play is questionable, advice from the physician may be requested.

Factors applicable to the healthy child at home should also be considered during hospitalization. Occasional play with younger children offers relief from competition with peers. However, continuous association with younger children tends to make children immature in their interests and behavior. Eventually they could fall behind their peers in physical skills and language. On the other hand, the child who is in the constant company of older children might feel inferior. This sets the pattern of submission to others. Older children tend to dominate and interfere with the friendships of younger children, which leads to bickering and disruption of play. When this is pronounced, the younger child loses friends and is unable to develop effective relationships with peers.

Potential dangers can be created by adults

through domination, indifference, and overconcern. The nurse or parent who directs all the child's activities, chooses friends, and plans and thinks for the child is doing the child a grave injustice. If one is indifferent to the social needs of preschool children, they will be lonely in the hospital, avoid peers, and remain friendless. Overly concerned adults cannot bear to have the child mistreated in any way during the normal give-and-take of childhood play. They scold the supposed offender and separate the children. This eventually isolates the child, making it impossible to form the social relationships needed for a healthy personality.

## PLAY AND THE RETARDED CHILD

The child who is mentally retarded needs more stimulation through play than the child who is not. The nurse must consider the mental age of the child rather than the chronologic age when selecting toys. Brightly colored objects should be strung across the crib for the infant. The environment should be as colorful and bright as possible. The child may be introduced to objects of various sizes and textures. Play with other children must be supervised because the poorer judgment of retarded children may get them into difficulty. They may be aggressive and may not realize their own strength. Adequate space in which to run is necessary. These children should be brought into group play gradually. Materials are presented one at a time.

Retarded children may have to be taught how to play, since they may have not had the preschool play experience of the unaffected child. Repetition of play experiences is necessary. Equipment and play materials need to be altered to accommodate the child's size and yet be suitable for the mental age. The nurse or teacher needs to improvise games and songs to meet the special needs of this group (Fig. 19–13).

## OTHER ASPECTS OF PLAY

**Therapeutic Play.** Play and toys can be of therapeutic value in retraining muscles, improving eye-hand coordination, and helping children to crawl and walk (push-pull toys). A musical instrument, such as the clarinet, promotes flexion and extension of the fingers. Blowing is an excellent prerequisite for speech therapy. Therapists supervise such activities. They leave specific instructions if they wish their work to be reinforced on the unit.

**Play Therapy.** The nurse may also hear the term *play therapy* used. This technique is used for the child under stress. A well-equipped playroom is provided. Children are free to play with whatever articles they choose. A counselor may be in the room observing and talking with the child, or the child may be observed through a one-way glass window. By using these as well as other methods, the therapist obtains a better understanding of the patient's struggles, fears, resentments, and feelings toward self and others. When children act out their feelings through "dramatic play," the feelings are externalized, which relieves tension. The interpretation of child behavior is complex and requires a great deal of time, study, and sensitivity to be fully understood.

**Art Therapy.** Ulman and Dachinger have defined art as "the meeting ground of the world inside and the world outside" (1975). Art therapy is useful in communicating with children and adults. It is becoming more widely utilized. The art therapist is specially trained to assist children to express their feelings and communicate through drawings, clay, and other media. Some hospitals with inpatient mental health units have art therapy departments. An example of art work created by a sexually abused child is depicted on page 899.

## OBSERVATIONS AND RECORDING

The nurse who is with children daily can describe their behavior. It is important to describe

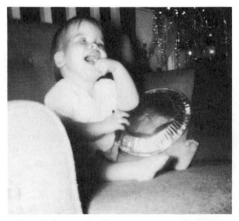

**Figure 19–13.** Improvised games and songs amuse Kelly.

good and poor behavior, conversations that seem pertinent, and the child's relationships with other children in the hospital. What is the approach to play? Do they join in freely or linger outside the group? Do they prefer active or quiet activities? Do they seem to tolerate frustrations? Can they talk with their playmates and convey their ideas? What kind of attention span do they have? These observations and charting are meaningful and promote better understanding and appropriate interventions by nurses and other personnel.

## KEY POINTS

- The child from 3 to 5 is often referred to as the "preschool child." During this period, the child grows taller and loses the chubbiness of the toddler period.
- Gross and fine motor skills become more developed, as evidenced by participation in running, skipping, and drawing pictures.
- Piaget refers to the preschool period as one in which symbolic thought processes and language emerge.
- Language ability develops rapidly, and the child is able to construct rather complicated sentences by the end of this period.
- Play is the business of children. It contributes to physical and mental well-being. Toys should be age-appropriate and safe.
- Social issues of the preschool period include learning to share and to control impulses.
- Common concerns of parents during this period include how to set limits, handle jealousy, and respond to thumb-sucking and masturbation.
- The preschool child is more fearful than the toddler.
- Careful evaluation of day-care and nursery school programs is important to ensure high-quality care.
- Accidents are still a major hazard for preschool children because of their increased locomotive skills and immature judgment.

# Study Questions

1. In what ways do the needs of the preschool child differ from those of the infant? The toddler?
2. Debbie, age 3, has a new baby brother. Discuss how you would prepare her for this situation.
3. What is meant by the term *discipline*? How do you feel about bodily punishment? Be prepared to discuss your answer in class.
4. Mrs. Welsh is wondering what to do with 4-year-old Freddie. She states, "Lately he just never bothers to come into the house to urinate." What do you think would be the most effective way to handle this situation?
5. How do you feel the preschool child would react to hospitalization? Give reasons for your answer.
6. Henry is 5 years old. His father died unexpectedly. What special problems might this present to him?
7. What are the characteristics of a good nursery school?
8. You have been observing nursery school children during the past week. How will this experience help you during your assignment to the pediatric unit?
9. Sandy, age 3, and Joan, age 2, are playing in the living room. There is a squabble, and when you appear, Sandy is snatching a book from Joan. Joan starts to cry. What do you do?

# Multiple Choice Review Questions

*Choose the most appropriate answer.*

1. Parents of the preschool child are taught that fear is
   a. rare in the preschool child
   b. abnormal in the preschool child
   c. heightened in the preschool child
   d. to be ignored in the preschool child

2. For the preschool child's behavior, parents serve as
   a. role models
   b. dictators
   c. buddies
   d. companions

3. Masturbation is
   a. uncommon during the preschool years
   b. common in both sexes during the preschool years
   c. a sign of extreme anxiety in the preschool child
   d. a sign of incompetent parenting

4. Another name for bedwetting is
   a. enuresis
   b. diuresis
   c. encopresis
   d. diaphoresis

5. A type of therapy that utilizes drawings to communicate with children is
   a. play therapy
   b. art therapy
   c. therapeutic play
   d. recreational therapy

## BIBLIOGRAPHY

Behrman, R.E. (1992). *Nelson textbook of pediatrics* (14th ed.). Philadelphia: W.B. Saunders.

Gellis, S.S., & Kagan, B.M. (1990). *Current pediatric therapy, 13.* Philadelphia: W.B. Saunders.

Graef, J., & Cone, T. (1985). *Manual of pediatric therapeutics* (3rd ed.). Boston: Little, Brown.

Howard, B. (1990). Growing together: Learning independence in the preschool years. *Contemporary Pediatrics, 7,* 11–26.

Levine, M.D., Carey, W.B., & Crocker, A.C. (1992). *Developmental-behavioral pediatrics* (2nd ed.). Philadelphia: W.B. Saunders.

Mott, S., James, S.R., & Sperhac, A.M. (1991). *Nursing care of children and families* (2nd ed.). Reading, MA: Addison-Wesley.

Pillitteri, A. (1992). *Maternal and child health nursing.* Philadelphia: J.B. Lippincott.

Rappaport, L. (1992). Enuresis. In M.D. Levine, W.B. Carey, & A.C. Crocker (1992).

Thompson, E.D., & Ashwill, J.W. (1992). *Pediatric nursing: An introductory text* (6th ed.). Philadelphia: W.B. Saunders.

Ulman, E., & Dachinger, P. (1975). *Art therapy.* New York: Schocken Books.

Whaley, L., & Wong, D. (1991). *Nursing care of infants and children* (4th ed.). St. Louis: C.V. Mosby.

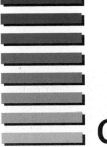

# Chapter 20

# The School-Age Child

# OBJECTIVES

*On completion and mastery of Chapter 20, the student will be able to*

■ Define each vocabulary term listed.
■ Describe the physical and psychosocial development of children from ages 6 to 12, listing age-specific events and type of guidance where appropriate.
■ Plan a diet that will provide adequate nutrition for the school-age child.
■ Discuss how to assist parents in preparing a child for entry into school.
■ List two ways in which school life influences the growing child.
■ Contrast two major theoretic viewpoints of personality development during the school years.
■ List two guidelines to help parents regulate television viewing by their children.
■ Discuss accident prevention in this age group.

## General Characteristics

School-age children from 6 to 12 differ from preschool children in that they are more engrossed in fact than in fantasy and are capable of more sophisticated reasoning (Fig. 20–1).

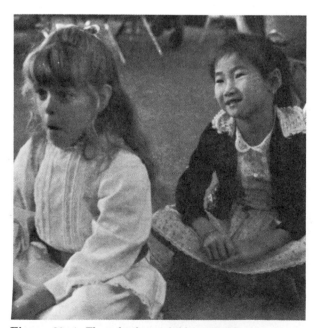

**Figure 20–1.** The school-age child is capable of more sophisticated reasoning.

They have an ardent thirst for knowledge and accomplishment and admire their teachers and adult companions, whom they consider wise. They use the skill and knowledge they obtain to attempt to master the activities they enjoy, including music, sports, and art. Thus, this phase is referred to by Erikson as the *age of industry*. Unsuccessful adaptations at this time can lead to a sense of inferiority. Children in school learn that they must cooperate with others. Participation in group activities heightens. Romantic love for the parent of the opposite sex diminishes, and children identify with the parent of the same sex. Freud refers to this period as a time of *sexual latency* (Box 20–1). The type of acceptance school children receive at home and at school will affect the attitudes they develop about themselves and their role in life. Piaget refers to the thought processes of this period as *concrete operations*. Reasoning is logical but limited to children's own experience; they understand cause and effect (Box 20–1; see also Table 16–4).

| BOX 20–1 | Features of Major Theories of Development During Later Childhood |
|---|---|

**Sigmund Freud**

- Child is in period of sexual latency
- Child's repression of sexuality makes it possible to form same-sex friendships; child assumes role of leader or follower
- Child is heavily influenced by parents and teachers, who can bolster self-image or more deeply repress sexuality

**Erik Erikson**

- Child's development is heavily influenced by others
- Child's leadership abilities and popularity depend on successfully controlling environment
- By learning to be productive, self-directing, and accepted at school and in society, child gains positive self-concept

**Jean Piaget**

- Younger school-age child can concentrate on only one aspect of a situation at a time
- Child becomes capable of limited reasoning, but thought is still limited to own experience
- Child understands cause and effect

Children of this age are aware that their parents are human and make mistakes. Conflicts may appear, particularly if what the child learns in school is different from what is practiced at home. Between 6 and 12, children prefer friends of their own sex and usually prefer the company of their friends to that of their brothers and sisters. Outward displays of affection by adults are embarrassing to them. Although they are now too big to cuddle on their parents' laps, they still require much love, support, and guidance.

## PHYSICAL GROWTH

Growth is slow until the spurt directly before puberty. Weight gains are more rapid than are increases in height. The average gain in weight per year is about 5.5–7 pounds or 2.5–3.2 kg. The average increase in height is approximately 2 inches, or 5.5 cm. Growth in head circumference is slower than before; between the ages of 5 and 12 years, the circumference increases from 20 to 21 inches. At the end of this time, the brain has reached approximately adult size.

Muscular coordination is improved, and the lymphatic tissues become highly developed. The skeletal bones continue to ossify. The body is supple, and sometimes skeletal growth is more rapid than is growth of muscles and ligaments. The child may appear gangling. There is a noticeable change in facial structures as the jaw lengthens. The sinuses are frequently sites of infection. The 6-year molars (the first permanent teeth) erupt. The gastrointestinal tract is more mature, and the stomach is upset less often. The heart grows slowly and is now smaller in proportion to body size than at any other time of life.

The shape of the eye changes with growth. The exact age at which 20/20 vision occurs, once believed to be about the age of 7, is now believed to be between 2 and 3 years of age. The capabilities of the child's sense organs, including hearing, have an important bearing on learning abilities.

The vital signs of the child of school age are near those of the adult. Temperature is 98.6°F; pulse is 85–100/min, and respiration is 18–20 min. The systolic blood pressure ranges from 90 to 108 mmHg, and the diastolic from 60 to 68 mmHg. Boys are slightly taller and somewhat heavier than girls until changes indicating puberty appear. The differences among children are greater at the end of middle childhood than at the beginning.

## GENDER IDENTITY

In some hospitals, before the newborn is aware that there are two sexes, he or she is placed in the nursery and covered with a blue or pink blanket. Male babies have always been highly valued, and in some cultures females have been killed at birth. Almost all societies perpetuate achievement and self-reliance in young boys, whereas young girls are taught obedience, nurturance, and responsibility.

Sex role development is greatly influenced by parents through differential treatment and identification. These two interdependent processes are at work in the family and in society. In infancy, boys and girls are cuddled somewhat differently. Later, their dress, the kinds of toys and games chosen for them, television, and the attitudes of family members serve to fortify gender identity.

The influence of the school environment is considerable. The teacher can directly foster stereotyping in the assignment of schoolroom tasks, the choice of textbooks, and disapproval of behavior that deviates from the child's sex role. Aggressive behavior is sometimes overlooked in boys but is discouraged in girls.

Although there is considerable talk about nonsexist socialization, most people have definite ideas about sex role deviance. The movement toward nonsexist upbringing seems to be stronger with regard to girls. Boys generally receive a more traditional sex socialization. A girl may be a "tomboy," but a boy should not be a "sissy."

Some adults are developing a sex role concept that incorporates both masculine and feminine qualities, sometimes termed *androgynous*. Because healthy interpersonal relationships depend on both assertiveness and sensitivity, the incorporation of traditionally masculine and feminine positive attributes may lead to fuller human functioning.

## SEX EDUCATION

Sex education is a lifelong process. Parents convey their attitudes and feelings about all aspects of life, including sexuality, to the growing child. Teaching is accomplished less by talking or formal instruction than by the whole climate of the home, particularly the respect shown to each family member. Sexuality is only one of the child's capacities and is not a fearful, isolated, episodic kind of experience.

Children's questions about sex are answered simply and at their level of understanding. Correct names are used to describe the genitals. The hospitalized child who complains, "My penis hurts," is understood by all. Private masturbation is normal and is practiced by both males and females at various times throughout their lives. It does not cause acne, blindness, insanity, or impotence. The young boy needs to be prepared for erections and nocturnal emissions (wet dreams), which are to be expected and are not necessarily due to masturbation. The young girl is prepared for menarche and is provided with the necessary supplies. This is particularly important to the early maturer because an elementary school may not provide dispensing machines in the restrooms.

Both sexes are concerned during the school years with the disproportion of their bodies, and they may be self-conscious when undressing. They may compare themselves with their friends. They need reassurance about their awakening sexuality, which affects their thoughts and behavior.

Sex education programs in the schools are still subject to various group and community pressures. Most are fragmented and provide only basic anatomy and physiology, with a general discussion of hygiene. When this is the case, and if children realize that parents are uncomfortable with the subject, they turn to peers, who often can supply only erroneous and distorted information. The Sex Information and Education Council of the United States, (SIECUS) maintains that every sex education program should present the topic from six aspects: biologic, social, health, personal adjustment and attitudes, interpersonal associations, and establishment of values.

Regardless of the practice setting, nurses can aid in the sex education of parents and children through careful listening and anticipatory guidance. They can teach decision-making skills and responsibility. When it is appropriate, they review normal developmental behavior and explain age-specific information, for example, sexual curiosity and masturbation. They provide families with useful written information that stresses sexuality as a healthful rather than as an illness-related concept. The nurse should consider cultural differences when counseling.

## Influences from the Wider World

### SCHOOL

Schools have a profound influence on the socialization of children. Children bring to school what they have learned and experienced in the home. Although some children come from healthy, intact families who are financially secure, many do not. The child may be disabled, retarded, or abused or may suffer from a chronic illness. Parents may be alcoholics, may be unemployed, or may suffer from numerous other physical or stress-related conditions. Nurses must remember these factors because they surface continually with this population. In addition, children may be unable to verbalize their needs; therefore, caretakers must become particularly astute in their observations.

Children may look similar, but what each can absorb intellectually is directly related to emotional health and, more often than not, to the family's emotional health. "Schools in different neighborhoods vary in style, expectations, and aspirations. Although they may have similar formal curricula, their subtle message and their milieu (environment) will vary significantly. They will reflect the social reality of the people living in the respective neighborhoods and communities" (Levine, M., et al. [1992]). School children are exposed to many new adults and peers whose values and expectations may be different from what they have experienced thus far.

Wright and Nader (1983) identified certain common stages or transitions in which predictable developmental crises may occur. These are school entry, the beginning of academic reading instruction, reading to learn at about third grade, start of middle school, and the period from junior to senior high school. In addition, children can no longer be protected from prejudices because of their beliefs, color, or ethnic background. The teacher becomes an impor-

## Nursing Brief

When discussing sexuality with school-age children, it is necessary to review slang or street terms. Most children hear the terms but may be confused about their meaning.

tant role model and influence, as do fellow students.

A holistic attitude of child care must focus not only on intellectual achievement and test scores but also on such qualities as artistic expression, creativity, joy, cooperation, responsibility, industry, love, and other attributes. The sensitive nurse can assist parents by affirming the individuality of children and by encouraging parents to share with their children the pride they are experiencing as the children learn and progress through the elementary grades. Box 20–2 is a summary of parental guidance that

---

**BOX 20–2 Parental Guidance for Children Starting School**

**Encourage parents to**

- Review normal growth and development of 5- to 6-year-olds
- Anticipate regression such as thumb-sucking, clinging behavior, occasional soiling
- Encourage children to express what they think school will be like
- Arrange for children to meet others who will be entering school with them
- Tour school with child
- Introduce child to school crossing guard, bus driver
- Teach child family name and telephone number
- Teach safety precautions about crossing street, strangers, "blue star" homes*
- Allow sufficient time in the morning to prepare for school
- Provide a cheerful send-off
- Instruct child as to where to go in case of emergency at home, e.g., neighbor or relative
- Walk to school until the child understands the route, or designate a bus stop
- Listen to child at end of day; become interested in school life
- Get to know the child's teacher; take an interest in the school
- Inform the teacher of sudden or unusual stress in the child's life

---

*Community-established "safe homes" for children in an emergency. Such houses are designated by a blue star or other symbol.
Data from Rogers, F., & Head, B. (1983). *Mister Rogers talks with parents.* New York: Berkley Books; and other sources.

---

the nurse may find useful in preparing children for the beginning of school.

By the time a child reaches middle school, anticipatory guidance should include dealing with peer abuse, vandalism, and substance abuse. The growing drug trade and the increased incidence of crime and victimization, particularly in inner-city schools, exposes children to assaults that have been unprecedented. The extent to which these situations affect the child and the learning process has yet to be explored.

The nurse assesses patterns of communication between parents and child and assists with specific behavioral problems. Parents may have a problem in "letting go." The nurse can support their endeavors in accordance with the child's maturity. The transition to junior high school generally means multiple classrooms, a series of teachers, and a change of buildings. The child is developing adult characteristics and has new feelings about the body and about parents, teachers, and peers. Anticipatory guidance includes a review of normal physiology and how it changes with puberty. Information concerning sexuality is reviewed, and the child is encouraged to ask questions at the time they arise.

A warm, ongoing relationship between parents and child helps to provide a safe atmosphere of caring. Adults should develop a heightened awareness for such things as school attendance problems, tardiness, and signs of loneliness or depression. They should continue to encourage children to discuss their school problems, feelings, and worries. Parents and children must set realistic goals. A good question for adults to contemplate periodically is, "When was the last time this child had a success?" Homework should be the child's responsibility, with a minimum of assistance from parents. For some children, visits to the nursing office may be their only continuous contact with a health-care worker. The nurse may be instrumental in establishing positive health patterns that may be carried into adulthood.

## TELEVISION

TV has a powerful influence on children. It has been called the "great baby-sitter" of our time. Some of the criticisms leveled at TV viewing by children are (1) it does not challenge the imagination, (2) it interferes with solitude and play, and (3) it promotes materialism and passivity. People on TV are frequently stereo-

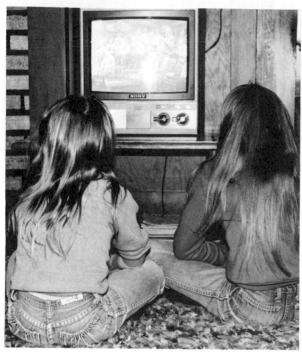

**Figure 20–2.** Parents need to supervise the amount and type of TV programs viewed by children.

**BOX 20–3** **Parental Guidance for Television Viewing by Children**

**Encourage parents to**

- Establish limits on viewing by day or week
- Establish limits on circumstances regarding viewing (no viewing during meals, no private sets in bedroom)
- Refrain from using TV as reward or punishment
- Be good role models
- Supervise or consult with children about various programs available
- Spend time watching TV with child; discuss feelings aroused
- Teach children to be critical of programs; help distinguish fact from fantasy
- Teach small children differences between program and commercials
- Encourage other activities, such as imaginative play, reading, active games

typed. Of particular concern is the continual violence and portrayal of unhealthy attitudes toward sex, nutrition, and drugs. There is often an unrealistic rapid resolution of problems. TV can also be a means of escape, shutting out the real world (Fig. 20–2). Noise levels and dissention over programming may affect family life.

Box 20–3 suggests ways in which the nurse can guide parents in regulating TV viewing by children. Some programs are educational and sensitive to the needs of children. Rogers and Head suggest that children's fears can be diminished by watching and discussing TV with them. They also suggest that we teach children to focus on "the helpers" of the story. Thus, they see volunteers and friends, who provide balance (Rogers & Head, 1983). The American Academy of Pediatrics suggests that parents limit their children's viewing to 1–2 hr/day. Concerned parents and educators can obtain more information about how they can help minimize TV's harmful effects from such organizations as Action for Children's Television (ACT) and the National Council for Children and Television.

Video games will also need to be evaluated because of their rise in popularity.

## LATCHKEY CHILDREN

A development of this generation is the large number of children left unsupervised after school closes. Many are asked to assume responsibilities for which they are not ready. Several factors contribute to this trend, most of which revolve around the changing nature of the family. There has been an increase in single-parent families headed predominantly by women whose income is at or near the poverty level. The high cost of living makes it necessary for both parents to work in order to make ends meet. In addition, the nuclear family is often separated geographically from the extended family; therefore, relatives are not available to care for children. There is a lack of assistance for intact families who are poor (McClellan, 1984).

Latchkey children are at increased risk for accidents due to mischief or immature judgment. They also show heightened evidence of fear and loneliness. They have fewer opportunities to socialize with friends because they may be instructed to remain alone in the house.

| BOX 20–4 | Guidance for Latchkey Families |
| --- | --- |

**Teach child about safety**

- Not to enter the house if the door is ajar or anything looks unusual
- Not to display keys; to keep door locked
- How to answer the telephone (parents are busy, not "out")
- First-aid techniques
- Fire safety rules and route of escape; walk through procedure with child
- Cooking rules; microwave ovens are safest
- Safe bathing methods (no electrical appliances around water); necessary when older children are watching younger children
- Weather-related safety (e.g., tornadoes, thunderstorms)
- The dangers of garage door openers

**Teach parents to**

- List emergency numbers and post near telephone
- Designate a neighbor who is usually home for help in emergencies
- Teach child own name, telephone number, address, and parents' name
- Leave work number with child
- Lock up firearms or remove from house
- Prepare a first-aid kit and designate location
- Address street safety with child when returning from school; include precautions with strangers
- Consider obtaining a pet for child
- Be home on time or call child
- Leave tape-recorded message to decrease loneliness of child, recommend specific activities rather than TV
- Help child feel successful and appreciated
- Assess home and neighborhood for hazards specific to their locale

*Data from McClellan, M. (1984). On their own: Latchkey children. *Pediatric Nursing*, 10, 200.

Box 20–4 shows parental and child guidance for latchkey children. Nurses should become aware of local resources, such as "Prepared for Today," a program sponsored by the National Boy Scouts of America, and Young Men's Christian Association (YMCA) and Young Women's Christian Association (YWCA) after-school activities. They can also assist in developing innovative programs such as cooperative baby-sitting, in which parents exchange child-care services. The nurse must spend time with parents, lend support, and help them explore their options.

## Physical, Mental, Emotional and Social Development

Table 20–1 provides an overview of the development of various competencies in the school-age child. The student should review it at this time in conjunction with the text.

### THE 6-YEAR-OLD

Children of 6 years burst with energy and are on the go constantly. They soon become overtired, and it is necessary to limit their activities. They like to start tasks but do not always finish them, for their attention span is fairly brief. They tend to be bossy and sometimes rude, but they are very sensitive to criticism. Sex investigations begun in earlier years may persist. Their conscience is active, and they find it difficult to make decisions.

One of the most obvious physical changes at this age is the loss of the temporary teeth (Fig. 20–3). The important 6-year molars also erupt. Children can jump rope, throw and catch a ball, tie shoelaces, and perform numerous other feats that require muscle coordination. Their language differs from that of the pre-school child. They use it for a purpose rather than for the pure joy of talking. Their vocabulary consists of about 2500 words. They require 11–13 hours of sleep a night.

Boys and girls play together at this age, although they begin to prefer to associate with children of the same sex. Certain activities, such as imaginative play, are common to both sexes (Fig. 20–4). Most children enjoy collecting objects such as shells, leaves, or stones. Play at this time usually reflects events that occur in the immediate environment.

Children of 6 need time and support to help them adjust to school. If they have nursery school or kindergarten experience, the transition may be more comfortable. Most children go to school expecting the same reception that they are accustomed to at home. If parents are critical or overprotective, children will assume

**Table 20–1.** SUMMARY OF SCHOOL-AGE CHILD GROWTH AND DEVELOPMENT AND HEALTH MAINTENANCE

| Age (Years) | Physical Competency | Intellectual Competency | Emotional-Social Competency |
|---|---|---|---|
| General: 6–12 | Gains an average of 2.5–3.2 kg/yr (5.5–7 lb/yr). Overall height gains of 5.5 cm (2 in)/yr; growth occurs in spurts and is mainly in trunk and extremities. Loses deciduous teeth; most of permanent teeth erupt. Progressively more coordinated in both gross- and fine-motor skills. Caloric needs increase with growth spurts | Masters concrete operations. Moves from egocentrism; learns he or she is not always right. Learns grammar and expression of emotions and thoughts. Vocabulary increases to 3000 words or more; handles complex sentences | Central crisis; industry versus inferiority; wants to do and make things. Progressive sex education needed. Wants to be like friends; competition important. Fears body mutilation, alterations in body image; earlier phobias may recur; nightmares; fears death. Nervous habits common |
| 6–7 | Gross-motor skill exceeds fine-motor coordination. Balance and rhythm are good—runs, skips, jumps, climbs, gallops. Throws and catches ball. Dresses self with little or no help | Vocabulary of 2500 words. Learning to read and print; beginning concrete concepts of numbers, general classification of items. Knows concepts of right and left; morning, afternoon, and evening; coinage; intuitive thought process. Verbally aggressive, bossy, opinionated, argumentative. Likes simple games with basic rules | Boisterous, outgoing, and a know-it-all; whiny; parents should sidestep power struggles, offer choices. Becomes quiet and reflective during 7th yr; very sensitive. Can use telephone. Likes to make things; starts many, finishes few. Give some responsibility for household duties |
| 8–10 | Myopia may appear. Secondary sex characteristics begin in girls. Hand-eye coordination and fine-motor skills are well established. Movements are graceful, coordinated. Cares for own physical needs completely. Constantly on move; plays and works hard; enforce balance in rest and activity | Learning correct grammar and to express feelings in words. Likes books he or she can read alone; will read funny papers, scan newspaper. Enjoys making detailed drawings. Mastering classification, seriation, spatial, temporal, and numeric concepts. Uses language as a tool; likes riddles, jokes, chants, word games. Rules guiding force in life now. Very interested in how things work, what and how weather, seasons, and the like are made | Strong preference for same-sex peers; antagonizes opposite-sex peers. Self-assured and pragmatic at home; questions parental values and ideas. Has a strong sense of humor. Enjoys clubs, group projects, outings, large groups, camp. Modesty about own body increases over time; sex-conscious. Works diligently to perfect skills he or she does best. Happy, cooperative, relaxed, and casual in relationships. Increasingly courteous and well mannered with adults. Gang stage at a peak; secret codes and rituals prevail. Responds better to suggestion than to dictatorial approach |
| 11–12 | Vital signs approximate adult norms. Growth spurt for girls; inequalities between sexes is increasingly noticeable; boys greater physical strength. Eruption of permanent teeth complete except for third molars. Secondary sex characteristics begin in boys. Menstruation may begin | Able to think about social problems and prejudices; sees others' points of view. Enjoys reading mysteries, love stories. Begins playing with abstract ideas. Interested in whys of health measures and understands human reproduction. Very moralistic; religious commitment often made during this time | Intense team loyalty; boys begin teasing girls and girls flirt with boys for attention; best-friend period. Wants unreasonable independence. Rebellious about routines; wide mood swings; needs some time daily for privacy. Very critical of own work. Hero worship prevails. Facts-of-life chats with friends prevail; masturbation increases. Appears under constant tension |

**Table 20–1.** SUMMARY OF SCHOOL-AGE CHILD GROWTH AND DEVELOPMENT AND HEALTH MAINTENANCE *Continued*

| Nutrition | Play | Safety |
|---|---|---|
| Fluctuations in appetite due to uneven growth pattern and tendency to get involved in activities. Tendency to neglect breakfast in rush of getting to school. Although school lunch is provided in most schools, child does not always eat it | Plays in groups, mostly of same sex; gang activities predominate. Books for all ages. Bicycles important. Sports equipment. Cards, board and table games. Most of play is active games requiring little or no equipment | Enforce continued use of seat belts during car travel. Bicycle safety must be taught and enforced. Teach safety related to hobbies, handicrafts, mechanical equipment |
| Preschool food dislikes persist. Tendency for deficiencies in iron, vitamin A, and riboflavin, 100 ml/kg of water/day, 3 gm/kg protein daily | Still enjoys dolls, cars, and trucks. Plays well alone but enjoys small groups of both sexes; begins to prefer same-sex peer during 7th yr. Ready to learn how to ride a bicycle. Prefers imaginary, dramatic play with real costumes. Begins collecting for quantity, not quality. Enjoys active games such as hide-and-seek, tag, jump rope, roller skating, kickball. Ready for lessons in dancing, gymnastics, music. Restrict TV time to 1–2 hr/day | Teach and reinforce traffic safety. Still needs adult supervision of play. Teach to avoid strangers, never take anything from strangers. Teach illness prevention and reinforce continued practice of other health habits. Restrict bicycle use to home ground; no traffic areas; teach bicycle safety. Wear helmet. Teach and set examples about harmful use of drugs, alcohol, smoking |
| Needs about 2100 calories/day; nutritious snacks. Tends to be too busy to bother to eat. Tendency for deficiencies in calcium, iron, and thiamine. Problem of obesity may begin now. Good table manners. Able to help with food preparation | Likes hiking, sports. Enjoys cooking, woodworking, crafts. Enjoys cards and table games. Likes radio and records. Begins qualitative collecting now. Continue restriction on TV time | Stress safety with firearms. Keep them out of reach and allow use only with adult supervision. Know who the child's friends are; parents should still have some control over friend selection. Teach water safety; swimming should be supervised by an adult |
| Male needs 2500 cal/day; female needs 2250 (70 cal/kg/day); both need 75 ml/kg of water/day; 2 gm/kg protein daily | Enjoys projects and working with hands. Likes to do errands and jobs to earn money. Very involved in sports, dancing, talking on phone. Enjoys all aspects of acting and drama | Continue monitoring friends. Stress bicycle and roller blade safety on streets and in traffic and use of helmet and other protective gear |

From Betz, C., Hunsberger, M., & Wright, S. (1994). *Family-centered nursing care of children* (2nd ed.). Philadelphia: W.B. Saunders.

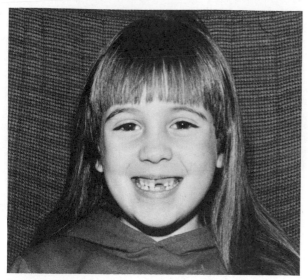

**Figure 20–3.** One of the most obvious physical changes of the 6-year-old is the loss of primary teeth.

that the teacher will be too. When the teacher's response differs markedly from their expectations, they feel insecure and may even be hostile toward the teacher. Parents need to observe children for signs of fatigue and stress. Not all children are ready for school merely because they reach the proper age. Even those who are ready need time and support from parents and teachers before they can settle down to the job at hand. Being in school exposes the child to infection more frequently than being at home.

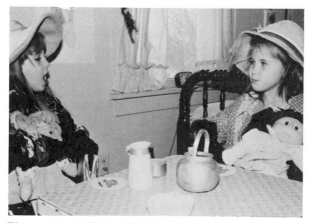

**Figure 20–4.** Young children prepare for various roles through imaginative play.

Preschool immunizations and a physical examination are indicated.

### THE 7-YEAR-OLD

At 7 children are generally less a problem than they were at 6. It is a quieter age, and the child does not go looking for trouble. Some educators have noted that second-graders are the easiest children to teach. They set high standards for themselves and for their families. They have a good sense of humor, tend to be somewhat of a "tease" (wiggle loose teeth to annoy adults), and are a little more modest than at an earlier age. They enjoy being active but also appreciate periods of rest. The second-grader may have a "crush" on a friend of the opposite sex.

These children know the months and seasons of the year and begin to tell time. They have a beginning concept of arithmetic, can count by twos and fives, and know that money is valuable. Their hands are steadier. Interest in God and heaven is heightened.

Active play is still important to both sexes. The boys are more apt to tease the girls than to participate in games such as jump rope or tag. Both sexes enjoy bike riding and table games (Fig. 20–5). Realistic toys, such as dolls that can be bathed and fed and trains that back up and whistle, appeal to the 7-year-old. Comic books are also popular. Becoming increasingly independent, the children imagine themselves accomplishing feats more adventurous than those of their parents. They cannot understand how Mom and Dad ever chose to lead such dull lives.

**Stealing.** One problem that may arise at this age is stealing. Repeated stealing is a signal of something lacking or a stressful event in the child's life. In many cases, children steal only to distribute their loot to neighborhood friends. This may be an attempt to buy friendship. Independence has separated them somewhat from their parents; if they cannot establish good relationships with their friends, they may feel left out. Sometimes stealing occurs because children do not have a sense of property rights, that is, what is theirs and what belongs to others.

Parents should tell a child who steals that they are aware of the fact and should insist on some form of restitution. They should not humiliate the child, but they must make it clear that stealing is not permitted. The nurse can be a resource to parents, helping them to assess the degree of a problem and to suggest methods of management

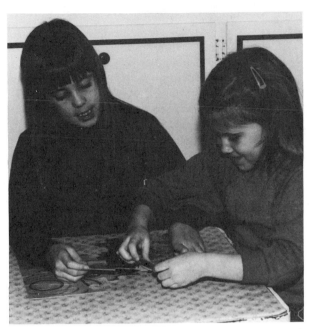

**Figure 20–5.** Competition between siblings is common in the school years.

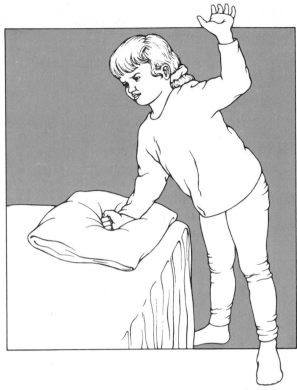

**Figure 20–6.** Punching a pillow is a good way for the child to release anger without hurting others.

that are not detrimental to the child's fragile self-esteem. As always, one accepts the child but not the deed, and then tries to understand the circumstances causing the behavior.

### THE 8-YEAR-OLD

The 8-year-old wants to do everything and can play alone for longer periods than the 7-year-old. The work of 8-year-olds is usually creative. They enjoy group activities, such as Brownies and Cub Scouts, and prefer companions of the same sex. They become interested in group fads. Eight-year-olds like to be considered important, particularly by adults. They may behave better for company than for the family. Hero worship is evident.

The arms and hands of the 8-year-old seem to grow faster than the rest of the body. The large and small muscles are better developed, and movements are smoother and more graceful. The child can write rather than print and understands the number of days that must pass before special events such as Christmas, birthdays, and discharge from the hospital.

The 8-year-old enjoys competitive sports but is generally a poor loser. Long, involved arguments frequently occur. A healthy way to teach a child to express anger is to have the child pound on a pillow (Fig. 20–6). Wrestling is frequent, and dramatic play is popular. Most children like to be the hero or heroine of their favorite program. Neighborhood secret clubs are organized, and all members must strictly adhere to the rules.

### THE 9-YEAR-OLD

The 9-year-old is dependable and is not as restless as the child of 8. Children of this age show more interest in family activities, assume more responsibility for personal belongings and for younger brothers and sisters, and are more likely to complete tasks (Figs. 20–7 and 20–8). They resist adult authority if it does not coincide with the opinions or ideals of the group. However, they are more able to accept criticism for their actions. Individual differences are pronounced.

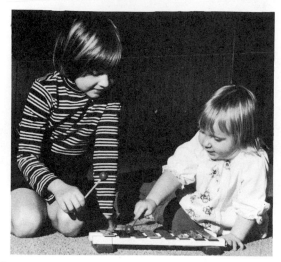

**Figure 20–7.** The child of school age entertains younger members of the family.

Worries and mild compulsions are common. Children avoid cracks in the pavement: "Step on a crack, break your mother's back." They realize that these actions are senseless but still feel obliged to repeat them. Nervous habits, sometimes referred to as tics, may appear and may vary widely. Eye blinking, facial grimacing, and shoulder shrugging are but a few examples. The child cannot help such actions and should not be scolded for them because they are mainly due to tension; they usually

## Nursing Brief

Mutual respect involves accepting the child's feelings. When helping children, identify feelings, start with the terms *mad*, *glad*, *sad*, or *scared*.

disappear when home and social life become more relaxed.

Hand and eye coordination is well developed, and manual activities are managed with skill. The child works and plays hard and becomes overtired. About 10 hours of sleep a night are needed. The permanent teeth are still erupting.

Competitive sports are still popular, as are reading, listening to the radio, and watching TV and movies. Contact sports should be limited in order to minimize permanent growth-related injuries. Girls play for long periods of time with dolls. An interest in music is shown, and the child may desire to take lessons (Fig. 20–9). Children know the date, can repeat months of the year in order, and can multiply and do simple division. They take care of their

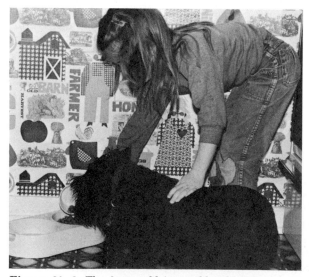

**Figure 20–8.** The 9-year-old is capable of caring for the family pet.

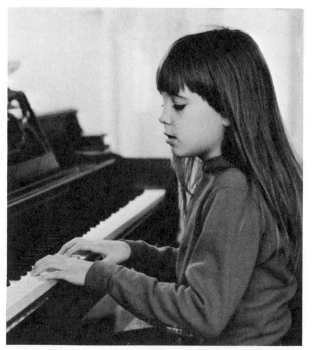

**Figure 20–9.** Outlets such as music help the child to express feelings in a positive way.

bodily needs, and by now their table manners are considerably improved.

## PREADOLESCENCE

### The 10-Year-Old

Age 10 marks the beginning of the preadolescent years. Girls are more physically mature than boys. The child begins to show self-direction, is courteous to adults, and thinks clearly about social problems and prejudices. The 10-year-old wants to be independent and resents being told what to do but is receptive to suggestions. The ideas of the group are more important than individual ideas. Interest in sex and sex investigations continue.

In general, girls are more poised than boys. Both sexes are fairly reliable about household duties (Fig. 20–10). Slang terms are used. The 10-year-old can write for a relatively long period of time and maintains good writing speed. The child uses fractions and knows

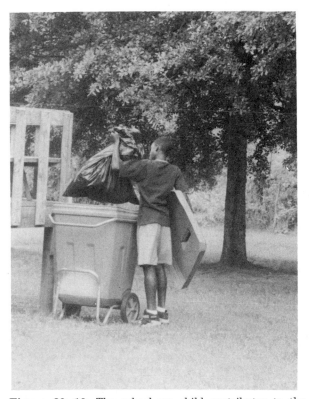

**Figure 20–10.** The school-age child contributes to the smooth running of the household by emptying the trash. (Reminders are frequently necessary!)

numbers over 100. Boys and girls begin to identify themselves with skills that pertain to their sex role. They are intolerant of the opposite sex. The play enjoyed by the 10-year-old is similar to that enjoyed by the 9-year-old. In addition, the child takes more interest in appearance.

### 11- and 12-Year-Olds

Adjectives that describe 11- and 12-year-olds include intense, observant, all-knowing, energetic, meddlesome, and argumentative. This period before the onset of puberty is one of complete disorganization. It begins earlier in some children; the onset and rate of physical maturity vary greatly. Before the end of this period, the hormones of the body begin to influence physical growth. Posture is poor. There are 24–26 permanent teeth.

The child has an overabundance of energy and is on the go every minute. Girls become "tomboyish" in their actions. Table manners are a thing of the past, and the refrigerator is constantly emptied. Children at this age are less concerned with their appearance. They seem to be often preoccupied, and this, along with physical activities and numerous anxieties, accounts for some of the decline seen in school grades. Ability to concentrate decreases, and parents complain that the child "never hears anything." When asked to do a new task, these children moan and groan.

Group participation is still important. Getting acquainted with peers can be scary and takes time (Fig. 20–11). Preadolescent children are not ready to stand alone, but they cannot bear the thought of depending on parents. They must overcome the problems they confront without parental help. Their attitude implies, "Can't you see that I'm not a child anymore?"

During preadolescence, children are interested in their bodies and watch for signs of growing up. Girls look forward to menstruation and wearing their first bra. Boys and girls tend to ignore the opposite sex, but really they are much aware of them. There is a tendency to tease one another. Their descriptions of each other are far from complimentary: "stupid," "crazy," and "nerd." Both sexes enjoy earning money by obtaining odd jobs. The preadolescent often seeks an adult friend of the same sex to idolize.

Guiding preadolescents is not easy. They need freedom within limits and recognition that

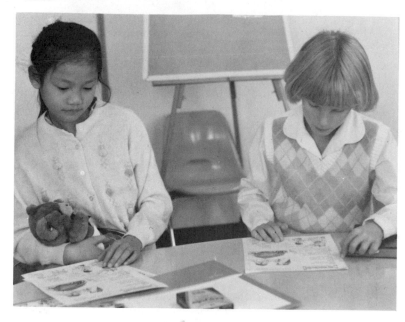

**Figure 20–11.** Getting acquainted is scary and takes time.

they are no longer babies (Fig. 20–12). They should know why parents make a decision. They should not be expected to follow household rules blindly. Their conscience enables them to understand and accept reasonable discipline. They ignore constant verbal nagging. They should be provided constructive opportunities to release pent-up emotions and energy. One can more easily accept their irritating behavior by realizing that much of it is indeed "just a phase."

## Physical Care

**Hygiene.** Children of school age are gradually able to accept more responsibility for personal hygiene. They need reminders and, in some instances, demonstrations of how to do the task correctly. They are able to dress, brush their teeth, comb their hair, and wash their face and hands. (Most children of this age tend to forget that they have ears and a neck.) They must be taught how to care for fingernails and toenails.

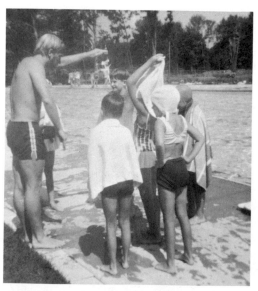

**Figure 20–12.** Children should be taught how to swim and should learn the rules of water safety.

## Nursing Brief

Provide protective equipment appropriate for any sport the child plays (e.g., helmets for bicycling, skateboarding, ice hockey).

**Clothing.** Clothing need not be expensive, but it should be simple in design and durable. Children are taught the proper way to care for their clothes, but parents should anticipate temporary regressions. Shoes must be sturdy and of the proper size. Boots and raincoats are necessary to protect the child from inclement weather. Socks should fit properly to prevent irritation of the feet. All valued clothes and articles taken to school are labeled. For potentially hazardous play, children should wear protective clothing (Fig. 20–13).

**Sleep.** Children of this age are so active during the day, physically and mentally, that they soon become exhausted. Children from 6 to 8 years average approximately 11–13 hours of sleep a night. As they grow older, a little less sleep is required. The 9- to 12-year-old averages about 10 hr/night. Parents can judge the amount of sleep children need by their behavior. If the child is eating and playing well and keeping up with school work, chances are that the amount of sleep is sufficient.

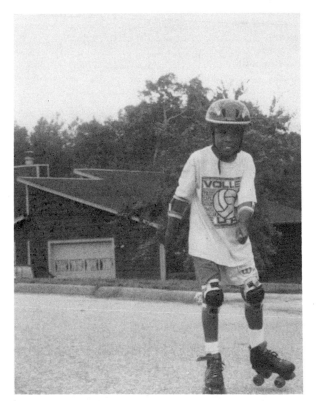

**Figure 20–13.** Protective clothing is necessary for potentially hazardous play.

**Health Examinations.** The yearly preschool physical examination is given in the spring preceding admission. This allows time to correct any problems that are found. Booster immunizations are given as needed; the child's teeth are examined and dental work is completed.

School health programs aimed at maintaining and promoting health are provided in most school systems. Nurses and other professional persons who take part in such programs can play an important role in counseling parents. They also help meet the needs of disabled children enrolled in their schools. A carefully taken health history provides the nurse with much-needed information (Fig. 20–14).

The eating habits of a child of this age should be basically sound, as long as a variety of nutritious foods are offered (Figs. 20–15 and 20–16). Food preferences occur. See Table 20–2 for recommended food intake for school-age children. A nutritious breakfast is important. The chief breakfast foods required are fruit, cereal, and milk. Eggs also add variety. Menus centered on these foods are more substantial than those consisting of doughnuts or sweet rolls and coffee.

The federal government has established the school breakfast program in many areas. The National School Lunch Program has been ongoing. Summer lunch programs are also available. These lunches must provide certain nutritional standards (the goal is to provide one-third of the recommended daily allowance of foods).

## Guidance

School children continuously need understanding from persons concerned with their care. Their past relationships are reflected in their behavior. They must know that they are wanted and loved and that their parents are proud of them and their accomplishments. They need approval for tasks well done and a minimum of criticism. They need assistance in recognizing and keeping in touch with their feelings and in managing success and failure. At this age, children are quite critical of themselves. They need help in self-acceptance. The judgment of school-age children improves with age. They need encouragement for their deci-

I. GENERAL INFORMATION
Name_____Date_____
Age and birth date _____Language _____
Grade _____Informant _____
Sex _____Parents' home and business,
Religion _____ phones _____

II. FAMILY PROFILE (health history of family members)
Mother _____
Father _____
Siblings _____
Paternal grandparents _____
Maternal grandparents _____
Life change events: death, divorce, new baby, moves of family, illness, separation, etc.
_____
_____

III. CHILD PROFILE
Newborn status: Did baby leave hospital with you? _____
Birth defects _____
Developmental history: Age for crawling_____sitting_____
 walking _____speech _____toilet training _____
Immunizations _____
Habits, general behavior in school _____ Home _____
Sleeping patterns _____ Fears _____
Exercise _____ Friends _____
Interests _____ Special skills _____

Previous illness or accidents _____
Is child taking any medications? _____
Hearing aid _____ Glasses _____
Dental care _____ Allergies _____
Typical foods consumed:
 breakfast _____
 lunch _____
 supper _____
 snacks _____
Eating problems _____ Elimination _____
Menses _____ Sexual maturation _____
Sex education _____ Personal hygiene _____
Review of systems _____
_____

IV. NURSE'S OBSERVATIONS AND COMMENTS
General physical description _____
_____
Results of screening procedures: vision _____ audiometer _____
Scoliosis _____ Other _____
Individual health education and guidance _____
_____
Problem-solving plan _____
_____

Interviewer _____

**Figure 20–14.** Health assessment summary of the school-age child.

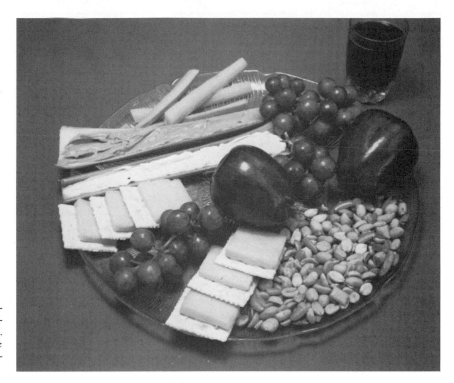

**Figure 20–15.** A variety of nutritious snacks for school-age children. (From Mahan, L., & Arlin, M. [1992]. *Krause's food, nutrition & diet therapy* [8th ed.]. Philadelphia: W.B. Saunders.)

sion-making capabilities (e.g., "That was a wise choice"). Some of their decisions will reflect their immaturity, and it may be necessary for parents to intervene if these are life-threatening or may cause injury. However, they learn from their mistakes. Parents and nurses who have empathy with school children can better understand their views.

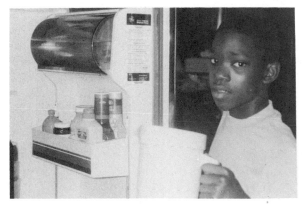

**Figure 20–16.** The eating habits of the school-age child are basically good as long as a variety of nutrients is available.

Preadolescents want to be accepted by their group; they imitate speech, manner of dress, actions, and activities (Fig. 20–17). Interest in organizations is at its peak. Children enjoy scouting and young people's groups. School children's social contacts may become a major topic of conversation. They have a growing understanding of relationships, which become major sources of feedback, pleasure, and self-esteem.

School children need time and a place to study. They require a desk in their own room or at least a private area of the house where they can concentrate. Their furniture should be of the proper size; lighting should be adequate. They must learn to take responsibility for their assignments and school supplies. Parents can

## Nursing Brief

Caution parents about the safe storage of firearms. Since 1979, more than 50,000 children in the United States have died from gunshot wounds. Most of these deaths occurred in the home, not the streets.

**Table 20–2.** RECOMMENDED FOOD INTAKE FOR GOOD NUTRITION ACCORDING TO FOOD GROUPS AND DAILY DIETARY ALLOWANCES: SCHOOL-AGE (7 TO 10 YEARS)

| Food Groups | Servings per Day | Serving Size |
|---|---|---|
| Bread Group | 6–9 | |
| • Bread | | 2 slices |
| • Cereal | | 1 oz |
| • Rice and pasta | | ½ C–¾ C |
| Vegetable Group | 3–5 total | |
| • Green-yellow vegetables (vitamin A source) | 1 or more | 4 tbsp |
| • Other vegetables | 2 or more | ⅓ C |
| Fruit Group | 3–4 total | |
| • Citrus fruits, berries, tomato, cabbage, cantaloupe (vitamin C source) | 1 or more | 1 medium orange |
| • Other fruits (apple, banana) | 2 or more | 1 medium |
| Milk Group | 2–3 | |
| • Milk/yogurt | | ½–1 C |
| • Cheese | | (1.5 oz cheese = 1 C milk) |
| Meat Group | 3 or more | |
| • Cooked lean meat, poultry, fish | | 4–6 tbsp |
| • Dry beans | | ½ C |
| • Egg | | 1 |
| • Peanut butter | | 2–3 tbsp |
| Fats, oils, sweets—USE SPARINGLY | | |

**Recommended Daily Dietary Allowances**

| Protein | Fat-Soluble | Vitamins | Water-Soluble | Vitamins | Minerals | | Energy Needs |
|---|---|---|---|---|---|---|---|
| 28 g | Vitamin A | 700 μg RE | Vitamin C | 45 mg | Calcium | 800 mg | 2000 kcal |
| | Vitamin D | 10 μg | Thiamine | 1.0 mg | Phosphorus | 800 mg | |
| | Vitamin E | 7 mg α—TE | Riboflavin | 1.2 mg | Magnesium | 170 mg | |
| | Vitamin K | 30 μg | Niacin | 13 mg NE | Iron | 10 mg | |
| | | | Vitamin B$_6$ | 1.4 mg | Zinc | 10 mg | |
| | | | Folate | 100 μg | Iodine | 120 μg | |
| | | | Vitamin B$_{12}$ | 1.4 μg | Selenium | 30 μg | |

From Betz, C., Hunsberger, M., & Wright, S. (1994). *Family-centered nursing care of children* (2nd ed.). Philadelphia: W.B. Saunders.

Adapted with permission from *Recommended Dietary Allowances: 10th Edition.* Copyright 1989 by the National Academy of Sciences. Published by the National Academy Press, Washington, D.C.; and U.S. Department of Agriculture, Human Nutrition Information Service (1992). *Food guide pyramid.* (Leaflet No. 572).Washington, D.C.: Author.

*Key:* RE, retinol equivalent; TE, tocopherol equivalent; NE, nicotine acid equivalent.

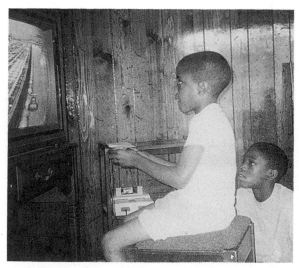

**Figure 20–17.** This child matches wits with an interactive video game while his brother coaches.

encourage school children by showing interest in what they are learning, by joining parent-teacher organizations, and by visiting periodically with the teacher. They must also vote on civic matters that will benefit the school system in their community.

At this age, an allowance or at least a means of earning money provides children with opportunities to learn its value. It takes time and encouragement for them to learn to spend money wisely. Such experiences aid in making the school childamoreresponsibleper-son.

Girls and boys need information and reassurance in advance about the changes that will take place in their bodies at puberty. This information is discussed in Chapter 21.

## KEY POINTS

- School age, from 6 to 12 years, is a time of increased independence when the child begins to incorporate, perfect, and process skills and information gained in early years.
- Erikson calls this stage the "stage of industry" or accomplishment.
- Freud describes this period as the sexual "latency stage," when the child's energy is directed toward cognitive and physical skills.
- Major changes occur in the child's cognitive-perceptual patterns. Piaget refers to this stage as the "concrete operational stage."
- Growth is slow until the spurt directly before puberty.
- School has an important influence on the socialization of child from 6 to 12.
- The child acquires a positive self-concept from the ability to be productive, self-directed, and accepted.
- Peers range from same-sex friends in the early years to opposite-sex friends around puberty. Group acceptance is important.
- Both sexes need accurate information and reassurance in advance about changes of puberty and reproduction.
- The availability of junk food hampers efforts to provide proper nutrition. Meals may be sporadic because of activities of the child and the parents' working schedules.
- Accident prevention is still extremely important. These children are prone to injuries from motor vehicles, bicycles, skateboards, swimming, and their tendency to be overactive and distracted.
- Parental concerns include how to protect children when they are unsupervised (the latchkey child) and issues such as stealing, lying, being irresponsible, and experiencing school-related stress.

# Study Questions

1. Identify the average range of vital signs for the school-age child.
2. Mrs. Thule has two children who are 6 and 9 years old. Chris, age 6, is a girl, and Brandon, age 9, is a boy. Select two games that both children might enjoy, and contrast their ability to use these games.
3. Melody, age 6, will be separated from her family for an overnight visit with friends. Suggest two ways in which her family might manage this experience so that it will be less threatening to her.
4. Leroy, age 11, is criticized by his siblings for cheating in a game. How would you advise his parents to handle this situation?
5. Carol, age 10, lied to her parents about her whereabouts after school. Discuss how you would advise her parents to handle this situation.
6. You are working the evening shift and visiting hours are over. When you enter the boys' unit, you find Freddie, age 10, and Don, age 12, engaged in a pillow fight. From your knowledge of this age group, would you consider this unreasonable behavior? How would you respond to this situation?

7. Discuss activities enjoyed by the child of 8. What diversions would you suggest for the long-term patient of this age?

8. Plan a day's menu for the school-age child. What foods should be included?

9. Nicole, age 7, is caught stealing change from her mother's purse. Discuss how you would advise her parents to handle this situation.

10. Plan an interview with a teacher in an elementary school. Determine what health needs she feels are being met and what areas could use improvement. Determine what resources are available in providing age-related health guidance.

# Multiple Choice Review Questions

*Choose the most appropriate answer.*

1. The pulse of the school age child is approximately
   a. 100–120 beats/min
   b. 95–120 beats/min
   c. 85–100 beats/min
   d. 60–80 beats/min

2. By age 12, the brain
   a. decreases in circumference
   b. reaches approximately adult size
   c. reaches approximately child size
   d. divides into cerebrum and cerebellum

3. Compared with the 6-year-old, the 7-year-old is generally
   a. quieter
   b. more anxious
   c. less happy
   d. not predictable

4. Steven, age 7, enters the house crying loudly; he says, "David left me flat to play with Eric." You would

a. call David's mother and express your feelings
b. ignore Steven's behavior, as you are busy
c. tell him not to be such a baby
d. encourage him to express his feelings about the event

5. Sandra, age 9, is practicing the piano. She continues to have difficulty in playing the theme from M*A*S*H. She starts to pound on the piano keys in frustration. You would enter the room and say
   a. "Just what do you think you're doing? That piano costs money!"
   b. "That's not difficult. Pull yourself together or you'll never amount to anything."
   c. "That piece sounds hard. I can see how you could be discouraged."
   d. "Here, let me show you how to play that."

## BIBLIOGRAPHY

Behrman, R.E. (1992). *Nelson textbook of pediatrics* (14th ed.). Philadelphia: W.B. Saunders.

Betz, C., Hunsberger, M., & Wright, S. (1994). *Family-centered nursing care of children* (2nd ed.). Philadelphia: W.B. Saunders.

Erikson, E. (1964). *Childhood and society.* New York: W.W. Norton.

Gellis, S.S., & Kagan, B.M. (1990). *Current pediatric therapy 13.* Philadelphia: W.B. Saunders.

Green, M., & Haggerty, R.J. (1990). *Ambulatory pediatrics IV.* Philadelphia: W.B. Saunders.

Greenwald, M. (1983). Visual development in infancy and childhood. *Pediatric Clinics of North America, 30,* 977.

Levine, M.D., Carey, W.B., & Crocker, A.C. (1992). *Developmental-behavioral pediatrics* (2nd ed.). Philadelphia: W.B. Saunders.

Mahan, L.K., & Arlin, M.T. (1992). *Krause's food, nutrition & diet therapy* (8th ed.).

McClellan, M. (1984). On their own: Latchkey children. *Pediatric Nursing, 10,* 198.

Mott, S., James, S.R., & Sperhac, A.M. (1990). *Nursing care of children and families* (2nd ed.). Reading, MA: Addison-Wesley.

Pillitteri, A. (1992). *Maternal and child health nursing.* Philadelphia: J.B. Lippincott.

Rogers, F., & Head, B. (1983). *Mister Rogers talks with parents.* New York: Berkley Books.

Thompson, E.D., & Ashwill, J.W. (1992). *Introduction to pediatric nursing* (6th ed.). Philadelphia: W.B. Saunders.

Whaley, L., & Wong, D. (1991). *Nursing care of infants and children* (4th ed.). St. Louis: C.V. Mosby.

Wright, G., & Nader, R. (1983). Schools as milieux. In M.D. Levine, W.B. Carey, A.C. Crocker, & R. Gross (Eds.). *Developmental-behavioral pediatrics.* Philadelphia: W.B. Saunders.

# Chapter 21

# The Adolescent

# OBJECTIVES

*On completion and mastery of Chapter 21, the student will be able to*

- Define each vocabulary term listed.
- Identify two major developmental tasks of adolescence.
- Discuss three major theoretic viewpoints on the personality development of adolescents.
- List five life events that contribute to stress during adolescence.
- Describe menstruation to a 13-year-old girl.
- Describe Tanner's stages of breast development.
- Identify two ways in which a person's cultural background might contribute to behavior.
- List three guidelines of importance for the adolescent participating in sports.
- Summarize the nutritional requirements of the adolescent.

---

**BOX 21–1** | **Features of Major Theories of Development During Adolescence**

**Sigmund Freud**

- Adolescent is in genital stage, the final stage of psychosexual development
- Self-love (narcissism) disappears; love for others (altruism) develops
- Peers and parents are less influential than before, but still provide love and support

**Erik Erikson**

- Adolescent's main concerns are self-definition and self-esteem
- Adolescent experiences identity crisis brought on by physical (including sexual) changes and conflict about future choices and expectations of others
- Adolescent must adapt to these changes and develop a new self-concept and appropriate vocational choices
- Adolescent learns to understand self in relation to others' perceptions and expectations

**Jean Piaget**

- Adolescent is in stage of formal operations, so has ability to reason logically and abstractly
- Adolescent is oriented toward problem-solving

---

# General Characteristics

*Adolescence* is defined as the period of life beginning with the appearance of secondary sex characteristics and ending with cessation of growth and emotional maturity. The term comes from the word *adolescere*, meaning "to grow up." Adolescence is often divided into early, middle, and late periods because the teenager of 13 varies a great deal from the 18-year-old. Middle adolescence appears to be the time of greatest turmoil for most families. Perhaps one of the most characteristic features of adolescence is its uncertainty. It is a period of life that in our culture lasts a comparatively long time and involves a great number of adjustments. Some of the major theories of development are summarized in Box 21–1.

Life is never dull when there are adolescents in the family. The surge toward independence becomes more and more pronounced, making it practically impossible for adolescents to get along with their parents, who represent authority. When adolescents submit to parental wishes, they may feel humiliated and childish. If they revolt, conflicts arise within the family. Parents and teenagers have to weather the storm together and try to come up with solutions that are relatively satisfactory to all.

Numerous other factors account for the restlessness of adolescents. Their bodies are rapidly changing, and they experience intense sexual drives. They want to be accepted by society, but they are not sure how to go about it. Adolescents question life and search to find what psychologists call their sense of identity: "Who am I?" "What do I want?" This is followed by the intimacy stage, in which teenagers must learn to avoid emotional isolation. They must face the fear of rejection in shared activities such as sports, in close friendships, and in sexual experiences. The older adolescent thinks about the future and is generally idealistic. Jean Piaget and other investigators indicate that during this time teenagers reach the final stages of abstract reasoning, logic, and other symbolic forms of thought, which increases sophistication in moral reasoning.

These facts sound complicated in themselves, but they are intensified by a world that is constantly changing. Even adults are confused by the rapid pace of living and the many advances in technology. The feminist movement has challenged the traditional roles of men and women in society. *Gender roles* are becoming less well defined in some households, which is likely to change parents' behavior as a model for their children. Many adolescents are living in single-parent homes or with working relatives, where little, if any, supervision is available.

Beall and Schmidt (1984) developed a Youth Adaptation Rating Scale to identify life events of adolescents that contribute to stress (Box 21–2). In their survey, students described the severity by ranking each item(0–5), with 0 being not stressful. A ratio value was then determined (figures in parentheses in Box 21–2). Six ethnic categories were identified and sampled, as were five communities of different sizes. A surprising result was that no significant differences existed among the ethnic groups or among the adolescents from communities of different sizes.

## Physical, Mental, Emotional, and Social Development

### PHYSICAL DEVELOPMENT

Preadolescence is a short period immediately preceding adolescence. In girls, it comprises the ages 10–13 and is marked by rapid changes in the structure and function of various parts of the body. It is distinguished by puberty, the stage at which the reproductive organs become functional and secondary sex characteristics develop. Both sexes produce male hormones, *androgens*, and female hormones, *estrogens*, in comparatively equal amounts during childhood. At puberty, the hypothalamus of the brain signals the pituitary gland to stimulate other endocrine glands—the adrenals and the ovaries or testes—to secrete their hormones directly into the blood stream in differing proportions (more androgens in the boy and more estrogens in the girl).

The age at puberty varies and is about 2 years earlier for girls than for boys. It is preceded by spurts in height and weight in both sexes. General appearance tends to be awkward, that is, long-legged and gangling; this growth characteristic is termed *asynchrony* because different body parts mature at different rates. The sweat glands are very active, and greasy skin and acne are common. Both sexes mature earlier and grow taller and heavier than in past generations (Fig. 21–1). Because of the gross motor development that occurs during adolescence, teenagers can gain satisfaction from sports (Fig. 21–2).

**Boys.** In boys, pubertal changes begin with enlargement of the testicles and internal structures but minimal enlargement of the penis. Erections and nocturnal emissions take place. The production of sperm begins between 13 and 14 years of age. The shoulders widen, and the pectoral muscles enlarge. The voice changes. Hair begins to grow on the chest, axillae, pubic areas (Fig. 21–3 and Box 21–3), and face. The genitals enlarge, and scrotal skin becomes darkly pigmented.

An athletic scrotal support (jock strap) is necessary for boys participating in sporting events, for dancers, and the like. It supports and protects the genitals and also prevents embarrassment from exposure. A support is purchased by size. Good personal hygiene is necessary because heat and friction may lead to jock itch, a ringworm infestation of the groin that is fungal. Sharing athletic supporters is discouraged.

The American Cancer Society recommends that boys examine their testes during or after a hot bath or shower. Each testicle is examined using the index and middle fingers of both hands on the underside of the testicle and the thumbs on the top of the testicle. The testicles are gently rolled between the thumb and the fingers. Testicular self-examinations are performed once a month. If a lump is discovered, it should be reported immediately to a health-care provider.

**Girls.** Puberty is easily recognized in girls by the onset of menstruation (Fig. 21–4). The first menstrual period is called the *menarche*. It commonly occurs about age 13, but this varies. It may occur as early as 10 or as late as 15 years of age. Secondary sex characteristics become more apparent before the menarche. Fat is deposited in the hips, thighs, and breasts, causing them to enlarge.

At this time, the teenager may need to be fitted for a bra. The lingerie department of a store has fitting rooms. Measurements need to be ascertained and various styles tried on for comfort.

---

**BOX 21–2** **Youth Adaptation Rating Scale**

- ☐ Graduation (.57)
- ☐ Pet dies (.55)
- ☐ Fights with parents (.67)
- ☐ Getting pressure about having sex (.63)
- ☐ Caught cheating or lying repeatedly (.73)
- ☐ Getting a major illness/injury/car accident (.81)
- ☐ Becoming religious or giving up religion (.63)
- ☐ Referral to the principal's office (.47)
- ☐ Getting acne/warts (.45)
- ☐ Trouble getting a date when it was not a problem before (.61)
- ☐ Problems developed with teachers/employers (.59)
- ☐ Making career decisions (college, majors, training, and the like) (.64)
- ☐ Starting to go to weekend parties/rock concerts (.35)
- ☐ First day of school (.37)
- ☐ Going on first date/starting to date (.53)
- ☐ Death of a parent/guardian (.95)
- ☐ Not getting promoted to next grade (.76)
- ☐ Getting caught using drugs (.86)
- ☐ Getting attacked/raped/beat up (.84)
- ☐ Getting a ticket or other minor problems with law (.58)
- ☐ Parents getting a divorce/separation (.83)
- ☐ Getting expelled/suspended (.71)
- ☐ Fad pressure (.43)
- ☐ Breaking up with boy/girlfriend (.57)
- ☐ Getting minor illness (cold, flu, and the like) (.30)
- ☐ Arguments with peers/brothers/sisters (.46)
- ☐ Starting to perform (speeches, presentations, musical or drama performances) (.60)
- ☐ Getting fired from a job (.63)

- ☐ Going into debt (.72)
- ☐ Being stereotyped/discriminated against/having rumors spread about you (.70)
- ☐ Death of a close family member (.94)
- ☐ Death of a boy/girlfriend/close friend (.94)
- ☐ Getting V.D. (.86)
- ☐ Getting someone pregnant/getting pregnant (.92)
- ☐ Taking finals/SAT (.61)
- ☐ Moving to a different town/school/making new friends (.67)
- ☐ Getting a car (.35)
- ☐ Trying to get a job/job interview (.49)
- ☐ Getting an award, office, and so on (.36)
- ☐ Making a team (drill, athletic, debate ) (.44)
- ☐ Getting married (.73)
- ☐ Getting beat up by parents (.86)
- ☐ Taking the driver's license test (.55)
- ☐ Getting a new addition to the family (.45)
- ☐ Going to the dentist or doctor (.37)
- ☐ Going to jail/reform school (.88)
- ☐ Starting to use drugs (.82)
- ☐ Getting braces (.45)
- ☐ Going on a diet (.41)
- ☐ Losing or gaining weight (.49)
- ☐ Changing exercise habits (.21)
- ☐ Pressure to take drugs (.71)
- ☐ Moving out of the house (.56)
- ☐ Falling in love (.66)
- ☐ Getting a bad haircut (.57)
- ☐ Getting glasses (.49)
- ☐ Family member moving out (.47)
- ☐ Getting a bad report card (.59)

## Scoring

5. Critical event in the life of a teenager. Very stressful. This would require a major change in one's life. Totally demanding
4. Semicritical event. Stressful. This would require changing one's life to adjust to the differences it would make
3. Moderately critical. This event causes stress, but one could take it without too great a change in living
2. Semimoderate. Stress is evidenced, but one could adjust fairly easily to this event without too much strain mentally, emotionally, or physically
1. Mild stress. Hardly any stress at all. One could make the changes that might be needed without much effort
0. Not stressful at all. Probably no change would be required in order to adjust to this event

From Beall, S., & Schmidt, G. (1984). Development of a youth adaptation rating scale. *Journal of School Health, 54*, 197. Copyright, 1984. American School Health Association, Kent, OH 44240.

Straps should fit so that they do not continually fall from the shoulders. Cups need to be large enough to support fullness near the underarms. The garment needs to fit across the back so that it is not uncomfortably tight. Teenagers generally like attractive undergarments that have some type of lace trim. Puberty is a good time to begin to teach breast self-examination (see

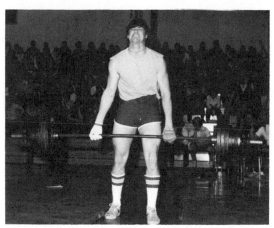

**Figure 21–1.** Young people today mature earlier than in past generations, and they are also taller and heavier. Many develop high levels of physical competence.

page 290). Informational materials are available through the American Cancer Society.

The external genitals grow. Hair develops in the pubic area (see Fig. 21–3 and Box 21–3) and

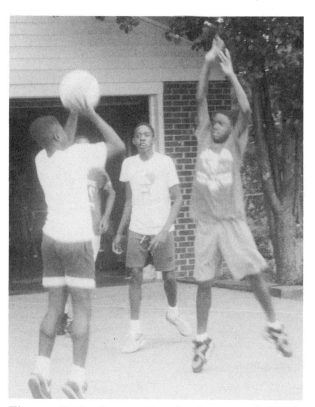

**Figure 21–2.** Gross motor development allows the teenager to develop and enjoy athletic skills with peers. He learns to become a team member.

## Nursing Brief

Although young women are often taught breast examination, young men are seldom instructed in examination of the testes.

the underarms. The body reaches its final measurements about 3 years from the onset of puberty. At this time, the ends of the long bones knit securely to their shafts, and further growth can no longer take place.

### SEXUAL BEHAVIOR

Sexual curiosity and masturbation are common among adolescents. There is also a need for the intimacy of close personal friendships. Seeking one person of the opposite sex to share confidences and feelings may lead to sexual intimacies. This may produce guilt feelings and can lead to isolation from friends and family. The breaking up of such romances is often a source of great emotional pain. Table 21–1 specifies growth tasks related to sexual drives and relationships, and to other areas, according to developmental phase.

Most of our knowledge about the sexual behavior of Americans comes from the pioneering efforts of Alfred Kinsey. Although his studies had flaws, they provided much in-depth information. One of his major findings was that premarital virginity was much rarer than most people thought. Today there is a general liberalization of sexual attitudes. A wide variety of sexual behavior is freely discussed and depicted in movies, in magazines, and on TV (Fig. 21–5). Music directed toward young people often centers on sexual themes. Premarital sexual activity has become much more widespread, and teenagers are initiating their sexual activity at increasingly younger ages. In 1989, a study by Orr et al. determined that 55% of adolescents in grades 7 through 9 were sexually active (Thompson & Ashwill, 1992).

**Sex Education.** In the past, sex education in the public schools tended to concentrate on the physiology of sex, on the reproductive systems, and on venereal disease. It was usually less informative about the psychologic and value aspects of sexuality and the facts about contraception. However, this is changing because

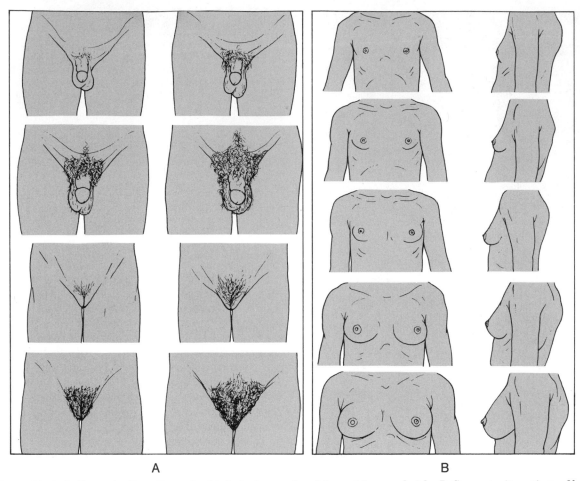

**Figure 21–3.** *A*, Sex maturity ratings of pubic hair changes in adolescent boys and girls. *B*, Sex maturity ratings of breast changes in adolescent girls. (Redrawn from photographs of J.M. Tanner, M.D., Institute of Child Health, Department of Growth and Development, University of London, England.)

of the acquired immunodeficiency syndrome (AIDS) crisis. More comprehensive curriculums, such as "Health Skills for Life," are being developed and utilized. They are geared to kindergarten through grade 12 and present information about all aspects of health, such as nutrition, dental care, how to avoid drugs, and AIDS. These are presented, as age-appropriate. Physiology of the reproductive systems is taught at about grade 5. By grade 8, such topics as coping skills for dating and sexuality, pregnancy, and birth are reviewed. Abstinence and contraception are discussed.

Decision-making is emphasized. Flow charts show the possible consequences of certain actions. The high school units include how to handle teenage pregnancy, prenatal and postnatal

care, and effective parenting techniques. The unit on intimate relationships is a series of discussions and activities designed to help students think about the nature of love. It covers ideas such as compromise, problem-solving, and communication skills. It emphasizes the many good reasons why teenagers should say "no" to casual sex.

These programs have met controversy. Some think they are too inclusive and that such private matters must be discussed in the family. Others think the AIDS crisis has made sexual education imperative. Regardless of one's viewpoint, it is evident that few adolescents can talk freely with their parents about sex, especially about their own sexual behavior and problems. Nonetheless, parents subtly convey sexual val-

| BOX 21-3 | Tanner's Stages of Sexual Maturity |
|---|---|

Sex maturity ratings (SMR) range from 1 to 5. A score of 1 represents the prepubertal child; 5 corresponds to adult status.

### Boys: Genital Development

Stage 1. Preadolescent; testes, scrotum, and penis are of about the same size and proportion as in early childhood
Stage 2. Enlargement of scrotum and testes; skin of scrotum reddens and changes in texture; little or no enlargement of penis at this stage
Stage 3. Enlargement of penis, which occurs at first mainly in length; further growth of testes and scrotum
Stage 4. Increased size of penis with growth in breadth and development of glands; testes and scrotum larger, scrotal skin darkened
Stage 5. Genitalia adult in size and shape

### Girls: Breast Development

Stage 1. Preadolescent: elevation of papilla only
Stage 2. Breast bud stage: elevation of breast and papilla as small mound; enlargement of areolar diameter
Stage 3. Further enlargement and elevation of breast and areola, with no separation of their contours
Stage 4. Projection of areola and papilla to form a secondary mound above the level of the breast
Stage 5. Mature stage: projection of papilla only due to recession of the areola to the general contour of the breast

### Both Sexes: Pubic Hair

Stage 1. Preadolescent; vellus over the pubes is not further developed than that over the abdominal wall, that is, no pubic hair
Stage 2. Sparse growth of long, slightly pigmented, downy hair, straight or curled, chiefly at the base of the penis or along the labia
Stage 3. Considerably darker, coarser, and more curled; hair spreads sparsely over the junction of the pubes
Stage 4. Hair now adult in type, but area covered is considerably smaller than in the adult; no spread to the medial surface of thighs
Stage 5. Adult in quantity and type with distribution of the horizontal (or classically "feminine") pattern; spread to medial surface of thighs, but not up linea alba or elsewhere above the base of the inverse triangle (spread up linea alba occurs and is rated stage 6)

Data from the standard illustrations in Tanner, J.M. (1962). *Growth of adolescence* (2nd ed.). Oxford: Blackwell Scientific.

ues, attitudes, and information by role modeling. In this way, parents initiate the learning of sex roles by their daughters and sons.

Factual and sensitive information provided by concerned parents is, of course, the ideal. However, too often peers provide erroneous material or parents postpone education until a crisis arrives. Children need to be told what bodily changes to expect and why these changes occur. *Two years too soon is better than 1 day too late.* Parents who have answered their children's questions truthfully throughout childhood offer a secure and natural foundation to build on.

**Concerns about Being "Different."** Adolescents have certain concerns that are specific to puberty. The girl who begins to experience physical changes at about the age of 10 may feel self-conscious, for she towers over her friends or has to wear a bra. She may be teased because she is different. The other extreme is the late-comer who feels abnormal and unattractive because her friends look more feminine.

Such problems are not limited to girls. Of particular concern is the boy on a slow schedule of development. Still a "shrimp" at 15, he is unable to compete for placement on school teams because of his size. He sees his male friends being admired for their height and strength, and this is a threat to him. Such fears are natural and usually are alleviated by reassurance that, although boys begin to grow later than girls, their growth spurt lasts longer and that, on the average, boys grow significantly taller than girls. During assessment, the nurse has an op-

1. The *pituitary gland* is a small gland at the base of the brain. It sends out chemical messengers through the blood to various parts of the body. These messengers, or hormones, are responsible for many steps of growth and change as we develop. When a girl reaches the age of puberty, the pituitary gland sends out a new hormone that affects the functions of a group of organs concerned with menstruation.

3. The *ovaries* are two small female organs that manufacture human egg cells. When a girl reaches the age of puberty, these little cells receive a signal from the pituitary gland and begin to grow. Each month a cell escapes from an ovary and starts to travel along a passageway—one of the fallopian tubes. This movement of the egg cell is called ovulation. If one of these cells becomes fertilized by a male cell, it can develop into a baby.

4. The *fallopian tubes*, into which the egg cells pass, lead toward the uterus.

5. The *uterus* is also called the womb. This is where the egg cell develops if it has been fertilized. Each month a soft, thick lining (the endometrium) of tissue and blood vessels forms inside the uterus.

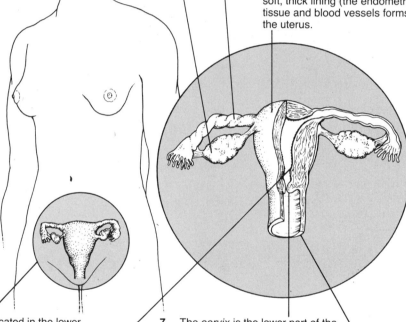

2. The *pelvic area* is located in the lower part of the body in the region of the hips. It is here that the organs associated with menstruation are located.

7. The *cervix* is the lower part of the uterus, which connects it with the vagina.

6. The *endometrium,* or uterus lining, serves as a warm nest to shelter and nourish the unborn child until it has grown enough to be ready to come into the world as a baby. But unless an egg cell has been fertilized and a baby started on its way toward birth, there is no need for the cell or for the blood and tissues of the endometrium. And so they are passed from the body.

8. The *vagina,* a passageway leading to the outside of the lower part of the body, carries away these materials in a flow of blood. This is called menstrual flow. When it occurs, it lasts for several days each month and is known as menstruation.

**Figure 21–4.** Menstruation.

**Table 21–1.** GROWTH TASKS BY DEVELOPMENTAL PHASE

| Tasks | Early: 10–13 Years | Middle: 14–16 Years | Late: 17 Years and Older |
|---|---|---|---|
| Independence | Emotionally breaks from parents and prefers friends to family | Ambivalence about separation | Integration of independence issues |
| Body image | Adjustment to pubescent changes | "Trying on" different images to find real self | Integration of a satisfying body image with personality |
| Sexual drives | Sexual curiosity; occasional masturbation | Sexual experimentation; opposite sex viewed as sex object | Beginning of intimacy and caring |
| Relationships | Unisexual peer group; adult crushes | Begin heterosexual peer group; multiple adult role models | Individual relationships more important than peer group |
| Career plans | Vague and even unrealistic plans ⟶ | | Specific goals and specific steps to implement them |
| Conceptualization | Concrete thinking ⟶ | | Ability to abstract |
| | | Fascinated by capacity for thinking | |
| Value system | Drop in superego; testing of moral system of parents | Self-centered ⟶ | Idealism; rigid concepts of right and wrong. Other-oriented; asceticism |

See accompanying text for further information on tasks.

From Levine M.D., Carey W.B., & Crocker A. (1992). *Developmental-behavioral pediatrics* (2nd ed.). Philadelphia: W. B. Saunders.

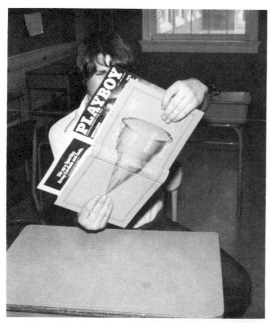

**Figure 21–5.** Teenagers' sexual attitudes are influenced by the media and by a general liberalization of society's attitudes toward sex.

portunity to support the adolescent concerned about normal growth and development.

**Gender Identity.** Gender identity is also being redefined. Traditional sex stereotypes define being "male" by activity and achievement and being "female" by sensitivity and interpersonal competence. Society's current trends toward equality of the sexes may affect these roles. Nevertheless, few adolescents escape the social pressures that dictate acceptable sexual attitudes and behavior for each gender.

In recent years, Jean Miller (*Toward a New Psychology of Women*, 1986) and Carol Gilligan and colleagues (*Women, Girls and Psychotherapy*, 1991) have raised many interesting questions about pressures that affect adolescent girls in a male-dominated society. They suggest that girls lose significant psychological ground during adolescence from a disavowing of the self. The messages girls receive are to be nice, not to be angry, and to submit. Girls begin to believe that by expressing themselves, they will disrupt their relationships. Because of these and other factors, girls are more apt to be depressed and to show more problems of self-esteem than are boys. Gilligan suggests that the cost of girls hiding their viewpoints and feelings may result in long-term psychological problems, particularly eating disorders. (Pillitteri, 1992).

**Homosexuality.** Homosexuality in adolescence is not uncommon. This experimentation is not a positive predictor of adult sexual preference; rather, it may merely indicate a desire to explore alternative lifestyles. However, most homosexuals do report having had homosexual experiences during adolescence (Levine, Carey, & Crocker, 1992). Homosexuality, although no longer classified as a disease, is nonetheless subject to great controversy. *Homophobia* refers to the fear or dislike of homosexuals. Many theories about the origins of homosexuality have been presented. These include a genetic basis, hormonal influences, and psychological and sociologic factors. None has yet been proved. Whether or not one is homosexual, unspoken suspicions during adolescence can create anxiety and turmoil for the young person and family. Gay and lesbian youths, in addition to handling the usual adolescent tasks, face problems of "coming out," rejection, and other issues.

Nurses must be sensitive to these issues when obtaining histories and working with young people. They must also be aware of their personal biases to determine their potential effectiveness with this population. Support groups for parents and friends of gay and lesbians are available. Those who question their sexual orientation are referred to counselors and health agencies that respond to their needs.

## PSYCHOSOCIAL DEVELOPMENT

**Sense of Identity.** The teenager's desire for freedom and independence is extremely important and necessary for developing individuality. To accomplish this, young persons must reject their childhood self and often the people most closely associated with it. Erikson identifies the major task of this group as *identity versus role confusion*. Emancipation is a critical element in the establishment of identity. Figure 21–6 is a picture drawn by a male teenager, illustrating his reaction to being told what to do.

Adolescents want to be people in their own right, and they "try on" different roles. *Self-concept* (one's view of oneself) fluctuates during this time and is molded by the demands of parents, peers, teachers, and others (Fig. 21–7). Interaction with others helps teenagers determine who they are and in what direction they want to proceed. This process is more difficult for low-income minorities and is complicated by many factors, such as illness, broken homes, and extent of formal education. Young persons who are unable to master confusion and establish an identity may become rigid in their actions, bewildered, or depressed, or they may cling to the conformity of peer groups long after the need should have passed. Some show an inordinate need for something "new and exciting." They may experience low self-esteem and alien-

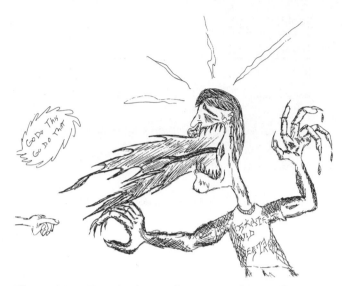

**Figure 21–6.** Drawing by a male teenager showing "how I feel when someone tells me what to do."

ation, and they may confront many other difficulties on entering the adult world.

**Sense of Intimacy.** Developing intimacy is closely entwined with resolving one's sense of identity. As adolescents move toward young adulthood, they become ready to take the risks of close affiliations and friendships and to establish relationships with the opposite sex (Fig. 21–8). Avoidance of this may lead to a deep sense of isolation. Adolescence is a period of trying and testing. Disagreements with parents often revolve around dating, the family car, money, chores, school grades, choice of friends, smoking, sex, and use of social drugs. The young person questions parental values and morals and is particularly sensitive to hypocrisy.

Adults who associate with teenagers should try to create an atmosphere of interest and understanding. Adolescents must know that adults care. They need practice in making deci-

## Nursing Brief

In adolescence, dependency creates hostility. Parents who foster dependence invite unavoidable resentment. Wise parents make themselves increasingly dispensable. Their language is sprinkled with such statements as "The choice is yours." "You decide about that." "If you want to." "It's your decision." "Whatever you choose is fine with me." *(Haim Ginott)*

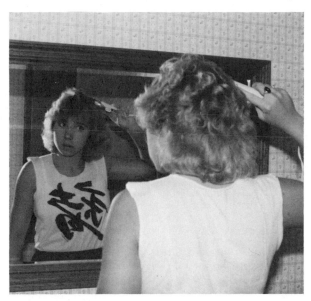

**Figure 21–7.** The teenager's self-esteem is influenced by how far her body image deviates from the mythic (body ideal).

sions, which need to be respected even if they make mistakes. Parents should set limits and expect them to be challenged but adhered to. Parents and nurses who see other people's intrinsic worth, feel good about themselves, and do not see the teenager's behavior as a reflection on their parenting or nursing provide a more secure environment for growth. Loving detachment is not easy, but it is an effective tool in dealing with adolescents.

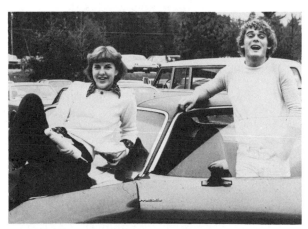

**Figure 21–8.** As adolescents move toward young adulthood, they become ready to take the risks of close affiliations and friendships and to establish relationships with members of the opposite sex.

**Cultural Considerations.** Americans are multicolored, multicultural, and multilingual. The value of independence as a goal of maturational and emotional development may not be adopted by all. Many immigrants and Americans of Asian-American background come from societies that are patriarchal and highly structured and that have distinct social roles. The good of the family takes precedence over personal goals. The protection of family image and neighborhood reputation is essential. The Chinese do not recognize the period of adolescence. There is no word for it in their language. Chinese children grow up in a society that offers little choice for mobility. A period of rebellion or the need to find an identity is incongruent with their system (Brown, 1983). The nurse's awareness of these and other cultural influences on the adolescent's behavior will help to provide holistic care (Fig. 21–9).

**Realistic Body Image.** In early adolescence, the young person must adjust to the dramatic changes of puberty. The focusing on bodily development during early and middle adolescence is one factor contributing to egocentrism, or self-centeredness. Young persons create what has been termed an "imaginary audience." They believe everyone is looking at them. This preoccupation with self is normal and accounts for the constant hair-combing and makeup-repairing frequently observed in a group of

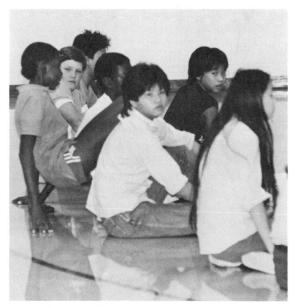

**Figure 21–9.** Understanding ethnic and cultural variations among teenagers is important in assessment planning.

teenagers. By late adolescence, most have completed their growth and are less self-conscious. Obesity, chronic illness, or anorexia nervosa may complicate or exacerbate unresolved problems of body image.

## COGNITIVE DEVELOPMENT

Piaget's theory of cognitive development holds that development is systematic, sequential, and orderly. Young adolescents are still in the concrete phase of thinking. They take words literally. A young teenage girl, if asked by the nurse, "Have you ever slept with anyone?" may not connect the question with a vaginal infection or sex. By middle adolescence, the ability to think abstractly has increased. Piaget calls this the stage of *formal operations*.

Older adolescents can see a situation from many viewpoints and can imagine or organize unseen or unexperienced possibilities. The failure to develop formal thoughts is cited by some as connected to the failure to develop a high level of moral reasoning. Adolescents who have developed both are most likely to evidence a high degree of morality and consistency in their behavior.

## PEER RELATIONSHIPS

Adolescent peer groups vary in number, interests, social background, and structure. They may consist of small groups of the same sex or both sexes, and, in late adolescence, of small groups of couples. The young person may belong to one or several groups. The peer group serves as a mirror for "normality" and helps determine where one "fits in." It is vitally important in helping adolescents define themselves. Acceptance by one's friends helps decrease the loneliness and sense of loss many teenagers experience on the road to adulthood (Fig. 21–10).

The social norms and pressures exerted by the group may cause problems. The selection of friends and allegiance to them may bring about confrontations within the family. Parents need help in understanding that the teenager's exaggerated conformity is necessary to moving away from dependence and obtaining approval from persons outside the nuclear family. Failure to develop social competence may produce feelings of inadequacy and low self-esteem.

Nurses can assist the family by supporting them and by educating them in the dynamics of this age group. They can direct them to such groups as peer helpers (for the adolescent) and

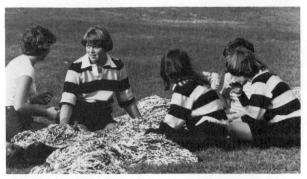

**Figure 21–10.** Immersion into a peer group helps adolescents free themselves from childhood dependence.

community educational programs sponsored by various agencies. Organizations such as Parents Without Partners might be another avenue. Teenagers who do not belong to the dominant system, for example, those from different cultural, social, or economic backgrounds, may see themselves as being quite different from their friends. For these teenagers, the utilization of family networks may prove helpful.

## CAREER PLANS

Some adolescents graduate from high school with a definite idea of what they would like to do. Many, however, are unsure of what they want. To choose a career that is best-suited for them, teenagers must first know themselves. What particularly interests them? What are they good at? What are their shortcomings?

By this time, adolescents have already taken some definite steps toward a goal. Choice of high-school curriculum and grades determines eligibility for college or preparation for a specific vocation. Parents should observe the interests of their children and encourage them to take advantage of their talents (Fig. 21–11). Whenever possible, a teenager should investigate various fields by talking to people who are involved in them.

Valuable information can also be obtained by career exploration, which is available at most colleges, and by pamphlets from professional organizations, the government, and other sources. The school guidance counselor administers aptitude tests as an additional guide and can work with the teenagers to expose them to as wide a selection of careers as possible (Fig. 21–12). The teenager must make the final decision. To be happy in their work, teenagers must choose

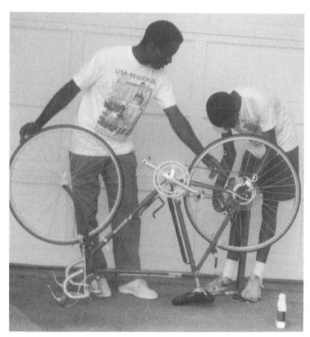

**Figure 21-11.** Mechanical skills will be useful in recreational or vocational pursuits.

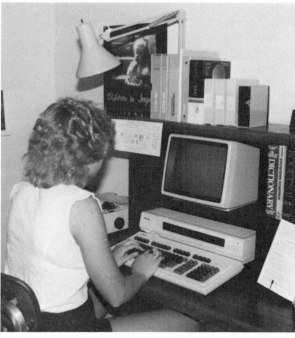

**Figure 21-12.** Technologic advances, such as the computer, are an integral part of the young person's learning process.

it of their own free will, not because their parents expect them to follow in their footsteps.

As a result of the feminist movement, more types of work are open to young women. Many are selecting careers that support an independent lifestyle, although they may choose to marry. Women also make up a larger proportion of the work force and are being introduced to more nontraditional occupations. Nevertheless, teenagers face more unemployment than do adults, and young women experience a higher rate of unemployment than do young men.

The job market today is extremely competitive and almost nonexistent for some people without skills or education. The unemployment rate is high among the general population, minorities, and the disabled. Certain fields of employment (high-tech industries) and certain geographic locations have fallen on hard times because of the economic recession. The causes of this are multifold, but the results are often feelings of hopelessness and decreased self-esteem in the individual.

Productive employment of young people needs to fit their life framework and offer an opportunity for personal growth. Some constructive aspects of employment include helping to build self-esteem, promoting responsibility, testing new skills, constructively chan-

neling energies, providing money for increased independence, engaging the young person in interactions with adults, and allowing them to assume an active rather than a passive role. In contrast, when adolescents are forced to take a job because of economic or personal pressures, they may have to drop out of school. With few skills and no experience, they may remain locked in low-level employment. This is often perpetuated from one generation to another.

## RESPONSIBILITY

Young people look forward to challenges. Parents must watch for ways to free their children to take on new responsibilities. Even routine jobs can be made more inspiring if youths are taught to see them in relation to a longer-term objective. Astronauts have a certain amount of dull routine in their jobs; so do doctors, nurses, and scientists. They are able to accept routine tasks because they contribute to the effectiveness of the entire project.

Young adolescents must also be taught the value of money. An allowance helps them learn management. If money is simply handed out as requested, it is more difficult to develop responsibility for finances. Allowances should be increased from time to time in order to comply with the age and needs of the teenager.

Middle and older adolescents who have jobs can be taught to use a checkbook and a savings account. Many find satisfaction in purchasing their own clothes. A teenager who buys an old car soon discovers that it takes money to run and repair it. Such experiences provide valu-

able lessons in finance. Among younger teenagers, a common means of earning money is baby-sitting. Many boys and girls begin to baby-sit at about 12 or 13 years of age. Baby-sitting courses are valuable because young people need to be prepared for this important responsibility. Box 21–4 outlines responsibilities of the baby-sitter.

---

| BOX 21–4 | Guidelines for Teenage Baby-sitters |
| --- | --- |

**Written Information**

- Address and phone number where parents can be reached
- What time will they be home?
- Emergency numbers, such as fire, police, neighbor, friend, doctor
- Bedtime (favorite blanket, toys, location of clothing)
- Special instructions (word for potty, medicine, and so on)
- Address of home where you are sitting
- Advise own parents of the above, including telephone number and approximate time you will return

**Telephone**

- Do not divulge that you are the sitter
- Convey to the caller that the person being sought cannot come to the phone
- Offer to take a message
- Write message down
- Limit personal phone calls

**Doors**

- Keep locked
- Ask parents if they are expecting anyone
- Attempted entry is rare in well-lighted home; if this occurs, keep calm, telephone police, do not hang up receiver

**Fire**

- Learn exits from house; know location of fire extinguisher
- Do not smoke cigarettes while baby-sitting
- Remove children immediately from building if fire apparent; stay together; do not reenter building
- Do not throw water on a grease fire; use baking soda
- If there is a lot of smoke, crawl along floor
- "Stop, drop, and roll" if clothing is ignited
- Call 911 or fire department immediately

**Responsibility and Privileges**

- Know where children are at all times
- Become interested in child; get to know habits
- No visitors unless cleared with parents
- Clarify hourly wage; have figured out in case you are asked
- Notify your parents if you will be later than expected; consult before accepting a job
- Do not sit if you are ill
- Do not hesitate to ask questions before parents leave; know what is expected of you; call parents when necessary
- Determine use of television, videocassette recorder, and availability of snacks
- Enroll in baby-sitting course as available in your area (American Red Cross, library, service agencies)

## WORRIES

Teenagers worry a lot. They are able to talk about fears that are not too intimate, such as school examinations or how they will look with a certain haircut. Nevertheless, they need assistance in understanding their emotions and in sorting out confused feelings. Adults must provide a confidential, accepting atmosphere in order to foster quality communication. One of the more difficult aspects of communicating with adolescents is their fluctuating attitude. They may vary from unconcern about deadlines to panic. They may wish to please but be overly critical of themselves and their own performance. They may try to control others by overtalkativeness and demonstrations of competence.

Physical symptoms such as stomachaches, dizziness, headaches, and insomnia surface and disappear periodically. Anxiety over future events, the possibilities of injury, relationships with peers, and meeting expectations of others are also prevalent. Age-mates often best understand their peers and so are well equipped to provide support (Fig. 21–13).

Teenagers often experience their parents' pain and feel tremendously responsible for the family's burdens and failures. For many, the image of what a family should be is derived from TV. Adolescents who have lifetime handicaps, alcoholic parents, physical or mental illness, or other serious problems, such as poverty, need the support of the medical community and other community resources. Bizarre behavior may be a call for long-overdue help.

## DAYDREAMS

Adolescents spend a lot of time daydreaming, in the solitude of their rooms or during a biology lecture. Most of this behavior is normal and natural for this age group. Daydreaming is usually considered harmless if the young person continues the usual active pursuits. It also serves several purposes. Adolescence is a lonely, in-between age; daydreaming helps fill the void. Imaginatively acting out what will be said or done in various situations prepares teenagers to deal with others, so that they are better able to cope with real situations. Daydreams are also a valuable safety valve for the expression of strong feelings.

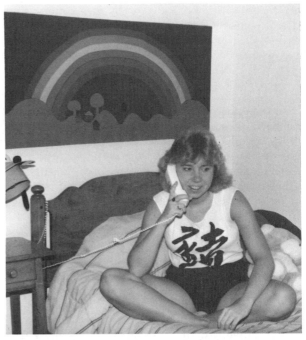

**Figure 21–13.** The teenager often finds that those who understand her best are age-mates. Communicating by telephone provides needed peer support.

## HETEROSEXUAL RELATIONSHIPS

Adolescents need to meet and become acquainted with members of the opposite sex. This may begin by admiration from afar, which is accompanied by daydreams as the young person attempts to attract the other's attention. Competition and rivalry may be keen. The adolescent may date a number of people or merely one. Dates may be frequent or sporadic.

The adolescent's cultural background influences patterns of dating. Conflict often arises when the teenager wants to be independent and quickly adopts American norms of dating while parents insist on strict traditional values. This is particularly noticeable with daughters.

Dating is one of the early social aspects of growing up. As such, it may become a battleground for the struggle for independence. Parental opposition is often based on their unspoken fears of rejection. They may also fear AIDS, sexual experimentation, or pregnancy. Parents may respond by imposing strict restrictions, such as curfews, chaperones, and limitations on use of the car. When these problems are not discussed openly, the adolescent may react by rebelling sexually or by other means for the purpose of testing injunctions of control, rather than for the prohibited act itself.

## Parenting

At times it is difficult for parents to cope with adolescents. The shift in parenting philosophies, from the rigid rules of discipline, to permissiveness, to the current middle-of-the-road position, has led to confusion. Some parents are unsure of their own opinions and may hesitate to exert authority. Others refuse to "let go" or change any of their beliefs to accommodate youth. Issues of privacy and trust abound, and conflict occurs as the adolescent desires more adult liberties. Some approaches to such problems are presented in Table 21–2.

The teenager who is the subject of heavy concentrations of parental attention can become overanxious. Mothers have a particular problem because they have to substitute other satisfactions for the dependent child. As adolescents

mature, they become more secure and are able to develop a new and more satisfactory relationship with their parents. In the meantime, one must keep the lines of communication open and realize that "this too shall pass" (Fig. 21–14). In spite of the problems parents face with their teenagers, throughout adolescence the family continues to play a major role in socialization (Fig. 21–15).

## Health Education and Guidance

### NUTRITION

Teenagers grow rapidly; therefore, they need foods that provide for their increase in height, body-cell mass, and maturation. Dietary deficiencies are more likely to occur at this age because of this acceleration and because eating patterns become more irregular. Nutritional requirements are more strongly correlated with sex maturity ratings (SMR) than with age.

**Table 21–2.** EFFECTIVE APPROACHES TO PROBLEMS

| Approach | Purpose | Example |
|---|---|---|
| Reflective listening | Showing you understand teenager's feelings. Used when teenager "owns" problem | "You're very worried about the semester exam?" "Sounds like you're feeling discouraged because the job's so difficult." |
| "I" message | Communicating your feelings about how teenager's behavior affects you. Used when you own problem | "When I'm ill and the dishes are left for me to do, I feel disrespected because it seems no one cares about me." "When you borrow tools and don't return them, I feel discouraged because I don't have the tools I need when there's a job to do." |
| Exploring alternatives | Helping teenagers decide how to solve problems they own<br>Negotiating agreements with teenager when you own problem | "What are some ways you could solve this problem?" "Which idea appeals to you most?" "Are you willing to do this until _____?"<br>"What can we do to settle this conflict between us?" "Are we in agreement on that idea?" "What would be a fair consequence if the agreement is broken?" |
| Natural and logical consequences | Permitting teenagers, within limits, to decide how they will behave and allowing them to experience consequences<br>Natural consequences apply when teenager owns problem. Logical consequences apply when either parent or teenager owns problem | *Natural:* teenager who forgets coat on cold days gets cold; teenager who skips lunch goes hungry<br>*Logical:* teenager who spends allowance quickly does not receive any more money until next allowance day; teenager who neglects to study for a test gets low grade |

Systemic Training for Effective Parenting of Teens, Parenting Teenagers © 1990, by Don Dinkmeyer and Gary D. McKay.

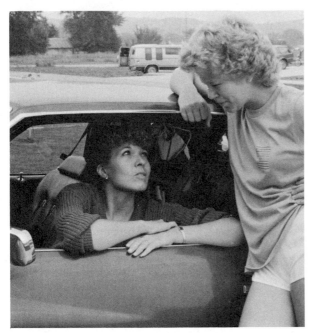

**Figure 21–14.** Listening is an important tool for establishing rapport.

Girls at SMR 2 and boys at SMR 3, for example, are close to their peak growth velocities. They require adequate intake of nutrients and calories, regardless of chronologic age.

The most noticeable changes in the adolescent's eating habits are skipped meals, more be-tween-meal snacks, and eating out more often. Breakfast and lunch are often omitted. Parttime jobs, school activities, and socialization may result in the teenager's eating little or nothing during the day and then "catching up" in the evening. Fast-food restaurants are inexpensive and provide food quickly for the busy adolescent. These foods tend to be high in calories, fat, protein, sugar, and sodium, and low in fiber. Most food chains have added salads and other more healthy foods, which is applauded. Carbonated drinks often replace milk, resulting in low intakes of calcium, riboflavin, and vitamins A and D. The few fruits and vegetables eaten provide insufficient fiber.

Foods should be selected from the basic food groups. In estimating calories, variables such as physical activity and gender must also be considered. Nutritional research pertaining to this age group is still meager, partly because studies must account for age as well as physical maturity. Minerals most likely to be inadequately supplied in the adolescent's diet are calcium and iron. Zinc is known to be essential for growth and sexual maturation and is therefore of great importance in adolescence. The retention of zinc increases, especially during the growth spurt, leading to more efficient use of sources of this nutrient in the diet (Mahan & Arlin, 1992). Good sources of zinc include meat, liver, eggs, and seafood, particularly oysters. Sources for vegetarians include nuts, beans, wheat germ, and cheese.

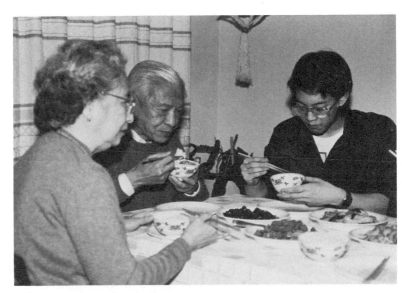

**Figure 21–15.** The family continues to be an important agent of socialization for the adolescent. (From Foster, R. Hunsberger, M., & Anderson, J.J. [1989]. *Family-centered nursing care of children*. Philadelphia: W.B. Saunders, p. 620.)

Calcium has a key role in bone formation. In both girls and boys, the daily recommended dietary allowance (RDA) for calcium increases from 800 mg at age 10 to 1200 mg during the growth spurt. The primary source of calcium is dairy products.

The need for iron increases in both sexes at this time. This increased need is primarily due to increases in muscle mass and blood volume in boys and, to a lesser degree, in girls. A menstruating female loses 15–30 mg of iron per cycle. Iron absorption varies in individuals. Good sources of iron include liver, poultry, fish, dried beans, vegetables, egg yolk, and enriched breads. The RDAs for adolescents are listed in Table 21–3.

**Vegetarian Diets.** A number of young people are becoming vegetarians. Lacto-ovo vegetarians include eggs and dairy products in their diets and generally have adequate nutrient intakes. This is one of the most common types of vegetarian diet.

However, total vegetarians (vegan), who eat no animal protein, eggs, or dairy products are at particular risk of developing deficiencies in protein, vitamin $B_{12}$, calcium, iron, iodine and possibly zinc. A total vegetarian diet can be adequate only if it is carefully planned.

**Sports and Nutrition.** The best training diet is one that contains foods from each of the basic food groups in sufficient quantities to meet energy demands and nutrient requirements. There is no evidence that eating large amounts of special foods or nutrients improves athletic performance. Protein supplements are not necessary and could even be harmful. Sweat must be replaced by drinking small amounts of fluid during a workout. Thirst is one guide for intake. Carbohydrates should not be used as the sole energy source, as they are stored in the body for a relatively short time. Sodium and potassium are usually replaced by eating a well-balanced diet.

Caffeine and alcohol deplete body water and are to be avoided. Anabolic steroids, used by some athletes to gain weight and increase strength, are detrimental to bone growth. Iron is particularly necessary for female athletes, who may be borderline or deficient in their intake of this mineral. On the day of the event, the athlete is advised to eliminate roughage, fats, and gas-forming foods.

**Fad Diets, Anorectic Drugs.** Fad diets, although popular with the teenager, provide little long-term success. Unsupervised weight loss can be dangerous. Anorectic drugs (sympathomimetic agents, diuretics, hormones) have limited effect on weight loss and can be harmful. The potential for stimulant-type drug abuse among teenagers is high, which makes avoidance of such self-medication even more important. Most fad diets tend to be monotonous. Liquid-protein diets can lead to a serious electrolyte imbalance. Diets that promote special food combinations tend to be unbalanced and expensive and difficult to maintain over a period of time. *Prolonged fasting can be life-threatening.*

A balanced weight reduction plan based on milk, meat, bread, fruits, and vegetables is best for losing weight gradually and maintaining the weight loss. It teaches the young person how to select nutritious foods and helps establish patterns that can be lifelong. Behavior modification techniques, such as keeping food diaries and learning to eat more slowly, and nonfood rewards, such as clothing and flowers, have also proved successful when combined with sensible eating. Weight reduction programs should also include an increase in regular physical activity. Group participation provides an opportunity for peer contact,

**Table 21–3.** RECOMMENDED DIETARY ALLOWANCES FOR THE ADOLESCENT AGED 11–18 YEARS

| Nutrient | Ages 11–14 Years | | Ages 15–18 Years | |
|---|---|---|---|---|
| | *Males* | *Females* | *Males* | *Females* |
| Kilocalories | 2500 | 2200 | 3000 | 2200 |
| Protein (gm) | 45 | 46 | 59 | 46 |
| Vitamin A (µg RE) | 1000 | 800 | 1000 | 800 |
| Vitamin D (µg) | 10 | 10 | 10 | 10 |
| Vitamin E (mg TE) | 10 | 8 | 10 | 8 |
| Vitamin C (mg) | 50 | 50 | 60 | 60 |
| Folate (µg) | 150 | 150 | 200 | 180 |
| Niacin (mg) | 17 | 15 | 20 | 15 |
| Riboflavin (mg) | 1.5 | 1.3 | 1.8 | 1.3 |
| Thiamine (mg) | 1.3 | 1.1 | 1.5 | 1.1 |
| Vitamin $B_6$ (mg) | 1.7 | 1.4 | 2 | 1.5 |
| Vitamin $B_{12}$ (µg) | 2 | 2 | 2 | 2 |
| Calcium (mg) | 1200 | 1200 | 1200 | 1200 |
| Phosphorus (mg) | 1200 | 1200 | 1200 | 1200 |
| Iodine (µg) | 150 | 150 | 150 | 150 |
| Iron (mg) | 12 | 15 | 12 | 15 |
| Magnesium (mg) | 270 | 280 | 400 | 300 |
| Zinc (mg) | 15 | 12 | 15 | 12 |
| Selenium (µg) | 40 | 45 | 50 | 50 |

From National Academy of Sciences–National Research Council. (1989). *Recommended Dietary Allowances* (10th ed.). Washington, DC.
Key: RE, retinol equivalent; TE, tocopherol equivalent.

acceptance, and support (see discussion of obesity, pp. 760–762).

## PERSONAL CARE

**Sleep.** Sleep requirements vary from individual to individual. Adolescents may obtain the 8 hours generally suggested, but often at irregular hours. Many employed young people have to work very late hours, particularly in the summer months. This necessitates sleeping later in the morning. Another trend is for the young people who have worked long hours during the day to try to make up for lost time after work. They seem either to sleep all the time or to burn the candle at both ends! Complaints of fatigue are heard more often at home than elsewhere. If teenagers stay up late at night, they will be tired in the morning. This is called "learning by natural consequences."

**Exercise.** Exercise has many benefits. One does not have to participate actively in sports per se to derive the benefits from a brisk walk, bike ride, or swim. Many teenagers who are not athletes can benefit from a less sedentary lifestyle. These patterns, when carried over into adulthood, contribute to good health.

**Hygiene.** The adolescent needs personal hygiene information because body changes require more frequent bathing and the use of deodorants. The nurse can help the young person sort out the various claims of reliability for hair removal, menstrual hygiene, and cosmetics products and procedures. Ear-piercing should be performed by an experienced person. The skin around the point of insertion of the earring is regularly inspected for signs of infection. Swapping of earrings is discouraged. Teenagers are warned not to use another's razor, particularly in light of the AIDS epidemic.

**Dental Health.** The prevalence of tooth decay has substantially decreased over the past few years. This is believed to result from the widespread use of fluorides, including community fluoridation, and dental products containing fluorides. Teenagers are nonetheless at risk for dental caries because of inadequate dental maintenance and frequent snacking on sucrose-containing candies and beverages. When dental hygiene is neglected, the period of greatest tooth decay in the permanent teeth is from ages 12–18 years. Lack of oral hygiene (inadequate brushing, flossing, and rinsing, particularly after meals) fosters the accumulation of plaque and food debris. Missing, aching, or decayed teeth contribute to poor nutrition. Young people with unattractive teeth may suffer from low self-esteem.

Healthy, white teeth are synonymous with popularity and sex appeal, according to media hype. A visit to the dentist twice a year is out of reach for many financially strapped young persons. For others it has low financial priority in the family. There is a need for more school dental programs and other innovative measures to reach a major proportion of our society. Dental insurance, although helpful, is generally available only for fully employed persons.

## SAFETY

The chief hazard to the adolescent is the automobile (Fig. 21–16). Road accidents kill and cripple teenagers at alarming rates. Many schools now offer driver training courses as an integral part of the educational program. Students learn how to drive and the accompanying responsibilities; however, this does not ensure compliance. Preventing motor vehicle accidents is of utmost importance to every community. Adolescents who ride motorcycles, motor scooters, or motorbikes should know the rules of the road and wear special safety equipment, such as helmets.

Young people should learn how to swim and swimming safety. Accidents result from diving into unsafe areas and from using alcohol or drugs while swimming. If adolescents are interested in hunting or similar sports that require a gun, they must be instructed in the proper safeguards.

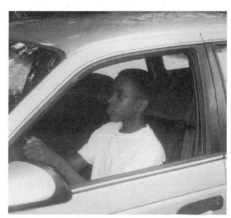

**Figure 21–16.** "I can't wait to get my driver's license." The teenager's search for independence also brings responsibilities.

The growing drug trade and the increase in vandalism and crime expose adolescents to unprecedented assaults in their schools and in their neighborhoods. Gang-related deaths from guns and knife wounds have escalated greatly. Seven out of ten homicides involve males. To parents and all who provide services to children, this growing menace is a source of great frustration and concern.

## PHYSICAL EXAMINATION

The prevention of illness in this age group, as in all others, is of primary importance. Yearly physical examinations are recommended for healthy adolescents. This is often a requirement for the young person wishing to enter a certain sport. Locker room physical examinations can vary greatly in their thoroughness. Immunizations need to be reviewed and updated. A rubella titer should be obtained from all girls. Those found to lack protective levels should be immunized, regardless of any history of infection or immunizations. The young woman is instructed to avoid pregnancy for at least 2 months after immunization. Many other screening programs are conducted in the school and community. Deficits of vision and hearing, scoliosis, or high blood pressure may be detected.

## TOXIC SHOCK SYNDROME

A menstrual history and gynecologic examination should be a routine part of the assessment of the adolescent girl. Toxic shock syndrome, although relatively rare, appears to be higher among adolescent females than other populations. Refer to page 284 for a more in-depth discussion of toxic shock syndrome.

## ADOLESCENT PREGNANCY AND SEXUAL RESPONSIBILITY

Approximately 1 million adolescent females become pregnant annually in the United States. Late prenatal registration for obstetric care of uninformed or frightened teenagers is common. The sequelae of adolescent pregnancy include a higher incidence of obstetric complications, as well as neonatal problems of prematurity and other infant risk factors. First intercourse experiences among young people are often characterized by the absence of effective contraception.

For the pregnant girl, concerns of body image become blurred, education is interrupted, and she may be separated from sources of support, such as her peer group. The father's studies may also be interrupted; he may become locked in low-paying employment; and he may face responsibilities for which he is ill-prepared.

Parenting classes, which provide guidance and support, and continued education regarding the normal processes of child growth and development are vital for these young people and for the health and welfare of their children. There is growing evidence that comprehensive programs for the pregnant teenager and her baby, especially those that emphasize continued schooling, are associated with fewer repeat pregnancies. Methods of contraception should be clarified to the adolescent who is at risk, even though there may be no guarantee that they will be put to use (Chapter 11). Many teenagers prefer to postpone intercourse. They need to understand that a choice exists and that delay is acceptable.

## KEY POINTS

- Adolescence is defined as the period of life beginning with the appearance of secondary sex characteristics and ending with cessation of growth and emotional maturity.
- According to Erikson, the major developmental task of adolescence is to establish a sense of identity.
- Freud considered adolescence as the last stage of psychosexual development. He termed this the *genital stage*.
- Jean Piaget suggests that the cognitive development during adolescence reflects abstract reasoning, and logic. He calls this stage the period of *formal operations*.
- The physical development seen during this period is distinguished by puberty, the stage at which the reproductive organs become functional and secondary sex characteristics develop.

- The first menstrual period is called the *menarche*.
- The teenager struggles with the development of a realistic body image.
- The epidemic of AIDS creates new demands for accurate, safe, and timely sex education.
- Adolescence is a time of conflict with parental authority and values. The influence of peers and heterosexual relationships increase.
- Motor vehicle accidents, homicide, and drownings are leading causes of mortality in this age group.

# Study Questions

1. Define the following: preadolescence, puberty, menstruation, menarche, and toxic shock syndrome.
2. Identify the physiologic changes that occur during puberty and adolescence.
3. Pedro and Maria are each beginning to establish a sense of identity. What does this mean? How might this development be reflected in their behavior?
4. Do you feel that you were well prepared for the changes that took place at puberty? How might you have been helped to meet this adjustment more satisfactorily?
5. At what age do you feel heterosexual relationships should begin? What anticipatory guidance is required to prepare young persons adequately for this event?
6. Plan a day's menu for 15-year-old Susan and 17-year-old Ron. What are their nutritional requirements for calories, protein, calcium, and iron?
7. Janet is 18 and a freshman in college. She has not selected a major field of study because she is not sure what she wants to do. What information would you need to know about Janet in order to guide her in making this decision?
8. Alice, age 16, spends a great deal of her time daydreaming. Of what value is this to her? How can it be detrimental?
9. Identify the common anxieties and fears of the adolescents, and suggest ways in which they might try to conceal them.
10. Review and discuss Table 21–2 on effective approaches to adolescent problems.

# Multiple Choice Review Questions

*Choose the most appropriate answer.*

1. One of the tasks of adolescence as defined by Erikson is
   a. finding an identity
   b. sexual latency
   c. heterosexuality
   d. concrete operations
2. Piaget defines the mid-adolescent as able to think in abstract terms. He refers to this as the
   a. sensorimotor stage
   b. preoperational stage
   c. stage of concrete operations
   d. stage of formal operations
3. Puberty can most accurately be defined as the period of life characterized by
   a. occurrence of sexual maturity and appearance of secondary sex characteristics
   b. substitution of adult interests and value systems for child interests
   c. the most rapid rate of physical and mental growth and development
   d. the awakening of sexual feelings and the initiation of sexual experience

4. Pat, age 16, towers over her companions. This bothers her, and she confides in you and says, "I just hate school—everyone is always staring at me." You answer
   a. "Don't pay any attention to it."
   b. "You just don't know how lucky you are to be tall."
   c. "This will resolve itself in time. Don't worry."
   d. "Tell me more about how this embarrasses you."

5. Raoul, age 17, approaches you for the family car. Which answer would help to increase his sense of responsibility and independence?
   a. "You know how much I worry when you take the car."
   b. "Forget it, I'll drive you."
   c. "You may have the car, but don't tell your father."
   d. "You may have the car, provided you refill the gas tank."

## BIBLIOGRAPHY

American Red Cross. Baby sitting course. Unpublished material. Des Moines, IA: American Red Cross.

Beall, S., & Schmidt, G. (1984). Development of a youth adaptation rating scale. *Journal of School Health, 54,* 197.

Behrman, R.E. (1992). *Nelson textbook of pediatrics* (14th ed.). Philadelphia: W.B. Saunders.

Brown, B. (1983). Growing up healthy: The Chinese experience. *Pediatric Nursing, 9,* 255.

Ching, C. (1984). Vietnamese in America: A case study in cross-cultural health education. *Health Values, 8,* 16.

Dinkmeyer, D., & McKay, G. (1990). *Parenting teenagers (STEP)* (2nd ed.). Circle Pines, MI: American Guidance Service.

Erikson, E. (1963). *Childhood and society* (2nd. rev. ed.). New York: W.W. Norton.

Gilligan, C., Rogers, A., & Tolman, D. (1991). *Women, girls and psychotherapy.* New York: Harrington Park Press.

Gizis, R. (1992). Nutrition in women across the life span. *Nursing Clinics of North America, 27,* 971.

Gortmaker, S., Walker, D., Weitzman, M., & Sobol, A. (1990). Chronic conditions, socioeconomic risks, and behavioral problems in children and adolescents. *Pediatrics, 85,* 267.

Levine, M.D., Carey, W.B., & Crocker, A.C. (1992). *Developmental behavioral pediatrics* (2nd ed.). Philadelphia: W.B. Saunders.

Mahan, L.K., & Arlin, M.T. (1992). *Krause's food, nutrition & diet therapy* (8th ed.). Philadelphia: W.B. Saunders.

Miller, J.B. (1986). *Toward a new psychology of women* (2nd ed.). Boston: Beacon.

Mott, S., James, S.R., & Sperhac, A.M. (1991). *Nursing care of children and families* (2nd ed.). Reading, MA: Addison-Wesley.

Orr, D., Wilbrandt, M., Brack, C., Rauch, S., & Ingersoll, G. (1989). Reported sexual behaviors and self-esteem among young adolescents. *American Journal of Disabilities in Children, 143,* 86.

Pillitteri, A. (1992). *Maternal and child health nursing.* Philadelphia: J.B. Lippincott.

Poleman, C.M., & Peckenpaugh, N.J. (1991). *Nutrition essentials and diet therapy* (6th ed.). Philadelphia: W.B. Saunders.

Thompson, E.D., & Ashwill, J.W. (1992). *Introduction to pediatric nursing* (6th ed.) Philadelphia: W.B. Saunders.

Whaley, L., & Wong, D. (1991). *Nursing care of infants and children* (4th ed.). St. Louis: C.V. Mosby.

# Unit 3

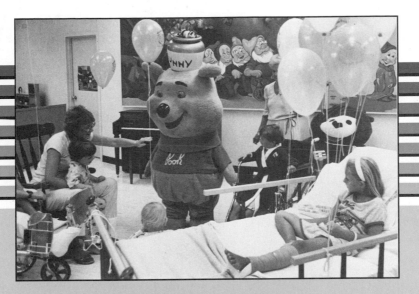

# The Child Needing Nursing Care

*Courtesy of Blank Memorial Hospital for Children, Des Moines, IA.*

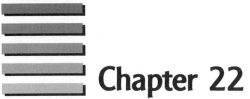

## Chapter 22

# The Child's Experience
# of Hospitalization

### VOCABULARY
**emancipated minor (552)**
**narcissistic (551)**
**peer (551)**
**rapport (547)**
**respite care (553)**
**rivalry (548)**
**role model (544)**
**separation anxiety (542)**
**sibling (542)**
**transitional object (546)**

The Hospitalized Infant
The Hospitalized Toddler
The Hospitalized Preschool Child
The Hospitalized School-Age Child
The Hospitalized Adolescent

# OBJECTIVES

*On completion and mastery of Chapter 22, the student will be able to*

■ Define each vocabulary term listed.
■ Describe three phases of separation anxiety.
■ Identify two problems confronting siblings of the hospitalized child.
■ List two ways in which the nurse can lessen the stress of hospitalization on the child's parents.
■ Contrast the child's and adult's expression of pain.
■ List four ways of providing sensorimotor activities for the infant.
■ Describe two ways to prepare the child emotionally for surgery.
■ Describe two milestones in the psychosocial development of the preschool child that contribute either positively or negatively to the adjustment to hospitalization.
■ Contrast the problems of the preschool child and school-age child facing hospitalization.
■ List three strengths of the teenager that the nurse might utilize when formulating nursing care plans.

Three major causes of stress for children of all ages are separation, pain, and fear of body intrusion. They are influenced by the patient's developmental age, the maturity of the parents, cultural and economic factors, religious background, past experiences, family size, state of health on admission, and other factors.

**Separation Anxiety.** Separation anxiety is most pronounced in the toddler. It is not as apparent before 4 months of age, but marked anxiety about a specific event may be seen thereafter. The stages of separation anxiety are presented on page 544. Because of their limited life experiences, children are more vulnerable to strange situations than adults. To make the hospital more "user friendly," the nurse can place age-appropriate books, toys, and crayons in the room before admission.

**Pain.** The negative physical and psychological consequences of pain are well documented. Patients in pain secrete higher levels of cortisol, have compromised immune systems, more infections, and delayed wound healing. Despite a greater national awareness of the need for pain relief, children's pain continues to be undertreated (Kachoyeanos & Friedhoff, 1993).

Nurses must maintain a high level of suspicion for pain when caring for children. Infants cannot show the nurse where it hurts, and frequently a child's report of pain is not given the credibility of an adult's report. Also, children may not realize they are supposed to report pain to the nurse. If children feel they will receive an injection in order to be more comfortable, they may refrain from complaining. Figure 22–1 lists four pain assessment tools. Chronically ill children in pain are frequently categorized as "demanding," "irritable," "manipulative," and worse. Their parents may be blamed for their behavior. Also of concern is the amount of emotional pain family members experience when a child is in physical pain.

Techniques such as drawing, distraction, imagery, relaxation, and cognitive strategies as well as *analgesia* provide necessary relief from symptoms. The child may draw "how the pain feels" and where it is located. Distractions such as story telling, quiet conversation, and puppet play are effective. Imagery techniques, such as having children imagine themselves in a safe place, relieves anxiety. Another technique is to have the child visualize an imaginary "magic glove" to lessen the discomfort of finger sticks. Kachoyeanos describes visualizing a "pain switch," similar to a light switch that can be turned off and on (Kachoyeanos & Friedhoff, 1993). Slowing down breathing and listening to relaxation tapes is effective in reducing pain in adolescents. Cognitive (thinking) techniques such as "thought stopping" are also helpful in older patients. In this technique, the patient is instructed to repeat the word *stop* in response to negative thoughts and worries. A back rub or hand massage is also relaxing, depending on the child's age and diagnosis.

**Fear.** Intrusive procedures, such as enemas, temperature-taking, intravenous (IV) lines, and blood tests, are fear-provoking. They disrupt the child's trust level and threaten self-esteem and self-control. They may require restriction of activity. *Care must be taken to respect the modesty, integrity, and privacy of each child.* Hospital personnel can provide an environment that supports the child's need for mastery and control. These interventions are discussed according to age in this chapter and throughout the text.

Siblings (brothers and sisters) are affected by the child's hospitalization. Their ability to cope is influenced by their age, their past expe-

1. Visual analog scale
   Child points to where the pain
   falls on the scale.

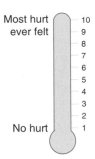

Most hurt — 10
ever felt — 9
— 8
— 7
— 6
— 5
— 4
— 3
— 2
No hurt — 1

2. Descriptive word scale
   Child chooses the word that describes the pain.

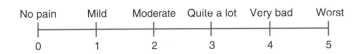

| No pain | Mild | Moderate | Quite a lot | Very bad | Worst |
|---------|------|----------|-------------|----------|-------|
| 0 | 1 | 2 | 3 | 4 | 5 |

3. Faces (Oucher) scale
   Child tells which face represents the pain at that moment.

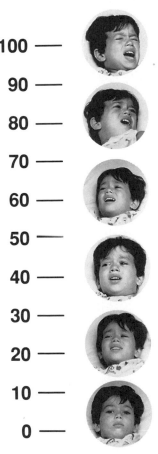

100 —
90 —
80 —
70 —
60 —
50 —
40 —
30 —
20 —
10 —
0 —

4. Poker chip
   a. Use 4 red poker chips  (color variations have also been cited)

   b. Place horizontally in front of child

   c. Say "These are pieces of hurt—one piece is a little,
      and four pieces are a lot."

   d. Ask "How many pieces of hurt do you have right now?"

   e. Record number on flow sheet (no pain equals zero)

**Figure 22-1.** Four pain assessment tools for children. (Oucher scale reproduced courtesy of Antonia M. Villarruel, Ph.D., R.N., and Mary J. Penyes, Ph.D., R.N., ©1990.)

rience, and the intactness of the family. Well siblings are included in visits to the hospital and given individual attention. They are provided knowledge of parents' whereabouts and the seriousness of the disease, as age-appropriate. Older children need to be made aware of parents' expectations of them if they are to assume increased responsibilities at home because of the disruption of routine. Selected nursing diagnoses for the hospitalized child and family are presented in Nursing Care Plan 22–1.

**Cultural Considerations.** Showing culturally sensitive attitudes toward families with hospitalized children decreases anxiety. Flexibility and careful listening are necessary to understand them. Studies of children in many different societies show that American middle-class culture is different from childhood environments derived from other traditions. An important consideration for the nurse admitting a child from a different cultural background is that the nurse is the one who seems different to the child and family (Pilliteri, 1992). Nurses must also be aware of their own cultural biases and how they might affect the assessment. In some cases, a translator may be required.

## The Hospitalized Infant

Hospitalization is frustrating for infants. During infancy, rapid physical and emotional development takes place. Infants are used to getting what they want when they want it, and they show their displeasure quickly when illness restricts satisfaction of their desires. Babies who were breast-fed at home may be unable to continue this regimen. They miss the continuous affection of their parents. Their daily schedule is upset. The infant who drinks well from a cup at home may refuse it entirely in the hospital.

Nursing personnel must try to meet the needs of these little patients by protecting them from excess frustration. It is not wise to expect them to develop new habits when they need energy to cope with their illness and the strange environment.

Assessing pain in newborns and preverbal children is difficult. In general crying becomes more intense, and there are increased body movements, skin changes (pale or flushed, diaphoresis), facial grimaces, and vital sign fluctuations. Changes in sleep and eating patterns may occur. Severely undernourished children become lethargic and quiet.

One of the nurse's major goals during this period is to assist with the parent-infant attachment process and to promote sensorimotor activities. This can be fostered by providing means for the infant and significant other to interact and by attempting to ease the tension of the parents. The nurse can serve as a role model by performing activities with the baby such as cuddling, rocking, talking, and singing. A swing, bath with squeeze toys, a pacifier, and a hanging mobile are also appropriate as the infant's condition permits.

Because the infant cannot understand explanations, the nurse administers uncomfortable procedures as gently as possible and returns the infant to the parents for consolation (Fig. 22–2). Liberal visiting hours are essential. When parents are not available, soothing support and gentle touch are provided; otherwise, the infant may learn to associate only pain with nursing care. Consistency of caretakers is also important at this stage of development.

## The Hospitalized Toddler

The toddler's world revolves around the parents, particularly mother (or significant caretaker). Hospitalization is a painful experience for toddlers. They cannot understand why they are separated from mother, and they become very distressed. Toddlers who have a continuous, secure relationship with mother react more violently to separation because they have more to lose. Nursing goals in the care of the hospitalized toddler are presented in Box 22–1.

Three stages of separation anxiety exist. These are *protest*, *despair*, and *denial*. Unless toddlers are extremely ill, their grief and sense of abandonment are obvious. They protest loudly. They watch and listen for their parents. Their cry is pitiful and continuous until they fall asleep in sheer exhaustion. They call, "Mommy, Mommy," and wonder why she does not answer. The second stage occurs as anger turns to despair. These children look sad and lonely and may refuse to eat. They are depressed and move about less. The third stage is

| NURSING CARE PLAN 22–1 | | |
| :---: | :---: | :---: |
| **Selected Nursing Diagnoses for the Hospitalized Child and Family** | | |
| **Goals** | **Nursing Interventions** | **Rationale** |

**Nursing Diagnosis:** Anxiety, related to nature of illness, possible separation, strange environment.

| | | |
| --- | --- | --- |
| Child's anxiety is reduced, as evidenced by a decrease in crying, clinging, regression, or maladaptive behaviors | 1. Provide as much consistency of personnel as possible | 1. Consistency is necessary in order to develop a sense of trust; although maladaptive behaviors may be normal in unfamiliar circumstances, if consistency and support are not given, coping abilities decrease |
| | 2. Direct attention to individual family members | 2. All family members are anxious when a child is hospitalized; decreasing family stress will help to foster feelings of security in the child |
| | 3. Recognize patient's separation behavior as age-appropriate | 3. Child's age is a factor in adjustment to separation |
| | 4. Assign foster grandparents as necessary | 4. Foster grandparents can provide individual attention to child; they promote intergenerational understanding |
| | 5. Suggest that family bring in photographs, familiar toys, tape-recorded family voices | 5. These activities will provide a link to home and promote security for child |
| | 6. Instruct parents to explain to the child when they will return as age-appropriate—for example, "after Sesame Street" | 6. This establishes trust and reassures child |
| | 7. Support parents by showing willingness to be available to them in order to answer questions and listen | 7. Nurse's availability to answer questions and to show interest in parents' concerns prevents problems and saves time later |
| | 8. Assess family knowledge | 8. Educating parents is an ongoing process; parental knowledge is important to ensure compliance with treatment protocol and to prevent complications |

**Nursing Diagnosis:** Pain, related to injury, illness, or treatments.

| | | |
| --- | --- | --- |
| Patient is able to verbalize relief of pain by Oucher scale, drawings, or other means, as age-appropriate | 1. Assessment tools are available that use self-reporting methods to help determine location and intensity of a child's pain | 1. Determining pain is difficult in small children because of their limited vocabulary |
| | 2. Administer pain-relieving medications as ordered | 2. Pain medication given at regular intervals around the clock prevents intensification of the pain cycle; nonverbal signs of pain in children are looked for, because children cannot always describe pain |
| | 3. Allow for expression of feelings | 3. Crying is acceptable, as are anger, jealousy, sadness, and fear |
| | 4. Explain use of equipment in age-appropriate terms | 4. Explanations decrease stress, which contributes to pain |
| | 5. Maintain child's contact with family; involve family in child's care | 5. Involving family members provides security for the child and a sense of purpose for the family |

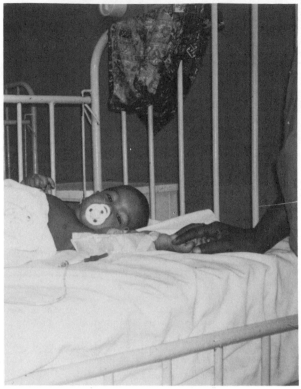

**Figure 22–2.** Having mother nearby and a pacifier comforts this hospitalized child.

one of denial. With further separation from the mother, children may try to deny their need for her and appear detached and uninterested in visits. On the surface it may seem that they have settled in, but this is only a disguise to prevent further emotional pain.

The nurse who comprehends the various separation stages sees parental visits as essential,

even though the process of separation and reunion is painful. A cohesive staff is essential to help tolerate the constant angry protest of these children. Education of the parents helps promote their continued visits and to decrease feelings of inadequacy.

Repetitive games that deal with disappearance and return are helpful. Peekaboo and hide-and-seek serve such a purpose. The use of a transitional object such as a blanket or a favorite toy promotes security. Pictures of the family and tape recordings of favorite stories are other measures that help the child to remain connected with the family. When the nurse or mother leaves, she explains when she will return in terms of the toddler's experience, for example, after naptime or lunch, and then she returns promptly at that time. If clinging and protest continue, try to distract the child in some way. A loving hug, good-bye, and prompt exit are then necessary. Parents should not wait until a child falls asleep to depart. This avoids confrontations but disturbs the child's sense of trust. The nurse assures the parents that she will remain with the child to comfort him. The continued reappearance of the parents as promised is of value in reducing the child's anxiety and reestablishing his or her sense of trust.

Rooming-in is highly desirable. When rooming-in is impossible, one nurse should be assigned to care for the child and the mother. The nurse indicates by her approach that she considers the mother's contributions extremely important to the patient's well-being. She interprets the stages of separation anxiety to the mother. The nurse must also realize that the mother is under stress and should not be asked to assume responsibilities beyond her capabilities. The nurse observes parents for signs of fatigue and suggests appropriate interventions.

Occasionally parents do not choose to care for their child; for example, "We feel that since we are paying for this, we should just be able to entertain him." In such instances, the parents' wishes are respected. Referral to the clinical nurse specialist might also be appropriate in order to facilitate communication and to understand better the underlying dynamics of the situation.

The home habits of the toddler are recorded and utilized. (One of our little patients liked her pacifier dipped in maple syrup!) A potty chair is provided if the child is trained. Some regression in behavior is to be expected. If the toddler still prefers bottles to cups, one should not attempt to change this in the hospital. Familiar

| BOX 22–1 | Nursing Goals in the Care of Hospitalized Toddlers |
|---|---|

Reassure parents, particularly the patient's mother

Maintain the toddler's sense of trust

Incorporate home habits of the patient into nursing care plans, for example, transitional objects

Allow child to work through or master threatening experiences through soothing techniques and play

Provide individualized, flexible nursing care plans in accordance with patient's development and diagnosis

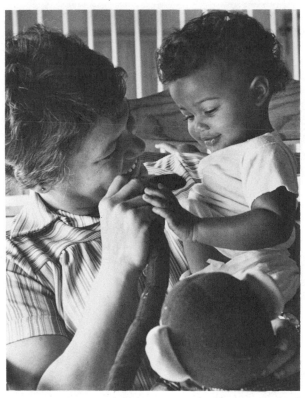

**Figure 22–3.** Establishing rapport with the hospitalized toddler. (Courtesy of Blank Memorial Hospital for Children, Des Moines, IA.)

toys and books are important. A steady, calm voice communicates safety (Figs. 22–3 and 22–4).

Children are forewarned about any unpleasant or new experience that they may have to undergo while in the hospital. This is done in keeping with their level of understanding. Being truthful about things that may hurt prevents the child from feeling betrayed. Preparation and explanation are done immediately before a procedure so that the child does not worry needlessly for an extended period of time. Crying and protesting when told about certain procedures are healthy expressions of feelings and relieve tension. Distractions such as blowing bubbles,

## Nursing Brief

Any time toddlers are left by their mother or primary caretaker, they experience some degree of separation anxiety, for example, when they are left with day-care personnel, baby-sitters, or relatives.

## Nursing Brief

Nursing students explain that they are going to "measure" the child's blood pressure and point to the scale on the sphygmomanometer. The phrase "to measure" is used rather than "to take," as the child may misinterpret the latter as meaning to remove something from the body.

looking through a kaleidoscope, and pop-up toys may help reduce anxiety and pain.

Supervised playroom activity contributes to intellectual, social, and motor development. Treatments in the playroom are avoided. Toddlers are encouraged to play with safe equipment used in their care, such as bandages, tongue blades, and stethoscopes. Whenever possible, they are allowed out of their cribs, as confinement is frustrating for little ones who have just begun to enjoy walking (Fig. 22–5).

There are indications that restraining the child's mobility by surgical and medical procedures involving splints, IV therapy, burn dressings, and so on may contribute to the development of emotional or personality problems or to speech and learning difficulties (Behrman, 1992). Therefore, when restraint is required, it must be accompanied by increased emotional support such as rooming-in, additional attention from nurses, and suitable diversion.

It is common for children to experience changes in behavior on their return home. They may be demanding and may cling to mother every minute. "He just won't let me out of his sight" is a common description. The mother should give the toddler extra attention and reassurance until trust is regained.

## The Hospitalized Preschool Child

Hospitalization is less threatening to the preschool child than to the toddler, and it is easier for patients who have had outside contact, such as nursery school and kindergarten, than for those who have never been separated from their parents. Because children of this age understand more, they can be better prepared for hospitalization. They are made to realize that it is not a punishment for something they have

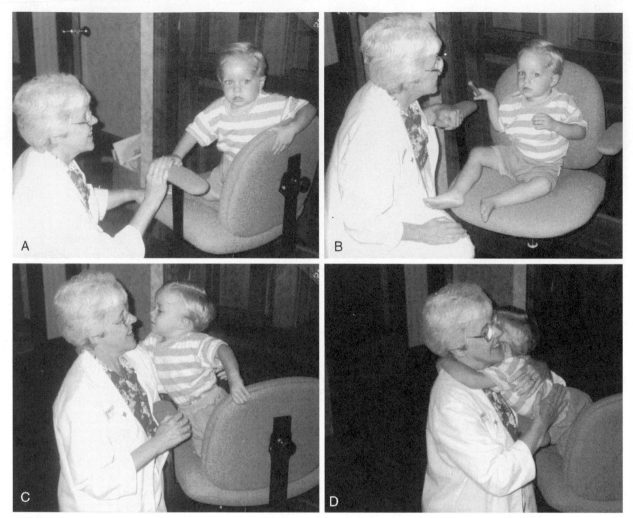

**Figure 22–4.** The clinical nurse specialist approaches the small child calmly, slowly, and at eye level. Note *A*, child's apprehension, *B*, contemplation, *C*, gaining of control, and *D*, beginning of trust.

done wrong. Children may feel guilty, particularly if an accident happens because of some mischief on their part, as in the case of burns or falls.

Preschool children are distressed when their mothers prepare to leave them, but unlike the toddler, they can understand time relationships through activities—at breakfast, after lunch, and the like. The nurse and parents must not tell the child that they will return unless they intend to do so.

Rivalry within a unit or in the playroom is common because the ages of the children are so varied. Younger children may wish to have the games or privileges that are allotted to the older children. They should be helped to understand that certain rights come with age. The nurse deals with each child according to specific needs. Some require more emotional support than others.

At this age, the child is afraid of bodily harm, particularly invasive procedures. The surgical patient needs to be shown the part of the body that requires surgery. The nurse can sketch a body outline and draw a circle around the operative site, giving simple information about the system that will be affected. It is stressed that only this area of the body will be involved. Patients also worry about other children on the unit who have physical deformities and

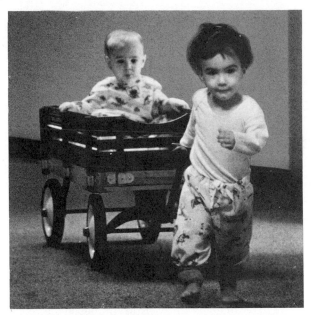

**Figure 22–5.** Although supervising the toddler out of his crib is at times harrowing, confinement is frustrating for children who have just learned to walk. (Courtesy of Blank Memorial Hospital for Children, Des Moines, IA.)

wonder if this will happen to them. Their questions about other children should not be ignored. Compliment children who show inquisitiveness; listen to them and correct any misinterpretations that they may have. Help the patient to increase self-esteem through praise. The child relieves tension through role playing. Tongue depressors, adhesive bandages (Band-Aids), and other materials related to everyday hospital life are relished by the sick child.

Parents are faced with a disrupted home life throughout the child's hospitalization. The mother cannot cope with everyday tasks when she is lonely for and worried about her child. The frequent trips to the hospital interfere with her daily routine and other children in the family may resent them. Contact with the physician is needed. Parents have a legal and ethical right to be informed of the benefits and risks of therapy and to be included in the decision-making process. When the child is finally discharged, he or she may be demanding and irritable. Parents need the kind support of hospital personnel to enable them to make informed decisions and meet these added strains.

# The Hospitalized School-Age Child

Children of school age are able to accept hospitalization more readily than the preschool child. They can endure separation from their parents if it is not prolonged. Children who have been cherished from birth can tolerate brief interruptions in their lives more easily than can those who have been denied a secure environment. To help these children, the nurse should find out as much about them as possible. Nurses who know a great deal about a patient are usually more interested in them as individuals. This is evidenced by the concern one has for children of friends or relatives who are hospitalized.

The nurse comes in contact with many school-age children who are chronically ill or disabled and are long-term or repeat patients. Unfortunately, some of them come from an unstable home environment or because of their illness or poor family relationships have been denied a healthy emotional development. They need help. Anyone can care for the cute, cooperative, well-adjusted patient. It takes an *exceptional* nurse to establish good rapport with a sulky, unruly, unhappy child.

At this age, children are trying to establish an image for themselves. They like to talk with adults and to feel that their opinions are respected and that they are important. Children seldom respond to direct questions from strangers. The student might try to establish rapport by engaging the patient in a competitive table game. As both patient and nurse become engrossed in the activity, the relationship becomes more relaxed and therapeutic communication is more easily established.

When students first enter a noisy unit and see school-age children bursting with pent-up energies, they may be puzzled as to how to proceed. Nurses should reject their first impulse to utilize negative discipline. Instead harmony may be fostered through mutual cooperation. Knowledge of growth and development in the school-age child assists in anticipatory guidance. Nurses can also enlist parents to determine what, if any, successful approaches they use in guiding the child. For specific patients whose behavior is unacceptable, the nursing care plan may need to be reassessed. Behavioral problems may be addressed by a team con-

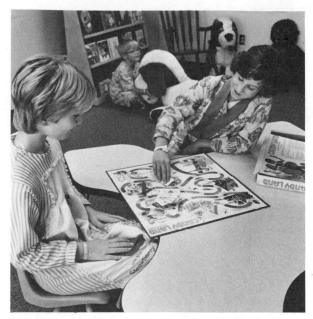

**Figure 22–6.** Socializing with peers is an important aspect of hospitalization for the school-age child. Furniture, games, and toys need to be appropriate for the child's age. (Courtesy of Blank Memorial Hospital for Children, Des Moines, IA.)

ference. Nurses who work with children should keep abreast of current trends and guidance approaches. Positive direction and consistency are tools of particular importance to the pediatric nurse.

The education of the school-age child must continue throughout any illness. This gives the child a sense of continuity with the outside world, provides periods of socialization (Fig. 22–6), and may reinforce weak academic areas. It involves the parents, who may act as liaisons between school and hospital. The teacher needs to be informed of the child's physical and emotional health in order to be effective. The nurse provides children with opportunities to study undisturbed so that they will be prepared for classes. Diagnostic tests and treatments should be scheduled around established school routines whenever possible.

## Nursing Brief

Observation of nonverbal clues, such as facial grimaces, squirming about, and finger-tapping, is important in determining pain relief and support for the child.

It is common for school-age children to be "brave," showing little, if any, fear in situations that actually upset them a good deal. Observation of body language may provide some clues to emotional states. The nurse's presence during unfamiliar procedures is comforting. Following treatments the nurse should encourage children to draw and talk about their drawings or to act out their feelings through puppet play.

## The Hospitalized Adolescent

Adolescents, in particular, experience feelings of loss of control on hospitalization. Daily routines are disrupted, and dependence-independence issues come to the foreground. The adolescent who is handicapped faces numerous social problems at this time. The child who has a chronic disease may find adolescence very threatening.

Since the 1960s, various clinics have been established for adolescents. They are quite diverse and range from university medical centers to inpatient units in general hospitals to storefront clinics to detention homes. Patients

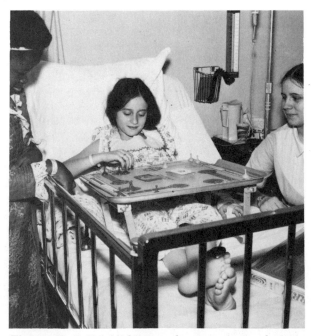

**Figure 22–7.** Establishing good communication between patient and nurse takes time and effort. (Courtesy of Rivier College/St. Joseph Hospital School of Practical Nursing, Nashua, NH.)

are also seen in private offices. A wide range of professionals provide services. The nurse who understands the biopsychosocial interaction of this age group and who enjoys working with teenagers can make an important contribution to this specialty (Fig. 22–7).

**Early Adolescence.** Nursing care plans need to be oriented to the adolescent's age. Illness during early adolescence, approximately 12–15 years of age, is seen mainly as a threat to body image. There is a narcissistic concern about height, weight, and sexual development. Patients are aware of heightened body sensations and often have numerous physical complaints. Intense relationships with members of one's own sex are prevalent; they precede heterosexual involvement. Patients in this age group are anxious about how the illness will affect their physical appearance, functioning, and mobility; however, they are not usually overwhelmed by forced dependence. Self-portrait drawings are effective at this time.

**Middle Adolescence.** During middle adolescence, approximately 15–18 years of age, teenagers are anxious about their ability to appeal to the opposite sex and to meet sex-role expectations. Physical growth is practically complete. The peer group assumes greater importance in determining acceptability and behavior. This period often begins with group dating, followed by "going together." These relationships are no longer narcissistic reflections but begin to show signs of mutual caring, affection, and responsibility. During middle adolescence, the struggle for emancipation from the family, although erratic, is at its peak. It is disturbing not only to the teenager but also to parents, who must relinquish much of their control and allow their children a certain amount of testing. They may also experience a real sense of loss. Because of the intensity of the emancipation process, which reflects the teenager's need for control and independence, hospitalization at this time can be extremely taxing.

**Late Adolescence.** Late adolescence, approximately 17–22 years of age, is mainly concerned with the task of education, career, marriage, children, community, and style of life. The dating partner becomes the person of primary importance. Hospitalization may pose the threat of postponement of career and future plans.

**Adjustment to Illness.** The adolescent has many intellectual strengths, including the ability to think abstractly and to solve problems. Adolescents can understand the implications of

their disease both in the present and in the future, and they are capable of participating in decisions related to treatment and care. The nurse who recognizes these skills and encourages their practice helps patients gain confidence in their intellectual abilities, thus increasing their sense of independence and self-esteem.

When hospitalization is necessary, it generates anxiety in proportion to the patient's past experiences and available strengths. The nature and treatment of the illness, the hospital environment, and the quality of support received from the medical staff, family, and peers all contribute to adjustment. How the illness is perceived is also a major factor—sometimes more so than the seriousness of the condition.

**Roommate Selection.** Roommate selection, although frequently overlooked, is extremely important for this age group. Teenagers usually do better with one or more roommates than in single rooms. Because few community hospitals have adolescent wings, it is helpful if the patients participate in the decision as to whether they are admitted to the pediatric or the adult unit. A few adjoining rooms at the ends of these units will suffice. One should avoid placing the teenager next to a senile, dying, or severely debilitated patient. Ideally, a recreation area should be provided for peer group association and privacy so that adult patients are not disturbed by the loud music and conversation typical of this age group.

**Admission to the Unit.** On the patient's arrival at the unit, the nurse introduces the patient to the staff; reviews routines, including any specific rules; and provides the patient with an information booklet. The nurse repeats the information periodically and has the patient verbalize understanding of it. The nurse acquaints the patient with the mechanics of the unit, for example, how to raise and lower the bed and use the call system, television, VCR, and intercom. Patients are helped to locate the bathroom, kitchen, and recreational facilities. Teenagers need a bedside telephone, and the dialing system is explained to them. They generally prefer their own clothes; however, some adolescent units keep scrub pants and tops in the unit, and the teenager may prefer them to conventional hospital garb.

The health assessment of the adolescent should include a complete psychosocial history as well as a physical examination. It may be difficult to obtain all the data in emergency situations, but it definitely should be completed within a day or two of admission. Such information is invaluable to the staff for anticipating behavior, identifying unmet health needs, planning care, assessing unhealthy reactions to adolescence, and determining just how the illness will affect the patient's maturation.

**Communication.** The nurse keeps patients informed as to what to expect. This includes personnel they will see and upcoming tests. Talking down to the patient is avoided. Time is allowed for questions and for the expression of feelings. The physician should discuss with the patient just what is wrong and what can be expected of therapy. When the prognosis is not predictable, the nurse shares uncertainty honestly while emphasizing that everyone is working together for the best possible outcome. Frequent staff conferences are needed in order to facilitate communication among professionals.

**Surgery.** Surgical patients need preoperative information. This includes such matters as what, if any, area of the body is to be shaved, why this needs to be done, and the likelihood of enemas, dietary restrictions, and medications. When possible, a visit to the recovery room is made in order to orient patients to postoperative surroundings. They are prepared in advance for waking up surrounded by life-support systems, bandages, casts, traction, or other apparatus following specific surgery. Also, one must explain to the patient and family the hospital's feedback system that will keep them informed of progress immediately following the operation. The inclusion of family and the sharing of feelings and ideas are extended throughout the confinement.

**Pain.** Adolescents are able to describe the location, intensity, and duration of pain. They can also request medication. Some teenagers have a heightened awareness of pain. Regression withdrawal, depression, and aggression are a few of the behaviors seen in adolescents. The nurse advises the patient of any anticipated discomfort from procedures and surgery. The nurse is also alert for "stoics" and reticent patients who could benefit from medication.

During early convalescence, the patient may feel the worst. Staff expectations should not exceed what the adolescent can do. As patients begin to take an interest in their surroundings, the nurse encourages self-care, ambulation, and socialization. Teenagers progress more slowly than their younger counterparts, and there is often a gap between how the adolescent per-

ceives progress and how the staff perceives it. It is unlikely, however, that the exuberant teenager will succumb to a life of bed rest if given an alternative!

**Behavioral Considerations.** Skillful management of adolescent behavior is best achieved through careful selection of nursing staff members. The nurses working with young people must be *flexible*. Often their patients compete for attention and can be manipulative. Adolescents may try to divide or come between staff members; this is termed staff "splitting." It is difficult to know how to handle the patient who instigates trouble, argues, uses profanity, or is manipulative. Personnel need frequent staff meetings during which they can air their concerns and develop awareness about their own reactions to certain aspects of behavior in their patients.

The nurse's role should be that of the person to whom the patient can relate in time of need. Young nursing personnel are apt to confuse this role by overidentifying with the patient and losing their objectivity. They may be unable to set limitations that the adolescent needs and wants. Working with this age group is a unique experience that carries its own rewards. The nurse who understands this and who is knowledgeable about the developmental and psychosocial considerations of adolescence contributes greatly to the patient's adjustment and recovery.

**Confidentiality and Legality.** Respecting the confidentiality of the teenager is important to establishing trust. In general, information should not be divulged or shared without consent. Many problems can be avoided if the confidentiality of the relationship is clearly defined during initial meetings. At this time, the nurse explains to teenagers that two conditions must be reported: plans to harm themselves and plans to harm someone else. Patient records must be carefully monitored in order to avoid loss or observation by unauthorized personnel. The nurse must avoid giving private information about the teenager to telephone callers or visitors. Appointment books in an office are kept closed rather than open on the clerk's desk.

*Emancipated minor* generally refers to an adolescent younger than 18 years of age who is no longer under the parent's authority. Married minors or minors in the military are automatically considered emancipated and may give consent for medical treatment for themselves and their children. The *mature minor role* recognizes that individuals mature at different rates. Many are able to understand the nature, potential risks, and benefits of proposed therapy. In such cases, medical personnel should document that the adolescent has acted in a responsible manner.

In some parts of the United States, the young adolescent may receive medical assistance without parental awareness for certain conditions, for example, sexually transmitted diseases, contraception, pregnancy, abortion, and drug abuse. These laws are designed to afford the young person immediate medical help without fear of reprisal. However, some are being challenged in the courts. In a *medical emergency*, a minor can be treated without the consent of parents if the situation is life-threatening. Most states require that an individual be 18 to give blood. *Organ donation* by a consenting minor usually requires adult consent as well as a court order.

Because laws vary from state to state, nurses must keep abreast of policies and legislation within their practice. Such information is available from the local medical or state nursing licensing boards. Most states do not specifically address the subject of responsibility for payment of medical care. In general, if the teenager is the sole consenter to a procedure, he or she has implied responsibility for payment.

**Chronic Illness.** Chronic illness during this period of life is in direct opposition to developmental needs. Specific programs that foster feelings of security and independence within the limits of the situation are essential. Behavior problems are lessened when patients can verbalize specific concerns with persons sensitive to their problems. If they feel rejected by and different from their peers, they may be prone to depression. To be in school and to be considered one of the group are important. Hospital school programs provide familiarity and enable patients to keep pace with their classmates. The recreational therapist may also be helpful in combating boredom and providing outlets for tension.

Nurses need to help patients to accept their body with all its strengths and imperfections. They must develop an awareness of the teenager's particular fears of forced dependence, bodily invasion, mutilation, rejection, and loss of face, especially within peer groups. The nurse anticipates a certain amount of reluctance to adhere to hospital regulations, which reflects the adolescent's need for self-determination. Recognizing this as an asset rather than a liability enables the nurse to respond creatively.

**Developmental Disabilities.** Adolescents who have a developmental disability that affects intellect or ability to cope face some unique difficulties. They may often be overprotected, unable to break away from supervision, and deprived of necessary peer relationships. The pubertal process with its emerging sexuality concerns parents and may precipitate family crisis. Most general hospital resources are not adequate to meet the many interdisciplinary needs of these adolescents and their families. However, a network of federal programs provides support and coordination of services to this population.

**Home Care.** Many teenagers with acute and chronic conditions are being cared for in the home. Home health care and other community agencies work together to provide holistic care. *Respite* care provides trained workers who come into the home for brief periods in order to relieve parents of the responsibility of caring for the child. This enables the parents to shop, do business transactions, or simply take a much-needed vacation. The school systems also share in the responsibility of care, which is crucial if a family is to be successful in home care. One mother, whose 13-year-old daughter has a severe developmental disability (cerebral palsy, blindness, scoliosis, mental retardation), offered these suggestions for the health-care worker assisting in the home:

- Observe how the parents interact with the child.
- Do not wait for the child to cry out for attention, as the youngster may be unable to communicate in this way.
- Watch for facial expression and body language.
- Post signs above the bed denoting special considerations, such as "Never position on left side" and "Do not feed with plastic spoon."
- Listen to the parents and observe how they attend to the physical needs of the youngster.
- Do not be afraid to ask questions or discuss apprehensions you may feel about your ability to care for the child.
- Be attuned to the needs of other children in the home.
- Be creative in exploring avenues for socialization, as these teenagers are seldom invited to birthday or slumber parties.
- Explore community facilities or support groups that might benefit the family.

## KEY POINTS

- Three major causes of stress for children of all ages are separation, pain, and fear of bodily harm.
- Separation anxiety is most pronounced in the toddler.
- Patients in pain secrete higher levels of cortisol and have compromised immune systems, more infections, and delayed wound healing.
- Nurses caring for children must maintain a high level of suspicion for pain, because they are often unable to verbalize discomfort.
- Techniques such as drawing, distraction, imagery, relaxation, and cognitive strategies as well as analgesia provide relief from pain.
- A culturally sensitive attitude toward families with hospitalized children decreases anxiety.
- Avoid treatments in the playroom.
- The surgical patient needs to be shown the part of the body that will be operated on. Children are assured that this is the only area of the body that will be involved.
- Education of the school-age patient must be continued, especially when the child is disabled or has a chronic illness that requires frequent absence from school.
- Respecting the confidentiality of the teenager is important to establishing trust.

# Study Questions

1. List and define the three stages of separation anxiety.
2. What problems confront siblings of the hospitalized child?
3. Illness and hospitalization of a child are stressful for parents as well as for the child. List two ways in which the nurse can lessen this stress for parents.
4. Identify some guidelines for establishing a trusting relationship with hospitalized children. Do these differ depending on the child's age?
5. List several factors that might influence a child's reaction to hospitalization.
6. What are some immediate problems that the child and family may experience at the time of admission to the hospital? Discuss nursing interventions for the problems cited.
7. List two developmental tasks of adolescence. How does immobilization interfere with these?
8. The need for confidentiality of patient knowledge is essential. Discuss confidentiality in terms of the health care of the adolescent.

# Multiple Choice Review Questions

*Choose the most appropriate answer.*

1. The stages of separation anxiety in the toddler are
   a. protest, despair, denial
   b. denial, dependence, submission
   c. protest, sadness, despair
   d. despair, anxiety, regression

2. An object such as a blanket or favorite toy is referred to as
   a. a transitory item
   b. a transitional object
   c. a transitional task
   d. a cuddly

3. Which of the following would you give priority to in terms of the adolescent's adjustment to hospitalization?
   a. view from room
   b. closeness to activity room
   c. roommate selection
   d. decor of room
4. Separation anxiety is most pronounced in the
   a. toddler
   b. preschooler
   c. school age child
   d. adolescent
5. The nurse must observe children for signs of nonverbalized pain, which might be signaled by
   a. fatigue, thumb-sucking
   b. fighting with other children
   c. regression, guarding of limb
   d. polyphagia, polydipsia

## BIBLIOGRAPHY

Acker, L., Goldwater, B., & Dyson, W. (1992). *AIDS-proofing your kids*. Hillsboro, OR: Beyond Words Publishing.

Behrman, R.E. (1992). *Nelson textbook of pediatrics* (14th ed.). Philadelphia: W.B. Saunders.

Hester, N., Jacox, A., Miaskowski, C., & Ferrell, B. (1992). The management of pain in infants, children, and adolescents undergoing operative and medical procedures. *MCN: American Journal of Maternal Child Nursing, 17*, 146–152.

Kachoyeanos, M., & Friedhoff, M. (1993). Cognitive and behavioral strategies to reduce children's pain. *MCN: American Journal of Maternal Child Nursing, 18*, 14–19.

Levine, M., Carey, W., & Crocker, A. (1992). *Developmental-behavioral pediatrics* (2nd ed.). Philadelphia: W.B. Saunders.

Mott, S., et al. (1991). *Nursing care of children and families* (2nd ed.). Reading, MA: Addison-Wesley.

Petrillo, M., & Sanger, S. (1980). *Emotional care of hospitalized children*. Philadelphia: J.B. Lippincott.

Pilliteri, A. (1992). *Maternal and child health nursing*. Philadelphia: J.B. Lippincott.

Scipien, G., et al. (1990). *Comprehensive pediatric nursing* (4th ed.). New York: McGraw-Hill.

Thompson, E.D., & Ashwill, J.W. (1992). *Pediatric nursing: An introductory text* (6th ed.). Philadelphia: W.B. Saunders.

Whaley, L., & Wong, D. (1991). *Nursing care of infants and children* (4th ed.). St. Louis: Mosby–Year Book.

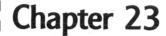

## Chapter 23

# Health-Care Adaptations
# for the Child and Family

## OBJECTIVES

*On completion and mastery of Chapter 23, the student will be able to*

- Define each vocabulary term listed.
- Describe the physical facilities of a children's unit and their significance to the patient's adjustment to hospitalization.
- List five safety measures applicable to the care of the hospitalized child.
- Describe how illness affects the child and family.
- Discuss three nursing measures to make hospitalization less threatening for the child.
- Describe the principles for using restraints for children.
- Devise a nursing care plan for a child with fever.
- Position an infant for a lumbar puncture.
- Contrast the administration of medicines to children and adults.
- Discuss two precautions necessary when a child is receiving parenteral fluids and the rationale for each precaution.
- Summarize the care of a child receiving oxygen.
- List the adaptations necessary when preparing a pediatric patient for surgery.
- Summarize isolation precautions and procedures relevant to preventing the transmission of infection on the children's unit.
- Discuss discharge planning for the pediatric patient.

# Health-Care Delivery Settings

## OUTPATIENT CLINIC

Many large hospitals today have well-organized outpatient facilities and satellite clinics for preventive medicine and care of the child who is ill. Although there are still substantial socioeconomic differences in access to routine preventive services, the advent of Medicaid and other such programs has made these services available to more low-income families. Within clinics, there may be specialty areas (particularly at children's facilities), such as cardiac clinics and orthopedic clinics, where the student can observe and assist. In some institutions, information is distributed, and brief classes are held for waiting parents.

**Types of Outpatient Clinics.** Satellite clinics are convenient and offer families flexible coverage. Some are located in shopping malls. Parents may browse with children and be contacted by a beeper when it is their turn to see the physician. This eliminates confining children in a small area and is less frustrating to caretakers. In many cities, a group of pediatricians practice in an office removed from the hospital, which aids in the distribution of health services and provides evening and weekend health coverage.

In some offices, the pediatricians or their nurses are available at certain hours of each day to answer telephone inquiries. The pediatric nurse practitioner may visit patients in the home, give routine physical examinations at the clinic, and otherwise work with the physician, so that a higher quality of individual care may be attained. The practitioner is frequently the primary contact person for children in the health-care system.

Another area of outpatient care is the pediatric research center, such as the one at St. Jude's Hospital in Memphis, Tennessee; this type of institution offers highly specialized care for patients with particular disorders, often at little or no expense to the patient. In the outpatient clinic, as in all other settings, documentation and record review are important parts of nursing assessment (Fig. 23–1).

**Outpatient Surgery.** Elective outpatient surgery for patients with uncomplicated conditions, such as a herniorrhaphy, is also being

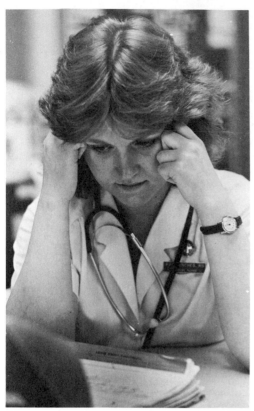

**Figure 23–1.** Documentation and record review are important parts of nursing assessment in all settings. (Courtesy of Iowa Methodist Medical Center, Des Moines, IA.)

done. Among the advantages of same-day surgery are reductions of nosocomial infection, hospital costs, and bed use. Outpatient clinics also eliminate the need to separate the child from the family, and thus the possibility of hospital trauma is avoided. In this type of program, careful preparation must be given, and assurance must be obtained that the child's home environment is adequate to meet recovery needs.

**Promoting a Positive Experience.** The attitude of nurses, receptionists, and other personnel in outpatient departments is of the utmost importance. It can make the difference between an atmosphere that is warm and kindly and one in which the patient is made to feel dehumanized. As more and more medical care is instituted in outpatient clinics, there will be an even greater reduction in the number of children who require hospitalization. For many, the only exposure to medical personnel will be through brief clinic appointments. We should all, therefore, make the encounters positive ones for patients and families.

## HOME

Because hospitalization is now brief for most children, the choice is not either hospital or home care but a combination of the two. They are becoming interdependent. Dramatic technical improvements and research in specific disease entities are also helping to advance the movement to home care (e.g., cryoprecipitate for hemophiliacs, Broviac catheters for chemotherapy, heparin locks, glucometers). Home care, however, is broader than in years past. It is not merely a matter of supplying appliances and nursing care but includes assessment of the total needs of children and their families. Families need to be linked to a wide variety of network services. This ideally involves a team approach headed by the physician or medical center.

The hospice concept for children is also under way and has received accolades from parents who have benefited from its service. Local and national support groups for specific problems afford opportunities for families to share and support one another and to learn from others' successes and failures. Special groups and camps for children with chronic illnesses are also well established. Group therapy for children under stress is equally important in preventing mental health problems (e.g., groups for children whose parents are divorced, Alateen for children of alcoholics). These and other programs not only have the potential for improving life for the child and family but may help reduce the high cost of medical care. At this writing, needed reform in the health-care system is being debated.

## CHILDREN'S UNIT

The student nurse may find the first day on the children's unit confusing because it is noisy and cluttered—it differs in many respects from adult divisions. The pediatric unit or hospital is designed to meet the needs of children and their parents. A cheerful, casual atmosphere helps to bridge the gap between home and hospital and is in keeping with the child's emotional and physical needs. Patients often wear their own clothing while they are hospitalized, and nurses wear colorful smocks or pastel uniforms. Colored bedspreads and wagons or strollers for transportation are also more homelike.

The physical structure of the division includes furniture of the proper height for the child, soundproof ceilings, and color schemes with eye appeal. There is a special treatment room for the doctor to examine the patient. In this way, the other children do not become disturbed by the proceedings. Some hospitals have a schoolroom. When this is not available, it is necessary for the teacher to visit each child individually. Today's modern general hospitals have separate waiting rooms for children. This is more relaxing for parents, since they do not have to worry about whether their child is disturbing adult patients, and it is less frightening to the child.

Most pediatric departments include a playroom in their structural plan (Fig. 23–2). It is generally large and light in color. Bulletin boards and blackboards are within reach of the patients. Mobiles may be suspended from the ceiling. Some playrooms are equipped with an aquarium of fish and blossoming plants because children love living things. A variety of toys suitable for different age groups are available. This room may be under the supervision of a play therapist or nursery school teacher. Parents usually enjoy taking their children to the playroom and observing the various activities. The assisting nurse should allow each child freedom to develop independently and should avoid excessive control or partiality. Further discussion on the value of play to the child is found in Chapter 19 (p. 490).

Some children are not able to be taken to the playroom because of their physical condition. In such cases, the nurse provides comfortable chairs for caretakers so that they are able to cuddle or read to the child.

Mealtimes on the children's unit differ from those on adult divisions. Patients whose conditions permit may be served together around small tables. This provides a homelike setting and offers the child a satisfying social experience.

The daily routine also differs widely for obvious reasons. Although rigid schedules are discouraged, children benefit from a certain amount of routine. Meals, rest, and play are carried out at approximately the same time each day. The number of nurses caring for the child should be minimal to promote security. Visiting hours on the pediatric unit are usually liberal. Parents are encouraged to stay with the child or to come as often as possible. They are considered an integral part of the child's recovery. Furniture that converts into beds for rooming-in is available.

## Safety Measures

The nurse must be especially conscious of safety measures on the children's division. *Accidents are a major cause of death among infants and children.* By demonstrating concern about safety regulations, the nurse not only reduces unnecessary accidents but also sets a good example for parents. Although the physical layout of each institution cannot be altered by personnel, many simple safety measures can be carried out by the entire hospital team. The following is a list of measures applicable to the children's unit.

### DOs

- Keep crib sides up at all times when the patient is unattended in bed (Fig. 23–3).
- Wash your hands before and after caring for each patient.
- Identify child by bracelet, not room number.
- Check wheelchairs and stretchers for flaws before placing patients in them.

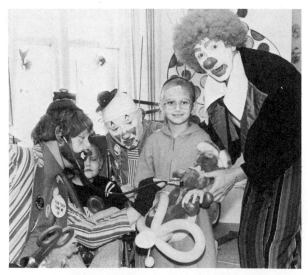

**Figure 23–2.** Special visitors to the playroom. (Courtesy of Blank Memorial Hospital for Children, Des Moines, IA.)

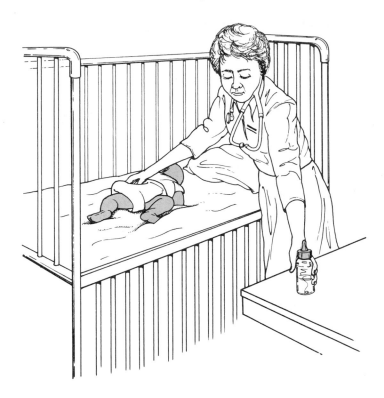

**Figure 23-3.** Maintain hand contact if you must turn your back on the infant or toddler. If you need equipment that is out of reach, raise the side of the crib before leaving the infant or child.

- Place cribs so that children cannot reach sockets and appliances.
- Inspect toys for sharp edges and removable parts.
- Apply restraints correctly in order to prevent constriction of a part.
- Keep medications and solutions out of reach of the child.
- Lock the medication cabinet when not in use.
- Identify the patient properly before giving medications.
- Keep powder, lotions, tissues, Chucks, disposable diapers, safety pins, and so on out of infant's reach.
- Check each thermometer for imperfections before inserting it, and remain with the small child while taking the temperature.
- Prevent cross-infection. Diapers, toys, and materials that belong in one patient's unit should not be borrowed for another patient's use.
- Restrain children in highchairs.
- Take proper precautions when oxygen is in use.
- Handle infants and small children carefully. Use elevators rather than stairs. Walk at the child's pace.

- Locate fire exits and extinguishers on your unit and learn how to use them properly. Become familiar with your hospital's fire manual.

**DON'Ts**

- Don't prop nursing bottles or force-feed small children. There is danger of choking, which may cause lung disease or sudden death.
- Don't allow ambulatory patients to use wheelchairs or stretchers as toys.
- Don't remove dressings or bandages unless specifically instructed.
- Don't leave an active child in a baby swing, feeding table, or highchair unattended.
- Don't leave a small child unattended when out of the crib.
- Remain with the child who uses the bathtub.
- Don't leave medications at the bedside.

Many other safety measures must be carried out as each student becomes more familiar with the hazards of individual units. Nurses must use their eyes to see with, not just to look at, and then must take the necessary precautions.

### TRANSPORTING, POSITIONING, AND RESTRAINING THE CHILD

The means by which the child is transported within the unit and to other parts of the hospital depends on age, level of consciousness, and how far one has to travel. Older children are transported in the same way as adults. Younger children are often transported in their cribs, in a wagon or wheelchair, or on a stretcher. The side rails on a stretcher are raised during transport. The nurse ensures that the patient's identification band is secured before leaving the division. A notation is made as to where the child is being taken and for what purpose. When a child is being permanently transferred, as from the intensive care unit (ICU) to a private room, the primary nurse should visit beforehand and meet the family.

Figure 23–4 depicts three safe methods for holding a baby. Head and back support are necessary for young infants. The movements of small children are often random and uncoordinated; therefore, they must be held securely. The football hold is useful when one hand needs to be free, such as for bathing the baby's head. Table 23–1 lists the principles for using restraints for children.

## The Child's Reaction to Hospitalization

The child's reaction to hospitalization depends on many factors such as age, amount of preparation given, security of home life, previous hospitalizations, support of family and medical personnel, and child's emotional health. These reactions are detailed according to age in Chapter 22. Many children cannot grasp what is going to happen to them even though they have been well prepared. At a time when children need their parents most, they may be separated from them, placed in the hands of strangers, and even fed different foods. Add to this a totally new environment and tummyache, and you have one frightened and unhappy child.

Each child reacts differently to hospitalization. One is demanding and exhibits temper tantrums, whereas another becomes withdrawn. The "good" child on the unit may be going through greater torment than the one who cries and shows feelings outwardly. The best-prepared nurse cannot replace the child's parents. However, hospitalization can be a period of growth rather than just an unpleasant interlude.

Children may see the nurse as someone who cares for them physically, as their parents would, and as a source of security and comfort.

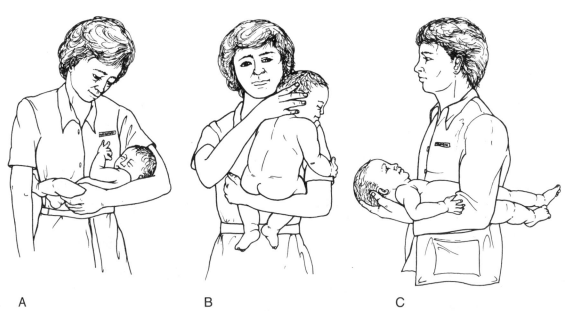

A          B          C

**Figure 23–4.** *A,* The cradle position. *B,* The upright position. *C,* The football position.

**Table 23–1.** PRINCIPLES FOR USING RESTRAINTS FOR CHILDREN

| Restraint and Use | Principles | Rationale | |
|---|---|---|---|
| Mummy<br>　Infants<br>　For comfort, scalp vein intravenous (IV), nasogastric (NG) tube | Arms in anatomic position as blanket or sheet is wrapped around each shoulder and arm; lower portion allows for leg extension<br><br>Position on side allows for oral drainage | Prevents undue discomfort and strain on arms and joints<br><br>Maximizes mobility within the restraint while still providing comfort of close wrapping<br>Secretions or vomitus could be aspirated if child's position prevents drainage | |
| Clove hitch<br>　Child of any age<br>　For restraining one or more extremities; for IV lines, NG tubes, and other tubes; for prevention of self-injury | Extremity must be padded under each restraint<br>Knot used must be a clove hitch<br><br><br>Nurse checks to see whether the knot will tighten with a child's resistance or pulling<br>Restraint attached to frame of crib or bed with a slipknot<br><br>Limb distal to the restraint checked every 15 min and restraint released frequently—all at once or one extremity at a time | Restraint could irritate skin without padding<br>Knot will not tighten as the child pulls against the restraint (other knots could tighten and reduce circulation)<br>Nurse needs to be certain the knot is correct<br><br>In emergency, nurse must be able to release the restraint quickly with one hand<br>Prevents circulatory compromisal<br>No pressure applied when side rail is lowered | |
| Jacket<br>　Child of any age<br>　Keeps child in crib or bed<br>　Can be used to prevent sitting or standing | Must fit well; ties in back<br>Attached to bed frame with a slipknot<br>Child must be checked every 15 min or be continually observed<br><br>Restraint released as much as possible | Child can slip out of a poorly fitting restraint<br><br>Airway can be totally occluded if a child wriggles to get out of tight but poorly fitting restraint<br>Prolonged immobility can lead to complications | |
| Elbow<br>　Child of any age<br>　Prevents flexion of elbows and thus the touching of face, scalp, IV line, other tubes, cleft lip or palate repair, skin conditions of face and upper trunk | Sleeves must fit well<br>Restraint must be secured with pins or straps<br>Color, sensation, and motion of fingers must be checked frequently<br>Restraints must be removed frequently for range of motion | Prevents flexion of elbow<br>Keeps restraint in place<br><br>Nerve damage is possible from pressure of restraint on the brachial area | |
| Bubble-top and net-top crib<br>　Older infant and young child<br>　Prevents falling and climbing out of crib | Bubble secured to ends of crib with clamps<br><br><br><br>Net tight and secured to frame and legs of crib<br><br>Side rails all the way up and secure | Firm attachment to frame of the crib allows child mobility and play without danger of dislodging the crib top<br>Tying to frame prevents pressure applied when side rail is lowered<br>With crib rails up and crib top tightly in place, child cannot climb out under the restraint | |

*Continued*

**Table 23–1.** PRINCIPLES FOR USING RESTRAINTS FOR CHILDREN *Continued*

| Restraint and Use | Principles | Rationale | |
|---|---|---|---|
| Bed cradle<br>　Older infant and older child<br>　Protects lower part of the<br>　　body from pressure of<br>　　bedding and from child's<br>　　hands | Cradle padded with a sheet or<br>　bath blanket secured with<br>　pins<br>Hospital gown may be spread<br>　over the cradle and pinned<br>　to cover | Protects child from metal of<br>　bed cradle and provides<br>　some privacy<br>Keeps gown off the child's<br>　body, provides privacy<br>Pinning gown may be enough<br>　to keep child's hands from<br>　touching surgical site or<br>　from scratching irritated<br>　skin | |
| Safety straps<br>　Child of any age<br>　Prevents child's falling from<br>　　a cart, chair, or frame | Folded sheet or strap firmly<br>　secured<br><br>Ends of strap tied in back of a<br>　chair (high chair or stroller)<br>Child checked very frequently | Child may climb or fall from<br>　go-carts, gurneys, high<br>　chairs, infant seats, feeding<br>　tables, orthopedic frames<br>Child cannot unfasten<br><br>Child may slip within the<br>　restraint, endangering<br>　airway or circulation | |

Modified from *Nursing care of children and families,* Second Edition, by S. Mott, S. James, and A. Sperhac. Copyright (©) 1990 by Addison-Wesley Nursing, a Division of the Benjamin/Cummings Publishing Company. Reprinted by permission.

They realize that the nurse sometimes administers strange treatments that can be painful. Older children soon discover the relationships among the nurse, parents, and doctor and realize that the nurse is a liaison between hospital and home. They may view the nurse as a health teacher and model to imitate. Children learn to know "their" nurses if the number of nurses caring for them is kept at a minimum.

# The Parents' Reactions to the Child's Hospitalization

When children are hospitalized, the whole family is affected. The parents of the hospitalized youngster need others to show interest in them as well. If they are frightened and tense, the child soon senses it. Some of the main reasons for their apprehension may be as follows.

**Guilt, Helplessness, and Anxiety.** Parents may feel that they are to blame for the child's illness; they may feel that they should have recognized the symptoms earlier or that they could have prevented an accident by closer supervision. Immunizations and other types of preventive care may also have been neglected.

Parents seldom are the cause for direct hospital admission of a child. Even in cases of child abuse or neglect, nothing is gained by blaming the parents. The nurse remains objective and empathetic. The nurse listens carefully to parental concerns and acknowledges the legitimacy of their feelings, for example, "It is understandable that you feel this way; everything happened so fast." Parents also frequently express feelings of helplessness at the loss of the parental role as protector. The nurse encourages and supports parents and other family members and stresses their importance to the child's recovery. They are involved in the care of the patient, as appropriate. The admission of a child to the hospital is anxiety-producing. The uncertainty of the situation can become overwhelming, causing feelings of panic. However, these feelings are usually temporary. The nurse remains relaxed, reassures the parents, and reinforces positive parenting. Information about the child's condition and treatment plan is given. Needs are assessed and interventions planned to meet specific needs.

**Fear of the Unknown.** Parents do not understand the functioning of a hospital. The child's disease may be relatively rare. Poor communication may also result in unnecessary fears. The nurse can explain in simple terms some of the equipment being used. Facilities available on the unit, such as the kitchen, washer, and dryer, need to be shown to the parents, and any instructions related to their use are carefully explained. The nurse listens attentively and tries to clear up misconceptions. Often parents are "left in the dark" about some of the simplest routines of the hospital merely because everyone assumes they have been informed.

**Fear of Improper Care.** The public realizes that many hospitals are crowded and understaffed. Parents may be unfamiliar with the physician. Trust takes time to build. Rooming-in may alleviate some of this distress. The nurse promptly and cheerfully attends to the needs of the child, which indicates to the parents that their child is in good hands.

**Fear of Financial Burden.** Hospital and doctor bills are expensive, particularly for long-term illness or treatment. Parents may also have to take time from work, especially if treatment involves travel to special centers. Ronald McDonald homes offer lodging and other familiar amenities at no cost for parents of patients with life-threatening illness. The availability of these facilities is explored. The social-service worker may be of help in such instances.

**Fear That the Child Will Suffer.** This may be due to the nature of the child's illness, or it may be fear of painful treatments or emotional deprivation. Parents need reassurance that their child will receive medication for pain whenever necessary. It is helpful to mention that although a lot of hospital equipment looks threatening—x-ray equipment, electrocardiograms, cast cutters—often their use presents little or no discomfort. If a procedure is known to be painful, patients are frequently anesthetized or given analgesics beforehand.

**Fear That Others in the Family Will Contract the Disease.** Parents may worry that the disease (eczema, for example) is infectious, when it is not. Reassurance by the nurse or doctor is indicated.

**Fear That Their Child Will Transfer Affection to Hospital Personnel.** This is more noticeable when parents are unable to assist with the child's care. Listening, supporting parenting skills, and clarifying information may allay some concerns. The nurse allows parents to assist or administer routine care to their child whenever possible.

## Nursing Brief

When a child is admitted to the hospital, every family member is affected.

The nurse must realize that parents are "not themselves" when they have such burdensome worries. Sometimes even the most mature and intelligent adult may ask questions that seem illogical. Parents may ventilate their feelings through anger, crying, or body language. If nurses could know the history of the parents who enter the hospital with a sick child, they would be in a better position to understand their behavior and accept them as individuals. Behavior is not only a response to the current situation but often involves attitudes resulting from early childhood experiences. The nurse must not be too quick to pass judgment on individuals whose behavior may seem demanding or unreasonable. *An understanding and acceptance of people and their problems are essential for the successful pediatric nurse.*

Siblings are also affected when a brother or sister is hospitalized. They may feel left out, guilty, or resentful of the attention focused on the ill child. Suitable interventions by the nurse include directing some attention to the siblings, supporting their efforts to comfort the family member, and engaging them in play or drawing pictures, such as "How it feels to have an ill brother or sister." They may also make cards and pictures for the patient.

## The Nurse's Role in Hospital Admission

As members of the nursing team, nurses are often called on to admit new patients. Besides performing the procedure skillfully, they must be prepared to meet the emotional needs of those involved. The impression the nurse gives, whether good or bad, definitely affects the patient's adjustment. When inexperienced students admit their first patient, they may be nervous and frightened. After completing the procedure, they should stop for just a moment, recall any anxieties, and realize that the parents and child are equally upset. The student will never have to do that procedure for the first time again, but almost every admission will bring contact with parents and a child undergoing an unfamiliar experience. Empathy in responding to the fears of the child and family members makes the admission procedure stimulating rather than merely a task to be completed.

A child must be prepared for hospitalization.

If possible, one should give the child and parents a tour of the pediatric unit before admission. This enables the parents to meet the people who will care for their child. Children and their families are often overwhelmed by the size of the institution and the fear of becoming lost.

Between ages 1 and 3, children are worried about being separated from their parents. After age 3, children may become more fearful about what is going to happen to them. Parents should try to be as matter-of-fact about this new experience as possible. Unless they have been hospitalized before, children can only try to imagine what will happen to them. It is not necessary to go into much detail, since the child's imagination is great and giving information that is beyond comprehension may create unnecessary fears. It is logical to dwell on the more pleasant aspects, but not to the extent of saying that hospitalization involves no discomforts. For example, one might mention that meals will be served on a tray, that baths will be taken from a basin at the bedside, and that the child will be with other children. The fact that there is a buzzer for calling the nurse may add to the child's sense of security. The parents may plan with the child what favorite toy or book to bring.

Perhaps more important than explaining certain occurrences is listening to how the child feels and encouraging questions. Parents should prepare them a few days, but not weeks, in advance. Never lure children to the hospital by pretending that it is some other place. In emergency situations, there is little time for preparation. The entire medical team must try to give added emotional support to the child in such cases.

The nurse prepares the equipment for the admission procedure in advance. This saves time and promotes secure feelings. Once the technical details are attended to, the nurse concentrates on the approach to the patient and family. The initial greeting should show warmth and friendliness—smile and introduce yourself.

Some hospitals allow the patient to be taken to the playroom for a short time before going to the room. When the parent tells the nurse the child's name, associating it with a familiar person who has the same name will help the nurse remember it. It creates a much warmer feeling to speak of "John" or "Susy" than "your little boy" or "your daughter."

When the child and parents are taken to the child's room, the nurse introduces them to the other children. The parent is seated comfortably. Explain the admission procedure carefully. Avoid discussing in front of children information that they will not understand. The parent is encouraged to do as much for the child as possible, for example, remove clothes. The nurse tries not to appear rushed. A matter-of-fact attitude must be maintained regardless of the patient's condition. A soft voice and quiet approach are less frightening to the child. A nurse's looking anxious causes unnecessary worry for everyone concerned. A troubled look may have nothing to do with the patient. Taking one step at a time is advised. Calmness is catching. The nurse remains available to answer questions that might arise. When there is a good relationship between parent and nurse, the child benefits from higher-quality care.

## Developing a Pediatric Nursing Care Plan

Developing the pediatric nursing care plan is similar to developing an adult care plan. The care plan is the result of the nursing process. It states specifically what is to be done for each child and keeps the focus on the child, not on the condition or therapy. An established list of accepted *nursing diagnoses* is available and in use. These serve as a standard for organizing data collection. They also serve as a vehicle by which one nurse can communicate with another. Nursing diagnosis for pediatric patients may require some modification. Assessing the child includes a knowledge of growth and developmental processes. It also includes evaluating the primary caretaker, who has a direct role in the safety and maintenance of the child's health. Nursing care plans are guides that need continual evaluation in order to determine if the goals for the individual child are being met. Some hospitals use a Kardex system (Fig. 23–5). Figure 23–6 shows a nurse entering assessment data, for later retrieval, into the unit computer.

## Nursing Brief

When explaining procedures to children, it is helpful to identify the child's role in the event: for example, "You will be asked to step on the scale."

12-1

| DIET 1800 calorie | Intake ✓ | IV's Heparin lock |
| Constant Carbohydrate | doctor's order 12-1 | for blood draws |
| | Output ✓ | |

Self Select __X__  Evenflo _____  Warm _____
Cup _____  Playtex _____  Cold _____   doctor's order 12-1

Date started 12-1
IV site Ⓛ hand
Needles #20 jelco
Tubing Change _____

| Activity | Bath | Safety Precautions |
|---|---|---|
| Bedrest _____ | Complete _____ | Crib Net _____ |
| Bathroom Priv. _____ | Partial _____ | Restraints _____ |
| May be held _____ | Tub/Shower 12-1 | Seiz. Prec. _____ |
| Up ad lib __X__  12-1 | Shampoo _____ | ID band on 12-1 |
| Playroom _____ | Special Instructions: | Name Tag |
| Other Pt to be up and dressed | | on Crib _____ |
| Interim Summary 12-5 | | Siderail release _____ |

Vital Signs  12-1
TPR Routine
BP Routine
Neuro Check _____
Growth Chart _____
OFC _____
Weight daily

| Special Equipment | Allergies | Resp. Therapy |
|---|---|---|
| Glucometer | none Known | |

Routine Lab Orders

Therapy Schedule
Exercise 1000 and
1400

| STANDING | MEDICATIONS | DATE | TREATMENTS |
|---|---|---|---|
| 12-1 | Sliding Scale Insulin  Sub-q  Give the following! | 12-1 | Blood glucose tests to be done at 0700, 1100, 1600, 2100, 0200 using dextrostix or chemstrips unless patient has own meter. Patient or parent to do testing except at 0200 |
| | 5 units Regular insulin acetone large | | |
| | 3 units Regular insulin acetone moderate | | |
| | 1 unit Regular insulin acetone small | | |
| | | 12-1 | Call resident if blood sugar is less than 50 or greater than 240 |
| | | 12-1 | Acetest all urines until negative or blood sugar below 240 |
| PRN 12-1 | Tylenol 325 mg q 3°-4° prn headache. | 12-1 | Oral treatment of insulin reaction 15 grams carbohydrate (6oz of orange juice) Repeat if signs or symptoms persist after rechecking. |

| Room | Name | Diagnosis | Assoc. Nurse | Primary Nurse | Doctor |
|---|---|---|---|---|---|
| 364-1 | Cory Johnson | Newly diagnosed diabetes mellitus | Peg T | Craig J | Roberts |

**Figure 23–5.** The Kardex serves as a reference to patient problems that require nursing intervention.

*Continued*

PEDIATRIC NURSING CARE PLAN

| Date | Patient Problems/Teaching Needs | Expected Outcomes | Nursing Orders | Initials |
|------|--------------------------------|-------------------|----------------|----------|
| 12-2 | Knowledge deficit related to newly diagnosed diabetes mellitus | Patient and patient's family will discuss disease and its treatment. | ① Show patient and family new equipment A. Syringes B. Insulin C. Glucometer D. Dextrosticks | CR |
| | | | ② Allow patient time to begin accepting disease | CR |
| | | | ③ Discuss resources outside hospital A. ADA B. JDF | CR |
| | | | ④ Be supportive to patient and family during learning process | CR |

| Age *13* | Birth Date *2-12-72* | Hospital # *73 91-85* | Religion *Methodist* | Service *PEDS* | Admission Date *12-1-85* | Time *1200* |
|---|---|---|---|---|---|---|

NURS 372 4/80 632034462

**Figure 23–5.** *Continued*

## Assessing the Child

### PULSE AND RESPIRATIONS

The nurse counting a pulse feels the wave of blood as it is forced through the artery. The pulse rate varies considerably in different children of the same age and size. The pulse rate and respiratory rate of the newborn are high (Tables 23–2 and 23–3). Both pulse and respiratory rates gradually slow down with age until adult values are reached.

The pulse of the older child is taken as that of an adult. Taking the pulse of the infant may seem more difficult at first. Apical pulses are often advised for children under age 5 years. The apical pulse is heard through a stethoscope at the apex of the heart. The nurse counts the rate for 1 full minute. Another common site is the radial pulse (at the thumb side of the wrist just above the radial artery). The temporal pulse

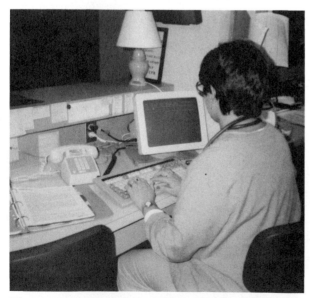

**Figure 23–6.** The nurse enters assessment data and retrieves information about the patient's progress on the unit computer. (Courtesy of Columbia/HCA Portsmouth Regional Hospital, Portsmouth, NH.)

**Table 23–2.** AVERAGE PULSE RATES AT REST

| Age | Lower Limits of Normal (Per Minute) | | Average (Per Minute) | | Upper Limits of Normal (Per Minute) | |
|-----|-----|-----|-----|-----|-----|-----|
| Newborn | 70 | | 125 | | 190 | |
| 1–11 mo | 80 | | 120 | | 160 | |
| 2 yr | 80 | | 110 | | 130 | |
| 4 yr | 80 | | 100 | | 120 | |
| 6 yr | 75 | | 100 | | 115 | |
| 8 yr | 70 | | 90 | | 110 | |
| 10 yr | 70 | | 90 | | 110 | |
| | *Girls* | *Boys* | *Girls* | *Boys* | *Girls* | *Boys* |
| 12 yr | 70 | 65 | 90 | 85 | 110 | 105 |
| 14 yr | 65 | 60 | 85 | 80 | 105 | 100 |
| 16 yr | 60 | 55 | 80 | 75 | 100 | 95 |
| 18 yr | 55 | 50 | 75 | 70 | 95 | 90 |

From Behrman, R.E., & Kliegman, R. (1992). *Nelson textbook of pediatrics* (14th ed.). Philadelphia: W. B. Saunders.

**Table 23–3.** NORMAL RESPIRATORY
RANGES FOR CHILDREN

| Age | Rate Per Minute |
|---|---|
| Birth to 1 mo | 30–40 |
| 1 mo to 1 yr | 26–40 |
| 1–2 yr | 20–30 |
| 2–6 yr | 20–30 |
| 6–10 yr | 18–24 |
| Adolescent | 16–24 |

may be taken if the child is asleep. Actually, the pulse may be taken in any area where a large artery lies close to the skin, especially if the artery runs across a bone and has little soft tissue around it. The following are the most common sites: radial, temporal (just in front of the ear), mandibular (on the lower jawbone), femoral (in the groin), and carotid (on each side of the front of the neck). The carotid pulse may not be appropriate in infants with chubby necks.

The child's respirations are taken in the same way as the adult's. For 1 minute the nurse notes the number of times the chest or abdomen rises and falls. The rate and character of respirations are important in determining the patient's general condition.

## BLOOD PRESSURE

Blood pressure is defined as the pressure of the blood on the walls of the arteries. It is an index of elasticity of arterial walls, peripheral vascular resistance, efficiency of the heart as a pump, and blood volume. Common sites for measuring blood pressure in children are the brachial artery, popliteal artery, and posterior tibial artery (Fig. 23–7).

There are several old and new methods for measuring blood pressure in newborns and children.

**Auscultation.** This is done as for an adult, using the pediatric stethoscope and cuff. The cuff should be long enough to encircle the extremity. It should cover two-thirds of the upper arm. The following sizes are suggested: birth to 1 year—1½ inches; 2–8 years—3 inches; 8–12 years—4 inches. Pressure is normally higher in the lower extremities. The American Heart Association designates the muffled tone as the most accurate index of diastolic pressure but recommends recording both that and the final distinct sound as the complete record; thus 120/80/78. Nurses should clarify this with the physician or the institution employed to ensure uniformity. To determine *pulse pressure*, the diastolic reading is subtracted from the systolic. This usually varies from 20 to 50 mmHg. Widening pulse pressure may be a sign of increased intracranial pressure.

**Palpation.** Palpation is one of the oldest methods. The cuff is applied and inflated above the expected pressure. The fingers are placed over the brachial or radial artery. The systolic pressure is recorded at the point when the pulse reappears. Diastolic pressure is unobtainable. This method is useful in newborns.

**Ultrasonographic (Doppler) Measurement.** This is a noninvasive type of blood pressure monitoring that ultrasonically detects motion of the arterial wall. A transducer with an attached cuff is secured over an artery, usually the brachial, femoral, or popliteal. The cuff is inflated above systolic pressure and then gradually reduced. The transducer transmits vascular sounds, and the measurement appears on a digital read-out. Both systolic and diastolic pressure are recorded. An accurate reading can be obtained only if the child's arm is held still. If the reading shows a major change, another reading is taken because the machines are sensitive to motion.

Some hospitals require blood pressure measurements for all children and others only for the older child. The width of the cuff should cover approximately two-thirds of the extremity used. Cuffs that do not fit can cause errors in readings. Thigh readings are slightly higher than arm readings. The nurse explains what is about to happen, for example, "This will hug your arm and feel tight for a few seconds." The child is allowed to examine the sphygmomanometer and cuff.

Blood pressure is lower in children than in adults. If a patient needs to have blood pressure measurements taken throughout hospitalization, the nurse observes the previous readings before charting the current one. Many factors account for variations in blood pressure. Included are time of day, sex, age, exercise, pain, and emotion. A blood pressure taken when a child is frightened or crying is not accurate. If a significant change is observed, recheck the blood pressure. Abnormal readings are charted and reported to the nurse in charge. Tables 23–4 and 23–5 show normal blood pressure readings for boys and girls, ages 1–18.

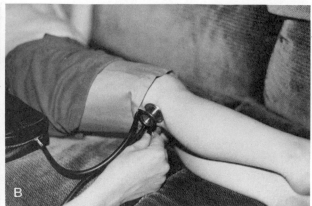

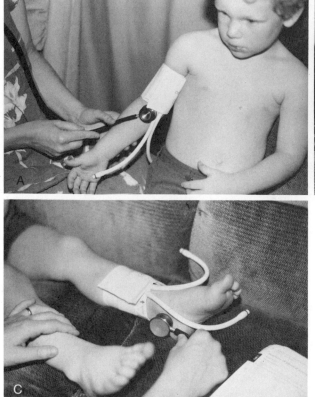

**Figure 23–7.** Common sites for measuring blood pressure in children: *A*, brachial artery, *B*, popliteal artery, and *C*, posterior tibial artery. (From Thompson, E., & Ashwill, J. [1992]. *Pediatric nursing: An introductory text* [6th ed.]. Philadelphia: W. B. Saunders.)

## TEMPERATURE

Body temperature measurement can be oral, rectal, axillary, or tympanic. There are several types of thermometers. Substitutes for the glass mercury thermometer now include the electronic thermometer, the plastic strip thermometer, and the tympanic membrane sensor. The electronic thermometer works quickly and is ideal because the plastic sheath is unbreakable. The plastic strip changes color according to sensed temperature changes. Newer electronic thermometers have a blunt tip that can be inserted into the ear. It records temperature from the tympanic membrane (eardrum) by an infrared emission. This site is of importance because both the hypothalamus (temperature-regulating center) and the eardrum are perfused by the same circulation.

**Oral Temperature.** The procedure is the same as for adults.

**Rectal Temperature.** The patient is placed in a comfortable position, either on the side with the knees slightly flexed or on the stomach.

Infants may be in the supine position with their legs firmly held around the ankles. This is not recommended for toddlers because they are stronger and the feet are in a good kicking position. Insert the lubricated thermometer a maximum of 1 inch. Electronic thermometers register within 15 seconds or less. Mercury rectal thermometers have a more rounded end and should remain in place for 3–5 minutes. Traditionally, the rectal temperature was considered 1°F higher than an oral reading. At this writing there is no consensus about how much rectal and axillary temperatures differ from oral temperatures. The rectal temperature is taken last because it may make the child cry, which influences pulse rate, respiratory rate, and blood pressure. Because this is an intrusive procedure, some institutions use only axillary temperatures for children unless contraindicated. Table 23–6 shows normal temperature ranges. Rectal temperatures are contraindicated in newborns because of the danger of rectal perforation. This method is not used for children who have had rectal surgery, are immune

**Table 23–4.** NORMAL BLOOD PRESSURE READINGS FOR BOYS

| Age in Years | Systolic Blood Pressure Percentile | | | | | Diastolic Blood Pressure Percentile | | | | |
|---|---|---|---|---|---|---|---|---|---|---|
| | 5th | 10th | 50th | 90th | 95th | 5th | 10th | 50th | 90th | 95th |
| 1 | 71 | 76 | 90 | 105 | 109 | 39 | 43 | 56 | 69 | 73 |
| 2 | 72 | 76 | 91 | 106 | 110 | 39 | 43 | 56 | 68 | 72 |
| 3 | 73 | 77 | 92 | 107 | 111 | 39 | 42 | 55 | 68 | 72 |
| 4 | 74 | 79 | 93 | 108 | 112 | 39 | 43 | 56 | 69 | 72 |
| 5 | 76 | 80 | 95 | 109 | 113 | 40 | 43 | 56 | 69 | 73 |
| 6 | 77 | 81 | 96 | 111 | 115 | 41 | 44 | 57 | 70 | 74 |
| 7 | 78 | 83 | 97 | 112 | 116 | 42 | 45 | 58 | 71 | 75 |
| 8 | 80 | 84 | 99 | 114 | 118 | 43 | 47 | 60 | 73 | 76 |
| 9 | 82 | 86 | 101 | 115 | 120 | 44 | 48 | 61 | 74 | 78 |
| 10 | 84 | 88 | 102 | 117 | 121 | 45 | 49 | 62 | 75 | 79 |
| 11 | 86 | 90 | 105 | 119 | 123 | 47 | 50 | 63 | 76 | 80 |
| 12 | 88 | 92 | 107 | 121 | 126 | 48 | 51 | 64 | 77 | 81 |
| 13 | 90 | 94 | 109 | 124 | 128 | 45 | 49 | 63 | 77 | 81 |
| 14 | 93 | 97 | 112 | 126 | 131 | 46 | 50 | 64 | 78 | 82 |
| 15 | 95 | 99 | 114 | 129 | 133 | 47 | 51 | 65 | 79 | 83 |
| 16 | 98 | 102 | 117 | 131 | 136 | 49 | 53 | 67 | 81 | 85 |
| 17 | 100 | 104 | 119 | 134 | 138 | 51 | 55 | 69 | 83 | 87 |
| 18 | 102 | 106 | 121 | 136 | 140 | 52 | 56 | 70 | 84 | 88 |

From the Second Task Force on Blood Pressure Control in Children, National Heart, Lung and Blood Institute, Bethesda, MD. Tabular data prepared by Dr. B. Rosner, 1987.

suppressed, or are receiving chemotherapy because it can irritate the rectal mucosa.

**Axillary Temperature.** Axillary temperatures are usually taken on newborns and preterms and/or according to unit policy. The thermometer is held in the axilla for 3 minutes with the baby's arm pressed against the side. Traditionally, an axillary temperature was considered 1°F lower than an oral temperature. More recently it has been demonstrated that it may be less than 1°F. Although this is subject to controversy, the nurse always records the route used.

**Table 23–5.** NORMAL BLOOD PRESSURE READINGS FOR GIRLS

| Age in Years | Systolic Blood Pressure Percentile | | | | | Diastolic Blood Pressure Percentile | | | | |
|---|---|---|---|---|---|---|---|---|---|---|
| | 5th | 10th | 50th | 90th | 95th | 5th | 10th | 50th | 90th | 95th |
| 1 | 72 | 76 | 91 | 105 | 110 | 38 | 41 | 54 | 67 | 71 |
| 2 | 71 | 76 | 90 | 105 | 109 | 40 | 43 | 56 | 69 | 73 |
| 3 | 72 | 76 | 91 | 106 | 110 | 40 | 43 | 56 | 69 | 73 |
| 4 | 73 | 78 | 92 | 107 | 111 | 40 | 43 | 56 | 69 | 73 |
| 5 | 75 | 79 | 94 | 109 | 113 | 40 | 43 | 56 | 69 | 73 |
| 6 | 77 | 81 | 96 | 111 | 115 | 40 | 44 | 57 | 70 | 74 |
| 7 | 78 | 83 | 97 | 112 | 116 | 41 | 45 | 58 | 71 | 75 |
| 8 | 80 | 84 | 99 | 114 | 118 | 43 | 46 | 59 | 72 | 76 |
| 9 | 81 | 86 | 100 | 115 | 119 | 44 | 48 | 61 | 74 | 77 |
| 10 | 83 | 87 | 102 | 117 | 121 | 46 | 49 | 62 | 75 | 79 |
| 11 | 86 | 90 | 105 | 119 | 123 | 47 | 51 | 64 | 77 | 81 |
| 12 | 88 | 92 | 107 | 122 | 126 | 49 | 53 | 66 | 78 | 82 |
| 13 | 90 | 94 | 109 | 124 | 128 | 46 | 50 | 64 | 78 | 82 |
| 14 | 92 | 96 | 110 | 125 | 129 | 49 | 53 | 67 | 81 | 85 |
| 15 | 93 | 97 | 111 | 126 | 130 | 49 | 53 | 67 | 82 | 86 |
| 16 | 93 | 97 | 112 | 127 | 131 | 49 | 53 | 67 | 81 | 85 |
| 17 | 93 | 98 | 112 | 127 | 131 | 48 | 52 | 66 | 80 | 84 |
| 18 | 94 | 98 | 112 | 127 | 131 | 48 | 52 | 66 | 80 | 84 |

From the Second Task Force on Blood Pressure Control in Children, National Heart, Lung and Blood Institute, Bethesda, MD. Tabular data prepared by Dr. B. Rosner, 1987.

**Table 23–6.** NORMAL TEMPERATURE RANGES FOR CHILDREN

| Method | Range |
|---|---|
| Oral | 36.4–37.4°C (97.6–99.3°F) |
| Rectal | 37.0–37.8°C (98.6–100.0°F) |
| Axillary | 35.8–36.6°C (96.6–98.0°F) |
| Ear | 36.9–37.5°C (98.4–99.5°F) |

**Tympanic Temperature.** The covered probe tip is placed gently in the outer portion of the ear. The temperature reading is obtained immediately. It is not affected by wax or infection in the ear (Weir & Weir, 1989). The normal range for children on an *Ivac* Corecheck is 36.9°–37.5°C (98.4–99.5°F).

The body temperature of a healthy child does not remain constant. Note range cited in Table 23-6. * When recording temperatures, the nurse notes the route utilized. If a great variation from normal is discovered, the nurse takes the temperature again, being sure that the mercury in a mercury-type thermometer is shaken down properly. If the same reading is obtained, it is immediately reported to the team leader or head nurse and entered on the chart. It is not uncommon for infants and young children to have convulsions from a high fever that would produce only chills in an adult. Managing fever in children is depicted in Nursing Care Plan 23–1.

The procedure for a sponge bath to reduce fever follows. Small children may be bathed in a tub or plastic basin. Alcohol is not used because it reduces body temperature too fast and may be absorbed. Shivering is to be avoided as it will increase the body temperature.

## WEIGHT

Weight must be accurately recorded on admission. The weight of a patient provides a means of determining progress and is necessary to determine the dosage of certain medications. The way in which the nurse weighs the child depends on the age.

The infant is weighed completely naked in a warm room. A fresh diaper or scale paper is placed on the scale. This prevents cross-contamination, that is, the spread of germs from one infant to another. The scale is balanced to com-

*A table of Celsius and Fahrenheit temperature equivalents appears in Appendix H.

## PROCEDURE FOR GIVING A SPONGE BATH TO REDUCE TEMPERATURE

### Equipment

Basin of tepid water
Three face cloths
Towel
Two bath blankets
Waterproof sheet

### Method

1. Assemble the equipment at the bedside. Explain the procedure to the patient.
2. Screen the child. Take and record temperature, pulse, and respiration.
3. Cover the patient with a bath blanket or sheet. Fanfold bedclothes to the foot of the bed. Place a waterproof sheet and bath blanket beneath the patient.
4. Remove the pillow from the bed. Remove the patient's gown.
5. Wash the patient's face and neck with tepid water.
6. Lift the corner of the bath blanket and bathe the child's body, part by part. Use long strokes. Expose one area of the body at a time.
7. Place moist, folded cloths over blood vessels that lie close to the skin (underarms and groin).
8. Turn the patient and repeat the procedure, beginning with the neck, and going to shoulders, back, and so forth.
9. Check color and pulse to be sure that the child is tolerating the procedure well.
10. If the child starts to shiver, raise the water temperature.
11. When the bath is completed, pat the skin dry and cover the patient with only a sheet.
12. Remove the waterproof sheet and blanket. Replace the hospital gown.
13. Arrange pillows and bedding for the patient's comfort.
14. Take the patient's temperature within 30 min of the time the procedure ended, and record. If the temperature has not started to go down, check to see if the procedure should be repeated. *Note:* The temperature is not expected to drop to normal but merely to a more reasonable level.
15. Chart the following: time procedure began, length of time administered, untoward reactions, patient's temperature before and after procedure.

| NURSING CARE PLAN 23–1 | | |
|---|---|---|
| **Selected Nursing Diagnoses for the Child with a Fever** | | |
| **Goals** | **Nursing Interventions** | **Rationale** |

**Nursing Diagnosis:** Fluid volume deficit: potential for dehydration due to increased metabolic rate.

| Goals | Nursing Interventions | Rationale |
|---|---|---|
| Child does not become dehydrated as evidenced by good skin turgor, moist mucus membranes, no weight loss | 1. Increase fluid intake; offer juice, water, Popsicles, yogurt, as age-appropriate | 1. Body's metabolic rate increases with fever; children have a higher proportion of body water; therefore, more water can be lost rapidly; body systems such as the kidneys are immature at some ages |
| Child's temperature will be between 36.5 and 37.4°C (97.4 and 99.4°F) | 1. Administer *tepid* sponge bath for fever of 40.0°C (104.0°F) | 1. Tepid baths help reduce fever and may make patient more comfortable |
| | 2. Assess vital signs prior to sponge bath | 2. Provides baseline data |
| | 3. Retake vital signs 30 min after procedure | 3. Retaking of vital signs will determine if fever is decreasing |
| | 4. Expose skin to air following procedure, prevent shivering | 4. Promotes evaporation and cooling of skin |
| | 5. Administer antipyretic medications according to physician's instructions | 5. Frequently child with a fever also has a headache and painful joints; antipyretic medications will relieve these discomforts as well as reduce fever |
| Child does not injure self as evidenced by absence of bruises | 1. Keep side rails raised | 1. Side rails provide safety from falls |
| | 2. Observe child frequently | 2. Frequent observation will detect subtle changes and possibly reduce complications |
| | 3. Remain with child if tub bath is given | 3. Threat of drowning is always present with small children and water |
| Parent understands and verbalizes nature and treatment of fever | 1. Explain nature of fever (not always bad); too-vigorous control may mask signs of illness | 1. Recently, potential benefits of fever have been cited; it is thought to enhance body's defense mechanisms and increase antibody activity |
| | 2. Emphasize removal of clothes when child has fever | 2. Removal of clothing cools child |
| | 3. Call physician if child looks sick or acts in a way different from normal | 3. Degree of fever does not always reflect severity of disease |
| Parent verbalizes understanding of how to read a thermometer | 4. Demonstrate how to read a thermometer | 4. This gives parents a sense of control; accuracy of fever will be ensured on discharge |
| Parent verbalizes understanding of potential for convulsion | 5. Discuss with parent potential for convulsion | 5. Only a small number of children convulse with fever; however, discussion is advisable |
| Parent knows how to give appropriate care during a convulsion | 6. Review management of a convulsion | 6. Knowledge allays anxiety |
| | 7. Discourage use of alcohol sponge baths, which may reduce temperature too fast, leading to convulsions | 7. Alcohol sponge bath may still be suggested by older relatives |
| | 8. Discourage use of cold water | 8. Cold water may cause shivering and raise body temperature |

pensate for the weight of the diaper. There are various ways of balancing scales; the nurse requests specific instruction for the particular scale used. The infant is placed gently on the scale. The nurse's left hand is held slightly above the infant to prevent falling. The nurse regulates the weights with the right hand. The scale is read when the infant is lying still. If the mother is present, she may distract the patient by speaking softly.

Once the exact weight is determined, the infant is removed from the scale, wrapped in a blanket, and soothed. The weight is immediately recorded. The scale paper is disposed of in the proper receptacle. An unsoiled diaper is returned to the patient's unit. Digital pediatric scales that provide read-outs in pounds and grams are used in many institutions. They do not require the regulation of weights.

The older child is weighed in the same manner as an adult. A paper towel is placed on the scale for the patient to stand on. The patient is generally weighed in a hospital gown. The shoes are removed. If the child is unable to stand on the scales, it may be necessary for the nurse to hold the child and read the combined weights. The nurse is then weighed and subtracts that number from the combined weight to obtain the patient's weight. Occasionally, a child is weighed while wearing a cast. The nurse records this as, for example, "weight 34 pounds with cast on right arm."

**Other Observations.** The child who has been undressed for weighing is observed for such objective symptoms as skin coloring, abrasions, rash, swelling, facial expressions (fear, pain, fatigue), discharge from nose or ears, dyspnea, condition of joints, odor of breath, condition of teeth, cough, or other abnormalities or markings.

## HEIGHT

The older child's height is measured along with weight. The infant's height must be measured while the infant is lying on a flat surface alongside a metal tape measure or yardstick. The knees should be pressed flat on the table. The measurement is taken from the top of the head to the heels and recorded.

## HEAD CIRCUMFERENCE

Head circumference increases rapidly during infancy as a result of brain growth. It is generally measured on infants and toddlers and on all children with neurologic defects. The tape measure is placed around the head slightly above the eyebrows and ears and around the occipital prominence of the skull. The measurement is recorded.

# Collecting Specimens

## URINE SPECIMENS

A urine specimen is obtained from the newly admitted patient. Certain general principles of collecting specimens are observed:

- Explain the procedure to the patient (as age-appropriate).
- Use a clean container or urine collection device.
- Check frequently for results.
- Label all specimens clearly and attach the proper laboratory slip.
- Record in nurses' notes.

---

**Figure 23–8.** Applying newborn and pediatric urine collectors. Two key points are as follows: (a) The skin must be clean and perfectly dry. Avoid oils, baby powders, and lotion soaps, which may leave a residue on the skin and interfere with the ability of the adhesive to stick. (b) Application must begin on the tiny area of skin between the anus and the genitals. The narrow "bridge" on the adhesive patch keeps feces from contaminating the specimen and helps position the collector correctly.

For girls, place the child on her back, spread her legs, and wash each skin fold in the genital area. A gentle bath soap is best. Do not use a scrub soap solution; it may leave a residue that interferes with adhesion. Wash the anus last. Rinse and dry. For boys, wash the scrotum first, then the penis; wash the anus last. Allow a few moments for air drying.

Remove protective paper from the bottom half of the adhesive patch. Most persons find it easier to keep the top half of the adhesive covered with paper until the bottom part has been applied to the skin. With a very active boy, you may want to keep all the paper in place until you have fitted the collector over the genitals.

For girls, stretch the perineum to separate the skin folds and expose the vagina. When applying adhesive to the skin, be sure to start at the narrow bridge of skin separating the vagina from the anus. Work outward from this point. For boys, begin between the anus and the base of the scrotum. Press adhesive firmly against the skin and avoid wrinkles. When the bottom part is in place, remove paper from the upper portion of the adhesive patch. Work upward to complete application. (Permission to reproduce this copyrighted material has been granted by the owner, Hollister, Inc., Libertyville, IL.)

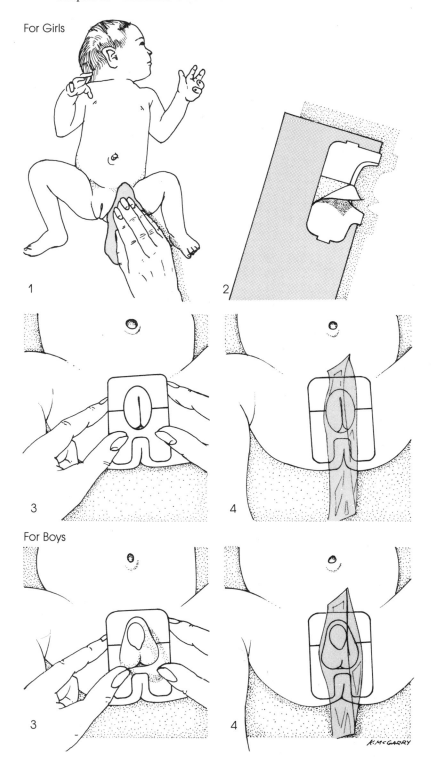

**Figure 23–8.** *See legend on opposite page.*

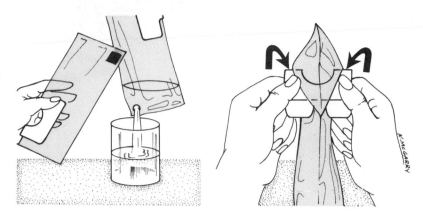

**Figure 23–9.** Recovering the specimen. You can drain the urine bag collector into a clean beaker or specimen bottle by removing the tab in the lower corner, or you can seal the specimen inside the collector itself by folding the sticky adhesive sides together. Then place the collector with specimen into a paper or plastic cup. (Permission to reproduce this copyrighted material has been granted by the owner, Hollister, Inc., Libertyville, IL.)

Figures 23–8 and 23–9 show how to apply newborn and pediatric urine collectors and how to recover a specimen.

**Obtaining a Clean-Catch Specimen.** Special sterile containers are available for clean-catch specimens; the manufacturer's directions should be followed. All require cleansing of the perineum with an antiseptic. Rinsing and drying of the perineum are important in order to prevent contamination of urine from the antiseptic. Wiping is done from front to back. After the urine stream has started, the midstream specimen is caught in the sterile container. The nurse's participation is either direct or supervisory, depending on the child's age or the availability of a parent. Adolescents, who may be embarrassed by carrying a urine specimen through the halls, may be given a bag or other suitable camouflage. If not tested immediately, the specimen is refrigerated because bacteria accumulate at room temperature.

**Obtaining Specimens by Catheterization.** Obtaining specimens by means of a catheter is seldom indicated in pediatric patients. If necessary the procedure is essentially the same as for adults except the size of the catheter is smaller (usually an 8 or 10 Foley). The nurse will require assistance because patients may resist. When required for surgical patients, the catheter may be inserted once the child has been anesthetized. This approach is less traumatic for children, who are usually frightened by the procedure.

**Obtaining a 24-Hour Specimen.** At times a 24-hour urine specimen may be requested in order to determine the rate of urine production and measure the excretion of specific chemicals from the body. The nurses on each shift must closely supervise this test to maintain its accuracy, as lost specimens necessitate restarting the test. Problems can arise if the collection device does not adhere to the skin properly; therefore, the nurse must be alert for this occurrence. Diversions suitable to the child's age are employed. Certain tests require that chemicals be added to the bedside collection receptacle. This requirement should be clarified before the procedure begins. A sign is attached to the infant's crib to alert personnel of a 24-hour urine collection. The average daily amount of urine excreted, by age, is given in Table 23–7.

**Determining Specific Gravity.** The nurse may be asked to measure the specific gravity of the urine. The normal range is 1.005–1.030.

Refractometers are used for this purpose in some hospitals. Urine can be obtained from some infants' diapers by utilizing a syringe without a needle. Only a few drops of urine are required.

**Table 23–7.** AVERAGE DAILY EXCRETION OF URINE

| Age | Fluid Ounces | Milliliters |
| --- | --- | --- |
| 1st and 2nd days | 1–2 | 30–60 |
| 3rd to 10th days | 3–10 | 100–300 |
| 10th day to 2 mo | 9–15 | 250–450 |
| 2 mo to 1 yr | 14–17 | 400–500 |
| 1–3 yr | 17–20 | 500–600 |
| 3–5 yr | 20–24 | 600–700 |
| 5–8 yr | 22–34 | 650–1000 |
| 8–14 yr | 27–47 | 800–1400 |

## PROCEDURE FOR DETERMINING URINE SPECIFIC GRAVITY

### Equipment

Urinometer, urine specimen

### Method

1. Fill the test tube three-fourths full of urine.
2. Insert the bobbin of the urinometer. Spin it gently to be sure that it is not touching the sides of the container.
3. Take the reading from the bottom of the meniscus.
4. Record the results.

**Testing for Albumin.** The nurse working in a doctor's office or clinic may also be requested to test urine for albumin, that is, protein. Normally, little or no albumin is found in the urine of a healthy child. Reagent strips especially intended for this purpose are available. The nurse dips the end of the strip into urine and compares the strip with a special color chart. Specific instructions accompany test materials.

## STOOL SPECIMENS

Stool specimens are obtained from older children as from adults. This is embarrassing for most children, who are "turned off" by the suggestion. The ambulatory child can use a bedpan placed beneath a toilet seat. It is difficult for a child to tell the nurse that the sample has been collected. The nurse can acknowledge these feelings by giving the child permission to express them without being critical, for example, "I know this must be embarrassing for you. It is for grown-ups too, but we need this because . . ." and so on. An infant's stool specimen can be obtained from the infant directly from the diaper if it has not been contaminated by urine. A rectal swab may also be ordered.

Some specimens must be sent to the laboratory while they are warm. The specimen is labeled properly, and the laboratory slip is attached. The nurse charts the time, color, amount, and consistency of the stool; the purpose for which it was collected, that is, blood, ova, parasites, or bacteria; and any related information.

## BLOOD SPECIMENS

Blood specimens are generally collected by the laboratory technician or by a specially trained nurse. The antecubital fossa is a common site for collection in children older than 2 years of age. Assistance may be required. Children are very frightened by this procedure. If the child struggles, the nurse avoids such statements as "be a good boy/girl," which are shame-based. Instead the nurse acknowledges that having blood drawn is difficult even for grown-ups.

**Positioning the Child.** Positioning the child for blood drawings is extremely important. The nurse is often asked to assist in these procedures. Figures 23–10 and 23–11 depict how to position the patient for jugular and femoral venipuncture. Both the jugular and the femoral veins are large; therefore, the patient is frequently checked to ensure that there is no

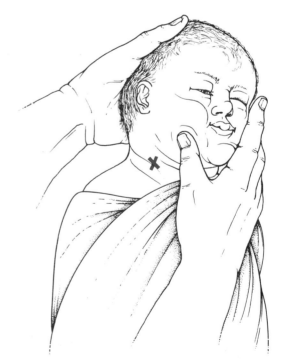

**Figure 23–10.** An infant prepared for jugular venipuncture. The head and shoulders are extended over a table or pillow.

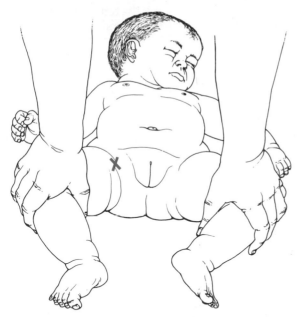

**Figure 23–11.** An infant positioned for femoral venipuncture. This position exposes the groin area.

bleeding. These sites are used mainly when other areas have been exhausted. The baby is soothed accordingly, as crying and thrashing may precipitate oozing. The nurse charts the site utilized, name of blood test, and any untoward developments.

## LUMBAR PUNCTURE

The nurse sometimes assists the physician with a lumbar puncture, which is also referred to as a "spinal tap." It is done to obtain spinal fluid for examination or to reduce pressure within the brain in such conditions as hydrocephalus or meningitis. Disposable lumbar puncture sets are available.

Normal spinal fluid is clear like water. The pressure ranges from 60 to 180 mmHg. It is somewhat lower in infants. The procedure for children is essentially the same as for adults. The main difference lies in the patient's ability to cooperate with positioning. The nurse explains that child must lie quietly and will be helped to do this. Sensations during a lumbar puncture include a cool feeling when the skin is cleansed and a feeling of pressure when the needle is inserted. The way in which the child is held can directly affect the success of the procedure.

The patient lies on the side with the back

parallel to the side of the treatment table. The knees are flexed, and the head is brought down close to the flexed knees. The nurse can keep the child in this position by placing the child's head in the crook of one arm and the knees in the crook of the other arm. The nurse's hands are then clasped together at the front of the child. The nurse leans forward, gently placing the chest against the patient (Fig. 23–12).

Once the child is positioned, the doctor prepares the lower back using sterile technique. A vial of 1% procaine hydrochloride (Novocain) may be necessary unless this is provided in the sterile set-up. The top of the vial is cleansed with an alcohol sponge. Once the area has been locally anesthetized, the doctor inserts a special hollow needle into the patient's lower back and collects the spinal fluid in two or three test tubes. When the procedure is completed, a sterile Band-Aid is placed over the injection site and the child is comforted. Specimens are labeled and taken to the laboratory with the appropriate requisition form.

Young children do not usually suffer from headaches following a lumbar puncture and may play quietly after the procedure unless

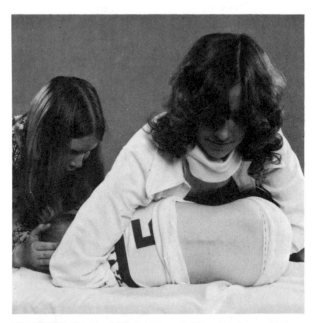

**Figure 23–12.** A child positioned for a lumbar puncture. Although the nurse may appear to be placing her weight on the child, the weight is actually placed on her elbows. If the parents are present during this procedure, they can give the child emotional support. (From Betz, C., Hunsberger, M., & Wright, S. [1994]. *Family-centered nursing care of children* [2nd ed]. Philadelphia: W. B. Saunders.)

ordered to do otherwise. The adolescent may avoid postlumbar puncture headache by lying flat for a period of time. The nurse charts the date and time of the lumbar puncture and the name of the attending physician. Also charted are the amount of fluid obtained; its character, for example, cloudy or bloody; whether or not specimens were sent to the laboratory; and the patient's reaction to the procedure. The nurse cleans and restocks the treatment room.

## Administering Medications

### VARIATIONS IN CHILDREN

The responsibility for giving medications to children is a serious one. Although the full description of technical details used in administering drugs is beyond the scope of this text, the following considerations and hazards applicable to pediatric patients are presented.

More than half of the drugs currently on the market are unsuitable for children because of their toxicity or because information about their effect on children is lacking. Children are smaller than adults, and their medications have to be adapted to their size and age. For instance, a student nurse who takes one adult as-pirin receives 5 grains. A mother who gives her 3-year-old child one baby aspirin is administering 1¼ grains, which is only one-fourth the dose taken by the nurse. Newborns and preterm infants are in particular jeopardy because of the immaturity of their body systems. In these patients, simply adjusting the dosage is insufficient. Drugs must be individualized and tailored to a multitude of factors (Fig. 23–13). Appendix F lists commonly used pediatric drugs.

Most pediatric medications are prescribed in milligrams per kilogram of body weight per 24 hours. A hospital drug formulary is usually available on the unit to enable the nurse to determine the safety of a particular dose. If there is any question, one may also consult another nurse, the physician who wrote the order, the hospital pharmacist, or the shift supervisor. The nurse should be undisturbed when preparing medications (Fig. 23–14).

At times, the physician needs to calculate a particular dosage of a medication for a certain child. One method, calculation by body surface area (BSA), is now considered to be the most accurate. In this method, a nomogram is used (Fig. 23–15). The child's height is located on the left scale, and weight on the right scale. A line is drawn between the two points. The point

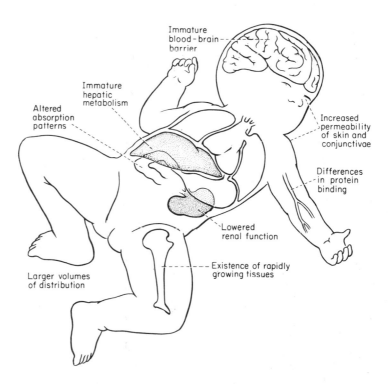

**Figure 23–13.** Some of the multiple factors that modify drug disposition in the newborn. (Adapted from Hirata, T. [1977]. In D. Smith [ed.], *Introduction to clinical pediatrics* [2nd ed.]. Philadelphia: W. B. Saunders.)

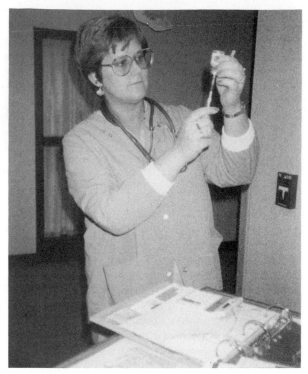

**Figure 23–14.** It is important that the nurse be undisturbed when preparing medications. (Courtesy of Columbia/HCA Portsmouth Regional Hospital, Portsmouth, NH.)

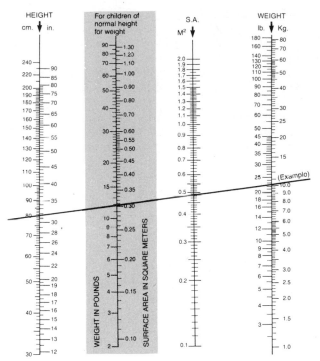

**Figure 23–15.** Nomogram for estimating surface area. The surface area is indicated where a straight line that connects the height and weight levels intersects the surface area column. If the patient is of average size, the surface area can be deduced on the basis of weight alone (see enclosed box). (Nomogram modified from data of E. Boyd by C. D. West. From Behrman, R., & Kliegman, R. [1992]. *Nelson textbook of pediatrics* [14th ed.]. Philadelphia: W. B. Saunders.)

at which the line transects the surface area (SA) gives the body surface area (BSA). If the patient's size is roughly average, the surface area can also be estimated from the weight alone by using the enclosed area. The results are inserted into a formula. The average adult BSA is approximately 1.7 m².

$$\frac{\text{BSA (child)}}{\text{BSA (adult)}} \times \text{average adult dose} = \text{child's dose.}$$

Besides knowing the correct amount and route of a drug, the nurse must also be aware of the toxic side effects that might occur. The absorption, distribution, metabolism, and excretion of drugs differ substantially in children, who also react more quickly and violently to medication. Drug reactions are therefore not as predictable as they are in adult patients. The drug's impact on normal growth and development must be considered. Drug circulars must be read carefully to determine suitability of a particular drug for children. *Drugs should be given only by the route indicated.*

One should double-check with another nurse if using calculated dosages or any drug or dosage that may cause concern. (Some hospitals specify double-checking for digoxin [Lanoxin], insulin, heparin, and certain other drugs.) *The child should be correctly identified by using the hospital identification band. The nurse must always know what medications the patient is receiving, whether or not the nurse personally administers them.* See Table 23–8 for further considerations about pediatric medications.

## ORAL MEDICATIONS

The administration of medication by mouth is preferred in children but is not always possible because of vomiting, malabsorption, or refusal. Children younger than 5 years find it difficult to swallow tablets or capsules, so many pediatric medications are available in liquid, suspension, or chewable tablets. Only scored tab-

**Table 23–8.** SELECTED CONSIDERATIONS IN GIVING MEDICATIONS TO CHILDREN

| Age | Consideration |
|---|---|
| Infant | Apply bib<br>Support and elevate head and shoulders<br>Plastic disposable syringe is accurate and safe for oral medications<br>Depress chin with thumb to open mouth<br>Slowly insert medication along the side of the infant's mouth; this helps prevent gagging<br>Allow time for swallowing<br>The recommended site for intramuscular (IM) injections is the vastus lateralis muscle<br>Avoid use of buttocks, as gluteal muscles are undeveloped in infants; danger of injury to sciatic nerve<br>As a rule of thumb, give no more than 1 ml of solution in a single site; if in doubt, confer with another nurse or physician<br>Soothe infant |
| Toddler | May require help of another person<br>May require some type of restraint if no assistance is available<br>Let child explore an empty medicine cup<br>Explain reasons for medication<br>Crush tablets if not chewable variety<br>If child is cooperative, may hold medicine cup<br>Allow child to drink at own pace<br>When giving IM medications, carry out injection quickly and gently<br>Be prepared to find that resistive behavior is at its peak, particularly kicking, crying, and thrashing about<br>Be prepared to be surprised, as some toddlers are very cooperative |
| Preschool | Chewable tablets and liquids are preferred<br>Regression in pill taking may be seen<br>Watch for loose teeth that may be swallowed<br>Avoid prolonged reasoning<br>Involve parents if appropriate<br>Provide puppet play to help child express frustrations concerning injections<br>Praise child following procedure |
| School Age | Can take pills and capsules; instruct child to place pill near back of tongue and immediately swallow water<br>Emphasize swallowing of fluid to distract child from swallowing of pill<br>Some children continue to have a difficult time swallowing pills, and other forms of the medication should be explored (many come in suspensions); never ridicule child<br>Child can be unpredictable from day to day in their cooperation; allow more time for giving pediatric medication<br>Always ascertain that child is fully awake (particularly after nap time and during night shift)<br>Always inform child of what you are about to do<br>Remain with fearful child after procedure until child regains composure<br>When this is not possible or appears prolonged, enlist help of auxiliary personnel |
| Adolescent | Prepare patient with explanations suitable to level of understanding<br>Always ensure privacy<br>Teach adolescent what side effects to report<br>Identify adolescents on contraceptives in order to avoid drug interactions (may have been too embarrassed to provide information during history or may be attempting to keep secret from significant others)<br>Remain with patient until medication is consumed (particularly if patient has a behavior disorder)<br>Anticipate mood swings in compliance<br>Consider possibility of adolescent addiction (drugs, alcohol) even though this may not be presenting problem; many medications would be altered by such conditions |

lets should be divided. Suspensions must be fully shaken before use.

Capsules may have to be emptied and the powder disguised in a pleasant-tasting medium. This is also necessary when the medication is bitter or otherwise unpalatable. Cherry syrup or jelly may be used. Use of important sources of nutrients, such as orange juice, for this purpose is discouraged because the child may develop a distaste for them. The medication is never referred to as "candy." Medication is administered slowly, especially if the child is crying. *The patient's head and shoulders are elevated to prevent aspiration.* Toddlers may attempt to push the medicine cup away. In anticipation of this response, the

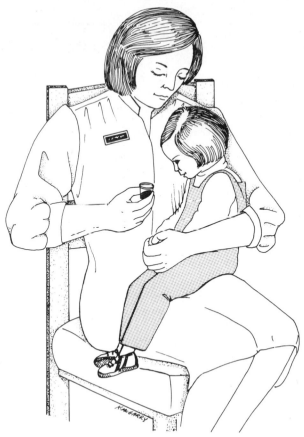

**Figure 23–16.** The cup method of administering medication. The nurse may hold the child on her lap and restrain the child's hands as shown, to prevent spilling of the medication.

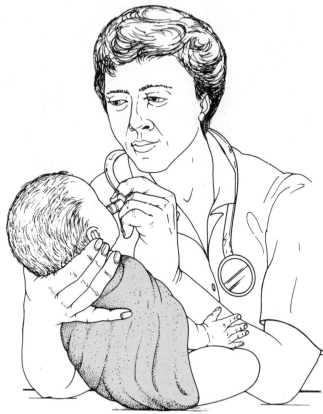

**Figure 23–17.** Medications can be administered to the infant by means of an oral syringe. The head of the infant must be elevated when oral medications are given.

nurse holds the child, with hands restrained, in the nurse's lap in a semisitting position (Fig. 23–16). "Chasers" of water, fruit juice, or carbonated beverage are appreciated. In choosing a chaser, the patient's age and diet are considered.

If a nasogastric tube is in place, the nurse tests for proper placement of the tube before pouring medication into the funnel. A small amount of water is administered afterward to cleanse the tube. The procedure is recorded on the intake and output (I & O) sheet.

For infants, an oral syringe is an excellent device for measuring small quantities (Fig. 23–17). It is easily transported, and medication can be given directly from the syringe. The syringe is inspected for rough edges before being used. The syringe is placed midway back at the side of the mouth. A bib is placed on an infant before performing the procedure. Med-

ication should not be placed in a bottle of juice or water; if some of the contents are refused, there is no way to determine how much of the drug was consumed.

A plastic medicine dropper is useful, and the drug manufacturer may provide one with the medication. It is used only for the medication specified—it is not intended for measuring other liquids. A drug ordered in teaspoons should be measured in milliliters to ensure accuracy (5 ml = 1 teaspoon). The nurse administering medications on the pediatric unit must keep the medicine tray or cart in sight at all times. This prevents other patients from upsetting or ingesting the contents.

## NOSE, EAR, AND EYE DROPS

Except for a few differences, the principles for administering nose, ear, and eye drops to children are essentially the same as for adults. Infants and small children need to be restrained.

## PROCEDURE FOR ADMINISTERING NOSE DROPS TO THE SMALL CHILD

**Equipment**
Sheet for restraint
Nose drops
Tissues

**Method**

1. Immobilize the infant with mummy restraint.
2. Wipe excess mucus from nose with a tissue.
3. Place infant on back with head over the side of the mattress or neck extended over a pillow.
4. Encircle infant's cheeks and chin with left arm and hand to steady.
5. Instill drops with right hand.
6. Keep infant in this position for ½–1 min to allow the drops to reach the proper area.
7. Remove restraints. Make infant comfortable.
8. Chart the following: time, name of nose drops, strength, number of drops instilled, how the patient tolerated the procedure, untoward reactions.

**Nose Drops.** The procedure for administering nose drops to a small child is listed above.

**Ear Drops.** The doctor may prescribe a drug to be instilled into the ear to relieve pain. If the drops were refrigerated, they are allowed to warm to room temperature. In the child under 3 years, the infected ear is drawn down and back to straighten the canal, and the correct number of drops are instilled. In the older child, the ear lobe is pulled upward and backward to obtain the same result. Gentle massage of the area in front of the ear may facilitate entry of the drops. If *sterile* cotton is to be placed in the ear, it must be inserted loosely in order to prevent infected material from being forced into the mastoid area. Some do not advise its use because they believe it interferes with free drainage. The patient remains supine for a few minutes to permit the fluid to be absorbed. The nurse charts the following: time, name of drug, number of drops administered, area (right or left ear), untoward reactions, and whether or not the patient obtained relief.

**Eye Drops.** Ophthalmic medication is administered to a child in the same manner as for the adult. The child is informed of the need for the medication. The patient is identified, and orders and the label on the bottle are checked for correct medication and concentration. The nurse ascertains which eye requires treatment, that is, right eye (O.D.); left eye (O.S.); or both eyes (O.U.). The hands are washed before and after the procedure. With the thumb and index finger, gentle pressure is applied in opposite directions to open the eye. The older child is instructed to "look up." Supporting the hand on the patient's forehead, the medication is instilled into the center of the lower lid (conjunctival sac) (Fig. 23–18). The child is instructed to close the eye but not to squeeze it, as this could expel some of the solution.

Ointment is applied in the same conjunctival sac as eye drops. When only one nurse is available and the patient is an infant, the mummy restraint is applied. Occasionally, children refuse to open their eyes. The nurse must use ingenuity to coax a reluctant patient. It may help to involve parents. Sometimes one fails. The nurse who is unable to complete a procedure because the child is uncooperative consults with appropriate personnel and records this information. Children have very little control in the hospital situation. Opportunities that afford them control are few and far between. Returning at another time, allowing the child to ventilate feelings via drawings or puppet play, or having the child administer pre-

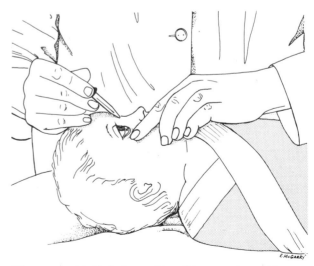

**Figure 23–18.** Technique of instilling eye drops. The eye drops should fall in the center of the lower conjunctival sac, never directly on the eyeball. Gloves are worn if there is infection or drainage from the eyes.

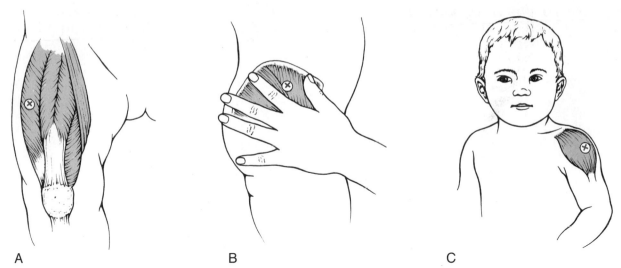

A       B       C

**Figure 23–19.** Appropriate sites for intramuscular injection in children. (*Note*: There is no universal agreement concerning sites. The vastus lateralis [A] is preferred in children under 3 years.)

tend eye drops to their stuffed toys may prove helpful.

## INTRAMUSCULAR INJECTIONS

The preferred injection site for children under 3 years of age is the vastus lateralis muscle (Fig. 23–19A). This is because it is the largest muscle in infants and small children and has few major nerves and blood vessels. After 3 years of age the ventrogluteal muscle may be used. The ventrogluteal site (Fig. 23–19B) is preferred over the dorsogluteal muscle because the dorsogluteal muscle is small and poorly developed in infants and there is danger of injuring the sciatic nerve. It is suggested that the dorsogluteal muscle not be used in any child who has not been walking for at least 2 years, and it is generally avoided in children under 6 years (Thompson & Ashwill, 1992). The deltoid muscle (Fig. 23–19C) may be used occasionally for small volumes of fluid in toddlers. However, some suggest this too should be avoided before 6 years (Betz et al., 1994). Sites are subject to controversy because of the current lack of research. Beecraft suggests in assessing the child for injection site that the child's size, musculature, skin condition, age, and medical diagnosis be taken into consideration (Beecraft & Redick, 1990). The practical nurse consults a registered nurse if she has any questions regarding site selection.

The size of the syringe and needle to be utilized varies with the size of the child, volume of medication prescribed, amount and general condition of the muscle tissue, frequency of injections, and viscosity (thickness) of the drug. A small needle gauge, such as 25–27, and a length of 0.5–1 inch is commonly used. As a general rule, 1 ml is the maximum volume to be given in one site to older infants and small children. Small or premature babies may require even less. For volumes less than 1 ml, a tuberculin syringe or low-dose syringe is preferred.

The nurse should anticipate some protest from children about injections. Whenever possible, a second person should assist by distracting and restraining the child. The child's first injection is particularly important because it establishes the pattern for future reactions (Fig. 23–20). Topical anesthetic creams applied to the skin at the injection site prior to administration of the medicine numb the area and decrease pain. The school-age child may assist in selection of the site, if possible. This helps to increase feelings of mastery and control. Injections are more of a threat to toddlers and preschool children, who are too young to understand the necessity for them. The nurse should not be offended or become indignant when children are hostile. The nurse remains with them until they calm down and can focus their attention elsewhere. Do not shame the uncooperative child. Fortunately, because most medications

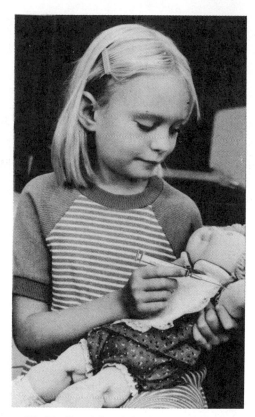

**Figure 23-20.** By giving injections to dolls or puppets, children can be prepared for this procedure and may be less frightened by it. (Copyright 1985, American Journal of Nursing Company. Reprinted with permission from Meer, P. [1985]. Using play therapy in outpatient settings. *MCN: American Journal of Maternal Child Nursing, 10,* 379).

can now be given orally, by rectum, or intravenously, the necessity for administering intramuscular injections is decreasing.

## INTRAVENOUS MEDICATIONS

Medications given by the intravenous (IV) route are being administered routinely in pediatric patients. In some cases it prevents repeated intramuscular injections, which are unpleasant. Other drugs are effective only if given by this method. The medication is also absorbed more rapidly, which is of value. Each hospital has its own policies about who may start IV lines or add medications to an established line. The nurse assesses the IV line carefully for infiltration, inflammation, and patency, particularly prior to the administration of medicine.

Compatibility of fluid and medication is always corroborated. If more than one medication is to be given, the others are also checked for compatibility. Medication is never administered via blood products being given intravenously. Sites for IV infusion in children are illustrated in Figure 23-21.

There are several ways to administer IV medications. Some vitamins and electrolytes are added directly to the IV bag or bottle. More often the medication is added to the calibrated burette (Soluset) (see p. 595) or is administered by precision-controlled syringe pumps (Autosyringe). In such cases, the medicine must be compatible with the IV solution. When it is not, a secondary or "piggyback" set-up is employed. A separate bag with the compatible solution with its own Soluset is utilized. Once this is attached and started, the original solution is stopped until the medication is absorbed and the tubing flushed.

Minibags of 50 to 100 ml of solution can be used if the IV does not have a Soluset. Antibiotics are frequently administered this way (Fig. 23-22).

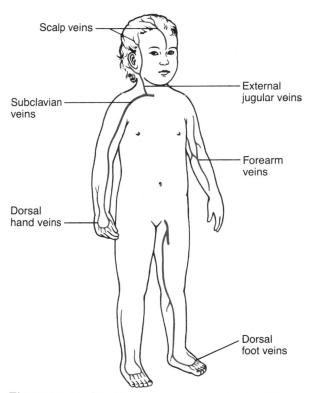

**Figure 23-21.** Sites for intravenous infusion in children.

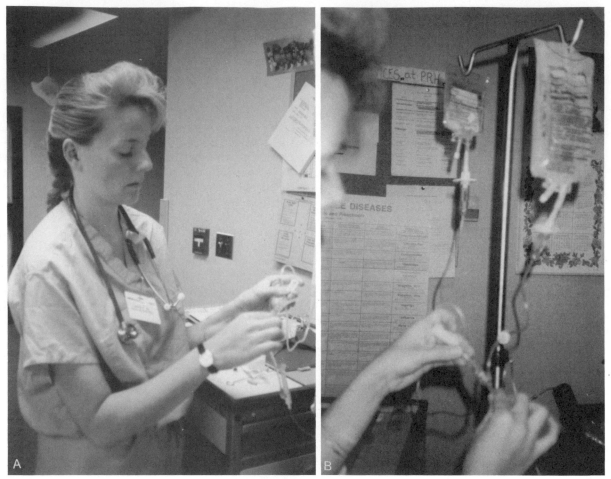

**Figure 23–22.** The nurse prepares a secondary (piggyback) set-up for the administration of an antibiotic. (Courtesy of Columbia/HCA Portsmouth Regional Hospital, Portsmouth, NH.)

In general, antibiotics should infuse within 1 hour. The line is flagged with the patient's name, the amount and time of medication, date, and the nurse's initials. When assigned to a patient receiving medication, the nurse observes the burette or minibag and reports its level to the medication nurse as appropriate. Continuous infusion pumps are used routinely to monitor flow and to prevent overload (see discussion of parenteral fluids, p. 588).

Although IV medications prevent the child from having to receive painful injections, they are not without discomfort. The initial insertion of the IV line and the limitations of immobilization are frustrating to children. Infiltration can cause damage to delicate tissues. Care is exerted when moving patients in order to avoid this complication.

## Long-Term Venous Access Devices (VAD)

**Heparin Lock.** A heparin lock is a device that keeps open a vein for long-term medicine administration. It allows children to be more ambulatory because they are free of IV tubing. When a patient has a heparin lock in place, repeated "sticks" can be avoided. The apparatus consists of an IV needle attached to a 3¼-inch plastic tube that is plugged by a resealable rubber insert. This rubber top allows the insertion of a needle so that blood can be drawn or medications administered. The original needle remains in place and is periodically flushed with heparin in order to prevent clotting. Parents and older children are taught to maintain the heparin lock at home. The patient is taught to allow only specially trained health professionals to draw blood or give medications in this fashion.

**Hickman, Groshong, and Broviac Catheters.** Hickman, Groshong, and Broviac catheters are tiny, flexible rubber tubes that can be inserted into a vein in the chest to establish a long-term IV site. Medications, chemotherapy, IV fluids, and blood products can be given through the catheter. They can also be utilized for hyperalimentation (see p. 589). The pediatric Broviac catheter is used for children. The line is inserted while the patient is under local or general anesthesia. It remains in the patient from 1 month to 1 year, or longer. The child or parents are taught how to care for the catheter during hospitalization so that they may continue the procedure at home. Some catheters are flushed daily with heparin. Activities of daily living are not curtailed; however, the physician should be contacted about any unusual change in activity, swimming, and the like.

**Implanted Ports.** Infusion ports that can be implanted under the skin are also available (port-A-Cath, MediPort, Infuse-A-Port, Groshong venous port). These small plastic devices are generally implanted under the chest skin beneath the clavicle. A small catheter is threaded from the port into a central vein. The procedure is done under local or general anesthesia. Blood samples can be obtained, and medicines injected by a puncture through the skin into the port. Special needles are provided by the manufacturer. The use of a local or topical anesthetic makes the skin puncture painless. The advantage is that nothing protrudes from the body that can be dislodged, and it is less apparent. This is especially important for the self-conscious young person.

### RECTAL MEDICATIONS

Some drugs, such as sedatives and antiemetics, come in the form of suppositories. Children's suppositories are long and thin in comparison with the cone-shaped types administered to adults. The nurse, wearing a rubber glove or finger cot, inserts the lubriated suppository well beyond the anal sphincter about half as far as the forefinger will reach. The nurse applies pressure to the anus by gently holding the buttocks together until the patient's desire to expel the suppository subsides.

## Principles of Fluid Balance in Children

Infants and small children have different *proportions of body water and body fat* than adults do (Fig. 23-23), and the water needs and water losses of the infant, per unit of body weight, are greater. In children under 2 years of age, *surface area* is particularly important in fluid and electrolyte balance because more water is lost through the skin than through the kidneys. The surface area of the infant is from two to three times greater than that of the adult in proportion to body volume or body weight. *Metabolic rate and heat production* are also two to three times greater in infants per kilogram of body weight. This produces more *waste products*, which must be diluted in order to be excreted. It also stimulates respiration, which causes greater evaporation through the lungs. Compared with adults, a greater percentage of body water in children under age 2 is contained in the *extracellular compartment*.

*Fluid turnover is rapid* and *dehydration* occurs more quickly in infants than in adults (Table 23-9 and Box 23-1). The infant cannot survive as long as the adult in the presence of continued water depletion. A sick infant does not adapt as rapidly to *shifts in I & O* because the *kidneys lack maturity.* They are less able to concentrate urine and require more water than an adult's kidneys in order to excrete a given amount of solute. Disturbances of the gastrointestinal tract frequently lead to vomiting and diarrhea. Electrolyte balance depends on fluid balance and cardiovascular, renal, adrenal, pituitary, parathyroid, and pulmonary regulatory mechanisms. Many of these mechanisms are maturing in the developing child and are unable to react to full capacity under the stress of illness.

### ORAL FLUIDS

Whenever possible, fluids are given by mouth. It is the most natural and satisfactory method. Nurses must use their ingenuity to coax sick children to take enough fluids because they may refuse food and water and do not understand their importance to recovery. Toddlers and infants are not capable of drinking by themselves. The busy nurse must find time to offer fluids and must be patient and gently persistent. Liquids are offered frequently and in small amounts. Brightly colored containers and

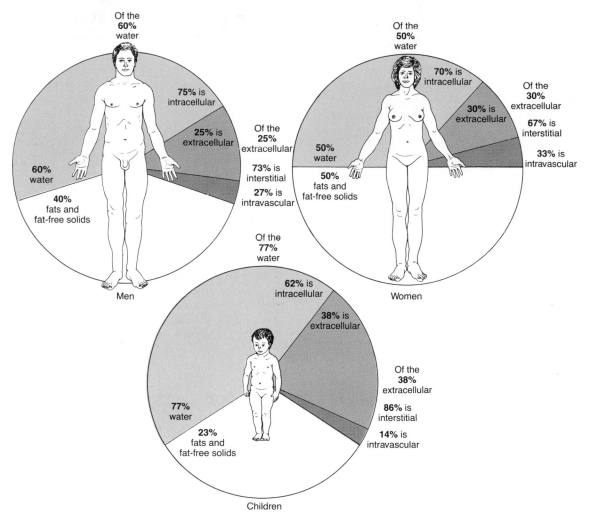

**Figure 23–23.** Relationship of body water and body solids to the body weight of the adult man and woman and the child.

**Table 23–9.** ESTIMATION OF DEHYDRATION

| | Degree | | |
|---|---|---|---|
| **Clinical Sign** | *Mild* | *Moderate* | *Severe* |
| Weight loss (%) | 5 | 10 | 15 |
| Behavior | Normal | Irritable | Hyperirritable to lethargic |
| Thirst | Slight | Moderate | Intense |
| Mucous membrane | May be normal | Dry | Parched |
| Tears | Present | +/− | Absent |
| Anterior fontanel | Flat | +/− | Sunken |
| Skin turgor | Normal | +/− | Increased |

From Graef, J., Cone, T. (1988). *Manual of pediatric therapeutics* (4th ed.). Boston: Little, Brown. With permission.

drinking straws may help. The nurse keeps an accurate record of the patient's I & O. The doctor cannot determine whether a child requires IV fluids with a partially completed chart. *One cannot overemphasize the importance of this particular responsibility on the pediatric unit.*

### PARENTERAL FLUIDS

Parenteral (*para*, "beside or apart from," and *enteron*, "intestine") fluids are those given by some route other than the digestive tract. They are necessary when sickness is accompanied by vomiting or loss of consciousness or when the gastrointestinal system requires rest. Paren-

---

| BOX 23–1 | **Initial Assessment of the Dehydrated Child** |
| --- | --- |

**History**

Urine output, weight change, infectious disease contacts, stool and vomiting frequency

**Clinical Examination**

Urine output, weight, skin turgor, mucous membrane moisture, fontanel fullness, mental state

**Laboratory Studies**

Complete blood count, serum $Na^+$ $K^+$, $Cl^-$, pH, $CO_2$, blood urea nitrogen, creatinine, osmolality, glucose, calcium

**Urinalysis**

Specific gravity, pH, glucose, ketones, amino acids, appropriate cultures
Water and electrolyte losses moderate to severe—see Table 23–9

Data from Graef, J., & Cone, T. (1985). *Manual of pediatric therapeutics* (3rd ed.). Boston: Little, Brown.

---

teral fluids are needed in severe cases of vomiting and diarrhea in which the loss of excessive water and electrolytes will lead to death if untreated. It also provides a means for the safe and effective administration of selective parenteral medications. Solutions given parenterally must be sterile in order to prevent a general or local infection. The nurse must be aware of the importance of parenteral therapy and the problems that might arise.

The infant or child receiving parenteral fluids needs the nurse's warmth and affection. Babies miss being held and are also deprived of the pleasures they receive from sucking. The doctor may recommend that a pacifier be used, if it is not contraindicated. Older children need suitable diversions and company.

**Fluids Given by Vein.** IV infusion presents certain problems in pediatric patients (Table 23–10). The procedure is more complicated and dangerous in infants and small children and is more taxing psychologically. The infant's veins are small and hard to locate. Often the veins of the scalp are used, which entails shaving the head. The baby must be effectively restrained

in order to prevent the needle from becoming dislodged. When fluids are given intravenously, regardless of the site, the infant must be *closely observed*. Fluids given by vein are passing into a closed space that can be distended only to a certain point without serious difficulties resulting. If the circulation becomes overloaded with fluid that is infused too rapidly, cardiac failure can result. The flow of a solution can become disturbed when an infant cries or wiggles. The nurse observes the child for

1. increase in the rate of flow of a solution
2. swelling at the needle site
3. slowing down or stopping of the drip
4. low volume in the bag or Soluset
5. pain or redness at the site of insertion
6. moisture at or around the site

A special hourly chart is kept for infants who are being given IV fluids (Fig. 23–24). The nurse charts such information as time, name and amount of the solution, amount absorbed, number of drops per minute, and amount of fluid remaining in the bottle.

Modern adapting devices are used to improve the accuracy and safety of IV fluids. In the past, it was difficult to slow down an IV infusion to 4–6 drops/min without stopping the flow completely. The "mini" or "micro" drop decreases the size of the drop and allows the patient to receive 50–60 "mini" or "micro" drops/milliliter rather than the usual 15 drops from the standard set-up. Another device uses a graduated control chamber (burette), which is attached to the IV bag in order to ensure that the child does not receive too much fluid too fast (Fig. 23–25). If the rate of the IV increases, only the amount in the drip chamber, and not the entire amount of the bag, would be infused. Parenteral fluid regulators such as the IVAC pump are used routinely to monitor infusions in children. An alarm sounds when difficulties arise. Such safeguards, nevertheless, do not replace close observation and charting by the nurse.

## TOTAL PARENTERAL NUTRITION

IV alimentation solutions are complex combinations of crystalline amino acids, dextrose, vitamins, and electrolytes. Conditions other than low birth weight that may require its use include severe burns, chronic intestinal obstruction, intractable diarrhea, irradiation, and other life-threatening maladies. Although the

**Table 23–10.** NURSING GUIDELINES FOR PEDIATRIC IVs AT VARIOUS STAGES OF CHILD'S DEVELOPMENT

| Developmental Characteristics* | IV Placement (Ideal Sites) | Preparation of Child | Family Involvement |
|---|---|---|---|
| **Infant (1st Year)** Dependent on others for all needs. Needs to feel physically safe through close relationship with one caretaking person (usually the mother). Trust develops through needs being met consistently. Mistrust and anxiety develop when needs are met inconsistently. Stranger anxiety begins at approximately 6–8 mo | Scalp vein (best site); foot, hand, forearm | Best not to feed infant immediately before IV insertion (vomiting and aspiration possible) | Prepare family about need for IV therapy, insertion procedure, appearance of infant with IV, and fluid needs. Encourage family to continue providing baby with tactile and verbal stimulation, and tender, loving care. Demonstrate safe ways to hold an infant with an IV. Encourage questions and clarify misconceptions |
| **Toddler (Ages 1–3)** Discovers and explores self and surrounding world. Enjoys new mobility skills. Develops egocentric thinking and need for parallel play. Tolerates short separations from mother. Transitional objects (security blanket, special toy) provide some comfort. Oppositional syndrome ("no" stage). Separation anxiety an important problem in hospitalized toddlers separated from mother, ages 8–24 mo | Hand, arm, foot. Important: From this age group on, the less dominant extremity should be used for the IV whenever possible. Determine handedness prior to IV insertion | Prepare child immediately before procedure (child has limited attention span and is likely to become more anxious if prepared sooner). Give very simple explanation in concrete terms. Show equipment to be used. Do not offer choice. See preparation for preschool age (below) and assess ability of each child to understand | Prepare family as to need for IV therapy, insertion procedure, and appearance of child with IV. Whether parents remain with the child during the procedure varies. If they stay with the child their role is to comfort rather than to assist with restraining. Demonstrate to parents how to safely handle child with IV |
| **Preschool (Ages 4–6)** Magical thinking, based on what the child would like to believe. Cannot always distinguish fantasy from reality. Fears intrusive procedures. Castration fears common. Develops conscience (guilt), while asserting independence and mastering new skills. Learning to share | Hand, forearm (less dominant) | Prepare child just prior to procedure. Using small bottle, tubing, and doll or stuffed animal, explain in literal terms the need for IV and insertion procedure. Allow child to see and touch equipment. Explain how child can help with procedure by cleaning site, opening packages, taping, and so on. Allow some degree of control in the situation. Say you will help child hold still and that it is O.K. to cry | As with toddlers, parents may or may not stay with the child during the procedure. If they stay, they should provide comfort and support, but they should not be asked to restrain the child for IV insertion. Reinforce child's need for honest, simple explanations. Reassure parents that child can still play and be active, even with IV |

**Table 23–10.** NURSING GUIDELINES FOR PEDIATRIC IVs AT VARIOUS STAGES OF CHILD'S DEVELOPMENT (*Continued*)

| Related Nursing Actions | Protection of IV Site | Mobility Considerations† | Safety Needs |
|---|---|---|---|
| Restrain during insertion. Comfort and cuddle during and after insertion. Observe carefully during insertion for problems of vomiting, aspiration, and so on. Firmly restrain extremity with IV (see next column). Use of pacifier diminishes stress, especially for infants given nothing by mouth (NPO) | IV may be secured with tape and is wrapped. Extremity may be restrained by using a small arm board, a sandbag, or wrist and ankle restraints | Keep restraints as loose as possible to allow for motion. Release any restrained extremities hourly for range of motion (ROM). Mitten hands with cotton and stockinette to prohibit infant's grasping IV. Restraining all extremities is *rarely* necessary. Remember infant's need for sensory stimulation | Maintain strict intake and output (I & O). Secure IV tubing out of range of kicking legs and flailing arms. Check restraints frequently for effectiveness and presence of adequate circulation |
| Restraining the toddler for an IV usually requires more than one person. Reassure child through verbal and tactile stimulation during procedure. Provide toys such as pegs to hammer, for therapeutic expression of anger, after procedure and throughout hospitalization | See that for infant (above). A securely anchored IV is essential for the normally active toddler. Even the best site protection will not remain effective unless it is coupled with close nursing supervision and distracting activities for the child | Toddlers cope with the world and learn about it through action. Therefore, minimum restraints should be used, and tying the child in bed is to be avoided. Parental presence during waking hours permits the child to be constantly supervised and makes restraints unnecessary in many cases. However, be careful to avoid setting up a situation in which the child associates parent's departure with punishment by restraint | Child is unaware of danger at this age; will not know that movement of IV causes pain. Constant supervision needed when out of bed. Remind frequently not to touch IV, but do not expect compliance. Distracting activities accomplish much more than does a scolding for handling the IV. Tape connections on tubing if child continues to handle tubing. Keep tubing clamps out of reach |
| Tell child IV is not being given as punishment. *Never* bribe or threaten with IVs (e.g., "Drink, or you'll get another IV.") Praise for cooperation or any efforts in that direction. Maintain patient privacy. Do not start an IV in view of other patients, visitors, or staff. Child needs support to cope with intrusiveness of this procedure. Show understanding | See that for infant (above). As with toddlers, securely anchored IVs are essential, but inadequate unless coupled with close supervision and age-appropriate activities | Preschoolers need maximum mobility to master surroundings. Provide a range of out-of-bed activities whenever possible | Child will be curious about IV. Is capable of understanding instructions to not touch it but needs frequent reminders. IV clamps should be out of reach or taped over. Constant supervision needed when out of bed. Child is liable to take off down the hall, heedless of pole, bottle, and so on. Short attention span limits duration of cooperation with instructions |

*Continued*

**Table 23–10.** NURSING GUIDELINES FOR PEDIATRIC IVs AT VARIOUS STAGES OF CHILD'S DEVELOPMENT *Continued*

| Developmental Characteristics* | IV Placement (Ideal Sites) | Preparation of Child | Family Involvement |
|---|---|---|---|
| **School Age (Ages 7–11))** Struggles between mastery of new skills and failure. Enjoys school, learning skills, games with rules. Needs to succeed. Fears body mutilation. May feel need to be brave. Can understand hospital rules. World now expanding beyond family. Peer group becomes important. Competitiveness | Hand, forearm (less dominant) | Prepare child ahead of time but on same day of insertion. Carefully explain and demonstrate equipment and reasons for IV therapy, letting patient watch you or help set up equipment. Ask child for questions about need for IV and procedure. Give child choices and let child help in procedure whenever possible. Tell child crying is O.K. because needles hurt, and you will help in holding still | Whenever possible, family and child should be prepared together so that family can reinforce what the child has been told. Stress to family the child's need for some independence in activities of daily living, even with an IV. Parental presence or participation in IV insertion may be appropriate, but child's preference should be considered primary |
| **Adolescent (Ages 12–18)** Vacillates between needs for independence and dependence. Adult cognitive abilities, deductive reasoning. Coping mechanisms: rationalization, intellectualization. Peer acceptance very important. Egocentric, rebellious at times, especially against parents and authority figures. Very concerned with body image, body changes, sexuality, and role. Searching for "who I am" | Hand, forearm (less dominant) | Prepare patient several hours to a day before procedure, if possible. Needs time between preparation and insertion to absorb explanations and ask questions. For most adolescents, approach discussions on an adult level. Explain need for IV therapy and expected duration, and show equipment. May need much support for acceptance of therapy | Explain therapy needs and duration as with patient. Decision regarding parental presence during procedure should be patient's, not parents'. Stress to family participation in decisions affecting child's care |

beginning student would not be given total responsibility for the child receiving total parenteral nutrition (TPN), all nursing personnel must be alert to the fact that this is not just the usual superficial vein infusion.

A Silastic catheter is passed directly into the superior vena cava by way of the jugular or subclavian vein, using careful surgical technique (Fig. 23–26). It is secured in place. A Millipore filter is attached to filter out bacteria and minimize contamination. An IV pump monitors the flow. The patient receiving TPN requires careful supervision and evaluation. Complications of this therapy can be serious and are related to both the catheter and the metabolism of the infusate. Contamination via catheter or solution is particularly dangerous because infectious organisms have direct access to body circulation. Thrombosis, dislodgment of the catheter, and

*extravasation* (the escape of fluid into surrounding tissue) can occur. Metabolic complications include hyperglycemia due to the high glucose content of the solution, osmotic diuresis, dehydration, and *azotemia* (the presence of nitogenous bodies in the blood). Laboratory assessments include complete blood count, blood urea nitrogen (BUN), glucose, and electrolytes. Home hyperalimentation (TPN) is now being successfully utilized for selected children. This requires specific instruction and demonstrations by specialty teams. Continuous support and supervision are vital to success. The parents' insurance policy must be investigated, because home hyperalimentation is costly.

Peripheral vein hyperalimentation is used for short-term therapy or as a supplement to IV alimentation. More diluted solutions are used. Infiltration is to be avoided, as severe tissue

**Table 23–10.** NURSING GUIDELINES FOR PEDIATRIC IVs AT VARIOUS STAGES OF CHILD'S DEVELOPMENT *Continued*

| Related Nursing Actions | Protection of IV Site | Mobility Considerations† | Safety Needs |
|---|---|---|---|
| Approach child expecting cooperation (this age group likes to please adults), but expect that child will need help holding still. Allow the child to clean the site with alcohol swab and to cut tape prior to insertion. Praise cooperative efforts. Give child step-by-step explanation of procedure as it progresses. Child may like to take some responsibility in keeping I & O | Will need less protection than younger children owing to interest in making IV work correctly. May naturally protect extremity with IV. Some children appreciate a warning sign—"Hands Off," on a piece of tape over the IV as a reminder. Utilize the child's natural curiosity and interest in learning. Tell child the rules of safe IV handling | Show patient and family how to safely manipulate IV for out-of-bed activities (walking in hall with pole, keeping tubing out of wheelchair wheels, and so on) | Remind patient periodically about necessary caution with IV. Show patient the clamps, and caution against handling them. Teach patient signs of IV problems. Enlist child's help in the interest of good compliance, but do not entirely depend on it. Tape tubing connections. Child may forget about IV. Emphasize need for caution in some activities, especially if play includes other children |
| Be aware of IV adding to patient's dependency status and need for some control. Encourage child to keep own I & O, help in counting drip rate, and so on | See that for school age (above). If patient is very active, will need well-protected, well-anchored IV, as movements may be more forceful and strength greater than those of younger patients | See that for school age (above). Encourage mobility as much as possible as a means of independence for the adolescent | Be aware of possibility of adolescent rebellion showing itself in lack of cooperation with therapy. These patients may rebel if feeling threatened, and may be very manipulative in testing behaviors. Consistent limits, clearly communicated to patient, parents, and staff, are needed. Instruct patient as to signs of infiltration, phlebitis, and so on |

Modified from Guhlow, L.J., & Kolb, J. (1979). Pediatric IVs: Special measures you should take. *RN*, 42, 40. Published in RN, the full-service nursing journal. Copyright © 1979 Medical Economics Company Inc, Oradell, NJ. Reprinted by permission.
*Each stage builds on the earlier ones, and during hospitalization many children regress to behaviors appropriate to earlier levels of development.
†No child should be restricted to bed simply because of having an IV!
IV refers to intravenous line, throughout table.

sloughing due to dextrose irritation may occur. Because hyperalimentation provides no fatty acids, solutions such as an Intralipid 10% may be ordered; this is administered via a peripheral line. Serum lipid concentrations are carefully monitored in these patients.

# Adaptation of Selected Procedures to Children

## NUTRITION, DIGESTION, AND ELIMINATION

**Gastrostomy.** A gastrostomy (*gastro*, "stomach," and *stoma*, "opening") is made for the pur-

pose of introducing food directly into the stomach through the abdominal wall. This is done by means of a surgically placed tube or button. It is used in patients who cannot have food by mouth because of anomalies or corrosive strictures of the esophagus or who are severely debilitated or in coma. Cleansing of the skin around the tube will prevent irritation from formula or gastric secretions. The nurse observes and reports vomiting or abdominal distention. Brown or green drainage may indicate that the tube has slipped through the pylorus into the duodenum. This could cause an obstruction and is reported immediately. Children who are on long-term feedings may have gastrostomy buttons im-

## Nursing Brief

One way of determining fluid loss in infants is to weigh the dry diaper, mark the weight on the outside of the diaper, and then weigh the wet diaper. This includes both urine and liquid stools (1 gm = 1 ml of output).

PEDIATRIC I.V. FLUID SHEET

DATE: Feb. 14, 1989

| TIME | SOLUTION | RATE cc/hr | AMT. IN BURETTE | AMT. ADDED BURETTE | TOTAL BURETTE | AMT. BOTTLE | AMT. ABS. | MED. | CUMU-LATIVE TOTAL | REMARKS | INITIAL |
|---|---|---|---|---|---|---|---|---|---|---|---|
| 0001 | 1000cc D5+⅛NS | 40 | — | 60 | 60 | 940 | — | ✓ | — | 250mg ampicillin added to burette | jnc |
| 0100 | | | 20 | 40 | 60 | 900 | 40 | | 40 | no redness or swelling at I.V. site | jnc |
| 0200 | | ↓ | 20 | 40 | 60 | 860 | 40 | | 80 | | jnc |
| 0300 | | 50 | 20 | 60 | 80 | 800 | 40 | | 120 | Rate changed to 50cc/hr. | jnc |
| 0400 | | | 30 | 50 | 80 | 750 | 50 | | 170 | | jnc |
| 0500 | | | 30 | 50 | 80 | 700 | 50 | | 220 | Sleeping | jnc |
| 0600 | | | 30 | 50 | 80 | 650 | 50 | ✓ | 270 | 250mg ampicillin add@ burette | jnc |
| 0700 | ↓ | ↓ | 30 | 50 | 80 | 600 | 50 | | 320 | →8 hr. Total | jnc |
| 0800 | D5½N.S. | 50 | 30 | 50 | 80 | 550 | 50 | | 50 | no redness or swelling @ site | PJW |
| 0900 | | 50 | 30 | 50 | 80 | 500 | 50 | | 100 | awake + alert | PJW |
| 1000 | | 50 | 30 | 50 | 80 | 450 | 50 | | 150 | | PJW |
| 1100 | | 50 | 30 | 50 | 80 | 400 | 50 | | 200 | | PJW |
| 1200 | | 30 | 30 | 20 | 50 | 380 | 50 | ✓ | 250 | Ampicillin 250mg Rate changed to 30 | PJW |
| 1300 | | 30 | 20 | 30 | 50 | 350 | 30 | | 280 | Dr. in for exam | PJW |
| 1400 | | 30 | 20 | 30 | 50 | 320 | 30 | | 310 | napping | PJW |
| 1500 | ↓ | 30 | 20 | 30 | 50 | 290 | 30 | | 340 | 8° Total | PJW |
| 1600 | D5½N.S. | 30 | 20 | 30 | 50 | 260 | 30 | | 30 | no redness or swelling @ I.V. site | E.T. |
| 1700 | | | 20 | 30 | 50 | 230 | 30 | | 60 | family visiting | E.T. |
| 1800 | | | 20 | 30 | 50 | 200 | 30 | ✓ | 90 | ampicillin 250mg added to burette | E.T. |
| 1900 | | | 20 | 30 | 50 | 170 | 30 | | 120 | | E.T. |
| 2000 | | | 20 | 30 | 50 | 140 | 30 | | 150 | | E.T. |
| 2100 | | | 20 | 30 | 50 | 110 | 30 | | 180 | Sleeping | E.T. |
| 2200 | ↓ | | 20 | 30 | 50 | 80 | 30 | | 210 | | E.T. |
| 2300 | 1000cc D5½N.S | | 20 | 30 | 50 | 970 | 30 | | 240 | 80cc discarded I.V. tubing changed | MEB |
| 2400 | ↓ | ↓ | 20 | 30 | 50 | 940 | 30 | | 270 | 8°Total | E.T. |

TOTAL AT 2400: 930cc          ADDRESSOGRAPH

**Figure 23–24.** Pediatric IV fluid sheet.

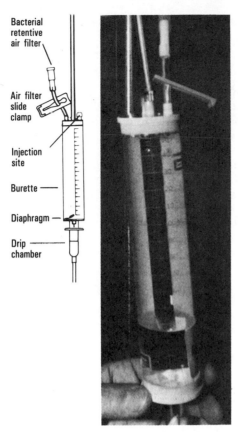

Bacterial
retentive
air filter

Air filter
slide
clamp

Injection
site

Burette

Diaphragm

Drip
chamber

**Figure 23-25.** The graduated control chamber delivers "micro" drops, making it easier to calculate the rate and amount of fluids absorbed. (Photograph from Betz, C., Hunsberger, M., & Wright, S. [1994]. *Family-centered nursing care of children* [2nd ed]. Philadelphia: W. B. Saunders; drawing modified with permission of Abbott Laboratories.)

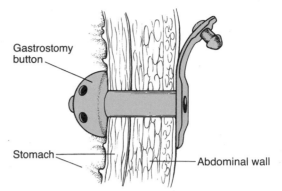

Gastrostomy
button

Stomach

Abdominal wall

**Figure 23-27.** The gastrostomy button allows feedings to be administered directly into the stomach through the abdominal wall.

planted (Fig. 23-27). Refer to the Procedure for Gastrostomy Tube Feeding.

**Enema.** Administering an enema to a child is essentially the same as for adults; however, the type, amount, and the distance for inserting the tube require modifications. In addition, a child's bowel is more easily perforated under pressure (Betz, 1994). An isotonic solution is used in children. Tap water enemas are contraindicated. Plain water is hypotonic to the blood and could cause rapid fluid shift and overload if absorbed through the intestinal wall. The type of solution intended is always ascertained. Commercial enemas specific for the child are commonly used. The amount of fluids varies somewhat in procedure recommendations. The smaller the pa-

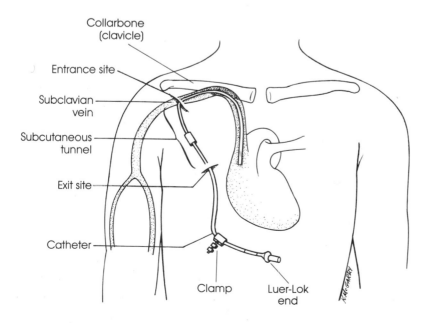

Collarbone
(clavicle)

Entrance site

Subclavian
vein

Subcutaneous
tunnel

Exit site

Catheter

Clamp

Luer-Lok
end

**Figure 23-26.** Catheter placement for total parenteral nutrition.

## PROCEDURE FOR GASTROSTOMY TUBE FEEDING

### Equipment

Tray
Warmed formula
Funnel or syringe barrel
Syringe for aspiration
15–30 ml of water to flush tube as ordered
*Note*: Equipment should be sterile for preterm and newborn infants.

### Method

1. Position child comfortably either flat or with head slightly elevated if not contraindicated. Provide pacifier in order to relax baby.
2. Check residual stomach contents by attaching syringe to gastrostomy tube and aspirating. If amount of residual is large (10–25 ml for newborns, over 50 ml for older children), replace residual and decrease present formula by equal amount or delay feeding for a short time. (This may vary according to the pediatrician's protocol.) Overloading the stomach can cause reflux and increases the danger of aspiration. If residual continues or increases, report this to the physician.
3. Attach syringe barrel (if not already present for continuous elevation) to gastrostomy tube. Fill with formula. Remove clamp. This prevents air from entering the stomach and causing distention.)
4. Elevate receptacle. Allow formula to flow slowly by gravity—force should not be used.
5. Continue to add formula to the syringe before it empties completely.
6. Clamp the tube as the final formula or water is passing through the lower part of the syringe. (*Note*: In infants, some physicians may prefer that the gastrostomy tube remain open at all times in order to produce a safety valve in the event that the baby vomits. In such cases, the tube is elevated above the patient's body.)
7. Whenever possible, hold the patient quietly after feeding. Reposition in the Fowler position or on right side to promote gastric emptying.
8. Record the type (gastrostomy feeding), the amount given, the amount and characteristics of residual, and how the patient tolerated the procedure. If the patient is on measured fluids, record this on the input and output section.

## PROCEDURE FOR ADMINISTERING AN ENEMA

### Equipment

Disposable irrigation bag with connecting tube and clamp. For smaller amounts, funnel or Asepto syringe and pitcher
Gloves
10–12-French catheter
Saline solution (1 teaspoon of salt to 1 pint of water)
Lubricant
Toilet paper
Waterproof sheet
Incontinent pad
Bedpan with cover
Extra diapers for infants

### Method

1. Assemble the equipment and take it to the bedside.
2. Place the waterproof sheet and incontinent pad beneath the child.
3. Pad the bedpan with a diaper. Place the child's pillow under the head and back.
4. Place the child on the bedpan. Restrain the legs by a diaper brought under the bedpan and pinned over the legs. Older children are positioned in the same manner as adults.
5. Allow the solution to run through the tubing to warm it and expel air.
6. Lubricate and insert the tube 1–4 inches into the rectum, depending on the age and size of the patient (1 inch for infants, gradually increasing to 4 inches for 11-year-olds).
7. Administer the prescribed amount. The temperature of the solution should range from 37.8–40.6°C (100–105°F).
8. Hold the irrigating bag not more than 18 inches above the level of the patient's hips. The solution should run slowly without pressure. Clamp the tubing at intervals and if the child experiences intestinal cramping.
9. Remain with the patient while the enema is being expelled. Small children may use the pot chair.
10. Remove the bedpan and pillow. Cleanse the buttocks.
11. Remove the waterproof sheet and incontinent pad.
12. Apply a clean diaper. Check to see if a stool specimen is desired.
13. Chart the following: time of procedure; name, amount, and temperature of solution

**Aftercare of Equipment**

Empty and cleanse the bedpan.

Discard disposable enema setup, tubing, and gloves.

**Oil-Retention Enema**

When giving an oil-retention enema, use prescribed amount, generally 60–100 ml of oil at 37.8°C (100°F). Apply gentle pressure over the anal area in order to prevent the oil from being expelled. A cleansing enema (saline) generally follows in ½–¾ hr.

---

tient, the less solution is used. The exact amount for infants should be prescribed by physician order. Guidelines range from a low of 50 ml for infants to a high of 500–750 ml for the adolescent. The nurse consults the procedure manual for the institution's guidelines. The tube is inserted from 1 to 4 inches, according to the size and age of the child. Infants and small children may be unable to retain the solution; therefore, it may be necessary to hold the buttocks together for a short time.

This is an invasive procedure for the patient; therefore, careful age-appropriate explanations are necessary. Other invasive procedures related to the gastrointestinal tract include barium enema, intestinal biopsy, endoscopy, and colonoscopy. These are performed by the gastroenterologist. Children must be allowed to express all concerns about these tests, and the nurse gives feedback to physicians about the difference in behavior between children who were well prepared and those who were not prepared. Refer to the Procedure for Administering an Enema.

## RESPIRATION

**Tracheostomy Care.** A tracheostomy is a surgical procedure in which an opening is made in the trachea to enable the patient to breathe. This artificial airway may be necessary in emergency situations, may be an elective procedure, or may be combined with mechanical ventilation. Some of the childhood conditions that may require tracheostomy are acute laryngotracheobronchitis, epiglottitis, head injury, burns, and any condition in which the patient is unconscious or debilitated for an extended period. Nursing care is indispensable to the survival of the patient, as blockage of the tube by mucus or other secretions can lead to suffoca-

tion. In many hospitals, the patient is placed in the ICU immediately following surgery, because this is a critical period requiring frequent suctioning and close observation. The patient is placed on heart and respiratory monitors. When the child's condition stabilizes, the patient is transferred to another unit.

The child is placed in an area of high visibility. This is important because small children communicate their needs by crying and the tracheostomy prohibits vocalization. Whenever possible, one person is assigned to the child and to work with the parents. The nurse reinforces preoperative teaching and explains what happened: for example, "You were having a lot of trouble breathing. This operation is called a tracheostomy and helps you to breathe easier. A small opening has been made in your neck. A hollow tube was inserted to keep the area open. It is frightening not to be able to speak. When you are better, the hole will close by itself and your voice will return." An explanation of suction might be, "We have to keep the area in your neck open. This tube goes into the throat and clears it." Use of suction can be shown in a glass of water. The child is prepared for the unfamiliar sound. "You might feel like gagging, but afterward you will feel better. I know this is difficult for you and I'm sorry there is no easier way." Another approach is to make up a story involving a favorite toy, which goes to the repair shop because the toy is having trouble breathing.

The nursing care of the child with a tracheostomy is a significant responsibility. The anatomic differences between children and adults and the small child's inability to communicate through writing increase the need for close observation. In addition toddlers often have short, stubby necks that become easily irritated. It may be helpful to place a reminder on the intercom at the clerk's desk or in other suitable areas, indicating that this patient cannot cry or speak. The nurse's touch and quiet voice and the presence of significant others help make the child feel secure. The nurse gives the parents permission to leave the child on occasion. The nurse also helps them prepare the patient for their departure in such a way as to promote trust. Familiar routines are incorporated by repeating effective stories. A favorite article, such as a blanket or toy, is kept nearby. A supply of teaching aids and dramatic play material is made available. Puppets are particularly valuable.

Room temperature should be comfortably warm. Moisture and humidity are added by a mist tent (Fig. 23–28), a special tracheostomy collar, or direct attachment to a mechanical ventilator. This is necessary because the nose and mouth no longer warm and moisten the inspired air. Adequate fluids are provided.

*Tracheostomy Tube.* Maintaining *patency* of the tracheostomy tube is of utmost importance. Plastic or Silastic tubes are generally used because they are flexible and reduce crust formation. They are lightweight and disposable, and most do not have inner cannulas. Cuffed tubes are not usually necessary in infants and small children, as their air passages are smaller and the tracheostomy tube provides a sufficient seal. The surgeon chooses a tracheostomy tube that is appropriate for the patient's neck size and condition. Administering oxygen by manual resuscitator (bagging) prior to or following the procedure helps prevent hypoxia.

*Suctioning.* Selection of a suction catheter is of importance. The nurse chooses one that does not block the tube during suctioning. The diameter should be about one-half the size of the tracheostomy tube. Hands are washed before proceeding. The nurse uses sterile gloves for the procedure, and all equipment used in the care of a tracheostomy should be sterile. Suction is applied as the catheter is withdrawn. The tube is rotated to allow removal of secretions on all sides. With Y-tube technique, suction is achieved by closing the port with the thumb. A drop of saline may be inserted before suctioning to aid in loosening secretions (this is subject to controversy). Ackerman suggests it induces violent coughing and may not actually aid in the removal of secretions (Ackerman, 1985). Because variations in this procedure exist and modifi-cations are frequently required, one must understand what is intended for the particular patient. The nurse asks for clarification and specific procedures of the institution where emloyed.

Suctioning is done periodically and when necessary. Indications for suctioning include noisy breathing, bubbling of mucus, and moist cough or respirations. During suctioning, patients can rapidly become hypoxic. Suctioning is limited to approximately 15 seconds. To judge timing, some nurses hold their own breath. Two or three breaths for reoxygenation are allowed between suctioning. The depth of suctioning is important. In general, suctioning is limited to the length of the tracheostomy tube or slightly beyond to stimulate coughing. The catheter is cleared with sterile water between insertions. Unnecessary suctioning is avoided. The suction catheter is discarded after use. Disposing of water after suctioning prevents the growth of *Pseudomonas*.

*Tracheal Stoma.* The tracheal stoma is treated as a surgical wound. The area is kept free of secretions and exudate in order to minimize the risk of infection. Cotton-tipped applicators dipped in half-strength hydrogen peroxide can be utilized to remove crusted mucus. Tapes around the child's neck should be loose enough to allow one finger to be easily inserted. The knot is placed

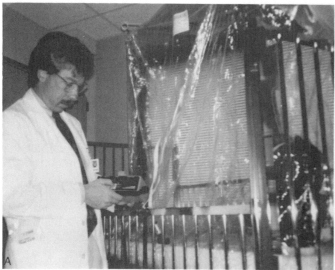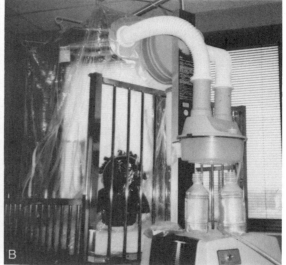

**Figure 23–28.** *A*, The respiratory therapist measures the oxygen concentration in the tent by an oxygen analyzer. *B*, The working unit of the mist tent. (Courtesy of Columbia/HCA Portsmouth Regional Hospital, Portsmouth, NH.)

to the side of the neck. The condition of the skin beneath the tape is assessed. The tape is changed as necessary. Two people are used for this procedure, one to hold the outer cannula and the other to change the tape. When feeding the infant, the nurse covers the tracheostomy with a bib or moist piece of gauze in order to prevent aspiration of food particles.

*Observing for Complications.* The nurse observes the patient for such symptoms as restlessness, rising pulse rate, fatigue, apathy, dyspnea, sternal retractions, pallor, cyanosis, and inflammation or drainage around the incision. Possible complications include tracheoesophageal fistula, stenosis, tracheal ischemia, infection, atelectasis, cannula occlusion, and accidental extubation. Baseline assessment of the patient is done on each shift and prior to suctioning. The patient's mental status, respirations, pulse rate and rhythm, and chest sounds are of particular importance. Accurate recording of observations is essential to evaluation. The time and frequency of suctioning, the character of secretions, the relief afforded the patient, the behavior, the appearance of the wound, and other pertinent data are recorded.

A sterile hemostat is kept at the bedside for emergency use. Accidental *extubation*, or expulsion of the tube, although uncommon, can occur from severe coughing if the tapes are too loose. Patency of the airway is maintained by spreading the edges of the wound with the sterile clamp until a duplicate tube is inserted. An extra tracheostomy tube and the equipment needed for its replacement are always kept in a visible, easily reached area at the bedside for use in such emergencies.

As the child's condition improves, he or she is weaned from the tube. The opening gradually closes by granulation. Children whose tubes must remain in place for a longer time require periodic tube changes.

*Additional Nursing Measures.* Additional nursing measures include frequent change of position, use of arm restraints, oral feedings unless contraindicated, and careful bathing to prevent water from entering the tube. Range-of-motion exercises are a must for long-term patients, and in acute cases arm restraints are removed one at a time in order to allow for passive exercises. The diet is ordered by the physician. Although patients may initially have nothing by mouth, as the condition improves they progress to a soft or normal diet. The Fowler position is preferred during feedings. The older child can cooperate by holding the head flexed with chin down. This decreases swallowing difficulties, as the esophagus opens and the airway narrows.

*Discharge.* Certain patients are discharged with a tracheostomy (Fig. 23–29). This is anticipated, and instruction and demonstration for the parents is begun early. Parents who are comfortable with the procedure during hospitalization will feel more secure when the child returns home. It is advisable that the parents spend one night with the child before discharge. Information about parent groups and visiting nurse and other referrals are made prior to discharge.

**Oxygen Therapy.** Table 23–11 covers selected considerations for the child receiving oxygen.

*Safety Considerations.* All equipment used for oxygen therapy must be inspected periodically in order to determine that materials are intact and that no pieces are missing. Combustible materials and potential sources of fire are kept away from oxygen equipment. These materials

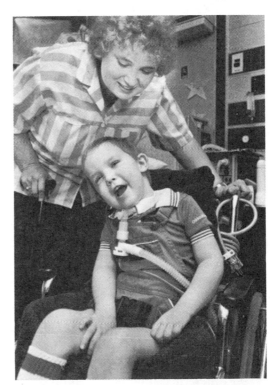

**Figure 23–29.** Tracheostomy. The acuity level of discharged patients is more intense today and necessitates education and support of family members in all aspect of care. This child is being discharged with a tracheostomy in place. (Courtesy of Blank Memorial Hospital for Children, Des Moines, IA.)

**Table 23–11.** SELECTED CONSIDERATIONS FOR THE CHILD RECEIVING OXYGEN

| Age | Comment |
| --- | --- |
| | *General Considerations:* Signs of respiratory distress include an increase in pulse and respiration, restlessness, flaring nares, intercostal and substernal retractions, and cyanosis. In addition, children with dyspnea frequently vomit, which increases the danger of aspiration. Maintain a clear airway by suctioning if needed. Organize nursing care so that interruptions are kept at a minimum. Observe children carefully, as your vision may be obstructed by mist, and young children are unable to verbalize their needs |
| Newborn | Oxygen may be provided via hood, which may be used in warming unit |
| | Oxygen may be provided via Isolette; keep sleeves closed to decrease oxygen loss |
| | Oxygen needs to be warmed in order to prevent neonatal stress from cold |
| | Analyze concentration carefully in order to avoid retrolental fibroplasia or pulmonary disease |
| | Parents are primary focus of preparations; help to develop good parenting skills, self-confidence in their ability to care for the child who is ill |
| Infant | Nose may need to be suctioned by bulb syringe in order to remove mucus |
| | Child may benefit from use of infant seat; secure seat to bed frame, watch for slumping in seat |
| | *Make sure crib sides are up; a canopy often gives the illusion of safety* |
| | Avoid the use of baby oil, A and D ointment, petroleum jelly (Vaseline) or other oil- or alcohol-based substances |
| | Anticipate stranger anxiety at around 6–8 mo; baby clings to parents, turns away from nurse |
| | An extremely irritable baby may benefit from comforting in parent's lap followed by sleeping in tent; clarify at report time |
| | Frequently, children can be removed from oxygen for bathing and eating; determine before proceeding |
| Toddler | Anticipate that a toddler will be distressed by a tent |
| | Anticipate regression |
| | When child is restless and fussy, she may pull tent and covers apart |
| | Toddler cannot tell nurse if tent is "too hot" or "too cold" |
| | Change clothing and bed linen when damp |
| | Child may be comforted by transitional object such as blanket |
| | Parents may have suggestions as to how to keep child happy in tent |
| Preschool | Tent plastic distorts view |
| | Because thought processes are immature in preschool children, reality and fantasy are inseparable |
| | Prepare child for all procedures in order to decrease fear |
| | Anticipate that child will feel lonely and isolated |
| | Child will enjoy stories, puppets, dramatic play |
| | If extremely restless and anxious, child may benefit from holding parent's hand through small opening in zippers |
| | Helpful if child can be out of tent for meals |
| School Age | School children usually are less frightened by tent; fears center around body mutilation and loss of control |
| | Preparation information continues to focus on what the child will see, hear, feel, and be expected to do |
| | Child may benefit from writing a story about the experience; nurse reviews story with child and clarifies misconceptions; posting story on unit affirms child's self-esteem and mastery (always ask permission to post) |
| | Allow child to make realistic choices before, during, and after procedures |
| | Draw "what it feels like to be in a tent" and discuss |
| Adolescent | Adolescent needs more time to process information, needs to know the results of blood studies and other tests |
| | Nurse remains available to the patient to answer questions as they arise |
| | Trust is extremely important as adolescent attempts to move beyond the nuclear family |
| | Anticipate problems of being restricted by apparatus |
| | May feel weird when visited by peers; wavers between feeling self-confident and feeling ineffective |
| | Reiterate no smoking and other safety precautions with patient and peers |
| | Include patient in therapy, may be able to manage own oxygen needs |
| | Review safe use of oxygen in the home if required for comfort and survival |

are essentially the same as for adults; for the child, however, friction toys are also to be avoided. Nylon or wool blankets are not to be used. One should know where the nearest fire extinguisher is located. Parents are alerted to the presence of "no smoking" signs.

Infection control is extremely important. It is imperative that cross-infection via unclean equipment be prevented. Humidifiers and nebulizers, which are warm and moist, serve as an excellent medium for the growth of disease-producing organisms. Although most masks, tents,

## PROCEDURE FOR ADMINISTERING OXYGEN BY TENT

### Equipment

Control cabinet
Plastic canopy
Distilled water
Oxygen flowmeter and tubing
Two bath blankets or extra sheet

### Method

1. Prepare bed and place bath blanket, rubber sheet, or absorbent pad over the mattress.
2. Select the tent according to the age and size of the patient. This information needs to be ascertained prior to admission for patients in acute respiratory distress.
3. Bring the canopy and control unit to the bedside and extend the overhead bar, and fold tent out along the bar.
4. Plug in control cabinet and turn on the unit. If there is a ventilation control on the refrigerator unit, set this halfway between low and high or according to the manufacturer's instructions.
5. Connect tubing to oxygen flowmeter and flush tent with oxygen for 2 min. Reset flowmeter to prescribed number of liters. Another method is to allow oxygen to flow at 15 liters for about 30 min. Analyze concentration.
6. Maintain a tight canopy. Provide nursing care through zippered openings; organize nursing care. Oxygen loss is greater at the bottom of the tent, because oxygen is heavier than air. The front of the tent may be secured with bath blanket or sheet.
7. Tent temperature is adjusted to 17.8–21.1°C (64–70°F). The patient should not appear too warm or too cold. Dress the child according to body temperature.
8. Inspect connecting tubes periodically for kinks, loose connections, or faulty apparatus. A hissing sound can be heard as oxygen passes through the tubing if lines are patent. This may also be tested by holding one finger over the end momentarily.
9. Empty condensation reservoir as needed.
10. Refill distilled water jar as appropriate.
11. Select toys that retard absorption and do not produce static electricity.

and cannulas that come into direct contact with the child are disposable, other pieces of mechanical equipment cannot be discarded. *They require periodic cleansing if therapy is extended and terminal cleansing according to product direction.*

Prolonged exposure to high oxygen concentrations can be toxic to some body tissues, for example, the retina in preterm infants and the lungs in the general population, but particularly in children with pulmonary diseases such as asthma or cystic fibrosis. It is therefore necessary to measure oxygen content at regular intervals with an *oxygen analyzer* (see Fig. 23–28). This is usually done by the respiratory therapist; however, the nurse needs to ensure that the procedure is carried out on assigned patients. Readings are obtained close to the child's head. The amount of oxygen administered depends on the child's arterial oxygen concentration. Frequent blood gas determinations ($Po_2$ and $Pco_2$) ensure safe and accurate therapy. Noninvasive techniques that measure blood oxygen tension via the skin are available.

Oxygen is a dry gas and requires the addition of moisture in order to prevent irritation of the respiratory tree. High-humidity concentrations may be achieved by the use of jet humidifiers on several oxygen units. *Compressed air rather than oxygen* may also be used for this purpose. *Oxygen therapy is terminated gradually.* This allows the patient to adjust to *ambient* (environmental) oxygen. The nurse slowly reduces liter flow, opens air vents in Isolettes, or opens zippers in croup tents. The child's response is constantly monitored. An increase in restlessness and in pulse and respirations indicates that the child is not tolerating withdrawal from the oxygen-enriched environment.

*Methods of Administration.* Oxygen is administered to children as age-appropriate via Isolette, nasal cannula, mask, hood, or tent. Regardless of the method used, the child is observed frequently in order to determine the effectiveness of the oxygen. *The desired goals include decreased restlessness and improved breathing, vital signs, and color.* The highest concentrations of oxygen are delivered by way of a plastic hood. Warmed, humidified oxygen is delivered directly over the child's head. It may be used in a warming unit.

Oxygen tents are available from various manufacturers. The directions for the specific apparatus are closely followed. Before assembling the tent, the plastic is carefully examined for tears. Tents consist of a plastic canopy suspended from an overhead rod that is attached to a cabinet containing a machine. When adjusted, the machine regulates the ventilation and temperature of the tent and may also provide increased humidity in connection with the oxygen flow. Read each manufacturer's instructions for individual variations. Refer to the Procedure for Administering Oxygen by Tent.

## PROCEDURES RELATED TO SURGERY

The child is particularly fearful of surgery and requires both physical and psychological preparation at the patient's level of understanding. Listening to the child is especially valuable in clarification of misunderstandings. The child is asked to point to the operative site on a body outline. "Show me what they are going to fix." Explain anesthesia and allow the child to play with a mask (Fig. 23–30). Children and adults need reassurance that they will not be awake during surgery. Nursing interventions following surgery are aimed at assisting the child to master a threatening situation and minimizing physical and psychological complications. (See Index for nursing care principles for specific surgery.) Table 23–12 and

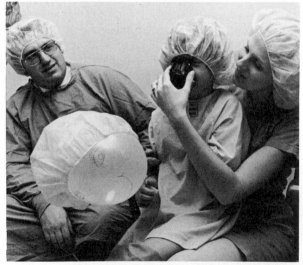

**Figure 23–30.** Preparing the child for the sights and sounds of surgery. (Courtesy of Blank Memorial Hospital, Des Moines, IA.)

23–13 summarize preparation for surgery and postoperative care.

**Sterile Dressings.** Sterile dressings may or may not be used, according to the preference of the surgeon. In many instances, *collodion* (a clear substance) is applied to the suture line. It keeps the wound visible and free from contamination. More extensive dressings may be preferred for wounds that require immobilization, or for draining wounds. Nursing intervention to promote healing may include changing dressings and observing the wound. All surgical dressings are done using aseptic technique.

When it is necessary to change a dressing on the surgical patient, the patient is brought to the treatment room, unless contraindicated. If the dressing is to be changed at the bedside, the patient is screened. Dusting, sweeping, or bed-making should not be allowed during the procedure. The windows and doors of the room are shut. Such measures lessen the chance of contamination of the wound by airborne bacteria. If the dressing is extensive, another person may be needed to assist. This is particularly important with children. Supplies vary according to the protocol of the physician. The nurse explains what will happen in terms that the child can understand. The term *bandage* may be more understandable to the pediatric patient.

The nurse prepares unsterile materials first. Adequate lighting is provided, and a newspaper, disposal bag, or kidney basin is positioned to receive the soiled dressing. Tape is cut into desired lengths. Most hospitals use individual disposable dressing trays and instruments. Prepackaged sterile sponges may also act as small sterile fields. Arrows indicate the direction in which to open. Sterile gloves are used to transfer the sponge from the package to the patient. Clean wounds are dressed before contaminated ones. The sterile field is arranged for ease in accessibility. The bedside stand or overbed table may be safer than the bed with children. The stand is positioned so that the nurse's back does not have to be turned on the sterile field. The older child is instructed not to touch the sterile field or the wound. Younger children may need to be restrained.

The hands are washed before beginning procedure. While the hand is protected with a clean glove, the outer tape and bandages are removed and discarded. If the wound needs to be bathed, sterile gloves are worn. Work around

**Table 23–12.** SUMMARY OF PREPARATION OF THE CHILD FOR SURGERY

| Procedure | Adult | Child | Modification |
|---|---|---|---|
| Consent | Yes | Yes | Parent or legal guardian |
| Blood work | Yes | Yes | Age-appropriate restraint |
| Urinalysis | Yes | Yes | Age-appropriate collection (U-bag) |
| | | | Assist school child |
| | | | Age-appropriate instructions |
| Evaluate for respiratory infection, nutritional status | Yes | Yes | Utilize more objective observations in infants and toddlers because of child's limited verbal skills |
| Allergies | Yes | Yes | Indicate clearly on chart |
| Nothing by mouth (NPO) | Yes | Yes | Increase fluids prior to NPO |
| | | | Length of time may vary with age and type of surgery (6–12 hr) |
| | | | If surgery is late, place appropriate notice on child: "Do not feed me" |
| | | | Remove goodies from bedside stand |
| | | | No gum |
| | | | Supervise hungry ambulatory patients carefully |
| Vital signs | Yes | Yes | Approach child carefully, explain, demonstrate |
| | | | Allow more time |
| Void before surgery | Yes | Preferred | Not always possible in infants and toddlers |
| Bath | Yes | Yes | Hospital gown, may wear underwear or pajama bottoms depending on age, type of surgery |
| Identification | Yes | Yes | Identification bracelet |
| Teeth | Yes | Yes | Check for loose teeth, orthodontic appliance |
| Skin preparation | Yes | Possible | May be done in operating room |
| Nails | Yes | Yes | Trim, remove nail polish |
| Glasses or contact lenses | Yes | Yes | Have children and adolescents remove glasses or contact lenses |
| Enemas | Possible | Possible | Not routine |
| Transportation | Yes | Yes | Crib or stretcher |
| | | | Parents may accompany to operating room door |
| Emotional preparation | Yes | Yes | Preoperative tour |
| | | | Group and individual puppet play |
| | | | Body drawings of parts involved |
| | | | Play selected by child as mode of expression |
| | | | Support parents during surgery |
| Sedation | Yes | Yes | Usually 20 min prior to surgery |
| Record all pertinent data | Yes | Yes | Essentially the same with pediatric modifications as indicated by the above |

drains is done gently. Dressings that stick are moistened with sterile saline solution. Cleansing with solution is done as ordered. The nurse should not reach across the sterile field or handle supplies unnecessarily. New sterile dressing is applied using forceps or sterile gloves and secured appropriately.

Following the procedure, the patient is comforted. The bedside unit is returned to normal. The type and amount of drainage on the soiled dressing is observed before being discarded. The procedure is recorded. Redness around the wound, increased drainage, or an elevation in temperature is reported to the physician. Additional notations include the time of the change, the area to which the dressing was applied, the color and amount of drainage (scant, moderate, profuse), the odor, the condition of the skin beneath the tape, medication if applied, any un-

usual findings, and how the patient tolerated the procedure.

## The Child with a Contagious Disease

Any patient suspected of having a contagious disease must be isolated until a definite diagnosis is established. A pediatric hospital has an isolation unit for this purpose. The smaller children's division of a general hospital may not have these facilities. The nurse admitting the patient must take certain precautions. The purpose of medical aseptic technique is to prevent the spread of the disease to the nurse and others. *Proper handwashing* cannot be overemphasized.

The patient is placed in a private room. All unnecessary furnishings are removed before

**Table 23–13.** SUMMARY OF POSTOPERATIVE CARE OF THE CHILD

| Procedure | Adult | Child | Modification |
|---|---|---|---|
| Return from recovery room | Yes | Yes | Notify parents<br>Smaller patients generally in crib<br>Age-appropriate safety precautions |
| Note general condition, alertness | Yes | Yes | Infant and toddler cannot verbalize fear or pain |
| Vital signs | Yes | Yes | Every 15–30 min until stable<br>Blood pressure is sometimes omitted for infant |
| Evaluate for shock | Yes | Yes | Essentially same |
| Assess operative site for bleeding, dressing intactness | Yes | Yes | Essentially same<br>Elevate casted extremities<br>Circle drainage |
| Restraints | Possible | Probable | May be necessary in order to protect IV<br>Remove periodically for range of motion |
| Connect dependent drainage (urinary catheter, Levin tubes, oxygen) | Yes | Yes | Prepare child for sight and noises of equipment, draw pictures to clarify purpose |
| Position patient | Yes | Yes | Prop on side unless contraindicated, no pillow |
| Intravenous (IV) | Yes | Yes | Should have pediatric adapting device and infusion pump<br>Monitor rate meticulously, as infants and small children respond quickly to fluid shifts<br>Measure and record intake and output |
| Assess elimination | Yes | Yes | Bowel and bladder |
| Relief of pain | Yes | Yes | Hold, comfort small children unless contraindicated<br>Be sensitive to behavioral changes such as increase in irritability, crying, regression, nail biting, passivity, withdrawal<br>Administer pain relievers<br>Involve parents in care<br>Provide transitional object such as blanket, favorite toy, pacifier<br>Be aware of transcultural considerations that provide familiarity and comfort |
| Nothing by mouth (NPO) | Yes | Yes | Until fully awake<br>Babies are started on clear fluids by bottle unless contraindicated<br>Avoid brown or red liquids, which may be confused with old or fresh blood<br>Monitor bowel sounds |
| Consider diet | Yes | Yes | Advance from clear to full liquids to soft to regular diet |
| Observe for complications | Yes | Yes | Turn, cough, deep breathe, dangle feet, ambulate early; less of a problem in children<br>Splint operative site with hands when child coughs |

the patient's arrival. Place an ample supply of paper towels and soap near the sink. A paper bag is attached to the bed for the patient to use as a wastebasket. Equipment for daily patient care is placed in the unit. This includes thermometer, bath equipment, bedpan, urinal, and tissues. Such equipment remains there until the patient is discharged, when it is treated by terminal disinfection. Disposable equipment is discarded in the proper receptacle. Linen is changed daily. An ample supply of gowns, masks, and newspapers saves much time and energy. A clean area is prepared according to hospital procedure. The floor is always considered contaminated. Anything that touches the floor must be discarded. Toys are tied to the bed with a short tape and must be washable.

When the blood pressure is taken, the patient's arm and the bed are protected by a clean gown or sheet in order to prevent contamination of the sphygmomanometer. Built-in wall units reduce the danger of contamination. When a flashlight, otoscope, or ophthalmoscope is used, it is protected by a technique paper. Any part that comes in direct contact with the patient must be disinfected. All the specimens that leave the room are marked "precaution" and are placed in a clean outer container according to hospital procedure. Trays necessary for general unit use are not brought into the patient's room. The necessary articles are removed and placed on a smaller paper tray, and the tray is carried to the bedside.

## PREVENTING INFECTION TRANSMISSION

### Medical Asepsis

The purpose of medical aseptic technique is to prevent the spread of infection from one child to another or from the child to the nurse. A person or object is considered *contaminated* if it has touched the infected patient or any equipment that has come in contact with the patient. People or articles that have had no contact with the patient are considered *clean*.

Articles that have come in direct contact with the patient must be disinfected before they can be used by others. When something is disinfected, microorganisms in or on it are killed by physical or chemical means. The autoclave, which uses steam under pressure, is considered effective in killing most germs when the article is adequately exposed and sterilized for the proper length of time.

Some materials, for example, the glass clinical thermometer, would be destroyed if autoclaved. A chemical disinfectant must be used instead. Before soaking an article in a disinfectant, the nurse must be sure that it has been properly washed in soap and water and rinsed. The strength of the disinfecting solution is generally determined by the hospital pharmacist and is dispensed to the units in suitable containers. Seventy per cent alcohol is an example of one type used. The article must be totally submerged and must remain in the solution for a *suitable length of time*. It is extremely important that articles in chemical solutions be marked with the time at which they are to be removed. If the nurse fails to do this, an unsuspecting person may assume that items are clean and may remove them before they are properly sterilized.

Disposable items are used whenever possible; they include diapers, tissues, needles, suction catheters, thermometers, suture sets, dishes, nursing bottles, and utensils. They are double-bagged and disposed of according to hospital procedure. *Used needles are not recapped but are placed in properly labeled puncture-proof containers* available in each patient's room (Fig. 23–31*D*).

Throughout this text, emphasis is placed on the role of the nurse in preparing a safe environment for the child and parents. Of all dangers in our surroundings, none is more serious than disease-bearing organisms. The nurse must understand the importance of protecting self and others from the isolated patient. This is accomplished by specific procedures, such as cleaning and disinfecting clothing, bedding, excreta, and hospital equipment. While doing this, the nurse must not, however, forget that the patient is the primary concern. As the student's confidence increases with repetition of the details of isolation, the approach to the patient and patient's problems will also be more effective. Isolation precautions are presented in Table 23–14. The communicable diseases are discussed in Chapter 34.

Because isolation procedures vary from hospital to hospital and from hospital to home, a minimum of specific procedures are presented here. An attempt is made to better acquaint the student with the underlying principles of medical aseptic technique so that the reliability of certain procedures can be judged. In general, measures of control are stricter for patients who have dangerous conditions than for those who have highly communicable but mild diseases. For example, the common cold is highly contagious, but patients are seldom isolated because of it. In contrast, meningococcal meningitis is now believed to be transmitted only by close contact with the infected person; nevertheless, most institutions carry out strict isolation procedures because of its seriousness.

### Specific Infections

**Universal Precautions.** Universal precautions are summarized in Appendix E. See also Table 23–14. They apply to all people regardless of known health status. Some materials used in procedures requiring universal precautions are illustrated in Figures 23–31 and 23–32.

**Respiratory Infections.** These include most common childhood diseases. Precautions must be taken against discharges from the eyes, nose, throat, and ears. Attendants wear gown and mask. Hands are washed between patients and after handling contaminated articles. Floors are damp-mopped to control dust.

**Wound Infections.** Organisms leave through the wound and may enter the body of the nurse through breaks in the skin, particularly of the hands. Germs may also become airborne when a wound is dressed. An infected wound is kept

**Table 23–14.** ISOLATION PRECAUTIONS

| Types and Examples* | Purpose | Private Room | Articles |
|---|---|---|---|
| *Strict* | | | |
| Herpes zoster<br>Varicella (chickenpox) | To prevent transmission of highly contagious organisms by both air and contact | Yes, *gowns, masks, and gloves,* door closed | Discard or wrap before being sent for decontamination and reprocessing<br>Bags are labeled or color designated in order to denote contaminated articles or infectious waste<br>*Hands must be washed after touching the patient or potentially contaminated articles and before taking care of another patient* |
| *Contact* | | | |
| Acute respiratory diseases in infants and young children: croup, bronchitis, bronchiolitis caused by various viruses, colds, viral pneumonia<br>Conjunctivitis, gonococcal in newborn<br>Eczema vaccinatum<br>Herpes simplex<br>Impetigo<br>Influenza, in infants and young children<br>Multiple resistant bacterial infection or colonization, i.e., *Pneumococcus* resistant to penicillin<br>Pediculosis<br>Pharyngitis<br>Rubella, congenital or other<br>Scabies<br>Skin wound or burn infection, including those infected with *Staphylococcus aureus* or group A streptococci | To prevent spread of highly transmissible diseases that do not warrant strict isolation, spread mainly by close or direct contact | Yes, during outbreaks, children with the same respiratory problem may share the same room<br>*Masks, gowns, and gloves* for direct contact | As for strict precautions |
| *Respiratory* | | | |
| Epiglottitis (*Haemophilus influenzae*)<br>Measles<br>Meningitis (*H. influenzae,* meningococcal)<br>Mumps<br>Pertussis<br>Pneumonia (*H. influenzae*) | To prevent airborne infection by droplets that are coughed, sneezed, or exhaled and are transmitted over a short distance | Yes, doors closed, *masks* | As previous page |

**Table 23–14.** ISOLATION PRECAUTIONS *Continued*

| Types and Examples* | Purpose | Private Room | Articles |
|---|---|---|---|
| *Tuberculosis*<br>(Acid-fast bacilli [AFB]) | Isolated category for patients with pulmonary tuberculosis with positive sputum or chest x-ray film that suggests active lesion; in general, infants and young children do not require isolation because they rarely cough and their bronchial secretions contain few AFB | Yes, special ventilation, door closed<br>*Masks* if patient is coughing, *gowns* as needed to protect clothing | As previous page<br>Articles are rarely involved in transmission of tuberculosis; must nevertheless be discarded or thoroughly cleaned and disinfected |
| *Enteric*<br>Coxsackievirus<br>Diarrhea<br>Encephalitis<br>Gastrointestinal upsets<br>Hepatitis (viral, type A)<br>Meningitis (viral)<br>Typhoid fever | To prevent transmission of infection by pathogens in feces | Yes, *gown and gloves* for direct contact | Articles contaminated with infective material should be discarded or bagged and labeled before being sent for decontamination and reprocessing<br>*Hands must be washed after touching the patient or potentially contaminated articles before taking care of another patient* |
| *Drainage/Secretion Precautions*<br>Minor or limited: burn infection, wound infection, abscess, decubitus ulcer, skin infection<br>Conjunctivitis | To prevent infections transmitted by direct or indirect contact with purulent material or drainage from an infected body site | No, *gown and gloves* for direct contact | Same as for enteric |
| *Blood/Body Fluid Precautions*<br>Acquired immunodeficiency syndrome<br>Arthropod-borne viral fevers (dengue, yellow, Colorado tick)<br>Hepatitis B<br>Hepatitis (non-A, non-B)<br>Syphilis (primary, secondary) | To prevent infections that are transmitted by direct or indirect contact with infected blood or body fluids | Yes, if patient hygiene is poor<br>*Gowns and gloves* for direct contact | As for enteric, plus:<br>*Avoid needle puncture injury*<br>Used needles are not recapped, broken by hand, or bent; instead are placed in properly labeled puncture-proof container designed specifically for such disposal<br>Wash hands immediately if potentially contaminated with blood or body fluids and before taking care of another patient<br>Clean blood spills promptly with solution of 5.25% sodium hypochlorite (bleach) diluted 1:10 with water |

*The examples cited are not intended to be all-inclusive. Data are adapted from the *CDC guidelines for isolation precautions in hospitals* (DHHS Publication No. [CDC] 83–8314). Washington, DC: U.S. Government Printing Office. Specific diseases are listed alphabetically in this publication and more detailed information is provided. (See Appendix F for univeral precautions.)

covered. If the nurse must handle the dressing, disposable gloves are worn. The contaminated dressings are disposed of according to the institution's procedure. Articles of clothing and bed linen that come in contact with the wound are treated as "precaution" linen. The nurse wears a gown and mask for dressing changes. Floors are damp-mopped to control dust.

**Skin Infections.** If the lesions cannot be covered, the patient is isolated, and bedding, clothes, and dishes are disinfected. The nurse wears a gown and gloves.

**Digestive Infections.** Precautionary measures are taken against all discharges from the mouth, stomach, and intestinal tract. Dishes, toilet articles, bedding, and clothing are considered contaminated. Stools may require added disinfection for some diseases. Glove and gown technique is employed.

**Genital Infections.** The danger of genital in-

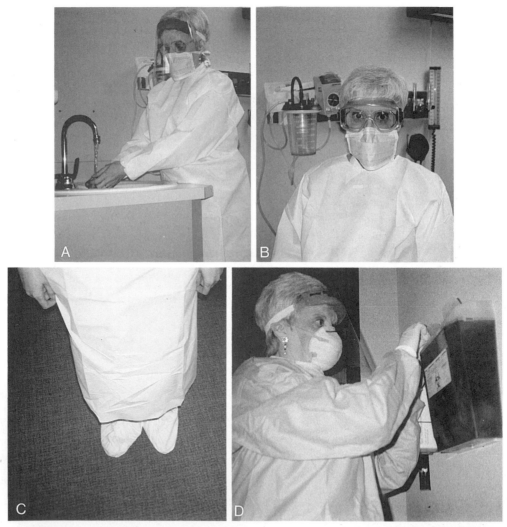

**Figure 23–31.** Some materials used in caring for patients who required universal precautions. *A,* Nurse wearing a face shield, disposable mask, and covergown and *washing hands thoroughly. B,* Protective goggles. *C,* Paper disposable boots to cover shoes in areas such as the delivery and operating rooms. *D,* Nurse wearing a mask, splash mask, and gloves. All sharp items are placed in puncture-resistant containers. (Courtesy, Columbia/HCA Portsmouth Regional Hospital.)

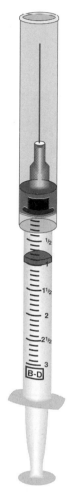

**Figure 23–32.** This syringe has a plastic sleeve that covers the needle after medication is administered. This helps protect the nurse from an accidental needle stick. (Redrawn from Becton Dickinson and Company, Franklin Lakes, NJ.)

fection lies in the discharge's coming in contact with the mucous membranes of the well person. The conjunctiva of the eye is particularly susceptible to infections of the same organisms that invade the genitals. Soiled dressings are disposed of according to hospital policy. Precautions should be used when handling clothing, bedding, dishes, and toilet facilities. Glove and gown technique is used.

## Specific Techniques

**Protective Isolation.** Protective isolation (also called reverse isolation or barrier technique) is used for patients with lowered resistance who are highly susceptible to infection. An article in the *New England Journal of Medicine* found that this simple procedure reduced the incidence of nosocomial (hospital) bacteria and fungal infection significantly in one pediatric intensive care unit (Klein, Perloff, & Maki, 1989). The patient is placed in a private room with the door closed. It is recommended that all persons wear gown, mask, and gloves when attending the child in isolation. (Masks can sometimes be omitted, depending on the patient's condition.) *Meticulous handwashing must be adhered to for the safety of the patient.* Some authorities suggest that plants, flowers, and water sources be removed from the environment in order to reduce the patient's contact with bacteria and fungi. Protective isolation units, such as life islands, are also available. Both the child and family need adequate explanations. The mechanics of isolation need to be periodically reinforced. It is not unusual for family members to feel distanced by the procedures. The nurse must determine the parents' perceptions of the child's illness, as guilt and denial may interfere with their cooperation.

**Handwashing.** Proper handwashing is essential to every procedure that the nurse performs, but it is doubly important in working with patients in isolation. A solution such as Hebiclens is used for handwashing with some immunocompromised patients.

**Mask Technique.** A supply of disposable masks is kept outside the patient's room. A fresh one is donned each time the nurse enters the room. A mask is used once and discarded. It is not allowed to hang around the neck and then be placed back over the face. It should cover the nose and mouth and should be changed at least once every hour. A mask is not touched once it is in place. It is removed after the gown when one leaves the unit, and the part that comes in contact with the face should not be touched. The mask is discarded in the room. Authorities disagree about the effectiveness of masks, so nurses follow the procedures of the hospital in which they are employed.

**Gown Technique.** Nurses wear gowns in order to protect their clothing from contamination when giving direct care to the child in isolation. If this were not done, organisms causing disease would be carried on the uniform, and the health of other patients could be endangered.

Sweaters are not worn in the isolation room. The nurse must be particularly conscientious on the children's unit because small children need to be held for feedings and comforting, and the nurse's relationship with the child is very direct.

Paper disposable gowns are now widely used. The gown is used once and discarded in a plastic isolation laundry bag held by a ringstand. The gown is put on and lapped over in the back (right side over left). The gown is removed by untying the waist strings, washing the hands, untying the neckband, and discarding the gown. The hands are rewashed. Technique papers are used to open the door, and these are discarded in the patient's room. The door of the room is closed. The nurse's shoes are always a source of contamination, and hands need thorough washing after touching them. Contaminated linen and trash are double-bagged and disposed of according to hospital procedure.

**Toys.** Toys must be washable. They may be kept in a special cloth bag tied to the patient's crib so that they will not drop to the floor. The string of the bag is kept short so that it will not become twisted around the child's neck. Because there is no satisfactory method of disinfecting books, reading is limited to magazines or materials that are not highly prized by the owner. In highly communicable diseases, reading material is burned during terminal disinfection of the unit.

**Educating the Family.** Visitors are usually restricted to members of the immediate family. This information is posted on the patient's door. Family members wear gowns and possibly masks while in the patient's room. Articles brought to the patient must be washable or disposable. After the visitor's gown has been removed and deposited in the laundry hamper, it must be washed. Visitors are not allowed to take articles from the room.

Education of family members is ongoing. Factors to be emphasized include the necessity for immunization of children, proper storage of food (particularly perishables), use of pasteurized milk, proper cooking of meats, cleanliness in food preparation, and proper handwashing. Review the ways in which infectious diseases are spread. Children need to be taught not to spit on others and to avoid using community hand towels. Other modes of transmission, such as crowded living conditions, insects and ro-

dents, and sandbox hazards, may also be discussed.

## Discharge Planning

### EDUCATING THE FAMILY

Preparation for the patient's discharge ideally begins on admission, for the goal of hospitalization is to return a healthier and happier child to the parents. An approach directed only toward good physical care of the patient's disease is not sufficient. The nurse must also consider the emotional growth of the child and the education of the patient and family. This will provide a positive learning experience for all involved.

If a patient requires specific home treatment, such as hyperalimentation, colostomy care, crutches, special diet, or insulin therapy, instructions are given to the parents gradually throughout their child's hospitalization. The instructions are written so that they may be referred to as needed. If the older child is to administer any self treatment, careful explanations and supervision will be required until both patient and parents are confident that they can carry out the procedure safely at home. This may require the home health services.

Parents also must be prepared for behavioral problems that may arise following hospitalization. Severe stress may be obvious during the patients' stay. The services of a children's counselor are helpful if nightmares and regression continue. Guidance suggestions include

- Anticipating behaviors such as clinging, regression in bowel and bladder control, aggression, manipulation, and nightmares.
- Allowing the child to become a participating family member as soon as possible.
- Taking the focus off the illness. Praising accomplishments unrelated to it.
- Being kind, firm, and consistent with misbehavior.
- Building trust by being truthful.
- Providing suitable play materials such as clay, paints, and doctor and nurse kits.
- Allowing time for free play.
- Listening to and clarifying misconceptions about the illness.

- Avoiding long periods of separation until a sense of security is regained
- Allowing the child to visit hospital staff during routine clinic visits if desired.

Whenever possible, parents are given at least 1 day's notice of their child's discharge from the hospital so that they can make necessary arrangements. This is particularly important if both parents work or if transportation is a problem. The physician writes the discharge order. The approximate hour of dismissal is relayed to the parents. The child is weighed and dressed, and all personal belongings are collected. Parents are given a written return appointment card when indicated. They are informed of any new habits the patient may have acquired during hospitalization. Necessary medications or materials that the parents have paid for are rendered.

Parents sign a release form and visit the hospital business office according to hospital procedure. In most cases, this is done on the way out. Nursing students inform the nurse in charge that they are leaving the unit with a patient.

According to condition, the child is placed in a hospital wagon, wheelchair, or stretcher for transport. The nurse assists the patient into the car seat or assists in fastening seatbelts. Charting includes when and with whom the patient departed, patient's behavior (smiling, alert, crying, and so on), method of transportation from the division, patient's weight, and any instructions or medications given to the patient or parents.

## DETERMINING CHILDREN AT RISK

The determination of children who may be at risk for child abuse, neglect, poverty, or a number of other conditions related to their particular disease condition or family lifestyle is of importance. Children who appear to be in jeopardy are referred to the hospital social service agency within 24 hours of admission. This is done in one hospital by filling out a high-risk profile sheet. It is also becoming more common for the nursing unit to telephone the family shortly after discharge in order to provide follow-up.

## KEY POINTS

- The nurse must be especially conscious of safety measures on the children's division, particularly of keeping crib sides up when the child is unattended, careful application of restraints, safe transport, and proper identification of the child.
- Include the parents in both planning and implementing care. Children are prepared for and encouraged to express their feelings about treatments.
- Weights must be accurate because medication is often estimated by patient weight.
- The correct-size blood pressure cuff must be used for children in order to obtain an accurate reading. It should cover two-thirds of the upper arm.
- Special urine collection devices are used for newborns and infants.
- Positioning of the child for jugular and femoral puncture is important. Because these are large veins, the infant is frequently checked for bleeding following these procedures.
- Medications for children have to be adapted to size, age, and body surface. The absorption, distribution, metabolism, and excretion of drugs differ substantially in children. Their reactions to drugs are less predictable.
- The recommended injection site for children under 3 years of age is the vastus lateralis.
- Careful observation of the child receiving intravenous fluids is necessary because overload of fluids in an infant can lead to cardiac failure. IVAC pumps are used to monitor infusions. Intake and output sheets must be accurate.
- Isolation technique must be carefully followed because small children need to be held and comforted, which increases the exposure of nurses.

# Study Questions

1. Observe a patient being admitted. How could the nurse have carried out this function more effectively?

2. Describe how and why measurement of blood pressure differs when the patient is a child.

3. Nine-year-old Chris Jones has just been admitted to the unit with a severe laceration of the leg. You are assigned to take his blood pressure. How would you explain this to Chris?

4. What is the purpose of the playroom?

5. Compile a list of safety measures that would be effective on the children's unit in your hospital. Underline measures that apply to the nurse.

6. List several ways in which children show their insecurities.

7. Of what value are visiting hours to the child, the parents, and the nurse?

8. Discuss how you would obtain a urine specimen from a 4-month-old baby.

9. Mrs. Lang, the head nurse, has just told you to prepare Room 101 for a newly admitted child suspected of having meningitis. The patient is a 6-year-old female. How would you do this?

10. What is the role of the nurse in assisting with a lumbar puncture?

11. What special precautions must be taken when giving medications to children? How and where are medications charted in your hospital?

12. Choose a drug that is administered to adults and children. Thoroughly investigate the use of the drug using the drug circular. What information is given about pediatric dosage and administration? Is this information adequate for your purposes? Present your findings to your classmates.

13. Rhonda, age 3, was admitted with acute laryngotracheobronchitis. She is crying anxiously in her Croupette. State the rationale for oxygen therapy. Devise a nursing care plan suitable to Rhonda's age and condition.

14. Rita, age 5, has been in isolation for meningitis for about a week. She is making satisfactory progress. How does her care differ from the care given to children who are not in isolation? List several diversions that appeal to the 5-year-old.

# Multiple Choice Review Questions

*Choose the most appropriate answer.*

1. The systolic blood pressure of a child is generally
   a. higher than an adult's
   b. lower than an adult's
   c. the same as an adult's
   d. not as important as an adult's

2. Three-year-old Ilze is admitted to the hospital for croup. Her orders include frequent observation as she is in a croup tent. This would include observing her for untoward signs, which would be
   a. increased restlessness, pulse, and respiration
   b. decreased restlessness, pulse, and respiration
   c. increase in blood pressure
   d. sleep disturbances, polyuria

3. Six-month-old Clair is admitted with diarrhea. An intravenous scalp infusion is running. The principal reason for careful regulation is to protect Clair from
   a. local skin infection
   b. heart failure
   c. abdominal distention
   d. alkalosis

4. Dehydration in Clair is evidenced by
   a. bradycardia
   b. poor skin turgor
   c. increased blood pressure
   d. excessive salivation

5. The clove hitch and mummy are forms of
   a. bandages
   b. restraints
   c. first aid
   d. fluid therapy

## BIBLIOGRAPHY

Ackerman, M.H. (1985). The use of bolus normal saline instillation in artificial airways; is it useful or necessary? *Heart and Lung, 14,* 505.

Beecroft, P., & Redick, S. (1990). Intramuscular injection practices of pediatric nurses; site selection. *Nurse Educator, 15,* 23–28.

Behrman, R.E., & Kliegman, R. (1992). *Nelson textbook of pediatrics* (14th ed.). Philadelphia: W. B. Saunders.

Betz, C., Hunsberger, M., & Wright, S. (1994). *Family centered nursing care of children.* (2nd ed.). Philadelphia: W. B. Saunders.

Bowlby, J. (1960). *Psychoanalytic study of the child* (Vol. 15). *Grief and mourning in infancy and early childhood.* New York: International.

Hayman, L., & Sporing, E. (1985). *Handbook of pediatric nursing.* New York: John Wiley & Sons.

*Hickman and Broviac catheters: A guide for patients.* (1983). Iowa City, IA: Department of Nursing, University of Iowa Hospitals and Clinics.

Klein, B., Perloff, W., & Maki, D. (1989). Reduction of nosocomial infection during pediatric intensive care by protective isolation. *New England Journal of Medicine, 320,* 1714.

Mott, S., James, S.R., & Sperhac, A.M. (1991). *Nursing care of children and families.* Reading, MA: Addison-Wesley.

Petrillo, M., & Sanger, S. (1980). *Emotional care of hospitalized children: An environmental approach* (2nd ed.). Philadelphia: J. B. Lippincott.

Pillitteri, A. (1992). *Maternal and child health nursing.* Philadelphia: J. B. Lippincott.

Thompson E. D., & Ashwill, J. W. (1992). *Pediatric nursing: An introductory text* (6th ed.). Philadelphia: W. B. Saunders.

Weir, M., & Weir, T. (1989). Are "hot ears really hot." *American Journal of Diseases of Children, 143,* 763–764.

Whaley, L., & Wong, D. (1991). *Nursing care of infants and children.* St. Louis: C.V. Mosby.

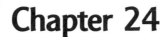

# Chapter 24

# The Child with an Ear, Eye, or Neurologic Condition

## VOCABULARY
athetosis (643)
humoral (618)
hyperopia (624)
hyphema (626)
idiopathic (637)
nystagmus (634)
postictal (637)
pupillary light reflex test (625)
retinoblastoma (626)
SIADH (632)

## OBJECTIVES

*On completion and mastery of Chapter 24, the student will be able to*

Define each vocabulary term listed.
■ Discuss the prevention and treatment of ear infections.
■ Outline the problems peculiar to the hospitalized child who is deaf.
■ Contrast amblyopia and strabismus.
■ Define *cataract.*
■ Determine when neural tube development occurs in fetal life.
■ List four tests used to determine neurologic problems.
■ Describe the child with symptoms of meningitis.
■ Discuss the various types of epilepsy.
■ Outline the symptoms, treatment, and nursing care for the child with Reye's syndrome.
■ Formulate a nursing care plan for the child in a coma.

Figure 24–1 summarizes ear, eye, and neurologic differences between children and adults.

## The Ears

The ear, which can be considered a part of the nervous system, contains the receptors of the eighth cranial nerve, the acoustic. The ear performs two main functions, hearing and balance. The three divisions of the ear are depicted in Figure 24–2. In the newborn, the tympanic membrane is almost horizontal and is more vascular than in the adult. It is also dull and opaque and has an inconsistent light reflex. The eustachian tube is horizontal at birth and shorter and straighter during infancy but gradually matures and lies at a 45-degree angle. Three functions of the eustachian tube are ventilation of the middle ear, protection from nasopharyngeal secretions and sound pressure, and drainage. Middle ear infections are common during childhood.

When nurses examine the ear, they observe both its exterior and its interior. Ear alignment is observed. The top of the ear should cross an imaginary line drawn between the eye and the back of the head. Low-set ears may be associated with Down syndrome and other disorders. The outer ear and the area around it are inspected for cleanliness and drainage. The inner ear is inspected with an otoscope. One method of restraint used when assisting with the examination of the inner ear is to lay the child on a table with the arms held alongside the head, which is turned to the side. The parent may also support the child in the lap.

**Ear Hygiene.** Teach parents to cleanse the ear with a wash cloth. Use swabs only on outer ear. Never probe with sharp objects. If wax (cerumen) is hard, it can be softened with a commercial product such as Debrox. If wax is persistent, consult with the physician during periodic checkups. Children sometimes poke objects into the ear. They need to be removed professionally to avoid wedging the object further or causing other damage.

### OTITIS MEDIA

**Description.** Otitis media (*ot,* "ear," *itis,* "inflammation of," and *media,* "middle") is an inflammation of the middle ear. The middle ear is a tiny cavity in the temporal bone. Its entrance is guarded by the sensitive tympanic membrane, or eardrum, which transmits sound waves through the oval window to the inner ear, which contains the organs of hearing and balance. The middle ear opens into air spaces, or sinuses, in the mastoid process of the temporal bone. It is also connected to the throat by a channel called the eustachian tube. These structures—the mastoid sinuses, the middle ear, and the eustachian tube—are lined by mucous membranes. As a result, an infection of the throat can easily spread to the middle ear and mastoid. The eustachian tube also protects the middle ear from nasopharyngeal secretions, provides drainage of middle ear secretions into the nasopharynx, and equalizes air pressure between the middle ear and the outside atmosphere. These protective functions are diminished when the tubes are blocked. Unequalized air within the ear creates a negative pressure that allows organisms to be swept up into the tube if it opens.

Otitis media may be secondary to an upper respiratory tract infection and may accompany communicable disease. After respiratory infections, it is the most prevalent disease of childhood. It occurs most often in patients of age 6–36 months, and again in those of age 4–6 years. It is more prevalent in males. It is caused by a variety of organisms. *Streptococcus pneumoniae* and *Haemophilus influenzae* are the most common causative agents. The complications of

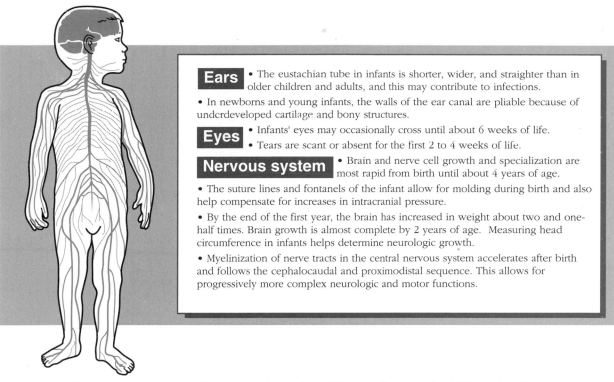

**Ears**
- The eustachian tube in infants is shorter, wider, and straighter than in older children and adults, and this may contribute to infections.
- In newborns and young infants, the walls of the ear canal are pliable because of underdeveloped cartilage and bony structures.

**Eyes**
- Infants' eyes may occasionally cross until about 6 weeks of life.
- Tears are scant or absent for the first 2 to 4 weeks of life.

**Nervous system**
- Brain and nerve cell growth and specialization are most rapid from birth until about 4 years of age.
- The suture lines and fontanels of the infant allow for molding during birth and also help compensate for increases in intracranial pressure.
- By the end of the first year, the brain has increased in weight about two and one-half times. Brain growth is almost complete by 2 years of age. Measuring head circumference in infants helps determine neurologic growth.
- Myelinization of nerve tracts in the central nervous system accelerates after birth and follows the cephalocaudal and proximodistal sequence. This allows for progressively more complex neurologic and motor functions.

**Figure 24–1.** Summary of ear, eye, and neurologic differences between the child and the adult.

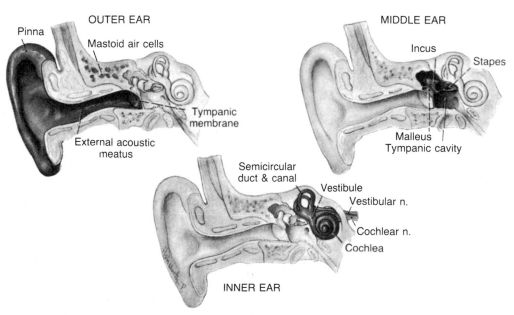

**Figure 24–2.** The three divisions of the ear. (From Jacob, S.W., Francone, C.A., & Lossow, W.J. [1982]. *Structure and function in man* [5th ed., p. 342]. Philadelphia: W.B. Saunders.)

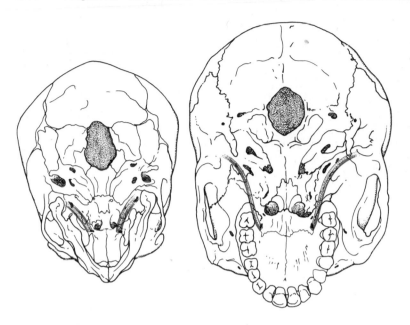

**Figure 24–3.** Diagram showing the position and direction of the eustachian tube in the infant and adult. The infant's eustachian tube is shorter, wider, and straighter.

acute otitis media and otitis media with effusion are significant health hazards for children.

Infants are more prone to ear infections than older children and adults, for their eustachian tube is shorter, wider, and straighter (Fig. 24–3). Because babies lie flat for long periods, microorganisms have easy access from the eustachian tube to the middle ear. The infant's humoral (*humor*, "body fluid") defense mechanisms are immature. Some studies suggest that feeding methods may have a bearing on infection (Teele et al., 1989). Breast-fed babies have fewer infections than do bottle-fed babies. This may result from immunity from the mother. In addition, the more slanted position of formula-fed infants during feeding allows formula to flow into the eustachian tubes. Passive smoking has also been implicated. Children in passive smoking environments have more respiratory infections and their attendant complications.

**Manifestations.** The symptoms of otitis media are pain in the ear, which is often very severe, irritability, and interference with hearing. Fever, which may run as high as 40°C (104°F), headache, and vomiting may also accompany it, as may diarrhea and febrile convulsions. The nurse may suspect an earache in the infant who rubs the ear frequently or pulls at it. The head may be rolled from side to side. The baby is fussy and cries. The older child can point to the place that is tender. Some patients are asymptomatic.

If an abscess forms, a rupture of the eardrum may result, and pus drains from the ear. When this happens, the pressure is relieved and the patient is more comfortable. Recurrent attacks can lead to complications. Otitis media is considered chronic if the duration persists for more than 3 months. A low-grade inflammatory reaction may lead to a foul-smelling exudate sometimes referred to as "glue ear." Mobility of the tympanic membrane is impaired. Although uncommon, this condition can lead to cholesteatoma (*chole*, "bile," *steato*, "fat," and *oma*, "tumor"), a cystlike sac filled with keratin debris. This may occlude the middle ear and erode adjacent ossicle bones, causing hearing loss. This condition is best treated by an otolaryngologist.

Other complications of an ear infection include deafness and mastoiditis. Partially treated otitis media may be the cause of meningitis in young children, although this is less common because of antibiotics. Prevention lies in prompt treatment of respiratory infections or infected tonsils and adenoids.

**Treatment and Nursing Care.** In examining the ears, one first observes their appearance and general hygiene. The lymph nodes about the ear are observed for swelling or tenderness. The patient's head is adequately stabilized in order to prevent injury to the ear canal from sudden, unexpected movement. The examiner ensures that no foreign bodies are lodged in the outer canal before inserting the otoscope. To straighten the canal and improve viewing, the ear is pulled *downward* and *backward* in infants and *upward* and *backward* in older children and adults.

There are certain landmarks within the ear.

If one imagines the external ear and the tympanic membrane as being superimposed on a clock face, it is easier to locate them. The otoscope is placed in the ear between the 3 o'clock and 9 o'clock positions, forward and downward. The canal is approximately 1 inch in length. The walls of the external canal are usually pink, and small hairs may be visible. The tympanic membrane appears as glistening, translucent, and pearly gray. At approximately 5–7 o'clock, the light of the otoscope should reflect in a characteristic cone shape. This is termed the *cone of light* or *light reflex*.

The *malleus*, commonly referred to as the "hammer bone," may also be visible. Absence of any of the usual landmarks may indicate bulging of the membrane from middle ear fluid or another condition. The drum may appear red in crying infants. Mobility of the eardrum (tympanic membrane) can be tested with a pneumatic device that is attached to the otoscope. Air is gently blown into the ear, and the tympanic membrane is observed for movement. A healthy membrane moves easily. The tympanogram is a graphic recording produced by a tympanometer. It is a more objective means of measuring function of the middle ear and motility of the tympanic membrane.

When an infection is evident, treatment is directed toward finding the causative organism and relieving the symptoms. A throat culture may be taken. Antibiotics are given initially until the specific organism is determined. These and the sulfonamides have proved very effective. Amoxicillin and ampicillin, broad-spectrum antibiotics, are given orally; when they are not effective, trimethoprim-sulfamethoxazole (Bactrim, Septra) may be given. Cephalothin (Keflin) may be used to combat chronic otitis media caused by *Staphylococcus*. Therapy is continued for at least 10 days. Analgesics are given to relieve pain. Nasal decongestants may be prescribed, although their use is controversial. Ear drops are no longer recommended because they obscure the tympanic membrane from view. Nursing Care Plan 24–1 specifies interventions for selected diagnoses pertaining to the child with otitis media.

**Surgical Treatment.** Surgical intervention may be necessary when medical treatment is unsuccessful. The physician may incise the tympanic membrane to relieve pressure and to prevent a tear by spontaneous rupture. This is called a myringotomy (*myringa*, "eardrum," and *otomy*, "incision of"). This procedure is not performed as routinely today as in the past because the availability of more effective antibiotics makes it unnecessary. Adenoidectomy may be indicated on some patients.

A *tympanic (TM)* button or tympanostomy ventilating tube may be inserted into the eardrum to act as a source of air and as a drain. This will eventually fall out spontaneously. In some patients, tubes must be reinserted to continue ventilation. Their use is controversial at this writing. Care is taken to avoid getting water in the ears while swimming and showering. Earplugs may be recommended. All children should be followed to ensure resolution of the condition.

**Local Heat or Cold.** An electric heating pad or covered hot water bottle may be applied locally (temperature of hot water bottle: 115°F). Because a heating pad may become overheated, it is placed on a low setting and observed frequently. If the eardrum has ruptured, the child is placed on the affected side with the ear on top of the heat source. Otherwise, position to avoid pressure on the ear. Cold may also be beneficial. An ice pack may reduce edema and pressure and increase the comfort of the child. The skin around the ears needs to be kept clean and protected from drainage in order to prevent it from breaking down. Parents are instructed not to use cotton swabs in the ears.

## HEARING IMPAIRMENT

**Description.** Hearing-impaired children present special challenges to the nursing team. Children are seldom seen in the hospital just for hearing impairment but more often are admitted because of other health problems. The student should have a basic knowledge of the problems that confront the hearing impaired in order to provide comprehensive nursing care.

The inner ear is fully formed during the early months of prenatal life. If an expectant mother contracts German measles or another viral infection during this period, the child may be born with a hearing loss, which is termed *congenital deafness*. Deafness can also be *acquired*.

## Nursing Brief

Instruct caretakers that the child's condition may improve dramatically after a few days on antibiotics. To prevent recurrence, they must continue to administer the prescription until the bottle is empty.

**NURSING CARE PLAN 24–1**

## Selected Nursing Diagnoses for the Child with Otitis Media

| Goals | Nursing Interventions | Rationale |
|---|---|---|
| **Nursing Diagnosis:** Pain related to pressure and inflammatory process. | | |
| Child does not express feelings or exhibit behaviors that denote pain or discomfort | 1. Position for comfort | 1. This will vary with the child; if tympanic eardrum has ruptured, child is placed with affected ear down to promote drainage; otherwise prevent pressure on infected ear |
| | 2. Observe behaviors that indicate pain; administer analgesic | 2. Infants may tug at ears, appear irritable, and cry |
| | 3. Apply external heat or cold | 3. Use heat pad at low setting for older responsible child; check frequently to avoid burns; a hot water bottle is covered and capped tightly; temperature of water 46°C or 115°F; a light ice compress placed over the infected ear may reduce edema and pressure; determine effectiveness of either procedure by asking child if it increases comfort; do not insist if there is resistance |
| | 4. Offer liquids and soft foods to avoid chewing | 4. Movement of eustachian tube while chewing may cause discomfort |
| | 5. Administer antipyretic medications to infants to avoid febrile convulsions | 5. Infants, in particular, may experience high fever and its associated discomforts |
| **Nursing Diagnosis:** Knowledge deficit regarding course and complications of "earache" or surgical intervention. | | |
| Parents and older child verbalize understanding of information and importance of compliance | 1. Stress importance of prescribed antibiotic routine, particularly completing regimen (child must take all medicine even though feeling much better); to promote compliance, make a medication reminder chart for full 10 days or time ordered; provide written instructions | 1. Usual course of antibiotics is 10–14 days; compliance is a problem, as most children show noticeable improvement within 48–72 hr |
| | 2. Promote early medical attention for upper respiratory infections, particularly if child has history of recurrent ear infections | 2. Otitis media is often a complication of an upper respiratory infection |
| | 3. Encourage breast feeding during infancy; hold infants upright for feedings | 3. A relationship between feeding methods of mothers and otitis media is suggested (see text); usual lying-down position of infants favors pooling of fluid in nasopharynx; breast feeding provides certain immunities, and infants experience fewer allergies |
| | 4. Discourage parents and baby-sitters from smoking near child | 4. Passive smoking contributes to upper respiratory infections |
| | 5. Discourage forceful nose blowing | 5. Forceful nose blowing causes infection to spread; instruct child to blow through both nostrils at same time to equalize pressure |

*Continued*

| NURSING CARE PLAN 24–1 *Continued* | | |
|---|---|---|
| **Selected Nursing Diagnoses for the Child with Otitis Media** | | |
| Goals | Nursing Interventions | Rationale |

**Nursing Diagnosis:** Knowledge deficit regarding course and complications of "earache" or surgical intervention.

| | Nursing Interventions | Rationale |
|---|---|---|
| | 6. Prevent contaminated water from entering ear (from baths, swimming, showers) | 6. Organisms may reinfect ears; fluid can cause pressure in ear |
| | 7. Investigate food allergies | 7. Food allergies may contribute to problem |
| | 8. Prepare family for surgical intervention if required (tube insertion, adenectomy) | 8. Preparation decreases anxiety levels |
| | 9. Instruct parents to notify health provider if grommet (tiny, white plastic spool-shaped tube) falls from ear | 9. No intervention required, but may be alarming to unprepared parent |
| | 10. Observe for hearing loss; stress importance of keeping follow-up appointments | 10. Hearing impairment may be a complication of otitis media |

Infectious diseases such as measles, mumps, chickenpox, or meningitis can result in various degrees of hearing loss. The common cold, some medications, certain allergies, and ear infections may also be responsible. Hearing problems can also be temporary because of wax accumulation.

The old adage "An ounce of prevention is worth a pound of cure" is particularly applicable to the invisible handicap of deafness. Excessive cleaning of the ear can be damaging, especially if one probes the canal with objects such as a hairpin. If a foreign object is trapped in the ear, consult a doctor. Trying to remove it may cause further damage.

The nurse must stress the importance of proper immunization during childhood in order to prevent many of the communicable diseases. Vaccines against regular measles (rubeola), mumps, and German measles (rubella) are now available. The child should be taken to the doctor for periodic health examinations. Early diagnosis and treatment of hearing-impaired children are important in order to prevent adverse physical and mental complications from developing. Members of the health team concerned with the child who is hearing impaired include the physician, otologist (ear specialist), audiologist, speech therapist, specially trained teacher, social worker, psychologist, nurse, and the child's family.

The various degrees of hearing loss range from complete *bilateral* (which affects both ears) to a loss so mild that the problem is never discovered. If loss is complete, the child misses all the pleasures of sound and has difficulty in communication, since children learn to talk by imitating what they hear. Behavior problems arise because these children do not understand directions. They may become aggressive with other children in their attempt to communicate. If ridiculed by playmates, personality development will be affected. Unless these children are helped, they will become socially isolated.

Partial bilateral deafness may be responsible for behavior problems and poor progress in school. It may be caused by chronic infections, such as otitis media, or by blockage of the eustachian tube. It may be a warning signal of more serious defects in later life. Children who have losses in one ear are less affected if hearing in the other ear is normal.

**Treatment and Nursing Care.** Early diagnosis and prompt treatment are primary requisites, regardless of the patient's age. *Evoked response audiometry* permits testing of newborns and children who cannot otherwise be tested. Figure 24–4 shows a newborn having a routine hearing test. Complete bilateral deafness is usually discovered during infancy. Partial deafness may be unrecognized until the child begins school. Many hearing problems are detected then by standard hearing tests. A machine called an *audiometer* is used. The child puts on an earphone that is connected to the audiometer. When the audiometer is turned on, it makes various noises and pitches of sound. The child raises the hand as the tone is heard.

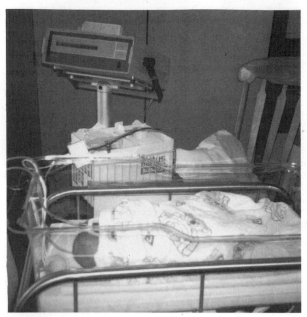

**Figure 24-4.** This newborn is having a routine hearing test. The baby must lie very still; therefore, feedings are given beforehand, and the baby is swaddled in a blanket.

When a test shows that the child has a hearing threshold deficit, a careful examination by an otologist is required. School children should be screened every 3 years.

Many hearing defects are amenable to medical or surgical treatment. Antibiotics are used for acute otitis media. Chronic otitis media may be helped by the insertion of *tympanostomy tubes*. Hearing aids can amplify sound waves in permanent *conductive* losses. Surgically placed *cochlear implants* are now used for some children with nerve damage. Children who suffer a severe loss of hearing need more extensive help from personnel at an auditory training center. These children need to begin treatment as soon as the loss is discovered.

Various methods are used to bring the child into the world of sound. Lip reading, sign language, writing, visual aids, music, and amplified sound are but a few examples. The hearing-impaired child is taught to speak so that others in the environment can comprehend. This is not accomplished overnight. If a hearing aid is indicated, the child is equipped with one and taught how to use it. Regular checkups ensure that the aid is working properly. A malfunctioning one may cause a child to lose interest in using it. The parents are instructed in means of communication that coincide with those used by the teachers.

**Role of the Nurse.** The nurse must be aware of the symptoms of deafness in the child. Newborns are observed for their response to auditory stimuli. The Brazelton Neonatal Behavioral Assessment Scale evaluates the infant's orientation response to the sound of a voice. Persistence of the Moro reflex beyond 4 months may also be an indication of deafness. The infant who makes no verbal attempts by the 18th month of life should undergo a complete physical examination. Poor school performance, indifference to sound, and behavior problems may also be signs of deafness. The nurse inquires into the facilities that are available in the community for such a patient.

Because prevention of this disorder is so important, the nurse takes advantage of opportunities to demonstrate and teach proper hygiene of the ears to the child and family. Nurses must stress the importance of infant immunization to parents with newborns. Proper safety measures must be taken to prevent injury to the ears from trauma to the head, especially during the toddler period. Mothers are instructed to avoid *ototoxic* drugs during pregnancy. Nurses should maintain a high index of suspicion in chronically ill children who may be on medications such as streptomycin, kanamycin, and neomycin. Sensorineural hearing loss can also be caused by noise pollution, such as loud rock music or target shooting. Symptoms include buzzing of the ears and muffled dull sounds immediately following exposure. To avoid discomfort during air travel, parents are instructed to feed the infant or to use a pacifier during take-off and landing.

The hearing-impaired child in the hospital needs the same opportunities to develop a healthy personality as the child who does not have this handicap. The nurse smiles when approaching the child. Body language communicates much to this patient, especially if there is a severe communication problem. The nurse faces the child when speaking and is positioned at eye level with the child. The nurse ensures being seen by, before touching, the child, to avoid startling the child. The nurse speaks in short sentences rather than separate words and speaks clearly in a natural tone. It is not neces-

## Nursing Brief

One person can make a difference.

sary to exaggerate speech. Nurses who are relaxed with the patient create an atmosphere that others will continue.

If the child is able to write, this can be used as a means of communication. The patient reads aloud what is written. This helps the nurse become better accustomed to the child's speech. Speech patterns may regress during hospitalization. The nurse does not assume that the child who is not talking a great deal does not understand what is being said. Certain statements are repeated or reworded, as would be done with any child.

The nurse determines whether or not the child fully understands what is asked. The hearing-impaired child tends to answer "yes" or "no" before grasping the complete meaning of the question. After explaining a procedure, the nurse asks questions to be sure that the child understands what is expected. This is pertinent to all small children in the hospital. Children respond to nurses who are interested and patient enough to listen to what they say.

Nurses are often called on to assist the physician in an ear examination. They hold the toddler in their lap with the head pressed against their chest. They place one hand on the child's forehead and the other securely around the body. The head is held still so that the delicate ear canal will not be injured by the *otoscope*. The ear *speculum* (a funnel-shaped device that comes in direct contact with the ear) must be washed and disinfected following each use.

A hearing aid is expensive and invaluable to the patient. It is put in a safe place when not in use. When the patient goes to surgery, it is placed in the hospital safe. The pockets of hospital gowns are checked before the gowns are placed in the laundry chute. The nurse can gain valuable information about the use of the hearing aid from the child's parents.

## The Eyes

The eye is the organ of vision. The anatomy of the eyeball is depicted in Figure 24–5. The eyes begin to develop as an outgrowth of the forebrain in the 4-week-old embryo. The newborn's sight is not mature, but the newborn can see. Visual acuity is estimated to be in the range of 20/400. This improves rapidly and may reach 20/30 to 20/20 by the age of 2 or 3 years (Behrman, 1992). The shape of the newborn's eye is less spherical than the adult's eye. The eyes may appear crossed in the early weeks of life. The ciliary muscles are immature, and the infant cannot fixate on an object for any length of time. Newborns are often tested by visually evoked response. This is done by placing electrodes on the head over the visual cortex. The eyes are stimulated by light, and recordings are taken. Depth perception does not begin to develop until about 9 months. Children are hyperopic (farsighted) until about 5 years of age.

On physical examination, the nurse observes the eyes to see if they are symmetric and an equal distance from the nose. Epicanthal folds (*epi*, "upon," and *canthus*, "angle") are present in children of Asian descent. Eyebrows and lashes are inspected for pigment or parasitic in-

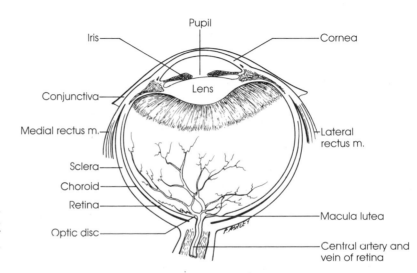

**Figure 24–5.** Structure of the eyeball. (From Marlow, D.R., & Redding, B.A. [1988]. *Textbook of pediatric nursing* [6th ed., p. 102]. Philadelphia: W.B. Saunders.)

fection. Pupils are observed for size, shape, and movement. Their reaction to light is observed by shining a penlight into the eye and quickly removing it. The healthy pupil constricts as the light approaches and dilates as it disappears. Older children are given explanations concerning the examination. They are allowed to hold the ophthalmoscope and turn it off and on.

## VISUAL ACUITY TESTS

There are a variety of visual acuity charts (Fig. 24–6). The Snellen alphabet chart and the Snellen E version, for preschoolers who have not learned the alphabet, are commonly used to assess the ability to see near and far objects. Picture cards are also useful for children who do not know letters.

The Titmus machine is frequently used for school children and adolescents. Directions for testing are standardized and must be carefully adhered to for proper results. Computerized tests, such as the random-dot stereogram, also show promise in the visual screening of children. Visual acuity is important in the learning process. *Developmental dyslexia* (*dys*, "difficult," and *lexis*, "diction") is a reading disability that is not caused by any defects in the eye or visual acuity. Nevertheless, an ophthalmologic evaluation of the child is helpful in differential diagnosis, correction of any ocular problems, and education of the parents. The following is a discussion of the more frequent eye conditions seen in

preterm children. Retinopathy of the premature (ROP) is discussed on page 322.

## AMBLYOPIA

**Description.** Amblyopia (lazy eye) is a reduction in or loss of vision that usually occurs in children who strongly favor one eye. If both retinas do not receive a clearly defined image, bilateral amblyopia may result. However, it is more common for one eye to be affected. The prognosis depends on how long the eye has been affected and the age of the child when treatment begins. The earlier the treatment, the better the results. One commonly accepted diagnostic sign is that vision in the normal eye is at least two Snellen lines (E charts) better than that in the affected eye. There are various types of amblyopia. Strabismus is the most common; however, dissimilar refractory errors can also result in this condition.

**Treatment and Nursing Care.** Early detection and prompt treatment are essential for the child with amblyopia. In infants this condition can be reversed in a matter of days or weeks. In an older child, months or years may be required. The goal of treatment is to obtain normal and equal vision in each eye. Treatment consists of glasses for significant refractive errors (hyperopia, myopia) and patching (occlusion) of the good eye. Daytime patching may be instituted. In some cases, part-time occlusion is sufficient. Occlusion therapy is often difficult to

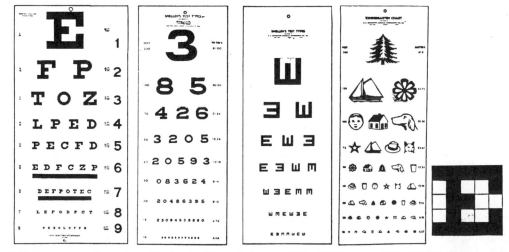

**Figure 24–6.** Various types of visual acuity charts. (From Behrman, R.E., & Kliegman, R.M. [1992]. *Nelson textbook of pediatrics* [14th ed.]. Philadelphia: W.B. Saunders.)

maintain. The nurse can be of help by explaining the importance of the procedure and by offering support. The child is often subject to ridicule by peers. Providing a safe place to express feelings is important to promoting a healthy self-image. In selected cases, an opaque contact lens or a contact lens of sufficiently high power to blur the vision in the better eye is used (Behrman, 1992).

## STRABISMUS

**Description.** Strabismus (cross-eye), also known as *squint*, is a condition in which the child is not able to direct both eyes toward the same object. There is a lack of coordination between the eye muscles that direct movement of the eye.

There are several kinds of strabismus. In *monocular* squint (*mono*, "one," and *oculus*, "eye"), one eye is continuously used for vision, and the other is turned inward or outward. In *alternating* squint, either eye may be used singly for vision, with the other eye crossed. Strabismus may be present at birth or may be acquired after a disease.

The *pupillary light reflex test*, done as part of a routine physical examination, is helpful in detecting strabismus. The examiner shines a penlight into the patient's eyes from a distance of about 18 inches. If the child is looking directly at the light, the reflection should be at the same point in each pupil. The *alternate cover test* is also useful in detecting strabismus. When quickly uncovered, the eye should not move; if it has to shift to focus on the light, malalignment is present. Muscle movement can be ascertained by having the patient follow the examiner's finger. Epicanthal folds can give a false impression of strabismus.

**Treatment.** When strabismus is seen during early infancy, the doctor may recommend that the unaffected eye be covered by a patch until the baby is old enough to wear glasses. The affected eye may improve through use and often becomes normal. Eye exercises and glasses are effective ways of treating the condition medically. If they do not help, surgery should be considered. It is generally performed when children are 3 or 4 years old; the condition should be corrected before they start school in order to prevent their becoming the subject of ridicule. Early correction is necessary in order to prevent amblyopia. If strabismus is left untreated, blindness may result because the

brain tends to obliterate the confusing double image.

**Nursing Care.** The child undergoing surgery for strabismus is hospitalized for only a brief period. Some doctors prefer not to have the child restrained following surgery because it is frightening and the child's struggles may increase. The surgery involves structures outside the eyeball; therefore, the child is allowed to be up and about postoperatively. Eye dressings are kept at a minimum, and elbow restraints may be sufficient to keep the child from touching the dressings.

If the doctor thinks that it is necessary to cover the eyes and restrain the patient's movement following surgery, the patient is told this before surgery and is assured that the bandages and restraints will be removed as soon as possible. Because this is frightening for patients, it is best that the parents remain with them. Since they cannot move or see, diversions such as stories and records are necessary. When nausea has ceased, the patient is placed on a regular diet. When feeding patients, the nurse tells them what they are about to eat. The nurse speaks to the children before touching them so that they are not startled.

*Prevention of Eyestrain.* The nurse stresses the importance of proper care of the eyes. Little children who are beginning to read need books with large type in which the letters are spaced far apart. The lighting must be adequate and without glare. Chairs and desks must be of the proper height.

Symptoms that may indicate eyestrain include inflammation, aching or smarting of the eyes, squinting, a short attention span, frequent headaches, difficulties with schoolwork, or inability to see the blackboard. They may occur suddenly. The child between 6 and 10 years of age often becomes nearsighted and has to hold books very close to the eyes to read. An eye examination and sometimes a complete physical examination are indicated.

## CONJUNCTIVITIS

Conjunctivitis (*conjungere*, "to join together," and *itis*, "inflammation") is an inflammation of the conjunctiva or the mucous membrane that lines the eyelids. It is caused by a wide range of bacterial and viral agents, allergens, irritants, toxins, and systemic diseases. It is common in childhood and may be infectious or noninfectious. The acute infectious form is commonly referred to as *pinkeye*. The common forms of conjunctivitis generally respond to warm compresses and topical antibiotic drops or ointment.

The nurse instructs parents to give the drops for the full 7 days or prescribed length of time to prevent recurrence. Parents and older children are taught to wipe secretions from the inner canthus downward and away from the opposite eye. Because conjunctivitis spreads easily, the affected child should use separate towels and be instructed to wash the hands frequently. Ophthalmia neonatorum, an acute conjunctivitis in the newborn, is discussed on page 234. Allergic conjunctivitis is often associated with allergic rhinitis (*rhin*, "nose," and *itis*, "inflammation") in patients with hay fever. Symptoms include itching, tearing of both eyes, and edema of the eyelids and periorbital tissues. The child may appear distracted and irritable.

## HYPHEMA

Hyphema, the presence of blood in the anterior chamber of the eye, is one of the most common ocular injuries. It can occur from either a blunt or a perforating injury. Blows from flying objects, such as a baseball or snowball, can cause this condition. These accidents are common among active school children. Hyphema appears as a bright-red or dark-red spot in front of the lower portion of the iris.

Treatment includes bed rest and topical medication. The head of the bed is elevated 30–45 degrees to promote settling and decrease intracranial pressure if there is an associated head injury. The condition generally resolves itself without damage. The child is closely observed for several days because the blood in the anterior chamber may elevate intraocular pressure, which can affect vision. In more severe cases, patching of the eyes may be required. This prevents movement of the eyes and pain. Analgesics are given for discomfort.

The nurse observes the patient for symptoms that may indicate complications. Diminished eyesight or flashes of light may indicate a detached retina. Sudden severe headache accompanied by nausea and vomiting may be a sign of glaucoma. These require immediate consultation with an ophthalmologist. The child is also observed for the usual clinical manifestations of head injury.

## CATARACTS

A cataract is any opacity (*opacitas*, "shadiness") of the transparent lens, located just behind the pupil (see Fig. 24–5). It prevents light from reaching the retina. When cataracts are severe, blindness results. Early developmental processes may be responsible for cataracts in children. Maternal disease, such as rubella, may cause congenital cataracts. They are seen in children with muscular dystrophy.

Prematurity, heredity, metabolic disease, and chromosomal defects are all implicated. Steroid medications are a major cause of cataracts in children. Cataracts are seen in child abuse and trauma to the eye.

Treatment depends on severity. Modern techniques to remove the lens have greatly reduced the risk of surgery and postoperative complications. Intraocular lens implant has successfully been used for some children who are unable to manage regular contacts. These techniques improve vision and appearance. Postoperatively, fluids are given cautiously to avoid increased ocular pressure by vomiting. Sedatives are administered to prevent crying, for the same reason, and to provide comfort. Parents are provided with support and education so that they can effectively carry out any procedures necessary on discharge.

## RETINOBLASTOMA

**Description.** Retinoblastoma is a malignant tumor of the retina of the eye. There are hereditary and spontaneous forms. Although considered rare in relation to other cancers, the tumor has an annual incidence of 3.4 in 1 million children. The average ages at diagnosis are 8 months for bilateral tumors and 26 months for unilateral tumors. (Behrman, 1992). Gene-mapping techniques have shown chromosome 13 to be affected in hereditary forms. These children may also evidence other congenital defects. Because of a dominant pattern of inheritance, the patient who survives retinoblastoma has a 90% chance of having a child with a tumor.

**Manifestations.** A yellowish-white reflex is seen in the pupil because of a tumor behind the lens. This is called the *cat's eye reflex* or *leukokoria* (*leuk*, "white," and *kore*, "pupil"). This may be accompanied by loss of vision, strabismus, hyphema, and in advanced tumors, pain. In unilateral tumors, metastasis to the second eye is common. When retinoblastoma is suspected in children, an examination under anesthesia is performed so that the eye specialist may carefully examine the fundus of the eye. As in other malignancies, a staging classification system is used to determine treatment.

**Treatment and Nursing Care.** The standard treatment for unilateral disease is enucleation (removal) of the eye. Irradiation may be used if the tumors are very small, but it is less common. Other treatments include cryosurgery (freezing the tumor to kill cells) and photocoagulation by laser to destroy the blood vessels supplying the tumor. On return from surgery for enucleation, the child has a large pressure dressing on the eye. Restraints may be necessary to prevent removal of the dressing. The bandage is observed for bleeding and vital signs are assessed. In a few days, the surgeon removes the dressing and an eye patch is applied. Other structures of the eye, such as the lids, lashes, and tear glands, are not affected. An eye prosthesis is fitted when the socket has healed. Instructions for care of the prosthesis are provided by the oculist. The prognosis is excellent in less advanced stages. Careful preparation and emotional support of the child and family are paramount. Because this is a major crisis, the services of the mental health clinician are advised.

# The Nervous System

The nervous system is the body's communication center; it receives and transmits messages to all parts of the body. It also records experiences (memory) and integrates certain stimuli (learning). The anatomy of the nervous system is depicted in Figure 24–7. Neural tube development occurs at about the 3rd or 4th week of fetal life. This eventually becomes the central nervous system (CNS). The fusing process of the neural tube is critical. Its failure to fuse may lead to such congenital conditions as spina bifida or anencephaly. Most neurologic disabilities in childhood result from congenital malformation (birth defects), brain damage, or infection. Parents of an infant who is born with or acquires a neurologic defect often fear the child's loss of intelligence or mobility.

Many sophisticated and simple tests are used to determine disorders of the nervous system. CNS dysfunction may be detected by skull x-ray films, ultrasound brain waves, computed tomography (CT), magnetic resonance imaging, electromyography, and other methods. The reflexes of the newborn are good indicators of neurologic health. In the ill child, level of consciousness is particularly significant. A patient's gait during play is another parameter. In the finger-nose test used to determine coordination, the child is asked to extend the arm and then to touch the nose with the index finger. This is done with the eyes opened and closed. The child may also be requested to balance on one foot.

The Denver Developmental Screening Test is another means of assessing neurologic development (see p. 449). The following is a discussion of the more frequent conditions of the nervous system encountered by children. Included are Reye's syndrome, bacterial meningitis, encephalitis, brain tumor, recurrent convulsive disorders, and cerebral palsy. Hydrocephalus, spina bifida, intracranial hemorrhage, and Down syndrome are discussed in Chapter 14.

## REYE'S SYNDROME

**Description.** Reye's syndrome (RS) is a disease characterized by a nonspecific encephalopathy with fatty degeneration of the viscera. It mainly affects the liver and brain. The cause is unknown, although it is probably a mitochondrial disease. Mitochondria (*mitos*, "thread," and *chondros*, "granule") are structures within the cytoplasm of cells. Damage to these structures impairs enzyme activity. This leads to hyperammonemia and fatty acidemia, which, along with other factors, are believed to account for brain swelling. The disease is triggered by a virus.

The number of cases of Reye's syndrome has been decreased dramatically because of increased awareness of the high association between the disorder and aspirin-containing medications. More recent studies appear to confirm this (Porter et al., 1990). Currently, it is mainly seen in adolescent aspirin users (Behrman, 1992). The exact incidence of the disorder is unknown. Reye's syndrome affects children under 18 years of age, with peaks during infancy and at ages 6–7 years. The younger the child, the

## Nursing Brief

Discourage the use of aspirin and other medications that contain *salicylates* in children with flu-like symptoms. Advise parents to read labels of medication carefully to determine ingredients.

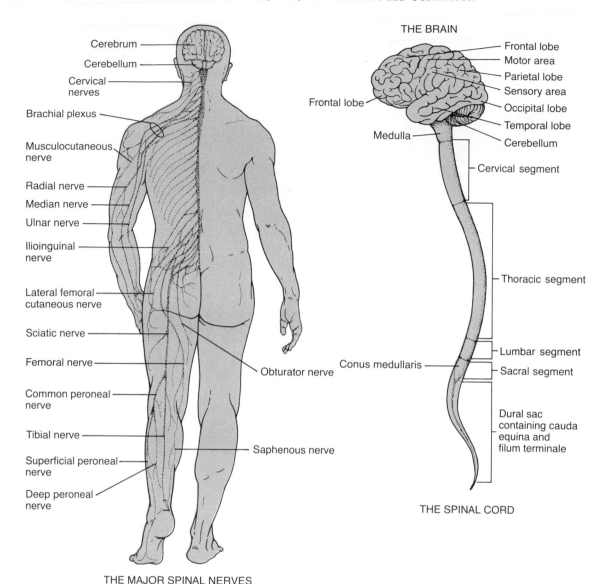

**Figure 24–7.** The nervous system consists of the brain, spinal cord, sense organs, and nerves. The nervous system is the principal regulatory system.

higher the morbidity and mortality rates. Prevention includes discouraging the use of aspirin and medications that contain *salicylates* (Pepto-Bismol) in children with virus-type symptoms. Early diagnosis is crucial because of the rapid, life-threatening course of the disease.

**Manifestations.** The clinical picture of Reye's syndrome is typical in that children have a viral infection from which they are recovering. This is generally influenza or chickenpox; however, other viruses have also been implicated.

The recuperation is interrupted by general malaise; persistent vomiting, which may continue for 24 hours; and lethargy (Table 24–1). Diagnosis is based on the patient's history, symptoms, and laboratory data. Examples of the latter include liver function tests, serum ammonia levels, blood glucose levels, and prothrombin times. Elevated serum liver enzyme levels and increased serum ammonia levels are indicative of the disorders. Metabolic acidosis and respiratory alkalosis may also be present. Liver biopsy may be done if the diagnosis is

**Table 24–1.** CLINICAL STAGING OF
REYE'S SYNDROME

| Grade | Symptoms at Time of Admission |
| --- | --- |
| I | Usually quiet, lethargic and sleepy; vomiting; laboratory evidence of liver dysfunction |
| II | Deep lethargy, confusion, delirium, combativeness, hyperventilation, hyperreflexia |
| III | Obtunded, light coma, ± seizures, decorticate rigidity, intact pupillary light reaction |
| IV | Seizures, deepening coma, decerebrate rigidity, loss of oculocephalic reflexes, fixed pupils |
| V | Coma, loss of deep tendon reflexes, respiratory arrest, fixed dilated pupils, flaccidity/decerebrate (intermittent); isoelectric electroencephalogram |

*Note*: Severity varies greatly; progression may stop at any point.

From Behrman, R.E. (1992). *Nelson textbook of pediatrics* (14th ed.). Philadelphia: W.B. Saunders.

questionable. A CT scan may be ordered to rule out a brain tumor. The prognosis depends on the severity of the illness. Most survivors recover completely; however, some suffer complications of neurologic sequelae.

**Treatment and Nursing Care.** The patient with Reye's syndrome is admitted to the intensive care unit (ICU). Treatment is supportive. Of particular priority is preventing brain insult, as the disease process in most other organs is reversible. Fluid management in conjunction with treatment of increased intracranial pressure (ICP) is crucial. Electroencephalograms (EEGs) are performed until stabilization is seen. Medications include osmotic diuretics (such as mannitol), sedatives, and barbiturates. Appropriate therapy for secondary infection is also instituted. Treatment programs are currently in a state of transition and vary with the severity of the illness.

The nursing care for patients with increased ICP is summarized on page 665. This is assumed by ICU nurses during the acute stage of the disease. Important aspects include elevating the patient's head to 30 degrees. The neck should not be compressed. Consider all procedures in terms of their effect on the child's ICP. Nursing care is performed gently to reduce agitation. The nurse anticipates and prepares for seizures. If the child is comatose, nursing measures to reduce secondary effects are considered. The Nursing Care plan for a comatose child is depicted on page 630. Respiratory status is evaluated frequently. The nurse is on the alert for drug incompatibilities. Overhy-dration is avoided, and the patient is observed for bleeding. A hypothermia pad may be used to prevent temperature elevations, which increase the demand for cerebral oxygen.

The rapid course of this disease is extremely frightening. Parents need information and reassurance. There is usually guilt. Family members may blame themselves for not recognizing the seriousness of the infection. Other children in the home may also be ill. The nurse addresses parental concerns and prepares parents for how the child looks, particularly if procedures with additional equipment have been introduced since their last visit. Parents are provided with a comfortable place to sleep. The nurse assesses family coping skills and refers family members to a chaplain, mental health clinician, social service, or Reye's Foundation. When the patients awake, they may be reserved, disoriented, and fearful of their environment. They may not recall any of the events surrounding hospitalization. Informing parents of this possibility decreases apprehension.

## BACTERIAL MENINGITIS

**Description.** Meningitis is an inflammation of the meninges, the covering of the brain and spinal cord. Different organisms cause bacterial meningitis in different age groups (Table 24–2). Organisms may invade the meninges indirectly by way of the blood stream from centers of infection such as the teeth, sinuses, tonsils, and lungs or directly through the ear (otitis media), from neurologic procedures, or from a fracture of the skull. Factors that may increase the risk of meningitis include CNS anomalies, humoral deficiencies, immunosuppressive therapy, sickle cell disease, and congenital or traumatic absence of the spleen.

Bacterial meningitis is often referred to as *purulent*, that is, pus-forming, because a thick exudate surrounds the meninges and adjacent structures. This can lead to certain sequelae, such as subdural effusion and, less frequently, hydrocephalus. The peak incidence for bacterial meningitis is between 6 and 12 months of age. It is less frequently seen in children older than 4 years. *Haemophilus influenzae* is the most common causative agent. Two *H. influenzae* type B vaccines are now available for infants. The approaches to nursing care for all types are similar.

**Manifestations.** The symptoms of purulent

| NURSING CARE PLAN 24–2 | | |
|---|---|---|
| **Selected Nursing Diagnoses for the Comatose Child** | | |
| **Goals** | **Nursing Interventions** | **Rationale** |

**Nursing Diagnosis:** High risk for injury, related to decreased sensorium, intracranial pathology.

| Goals | Nursing Interventions | Rationale |
|---|---|---|
| Child's vital and neurologic signs remain within normal parameters | 1. Monitor vital signs | 1. Heart rate and blood pressure must be maintained in order to prevent hypoxia; hypoxia can lead to hypercapnia, an increased amount of carbon dioxide in blood; to compensate, blood vessels dilate, which causes local swelling leading to cerebral edema and increased intracranial pressure (ICP) |
| | 2. Monitor intake and output | 2. Fluid restrictions may be required in order to decrease central and therefore cerebral blood volume; observe mechanical pump and burette to avoid accidental fluid overload; be alert also for hypovolemia (decreased blood volume) |
| | 3. Check pupils for size, reaction to light, accommodation, equality | 3. Monitoring changes in neurologic status helps alert nurse to progress or deterioration of patient's condition |
| | 4. Measure head of infants, assess fontanel, that is, full, tense, or soft | 4. Head measurements determine amount of swelling; in infants, cranial sutures are still open, so fontanels may bulge |
| | 5. Elevate head of patient 15–30 degrees to reduce ICP | 5. An upright position promotes venous outflow from brain by gravity into neck veins |
| | 6. Softly talk to patient while attending; refrain from inappropriate discussion within patient's hearing | 6. Crying increases ICP; even though patient appears unconscious or may be on pancuronium bromide (Pavulon) or barbiturates, sensory function is intact |
| | 7. Organize nursing procedures to prevent overstimulation | 7. Overstimulation can result in peripheral vasoconstriction, which may contribute to increased ICP; range-of-motion exercises are not performed vigorously |
| | 8. Observe and record response of patient, resistance to care | 8. Patient response may indicate return to consciousness or deepening coma |

**Nursing Diagnosis:** High risk for physical injury, related to seizure activity.

| Goals | Nursing Interventions | Rationale |
|---|---|---|
| Child's skin remains intact, no additional bruises are observable, and signs of seizure activity are absent | 1. Pad side rails of bed | 1. Padding side rails will protect restless patient |
| | 2. Instigate seizure precautions; administer anticonvulsants or sedatives as prescribed | 2. Neurologic insult may result in seizures or muscle spasms |

meningitis result mainly from intracranial irritation. They may be preceded by a cold. There are severe headache, drowsiness, delirium, irritability, restlessness, fever, and vomiting. Stiffness of the neck and spine is yet another symptom. In infants, a characteristic high-pitched cry is noted. Convulsions are common. Coma may occur fairly early in the older child. In severe cases, involuntary arching of the back due to muscle contractions is seen. This condition is called *opisthotonos* (*opistho*, "backward," and *tonos*, "tension"). The presence of *petechiae*—

### Selected Nursing Diagnoses for the Comatose Child

| Goals | Nursing Interventions | Rationale |
|---|---|---|
| **Nursing Diagnosis:** Ineffective airway clearance. | | |
| Child's airway remains patent; patient breathes easily | 1. Closely observe and evaluate breathing of patient; suction as necessary<br>2. Review blood gases and pH | 1. A clear airway is vital for oxygenation<br>2. Blood gas measurements are sensitive indicators of respiratory status; they provide information concerning lung function and tissue perfusion; they assist physician in determining interventions such as adjustments on a ventilator, chest physical therapy, and inhalation therapy |
| | 3. Change position of patient at least every 2 hr<br>4. Give chest physiotherapy if ordered | 3. Prevents lung infection and skin breakdown<br>4. Helps remove secretions from child's lungs |
| **Nursing Diagnosis:** Impaired physical mobility. | | |
| Patient retains flexibility of limbs and full range of motion; contractures are absent | 1. Perform passive range-of-motion exercises gently<br>2. Apply splints as ordered | 1. Prevents contractures of joints; increases muscle tone<br>2. Prevents contractures by positioning extremity |
| **Nursing Diagnosis:** Self-care deficit: feeding, bathing, and hygiene. | | |
| Child is well nourished as determined by nutritional parameters<br>Child appears clean and well-groomed | 1. Provide nourishment suitable to child's condition | 1. Unconscious child is generally fed through a nasogastric or gastrostomy tube; posturing and seizures may cause food to reflux through tubing |
| | 2. Consult nutritionist on regular basis | 2. Caloric needs are calculated to ensure adequate nutrition and prevent muscle wasting; overfeeding is avoided as metabolism is decreased; a catabolic state interferes with patient recovery |
| | 3. Bathe daily and as necessary | 3. Personal hygiene is important for good health; a bath adds to patient's comfort, prevents skin irritation, provides periods of observation of child's skin and muscles |
| | 4. Wash, comb, and style hair as appropriate | 4. Improves comfort of patient; encourages family about quality of care patient is receiving |
| | 5. Cleanse genital area daily and as necessary; diaper as needed | 5. Prevents irritation and infection |

small hemorrhages beneath the skin—is suggestive of meningococcal infection.

**Treatment.** At the first indication of meningitis, the physician performs a spinal tap (lumbar puncture) (see p. 578). In the early stages of the illness, the fluid may be clear, but it rapidly becomes full of pus. The pressure is increased, and further laboratory analysis indicates many white cells, sometimes too numerous to count. There is an increase in protein and a decrease in glucose.

The patient is placed in isolation for 24 hours after antibiotic therapy. An intravenous (IV) line is established. The fluid serves as a vehicle

**Table 24–2.** ORGANISMS CAUSING BACTERIAL
MENINGITIS IN VARIOUS
AGE GROUPS

| Age | Organism |
|-----|----------|
| Birth to 2 mo | *Escherichia coli*, group B streptococci |
| 2 mo to 3 yr | *Haemophilus influenzae* type B, *Streptococcus pneumoniae Neisseria meningitidis* (meningococci) |
| 3–16 yr | *N. meningitidis, S. pneumoniae* |

*Note:* Other bacteria may also cause meningeal infection
when the patient has a disorder that compromises the
defense mechanisms or when there has been a penetrating trauma.

for the administration of antibiotics, which
need to be quickly assimilated, and also aids in
the restoration of fluids and electrolytes.
Antibiotics are given in combination and are
adjusted on the basis of culture and sensitivity
reporting. The initial choice is dictated by the
CSF Gram-stained smear and the patient's age.
They are given according to the patient's
progress but are always administered for a
minimum of 10 days. Chloramphenicol in combination with ampicillin has proved effective in
babies over 2 months of age. More recent drugs
with broad-spectrum coverage, such as the
third-generation cephalosporins, are widely utilized. Newborns may be treated with ampicillin, gentamicin, kanamycin, and other combinations. A sedative, such as phenobarbital, may
make the patient less restless. An anticonvulsant such as phenytoin (Dilantin) may also be
required.

Prospective studies have shown that almost
60% of children with bacterial meningitis develop the syndrome of inappropriate secretion
of antidiuretic hormone (SIADH). In order to
determine the presence of SIADH, body weight,
serum electrolytes, and serum and urine osmo-
larities should be measured at the time of hospital admission. If SIADH is detected, the patient is best treated by fluid restriction.

Initially, the patient is given nothing by
mouth. An accurate record is kept of fluid intake and output, and vital signs and pupils are
checked hourly. Oxygen is ordered when necessary. It is uncommon for others in the family to
contract the disease, but the doctor will order
preventive medicines if necessary. New or persistent fever requires reevaluation. A CT scan
may be helpful in pinpointing secondary sites of
infection.

**Nursing Care.** The nursing care of the child
with meningitis is extensive. The isolation room
is prepared in accordance with hospital procedure. Articles used by the physician are treated
as contaminated. They are left in the room for
further use, discarded, or sterilized for safe
reuse. Particular attention is given to materials
used during the spinal tap and to those that
have come in contact with secretions from the
nose, mouth, and ears. Disposable equipment is
utilized whenever possible. The room is kept
cool and as clean and orderly as time permits.

Because the patient is overly sensitive to stimuli, indirect lighting is used. Shades are drawn on
a bright day. The nurse carefully raises and lowers
crib sides to avoid jarring the bed. Padded side
rails ensure that the patient will not be injured in
the event of a convulsion. The nurse avoids startling the patient by using a gentle touch when
waking and by speaking in a low voice. This precaution is also explained to parents.

The patient is placed on the side to avoid aspiration of vomitus. Since a minimum of handling
is necessary during the acute stage, the nurse
organizes care so that the patient is disturbed
as little as possible yet still receives the treatment necessary for survival and recovery.
Frequent change of position is required in order
to prevent pneumonia and to avoid breakdown
of the skin. However, careful planning and con-
solidation of nursing procedures can minimize
activity about the patient. As the child's condition improves, nursing care plans include range-
of-motion exercises (easily done during bath
time) to prevent painful contractures. In long-
term patients, splinting of the extremities may
also be necessary to avoid this complication.

Frequent monitoring of the patient's vital
signs is necessary. A slowed pulse rate, irregular respirations, and an increase in blood pressure are reported immediately, as they could indicate increased ICP. Fever may be controlled
by antipyretics, sponge baths, and a water
mattress. The nurse observes the child for
additional or subtle signs of increased ICP,
especially a change in alertness or muscle
twitchings. She also observes the joints for
swelling, pain, and immobility. Oxygen is given
as needed.

The patient's intake and output are carefully
observed and recorded. *Careful attention is
given to maintaining the IV line.* If SIADH occurs, there may be fluid restriction. Good oral
hygiene is essential during this stage, when the
patient is receiving nothing by mouth. As the

# Nursing Brief

Encephalitis may occur as a complication of childhood diseases such as measles, mumps, or chickenpox. It is crucial that children receive the immunizations available for the diseases that are preventable.

---

patient's condition improves, the diet progresses from clear fluids to house diet. A special formula may be given when nasogastric feedings are necessary. During the convalescent period, oral fluids are forced, unless contraindicated, as the patient's urine tends to be highly concentrated. The nurse promptly reports a decrease in output of urine, which could signal *urinary retention*. Bowel movements are recorded each day in order to detect constipation and avoid fecal impaction (an accumulation of feces in the rectum). The nurse watches for signs of residual effects from the disease, such as weakness of limbs, speech difficulties, mental confusion, and behavior problems.

The nurse's approach to the patient and the patient's reaction to isolation are discussed on page 605. The diagnosis of meningitis is very frightening to parents, as is the prospect of the child's having to undergo a spinal tap. There is also concern for the health of other members of the family. The nurse directs attention to the parents, finding a quiet corner for them, indicating where rest rooms and telephones are located, and explaining visiting hours. Parents are advised to stay as long as they wish but to notify the charge nurse or unit clerk before they leave the hospital.

## ENCEPHALITIS

**Description.** Encephalitis (*encephalo*, "brain," and *itis*, "inflammation") is an inflammation of the brain. When the spinal cord is also infected, the condition is known as encephalomyelitis (*myelo*, "spinal cord"). This disorder can be caused by arboviruses (RNA viruses) and herpesvirus types 1 and 2; it can be the aftermath of disorders such as upper respiratory tract infections, German measles, or measles, or, rarely, an untoward reaction to vaccinations such as diphtheria, pertussis, and tetanus (DPT); or it may result from lead poisoning. Other less common etiologic agents are bacteria, spirochetes, and fungi. More than half of the cases of encephalitis

in the United States are caused by unknown complexes.

This disease also affects horses, and during epidemics, newspapers specify the equine variety if this is the case. If the specific virus is determined, it is given the name of the geographic location in which it is found, for example, eastern (United States), western (United States), St. Louis, and California. The infection is transmitted to horses and humans by mosquitoes and ticks.

**Manifestations.** The symptoms of encephalitis result from the CNS response to irritation. In general, the viruses invade the lymphatic system and multiply. The blood stream becomes affected, and consequently, various organs are also involved. Characteristically, the history is that of a headache followed by drowsiness, which may proceed to coma. Because coma is sometimes prolonged, encephalitis is sometimes referred to as "sleeping sickness." Convulsions are seen, particularly in infants. Fever, cramps, abdominal pain, vomiting, stiff neck, delirium, muscle twitching, and abnormal eye movements are other manifestations of the disease. The patient's history is of particular significance. Recent illness, injections, travel, and geographic location are recorded.

**Treatment and Nursing Care.** At this time, no specific medication is known, with the exception of adenine arabinoside for herpesvirus encephalitis. Some vaccines are available but are not generally used for human patients. Mosquitoes and ticks should be destroyed in known infested areas where encephalitis is prevalent. A brain scan, EEG, and CT may be useful in determining the diagnosis. A lumbar puncture may be done. Intracranial monitoring may also be employed.

The treatment is supportive and is aimed at providing relief from specific symptoms. Sedatives and antipyretics may be prescribed. Seizure precautions are taken. Adequate nutrition and hydration via gavage or IV therapy, control of convulsions, and catheterization for urinary retention may also be required. The nurse provides a quiet environment, good oral hygiene, skin care, and frequent change of position. Oxygen is given as needed, and the mouth and nose are kept free of mucus by aspiration. Bowel movements are recorded daily, as the patient may be constipated from lack of activity. Preventing this and other secondary effects of immobility is paramount. Physical therapy may also be indicated.

The nurse closely observes the patient for neurologic changes. Fatality rates and residual effects are higher among infants than older children. Speech, mental processes, and motor abilities may be slowed, and permanent brain damage and mental retardation can result. Parents are encouraged to help with the care of the child as soon as the condition is stable. They are instructed in the nursing procedures required for home care. In long-term cases, the services of the public health nurse and related agencies are invaluable.

## BRAIN TUMORS

**Description.** Brain tumors are the second most common type of neoplasm in children (the first is leukemia). The majority of childhood tumors occur in the lower part of the brain (cerebellum or brain stem) (Fig. 24–8). The etiology of these tumors is unknown. They occur most commonly in school-age children. Diagnosis is difficult because of the insidious onset. Metastatic tumors of the brain are rare in children. A synopsis of brain tumors in children is listed in Table 24–3.

**Manifestations.** The signs and symptoms are directly related to the location and size of the tumor. Most tumors create increased ICP with the hallmark symptoms of headache, vomiting, drowsiness, and seizures (see pp. 339–340). *Nystagmus* (constant jerky movements of the eyeball), strabismus, and decreased vision may be evidenced. *Papilledema* (edema of the optic nerve) may be seen. Other symptoms include ataxia, head tilt, behavioral changes, and cerebral enlargement, particularly in infants. Disturbances in vital signs are noticeable when the tumor presses on the brain stem.

**Treatment and Nursing Care.** The treatment and nursing care are highly specific and transcend pediatric nursing into the fields of oncology, neurology, and other specialties. In general, nursing care falls into several phases: diagnosis, preoperative care, postoperative care, radiation therapy and chemotherapy, and convalescence. The objectives for each area are specific but also overlap. One pervading theme is the continual emotional support for the child and family during this taxing ordeal. Diagnosis is determined by clinical manifestations, laboratory tests, CT, MRI, and myelogram. Angiography is used to assist in the surgical approach by identifying the tumor's blood supply. At times the pathologist must perform special tests on the excised tissue. This results in a waiting period that increases the anxiety level of the entire family.

Nursing care parallels the phase of treatment. Preoperative emphasis is placed on careful explanation of various procedures and on familiarizing the patient and family with the recovery room, ICU, and hospital personnel. The nurse explains that the patient will have the head shaved. The nurse anticipates anxiety and provides empathy and support. The size of the postoperative dressing is carefully explained. Applying a similar dressing to a doll may be helpful.

The postoperative care is that given the criti-

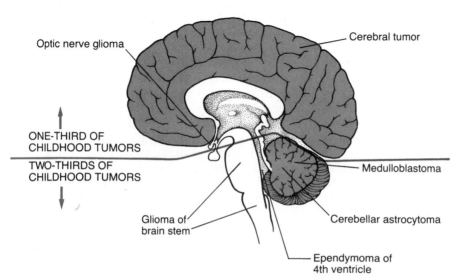

**Figure 24–8.** Location of brain tumors in children.

Table 24–3. CHARACTERISTICS AND PEAK AGE OF OCCURRENCE OF CHILDHOOD BRAIN TUMORS

| Tumor | Peak Age | Characteristics |
|---|---|---|
| Cerebellar astrocytoma | 5–8 yr | Slow-growing, cystic tumor; very high rate of cure with surgery (90%) |
| Medulloblastoma | 2–6 yr | Rapid-growing, highly malignant; occurs more often in boys; treatment—surgery, craniospinal irradiation, chemotherapy; prognosis—improved |
| Glioma of brain stem | 6–8 yr | Slow-growing; cannot be removed by surgery; affects cerebral pathways, cranial nerves; treatment—site irradiation to shrink tumor; prognosis—poor |
| Ependymoma of fourth ventricle | 2–6 yr | Tumors grow at various speeds; because of location, invade vital centers, obstruct flow of cerebrospinal fluid; treatment—partial surgical removal, irradiation of entire cerebrospinal axis; prognosis—few long-term survivors |

## Nursing Brief

The timing of information is important when preparing the child for various procedures.

cally ill child. Student nurses may assist but are not expected to assume full responsibility. Adjuncts to care may include the use of a hypothermia blanket or a mechanical respirator. Parents must be prepared for the appearance of the child following surgery. The patient may be unconscious for a while, or there may be facial edema. In supporting the family, several common issues may need to be addressed. These are the fear of pain, truthfulness versus withholding facts, feelings of helplessness and guilt, and concerns about the future. In addition, the fear of loss is always present. Depending on the circumstances, supportive care for the terminally ill child and for the family may be necessary. Oncology support groups are particularly helpful. The families identify with one another and share common concerns.

Radiation treatment requires preparation. The radiologist outlines the areas to be treated. These marks are not washed off. Small doses of radiation are given over a period of weeks. The nurse determines what the radiologist has told the patient. Support is given to the child, who may fear being burned. The nurse explains that the child will be alone in the room but will retain voice contact. The patient is given a tour of the facility. Physical symptoms of fear are noted, such as dry mouth, pupillary dilation, trembling, and clinging. Untoward effects of treatment may begin about the end of the 1st week. Headaches, anorexia, nausea and vomiting, diarrhea, and general lethargy may ensue. More severe effects include leukopenia, decrease in platelets, skin breakdown, and hair loss. The family is reassured that the hair will grow back but that it may be a different color or texture. Medication may be prescribed to help alleviate symptoms. Nutritious foods in small quantities are offered. A pleasant environment is provided, one that is free of odors, sounds, and sights that might induce nausea.

**Chemotherapy Regimens.** Chemotherapy regimens are individualized and various combinations of medication are utilized. The child and family are prepared for the possible side effects of medications. This is initially done by the physician in charge of treatment. Ongoing education by nurses is necessary, as distraught parents can incorporate only so many facts. The nurse stresses the importance of return visits to monitor bone marrow depression and other parameters. Children need to know that the medicine is designed to make them feel better but that they may feel sicker at first. The nurse frequently observes the sleeping child who has experienced nausea and vomiting. The patient is positioned to avoid aspiration. Prolonged vomiting may be an indication that the medicine should be withheld or reduced. In cases in which therapy is being administered on an outpatient basis, careful instruction of parents or guardians is paramount.

The period of convalescence is punctuated by frequent clinic visits that are anxiety-provoking. "Will the blood tests be all right?" "She's lost so much weight." "I hope he won't have to go back on medication." Some parents have to commute long distances to medical facilities. These problems involve all aspects of care of the chronically ill child. Some nurses try to maintain contact with discharged patients by mail, reunions at the clinic, and involvement in cancer camps.

The community health nurse and school nurse become significant persons on discharge. The child must maintain adequate nutrition and hydration. The child is assisted in relating to a new body image. This may be augmented with caps, wigs, or head scarfs. Residual effects depend on the type and extent of the tumor. It is not unusual for information, such as the death of a loved child, to reach persons who were directly involved with the child's care. This news can create grief, which must be dealt with by the medical persons involved (see p. 889).

## NEUROBLASTOMA

**Description.** Neuroblastoma is considered the most common malignant solid tumor of infancy and childhood. The median age at the time of diagnosis is about 2. "Deletions in chromosome 1 are commonly found in tumor tissue" (Behrman, 1992). The neuroblastoma occurs during embryonic development and may be evidenced wherever sympathetic nervous tissue is found. Although it may originate anywhere along the craniospinal axis, it is most often seen in the abdomen, in which case it may arise from the adrenal medulla. It is also seen in the head, neck, chest, or pelvis.

**Manifestations.** The primary tumor is often discovered as a mass in the upper abdomen. Urinary frequency may be noticed if there is compression on the ureters or bladder. Pressure on the adrenal gland from the tumor may cause excessive perspiration, flushed face, and hypertension. Other primary tumors cause symptoms associated with their location, such as weakness of the extremities, respiratory embarrassment, supraorbital ecchymoses, or *proptosis* (protruding eye). In addition, general systemic manifestations such as lethargy, anorexia, and weight loss may be evidenced. Disseminated disease is common at the time of diagnosis.

**Treatment and Nursing Care.** Neuroblastoma must be differentiated from Wilms' tumor, cystic kidneys, and hydronephrosis. Emphasis is placed on locating the primary site and any areas of metastasis. Cerebral and thoracic CT scans, angiography, and bone scans are useful. Urinary and plasma catecholamines may be elevated. Surgery, chemotherapy, and irradiation

**Table 24–4.** CRITERIA FOR STAGING OF NEUROBLASTOMA

| Stage | Criteria |
|-------|----------|
| I | Localized tumor, well encapsulated, confined |
| II | Extended to local lymph nodes, not midline |
| III | Extensive tumor spread across midline |
| IV | Distant metastasis with involvement of bone |
| IVS* | Patient who otherwise would be stage I or II with small tumor; metastasis confined to liver, skin, or bone marrow; not bone |

*S, special.

are used for therapy. Table 24–4 lists the staging systems used in planning treatment and determining progress. Spontaneous regression may occur, particularly in children under 1 year of age who have stage I or stage IVS disease.

Nursing considerations are similar to those for children with other neoplasms. When a 24-hour urine specimen is collected for catecholamines, their end products, vanillylmandelic acid and homovanillic acid, are measured. A 24-hour urine specimen is collected in a refrigerated brown bottle to which the preservative hydrochloric acid has been added. Two days before collection, the patient is restricted from eating such foods as ice cream, bananas, and foods containing vanilla flavoring. The nurse checks laboratory procedure manuals for these restrictions and also for exercise limitations. Treatment success depends heavily on the child's age and stage of disease. Bone marrow transplants for these patients have commenced. Because this diagnosis is so threatening, every effort is made to support the child's family and to offer home care and hospice services as indicated.

## SEIZURE DISORDERS (EPILEPSY)

**Description.** The term *epilepsy* (chronic recurrent convulsions) comes from the Greek *epilepsia*, which means "seizure." It is the name of a very old and misunderstood disease. Over 2 million Americans have the disorder. Three of four cases begin in childhood. Education of the patient and family is a prime consideration in developing nursing care plans. In the past, words such as "fit," "spell," and "blackout" were used to describe this entity. These are nonspecific and create confusion. Children who state that they are subject to seizures indicate that they are aware of their condition and encourage others to relate to them in a mature way.

Epilepsy is characterized by recurrent paroxysmal attacks of unconsciousness or impaired consciousness that may be followed by alternate contraction and relaxation of the muscles or by disturbed feelings or behavior. It is a disorder of the CNS in which the neurons or nerve cells discharge in an abnormal way. These discharges may be focal or diffuse. The site of general discharge can sometimes be ascertained by observing the patient's symptoms during the attack. The international classification of epileptic seizures is condensed in Table 24–5. It provides a framework on which medical therapy may be based. When the cause is unknown, the term *idiopathic* (spontaneous) or *cryptogenic* (hidden) is used. If a cerebral abnormality is found, the patient may be said to have *organic* or *symptomatic* epilepsy.

Idiopathic epilepsy is the most common cause of recurrent convulsions in children older than 3 years of age. It is possible that some specific genetic defect in cerebral metabolism is responsible in many children. It has been pointed out that electroencephalographic abnormalities (cerebral dysrhythmias) are more likely to be found in parents and siblings of affected children than in the population at large.

Organic epilepsy may be caused by a number of conditions or injuries that have impaired the brain. Many genetically determined conditions, such as phenylketonuria (PKU), hydrocephalus, and tuberous sclerosis, are associated with seizures. Convulsions may also occur as a result of brain injury during prenatal, perinatal, or postnatal periods. Acute infections may be responsible for epilepsy in infants and toddlers. There are also contributing conditions that can alter the convulsive threshold. If the patient becomes overtired or overexcited or faces a stressful situation, a seizure may occur. An alteration in serum and brain concentrations of sodium, potassium, and water due to fluid retention can be a precipitating factor. Hormonal changes during puberty, excess fluid intake, and photogenic stimulation have also been suggested as causes.

Prevention of organic epilepsy is fostered by nurses who promote good prenatal and postnatal care and healthful living for children. Parents need to be educated about the importance of providing a safe environment and supervision for small children. Play areas need to be properly supervised, poisonous substances must be stored away from little hands, and proper seat belts should be worn in automobiles to prevent head injury. Early diagnosis and treatment for conditions such as PKU, meningitis, Reye's syndrome, and encephalitis are also crucial in minimizing irreversible brain damage. Children must be immunized against childhood diseases that could foster epilepsy. The abuse of drugs, including alcohol, and drug combinations by teenagers can result in cerebral anoxia and convulsions, and this danger should be stressed in comprehensive health teaching for this age group.

It is not possible or desirable to shield children from every stressful situation, but adults can assist growing children by helping them to make wise decisions at their level of competence and by being supportive. The response of parents and nurses in stressful situations is also important as role modeling.

**Types and Manifestations.** Symptoms vary according to the type of seizure. Mixed seizures may also occur in epileptics. Seizures may be convulsive or nonconvulsive.

*Tonic-Clonic (Grand Mal).* This is the most common type of seizure and probably the most dramatic. It is centrencephalic, emanating from the central portion of the brain. It is a generalized convulsion, usually with *tonic* and *clonic* phases. Onset is abrupt. During the tonic phase, the body stiffens; the patient may simultaneously lose consciousness and may drop to the floor if sitting or standing. This may be preceded by an aura, which is a particular sensation, such as dizziness, visual images, nausea, headache, or an ascending feeling of abdominal discomfort. This phenomenon is not as well established in children, who may be unable to describe it.

The face becomes pale at first and then cyanotic because of the arrest of respiratory movements. The eyes roll upward or to one side. The child may utter a brief cry as air is forced out of the lungs across tightly closed vocal cords. The head, back, and legs stiffen. This phase lasts about 20–40 seconds and is followed by the clonic phase, which lasts for variable periods. Jerking movements of the trunk and extremities begin. Frothing at the mouth, biting of the tongue, and urinary or fecal incontinence may occur. Muscle contraction and relaxation gradually subside, and the child enters the postictal (*post*, "after," and *ictus*, "a sudden stroke") state. The patient appears dazed and confused and generally sleeps for a while.

On awakening, the patient may complain of a headache and may perform more or less auto-

**Table 24–5.** SEIZURE RECOGNITION AND FIRST AID

| Seizure Type | What It Looks Like | Often Mistaken for | What to Do | What Not to Do |
|---|---|---|---|---|
| Generalized tonic-clonic (also called grand mal) | Sudden cry, fall, rigidity, followed by muscle jerking, shallow breathing or temporarily suspended breathing, bluish skin, or possible loss of bladder or bowel control; usually lasts a couple of minutes; normal breathing then starts again; may be some confusion or fatigue, followed by return to full consciousness | Heart attack Stroke | Look for medical identification Protect from nearby hazards Loosen ties or shirt collars Protect head from injury Turn on side to keep airway clear Reassure when consciousness returns If single seizure lasted less than 5 min, ask if hospital evaluation is wanted If multiple seizures, or if one seizure lasts longer than 5 min, call ambulance If person is pregnant, injured, or diabetic, call for aid at once | Do not put any hard implement in the mouth Do not try to hold tongue; it cannot be swallowed Do not try to give liquids during or just after seizure Do not use artificial respiration unless breathing is absent after muscle jerks subside, or unless water has been inhaled Do not restrain |
| Absence (also called petit mal) | A blank stare, beginning and ending abruptly, lasting only a few seconds; most common in children; may be accompanied by rapid blinking, some chewing movements of the mouth; child is unaware of what is going on during the seizure, but quickly returns to full awareness once it has stopped; may result in learning difficulties if not recognized and treated | Daydreaming Lack of attention Deliberate ignoring of adult instructions | No first aid necessary, but if this is first observation of seizure(s), medical evaluation should be recommended | |
| Simple partial (also called jacksonian) | Jerking may begin in one area of body, arm, leg, or face; cannot be stopped, but patient stays awake and aware; jerking may proceed from one area of the body to another and sometimes spreads to become a convulsive seizure | Acting out, bizarre behavior Hysteria Mental illness Psychosomatic illnes Parapsychological or mystical experience | No first aid necessary unless seizure becomes convulsive, then first aid as indicated; no immediate action needed other than reassurance and emotional support; medical evaluation should be recommended | |

**Table 24–5.** SEIZURE RECOGNITION AND FIRST AID *Continued*

| Seizure Type | What It Looks Like | Often Mistaken for | What to Do | What Not to Do |
|---|---|---|---|---|
| Simple partial (also called sensory) | May not be obvious to onlooker, other than patient's preoccupied or blank expression; patient experiences a distorted environment; may see or hear things that are not there, may feel unexplained fear, sadness, anger, or joy; may have nausea, experience odd smells, and have a generally "funny" feeling in the stomach | Hysteria<br>Mental illness<br>Psychosomatic illness<br>Parapsychological or mystical experience<br>Drunkenness<br>Intoxication on drugs<br>Mental illness | No action needed other than reassurance and emotional support | |
| Complex partial (also called psychomotor or temporal lobe) | Usually starts with blank stare, followed by chewing, followed by random activity; person appears unaware of surroundings, may seem dazed and mumble, is unresponsive; actions clumsy, not directed; may pick at clothing, pick up objects, try to take off clothes; may run, appear afraid; may struggle or flail at restraint; once pattern established, same set of actions usually occurs with each seizure; lasts a few minutes, but postseizure confusion can last substantially longer; no memory of what happened during seizure | Disorderly conduct | Speak calmly and reassuringly to patient and others<br>Guide gently away from obvious hazards<br>Stay with person until completely aware of environment<br>Offer to help getting home | Do not grab hold unless sudden danger (such as a cliff edge or an approaching car) threatens<br>Do not try to restrain<br>Do not shout<br>Do not expect verbal instructions to be obeyed |
| Atonic seizures (also called drop attacks) | A child or adult suddenly collapses; after 10 sec to 1 min, child recovers, regains consciousness, and can stand and walk again | Clumsiness<br>Normal childhood stage<br>In a child, lack of good walking skills<br>In an adult, drunkenness, acute illness | No first aid needed (unless hurt during fall), but the child should be given a thorough medical evaluation | |

*Continued*

**Table 24–5.** SEIZURE RECOGNITION AND FIRST AID *Continued*

| Seizure Type | What It Looks Like | Often Mistaken for | What to Do | What Not to Do |
|---|---|---|---|---|
| Myoclonic seizures | Sudden brief, massive muscle jerks that may involve whole body or parts of body; may cause person to spill what was holding or fall off a chair | Clumsiness Poor coordination | No first aid needed, but should be given a thorough medical evaluation | |
| Infantile spasms | These are clusters of quick, sudden movements that start between 3 mo and 2 yr; if child is sitting up, head falls forward, and arms flex forward; if child is lying down, knees are drawn up, with arms and head flexed forward as if baby is reaching for support | Normal movements of baby, especially if they happen when baby is lying down | No first aid, but prompt medical evaluation is needed | |

From Epilepsy Foundation of America. (1989). *Seizure recognition and first aid.* Landover, MD: Author.

matic acts. This is believed to be due to malfunctioning of the neurons, which may not be fully recovered. There is no recollection of the seizure. *Status epilepticus* is a series of convulsions rapidly following one another. The most common cause is abrupt withdrawal of anticonvulsant medication. It is an emergency situation because death can result from respiratory failure and exhaustion.

Table 24–5 describes the first aid treatment for various types of seizures. The nurse observes and records the following: the child's activity immediately before the seizure; body movements; changes in color, respiration, or muscle tone; incontinence; and the parts of the body involved. When possible, the seizure is timed. The child's appearance, behavior, and level of consciousness following the seizure are also documented.

*Absence (Petit Mal).* These seizures are characterized by transient loss of consciousness. They originate from the central portion of the brain and cortex and last less than 30 seconds. There may be associated upward rolling of the eyes, rhythmic nodding of the head, or slight quivering of the limbs. This condition is rarely seen in children less than 3 years old and often disappears by puberty. The patient seldom falls but may drop articles being held. These episodes are often referred to by parents as "lapses," "absences," or "dizzy spells." The condition is more common among girls. Attacks vary in frequency. Following the attack, the child is alert and appears normal, as if nothing had happened.

*Atonic (Akinetic).* Also called "drop seizures," akinetic seizures are characterized by a sudden loss of postural muscle tone. The patient loses consciousness momentarily and if standing may fall to the ground. Some patients experience only a dropping forward of the head and neck. The episodes may occur frequently during the day.

*Myoclonic.* These are brief, shocklike contractions that may involve the entire body or be confined to the face, trunk, or extremities.

*Infantile Spasms.* Infantile spasms usually start between 3 months and 2 years. There may be a sudden dropping of the head and flexion of the arms. Clonic movements of the extremities may also be seen. The episodes last only a few seconds and vary in frequency. They are the most common type of seizure seen in infancy, with the exception of febrile convulsions. When spasms occur before 4 months of age, a congenital cerebral defect is most likely. There may be significant developmental retardation. Infantile spasms disappear at about 4 years of age but are often replaced by major motor seizures.

*Simple Partial.* Focal or partial cortical seizures may arise from any area of the cerebral cortex but usually affect the frontal, temporal, or parietal lobe. They may be either motor or sensory in nature. Focal seizures may sometimes become generalized. Minor one-sided tonic or clonic seizures are most common in children.

*Complex Partial (Psychomotor).* This type of seizure is more common in adults but is also seen in children over 3 years of age. It is localized to the temporal lobe of the cerebrum and is characterized by an altered state of consciousness. The patient appears to be in a dreamlike state. The child may perform *automatisms,* such as lip smacking, grimacing, or repeating words. The young child may cry out and run to an adult. There are generally no clonic or tonic movements, although the patient may gently collapse to the floor. A brief period of unconsciousness may follow. On awakening, the patient resumes normal activities. Some patients sleep for a period of time. These seizures are difficult to recognize and control. Electroencephalographic patterns remain normal except when the EGG is taken during an attack.

**Treatment and Nursing Care.** Initially, treatment is aimed at determining the type, site, or cause of the disorder. Diagnostic measures include a complete history and physical and neurologic examinations. Skull radiography and CT are employed to establish the presence or absence of tumors, skull abnormalities, hematomas, and intracranial calcifications. MRI may be utilized. The EEG is also a valuable tool in evaluating seizures. It is especially helpful in differentiating between an absence seizure and a complex partial seizure. Video EEG recordings can detect more subtle manifestations and provide a permanent record for playback. Prolonged ambulatory EEG monitoring (24 hours) is another advanced technique.

Laboratory studies such as complete blood count (CBC) and determinations of serum calcium and blood urea nitrogen (BUN) may detect acute infections, lead poisoning, or other metabolic disorders. A spinal tap may be ordered when encephalitis or meningitis is suspected. If the seizure is related to any such underlying cause, appropriate therapy is begun. Anticonvulsive drug therapy is begun only after all such causes have been excluded. Several neurosurgical procedures are available for selected cases.

**Table 24–6.** PROPERTIES OF SOME COMMONLY USED ANTICONVULSANT DRUGS

| Drug | Side Effects | Comments |
|---|---|---|
| Tegretol (carbamazepine) | Blurred vision, diplopia, drowsiness, vertigo | Few side effects, fewer sedative properties |
| Luminal (phenobarbital) | Drowsiness, irritability, hyperactivity | Safest overall medication; bitter, often combined with other drugs |
| Dilantin (phenytoin) | Ataxia, insomnia, motor twitching, gum overgrowth, hirsutism (hairiness), rash, nausea, vitamin D and folic acid deficiencies | Generally effective and safe; regular massaging of gums decreases hyperplasia; used in combination with phenobarbital or primidone |
| Depakene (valproic acid) | Gastrointestinal disturbance, altered bleeding time, liver toxicity | Monitor blood counts; take with food or use enteric-coated preparations; potentiates action of phenobarbital and other drugs |
| Mysoline (primidone) | Ataxia, vertigo, anorexia, fatigue, hyperirritability, dermatitis | May be used alone or in combination; side effects minimized by starting with small amounts |
| Valium (diazepam) | Headache, tremor, fatigue, depression | Used in combination or alone |
| Clonopin (clonazepam) | Behavior changes, ataxia, anorexia, nystagmus | Effective for most minor motor seizures |

*Note:* The physician determines the child's medication by the type of seizure and other factors. The goal is to achieve the best control with the minimum dosage and the least number of side effects. An important aspect of nursing intervention includes reinforcing the need for drug supervision and compliance.

Some common anticonvulsants and their side effects are listed in Table 24–6. The duration of therapy is individual. Initially, the doctor prescribes the lowest dose likely to control the seizures. The doctor may have to experiment with a combination of drugs. Drowsiness, a common side effect of many anticonvulsants, can interfere with the child's activities and requires regulation. Careful recording of seizure activity and adherence to the drug regimen are of particular importance in determining a suitable program. The medication is not addictive when used as prescribed. Tablet form is preferable to suspensions, which are more expensive and tend to separate if not shaken well. Most small children can ingest the tablet when it is administered in a teaspoon with a small amount of applesauce. Medication is given at the same time each day, generally with meals or at bedtime.

If it is necessary for the child to take medication during school hours, the parents sign a consent form so that the school nurse can monitor administration. This provides the child and the nurse opportunities to get acquainted and share their knowledge of the disease. Nurse and teacher response, particularly during and after a seizure, will have a significant effect on the attitude of classmates toward the disease.

Medication must be reduced gradually under a physician's supervision, because abrupt withdrawal of medications is the most common cause of status epilepticus. In the hospital, the nurse consults the physician as to whether anticonvulsants are to be withheld if the patient is to consume nothing by mouth. As in any long-term drug therapy, periodic blood and urine tests are performed to detect subtle side effects. When children are old enough, they can assume responsibility for their own medications. They should wear a Medic-Alert bracelet. During puberty and adolescence, dosages may have to be adjusted to meet growth needs. Premenstrual fluid retention in girls can sometimes trigger seizures. Surgery is being performed on children who are unresponsive to anticonvulsants and who have a well-defined focus of seizure activity in the brain. It does not eliminate the need for medication.

The ketogenic diet is sometimes prescribed for children who do not respond well to anticonvulsant therapy. It is high in fats and low in carbohydrates and produces ketoacidosis in the body, which appears to have a calming effect. The use of medium-chain triglycerides is more flexible and palatable. It simulates fasting, which has been used for years to control grand mal seizures. Reduction of fluid intake tends to increase its ketogenic effect. Use is limited because the diet is boring and requires strict adherence to intake. Ketogenic diets lose some of their anticonvulsant effects over time (Mahan & Arlin, 1992).

Rebellion against medical routine is not uncommon during adolescence. Some states do not allow controlled epileptics to obtain a driver's license, which is disheartening to the patient. Other states have stipulations as to the amount of seizure-free time required before licensing. Obtaining insurance may be difficult. Excess intake of fluids, particularly alcoholic beverages, can be a source of contention. Parents can obtain valuable information and support from the Epilepsy Foundation of America. Other major resources include the Department of Vocational Rehabilitation, the Department of Public Health, the Department of Social Services, and the Department of Mental Health. The greatest untapped resource for persons with epilepsy is often within themselves. In a comprehensive treatment approach, team members help the persons mobilize their inner resources. The need for public education to dispel the myths surrounding the disease is paramount (Epilepsy Foundation of America, 1992).

A fundamental principle of comprehensive epilepsy management is that the person become an active member of the team. The well-controlled patient can lead a normal life with a few safety restrictions. A family assessment is helpful in establishing rapport and setting realistic short-term and long-term goals. Too much attention to seizures by well-meaning adults can make control difficult. The child may also learn to use the threat of a seizure to manipulate caretakers. Patients can participate in selected athletic and recreational activities. Death or serious injury rarely occurs from a seizure, and it does not cause mental deterioration. The Individuals with Disabilities Education Act (IDEA) guarantees children with disabilities the right to publicly financed educational programs in the least restrictive environment. Most patients under proper treatment can lead full and productive lives.

## CEREBRAL PALSY

**Description.** Cerebral palsy refers to a group of nonprogressive disorders that affect the motor centers of the brain. It is not fatal in itself, but at present there is no cure. It is one of the most common handicapping conditions seen in children; there are at least 300,000 affected children in the United States. This disease is caused by many factors, some of which are birth injuries, neonatal anoxia, subdural hemorrhage, and infections such as meningitis and encephalitis. Studies indicate that more than one-third of children with cerebral palsy weighed less than 2500 gm at birth. Lead poisoning, head injuries, and febrile illness are sometimes responsible during the toddler period. In some patients, no single cause can be found.

**Manifestations.** The symptoms of cerebral palsy vary with each child and may range from mild to severe. Mental retardation sometimes accompanies this disorder; however, many victims have normal intelligence. The disease is suspected during infancy if there are feeding problems, convulsions not associated with high fever, and physical retardation. (The child cannot sit, crawl, creep, stand, and so forth at the approximate age level expected.) *Ataxia*, or lack of muscle coordination, may be seen. Diagnostic tests may include spinal tap, electroencephalography, pneumoencephalography, CT, and screening for metabolic disorders. Brain tumors must also be ruled out. Early recognition is important.

There are many types of cerebral palsy (Table 24–7). Two of the more common are those marked by spasticity and athetosis (Fig. 24–9). These conditions occur in about 75% of the cases. Spasticity is characterized by tension in certain muscle groups. The stretch reflex is present in the involved muscles. When the child tries to move the voluntary muscles, jerky motions result, and eating, walking, and other coordinated movements are difficult to accomplish. The lower extremities are usually involved. The legs cross and the toes point inward. The arms and trunk may also be affected. In *athetosis*, the patient has involuntary, purposeless movements that interfere with normal motion. Speech, sight, and hearing defects and convulsions may be complications. Emotional problems sometimes present more difficulties than does the physical disability.

**Treatment and Nursing Care.** The objective of treatment of children with cerebral palsy is to assist them in making the most of their assets and to guide them in becoming happy, well-adjusted adults performing at their maximum ability. Both short-term and long-term goals must be realistic. Parents need help in accepting the child and should not be deceived into expecting miraculous cures from treatment.

**Table 24–7.** CLASSIFICATION OF CEREBRAL PALSY

| Type | Comment |
| --- | --- |
| Spastic | Most common, approximately 65% of patients |
| Also classified by distribution of muscles involved: | |
| Hemiplegia | Limited to one side of the body |
| Paraplegia | Involves legs only |
| Quadriplegia | Involves all four extremities (upper and lower limbs equally affected) |
| Athetosis | Second most frequent type |
| Ataxia | Least common form, approximately 1–10% of patients; characterized by imbalance, nystagmus, lurching |
| Mixed types | Most often athetosis and spasticity |
| Degree of severity | |
| Mild | Affects fine precision |
| Moderate | Affects gross and fine movements and speech; patient is able to perform usual activities of daily living |
| Severe | Patient is unable to perform usual activities of daily living |

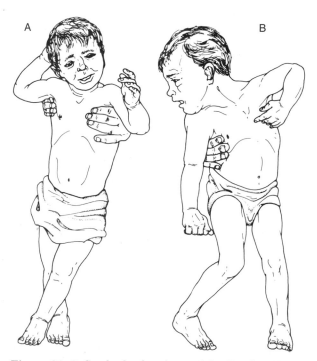

**Figure 24–9.** Cerebral palsy: *A*, spasticity. *B*, athetosis.

The sooner the case is diagnosed, the fewer the physical and emotional problems.

Parents must be informed of community resources available to them. The patient's religious affiliation should not be overlooked, as it can be a source of support and help during times of stress. The long course of this disability is a financial burden. Caretakers need respite care from time to time so that they can refresh their outlook on life.

The specific treatment is highly individualistic, depending on the severity of the disease. It is not uncommon for the parents of children with cerebral palsy to become the experts in caring for their child. Therefore, it behooves medical personnel to listen and incorporate parents' suggestions when developing nursing care plans.

Good skin care is essential for the patient with cerebral palsy. The nurse observes the skin for redness and other evidence of pressure sores. The bedclothes are kept clean, dry, and free of wrinkles.

All precautions are taken to prevent the formation of *contractures* (degeneration or shortening of the muscles due to lack of use). The damage may be permanent, resulting in a loss of function of the part involved, for example, leg, arm, or finger. A common expression in relation to this is "What you don't use, you lose." Knowing this, the nurse represses a natural desire to help the patients and encourages them to do as much as they can for themselves. When patients take their own bath in the morning, they put their muscles and joints through the normal range of motion. When nurses give the bath, they put *their* muscles through the necessary movements, not the patient's. Of course the nurse must use judgment in assessing the patient's capabilities.

Other measures necessary to prevent deformities include frequent change of position, the use of splints, and the carrying out of passive, range-of-motion, and stretching exercises. The nurse must also ensure that the patient maintains good posture while in bed. This is done through the use of footboards and the proper positioning of pillows and other comfort devices. The principles involved in preventing contractures can be applied to the nursing care of all long-term patients. The physical therapist spends many hours with the patient. Instructions must be carried out by unit personnel to ensure continuity of care.

Braces are frequently used in the treatment of this disability. A brace is a mechanical aid that strengthens or supports weakened muscles or limbs. All braces are checked from time to time for correct alignment, loose or missing parts, and condition of the straps and buckles. The child needs assistance to adjust to this unfamiliar device. Wheelchairs and crutches are designed to the size of the patients.

Orthopedic surgery may be indicated. It may be followed by an extensive period of hospitalization. The nurse must remember that the child is in a continuous state of psychological as well as physical growth during this period. Interest, or lack of it, may have a decided effect on the personality of the child in later years. The nursing care of the patient with a cast is discussed on page 345.

Feeding problems can lead to nutritional deficiencies. Vitamin, mineral, or protein supplements may be indicated for some children. Swallowing and sucking may be difficult. Vomiting is frequent because the gag reflex is overactive. The entire body may become tense. The nurse must be especially careful to feed the child slowly in order to prevent aspiration. It is difficult for these infants to adjust to solid foods, and it takes a great deal of patience on the part of parents and nurses to help them adapt to this new experience. As the children grow, they can be taught to manage special feeding equipment so that they are able to eat independently. They are also taught such activities as dressing and combing their hair.

The physically challenged child needs opportunities to play alone and with other children. Games suited to ability, such as finger painting, are fun and allow freedom of expression. Activities that require fine muscular movements of the hand cause frustration in the child whose arms and hands are affected by the disease. The nurse can learn a great deal from the parents about types of play the child enjoys.

Children with cerebral palsy tire easily but find it difficult to relax. They are under a constant strain to accomplish the simplest of tasks. They do not respond well to being hurried or overstimulated. The nurse must see that they take frequent naps in a quiet room. They should not become overexcited before bedtime.

Educational opportunities geared to the patient's abilities are essential. Public law 94-142 mandates that public schools provide education for handicapped children. The patient's mental capacity is determined not just in the light of IQ itself but also by the demonstrated potential of the individual. Mental ability is difficult to evaluate because the type of brain injury associated with cerebral palsy interferes with both verbal and motor expression.

Nursery schools are available. Summer camps for exceptional children are becoming more numerous. These programs vary in the quality and the extent of services provided. Parents need the nurse's and physician's aid in determining the best type of program for their child. Parents are also referred to the United Cerebral Palsy Association, a national organization that provides education and support services. The expanding role of nurses in the home may further involve them in mainstreaming these children into social situations once denied them.

Children with cerebral palsy may appear to be emotionally unstable. This is not surprising when one considers the number of activities denied them that are associated with normal growth and development. Take for instance the task of tying a shoe. Well children become frustrated when they cannot make a bow from the laces. They try over and over again. Mastering this simple task is a source of pride and accomplishment. The handicapped child finds the same procedure overwhelming. It is a continual source of failure. Successful experiences help to improve a child's self-concept; repeated failures are demoralizing and may lower self-esteem. The cerebral palsy team works to bring satisfaction to these patients by making it possible for them to succeed. The amount of confidence and self-respect that a disabled person has depends a great deal on a supportive environment. Although some emotional instability generally accompanies disorders of the nervous system, much of it results from the kind of guidance the person has had, particularly during the formative years.

**Mental Health Needs of the Physically Challenged Child.** The requirements for good mental health in the physically challenged child do not differ greatly from those for all persons. They need to have their basic human drives satisfied and people who are genuinely interested in them. As children grow, they need social experience with both sexes to help them adjust to adolescence (Fig. 24–10). The disabled child needs to participate to the fullest extent in family, school, and community activities. Friendships with other handicapped and nonhandicapped peers are encouraged. Extended family and the community are important resources or sources of stress. Frequently families are isolated or stigmatized because of fear and lack of knowledge on the part of the public. Educational programs are attempting to integrate the handicapped more fully into the community. Barrier-free buildings and modifications that improve accessibility contribute positively to these efforts.

**Attitude of the Nurse.** Inexperienced nurses may find that they are not immediately attracted to children who are physically challenged and who may be unattractive. They may feel inadequate and may not know how to approach or assist them. Fear of the unknown is natural. Focus may be on the abnormalities of the child rather than on the child as a person. The nurse's first problem may be to think of what to say to the child. The best advice is the easiest: Be natural and treat the child in a natural manner. Listen to what is being said. Do not be overly kind and solicitous, for this increases dependence. Let the child do as much for the self as possible. Be there to assist if necessary but do not wait on the child hand and foot. The child is happier without pity. Limit setting is essential and provides security. Even patients with the most serious defects can grow up to be happy and self-reliant if they are accepted as they are and are encouraged to perform the tasks they are capable of doing.

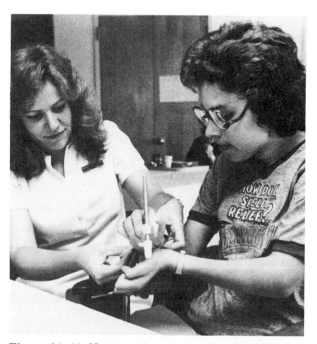

**Figure 24–10.** New experiences await the physically challenged adolescent. Positive encouragement from an early age on helps the youngster develop a healthy self-concept. (Courtesy of Blank Memorial Hospital for Children, Des Moines, IA.)

## KEY POINTS

- Infants are more prone to ear infections than are older children because their eustachian tube is shorter, wider, and straighter.
- Complications of ear infection include deafness, mastoiditis, and chronic otitis media. Partially treated infection can lead to meningitis in young children.
- Proper immunization of infants and children against communicable diseases is a major measure in preventing deafness and other sequelae.
- When amblyopia is treated promptly in infants, it can be corrected in days or weeks. In older children, it may take months or years.
- Do not give aspirin or other salicylates to children with symptoms of influenza or chickenpox because the drug is linked to the cause of Reye's syndrome, a serious and life-threatening illness.
- Level of consciousness is the most important indicator of neurologic health.
- Nursing care of the unconscious child includes assessing the patient for increased intracranial pressure, maintaining an open airway, providing adequate nutrition and fluids, positioning and maintaining flexibility of joints, and preventing injury.
- Meningitis is an inflammation of the meninges, the covering of the brain and spinal cord.
- A seizure is a symptom of underlying pathology.
- Grand mal seizures have tonic and clonic phases.

# Study Questions

1. Peggy, age 11 months, is admitted to the hospital with the diagnosis of meningitis. List the symptoms of meningeal irritation.
2. What facilities are available in your community for patients with cerebral palsy? Deafness?
3. Billie, age 4, has alternating strabismus. What is the cause and treatment of this condition? List two methods of detection.
4. You are requested to give a talk on epilepsy to a group of school children, ages 10–12. What facts about this disease would you emphasize? Why?
5. Angela, age 2, has an ear infection. How might one determine the symptoms of an earache in a child this age?
6. List the initial symptoms of Reye's syndrome and summarize its progressive stages.
7. Outline the nursing care for a 3-year-old girl with encephalitis.
8. List the signs and symptoms of a brain tumor.
9. How is encephalitis transmitted?
10. In what condition is leukokoria (cat's eye reflex) seen?

# Multiple Choice Review Questions

*Choose the most appropriate answer.*

1. Symptoms of an earache in an infant include
   a. external drainage, pain, decrease in temperature
   b. tugging at the ear, rolling head from side to side
   c. crying, pointing to affected ear
   d. redness of the cheeks, cyanosis of ear

2. The medical term for crossed eyes is
   a. strabismus
   b. amblyopia
   c. myopia
   d. PERRLA
3. Reye's syndrome affects the
   a. stomach and intestine
   b. islet of Langerhans
   c. liver and brain
   d. heart and blood vessels

4. Following an epileptic seizure, the patient is likely to be
   a. confused
   b. delirious
   c. hostile
   d. talkative
5. The seizure in which the child cries out, falls to the floor, becomes rigid, and then has a convulsion is termed
   a. petit mal
   b. jacksonian
   c. grand mal
   d. atonic

## BIBLIOGRAPHY

Behrman, R.E. (1992). *Nelson textbook of pediatrics* (14th ed.). Philadelphia: W.B. Saunders.

Epilepsy Foundation of America. (1989). *Seizure recognition and first aid*. Landover, MD: Author.

Epilepsy Foundation of America. (1992). *The comprehensive clinical management of the epilepsies*. Landover, MD: Author.

Epilepsy Foundation of America. (1992). *How to recognize and classify seizures and epilepsy* (2nd ed.). Landover, MD: Author.

Gellis, S., & Kagan, B. (1990). *Current pediatric therapy 13*. Philadelphia: W.B. Saunders.

Graef, J., & Cone, T. (1985). *Manual of pediatric therapeutics*. Boston: Little, Brown.

Hayman, L., & Spring E. (1985). *Handbook of pediatric nursing*. New York: John Wiley & Sons.

Lockman, L. (1989). Absence, myoclonic, and atonic seizures. *Pediatric Clinics of North America*, 35:331–341.

Mahan, L.K., & Arlin, M.T. (1992). *Krause's food, nutrition & diet therapy* (8th ed.). Philadelphia: W.B. Saunders.

Mott, S., James, S.R., & Sperhac, A.M. (1991). *Nursing care of children and families*. Reading, MA: Addison-Wesley.

Pillitteri, A. (1992). *Maternal and child health nursing*. Philadelphia: J.B. Lippincott.

Porter, J.D., et al. (1990). Trends in the incidence of Reye's syndrome and the use of aspirin. *Archives of Disease in Childhood*, 65, 826.

Teele, D.W., et al. (1989). Epidemiology of otitis media during the first seven years of life in children of greater Boston: A prospective cohort study. *Journal of Infectious Diseases*, 160, 83–94.

Thompson, E.D., & Ashwill, J.W. (1992). *Pediatric nursing* (6th ed.). Philadelphia: W.B. Saunders.

Whaley, L., & Wong, D. (1991). *Nursing care of children* (4th ed.). St. Louis: C.V. Mosby.

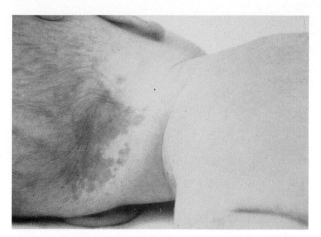

**Figure 1.** Stork bites (telangiectatic nevi). These flat, red areas are seen on the nape of the neck and on the eyelids. They result from the dilation of small vessels. (Courtesy of Jane Deacon, MS, RN, NNP, The Children's Hospital, Denver, CO.)

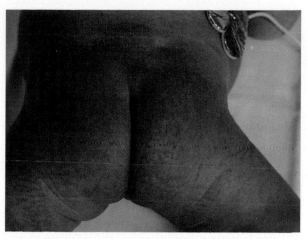

**Figure 2.** Mongolian spots (hyperpigmentation) are bluish discolorations of the skin, found mainly in newborns with dark skin tones. The sacral and gluteal areas are the usual sites. (From Gorrie, T. S., McKinney, E. S., Murray, S. S. [1994]. *Foundations of maternal newborn nursing.* Philadelphia: W. B. Saunders.)

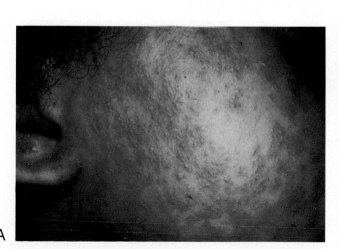

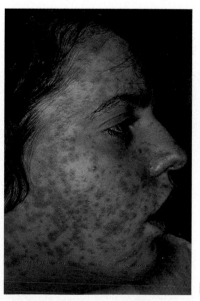

A           B

**Figure 3.** Measles (rubeola). Red-purple maculopapular blotchy rash in dark skin (*A*) and in light skin (*B*) appears on third or fourth day of illness. Rash appears first behind ears and spreads over face, then over neck, trunk, arms and legs; looks "coppery" and does not blanch. Also characterized by Koplik's spots in mouth—bluish white, red-based elevations of 1 to 3 mm. (*A*, From Feigin, R. D., & Cherry, J. D. [1987]. *Textbook of pediatric infectious diseases* [2nd ed.]. Philadelphia: W. B. Saunders, p. 807. *B*, From Hurwitz, S. [1981]. *Clinical pediatric dermatology: A textbook of skin disorders of childhood and adolescence.* Philadelphia: W. B. Saunders, p. 350.)

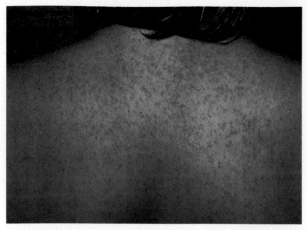

**Figure 4.** German measles (rubella). Pink papular rash (similar to measles but paler) first appears on face, then spreads. Distinguished from measles by presence of neck lymphadenopathy and absence of Koplik's spots. (From Hurwitz, S. [1993]. *Clinical pediatric dermatology: A textbook of skin disorders of childhood and adolescence* [2nd ed.]. Philadelphia: W. B. Saunders, p. 356.)

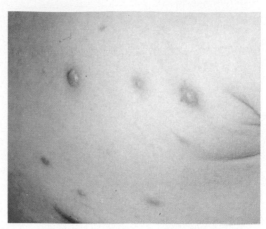

**Figure 5.** Chicken pox (varicella). Small tight vesicles first appear on trunk, then spread to face, arms, and legs (not palms or soles). Vesicles erupt in succeeding crops over several days, then become pustules, and then crusts. Intensely pruritic. (From Feigin, R. D., & Cherry, J. D. [1987]. *Textbook of pediatric infectious diseases* [2nd ed.]. Philadelphia: W. B. Saunders, p. 807.)

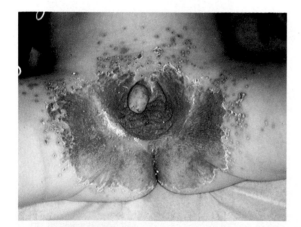

**Figure 6.** Intertrigo (candidiasis). Red, moist patches with sharply demarcated borders, some loose scales. Usually in genital area extending along inguinal and gluteal folds. Infectious disease aggravated by urine, feces, heat, moisture. (From Hurwitz, S. [1993]. *Clinical pediatric dermatology: A textbook of skin disorders of childhood and adolescence* [2nd ed.]. Philadelphia: W. B. Saunders, p. 36.)

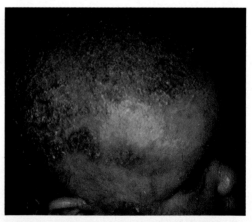

**Figure 7.** Seborrheic dermatitis (cradle cap). Thick, yellow, greasy, adherent scales on scalp and forehead; very common in early infancy. Resembles eczema lesions except cradle cap is distinguished by absence of pruritus, "greasy" yellow-pink lesions, and negative family history of allergy. (From Hurwitz, S. [1993]. *Clinical pediatric dermatology: A textbook of skin disorders of childhood and adolescence* [2nd ed.]. Philadelphia: W. B. Saunders, p. 17.)

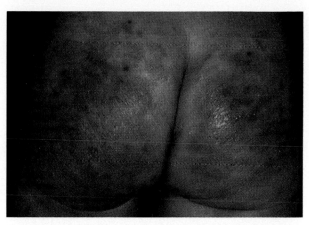

**Figure 8.** Diaper dermatitis. Red moist maculopapular patch with poorly defined borders in diaper area, extending along inguinal and gluteal folds. History of infrequent diaper changes or occlusive coverings. Inflammatory disease due to skin irritation from ammonia, heat, moisture, occlusive diapers. (From Hurwitz, S. [1993]. *Clinical pediatric dermatology: A textbook of skin disorders of childhood and adolescence* [2nd ed.]. Philadelphia: W. B. Saunders, p. 37.)

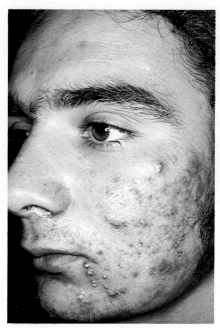

**Figure 9.** Acne. Acne is the most common skin problem of adolescence. An increase in sebaceous gland activity creates increased oiliness. Almost all teens have some acne, even if it is the milder form of open comedones (blackheads) and closed comedones (whiteheads). Severe acne includes papules, pustules, and nodules. The lesions usually appear on the face and sometimes on the chest, back, and shoulders. (From Hurwitz, S. [1993]. *Clinical pediatric dermatology: A textbook of skin disorders of childhood and adolescence* [2nd ed.]. Philadelphia: W. B. Saunders, p. 137.)

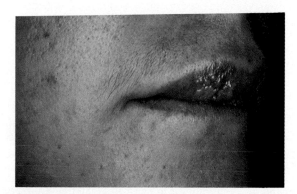

**Figure 10.** Herpes simplex (cold sores). Begins with skin tingling and sensitivity. Erupts with tight vesicles, then pustules, then crust. Common location is upper lip; also appears in genitalia. (From Hurwitz, S. [1993]. *Clinical pediatric dermatology: A textbook of skin disorders of childhood and adolescence* [2nd ed.]. Philadelphia: W. B. Saunders, p. 321.)

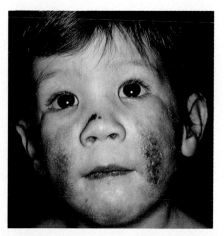

**Figure 11.** Infantile eczema (atopic dermatitis). Erythematous papules and vesicles, with weeping, oozing, and crusts. Lesions usually on scalp, forehead, cheeks, forearms and wrists, elbows, backs of knees. Paroxysmal and severe pruritus. Family history of allergies. (From Hurwitz, S. [1993]. *Clinical pediatric dermatology: A textbook of skin disorders of childhood and adolescence* [2nd ed.]. Philadelphia: W. B. Saunders, p. 280.)

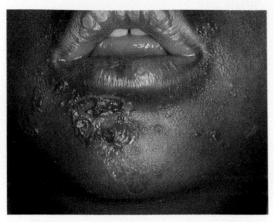

**Figure 12.** Impetigo. Moist, thin-roofed vesicles with thin erythematous base. Rupture to form thick honey-colored crusts. Contagious bacterial infection of skin; most common in infants and children. (From Hurwitz, S. [1993]. *Clinical pediatric dermatology: A textbook of skin disorders of childhood and adolescence* [2nd ed.]. Philadelphia: W. B. Saunders, p. 280.)

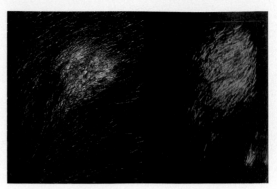

**Figure 13.** Tinea capitis (scalp ringworm). Rounded patchy hair loss on scalp, leaving broken off hairs, pustules, and scales on skin. Due to fungal infection; lesions fluoresce under Wood's light. Usually seen in children and farmers; highly contagious. (From Lookingbill, D. P., & Marks, J. G. [1993]. *Principles of dermatology* [2nd ed.]. Philadelphia: W. B. Saunders, p. 282.)

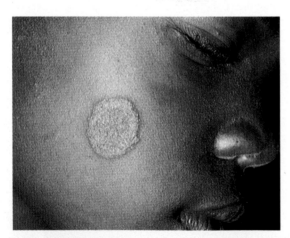

**Figure 14.** Tinea corporis (ringworm of the body). Scales—hyperpigmented in whites, depigmented in dark-skinned persons—on chest, abdomen, back of arms, forming multiple circular lesions with clear centers. (From Hurwitz, S. [1993]. *Clinical pediatric dermatology: A textbook of skin disorders of childhood and adolescence* [2nd ed.]. Philadelphia: W. B. Saunders, p. 380.)

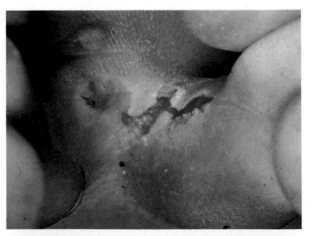

**Figure 15.** Tinea pedis (ringworm of the foot). "Athlete's foot," a fungal infection, first appears as small vesicles between toes, sides of feet, soles. Then grows scaly and hard. Found in chronically warm moist feet: children after gymnasium activities, athletes, aging adults who cannot dry their feet well. (From Feigin, R. D., & Cherry, J. D. [1987]. *Textbook of pediatric infectious diseases* [2nd ed.]. Philadelphia: W. B. Saunders, p. 813.)

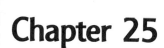

# Chapter 25

# The Child with a Musculoskeletal Condition

## VOCABULARY
arthroscope (650)
Buck extension (656)
compound fracture (654)
epiphyses (653)
ischemia (655)
Milwaukee brace (669)
nuchal rigidity (667)
osteochondroses (652)
retrograde amnesia (665)
shin splint (671)

Duchenne's Muscular Dystrophy
  (Pseudohypertrophic)
Legg-Calvé-Perthes Disease (Coxa Plana)
Traumatic Fractures and Traction
Osteomyelitis
Osteosarcoma
Ewing's Sarcoma
Juvenile Rheumatoid Arthritis
Head Injuries
Torticollis (Wry Neck)
Scoliosis
Sports Injuries

# OBJECTIVES

*On completion and mastery of Chapter 25, the student will be able to*

- Define each vocabulary term listed.
- List two symptoms of Duchenne's muscular dystrophy.
- Name a procedure commonly performed on an injury to the knee.
- Differentiate between Buck extension and Russell traction.
- Describe two topics of discussion applicable at discharge for the child with juvenile rheumatoid arthritis.
- Describe the symptoms, treatment, and nursing care for the child with Legg-Calvé-Perthes disease.
- Compile a nursing care plan for the child who is immobilized by traction.
- Describe the signs of increased intracranial pressure in the child suffering from a head injury. Include nursing observations necessary to establish a baseline of information.
- Describe three nursing care measures required to maintain skin integrity in a 14-year-old child casted for scoliosis. Provide the rationale for each measure.

The musculoskeletal system supports the body and provides for movement. The muscular and skeletal systems work together to enable a person to sit, walk, and remain upright. In addition, muscles move air into and out of the lungs, blood through vessels, and food through the digestive tract. They also produce heat, which aids in numerous body chemical reactions. Bones act as levers and provide support. Red blood cells are produced in the bone marrow, and minerals such as calcium and phosphorus are also stored there. Figure 25–1 describes the differences between the child's and adult's skeletal and muscularsystems.

The musculoskeletal system arises from the mesoderm in the embryo. A great portion of skeletal growth occurs between the 4th and 8th weeks of fetal life. As the limbs elongate prior to birth, muscle masses form in the extremities. The Dubowitz scoring system (see p. 449) is one measure of assessing neuromuscular maturity at birth. Testing various reflexes is another. Locomotion develops gradually and in an orderly manner in the growing child. A marked slowing down of growth is always a signal for investigation.

A thorough history is necessary to determine the basis for musculoskeletal problems, which are often insidious in nature. The nurse determines when symptoms started; location of pain; history of injury; any weakness, numbness, or loss of function in an extremity; and whether the problem is affecting the daily activities of the child. Diagnostic procedures may include x-ray studies, blood tests, pulmonary function tests (scoliosis may cause breathing problems), bone scans, and myelograms. Arthroscopies are commonly done on adolescents with sports injuries. The physician is able to look inside the joint (usually the knee) in order to determine the extent of injury. The area is inspected, foreign particles removed, or repairs made to the torn menisci. Muscle biopsy may detect muscular dystrophy. A bone biopsy may reveal a malignancy.

Traction, casting, and splints are used in accordance with the patient's needs. Three types of skin traction are frequently used for the lower extremities of children. These are Bryant traction, Buck extension, and Russell traction (see Figs. 25–5 to 25–7). Children with musculoskeletal disorders may require lengthy hospitalization. Immobility causes a slowing down of body metabolism. Nursing intervention is focused on maintaining body mobility. Range-of-motion exercises and the use of a trapeze prevent muscle atrophy. Foods high in roughage stimulate the digestive tract and prevent constipation. Respiratory exercises prevent pneumonia. These and other measures can prevent complications that can lengthen hospitalization for the child. The following is a discussion of musculoskeletal conditions seen in children. These include Duchenne's muscular dystrophy, Legg-Calvé-Perthes disease, traumatic fractures, osteomyelitis, osteosarcoma, Ewing's sarcoma, juvenile rheumatoid arthritis, head injuries, torticollis, scoliosis, and sports injuries. Clubfoot and congenital hip dysplasia are discussed on pp. 345–346. Rickets is discussed in Chapter 32. General information on cast care is also found on p. 345.

# Duchenne's Muscular Dystrophy (Pseudohypertrophic)

**Description.** The muscular dystrophies are a group of disorders in which progressive muscle degeneration occurs. The childhood form (Duchenne's muscular dystrophy) is the most common type, with an incidence of about 0.14 in 1000 children. It is a sex-linked inherited

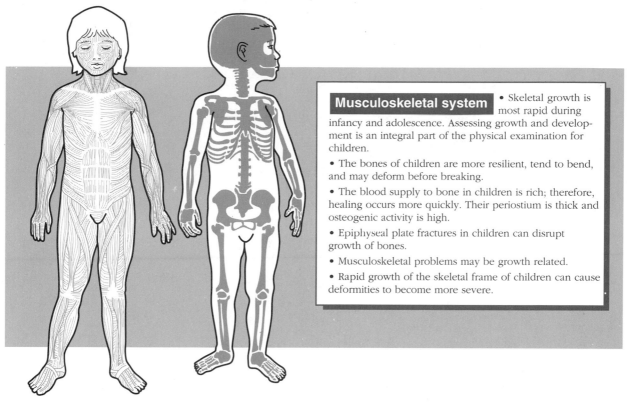

**Musculoskeletal system**
- Skeletal growth is most rapid during infancy and adolescence. Assessing growth and development is an integral part of the physical examination for children.
- The bones of children are more resilient, tend to bend, and may deform before breaking.
- The blood supply to bone in children is rich; therefore, healing occurs more quickly. Their periosteum is thick and osteogenic activity is high.
- Epiphyseal plate fractures in children can disrupt growth of bones.
- Musculoskeletal problems may be growth related.
- Rapid growth of the skeletal frame of children can cause deformities to become more severe.

**Figure 25–1.** Summary of musculoskeletal system differences between the child and the adult. The muscular system consists of the large skeletal muscles that enable us to move as well as the cardiac muscle of the heart and the smooth muscle of the internal organs. The skeletal system consists of bones and cartilage. This system helps to support and protect the body.

disorder occurring only in boys. Mothers are likely carriers for the disease; however, spontaneous mutations also occur. Individuals at risk in the female bloodline may choose to be evaluated and counseled about the carrier state.

**Manifestations.** The onset is generally between 2 and 6 years of age; however, a history of delayed motor development during infancy may be evidenced. It primarily affects muscles of the shoulders and pelvis. A waddling gait, slowness in running or climbing, and enlarged, rubbery muscles are indicative of this disorder. The calf muscles in particular become hypertrophied. The term *pseudohypertrophic* (*pseudo*, "false," and *hypertrophy*, "enlargement") refers to this characteristic. Other signs include frequent falling, clumsiness, contractures of the ankles and hips, and the Gowers' maneuver (a characteristic way of rising from the floor) (Fig. 25–2).

Laboratory findings show marked increases in blood creatine phosphokinase. Muscle biopsy reveals degeneration of muscle fibers and their replacement by fat and connective tissue. An electromyogram (a graphic record of muscle contraction as a result of electrical stimulation) shows decreases in amplitude and duration of motor unit potentials. Electrocardiographic abnormalities are also common. The disease becomes progressively worse, and wheelchair confinement occurs when the child is about 12 years old. Death is usually due to cardiac failure or respiratory infection. Mental retardation is not uncommon.

**Treatment and Nursing Care.** Treatment at this time is mainly supportive. It consists of passive exercises to prevent joint contractures, bracing, weight control, surgery for joint contractures, and referrals to appropriate social agencies. Psychological considerations revolve about the chronic and progressive nature of the disease and its fatal outcome. Family denial of the diagnosis is common early in the disease, when symptoms are fairly benign.

If the patient is hospitalized for diagnosis, parents and child are prepared for muscle

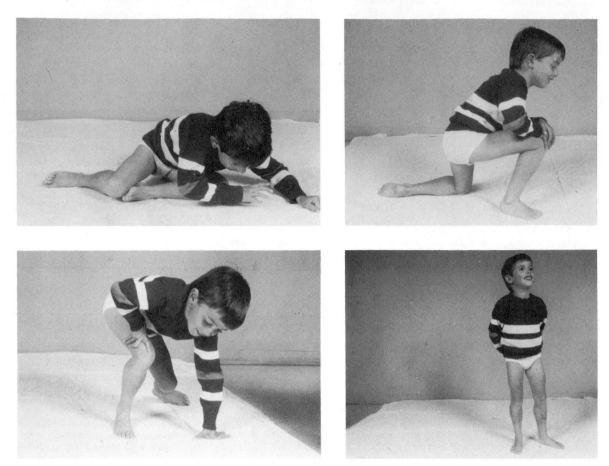

**Figure 25-2.** Gowers' sign in a boy with hip girdle weakness from Duchenne type muscular dystrophy. (From Behrman R. E., & Kliegman, R.M. [1992]. *Nelson textbook of pediatrics* [14th ed., p. 1478]. Philadelphia: W.B. Saunders.)

biopsy and electromyography. During the biopsy, a small piece of muscle is removed for examination. Vital signs and drainage from the incision are monitored following the procedure. During electromyography, small needles are placed in the muscles to record contractions. Muscles examined may ache slightly following the test, but this is temporary. There is no special preparation for electromyography. Whenever possible, the nurse remains with the child during the test.

Compared with other children with disabilities, some children with muscular dystrophy may appear passive and withdrawn. Early on, depression may be seen because the child is unable to compete with peers. Social and emotional pressures on the child and family are great. Financial pressures become magnified as medical and surgical costs escalate. In addition, expensive alterations to the family home and vehicles are sometimes necessary.

The nurse functions as a team member along with personnel from many other disciplines in the care of the child with muscular dystrophy. The child is encouraged to be as active as possible in order to delay muscle atrophy. Support is provided for the many daily issues that occur by placing parents in touch with other parents, camp programs, respite care, the Muscular Dystrophy Association, public health nurses, home health agencies, family therapists, and eventually hospice care.

## Legg-Calvé-Perthes Disease (Coxa Plana)

**Description.** Legg-Calvé-Perthes disease is one of a group of disorders called the osteochondroses (*osteo*, "bone," *chondros*, "cartilage," and *osis*, "disease"), in which the blood supply to the epiphyses, or end of the bone, is disrupted. The tissue death that results from the inadequate blood supply is termed avascular necrosis (*a*, "without," *vasculum*, "vessels," and *nekros*, "death"). Legg-Calvé-Perthes disease affects the development of the head of the femur. Its cause and incidence are unknown. The disease is age-related and is seen most commonly in boys between ages 5 and 9, although children between ages 3 and 11 may be affected. It is more common in Caucasians than in African Americans. This disease is unilateral in about 85% of cases. Healing occurs spontaneously over 2–4 years; however, marked distortion of the head of the femur may lead to an imperfect joint or degenerative arthritis of the hip in later life. Symptoms include limping, pain that may be referred to the knee, and limitation of motion. A number of cases are diagnosed in sports clinics. Legg-Calvé-Perthes disease may or may not be preceded by trauma or infection. X-ray films and isotopic bone scans confirm the diagnosis.

**Treatment.** In general, the earlier the age of onset, the better the results of treatment. In recent years, extensive confinement of the child and weight-relieving methods have been replaced by allowing weight bearing and by keeping the femoral head deep in the hip socket while it heals. This is accomplished through the use of ambulation-abduction casts or braces that prevent subluxation (*sub*, "beneath," and *luxatio*, "dislocation") and enable the acetabulum to mold the healing head in such a way that it does not become deformed. This treatment may be preceded by bed rest and traction. Newer surgical reconstruction and containment methods show promise in shortening the length of treatment. The prognosis in Legg-Calvé-Perthes disease is fair. Some affected people may require joint replacement procedures as adults.

**Nursing Care.** Nursing considerations depend on the age of the patient and the type of treatment. When immobilization of the child is necessary, the general principles of traction, cast, and brace care are employed. Teaching and counseling are directed toward a holistic understanding of and interest in the individual child and family. Total immobility or partial mobility is particularly trying for children. Braces and casts hinder the patient's movement toward independence; the child is deprived of the many natural outlets for relieving stress. The natural inclination to compete physically is thwarted.

When hospitalization is required, environmental stimuli and peer interaction are limited.

The danger that the child might develop a sense of inferiority and inadequacy is heightened unless thoughtful nursing intervention is employed. The nurse provides support for the parents and includes their input when designing care plans. Inquiring about the welfare of siblings at home may aid parents in understanding the impact of one child's illness on the total family.

# Traumatic Fractures and Traction

**Definitions.** A fracture is a break in a bone and is mainly caused by accidents. It is characterized by pain, tenderness on movement, and swelling. Discoloration, limited movement, and numbness may also occur. In a simple fracture, the bone is broken, but the skin over the area is not. In a compound fracture, a wound in the skin leads to the broken bone, and there is an added danger of infection. A greenstick fracture is an incomplete fracture in which one side of the bone is broken and the other is bent. This type of fracture is common in children because their bones are soft, flexible, and more likely to splinter. In a complete fracture, the bone is entirely broken across its width. Figure 25–3 illustrates various types of fractures.

Healing of a fracture in a child is more rapid than it is in an adult. The child's periosteum is stronger and thicker, and there is less stiffness on mobilization. Injury to the cartilaginous epiphyseal plate, found at the ends of long bones, is serious if it happens during childhood because it may interfere with longitudinal growth.

**First Aid.** If a fracture is suspected, the child is not allowed to use the limb or part, and the nurse does not move it either. The child who is in a safe place is not moved and is kept warm. The nurse calls for emergency assistance. A covered ice pack applied to the injured part may minimize swelling. When the fracture is compound, the injury is lightly covered with a sterile dressing. If it is necessary to move the child, a splint is applied. The joints above and below the break are immobilized by a rolled newspaper or bath towels and tied beyond the injury. If the arm is injured, it is kept elevated by a sling in order to reduce swelling and hemorrhage. This is also necessary once the arm is casted (Fig. 25–4). If a back or neck injury is evident, the child is not moved unless it is a dire neces-

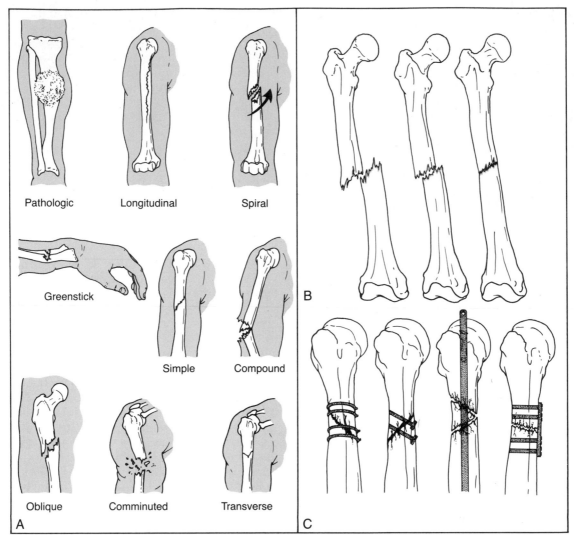

**Figure 25–3.** *A,* Types of fractures. *B,* Reduction of a fractured bone. A gradual pull is exerted on the distal (lower) fragment of the bone until it is in alignment with the proximal fragment. *C,* Various methods of internal fixations, using plates, pins, nails, and screws to hold fragments of bone in place. (Redrawn from deWit, S.C. [1992]. *Keane's essentials of medical-surgical nursing* [3rd ed.]. Philadelphia: W.B. Saunders.)

sity. The nurse calls for an ambulance immediately.

**Fractures of the Femur in Early Childhood.** The femur, the thigh bone, is the largest and strongest bone of the body. Children may fracture this bone in a severe fall or an automobile accident. It is one of the most prevalent serious breaks that occur during early childhood. The child complains of pain and tenderness when the leg is moved and cannot bear weight on it. Clothes are gently removed, starting at the uninjured side and proceeding to the injured side. It may be necessary to cut the clothes. X-ray films confirm the diagnosis. Skin traction is used to reduce the fracture, to keep the bones in proper place, and to immobilize both legs.

Bryant traction is used for treating fractures of the femur in children under 2 years of age or under 20–30 pounds. Weights and pulleys extend the limb as in Buck extension; however, the legs are suspended vertically (Fig. 25–5). The weight of the child supplies the countertraction.

The nurse observes the traction ropes to be sure that they are intact and in the wheel grooves of the pulleys and that the child's body

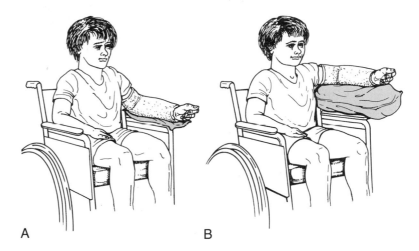

**Figure 25–4.** Correct and incorrect positions for a child in a wheelchair. *A*, In the incorrect position, the support is too low to relieve local edema. *B*, Correctly positioned, the arm is elevated, the wrist is higher than the elbow, and the elbow is higher than the shoulder. (Redrawn from Leifer, G. [1982]. *Principles and techniques in pediatric nursing* [4th ed., p. 180]. Philadelphia: W.B. Saunders.)

is in good position. The legs should be at right angles to the body, and the buttocks raised sufficiently to clear the bed. Elastic bandages should be neither too loose nor too tight. A restraint jacket may be used to keep the child from turning from side to side. The weights are not removed once applied. Continuous traction is necessary. The weights must hang free, and the pull of the weights must not be obstructed by bedroom furnishings, such as a chair. The weights are *not* supported when the bed is moved. The nurse frequently checks the child's toes to see that they are warm and that their

color is good. Cyanosis, numbness, or irritation from attachments, tight bandages, severe pain, or absence of pulse in the extremities is reported immediately to the nurse in charge. A specific and serious complication of Bryant traction is *Volkmann's ischemia* (*ischein*, "to hold back," and *haima*, "blood"), which occurs when the circulation is obstructed. Because the legs are elevated overhead, there is gravitational vascular drainage. Arterial occlusion can cause anoxia of the muscles and reflex vasospasm, which when unnoticed could result in contractures and paralysis.

The child is bathed daily, and the back is frequently rubbed in order to prevent ulceration. The nurse reaches under the patient's body to rub the back and buttocks. A sheepskin padding may also be utilized. The sheets are pulled taut and are kept free of crumbs. The jacket restraint is changed when it is soiled. The child is encouraged to drink lots of fluids and to eat foods that are high in roughage in order to prevent constipation due to lack of exercise. Stool softeners may be necessary. A fracture pan is used for bowel movements, and a careful record is kept of eliminations. Deep-breathing exercises are encouraged to prevent collection of fluids in the lungs owing to the child's immobility. These exercises may be done by blowing bubbles or blowing a pinwheel.

Diversional therapy is important, as hospitalization may be lengthy. Toys may be suspended over the child's head within reach. The nurse watches for the possibility of strangling from the suspension device. The child's crib is taken to the playroom when possible so that the child

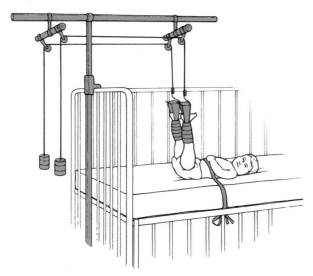

**Figure 25–5.** Bryant traction is used for the young child who has a fractured femur.

may experience the excitement of the activities there. Records, stories, and other forms of entertainment are essential to a total nursing care plan. Parents are encouraged to visit the patient as often as possible. With proper treatment, the prognosis for the child with this condition is good.

**Fractures and Traction in the Older Child.** The active school-age child is often subject to traumatic injury to the extremities due to bicycle accidents, sports injuries, or falls on the playground. Traction is used when the immobilization required is more than what could be obtained by casting. Skeletal muscles act as a splint for the fracture. Traction extends the injured extremity by the use of weights and countertraction. Immobilization is maintained until the bones fuse.

*Buck extension* (Fig. 25–6) is a type of skin traction used in fractures of the femur and in hip and knee contractures. It pulls the hip and leg into extension. Countertraction is supplied by the child's body; therefore, it is essential that the child not slip down in bed. Buck extension is sometimes used preoperatively, either unilaterally or bilaterally, to reduce pain and muscle spasm associated with a slipped capital femoral epiphysis. *Russell traction* is similar to Buck extension; however, in the former a sling is positioned under the knee, which suspends the distal thigh above the bed (Fig. 25–7A). Skin traction is applied to the lower extremity. Pull is in two directions—vertically from the knee sling and longitudinally from the footplate. This prevents posterior subluxation of the tibia on the femur, which can occur in children in traction. *Split Russell traction* (Fig. 25–7B) uses two sets of weights, one suspending the thigh and the other exerting a pull on the leg. Note the weights at head and foot of the bed.

In *skeletal traction*, a Steinmann pin or Kirschner wire is inserted into the bone, and

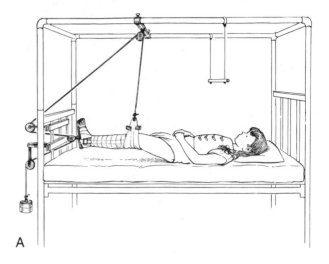

A

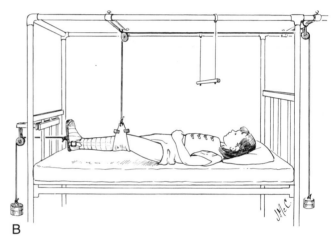

B

**Figure 25–7.** Russell skin traction (*A*) and split Russell traction (*B*). (Modified from Tachdjian, M. [1972]. *Pediatric orthopedics*. Philadelphia: W.B. Saunders. Reprinted from Betz C., et al. [1994]. *Family-centered nursing care of children* [2nd ed., p. 1827]. Philadelphia: W.B. Saunders.)

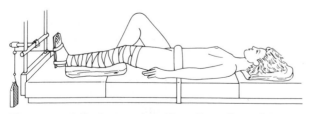

**Figure 25–6.** Buck extension. (From Betz, C., et al. [1994]. *Family-centered nursing care of children* [2nd ed., p. 1826]. Philadelphia: W.B. Saunders.)

traction is applied to the pin. Ninety-ninety traction with a boot cast or sling on the lower leg may be used (Fig. 25–8). *Crutchfield* or *Barton tongs* may be used in the skull to provide cervical traction (Fig. 25–9). Skeletal traction carries the added risk of infection from skin bacteria that may cause osteomyelitis. *Suspension therapy* elevates or suspends an extremity above the bed. It can be utilized by itself or with skin or skeletal traction. Suspension therapy reduces edema and increases the patient's comfort. Balanced suspension, employing the *Thomas splint* and *Pearson attachments* (Fig. 25–10) is used to treat diseases of the hip as well as fractures in older

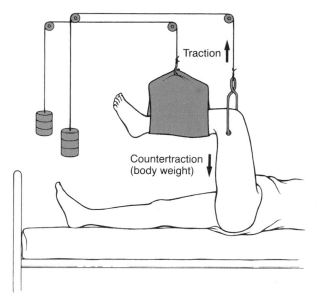

**Figure 25–8.** 90 degree–90 degree skeletal traction. A wire pin is inserted into the distal segment of the femur. The lower leg may be placed in a boot cast or is supported by a sling.

children and adolescents. It may be used both before and after surgery. Nursing Care Plan 25–1 describes interventions for the child in traction. The child in traction experiences certain effects as a result of immobilization; these are illustrated in Figure 25–11. Visitors are important to the child in traction (Fig. 25–12).

## Osteomyelitis

**Description.** Osteomyelitis is an infection of the bone that generally occurs in children younger than 1 year and in those between 5 and 14 years of age. It is more common in boys than in girls. *Staphylococcus aureus* is the organism responsible in 75–80% of cases. Other organisms include group A streptococci, pneumococci, and *Haemophilus influenzae*. *Salmonella* is frequently seen in patients with sickle cell anemia. It may be preceded by a local injury to the bone, such as an open fracture, burn, or contamination during surgery. It may also follow a furuncle, impetigo, and abscessed teeth. The incidence of osteomyelitis has decreased as a result of antibiotics. Infective emboli may travel to the small arteries of the bone, setting up local destruction and abscess. For this reason, a careful search for

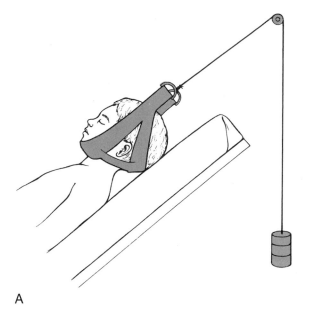

A

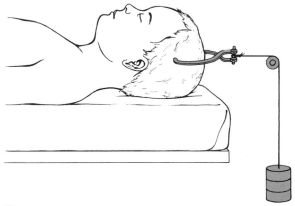

B

**Figure 25–9.** *A,* Cervical traction. *B,* Crutchfield tong traction.

infection in other bones and soft tissues is necessary.

**Manifestations.** The illness begins abruptly with fever, rapid pulse, and dehydration. It localizes most often in the long bones. There may be associated swelling and tenderness and decreased movement. There is an elevation in white blood cell count and sedimentation rate. X-ray films fail to reveal infection until about 10 days later. Tomography may detect it earlier. Blood cultures are taken in order to determine the causative organism.

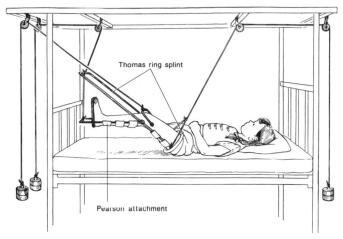

**Figure 25–10.** Suspension traction with wire through the distal femur with a Thomas ring splint and Pearson attachment. (Modified from Tachdjian, M. [1972]. *Pediatric orthopedics.* Philadelphia: W.B. Saunders. Reprinted from Betz, C. [1994]. *Family-centered nursing care of children* [2nd ed., p. 1828]. Philadelphia: W.B. Saunders.)

**Treatment and Nursing Care.** As most pediatric cases of osteomyelitis are caused by staphylococci, large doses of penicillin G are administered intravenously along with other antibiotics. This is continued for about 4–6 weeks. The child is placed on bed rest, and the extremity is cradled in a bivalved cast in order to limit the spread of infection and maintain alignment of the bones if a fracture is present. Surgical drainage may be considered in order to prevent abscess formation and remove dead bone. Sterile technique must be meticulously adhered to during dressing changes in order to avoid contamination of the wound by new organisms. Healing is complicated because the blood supply to the affected area is reduced, which also decreases antibiotic transport. The nursing considerations for osteomyelitis are outlined in Nursing Care Plan 25–2.

# Osteosarcoma

**Description.** Osteosarcoma (*osteo*, "bone," *sarx*, "flesh," and *oma*, "tumor") is a primary malignant tumor of the long bones. The two most common types of bone tumors are osteosarcoma and Ewing's tumor. Bone tumors are second only to lymphomas as the most frequently occurring neoplasms in adolescents (Pillitteri, 1992). The mean age of onset of osteosarcoma is 15 years. It is seen in both girls and boys; however, the incidence increases for older boys, whereas that for girls appears to

| NURSING CARE PLAN 25–1 | | |
| :---: | :---: | :---: |
| **Selected Nursing Diagnoses for the Child in Traction** | | |
| **Goals** | **Nursing Interventions** | **Rationale** |

**Nursing Diagnosis:** Impaired physical mobility related to fixation devices.

| | | |
| --- | --- | --- |
| Child demonstrates how to obtain help via call bell<br>Child will not develop complications of immobility as evidenced by intact skin and absence of respiratory and urinary infections<br>Child will have a bowel movement each day or according to previous routine | 1. Draw picture of fracture for child, explain; explain traction apparatus<br><br>2. Designate call bell<br><br>3. Change position as traction allows every 2 hr<br><br>4. Encourage exercise through play (throwing foam balls, bean bags, pull-ups on trapeze)<br><br>5. Institute range-of-motion exercises to avoid muscle atrophy or contractures | 1. An understanding of condition and traction used reduces anxiety and promotes compliance with treatment protocol<br>2. It is frightening to be immobilized; a call bell provides reassurance that help is at hand<br>3. Type of traction and amount of movement allowed are explained to child<br>4. Immobilization lowers body's metabolic rate and oxygen consumption and affects all body's systems<br>5. Although it is important that traction is not disrupted, unaffected limbs need exercise in order to prevent stiffness, muscle atrophy, and deformities; moving patient promotes respiration, circulation, and elimination and avoids pressure on areas of the skin |

*Continued*

## Selected Nursing Diagnoses for the Child in Traction

| Goals | Nursing Interventions | Rationale |
|---|---|---|
| **Nursing Diagnosis:** Impaired physical mobility related to fixation devices. | | |
| | 6. Encourage self-care | 6. Self-care provides self-movement and self-control |
| | 7. Encourage blowing of harmonica or bubbles as lung exercise | 7. Lung exercise prevents pneumonia and other complications |
| | 8. Anticipate urinary tract infection | 8. Kidney filtration slows down with immobilization; immobility causes minerals (e.g., calcium) to leave bones and pool in renal pelvis; stasis of urine is likely to occur, causing renal calculi |
| | 9. Provide roughage foods to prevent constipation | 9. Roughage prevents constipation, which is one of most frequent effects of immobilization; high-fiber diets and stool softeners are helpful |
| | 10. Provide adequate fluids; monitor intake and ouput | 10. Increased fluids are necessary to hydrate body |
| **Nursing Diagnosis:** Pain due to tissue trauma. | | |
| Child will be comfortable, as evidenced by a decrease in irritability, crying, body posturing, anorexia<br>Older child verbalizes relief of pain | 1. Administer pain medication before pain begins or escalates | 1. Child may be unable to verbalize pain |
| | 2. Allow child to choose method of pain relief, if possible | 2. Allowing child some choice, if there is one, promotes self-control |
| | 3. Encourage child to hold favorite possession; provide pacifier for toddler | 3. Favorite possessions and a pacifier are comforting, particularly to small child |
| | 4. Distract with music box or tapes, as age-appropriate | 4. Distraction from a problem reduces stress and tension |
| | 5. Listen and communicate with child | 5. Listening to child gives nurse clues as to amount of pain; nonverbal cues are important in infants and toddlers |
| | 6. Use touch as a comfort measure | 6. Touch is particularly important in infants and toddlers but is comforting for all ages; proceed with caution if there is reason to suspect abuse |
| | 7. Involve family in supporting child's ability to cope with pain | 7. Child trusts family; family members may be able to suggest favorite types of comfort for child |
| | 8. Consider cultural background in relation to pain expression | 8. In some cultures, showing pain is considered cowardly |
| | 9. Determine vital signs | 9. Heart rate and respirations increase with pain; these should improve after medication or comfort measure |
| | 10. Evaluate pain management techniques daily | 10. Discussing comfort measures during conferences pools ideas |
| | 11. Anticipate patient's pain as a stressor for family members | 11. It is difficult for parents to observe their child in pain; parents need support at this time |

*Continued*

| NURSING CARE PLAN 25–1 *Continued* | | |
| --- | --- | --- |
| **Selected Nursing Diagnoses for the Child in Traction** | | |
| **Goals** | **Nursing Interventions** | **Rationale** |

**Nursing Diagnosis:** High risk for impaired skin integrity related to immobility, traction, poor circulation.

| Goals | Nursing Interventions | Rationale |
| --- | --- | --- |
| Skin remains intact with no evidence of breakdown<br>Circulation of affected extremity is adequate as evidenced by normal capillary refill, equal and strong peripheral pulses, and sensation and motion in extremity | 1. Inspect skin regularly | 1. Preventing skin breakdown is first concern, as bedsores are difficult to heal |
| | 2. Check capillary refill of nailbeds in affected extremity every 4 hr or as ordered | 2. When blood supply to a part is impeded, circulation decreases; careful monitoring leads to early intervention; by pressing on each nailbed, releasing, and observing return of color, nurse is able to evaluate capillary refill; it should be immediate and comparable to that of unaffected extremity |
| | 3. Measure peripheral pulses when checking refill | 3. A normal pulse distal to traction should be present |
| | 4. Have child wiggle toes or fingers of affected extremity to determine sensation and motion | 4. Wiggling toes and fingers determines mobility and sensation |
| | 5. Assess restraining devices and elastic bandages for wrinkles or looseness | 5. Excessive tightness or wrinkles in bandages can cause swelling and irritation of underlying tissue |
| | 6. Utilize sheepskin underneath hips and back | 6. Sheepskin may protect susceptible areas, such as bony prominences about sacrum |
| | 7. Monitor traction and pulleys for intactness, rubbing on skin surfaces, patient comfort | 7. Areas exposed to frequent friction may break down |
| | 8. Maintain body alignment, massage skin | 8. Gentle massage stimulates circulation |
| | 9. Inspect pin sites for redness, bleeding, infection | 9. These are focal points for irritation and infection |

**Nursing Diagnosis:** Diversional activity deficit related to boredom and restriction of activity by treatment apparatus.

| Goals | Nursing Interventions | Rationale |
| --- | --- | --- |
| Child's developmental level is maintained<br>Child will participate in one enjoyable activity | 1. Allow child to chose age-appropriate games, regulate daily schedule | 1. Allowing child to choose activities increases self-confidence and self-control |
| | 2. Promote self-care activities as appropriate | 2. Self-care leads to independence |
| | 3. Encourage peer contact and interaction with new hospital friends | 3. Children, particularly those of school age and adolescents, must remain in contact with their peers to prevent feeling isolated |
| | 4. Assist in decorating environment | 4. Personalizing the environment is fun and creative, and it affords a place of one's own |
| | 5. Involve child-life specialist, play therapist, volunteers to visit and interact with child | 5. Boredom and inactivity can lead to depression |

plateau around age 13. Children who have had radiation therapy for other types of cancer and children with retinoblastoma have a higher incidence of this disease. Metastasis occurs quickly because of the high vascularity of bone tissue. The lungs are the primary site of metas-tasis; brain and other bone tissue are also sites of metastasis.

**Manifestations.** The patient experiences pain and swelling at the site. In adolescents this is often attributed to injury or "growing pains." The pain may be lessened by a flexed position of

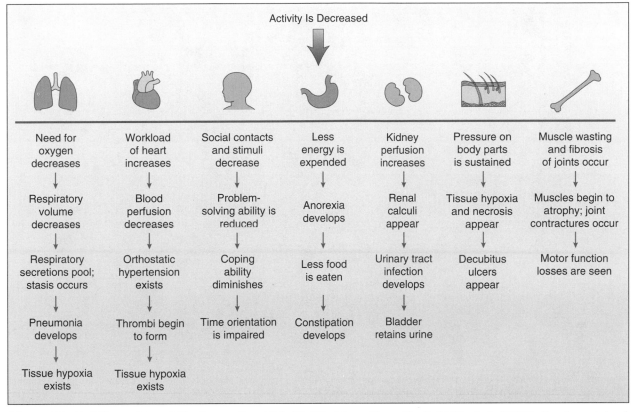

**Figure 25–11.** Effects of immobilization on the child. (Modified from Kemp, B., & Pillitteri, A. [1989]. *Fundamentals of nursing.* Boston: Little, Brown.)

the extremity. Later a pathologic fracture may occur. Diagnosis is confirmed by biopsy. A complete physical examination including computed tomography (CT) and bone scans is done. Radiologic studies are characteristic for each type of tumor.

**Treatment and Nursing Care.** Treatment of the patient with osteosarcoma consists of surgery. This may include amputation of the limb or wide local excision of a flat bone. Internal prostheses are now available for most sites, and amputation is avoided whenever possible. A thoracotomy may be performed to remove sites of metastasis to the lungs. Chemotherapy may be given prior to surgery. In the past this condition was considered fatal. Long-term survival is now being seen, particularly with early diagnosis and treatment.

The nursing care is similar to that for other types of cancer. Problems of body image are particularly important to the self-conscious teenager. If amputation is necessary, the family and patient will need much support. The nurse

anticipates anger, fear, and grief. Immediately following surgery, the stump dressing is observed frequently for bleeding. Vital signs are ascertained. The child's position is as ordered. *Phantom limb pain* is likely to be experienced. This is the continued sensation of pain in the leg even though the leg is no longer there. It occurs because nerve tracts continue to report pain. This pain is very real and an analgesic may be necessary. Rehabilitation measures follow surgical recovery.

## Ewing's Sarcoma

**Description.** Ewing's sarcoma was first described in 1921 by Dr. James Ewing. It is a malignant growth that occurs in the mid-shaft of long bones and in flat bones such as the pelvis, scapulae, and ribs. Tissue samples of this tumor show round cells rather than the characteristic large spindle cells of osteosarcoma. It occurs mainly in older school children and early

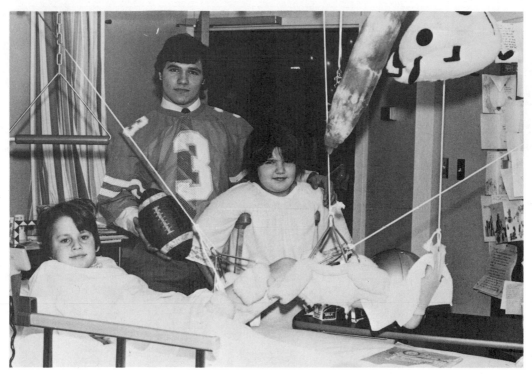

**Figure 25–12.** Children with orthopedic conditions enjoy visitors. Note how this child has personalized his environment. (Courtesy of Blank Memorial Hospital for Children, Des Moines, IA.)

adolescence. When metastasis is present on diagnosis, the prognosis is poor. Without metastasis there is a 60% survival rate. Primary sites for metastasis are the lungs and bones.

**Treatment and Nursing Care.** The initial symptom is pain that may be accompanied by fever and tenderness at the site. It is sometimes mistaken for osteomyelitis. Confirmation requires surgical biopsy. Amputation is not generally recommended for Ewing's sarcoma because the tumor is sensitive to radiation therapy and chemotherapy. This is a relief to the patient and family. Patients are warned against vigorous weight bearing by the involved bone during therapy to avoid pathologic fractures. They need to be prepared for the effects of radiation therapy and chemotherapy. The nurse supports the family members in their efforts to gain equilibrium following such a crisis.

## Juvenile Rheumatoid Arthritis

**Description.** Juvenile rheumatoid arthritis (JRA) is the most common arthritic condition of childhood. It is a systemic inflammatory disease or group of diseases that involve the joints, connective tissues, and viscera. JRA is not a rare disease, as an estimated quarter million children in the United States have the disorder (Behrman, 1992). The exact cause is unknown, but infection and an autoimmune response have been implicated.

**Manifestations and Types.** This disease varies from one patient to the next and has three distinct methods of onset: systemic (or acute febrile), polyarticular, and pauciarticular. The *systemic* form is manifested by fever, rash, abdominal pain, pleuritis, pericarditis, and enlarged liver and spleen. It occurs most frequently in children 1–3 and 8–10 years of age. Joint symptoms may be absent at onset but will develop in most patients. The *polyarticular* form can involve any of the joints, which become swollen, warm, and tender. This form occurs throughout childhood and adolescence and predominantly affects girls. Approximately 40% of patients with JRA have the polyarticular type. The *pauciarticular* form is limited to four or fewer joints, generally the larger ones such as the hips, knees, ankles, and elbows. It occurs in children under age 3 years (mostly in girls)

| NURSING CARE PLAN 25-2 |
|---|

## Selected Nursing Diagnoses for the Child with Osteomyelitis

| Goals | Nursing Interventions | Rationale |
|---|---|---|
| **Nursing Diagnosis:** Pain related to swelling, hyperthermia, infectious process of the bone.. | | |
| Child shows decrease in restlessness, irritability, body posturing, complaints | 1. Administer antipyretics as ordered<br><br>2. Administer pain medication before pain escalates<br><br>3. Position for comfort | 1. Reduction of fever increases child's comfort<br>2. Behavioral responses to pain vary with age; when pain increases, recommended dosage may not be effective<br>3. Child may be afraid to move in bed because of pain; joints need to be supported above and below affected area |
| **Nursing Diagnosis:** High risk for impaired skin integrity related to wound dressings, mechanical irritation of cast or splint. | | |
| Healing of wound is evidenced by amount and character of drainage, approximation of edges<br>Skin integrity is maintained, as evidenced by good circulation, sensation, and lack of signs of inflammation | 1. Monitor intravenous antibiotics; check for compatibility<br>2. Assess wound for swelling, heat, tenderness<br>3. Note character and amount of wound drainage<br>4. Maintain aseptic technique<br>5. Perform wound irrigations if prescribed<br><br>6. Utilize wound precaution according to hospital protocol<br>7. Inspect skin regularly for breakdown<br>8. Check area surrounding cast for neurovascular complications | 1. Antibiotics are instituted; because more than one may be used, compatibility is ascertained<br>2. These are signs of infection or inflammation<br>3. Increased amounts of drainage and odor indicate chronic bone infection<br>4. Aseptic techniques prevent further infection<br>5. Abscess formed in bone needs to be surgically drained and curetted; direct application of antibiotics hastens healing<br>6. Prevent spread of pathologic organisms<br>7. Early detection of minor skin irritations prevents skin breakdown<br>8. Compression from cast may cause pallor, puffiness, pain, loss of sensation, loss of pulse, paresthesia |
| **Nursing Diagnosis:** High risk for constipation related to inactivity. | | |
| Child will have a bowel movement each day or according to previous routine | 1. Check frequency and consistency of bowel movements<br>2. Report absence, abdominal pain, hard stools<br>3. Administer stool softeners as indicated<br>4. Offer bedpan after breakfast if age-appropriate; provide privacy while patient is on bedpan<br>5. Maintain adequate fluids and fiber | 1. Immobility may lead to constipation<br>2–5. These measures promote regularity of bowel movements and prevent complications of discomfort or intestinal blockage |

and in those over age 13 years (mostly in boys). Approximately 35% of patients with JRA have the pauciarticular form.

*Iridocyclitis.* Children with pauciarticular disease are at risk for iridocyclitis (*irido,* "iris," *cycl,* "circle," and *itis,* "inflammation"), an inflammation of the iris and ciliary body of the eye. Symptoms include redness, pain, photophobia, decreased visual acuity, and nonreactive pupils. This disease occurs most frequently in young girls (in a 7:1 ratio). There is no parallel between the eye inflammation and the joint disease (Nelson, 1991). The course is unpredictable. All children with pauciarticular arthritis need slit-lamp eye examinations periodically. Distortion of the pupil and cataracts may occur. The long-term visual prognosis is uncertain.

**Treatment.** There are no specific tests or cures for JRA. The duration of the symptoms is important, particularly when they have lasted longer than 6 weeks. Diagnosis is determined by clinical manifestations, x-ray studies, laboratory results, and exclusion of other disorders. Aspirated joint fluid is yellow to green and cloudy and has a low viscosity. The goals of therapy are to reduce pain and swelling, to promote mobility, to preserve joint function, to educate the patient and family, and to help the child and family adjust to living with a chronic disease.

Treatment is supportive. Drug therapy and exercise are the mainstays of therapy. The three principal medications used in this condition are aspirin, the corticosteroids, and nonsteroidal antiinflammatory agents, such as indomethacin or naproxen. Gold compounds are used when other measures prove ineffective. Regular monitoring of all medications is imperative.

Aspirin is given with meals in order to avoid gastric irritation. Parents are informed of the side effects of aspirin, which include tinnitus, lethargy, hyperventilation, dizziness, headaches, nausea, and vomiting. Aspirin is discontinued if the prothrombin time is prolonged excessively. Acetaminophen (Tylenol) does not have antiinflammatory properties; therefore, it cannot be substituted for acetylsalicylic acid for these patients. This is explained to parents because aspirin is associated with Reye's syndrome. Although children without JRA should receive Tylenol for fevers, the child with JRA needs aspirin because its antiinflammatory effect is important in preventing pain. If the parents have a question concerning a particular episode or symptoms, they should call their physician. Chewable aspirin has been linked to dental caries (Brewer, 1990); therefore, brushing after ingestion is recommended.

The corticosteroids have to be closely screened. Opportunistic infections may occur, as advanced warning of serious infections may be masked by steroids. Gold compounds are given intramuscularly. The effect of these compounds occurs slowly. Liver function tests, blood urea nitrogen, creatinine, complete blood count, platelet count, and urinalysis are checked prior to initiation of gold compounds. The patient is warned to avoid exposure to strong sunlight. The skin and mucous membranes are inspected before each injection for rash, stomatitis, or itching. The nurse reads the manufacturer's circular carefully because test doses are required.

**Nursing Care.** The nurse functions as a member of a team that includes the pediatrician, rheumatologist, social worker, physical therapist, occupational therapist, psychologist, ophthalmologist, and school and community nurses. The child may be hospitalized during an acute episode or for an unrelated illness. Treatment consists of the administration of medications, warm tub baths, joint exercises, and rest. The physical therapist oversees the type and amount of exercise performed. Daily range-of-motion exercises and play activities that incorporate specific routines help preserve function, maintain muscle strength, and prevent deformities. One must be careful to avoid traumatizing an inflamed joint. Morning tub baths and the application of moist hot packs help lessen stiffness. Resting splints may be ordered to prevent flexion contractures and preserve functional alignment. Proper body alignment with regular change to the prone position (unless contraindicated) facilitates comfort. Either no pillow or a small flat pillow is advocated. Measures to alleviate boredom are instituted.

**Home Care.** The patient is discharged with written instructions for home care. These are reviewed with family members in order to determine their level of understanding. A firm mattress or bed board is necessary to prevent joints from sagging. Age-appropriate tricycles and pedal cars promote mobility and exercise. Modifications in daily living, such as elevation of toilet seats, installation of hand rails, Velcro fasteners, and so on, may be necessary. Swimming is an excellent form of exercise. Assist parents in planning nutritional meals. Weight gain is to be avoided, as it places further stress on the joints. The importance of regular eye examinations is emphasized. Unnecessary physical restrictions should be avoided, as these can lead to rebellion.

School attendance is encouraged. Excessive absence from school, particularly for nonspecific complaints, may suggest that the child is depressed or overly preoccupied with the illness. In such cases, the meaning of the illness to the child and family and its effect on daily life need to be explored. Parents need assistance in es-

## Nursing Brief

The child may see a whirlpool bath as "boiling water." Reassure the patient that immersion into the tank will not cause burns.

---

tablishing limits. Consistently negative behavior in social situations can present more problems than the actual disability. Overindulgence and preferential treatment often compromise the child's potential for happiness and independence. Siblings of chronically ill children may resent the special attention given to the patient. They may be torn by loyalty to the brother or sister and their own need to be with others. Parents need ongoing counseling and the services of various community resources. One resource is the Arthritis Foundation, which sponsors the American Juvenile Arthritis organization. The child may benefit from association with other arthritic children.

This long-term disease is characterized by periods of remission and exacerbations. There is no known cure for JRA at this writing. Nurses can serve as advocates for the child, that is, they can help alleviate stress by recognizing the impact of the disease and by openly communicating with the child, the family, and other members of the health-care team. Nurses support the child and family members and instill hope.

## Head Injuries

The incidence of head injury among children is high. About 200,000 children are admitted to hospitals each year. Head injuries occur twice as often in boys as in girls and are very prevalent in adolescents. A *concussion* is a temporary disturbance of the brain that is immediately followed by a period of unconsciousness. It jars the brain stem and is often accompanied by loss of memory of events that occurred immediately before (retrograde amnesia), during, and after the accident. A *skull fracture* can result from a severe head injury. In this condition, the cranium is actually broken. Bleeding may occur, and pressure may be exerted on the brain.

The toddler is famous for incurring head injuries. If the child stops crying shortly after a blow to the head, retains consciousness, maintains good color, and does not vomit, there is little chance that the brain has been injured. A lump may result from broken blood vessels beneath the skin, but this is not meaningful if no other symptoms are present. A covered ice pack is applied to the site. During the first night following a bump on the head, parents are advised to be sure that they can arouse the child at least once, because intracranial bleeding occasionally occurs from a minor injury. If the child appears confused, has trouble seeing or speaking, or walks unsteadily, contact a physician.

The major complications of head injury are hemorrhage, infection, cerebral edema (swelling of the brain), and compression of the brain stem. The brain and its interrelated compartments are tightly confined by the skull. Enlargement of any intracranial component (brain or subarachnoid, venous, or arterial space) may increase intracranial pressure (ICP), which can lead to permanent brain damage or death. Aggressive medical management, CT, and intensive therapy to counter increased ICP have dramatically altered morbidity and mortality in pediatric head injury.

Frequently, a child who has suffered a blow to the head is brought to the hospital for overnight observation in order to rule out or confirm the diagnosis. The patient may experience all or some of the following symptoms: headache (manifested by fussiness in toddler), drowsiness, blurred vision, vomiting, and dyspnea. In severe cases, the patient may be completely unconscious. Decerebrate or decorticate posturing may be evident (Fig. 25–13). In decerebrate rigidity all four limbs are extended. In decorticate rigidity the arms, wrists, and fingers are flexed. Plantar flexion occurs in the feet. Both pathologic postures are sometimes seen in severe brain injury if the patient is startled.

A careful history is obtained in order to determine any preexisting conditions and to ascertain the exact circumstances of the accident. Of particular importance is the patient's state of consciousness immediately following the occurrence.

Patients are handled gently and are inspected for injuries to other areas. They are placed in a crib or bed in accordance with their size. Side rails are raised, as seizures are not uncommon. The headrest is slightly elevated in order to decrease cerebral edema. Figure 25–14 shows a type of crib used in hospitals to protect small children from falls.

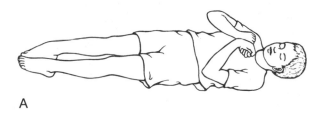

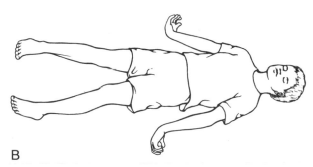

**Figure 25–13.** Pathologic posturing that may occur in the patient with severe brain damage. *A*, Decorticate posturing. *B*, Decerebrate posturing.

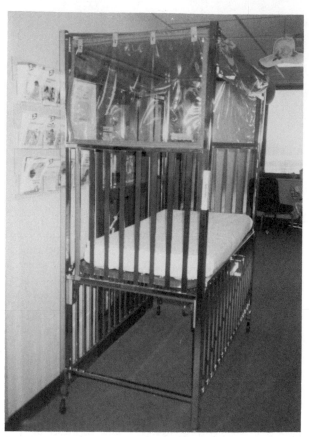

**Figure 25–14.** One type of crib used in the hospital to protect toddlers and small children from falls. (Courtesy of Columbia/HCA Portsmouth Regional Hospital, Portsmouth, NH.)

The nurse observes the patient for signs of increasing ICP. Four components of a cranial or neurologic check are (1) level of consciousness, (2) pupil and eye movement, (3) vital signs, and (4) motor activity.

**Level of Consciousness.** Changes in level of consciousness are particularly meaningful and require immediate medical attention. The child's alertness on admission is recorded for use as baseline data. Response should be correlated with the developmental age of the patient. Parents can be helpful in providing information about the child's usual capabilities. In general, patients should be oriented to person, time, and place (may not be accessible in the toddler). The nurse asks, "What is your name?" and "Where are you?" Older children may know the day of the week. The patient should recognize parents. The nurse points to the mother and asks, "Who is this?" The child should be able to follow simple commands, such as "turn over."

When the patient does not respond to verbal stimuli, the upper arm is gently pinched and the response observed. The presence or absence of crying or speech is noted. It is not unusual for children to fall asleep, but they should be easily aroused. The nurse records changes in sleeping posture, movements of extremities, and any signs of tremors or restlessness. The

bladder is observed for distention, which can contribute to irritability. Incontinence in the child who is toilet-trained is significant. Behavior is described in the nurse's notes.

The Glasgow Coma Scale (Table 25–1) is valuable in determining various levels of consciousness. It consists of three parts: eye opening, motor response, and verbal response. A numeric value of 1–5 is assigned to each part. The lower the score, the deeper the coma. Table 25–2 shows a verbal scale modified for infants.

**Pupil and Eye Movement.** When observing the patient's eyes, the nurse notes size, shape, and equality of pupils and their reaction to light and extraocular movements. (Have the patient follow your finger from side to side and up and down in order to detect movement.) Strabismus, nystagmus, and inability to move eyes in all four quadrants indicate abnormality.

**Table 25–1.** THE GLASGOW COMA SCALE

| Response | Degree |
|---|---|
| Eye opening | 4. Spontaneous |
| | 3. To speech |
| | 2. To pain |
| | 1. None |
| Best verbal response | 5. Oriented |
| | 4. Confused |
| | 3. Inappropriate |
| | 2. Incomprehensible |
| | 1. None |
| Best motor response | 6. Obeys commands |
| | 5. Localized pain |
| | 4. Withdraws |
| | 3. Flexion to pain |
| | 2. Extension to pain |
| | 1. None |

From Zimmerman, S.S., & Gildea, J.H. (1985). *Critical care pediatrics*. Philadelphia: W.B. Saunders.

The patient should be able to blink the eyes. If ICP is increasing, pupils become sluggish to light stimulus, dilated, and eventually fixed.

**Vital Signs.** An increase in blood pressure and a decrease in pulse and respiration are evidence of ICP. Temperature elevations may be due to inflammation, systemic infection, or damage to the hypothalamus, which regulates body temperature. Mild elevations due to trauma are not uncommon during the first 2 days.

**Motor Activity.** Because nerves energize the muscle tissue, any damage to the nervous system affects body movement. The quality and strength of muscle tone are observed in all four extremities. The patient should be able to squeeze the nurse's hands. The grip should be equal in both hands. The patient should be able to move the legs and push against the nurse's hands with both feet. The face should be symmetric. The patient can smile and frown. Drooping of the eyes, ptosis, inability to close the eyes tightly, and drooping of the corner of the mouth are considered adverse signs. The patient should be able to raise the arms and extend the palms upward and downward. Abnormal posturing is described and recorded.

**Other Nursing Observations.** Other factors include examination of wound swelling if a laceration of the head is present. The type and amount of drainage from the ears and nose are recorded. The nurse checks for *nuchal* or neck rigidity, which might indicate infection. Occipital frontal circumference is monitored in

**Table 25–2.** THE GLASGOW COMA SCALE MODIFIED FOR INFANTS

| Age in Months | Response |
|---|---|
| 1 | 1. None |
| | 2. Crying to stimuli |
| | 3. Crying spontaneously |
| | 4. Blinks when eyelashes touched |
| | 5. Throaty noises |
| 2 | 1. None |
| | 2. Crying to stimuli |
| | 3. Shuts eyes to light |
| | 4. Smiles when caressed |
| | 5. Babbles—single vowel sounds |
| 3 | 1. None |
| | 2. Crying to stimuli (moans) |
| | 3. Stares to response and looks at environment |
| | 4. Smiles to sound stimulation |
| | 5. Coos, chuckles, *vowels* in a prolonged way |
| 4 | 1. None |
| | 2. Crying to stimuli (moans) |
| | 3. Turns head to sound |
| | 4. Smiles spontaneously or when stimulated, laughs when socially stimulated |
| | 5. Modulating voice and perfect vocalization of vowels |
| 5 and 6 | 1. None |
| | 2. Crying to stimuli (moans) |
| | 3. Localizes general direction of sound |
| | 4. Discriminates family members |
| | 5. Babbles to people, toys |
| 7 and 8 | 1. None |
| | 2. Crying to stimuli (moans) |
| | 3. Recognizes familiar voices and family |
| | 4. Babbles |
| | 5. "Ba," "Ma," "Da" |
| 9 and 10 | 1. None |
| | 2. Crying to stimuli (moans) |
| | 3. Recognizes (smiles or laughs) |
| | 4. Babbles |
| | 5. "Mama," "Dada" |
| 11 and 12 | 1. None |
| | 2. Crying to stimuli (moans) |
| | 3. Recognizes—smiles |
| | 4. Babbles |
| | 5. Words (specifically "Mama" and "Dada") |

From Zimmerman, S.S., & Gildea, J.H. (1985). *Critical care pediatrics*. Philadelphia: W.B. Saunders.

infants, as are tension of the fontanels and presence of a high-pitched cry. Fluids are carefully monitored in order to control *cerebral edema*. Overhydration increases the amount of cerebral fluid. Feeding difficulties should be noted as the child's diet is increased. Patients are observed for signs of shock, which can also occur. Patients whose condition has remained stable are discharged. Parents are instructed about any additional observations and follow-up care.

## Torticollis (Wry Neck)

**Description.** Torticollis (*tortus*, "twisted," and *collium*, "neck") is a condition in which neck motion is limited because of shortening of the sternocleidomastoid muscle. It can be either congenital or acquired. It can also be either acute or chronic. The most common type is a congenital anomaly in which the sternocleidomastoid muscle is injured during birth. It is associated with breech and forceps delivery and may be seen in conjunction with other birth defects, such as congenital hip.

**Manifestations.** In congenital torticollis the symptoms are present at birth. The infant holds the head to the side of the muscle involved. The chin is tilted in the opposite direction. There is a hard palpable mass of dense fibrotic tissue (fibroma). This is not fixed to the skin and resolves by 2–6 months. The value of passive stretching exercises is controversial (Behrman, 1992). Feeding and playing with the infant can encourage turning to the desired side for correction. Operative correction is indicated if the condition persists beyond 2 years.

Acquired torticollis is seen in older children. It may be associated with injury, inflammation, neurologic disorders, and other causes. Nursing intervention is primarily that of detection. Infants who have limited head movements require further investigation.

## Scoliosis

**Description.** The most prevalent of the three skeletal abnormalities shown in Figure 25–15 is scoliosis. Scoliosis refers to an S-shaped curvature of the spine (Fig. 25–16). During adolescence, scoliosis is more common in girls. Many curvatures are not progressive and may require only periodic evaluation. Untreated progressive scoliosis may lead to back pain, fatigue, disability, and heart and lung complications. Skeletal deterioration does not stop with maturity and may be aggravated by pregnancy.

**Causes.** There are two types of scoliosis—

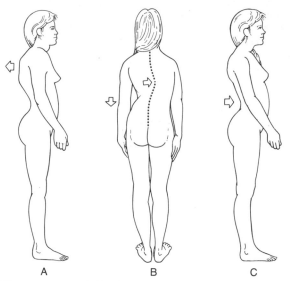

**Figure 25–15.** *A,* Kyphosis involves a hunched back and outward curvature of the spine. *B,* In scoliosis, the spine has an S shape. *C,* In lordosis, the spine is curved in such a way that the pelvis tilts forward. (From Betz, C., et al. [1994]. *Family-centered nursing care of children* [2nd ed., p. 1853]. Philadelphia: W.B. Saunders.)

functional and structural. Functional scoliosis is usually caused by poor posture and not by spinal disease. The curve is flexible and easily correctable. Structural or fixed scoliosis is due to changes in the shape of the vertebrae or thorax. It is usually accompanied by rotation of the spine. The hips and shoulders may appear uneven. The patient cannot correct the condition by standing in a straighter posture.

There are many causes of structural scoliosis. Some are congenital and develop in utero. These are noticeable at birth or during periods of rapid growth. *Neuromuscular* scoliosis is the result of muscle weakness or imbalance. It is seen in children with cerebral palsy, muscular dystrophy, and other conditions. The cause of *idiopathic* scoliosis is unknown. A person who has scoliosis has an increased chance of having children with the condition. Current evidence indicates it is transmitted as an autosomal dominant trait.

**Treatment.** Treatment is aimed at correcting the curvature and preventing more severe scoliosis. Curves up to 20 degrees do not require treatment but are carefully followed. Curves between 20 and 40 degrees require daily exercise

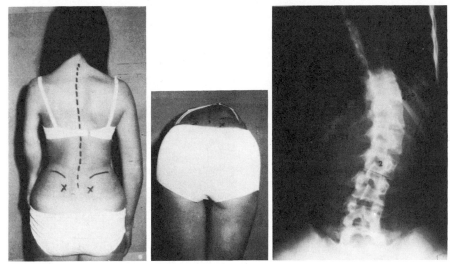

**Figure 25-16.** Scoliosis. The spine rotates as it curves, with the spinous processes moving toward the concavity. The severe curve of 46 degrees seen by roentgenogram on the right is only partly recognizable when the patient stands upright. However, examination with the child's spine flexed shows the rotation on the right that indicates a structural scoliosis. (From Behrman R.E., & Kliegman, R.M. [1992]. *Nelson textbook of pediatrics* [14th ed., p. 1711]. Philadelphia: W.B. Saunders.)

and the use of a Milwaukee brace (Fig. 25-17). This apparatus exerts pressure on the chin, pelvis, and convex (arched) side of the spine. It is worn approximately 23 hours a day and is worn over a T-shirt to protect the skin. An underarm modification of the brace (the Boston brace) is proving effective for patients with low curvatures. It is less cumbersome and more acceptable to the self-conscious young person. The use of a TENS unit (electrical stimulation) to prevent progression of the disorder in mild to moderate cases has shown some success. Its use is controversial.

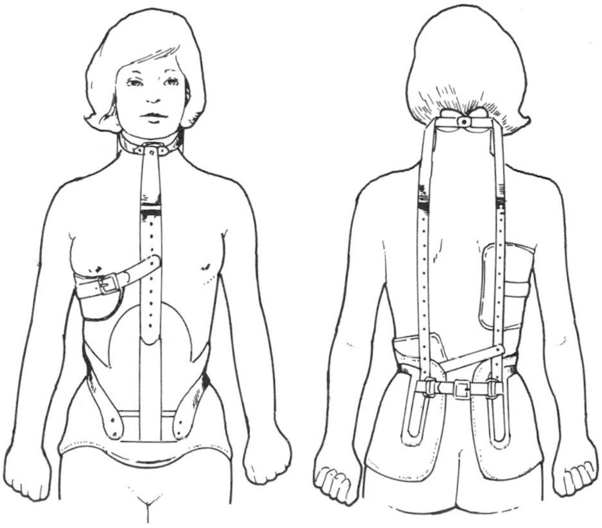

For curves of more than 40 degrees and for patients in whom conservative measures are not successful, hospitalization is required. A spinal fusion is performed. This is sometimes done in stages. A Harrington rod, Dwyer instrument, or Luque wires may be inserted for immobilization during the time required for the fusion to become solid. Halo traction may be used when there is associated weakness or paralysis of the neck and trunk muscles (Fig. 25-18); it is also used in treating cervical fractures and fusions.

**Figure 25-17.** The Milwaukee brace.

## Nursing Brief

Insertion of a Harrington rod or other metal device will delay a patient at an airport security scanner, as the metal activates the alarm. The physician can supply a note to be used as clearance for air travel.

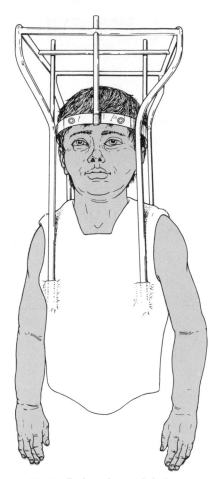

**Figure 25–18.** Body jacket with halo apparatus.

### Nursing Care

*Community Nursing.* The management of scoliosis begins with screening. This is done in middle school. It should be a part of every yearly physical examination given to prepubescent youngsters. Camp nurses also need to be aware of symptoms. Early recognition is of utmost importance in detecting mild cases amenable to nonsurgical treatment. When screening is conducted within a school system, consent forms are obtained from parents and inservice training sessions of personnel are held.

The school nurse and the physical education teacher work as a team to screen the students, usually during regular physical education classes. They prepare the students by explaining the purpose of the procedure and by reassuring them that it merely entails observation of the back while standing and while bending forward. Students need to know that it is simple, quick, and painless and that privacy will be afforded. They are instructed to wear clothing that is easy to remove, such as a pullover top. Boys disrobe to the waist, girls generally to the bra. No slip or undershirt should be worn.

The procedure consists of examining the spine from the front, side, and back while the student stands erect and then observing the back as the student bends forward. One looks initially for general body alignment and *asymmetry* (lack of proportion). In scoliosis, one shoulder may be higher than the other, a scapula may be prominent, the arm-to-body spaces may be unequal, or a hip may protrude; one arm may appear longer than the other when the person bends forward. Sometimes the patient complains of a "crooked back," uneven hemline, and difficulty in fitting of clothes. Fourth-grade boys are especially lordotic; therefore, developmental patterns at various ages must be considered. Referrals are made as indicated. Because of the familial tendencies of this condition, brothers and sisters of patients should be examined. Community understanding of scoliosis will benefit those who must obtain further treatment.

*Hospital Care.* Nursing care for hospitalized patients coincides with treatment programs. Patients may be admitted overnight for a cast change or may require more extensive correction by spinal fusion. The nurse's knowledge of preadolescent and adolescent developmental tasks is imperative, because therapy often conflicts with these tasks.

Basic cast care is described on page 345. The adolescent in a body cast has many adjustments to make as a result of its weight and its restrictions on mobility. Ambulation is difficult, as is sleeping. Modifications must be made in bathing, shampooing, dressing, and eating, and these can be frustrating. Teenagers are concerned about how they look in the cast, and clothes made especially for them boost their morale.

The usual *preoperative nursing care* of the patient is necessary for casting or spinal fusion. This includes instructing the patient and family about the purpose and extent of the cast, postoperative traction, and the use of frames and other apparatus. It is important that the nurse evaluate and document the patient's neuromuscular status at this time so that it may be used as a basis for comparison after the procedure. All four extremities are observed for color, temperature, capillary filling, edema, sensation, and motion. The nurse explains to the patient that breathing exercises and frequent change of position are necessary in order to prevent heart and lung complications. If postoperative log-rolling is anticipated, it can be practiced before surgery, or when possible, the patient may watch the procedure being done on another patient.

Much of the *postoperative nursing care* is directly related to combating the physical results of immobilization (see Fig. 25–11). The body systems become sluggish because of inactivity. This is evidenced in the gastrointestinal tract by anorexia, irregularity, and constipation. Allowing the adolescent to select foods with the aid of the dietitian is helpful in improving appetite. Increasing fluid intake reduces constipation; laxatives and enemas are sometimes required as supplemental aids. Juices, gelatin, cola drinks, soup, and noncarbonated beverages promote kidney function. The limitation of milk and milk products is controversial at this writing. Cranberry juice helps neutralize the alkaline content of urine and decrease the possibility of bladder infection.

Cardiopulmonary slowdown is counteracted by frequently changing position, exercising, and allowing the patient to do as much as possible. Range-of-motion exercises help maintain muscle tone. Activities to stimulate mental awareness are of equal importance. Emotional reaction to confinement should be anticipated. In particular, the patients fear for their safety.

When pins and wires are used, they are inspected daily to detect redness, heat, drainage, or slippage. Such symptoms are immediately reported, as the danger of bone infection is great. Instructions for home care are begun early in treatment. These should be written, and their importance should be carefully explained.

## Sports Injuries

A high percentage of adolescent males and females participate in athletic activities. Authorities disagree about what constitutes a good sports physical examination; however, they are unanimous about the necessity for precompetition medical examinations. The American Academy of Pediatrics recommends that a complete physical examination be given at least every other year during adolescence and that sports-specific examinations be given for those involved in strenuous activity on entry into junior or senior high school. Such examinations should be updated by an annual questionnaire. The family history and an orthopedic screening are important in identifying risk factors.

**Prevention.** Several factors help prevent sports injuries. Some of these are adequate warm-up and cool-down periods; year-round conditioning; careful selection of activity according to physical maturity, size, and skill necessary; proper supervision by adults; safe, well-fitting equipment; and avoidance of participation when in pain. Proper diet and fluids are also necessary. A few of the more common injuries are listed in Table 25–3. The nurse has a major role in educating and directing parents to sources of accurate information to ensure that the physical, emotional, and maturational levels of the adolescent are appropriate for the activity. Parents are encouraged to inquire as to the capabilities of personnel and availability of

**Table 25–3.** SOME OF THE MORE COMMON SPORTS INJURIES

| Type | Comment |
|---|---|
| Concussion | Any blow to the head followed by alterations in mental functioning should be treated as a possible concussion; observe carefully for sequelae |
| "Stingers" or "burners" | A common neck injury when a player hits another with the head in such sports as football or rugby; due to brachial plexus trauma; feels like an electrical jolt; usually mild, disappears suddenly; restrict sports activity until symptoms disappear; reassess protective gear |
| Injured knee ligaments | Usually a result of stress on the knee; potentially serious; should be evaluated by an experienced trainer or physician; may require arthroscopy |
| Sprain or strained ankle | May injure growth plate; x-ray films important in adolescents |
| Muscle cramps | Due to injury, alterations in blood flow, electrolyte deficiencies; important to warm up before activity; ensure fluid intake is adequate |
| Shin splints | Pain and discomfort in lower leg due to repeated running on a hard surface such as concrete; avoid such activity; use well-fitting shoes; decrease inflammation by rest |

emergency services prior to the beginning of the competition.

**Considerations for Female Athletes.** Irregular menses and amenorrhea are relatively common with any heavy exercise. This may be due to a decrease in the percentage of body fat. Weight loss, thinness, and physical and emotional stress may also precipitate such irregularities. It is suggested that teenage girls who stop menstruating for 2 months or more and those who menstruate irregularly be examined. Amenorrhea that is exercise-induced can be confused with pregnancy by the teenager. Although breast injuries are not common, several sports bras are available that provide support.

## KEY POINTS

- Immobility causes a slowing down of body metabolism.
- Injury to the epiphyseal plate at the ends of long bones is serious during childhood because it may interfere with longitudinal growth.
- Legg-Calvé-Perthes disease affects the development of the head of the femur.
- In a compound fracture, a wound in the skin leads to the broken bone, and there is added danger of infection.
- A complication of Bryant traction is an arterial occlusion termed Volkmann's ischemia.
- Juvenile rheumatoid arthritis is the most common arthritic condition of childhood.
- The major complications of head injury are hemorrhage, infection, swelling of the brain, and compression of the brain stem.
- The Glasgow Coma Scale is valuable in determining various levels of consciousness.
- Medical treatment of scoliosis includes bracing, exercise, and the use of TENS electrical stimulation.
- Adolescents who participate in sports are subject to injuries, such as concussions, and ligament injuries. Activities need to be selected carefully according to physical maturity, size, and skill required.

# Study Questions

1. List four symptoms of Duchenne's muscular dystrophy.
2. What structures are affected by Legg-Calvé-Perthes disease?
3. Ann, age 4, suffered a fractured femur in a fall from a tree. She has been hospitalized for 3 weeks in Bryant traction. What factors would you consider in planning her daily care?
4. Angela, age 9, was hit by a car while riding her bicycle in her neighborhood. What information about bicycle safety do children require? Be prepared to discuss your answer in class.
5. Angela's left leg is in Buck extension. Describe this apparatus and the nursing considerations necessary in caring for Angela. Provide the rationale for your answer.
6. List five diversions suitable for the school-age child who is immobilized.
7. Describe three methods of onset of juvenile rheumatoid arthritis.
8. What factors would you consider when providing discharge instructions for the child with juvenile rheumatoid arthritis?
9. List the symptoms of increased intracranial pressure in the small child. How does determining level of consciousness differ in children?

# Multiple Choice Review Questions

*Choose the most appropriate answer.*

1. A disorder in which the blood supply to the epiphyses of the bone is disrupted is called
   a. muscular dystrophy
   b. cerebral palsy
   c. congenital hip dysplasia
   d. Legg-Calvé-Perthes disease
2. The term used when the circulation to a part of the body is obstructed is
   a. ischemia
   b. ischesis
   c. anemia
   d. infarction
3. Buck extension is an example of
   a. skin traction
   b. skeletal traction
   c. balanced traction
   d. Bryant traction
4. An S-shaped curvature of the spine seen in school-age children is
   a. sclerosis
   b. sciatica
   c. scabies
   d. scoliosis
5. Marie, age 14, is admitted for insertion of a Harrington rod in her spine. This is
   a. a metal device used to immobilize the spine
   b. a wooden device used to immobilize the spine
   c. useful in curves up to 20 degrees
   d. similar to a Milwaukee brace

## BIBLIOGRAPHY

Behrman, R.E., & Kliegman, R.M. (1992). *Nelson textbook of pediatrics* (14th ed.). Philadelphia: W.B. Saunders.

Betz, C., et al. (1994). *Family-centered nursing care of children* (2nd ed.). Philadelphia: W.B. Saunders.

Brewer, E.J. (1990). Collagen vascular disease. In S.S. Gellis & B.M. Kagan (Eds.). (1990). *Current pediatric therapy 13.* Philadelphia: W.B. Saunders.

DeRosa, G. (1990). Musculoskeletal disorders: Congenital, developmental, and nontraumatic. In M. Green & R.J. Haggerty (Eds.), *Ambulatory pediatrics IV* (pp. 333–347). Philadelphia: W.B. Saunders.

Dickerman, J.D., & Lucey, J.F. (1984). *Smith's the critically ill child* (3rd ed.). Philadelphia: W.B. Saunders.

Graef, J., & Cone, T. (1985). *Manual of pediatric therapeutics.* Boston: Little, Brown.

Green, M., & Haggerty, R.J. (1990). *Ambulatory pediatrics IV.* Philadelphia: W.B. Saunders.

Mott, S., James, S.R., & Sperhac, A.M. (1991). *Nursing care of children and families* (2nd ed.). Reading, MA: Addison-Wesley.

Neinstein, L. (1984). *Adolescent health care.* Baltimore: Urban & Schwarzenberg.

Nelson, L.B., Calhoun, J.H., & Harley, R.D. (1991). *Pediatric Ophthalmology* (3rd ed.). Philadelphia: W.B. Saunders.

Pillitteri, A. (1992). *Maternal and child health nursing.* Philadelphia: J.B. Lippincott.

Stewart, D., & Neinstein, L. (1984). Guidelines in sports medicine. In L. Neinstein (Ed.), *Adolescent health care.* Baltimore: Urban & Schwarzenberg.

Whaley, L., & Wong, D. (1991). *Nursing care of infants and children* (4th ed.). St. Louis: C.V. Mosby.

Wisoff, J., & Epstein, F. (1985). Management of pediatric head trauma. In S.S. Zimmerman & J.H. Gildea (Eds.), *Critical care pediatrics.* Philadelphia: W.B. Saunders.

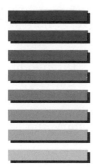

# Chapter 26

# The Child with a Circulatory or a Respiratory Condition

## VOCABULARY
**dysphagia (696)**
**hydration (703)**
**hypothermia (677)**
**laryngeal spasm (696)**
**meconium ileus (710)**
**osteoporosis (711)**
**Pleur-Evac (685)**
**status asthmaticus (705)**
**stenosis (680)**
**sternotomy (678)**

# OBJECTIVES

*On completion and mastery of Chapter 26, the student will be able to*

■ Define each vocabulary term listed.
■ Define or identify each vocabulary term listed.
■ List the general signs and symptoms of congenital heart disease.
■ Differentiate among patent ductus arteriosus, coarctation of the aorta, atrial septal defect, ventricular septal defect, and tetralogy of Fallot.
■ Discuss six nursing goals relevant to the child with heart disease.
■ Discuss hypertension in childhood.
■ Differentiate between primary and secondary hypertension.
■ List the symptoms of rheumatic fever.
■ Outline the nursing observations and care necessary for a 2-year-old child with pneumonia who requires the use of a mist tent.
■ Discuss the preoperative and postoperative care of 5-year-old Jeanine, who is scheduled for removal of her tonsils and adenoids.
■ List three topics the nurse might address in teaching self-care to the 7-year-old asthmatic child.
■ Devise a nursing care plan for the child with cystic fibrosis, including family interventions.
■ Teach a 5-year-old asthmatic child pursed-lip breathing.
■ List three medications used for asthma.
■ Discuss the role of exercise in the patient with a respiratory condition.
■ List two restrictions in the diet of a child with cystic fibrosis.

# Cardiovascular System

The cardiovascular system consists of the heart, the blood, and the blood vessels. As the heart beats, blood, oxygen, and nutrients are transported to all the tissues of the body, and waste products are removed. Because of anatomic and physiologic immaturity, the cardiovascular system of the child differs from that of the adult. Figure 26–1 summarizes these differences.

The cardiovascular system develops from the 3rd to 8th weeks of gestation. It is the first system to function in intrauterine life. When cardiovascular development is incomplete, heart defects occur. Fetal circulation is designed to serve the metabolic needs during intrauterine life and also to permit safe transmission to life outside the womb. The heart and the circula-

tory and respiratory systems work together to keep one alive. When problems arise from the heart, hemodynamics, or blood flow, is disrupted. Normal blood flow may be impaired because blood flows through openings that should have closed or because of strictures or pressure build-up within various chambers of the heart. There may also be an abnormal connection between the pulmonary and the systemic circulations.

The congenital heart defects (CHDs) discussed in this chapter are atrial septal defects (ASDs), ventricular septal defects (VSDs), patent ductus arteriosus (PDA), coarctation of the aorta, and tetralogy of Fallot. These conditions are generally recognized during the newborn period. Some acquired diseases such as congestive heart failure (CHF), rheumatic fever, systemic hypertension, and hyperlipidemia are also presented.

## CONGENITAL HEART DISEASE

**Description.** A baby born with CHD has a defect in the structure of the heart and/or one or more of the large blood vessels that lead to and from the heart. The heart or vessels have failed to develop properly. The incidence of CHD is approximately 8 in 1000 live births. The heart of the fetus is completely developed during the first 8 weeks of pregnancy (see page 400). A mother who contracts German measles early in her pregnancy or who is poorly nourished may bear a child with a faulty heart. Other prenatal or maternal factors associated with increased risk include alcoholism, exposure to coxsackievirus, diabetes mellitus, ingestion of lithium salts, and advanced maternal age. Patients with genetic factors such as a history of CHD in other family members, patients with Down syndrome or other chromosomal aberrations, and patients who have other congenital defects often contribute to the incidence of CHD.

Research indicates that most congenital heart lesions are produced by a genetic-environmental interaction, that is, they are multifactorial. In other words, CHDs are not all one disease; a hereditary predisposition is determined by many genes, and an environmental factor "pushes" the predisposed fetus over the threshold from normal to abnormal development.

Of the congenital anomalies, heart defects are the principal cause of death during the 1st year of life. Therefore, nurses must stress the need for good prenatal care and impress on par-

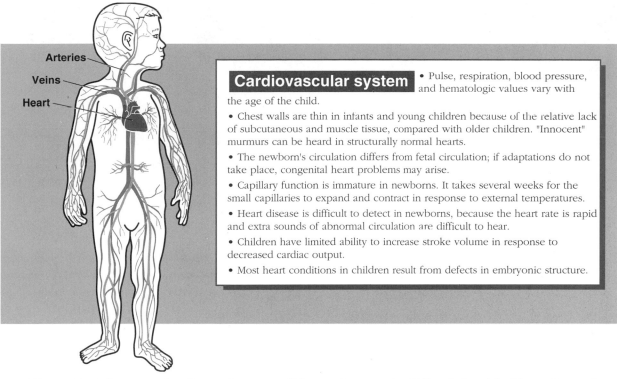

Arteries
Veins
Heart

**Cardiovascular system**

• Pulse, respiration, blood pressure, and hematologic values vary with the age of the child.

• Chest walls are thin in infants and young children because of the relative lack of subcutaneous and muscle tissue, compared with older children. "Innocent" murmurs can be heard in structurally normal hearts.

• The newborn's circulation differs from fetal circulation; if adaptations do not take place, congenital heart problems may arise.

• Capillary function is immature in newborns. It takes several weeks for the small capillaries to expand and contract in response to external temperatures.

• Heart disease is difficult to detect in newborns, because the heart rate is rapid and extra sounds of abnormal circulation are difficult to hear.

• Children have limited ability to increase stroke volume in response to decreased cardiac output.

• Most heart conditions in children result from defects in embryonic structure.

**Figure 26–1.** Summary of cardiovascular system differences between the child and the adult. The cardiovascular system consists of the heart, blood, and blood vessels. As the heart beats, blood, oxygen, and nutrients are transported to all the tissues of the body, and waste products are removed.

ents the value of regular checkups at baby clinics. Many organic heart murmurs have been detected early in infancy at periodic checkups. A careful health history is particularly useful. The symptoms, as indicated in Box 26–1, depend on the location and type of heart defect. Some patients have mild cases and can lead a fairly normal life under medical management. Others are treated medically until the optimal time for surgery.

**Surgical and Diagnostic Progress.** Many exciting advances are being made in the field of cardiac surgery (Fig. 26–2). Better techniques and finer monitoring devices are being perfected. The thoracotomy is now widely performed with fewer complications; thus, the risks associated with entering the chest cavity are decreased. Cardiac catheterization is routinely performed and is being scheduled on an outpatient basis in some hospitals (Table 26–1). The cardiopulmonary bypass machine takes over the function of the heart and lungs. By keeping other vital tissues of the body alive, this machine gives the surgeon more time and a clearer field in which to operate. Another technique used in heart surgery is hypothermia (*hypo,* "under," and *therme,* "heat"). This procedure reduces the temperature of body tissues, which in turn decreases their need for oxygen. Hypothermia may be done by using cooling agents in the heart-lung machine. Complete heart transplantation offers another avenue of hope for the child with a CHD that is incompatible with life.

**Classification.** Formerly, congenital heart defects were divided into two categories: cyanotic and acyanotic. This classification is somewhat misleading because patients do not always fall into the two categories but display mixed or alternate features that do not fit the clinical picture. A more accurate classification is based on the effect of the defect on blood circulation. The study of blood circulation is termed *hemodynamis* (*hemo,* "blood," and *dynamics,* "power"). Blood always flows from an area of high pressure to an area of low pressure and takes the path of least resistance. Physiologically, defects can be organized into (1) lesions that increase

| BOX 26–1 | Manifestations of Congenital Heart Abnormalities in Infants and Children |
|---|---|

**Infants**

Dyspnea
Difficulty with feeding
Stridor or choking spells
Pulse rate over 200 beats/min
Recurrent respiratory infections
Failure to gain weight
Heart murmurs
Cyanosis
Cerebrovascular accidents
Anoxic attacks

**Children**

Dyspnea
Poor physical development
Decreased exercise tolerance
Recurrent respiratory infections
Heart murmur and thrill
Cyanosis
Squatting
Clubbing of fingers and toes
Elevated blood pressure

From Ross Laboratories. (1986). *A study guide to congenital heart abnormalities.* Reproduced with permission of Ross Laboratories, Columbus, Ohio 43216. © 1986, Ross Laboratories.

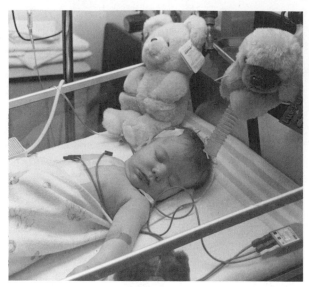

**Figure 26–2.** An infant recovering from repair of a congenital heart defect. (Courtesy of Mercy Hospital Medical Center, Des Moines, IA.)

pulmonary blood flow, (2) lesions that obstruct blood flow, and (3) lesions that decrease pulmonary blood flow. There are also mixed lesions. A *shunt* refers to the flow of blood through an abnormal opening between the right and left sides of the heart, or between two vessels of the heart. Figure 26–3 illustrates some of these defects.

### Defects That Increase Pulmonary Blood Flow

**Atrial Septal Defect.** In ASD, there is an abnormal opening between the right and the left atria. Blood that contains oxygen is forced from the left atrium to the right atrium. This type of arteriovenous shunt does not produce cyanosis unless the blood flow is reversed by heart failure. The incidence is higher in girls than in boys. Most patients do not have symptoms. The defect may be recognized during a routine health examination, when a murmur is heard. Cardiac catheterization, electrocardiogram, and echocardiography may be performed to assist in determining diagnosis. The surgical repair involves a median sternotomy (*sternum* and *otomy*, "cutting"). Closure is similar to that for VSD (see the following discussion). Continued cardiology follow-up is necessary. Prognosis is excellent.

**Ventricular Septal Defect.** VSD is the most common heart anomaly. It accounts for 25% of CHDs (Behrman, 1992). As the name suggests, there is an opening between the right and left ventricles of the heart. Increased pressure within the left ventricle forces blood into the right ventricle. A loud, harsh murmur combined with a systolic tremor is characteristic of this defect. The condition may be mild or severe. It is frequently associated with other defects. Many children with small defects may experience spontaneous closure during the 1st year of life as a result of growth.

Treatment includes close observation of the growing child. Prophylactic antibiotics may be given to prevent bacterial endocarditis. If closure does not occur, open heart surgery is performed under hypothermia. With the use of the heart-lung bypass machine, the condition can

**Table 26–1.** VALUE OF DIAGNOSTIC TESTS USED IN CONGENITAL HEART DEFECTS

| Test | Definition | Value |
|---|---|---|
| Angiocardiography (selective) | Serial x-ray films of the heart and great vessels following injection of an opaque substance; a radiopaque catheter is moved into the heart chambers, and contrast medium is injected in specific areas | Abnormal communications in the heart can be observed; the course of the blood through the heart and great vessels can be traced |
| Aortography | X-ray films of the aorta after the injection of an opaque material | Useful in revealing patent ductus arteriosus |
| Radionuclide angiocardiography | Noninvasive nuclear procedure that permits visualization of the course of blood through the heart | May be used as a pre-cardiac catheterization screening study; provides assessment of congenital and acquired cardiovascular lesions and monitors the effects of therapy; an intravenous device is necessary to permit injection of the radionuclide |
| Barium swallow | Barium given by mouth | Shows indentation of the esophagus by the aorta or other vessels |
| Cardiac catheterization | A radiopaque catheter is passed through a cutdown site directly into the heart and large vessels | Reveals blood pressure within the heart; doctors can examine the heart closely with the tip of the catheter to detect abnormalities; blood samples can be obtained in order to determine oxygen content |
| Chest x-ray film | — | Provides a permanent record; shows abnormalities in shape and position of heart |
| Cineangiocardiography | Motion pictures of images recorded by fluoroscopy | Useful record and monitoring device |
| Echocardiography | The use of ultrasound to produce an image of sound waves of the heart; transducer placed directly on chest; sounds are analyzed on paper | Noninvasive procedure; localizes murmurs; determines if heart is structurally normal |
| Electrocardiogram | Tracing of heart action by electrocardiography | Detects variations in heart action and shows the condition of the heart muscle; may also be used as a monitoring device during cardiac catheterization |
| Magnetic resonance imaging | Noninvasive imaging technique that uses low-energy radio waves in combination with a magnetic field to generate signals that produce tomographic images | Very useful in diagnosing coarctation of the aorta |

be corrected in a fairly dry or bloodless field. The hole is ligated with sutures or a synthetic patch. "The patch is not rejected because it is an inert substance and cardiac tissue completely covers the patch within 6 months after surgery" (Daberkow-Carson & Smith, 1994). A staged banding procedure by way of closed heart surgery is sometimes done on babies who are too ill to risk open heart surgery. This procedure provides relief from symptoms until the optimal time for definitive surgery arrives. The long-term prognosis after surgery is excellent.

**Patent Ductus Arteriosus.** The circulation of the fetus differs from that of the newborn in that most of the fetal blood bypasses the lungs.

The ductus arteriosus is the passageway through which the blood crosses from the pulmonary artery to the aorta and avoids the deflated lungs. This vessel closes shortly after birth; however, when it does not close, blood continues to pass from the aorta, where the pressure is higher, into the pulmonary artery. This causes oxygenated blood to recycle through the lungs, overburdening the pulmonary circulation and making the heart pump harder.

The symptoms of PDA may go unnoticed during infancy. However as the child grows, dyspnea is experienced, the radial pulse becomes full and bounding on exertion, and there is an unusually wide range between systolic pressure and diastolic pressure. This is referred to as the pulse pressure. The classic "machinery type" murmur may be heard. A two-dimensional echocardiogram is useful in visualizing and determining blood flow across the PDA.

PDA is one of the most common cardiac anomalies. It occurs twice as frequently in girls as in boys. Closed heart surgery is performed in all diagnosed patients if there are no other complications. If this condition is left uncorrected, the patient could eventually develop CHF or endocarditis. The opening is closed by ligation or by division of the ductus. Indomethacin has been used medically to close the ductus in premature babies. The prognosis is excellent.

## Obstructive Defect: Coarctation of the Aorta

The word *coarctation* means "a tightening." In coarctation of the aorta, there is a constriction or narrowing of the aortic arch or of the descending aorta (the blood meets an obstruction). Hemodynamics consists of increased pressure proximal to the defect and decreased pressure distally. The classic symptoms are a marked difference in the blood pressure and pulses of the upper and lower extremities. The patient may not develop symptoms until late childhood. Treatment depends on the type and severity of the defect. Infants who have associated CHF are treated medically until the optimal time for surgery.

The surgeon resects the narrowed portion of the aorta and joins its ends. The joining is called an *anastomosis*. If the section removed is large, an end-to-end graft using tubes of synthetic polyester (Dacron) or similar material may be necessary. Because the graft will not grow but the aorta will, the best time for surgery is between the ages of 2 and 4 years. As in PDA, closed heart surgery is performed because the structures are outside the heart. The prognosis is good if there are no other defects and the child's physical condition is favorable at the time of surgery. Newer surgical techniques are being perfected for infants in whom a high incidence of restenosis occurs.

## Defect That Decreases Pulmonary Blood Flow: Tetralogy of Fallot

*Tetra* means "four." In this condition, there are four defects: (1) stenosis or narrowing of the pulmonary artery, which decreases the blood flow to the lungs; (2) hypertrophy of the right ventricle, which enlarges because it has to work harder in order to pump blood through the narrow pulmonary artery, (3) dextraposition (*dextra*, "right," and *position*) of the aorta, in which the aorta is displaced to the right and blood from both ventricles enters it; and (4) VSD (see Fig. 26–3).

When venous blood enters the aorta, the infant displays severe heart trouble. Cyanosis increases with age, and clubbing of the fingers and toes is seen. The child rests in a "squatting" position to breath more easily. This position increases systemic venous return. Feeding problems, growth retardation, frequent respiratory infections, and severe dyspnea on exercise are prevalent. The red blood cells of the body increase, causing polycythemia (*poly*, "many," *cyt*, "cells," and *hema*, "blood") in an effort to compensate for the lack of oxygen.

All children with cyanotic CHD are at risk for neurologic sequelae, such as cerebrovascular accident. Tetralogy spells characterized by cyanosis, irritability, pallor, blackouts, and convulsions may occur. Iron-deficiency anemias, due to poor appetite, are common. In some cases, mental retardation develops because too little oxygen reaches the brain. The child is medically treated until the optimal time for surgery. Staged surgery may be done to increase the flow of blood to the lungs. With the advent of microvascular surgery, these procedures can be successfully carried out in the newborn period. Open heart surgery is performed for permanent correction of the defect. The surgical risk of total correction is currently under 5% (Behrman, 1992). After successful total correction, patients are able to lead unrestricted lives.

## ACQUIRED HEART DISEASE

### Congestive Heart Failure

**Description.** An infant with a severe heart defect may develop CHF. When this occurs, the heart enlarges and is unable to pump an adequate supply of blood throughout the body. In the older child CHF may be caused by arrhythmias, anemia, myocarditis, sepsis, or hypertension.

**Manifestations.** Manifestations depend on the side of the heart affected (Fig. 26–4). Signs differ somewhat and are more subtle in infants. Some of these signs are cyanosis, pallor, rapid respiration, rapid pulse, feeding difficulties,

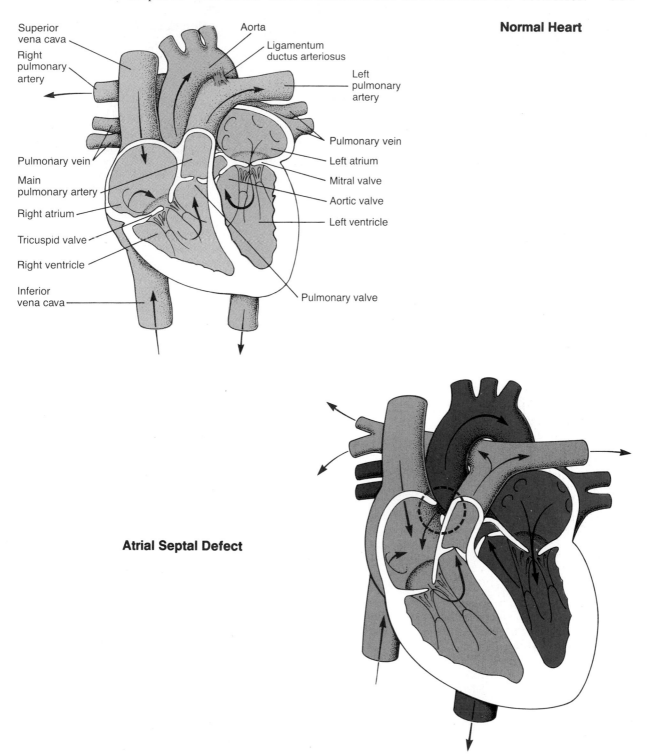

**Normal Heart**

Superior vena cava

Right pulmonary artery

Aorta

Ligamentum ductus arteriosus

Left pulmonary artery

Pulmonary vein

Left atrium

Mitral valve

Aortic valve

Left ventricle

Pulmonary vein

Main pulmonary artery

Right atrium

Tricuspid valve

Right ventricle

Inferior vena cava

Pulmonary valve

**Atrial Septal Defect**

**Figure 26–3.** The normal heart and hearts with congenital defects. (Modified from Betz, C., Hunsberger, M., and Wright, S. [1994]. *Family-centered nursing care of children* [2nd ed.]. Philadelphia: W.B. Saunders.)

*Continued*

**Ventricular Septal Defect**

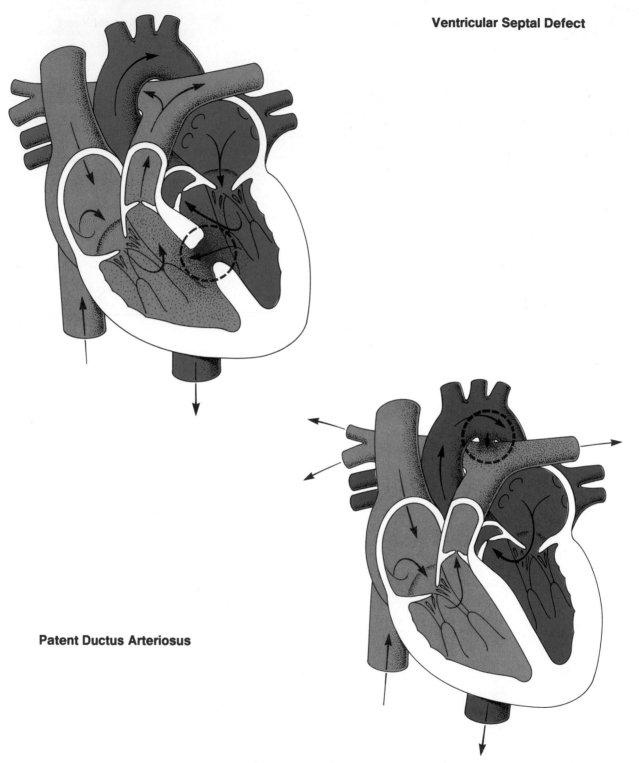

**Patent Ductus Arteriosus**

**Figure 26–3.** *Continued*

**Coarctation of the Aorta**

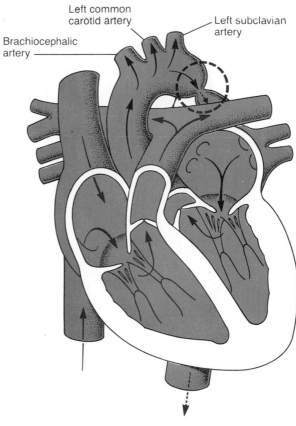

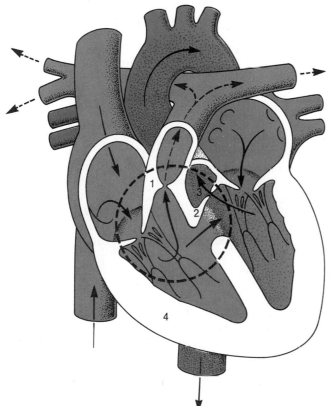

**Figure 26–3.** *Continued*

**Tetralogy of Fallot**

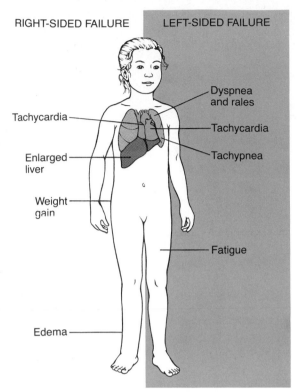

RIGHT-SIDED FAILURE      LEFT-SIDED FAILURE

Tachycardia

Enlarged liver

Weight gain

Edema

Dyspnea and rales

Tachycardia

Tachypnea

Fatigue

**Figure 26–4.** Manifestations of congestive heart failure. (Redrawn from Pillitteri, A. [1992]. *Maternal and child health nursing: Care of the childbearing and childrearing family.* Philadelphia: J.B. Lippincott.)

fatigue, failure to gain weight, edema, and frequent respiratory infections.

*Cyanosis.* When observing color, the nurse notes whether the cyanosis is general or localized. If it is localized, the exact location is recorded in the nurse's notes, for example, hands, feet, lips, or around the mouth. Is the cyanosis deep or light? Is it constant or transient? Sometimes color improves during crying, and sometimes it gets worse; this is significant. If overt cyanosis is not apparent in the African-American infant, the palms of the hands and bottoms of the feet are observed. Clubbing of the fingers and toes as a result of blood pooling in the capillaries of the extremities may be evident. The skin may be very pale or may be mottled. Sweating, particularly of the head, may be evidenced.

*Rapid Respiration.* Rapid respiration is *tachypnea.* Over 60 breaths/min in a newborn at rest indicates distress. The amount of dyspnea does vary. In more acute cases, dyspnea is accompanied by flaring of the nostrils, mouth breathing, grunting, and sternal retractions.

The baby has more trouble breathing when flat in bed than when held upright. Air hunger is indicated if the patient is irritable and restless. The cry is weak and hoarse.

*Rapid Pulse.* Rapid pulse is termed *tachycardia.* An increase in pulse rate is one of the first signs of CHF. The heart is pumping harder in an effort to increase its output and provide increased oxygen to all the tissues of the body. Cardiac output can be increased by one of two mechanisms—tachycardia or increased *stroke volume.* Stroke volume is the amount of blood ejected during one contraction. Because infants and small children have a limited ability to increase stroke volume, their heart rate increases. The heart is pumping harder in an effort to get sufficient oxygen to all parts of the body.

*Feeding Difficulties.* When the nurse tries to feed these infants, they tire easily. They may stop after sucking a few ounces. When placed in the crib, they cry and appear hungry. They may choke and gag during feedings; the pleasure of sucking is spoiled by their inability to breathe.

*Poor Weight Gain.* The patient fails to gain weight. A sudden increase in weight may indicate the beginning of heart failure.

*Edema.* Blood flow to the kidneys is decreased, and the glomerular filtration rate slows. This causes both fluid and sodium to be retained. The nurse watches for puffiness about the eyes and, occasionally, in the legs, feet, and abdomen. Urine output may decrease.

*Frequent Respiratory Tract Infections.* Resistance is very low. Slight infections can be highly dangerous, because the heart and lungs are already compromised. Immunizations are reviewed and updated as needed. The nurse prevents exposure to other children who have upper respiratory tract infections, diarrhea, and the like.

**Treatment and Nursing Care.** The nursing goals significant to the care of children with heart defects are (1) to reduce the work of the heart, (2) to improve respiration, (3) to maintain proper nutrition, (4) to prevent infection, (5) to reduce the anxiety of the patient, and (6) to support and instruct the parents.

The nurse must organize care so that the baby is not unnecessarily disturbed. The patient needs a great deal of energy. A complete bath and linen change are luxuries that an infant with a serious heart defect cannot afford.

The infant is fed early if crying and late if asleep. The physician orders the position in which the infant is placed. In some cases, the knee-chest position facilitates breathing; in other cases, a slanting position with the head elevated may be helpful. Older babies may be placed in infant seats.

Feedings are small and frequent. A soft nipple with holes large enough to prevent the infant from tiring is provided. Older children generally tolerate a "no added salt" diet with a restriction on high-sodium foods. In some cases, nasogastric tube feedings are advantageous because they are less tiring for the patient. Oxygen is administered in order to relieve dyspnea. As breathing becomes easier, the baby begins to relax. A soft voice and gentle care soothe the patient. Whenever possible, the infant is held and shown love during feedings.

Digitoxin and digoxin (Lanoxin) are common oral digitalis preparations. In pediatric patients, Lanoxin is preferred because of its rapid action and shorter half-life. These agents slow and strengthen the heartbeat. The nurse counts the patient's pulse for 1 full minute before administering them. A resting apical pulse is most accurate. As a rule, if the pulse rate of a newborn is below 100 beats/min the medication is withheld and the physician is notified. In older children, the pulse rate should be above 70 beats/min. Because the pulse rate varies with the age of the child, it is ideal for the physician to specify in the written drug order at what heart rate the nurse should withhold the drug. When this is not done the nurse obtains clarification. The physician is notified when the drug is withheld.

If the patient vomits the physician is contacted. Digitalis administration is not repeated until the physician confirms it is safe to do so. Tachycardia and irregularities in the rhythm of the pulse are significant and should be reported. Symptoms of toxicity include nausea, vomiting, anorexia, irregularity in rate and rhythm of the pulse, and a sudden change in pulse. If the baby is discharged while still receiving medication, the parents are taught how to take the pulse and what signs to be alert for when administering the drug.

Diuretics such as furosemide (Lasix) or chlorothiazide (Diuril) are useful in reducing edema. Careful monitoring of serum electrolyte levels prevents electrolyte imbalance, particularly potassium depletion. Parents of older patients are taught to recognize foods high in potassium, such as bananas, oranges, milk, potatoes, and prune juice. Diapers are weighed in order to determine urine output. Daily weighing of the baby also helps the physician determine the effectiveness of the diuresis.

Complications other than cardiac decompensation (heart failure) may arise before or after surgery. Because of the increase in numbers of red blood cells circulating within the body (polycythemia), the blood becomes sluggish and prone to clots. When this is accompanied by dehydration, the threat of cerebral thrombosis may become a reality.

An accurate record of intake and output is essential. Signs of dehydration, such as thirst, fever, poor skin turgor, apathy, sunken eyes or fontanel, dry skin, dry tongue, dry mucous membranes, and decrease in urination, should be brought to the immediate attention of the nurse in charge. Pneumonia can occur rapidly. Fever, irritability, and increase in respiratory distress may indicate this condition. The patient's position is changed regularly in order to help prevent this setback.

Chest tubes may be used postoperatively to remove secretions and air from the pleural cavity and to allow reexpansion of the lungs. These are attached to underwater-seal drainage bottles or a commercially manufactured disposable system, such as Pleur-Evac. Units for infants and older children are available. This system must be *airtight* in order to prevent collapse of the lung. Drainage bottles are always kept below the level of the chest to prevent backflow of secretions. This is especially important during transportation. Two rubber-shod Kelly clamps are available at all times for emergency clamping of tubes. These are applied to the tubes as close as possible to the child's chest if a break in the system occurs.

The nurse working in a cardiac unit assesses the patient frequently for complications of cardiac and respiratory arrest (Fig. 26–5) and should be competent in cardiopulmonary resuscitation techniques and the necessary modifications required for pediatric patients (see p. 468).

The parents of the child need support and understanding over a long period of time. A mother's fears and dependencies come to the surface when she gives birth to a baby with a defect. Because the heart is the body's major vital organ, this type of diagnosis causes much apprehension (Fig. 26–6). The physician has to reassure the parents without minimizing the

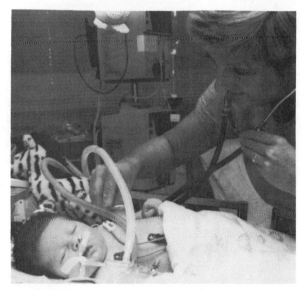

**Figure 26–5.** A registered nurse assesses a critically ill infant in the cardiac intensive care unit. Parents need to be prepared for the intrusive mechanical devices required in the patient's care. (Courtesy of Mercy Hospital Medical Center, Des Moines, IA.)

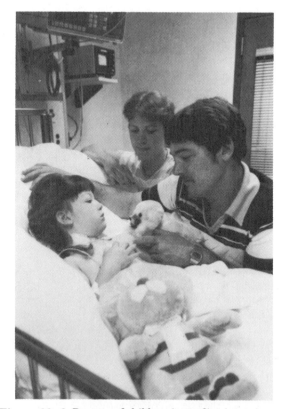

**Figure 26–6.** Parents of children in cardiac intensive care units experience a great deal of anxiety, because the heart is such a vital organ. (Courtesy of Mercy Hospital Medical Center, Des Moines, IA.)

danger involved. If the condition permits, the infant is sent home under medical supervision until the preferred age for surgery. The family must make every effort to provide the child with a normal environment within the necessary limits. It is easy for parents to become overpermissive because they do not wish the child to become unnecessarily excited. The child senses this and soon gains control of the home. This situation is difficult for everyone but is especially exhausting and confining for the mother. Disciplining the child, such as with a 5-minute time-out (chair time), is beneficial if done with consistency.

The patterns formed during infancy can build the framework of a healthy personality for the patient. Children with heart conditions who are well integrated into family life have a decided advantage over children who are made to think they are invalids. Routine naps and early bedtime provide adequate rest for most patients. As patients grow, they usually set their own limits on the amount of activity they can handle. Substitutions can be made for strenuous activities, such as bicycle riding, and for rigorous competitive games. The child receives the usual childhood immunizations. Prompt treatment of infections is important. A suitable diet with adequate fluids is necessary. Eating iron-rich foods is encouraged. Dental care should be regular. All-day attendance in school may be too tiring for the child; therefore, special provisions may be necessary. The child needs careful evaluation before any type of minor surgery is performed.

Some children will need occasional hospitalization for various tests or problems. They must be given simple explanations about their condition. They should be allowed to handle and to see hospital equipment before it is used whenever feasible. Cardiac surgery is generally performed at a regional medical center where the necessary costly equipment is available. The American Heart Association has established standards and recommendations for centers that care for children with CHDs. To provide a continuum of nursing care, one nurse per shift is assigned to each child. Detailed discharge planning and coordination of community services are of value to the family. Over the years, the financial burden to the parents for medical and surgical necessities is phenomenal. All avenues for financial aid should be explored by qualified personnel. Nursing Care Plan 26–1 specifies interventions for the infant with a CHD complicated by CHF.

## Selected Nursing Diagnoses for the Infant with a Congenital Heart Defect Complicated by Congestive Heart Failure

| Goals | Nursing Interventions | Rationale |
|---|---|---|
| **Nursing Diagnosis:** High risk for altered cardiac output: decreased related to the heart's inability to pump enough blood to meet the metabolic needs of the body. | | |
| Infant has adequate rest that is reflected by improved cardiac status (vital signs, laboratory results) | 1. Reduce workload on heart by maintaining a quiet environment; organize treatments so as to decrease disturbance; monitor vital signs carefully | 1. Optimum rest will decrease demands on heart; pulse rate increases dramatically during congestive heart failure and may be one of the first signs of heart failure in the absence of fever |
| | 2. Assess response to digoxin (if administered) | 2. Digoxin is very effective in improving workload of heart by increasing ventricular contractility and decreasing heart rate, but it is also lethal if levels become too high |
| | 3. Use larger-holed nipples to minimize energy needed for sucking | 3. Feeding difficulties are frequent because infants are subject to dyspnea, choking, and fatigue |
| Infant does not become chilled or overheated as evidenced by temperature evaluation of body and environment | 4. Avoid chilling by dressing infant appropriately for ambient temperature | 4. Thermoregulation is important because extremes could increase body's metabolic rate and oxygen requirements |
| | 5. Report temperature increases | 5. Could indicate infection |
| **Nursing Diagnosis:** High risk for impaired gas exchange related to excessive pulmonary congestion and anxiety. | | |
| Infant balances energy demands with cardiac output as evidenced by stable vital signs and pink, warm skin | 1. Monitor respiratory status frequently | 1. Arterial blood gases or pulse oximetry provides important information as to respiratory status; pulmonary edema is manifested by tachypnea and decreased tidal volume |
| | 2. Note color of extremities, lips, nail beds | 2. Cyanosis of extremities, lips, and nail beds is a sign of decrease in peripheral tissue perfusion |
| Infant expends less effort and does not use accessory muscles to breathe | 3. Note sternal retractions | 3. Sternal retractions indicate a progression in respiratory distress; Cheyne-Stokes respirations indicate worsening heart failure |
| | 4. Place in semi-Fowler position | 4. Prevents abdominal organs from pressing on diaphragm (unless contraindicated because of other congenital defects) |
| | 5. Assess for signs of respiratory infection, such as cough, increased dyspnea, fever, congestion, sneezing | 5. Children with heart disease are subject to frequent respiratory infections; infection increases oxygen demand |
| | 6. Avoid restrictive clothing | 6. Restrictive clothing can inhibit breathing |
| | 7. Administer oxygen to reduce stress on heart; monitor via pulse oximetry or arterial blood gases | 7. Infants with congestive heart failure have decreased oxygenation of their tissues because of inadequate circulation; oxygen is given to increase the amount of $O_2$ in blood and to reduce hypoxia; suctioning and positioning can also improve tissue oxygenation |

*Continued*

| NURSING CARE PLAN 26–1 *Continued* | | |
|---|---|---|
| **Selected Nursing Diagnoses for the Infant with a Congenital Heart Defect Complicated by Congestive Heart Failure** | | |
| **Goals** | **Nursing Interventions** | **Rationale** |

**Nursing Diagnosis:** Altered nutrition: less than body requirements due to inadequate caloric intake related to fatigue, immature digestive tract, poor sucking ability.

| Goals | Nursing Interventions | Rationale |
|---|---|---|
| Infant ingests adequate calories for growth by 24 hr<br>Regurgitation decreases in frequency and amount | 1. Feed at first sign of hunger; crying wastes energy<br>2. Provide adequate rest before and after feeding | 1. Decrease energy expenditures<br>2. Infants tire easily; many babies are physically undeveloped—preterm infants and the like; gavage feedings may be ordered to ensure adequate nutrients while decreasing energy requirements; avoiding procedures following feedings may prevent regurgitation |
| Infant gradually ingests greater quantities of food | 3. Provide small, frequent feedings<br><br>4. Weigh daily | 3. Capacity of infant's stomach is small; frequent small feedings prevent regurgitation<br>4. Decreased renal perfusion results in salt and water retention, which leads to edema; daily weighings assist in determining effectiveness of treatment (many infants are on diuretics), nutritional status, and growth; also important in determining dosage of digoxin |
| Infant's weight begins to stabilize | 5. Administer potassium, if ordered, if infant is on diuretic or digoxin to prevent hypokalemia<br><br>6. Monitor electrolytes<br><br><br><br><br><br><br><br><br><br><br>7. Administer vitamins<br><br><br><br><br><br>8. Keep accurate record of intake and output; weigh diapers | 5. Diuretics decrease salt and water retention related to decreased renal perfusion; since potassium may be lost during diuresis, hypokalemia may occur<br>6. Diuretic agents may cause profound changes in electrolyte composition; therefore, frequent electrolyte evaluations are made; potassium depletion, especially in digitalized patient, is very dangerous; anatomic and physiologic makeup of infants and small children makes them vulnerable to imbalances in fluid and electrolytes, particularly during illness<br>7. In severe heart failure, child is less likely to eat and may become malnourished from a decreased intake of nutrients; children in process of growth may require additional vitamins<br>8. Diuretic therapy is used when edema and pulmonary congestion are associated with retention of sodium by kidneys; an accurate intake and output sheet determines necessity for hydration and reaction to medication and treatment protocol |

### Selected Nursing Diagnoses for the Infant with a Congenital Heart Defect Complicated by Congestive Heart Failure

| Goals | Nursing Interventions | Rationale |
|---|---|---|
| **Nursing Diagnosis:** High risk for altered family processes due to misunderstanding, feelings of helplessness, fatigue. | | |
| Parents verbalize fears, ask questions | 1. Assess parents' understanding of all treatments and procedures | 1. Good teaching begins with exploring what person understands and building on the known |
| | 2. Assess need for information | 2. Pick opportune time to teach; if family is very stressed, little will be retained |
| Parents participate in the care of their infant if they wish and as feasible | 3. Encourage parents to participate in baby's care | 3. Active participation by family helps decrease anxiety |
| | 4. Educate parents in procedures related to daily care, signs of congestive heart failure, conservation of baby's energy, feedings, medications (*Note:* Digoxin can be fatal if taken accidentally; inform parents not to leave drug where siblings could reach it) | 4. Discharge planning begins on admission; hospitalization is often briefer, necessitating an early start; ensures uninterrupted care |
| | 5. Allow siblings to visit | 5. Sibling visits promote bonding, allay fears, and help children feel a part of what is occurring |
| | 6. Provide homelike atmosphere | 6. Homelike atmosphere helps reduce anxiety |
| | 7. Educate as to local support groups | 7. Because this disease is so frightening, support by others who have experienced similar crises is helpful |
| Parents verbalize the importance of managing their own stress | 8. Discuss necessity for parents to relieve their stress by exercise, meditation, communicating with one another, obtaining sufficient rest | 8. Family's intactness is crucial for infant's health and happiness |

## Rheumatic Fever

**Description.** Rheumatic fever is a systemic disease involving the joints, heart, central nervous system, skin, and subcutaneous tissues. It belongs to a group of disorders known as *collagen diseases*. Their common feature is the destruction of connective tissue. Rheumatic fever is particularly detrimental to the heart. It is rare in the first 3 years of life, but reaches its peak incidence between the ages of 5 and 15. The first attacks occur most often between 6 and 8 years of age. Rheumatic fever has a high family incidence and is more common world wide in lower-income groups and where overcrowded conditions exist. It is more prevalent during the winter and spring, and carrier rates among school children are believed to be in-creased during these seasons. Genetic factors have been implicated.

Rheumatic fever is an autoimmune disease that occurs as a reaction to a group A beta hemolytic streptococcus infection of the throat. The exact pathogenesis is unclear. The body becomes sensitized to the organism after repeated attacks and develops an allergic response to it. During the 1960s and 1970s, the disease almost disappeared; however in the late 1980s, a resurgence occurred in the United States. This has emphasized the need for better understanding of its origin and transmission so that appropriate public health measures can be instituted.

**Manifestations.** Symptoms of rheumatic fever range from mild to severe and may not occur for several weeks after a "strep throat" (Fig. 26–7).

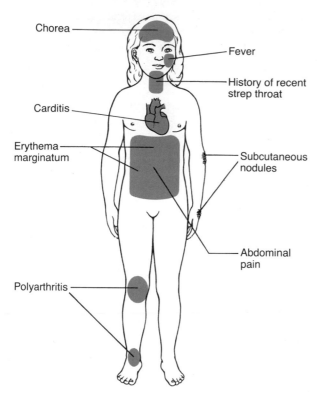

**Figure 26-7.** Manifestations of rheumatic fever.

The classic symptoms are *polyarthritis* (wandering joint pains), *skin eruptions*, *chorea* (a nervous disorder), and *inflammation of the heart.* Subcutaneous nodules may appear beneath the skin but are less common in children. Abdominal pain, often mistaken for appendicitis, sometimes occurs. Fever varies from slight to very high. Pallor, fatigue, anorexia, and unexplained nosebleeds may be seen. Rheumatic fever has a tendency to *recur*, and each attack carries the threat of further damage to the heart. The recurrences are most frequent during the first 5 years following the initial attack, and they decline rapidly thereafter.

*Polyarthritis.* The polyarthritis (*poly*, "many," *arthr*, "joint," and *itis*, "inflammation of") seen in rheumatic fever is distinctive in that it does not result in permanent deformity to the joint. It involves mainly the larger joints: knees, elbows, ankles, wrists, and shoulders. The joints become painful and tender and are difficult to move. The symptoms last for a few days, disappear without treatment, and frequently return in another joint. This pattern may continue for a few weeks. The symptoms

tend to be more severe in older children. The joint may be visibly swollen and inflamed. On diagnosis salicylates are administered to relieve the pain.

*Skin Eruptions. Erythema marginatum,* the rash seen in rheumatic fever, consists of small red circles and wavy lines appearing on the trunk and abdomen. They appear and disappear rapidly and are significant in diagnosing the disease.

*Sydenham's Chorea.* This is a disorder of the central nervous system characterized by involuntary, purposeless movements of the muscles. It may occur as an acute rheumatic involvement of the brain. Sydenham's chorea is primarily seen in prepubertal girls.

Attacks of chorea, which begin slowly, may be preceded by increased tension and behavioral problems. The child may stumble and spill things, and may have difficulty buttoning clothes and writing. When the facial muscles are involved, grimaces occur. The child may laugh and cry inappropriately. In severe cases, the patient may become completely incapacitated, and deterioration in speech may be noticeable. Treatment of Sydenham's chorea is directed toward the relief of symptoms by physical and mental rest. Medication may also be required.

*Rheumatic Carditis.* Inflammation of the heart, a manifestation of rheumatic fever, can be fatal. It occurs more often in the young child. The tissues that cover the heart and the heart valves are affected. The heart muscle—the myocardium—may be involved, as may the pericardium and endocardium. The *mitral valve,* between the left atrium and left ventricle, is frequently involved. Vegetations form that interfere with the proper closing of the valve and disturb its normal function. When this valve becomes narrowed, the condition is called *mitral stenosis.* Myocardial lesions called *Aschoff's bodies* are also characteristic of the disease. The burden on the heart is great because it has to pump harder to circulate the blood. As a result, it may become enlarged. Symptoms of poor circulation and heart failure may appear.

The patient has an irregular low-grade fever, is pale and listless, and has a poor appetite. Moderate anemia and weight loss are apparent. The child may experience dyspnea on exertion. The pulse and respiration rates are out of proportion to the body temperature. The physician may detect a soft murmur over the apex of the heart.

**Diagnosis.** The diagnosis of rheumatic fever

**Table 26–2.** MODIFIED JONES CRITERIA

| Major Criteria | Minor Criteria |
|---|---|
| Carditis | Fever |
| Polyarthritis | Arthralgia |
| Erythema marginatum | Previous history of rheumatic heart disease |
| Chorea | Elevated erythrocyte sedimentation rate |
| Subcutaneous nodules | Leukocytosis |
| | Altered P-R interval on electrocardiogram |
| | Positive C-reactive protein |

A positive diagnosis of rheumatic fever cannot be made without the presence of two major criteria, or one major and two minor criteria, plus a history of streptococcal infection.

is difficult to make, and for this reason the *Jones criteria* have been developed and modified over the years (Table 26–2). The presence of two major criteria or one major and two minor criteria, supported by evidence of recent streptococcal infection, indicates a high probability of rheumatic fever. A careful physical examination is done, and a complete history of the patient is taken. Certain blood tests are helpful. The erythrocyte sedimentation rate is elevated. Abnormal proteins, such as C-reactive protein may also be evident in the serum. Leukocytosis may occur but is not regularly present. Antibodies against the streptococci (measured by ASO titer) may also be detected. Additional studies may include chest x-ray films, throat culture, and lung tests. The electrocardiogram, a graphic record of the electrical changes caused by the beating of the heart, is very useful. Changes in conductivity, particularly a prolonged P-R interval (first-degree heart block), may indicate carditis. These tests are repeated throughout the course of the disease so that the doctor may determine when the active stage has subsided.

**Treatment and Nursing Care.** Treatment is aimed at preventing permanent damage to the heart. This is accomplished by antibacterial therapy, physical and mental rest, relief of pain and fever, and management of cardiac failure should it occur. Initial antibacterial therapy is directed toward elimination of the streptococcal infection. Penicillin is the drug of choice unless the patient is sensitive to it, in which case erythromycin is substituted.

Elimination of infection through medication is

followed by long-term *chemoprophylaxis* (prevention of disease by drugs); intramuscular benzathine penicillin G is given monthly to patients with a history of rheumatic fever or evidence of rheumatic heart disease to prevent recurrence. Oral administration is considered for patients with minimal involvement whose reliability about taking medications can be ascertained. The duration of therapy is generally the lifetime of the patient. Sulfadiazine or erythromycin is recommended for long-term therapy for patients who cannot tolerate penicillin. Financial assistance is available to patients. Local heart associations, rehabilitation services, and state and municipal health departments are sources of such aid.

Antiinflammatory drugs are used to decrease fever and pain. Aspirin is the drug of choice for joint disease without evidence of carditis. The use of steroids is controversial. Concerns during therapy include aspirin toxicity and the effects of aspirin on clotting of the blood. Mild signs of Cushing's disease, such as moonface, acne, and hirsutism (increased hairiness), should be anticipated with the use of steroids. More severe reactions, such as gastric ulcer, hypertension, overwhelming infection, and toxic psychosis, should be guarded against. Phenobarbital is effective in reducing chorea. Padded side rails are used to protect the patient having spasms. If CHF occurs, measures to reduce its effects are taken.

Bed rest during the initial attack is recommended, especially if carditis is present. The amount of work the heart has to do must be limited by resting the entire body. In this way, the circulation of the heart is slower, and the heart does not have to work as fast or as hard as when a patient is active. The nurse clarifies the amount of confinement desired with the physician. This issue has added importance now that more rheumatic patients are treated at home.

A schedule of daily events is discussed with the child and parents, and the need for bed rest is emphasized. To minimize boredom, parents and siblings might set aside a special time daily to spend with the patient. They should be prepared for periods of withdrawal or rebellion, which are common to all children whose activities are curtailed. In the hospital, the patient may benefit from having a roommate who is similarly confined. On recovery, no restrictions on physical activity are usually required except in cases of cardiac enlargement.

Nursing procedures are carried out quickly and skillfully to minimize discomfort. They should be organized to ensure as few interruptions as possible to prevent tiring the patient. A bed cradle is used to prevent pressure on painful extremities. The nurse supports the joints with the hands when moving the patient. Care includes special attention to the skin, especially over bony prominences; back care; good oral hygiene; and small frequent feedings of nourishing foods. Maintenance of healthy teeth and prevention of cavities are of special importance. The patient with rheumatic fever is particularly susceptible to *subacute bacterial endocarditis*, which can occur as a complication of dental or other procedures likely to cause bleeding or infection. Nutrition consists of small servings from the basic food groups. These are increased as the child's appetite improves. Avoid overfeeding, which can lead to weight problems. A record of fluids is kept, as overhydration may tax the heart. All efforts are made to provide emotional support for the child and family. Provisions are made for the child to continue school studies.

**Prevention.** The nurse may be involved in the prevention of rheumatic fever through routine throat culture screening programs. Any child with symptoms who has been exposed to scarlet fever or another person with strep throat requires investigation. Examination of family contacts is also important. Once diagnosis is established, the nurse stresses the need to complete antibiotic therapy to prevent relapse. Close medical supervision and follow-up care are essential. The prognosis is favorable.

### Systemic Hypertension

**Description.** Hypertension, or high blood pressure, is being seen more frequently during childhood and adolescence. Blood pressure is a product of peripheral vascular resistance and cardiac output. An increase in cardiac output or peripheral resistance results in an increase in blood pressure. Systemic blood pressure increases with age and is correlated with height and weight throughout childhood and adolescence. *Significant hypertension* is considered when measurements are persistently between the 95th and 99th percentiles for the patient's age and sex. *Severe* hypertension is a blood pressure persistently at or above the 99th percentile for age and sex. When the cause of the increase in pressure can be explained by a dis-

ease process, the hypertension is referred to as *secondary*. Renal, congenital, vascular, and endocrine disorders represent the majority of illnesses that account for hypertension. *Primary* or *essential* hypertension implies that no known underlying disease is present. Nevertheless, heredity, obesity, stress, and salt intake can contribute to hypertension.

There is increasing evidence that essential hypertension, although not generally seen until adolescence or adulthood, may have its roots in childhood. The prevention of this is significant in reducing stroke or myocardial infarction as a person ages. The cause of essential hypertension is unknown. Patients rarely show symptoms. There is reason to believe that genetics and environment play a role in this transmission. Hypertension is more prevalent in children whose parents have high blood pressure. African Americans show a higher incidence of hypertension than do Caucasians. The disorder also appears at a younger age among African Americans and is more severe.

**Manifestations.** As was previously mentioned, the child with high blood pressure rarely exhibits symptoms. Frequent headaches, vision problems, and dizziness may or may not be related to hypertension but should be investigated. Whaley and Wong also report symptoms of irritability, excessive head banging, and nighttime terrors seen in some infants and small children who are found to have hypertension (Whaley & Wong, 1991).

**Treatment and Nursing Care.** The revelation of such data indicates the necessity for routine blood pressure measurements in young children. The National Heart, Lung, and Blood Institute's Task Force on Blood Pressure Control in Children recommended that a blood pressure sustained above the 95th percentile on three separate occasions be investigated further. The pressure is taken in the right upper extremity while the child is seated.

Measuring blood pressure in young children requires careful attention to cuff size (see p. 569). The examination may cause stress, which also leads to inaccuracy. An adolescent who shows consistently high readings should be given a complete physical examination. Eating habits need to be carefully reviewed. The use of medicine to control hypertension is controversial because the long-term effects on the hormonal cycles of growing children are unknown. In selected patients, diuretics and beta-adrenergic blockers, such as propranolol hydrochlo-

## Nursing Brief

Children younger than 2 years of age should not be put on low-fat diets.

ride (Inderal) or angiotensin-converting enzyme (ACE) inhibitors such as Captopril may be indicated. Good health habits, such as exercise, limitation of salt in the diet, weight control, and stress reduction, are emphasized. If the adolescent smokes or takes contraceptives or other drugs that might raise the blood pressure, additional counseling and education are necessary. Therapy for secondary hypertension involves diagnosis and treatment of the underlying cause.

### Hyperlipidemia

Hyperlipidemia refers to excessive lipids (fat and fatlike substances) in the blood. Because there is evidence that the factors responsible for degenerative vascular disease may begin in childhood and that they may be somewhat controllable, considerable interest has developed in screening children for risk factors and in attempting to change these risks. Children whose parents or grandparents had early coronary artery disease appear to be at highest risk. The American Academy of Pediatrics (AAP) suggests that children with this heritage be regularly screened for cholesterol levels beginning at age 2 (American Academy of Pediatrics, Committee on Nutrition, 1986). During infancy, fatty streaks or abnormal lipid accumulations may begin to appear in the aorta. These streaks may disappear, remain unchanged, or later develop into atherosclerotic plaques. Because fatty acids are essential to myelinization (formation of the myelin sheath around certain nerves), which continues after birth, the AAP

## Nursing Brief

Hospitalization provides an excellent opportunity for the nurse to review heart-healthy information. Reviews of family history, lifestyle, and eating patterns are suitable interventions, even in the absence of high risk.

cautions against restrictive diets for children but suggests instead a prudent lifestyle. Their recommendations are presented in Table 26–3. The dietary practices of children in the United States are poor. Children and preadolescents often consume high-fat, low-fiber diets with a minimum amount of complex carbohydrates, vegetable protein and fat, and potassium.

Atherosclerosis, hypertension, hyperlipidemia, hypercholesterolemia, and cigarette smoking are risk factors associated with adult coronary artery disease. Children who are identified as high-risk should not be labeled "ill." Instead, the nurse emphasizes the value of a healthy lifestyle in decreasing the possibility of coronary artery disease in adulthood(see also Box 16–4).

## Respiratory System

Pulmonary structures differentiate in an orderly fashion during fetal life. This makes it possible to determine at what point a particular defect occurred. The laryngotracheal groove appears at 2–4 weeks of gestation. The lower respiratory tract begins development as a branch from the upper digestive tract. Gradually the esophagus and trachea completely separate. The trachea branches to form the right and left bronchi and eventually differentiates into the alveoli. During fetal life the respiratory tract produces a fluid that fills the lungs. Gaseous exchange occurs at the placental interface. The lungs do not function until birth. At about 21–24 weeks, the lungs begin to mature and produce surfactant. This slippery lipoprotein makes it easier for the newborn to breath after birth by keeping the alveoli from collapsing. The anatomy of the respiratory system and the differences between the child and adult systems are depicted in Figure 26–8. Respiratory problems are more common than heart problems in young children, although the latter may cause or contribute to impaired respiration. If the lungs do not adapt to extrauterine life, the newborn will experience respiratory distress. Respiratory distress syndrome, also called hyaline membrane disease, and atelectasis are discussed on page 319.

Procedures that may be performed on the child with a respiratory condition include throat and nasopharyngeal cultures, bronchoscopy, lung biopsy, arterial blood gas analysis ($PO_2$, $PCO_2$) and pH, pulse, and ear oximetry, transcutaneaus monitoring, and various pul-

**Table 26–3.** HEART-HEALTHY GUIDELINES FOR CHILDREN

| Age | Guidelines |
|---|---|
| Infants | Breast milk or formula for 1 yr |
| | Rice or other single-grain cereal from 4–6 mo |
| | Balanced mixture of cereal, vegetables, fruits, and meats for second 6 mo of life |
| | Baby foods are labeled as to calories and nutrient composition; avoid foods with added sugar or salt; most baby foods with the exception of combined foods and desserts do not have these additives |
| | Babies do not need desserts to grow; infant fruits are more nutritious |
| | Fats do not need to be restricted in healthy infants |
| Toddlers and preschoolers | Avoid excessive fats, salt, and refined sugars |
| | Avoid salty snacks and sweet desserts |
| | Offer heart-healthy snacks of vegetables, fruits, finger foods |
| | Offer a variety of foods from the basic food groups |
| | Discourage the consumption of large amounts of milk, which can lead to nutritional imbalances |
| School-age children | Provide heart-healthy school lunches |
| | Role model good daily exercise |
| | Screen children with family history of congenital heart disease* (cholesterol, triglycerides, blood pressure) |
| | Avoid obesity |
| | Discourage smoking |
| Adolescents | Emphasize importance of heart-healthy foods to improve endurance, good body image |
| | Avoid sedentary lifestyle |
| | Discourage excessive intake of dietary saturated fat, sodium, sugar, and excess calories |
| | Be a nonsmoking parent |
| | Assess stress management capabilities, counsel accordingly |
| | Screen periodically for serum cholesterol elevations, blood pressure |
| | Serial monitoring of adolescents deemed high risk (sustained high blood pressure readings on at least three separate occasions) |

*Children over the age of 2 years with a family history of hyperlipidemia or early atherosclerotic heart disease should undergo routine screening for hyperlipidemia.

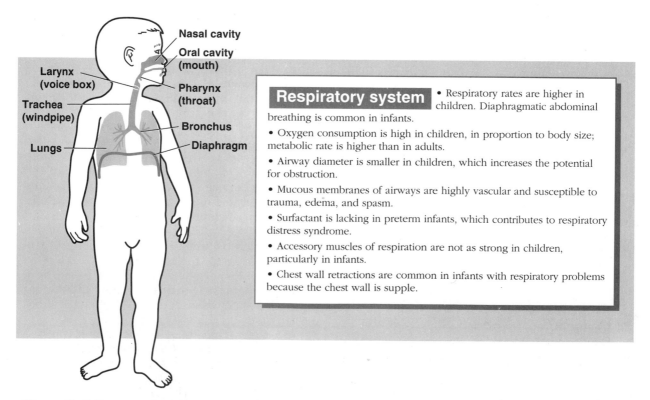

**Respiratory system**

• Respiratory rates are higher in children. Diaphragmatic abdominal breathing is common in infants.

• Oxygen consumption is high in children, in proportion to body size; metabolic rate is higher than in adults.

• Airway diameter is smaller in children, which increases the potential for obstruction.

• Mucous membranes of airways are highly vascular and susceptible to trauma, edema, and spasm.

• Surfactant is lacking in preterm infants, which contributes to respiratory distress syndrome.

• Accessory muscles of respiration are not as strong in children, particularly in infants.

• Chest wall retractions are common in infants with respiratory problems because the chest wall is supple.

**Figure 26–8.** Summary of respiratory system features in children. The respiratory system warms and moistens air brought to the alveoli. Its function is to oxygenate arterial blood and remove carbon dioxide from venous blood.

monary function tests. Chest x-ray films, computed tomography, radioisotope scan, bronchogram, and angiography may prove useful, depending on symptoms. Inspection, percussion, and auscultation procedures done by the nurse are of utmost value. The following is a discussion of children with nasopharyngitis, acute pharyngitis, croup, epiglottitis, bronchitis, pneumonia, tonsillitis and adenoiditis, asthma, and cystic fibrosis.

## NASOPHARYNGITIS

**Description.** A cold, also known as acute coryza, is the most common infection of the respiratory tract. It is caused by one or a number of viruses, principally the *rhinoviruses*, which are spread from one child to another by sneezing, coughing, and direct contact. Group A beta-hemolytic streptococci are the prominent bacterial offenders. Droplets remain suspended in the air and on dust particles for short periods of time. The infection is transferred mainly during the initial stage. In the second phase of a cold, nasal drainage becomes thicker and purulent. Factors that contribute to the individual's susceptibility include age, state of nutrition, general health, fatigue, and emotional upsets.

As the child becomes exposed to more children, the number of colds contracted increases. Parents may notice this, particularly during the child's first few years of day care or school, because the child has had little opportunity to build up resistance. Older children are better able to resist infection. In temperate climates, the incidence of rhinoviral infection peaks in September and again in April or May.

To prevent a cold, the child's exposure to those with this virus is avoided to the extent possible. Infants less than 6 months of age can acquire this infection, so they too must be protected from infected persons. The child should eat nourishing foods and get sufficient rest.

**Manifestations.** The symptoms of a cold in an infant or small child are different from those in an adult. Children's air passages are smaller and more easily obstructed. Fever as high as 40°C (104°F) is not uncommon in children under 3 years of age. Nasal discharge, irritability, sore throat, cough, and general discomfort are present, and there may be vomiting and diarrhea. The diagnosis is complicated by the fact that many infectious diseases resemble the common cold during their onset. Complications of a cold include bronchitis, pneumonitis, and ear infections.

**Treatment and Nursing Care.** There is no cure for the common cold. When a cold is suspected, treatment should begin early. The treatment is designed to relieve the symptoms. Rest, fluids, and proper diet are important. Parents are taught to watch the child for signs of dehydration. If anorexia is present, food should not be forced. The appetite will gradually improve as the condition subsides. When high fever accompanies a cold, the doctor must be consulted.

Acetaminophen (Tylenol) reduces the temperature, but the correct dosage should be prescribed, particularly in patients under 1 year of age. Aspirin is not recommended because of its implication in Reye's syndrome. Aqueous nose drops will relieve nasal congestion. The older child can help squeeze the bulb of the dropper when they are instilled. The infant needs nose drops mainly before feedings and at bedtime. When drops are instilled 10–15 minutes before nursing, the nasal passages clear so that sucking is easier. Each child needs an individual bottle of nose drops to prevent cross-infection.

Moist air soothes the inflamed nose and throat. An electric cold air humidifier is safe and convenient. It is cleaned and disinfected regularly. If a great deal of moisture is indicated, as in croup, the infant may be taken to a small room, such as the bathroom, and all the hot water faucets can be turned on to produce sufficient steam.

The older child is taught the proper way to remove nasal secretions from the nose. The mouth is opened slightly and secretions are gently blown through both nostrils at the same time. This method prevents infection from being forced into the eustachian tubes. When there is a large amount of nasal discharge, the nurse or parent protects the upper lip by applying cold cream or petroleum jelly.

During the initial stage of the fever children are kept quiet. It is difficult to keep a child with a cold away from other members of the family. They must be taught to cover the mouth and nose when sneezing and to wash the hands afterward. Tissues must be properly discarded and burned. Parents need not be embarrassed at turning the neighborhood children away from the door when their child has a cold. They are not only doing the neighbors a favor but are also protecting their sick child from further infection.

The child should not be allowed to become fatigued immediately after a cold. If fever persists beyond 48–72 hours or if it occurs 3 or 4 days following a cold, a physician is consulted because this may indicate bacterial complications. A day or two is reserved for convalescence.

## ACUTE PHARYNGITIS

Acute pharyngitis is an inflammation of the structures in the throat. When it includes the tonsils and pharynx, it is referred to as pharyngotonsillitis. This infection is common among children between ages 5 and 15. In 80% of cases the causative organism is a virus. Group A beta-hemolytic streptococcus (strep throat) occurs in 20% of the cases. In children under age 3, the bacterium *Haemophilus influenzae* is common.

**Manifestations, Treatment, and Nursing Care.** Symptoms include fever, malaise, dysphagia (*dys*, "difficult," and *phagia*, "swallowing"), and anorexia. It is difficult to distinguish viral from bacterial types by symptoms only. A strep throat is determined by throat culture. When the culture is positive, antimicrobial therapy (penicillin) is administered. It is prescribed orally for 10 days. Compliance is a problem; therefore, the nurse carefully explains to parents the need for the child to finish all of the medication. If the child is allergic to penicillin, erythromycin may be used. Acetaminophen (Tylenol) may be taken to relieve soreness of the throat. If the child is old enough to gargle, a solution of warm water and salt may be used.

Prompt treatment of strep throat is important in order to avoid serious complications such as rheumatic fever, glomerulonephritis, peritonsillar abscess, otitis media, mastoiditis, meningitis, osteomyelitis, or pneumonia. Persistence of positive streptococcal culture after careful follow-up and therapy may indicate that the child is a group A beta-hemolytic streptococci carrier. Generally, however, it means that the child did not complete the 10-day course of medication or that a penicillin-resistant organism has evolved. No immunization is presently available to prevent this condition.

## CROUP SYNDROME

**Description.** Croup is a nonspecific term applied to a number of conditions whose chief symptom is a brassy (croupy) cough and varying degrees of inspiratory stridor (a harsh, high-pitched sound). When the larynx is involved, the clinical picture becomes more intense because of possible alterations in respiratory status, for example, airway obstruction, acute respiratory failure, and hypoxia. Acute spasmodic laryngitis is the milder form of the syndrome. Acute laryngotracheobronchitis is the most common. It is also referred to as subglottic croup, as edema occurs below the vocal cords.

Respiratory infections are common in pediatric patients, especially in children under 5 years of age. Children have smaller air passages than adults and experience more narrowing with inflammation. Acute infections of the larynx are common in the toddler. Involvement of other parts of the respiratory tract is frequent. A wide variety of organisms cause croup, but most often the infectious agent is a virus. The patient's history is valuable in diagnosis, as there appears to be a familial tendency. The incidence is higher in boys than in girls, and some have suggested that psychogenic and allergic factors may be important.

**Manifestations.** Croup is characterized by a hoarse cough and dyspnea. It occurs suddenly during the night, often without earlier symptoms of a cold. The child sits up in bed frightened and struggles to breathe. The infant prefers to be held upright. Inspiration is difficult and is accompanied by stridor. The spasms last for a few hours and may recur later in the night. They may return again on the 2nd and 3rd nights but are less severe. Although croup is alarming to the child and parents because the child is distressed, most cases are mild. Croup is not considered a communicable disease and can usually be managed at home.

**Treatment and Nursing Care.** The treatment is directed toward reducing laryngeal spasm. The patient is placed in an atmosphere of high humidity to aid in liquefying secretions and to reduce spasm. In the home, the child is taken into the bathroom and the hot water in the shower and basin is turned on. The child inhales the moist air. This often reduces distress within minutes. Parents are instructed to use an electric cold water humidifier in the child's room. The vaporizer is regularly disinfected. If the use of moisture does not relieve symptoms and if it is the middle of the night, the child is transported to the nearest emergency center for evaluation.

The toddler admitted to the hospital with respiratory distress is anxious and fatigued. The nurse remains calm while preparing the mist tent. Children enjoy special hideaways, and using the tent may appeal to the patient. The nurse also directs attention to the parents, who need reassurance. As the parents become more relaxed, the patient also becomes less apprehensive. Parents remain with the child to provide security. Restraining a child who has respiratory distress keeps the patient in one position too long, and complications can develop more easily. Fluids are encouraged and in some instances an intravenous may be started.

Medications used in the treatment of croup include corticosteroids and racepinephrine (Vaponefrin). Although controversy remains about the use of corticosteroids, they have proved helpful in avoiding intubation in more seriously ill children. Vaponefrin is inhaled via a face mask. It decreases edema by vasoconstriction and provides immediate relief, although this may be temporary. Vaponefrin may be repeated in several hours if necessary. A single inhaled dose peaks in 10–30 minutes, with an overall duration of 2 hours. *Close observation is necessary because some patients may experience a rebound effect and become more obstructed.*

The nurse observes and records temperature, pulse, respiration, and blood pressure if ordered. Particular attention is given to the type and rate of respirations. The child's color and degree of restlessness and anxiety are also observed (Fig. 26–9). Respiratory distress should

## Nursing Brief

Respiratory illness is always potentially more serious in children than in adults.

begin to diminish as the child remains in the tent. An increase in respiratory distress is reported immediately because complications may arise that necessitate endotracheal intubation or tracheotomy (*trachea*, and *otomy*, "incision of") (see Fig. 26–9). Specific nursing care is indicated in such cases (see p. 597). Children who progress well are gradually weaned from the croup tent.

### EPIGLOTTITIS

Epiglottitis is a swelling of the tissues *above* the vocal cords, that is, supraglottic swelling. This results in narrowing of the *airway inlet*, with the possibility of total obstruction. It is caused by *Haemophilus influenzae* type B and occurs in the child of age 3–6 years. It can occur in any season. The course is rapid and progressive. Epiglottitis is a life-threatening medical emergency. Blood gases fluctuate, and there is leukocytosis. Bacteremia is often present. *if epiglottitis is suspected, one should not examine the pharynx (back of the throat), as laryngospasm may occur, followed by respiratory ar-*

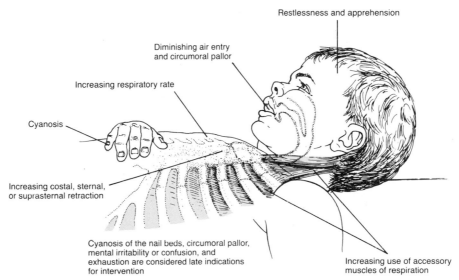

Restlessness and apprehension

Diminishing air entry and circumoral pallor

Increasing respiratory rate

Cyanosis

Increasing costal, sternal, or suprasternal retraction

Cyanosis of the nail beds, circumoral pallor, mental irritability or confusion, and exhaustion are considered late indications for intervention

Increasing use of accessory muscles of respiration

**Figure 26–9.** The primary indication for tracheotomy is progressive respiratory obstruction.

*rest.* The diagnosis can be confirmed by a lateral x-ray film of the neck.

Prophylactic placement of an artificial airway is the treatment of choice, and a skilled endoscopist is required. Nasotracheal intubation is generally selected. Nursing care is the same as that given to the critically ill child. Prevention includes the administration of *Haemophilus influenzae* type B conjugate vaccine, which can be given at 2 months of age. As this vaccine is administered more routinely, the incidence of epiglottitis should decrease.

## BRONCHITIS

**Description.** A study of the respiratory system reveals that the air tubes leading to the lungs resemble an upside-down tree. The trachea is the main trunk, with the bronchi, bronchioles, and alveoli as branches. These passages proceed from large to small and are lined with a continuous membrane. If there is an infection of the bronchial tree, it is seldom confined to one area but more often involves other structures. The physician designates the exact passages involved. The student nurse may see terms such as acute tracheobronchitis, bronchiolitis, and laryngotracheobronchitis. The more extensive the infection, the sicker the child. The nursing care problems are basically the same, but the degree of attention required is different. A discussion of acute bronchitis follows; however, the author has extended the nursing care section to allow for adaptations by the nurse to patients who have more involved infections.

Acute bronchitis is an infection of the bronchi. It seldom occurs as a primary infection—it is usually secondary to a cold or communicable disease. It is caused by a variety of organisms. Poor nutrition, allergy, and chronic infection of the respiratory tract may precipitate this condition (Table 26–4). Age is an important factor; most patients are under 4 years old. The patient may have a family history of acute bronchitis.

**Manifestations.** The most noticeable symptom is a dry cough that becomes looser as the disease advances. Large amounts of sputum develop. Sputum may be raised by the older child but is frequently swallowed by the infant and is sometimes aspirated into the trachea and bronchi. Vomiting may occur. The child has a moderate fever, usually not over 39°C (102°F). Older children may complain of a dry throat and sore chest.

**Treatment and Nursing Care.** Uncomplicated acute bronchitis can usually be treated at home if the child is healthy. The patient must rest, drink plenty of fluids, and take the prescribed medications. Acetaminophen (Tylenol) is used to relieve discomfort and quiet the child. Increased humidity is helpful. A warm, moist wash cloth placed over the sinus area may help loosen the secretions. Postnasal drip may precipitate coughing at night. Sometimes relief may be obtained by providing sips of water. Nose drops may be prescribed by the physician, especially before feedings. The mother is instructed to purchase a small bottle

**Table 26–4.** CAUSATIVE AGENTS, MANIFESTATIONS, AND TYPICAL AGE OF ONSET OF BRONCHIAL INFECTIONS

| Infection | Causative Agent | Manifestations | Typical Age of Patient | Comment |
|---|---|---|---|---|
| Asthmatic bronchitis | Virus | Wheezing<br>Coughing | Toddler or young child | Preceded by upper respiratory infection |
| Bronchitis | Virus<br>Air pollution<br>Other agents | Low-grade fever<br>Dry cough, later becoming productive<br>Sore chest | 1–4 yr | Usually accompanied by some degree of tracheitis |
| Bronchiolitis | Respiratory syncytial virus | Wheezing<br>Coryza<br>Cough<br>Dyspnea<br>Intercostal and substernal retractions<br>Flaring of nares | Under 1 yr | Affects smaller airways<br>Incidence decreases after 18 mo of age |

of nose drops and to discard it after the illness. Cold air irritates the respiratory tract; therefore, the child must remain indoors during inclement weather.

Pneumonia is seldom a complication since the advent of the newer antibacterial drugs. The acute symptoms last for about a week, but a cough and expectoration remain for another week or two. The child who suffers from repeated attacks of bronchitis should be thoroughly examined so that the possibility of infected tonsils and adenoids, cystic fibrosis, allergy, tuberculosis, and other disorders may be ruled out.

The patient who is admitted to the hospital requires more extensive observation and care. Infants' respiratory passages are smaller than those of adults; therefore, when these passages swell, real respiratory distress occurs. In addition, a young child's cough reflex is not too effective in raising sputum, the immune mechanism may be poorly developed, and the wide, straight eustachian tubes invite ear infection. Nurses must organize their work so that they do not disturb the patient unnecessarily. Sometimes coughing is reduced by giving sips of water. When the patient has a coughing spell, the nurse places the child in a sitting position; the nurse's hands support the child's chest and back. If persistent coughing disturbs the patient's sleep, the doctor is notified.

The baby breathes more easily when sitting up. In this position, the organs of the abdomen do not press against the diaphragm. The infant in an Isolette may have the head and shoulders raised by elevating one end of the mattress. Babies in large cribs benefit from the use of an infant seat. This is supported by a pillow at the back and is secured to the crib. Supporting a baby with an infant seat is better than propping with pillows because the baby does not slump.

The infant seat can be placed in a Croupette if necessary. The Croupette, mistifier, Universal tent, or similar apparatus is used to provide the necessary increase in humidity. The nurse notes on the flow sheet the date and time at which the infant is put into and taken out of the apparatus. If the patient's condition prevents removal from the oxygen apparatus, a notation is made by a nurse on each shift that the therapy has been maintained. Babies who suck their thumbs become frustrated, since they cannot suck and breathe at the same time. Mucus is cleansed from the nose as needed, and aqueous nose drops are administered as directed.

Solid foods may be refused. Foods such as gelatin, Pedialyte, Gatorade, and Popsicles may be offered. Dairy products are to be avoided because they produce mucus. Fluids are forced, and the intake and output are recorded. A good urinary output is necessary for the excretion of medications. Parenteral fluids may be indicated. Medications and fluids are given slowly. The nose is cleansed or suctioned prior to bottle feedings because the baby cannot suck and breathe at the same time. The baby sucks briefly, pulls away, and cries in frustration. Frequent, small feedings are offered; the patient should not be hurried.

Careful observation and charting are paramount. The nurse watches for signs of dyspnea, such as mouth breathing, flaring of the nostrils, sternal retractions, and stridor. The nurse notes whether the difficulty occurs on inspiration or expiration, or both. The skin, mucous membranes, and fingernails of the patient are observed to determine color, that is, pink, white, gray, blue. In the African-American child, the palms of the hands, soles of the feet, and lower lids of the eyes may be observed for signs of pallor and anoxia. Restlessness, an indication of air hunger, is reported and charted. The general behavior of the child is significant and should be recorded in the nurse's notes, that is, "cranky," "listless," "irritable," or "content."

The psychological factors involved in caring for the infant and small child are closely intertwined with the physical care the nurse administers. A nurse's genuine interest in the patient is reflected in every procedure that is done. A kind and gentle manner in giving the morning bath, a sense of humor, and an eagerness to help—these qualities promote feelings of security, belonging, and love. On the other hand, lack of warmth and attention by the nurse may promote hostility, depression, and a negative attitude on the part of the patient.

If the patient's condition permits, the child should be removed from the Croupette at least once during every shift to be played with, rocked, and cuddled. When this is contraindicated, the nurse visits the child, pats or touches the child in a loving way, and provides toys for diversion. The child with respiratory distress is apprehensive; therefore, the nurse's presence is reassuring. This is true even in the youngest of children. The parents also need continuous reassurance. Nothing is more frightening than to see one's child gasping for every breath of air.

The nurse directs attention to the parents during visiting hours, listens to them, and in general treats them with as much consideration as time allows.

## PNEUMONIA

**Description.** Pneumonia or pneumonitis is an inflammation of the lungs in which the *alveoli* (air sacs) become filled with exudate. The affected portion of the lung does not receive enough air. Breathing is shallow. As a result, the blood stream is denied sufficient oxygen.

Pneumonia may occur as the initial or *pri-*mary disease, or it may complicate another illness, in which case it is termed *secondary* pneumonia. Secondary pneumonia may accompany various communicable diseases or may follow surgery. It is more serious than primary pneumonia because the patient is already weak.

There are many types of pneumonia. Classification may be by causative organism (i.e., bacterial or viral) or by the part of the respiratory system involved (i.e., lobar or bronchial), or by other methods. Table 26–5 provides a classification scheme.

The pneumococcus was the chief organism causing pneumonia in infants and children be-

**Table 26–5.** AGE OF ONSET OF VARIOUS TYPES OF PNEUMONIA IN CHILDREN

| Type | Age of Onset | Comment |
|---|---|---|
| *Primary* | | |
| Bacterial | | |
| Pneumococcal | First 4 yr (peak), occurs also in older children and adolescents | Most common bacterial pathogen, occurs in late winter to early spring; pneumococcal vaccine now licensed for high-risk children over 2 yr |
| Group A streptococcal | 3–5 yr of age | Less frequent |
| Group B streptococcal | Newborns | Leading cause of septicemia and meningitis in newborns |
| Staphylococcal | Newborns, infants | Transmitted primarily by direct contact; pay strict attention to handwashing; most serious, rapid progression |
| *Haemophilus influenzae* (type B) | Infants, young children under 5 yr of age | Occurs more often in boys; complications frequent (bacteremia, pericarditis, meningitis, others); vaccine now available |
| *Mycobacterium tuberculosis* | More severe in younger children | Continues to be important because of immigrant flux, poverty, acquired immunodeficiency syndrome (AIDS) |
| Nonbacterial | | |
| Respiratory syncytial virus | More serious in infants | Responsible for the largest percentage of cases |
| Influenza virus | | |
| Adenovirus | | Less common |
| Other | | |
| *Mycoplasma pneumoniae* (primary atypical) | School-age children Adolescents Young adults | More common in fall and winter; crowded conditions |
| *Secondary* | | |
| *Pneumocystis carinii* | Infants 3–5 wk old Immunocompromised children | Being seen as more children with malignancies are surviving; immunodeficiency diseases (especially under 1 yr of age); AIDS patients |
| Aspiration | Infants Toddlers | Avoid feedings that overdistend the stomach, particularly in gavage-fed infants; gastroesophageal reflux occurs in some babies; inhaled foreign bodies occlude airways. Many chemicals (kerosene, gasoline) cause edema, inflammation, and the like |
| Hypostatic | Immobile child of any age | Prevention is highly important (turning, coughing, deep breathing) |

fore the advent of antibiotics and sulfonamides. Today, respiratory viruses cause a number of cases of pneumonia, particularly in children under 5 years of age. *Staphylococcal* pneumonia is particularly dangerous because strong strains of this organism do not respond to antibiotic therapy. It may begin as a skin infection in the newborn nursery, pediatric unit, or home. The patient may then carry the germs in the nasal passages until a later date, when the child or a close associate contracts the disease. *Immunocompromised* children frequently develop pneumonia caused by gram-negative organisms such as *Pneumocystis carinii* and fungi.

Some types of pneumonia occur primarily in certain age groups. Pneumonia in the newborn may be directly connected with the birth process, that is, aspiration of infected amniotic fluid, or may result from exposure to infected personnel. Toddlers frequently aspirate small objects such as peanuts or popcorn and develop pneumonia as a result; therefore, such foods are to be discouraged for this age group. *Lipoid* pneumonia occurs when the baby inhales an oil substance into the airways. It is less common today as children are seldom given cod liver or castor oil routinely, as they were in the past. Nose drops with an oil base are dangerous. The toddler who drinks kerosene may also develop a type of pneumonia. *Hypostatic* pneumonia may occur in patients who have poor circulation in their lungs and remain in one position too long. The child recovering from anesthesia needs to be turned frequently in order to stimulate circulation through the lungs. Early ambulation also accomplishes this.

**Manifestations.** The symptoms of pneumonia vary with the age of the patient and the causative organism. They may develop suddenly or may be preceded by an upper respiratory tract infection. The cough is dry at first, but it gradually becomes productive. Fever rises as high as 39.5–40°C (103–104°F) and may fluctuate widely during a 24-hour period. The respiration rate may increase to 40–80 times/min in infants, and in older children to 30–50 times/min. Respirations are shallow in an attempt to reduce the amount of chest pain. *Sternal retractions* may be seen as the assisting muscles of respiration are used. The nostrils may flare. The child is listless and has a poor appetite. The patient tends to lie on the affected side.

**Treatment.** The patient is given a complete physical examination. A tuberculosis skin test is administered as indicated. The doctor pays particular attention to the examination of the child's chest. X-rays films confirm the diagnosis and determine whether there are complications. A differential white blood cell count is routinely done. Blood specimens show a marked increase in the number of white blood cells (16,000–40,000/mm$^3$). The number of red blood cells and the amount of hemoglobin may be slightly reduced. The urine is dark amber, and there is a decrease in the amount voided. The specific gravity is high. Cultures may be taken from the nose and throat. Tracheal cultures may also be indicated.

Treatment depends on the causative organism. Bacterial pneumonia is treated with antibiotics. In cases of viral pneumonia antibiotics are not effective. Treatment is mainly supportive. In cases caused by the respiratory syncytial virus, ribavirin, an antibiotic specific for the virus, is given by nebulizer. Antipyretics are given to reduce fever. Oxygen is administered for dyspnea or cyanosis. When this treatment is begun early, the child is less restless and does not require as many sedatives or drugs to relieve pain. Since drug therapy has become so effective, many uncomplicated cases can be treated at home. Fluid intake should be increased, particularly clear fluids and "flattened" soft drinks.

**Nursing Care.** Nursing care in all types of pneumonia is basically the same. The age of the patient determines the nurse's approach and the type of equipment used. (The newborn receives oxygen in the Isolette, whereas the older child requires a Croupette or a larger tent.) Rest is an important part of the treatment. The nurse must be organized so that the child is not disturbed unnecessarily. Planned, quiet activities for the child are recommended (Fig. 26–10).

The nurse checks the vital signs at regular intervals. During the acute stages, the temperature may rise as high as 39.5–40°C (103–104°F). When a child is flushed with fever, *heavy clothing and blankets should be removed.* The nurse may be asked to give the child tepid sponge baths to help reduce the fever (this procedure is presented on page 572). Smaller children are bathed in a tub or basin. The nurse offers the older patient the bedpan before the procedure begins.

The nurse encourages the child to take fluids. Small sips of water are offered frequently (at least every hour). If vomiting persists, parenteral fluids are given. The appetite of the child improves as the condition does.

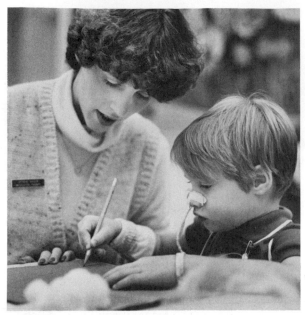

**Figure 26–10.** Planned quiet activities aid the hospitalized child to gain self-control following invasive procedures. (Courtesy of Blank Memorial Hospital for Children, Des Moines, IA.)

The patient is turned *regularly*. Although this is painful, it is essential to total recovery. The child will probably prefer to lie on the affected side because it is more comfortable. The doctor prescribes an analgesic to increase the patient's comfort. The nurse assists and encourages the patient to walk about the room and in the hallways when such activity is prescribed. Small children can exercise their lungs by blowing bubbles through a straw. The physical therapist may provide chest clapping and postural drainage exercise.

The nurse observes the patient for unfavorable symptoms, such as a weak and rapid pulse, cyanosis, abdominal distention, constipation, and disorientation. Although today recovery from uncomplicated pneumonia is dramatic, recuperation takes time. Upon discharge from the hospital, parents receive written instructions concerning diet, activity, medication, return appointments, and so on. It is helpful if the parents repeat these instructions to the nurse.

## TONSILLITIS AND ADENOIDITIS

**Description.** The tonsils and adenoids, located in the pharynx (throat), are made of lymph tissue and are part of the body's defense mechanism against infection. The tonsils and adenoids were formerly blamed for causing many illnesses, and for a time it was thought that having them removed was part of growing up. Today, doctors stress that *not all* children need to have them removed. A careful physical examination and an evaluation of the patient's history are made in order to rule out other diseases. Enlargement of tonsils is not sufficient reason for removal. These structures are normally larger in early childhood than in later years. The current trend is to treat the conditions as separate problems, according to individual criteria (Box 26–2).

**Treatment.** The removal of the tonsils and adenoids, referred to as a "T & A," is not usually recommended for the child under 3 years of age. It is thought that if surgery is postponed, the condition may correct itself, since the tis-

---

**BOX 26–2** | **Indications for Tonsillectomy and Adenoidectomy**

**Some Indications for Tonsillectomy**

Recurrent tonsillitis with documented streptococcal infection (at least four or more infections in 1 yr)
Marked hypertrophy that results in difficult swallowing, disturbances in speech, or apneic episodes while asleep
Malignancy of tonsils
Diphtheria carrier
Cor pulmonale due to obstruction of airway
Recurrent peritonsillar abscess (rare today)

**Some Indications for Adenoidectomy**

Hypertrophy leading to obstruction of airway and impaired breathing (hypoxia, pulmonary hypertension, cor pulmonale)
Chronic otitis media or hearing loss due to hypertrophy, severe speech impediment
Persistent mouth breathing and recurrent rhinitis and sinusitis that appear to be related to infected adenoids

**Contraindications**

Cleft palate
Under 3 yr of age
Blood conditions such as leukemia, purpura, hemophilia

*Note:* Controversy still exists among practitioners as to the indications for surgery.

sues become smaller as the child grows. It is also easier for an older child to cope with hospitalization. Fears, especially those of separation, are less intense.

Determining whether surgery is required is perhaps the single most important medical decision. Same-day surgery is becoming common. Administration of antibiotics during acute infections has reduced the need for surgery. Ideally the patient is free of symptoms for at least 2 weeks before an operation is attempted. If the infection is persistent, the child is given antibiotics for a few days before and after surgery. They are also administered to children with a history of rheumatic fever, regardless of the presence of infection.

### Nursing Care

*Preoperative Care.* The child is prepared in advance for hospitalization. Children need to know that the tonsils are two small lumps located in the back of the mouth. Because they are causing the throat to be sore (or whatever symptoms the child is experiencing), they need to be fixed. The doctor will do this by taking them out. This is done through the mouth. The doctor will not operate on any other part of the body. Children are also informed that they will receive a special medicine that will make them go to sleep and will keep them asleep until the operation is over. *Then they will wake up.*

Medical personnel and parents must be alert to the young child's fantasies and anxieties. They must answer questions honestly and at a level suitable to the age of the child. One concern uncovered by the television personality Mister Rogers is that many young children fear that an operation will change them into a completely different person (Rogers & Head, 1983). Children need to know that medical personnel understand their feelings. They need someone they know and trust to be close by. The child's parents are included in discussions and encouraged to stay with the child. Many hospitals have special programs to prepare children for surgery. These include videotapes, prehospital tours, and opportunities to handle supplies.

A complete physical examination and urinalysis are performed before surgery. Blood work includes hemoglobin, hematocrit, prothrombin time, and partial thromboplastin time. The latter tests are done because bleeding is anticipated. These procedures are usually performed prior to admission. The child is inspected for loose teeth and signs of upper respiratory tract infection. It is also important to determine any family bleeding tendencies, any history of chronic illness (such as rheumatic fever), elevations in temperature, and recent exposure to communicable diseases. The child is encouraged to drink fluids on the evening before surgery in order to maintain hydration; however, food and fluids are withheld for several hours prior to surgery in order to prevent aspiration from vomitus.

In the hospital, the child's bed is tagged with a "nothing-by-mouth" sign; in some hospitals, a sign is attached directly to the child's clothing. The nurse checks the patient's bedside stand for candy or gum and removes it. Preoperative medication of atropine and one of the barbiturates may be given. Some facilities use rectal induction, which allows the child to go to sleep in the parent's arms (Thompson & Ashwill, 1992). The nurse checks to see that the child's identification band is securely attached to the wrist. The patient should void before leaving the unit. Review postoperative procedures with the parents, including what to expect in the recovery room or on return to the unit (e.g., color, bleeding, possible use of an intravenous tube, vomiting, irritability). Explain how and when they will be notified of the results of the surgery.

*Postoperative Care.* Immediately following surgery, to facilitate drainage, the child is placed partly on the side and partly on the abdomen, with the knee of the uppermost leg flexed to hold the position. The child is watched carefully for evidence of bleeding, that is, an increase in pulse and respirations, restlessness, frequent swallowing (which may be from blood trickling down the back of the child's throat), and vomiting of bright red blood. An ice collar may be applied for comfort. An emesis basin and tissues are provided. The child's face and hands are wiped with a warm face cloth, and the hospital gown and linen are changed whenever necessary. Small amounts of clear liquids are given when the vomiting has ceased. Synthetic fruit juices are used because they are not as irritating as natural juices. A Popsicle may appeal to the child. If these are well tolerated, progression to a soft diet is begun. The child is kept quiet for the remainder of the day. A small child may nestle on a parent's lap.

Hemorrhage is the most common postoperative complication. The nurse should not assume that because surgery is minor it does not involve certain risks. Because bleeding after this type of surgery is concealed, the nurse must watch carefully for evidence of hemorrhage. When bleeding is suspected, packing and sometimes ligation are indicated. Lung abscesses and pneumonia are infrequent complications.

***Hospital Discharge.*** Written instructions are given to the parents when the child is discharged. The child should be kept quiet for a few days and should receive nourishing fluids and soft foods. After this, children may continue to take a nap or have a rest period so that they have sufficient convalescent time. Acetaminophen (Tylenol) may be given to reduce discomfort in the throat. The child needs to be protected from exposure to infections. Fresh bleeding, chest pain, or persistent cough should be reported to the physician. Earache may follow a T & A, and slight fever (37.2–37.8°C or 99–100°F) may occur for 1 or 2 days. A follow-up appointment is made because the surgeon will wish to check the operative site after it has healed.

### ASTHMA

**Description.** Asthma is the principal cause of chronic illness in children. It is the leading cause of school absenteeism, emergency room visits, and hospitalization. Although it may occur at any age, about 80% of asthma sufferers have their first symptoms before 5 years of age. Prior to puberty, about twice as many boys as girls are affected; thereafter, the sex incidence is equal. The course and severity of asthma are difficult to predict. Asthma is a complex disease in which biochemical, autonomic, immunologic, infectious, endocrine, and psychological factors occur in varying degrees in different individuals (Behrman, 1992).

Although death from asthma is uncommon, the incidence is increasing world wide, particularly among teenagers. The exact cause of this is uncertain. Some have suggested that poor access to care, and failure of families and practitioners to recognize the severity of the disease may have a bearing.

Asthma is a recurrent and reversible obstruction of the airways in which bronchospasm, mucosal edema, and secretion and plugging of mucus contribute to significant narrowing of the airways and subsequent impaired gas exchange (Fig. 26–11). Both large (>2 mm) and small (<2 mm) airways may be involved. The onset of asthma may be triggered by house dust, animal dander, wool, feathers, pollen, mold, passive smoking, strong odors (as from wet paint, wood stoves, fireplaces), and certain foods (Fig. 26–12). Vigorous physical activity, especially in cold weather, may precipitate an attack, as may rapid changes in temperature and humidity. Viral infections are also responsible. Emotional upsets, which affect smooth muscle and vasomotor tone (*vas*, "vessel," and *motor*, "mover"), are closely intertwined with the condition. Whatever the precipitating cause, the response of the airways is similar. As the attack worsens, arterial blood gases change. $PCO_2$ rises and the blood pH falls, increasing respiratory acidosis and producing a strain on the heart. Children who are prone to allergies often trade one sensitivity for another. Some children who suffer from infantile eczema (see p. 812) develop asthma as they grow older. A family history of allergies is often seen, although the patient may suffer from a different manifestation.

**Manifestations.** The symptoms of asthma may begin slowly or abruptly. They may be

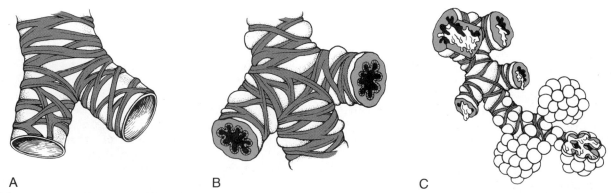

**Figure 26–11.** Obstruction of bronchial asthma. *A,* Cross-section of normal bronchi. *B,* Asthmatic bronchi. *C,* Constriction, inflammation, and increased production of mucus.

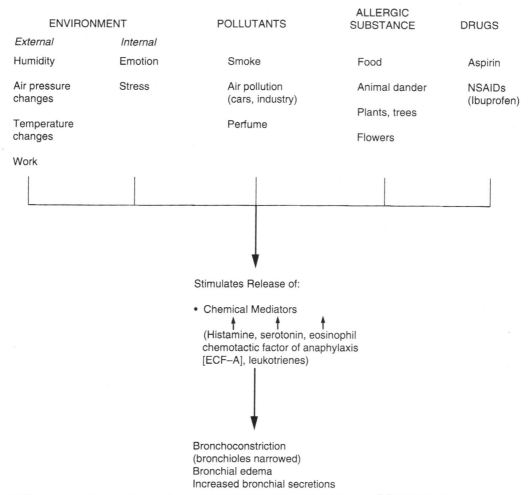

**Figure 26–12.** Factors contributing to bronchoconstriction. (From Kee, J.L., & Hayes, E.R. [1993]. *Pharmacology: A nursing process approach*. Philadelphia: W.B. Saunders.)

mild, moderate, or severe. In acute episodes, the patient coughs, wheezes, and has difficulty breathing, particularly during expiration. The child may complain that the chin, neck, or chest itches. Signs of air hunger, such as flaring of the nostrils, cyanosis, and use of the accessory muscles of respiration, that is, chest and abdominal muscles, may be evident. Orthopnea appears. The child is restless, perspires, and sometimes complains of abdominal pain. Vomiting may occur. Pulse and respirations are increased, and rales, abnormal respiratory sounds, may be heard in the chest. Inflammation of the nose and sinuses may accompany asthma.

These attacks often happen during the night and are frightening for the child and parents. Repeated attacks over a long period may lead to emphysema. Complications include pneumonia, atelectasis, mucus plugs in the bronchi, and *status asthmaticus*. Chronic asthma is manifested by discoloration beneath the eyes (allergic shiners), slight eyelid eczema, and mouth breathing.

Status asthmaticus is a medical emergency in which the attack does not respond to usual treatments. Because hypoxia and acid-base disturbances may cause cardiac arrhythmias and since theophylline and adrenergics can be potentially toxic to the heart, cardiac monitoring is indicated. If untreated, respiratory failure and death may result.

**Treatment.** The physician obtains the child's history in detail. Skin tests may be administered to determine if allergy is a cause. It is then necessary to eliminate the offender, whether it is an environmental agent or food. Depending on the severity, pulmonary function tests may be ordered. These will reflect the obstructive process of the small bronchioles. The education and cooperation of the parents and child are important because the treatment program needs to be carried out over a prolonged period.

Patients can be taught to monitor their own lung function. This is accomplished by the use of a portable, hand-held peak flowmeter. Patients are encouraged to take a reading at the same time every day. The age and size of the patient have a bearing on the reading, but readings below 100 ml/sec generally indicate a problem. Adequate rest, good health habits, exercise, and a generous amount of fluid may prevent an attack. The patient must try to avoid situations that cause emotional upset. For re-

lief of an acute attack, aqueous epinephrine (Adrenalin), a vasoconstrictor, is used. It relaxes the smooth muscles of the respiratory tract and provides immediate relief. Its absorption is increased by massaging the injection site. Terbutaline sulfate is an alternative drug that has longer action and causes less tachycardia. Other medications and their side effects are listed in Box 26–3.

In more severe attacks the child is hospitalized. The nurse limits conversation with the patient during the emergency period to questions that can be answered "yes" or "no." Oxygen will reduce hypoxia and improve the patient's color. It is administered by nasal prongs, hood, or mask. Albuterol given by nebulizer is also effective in relieving symptoms. Aminophylline is

| BOX 26–3 | Common Bronchodilators Used in Management of Asthma | | |
|---|---|---|---|
| **Beta-adrenergics** | **Action** | **Common Side Effects** | **Nursing Considerations** |
| Albuterol (Ventolin) (Proventil) Isoetharine (Bronkosol) (Bronkometer) Metaproterenol (Alupent) (Metaprel) Terbutaline (Brethine) (Brethaire) | Relaxes constricted airways by stimulating beta-adrenergic receptors | Gastrointestinal (GI) upset, increase in heart rate, shakiness, dry mouth | Contraindicated in seizure disorders If given by metered-dose inhaler, instruct patient as to use Explain that excessive use may lead to tolerance and loss of drug effectivenesss |
| **Xanthine Derivative** | **Action** | **Common Side Effects** | **Nursing Considerations** |
| Theophylline (Theo-Dur) (Slo-phyllin) | Relaxes smooth muscles of respiratory tract by inhibition of the breakdown of cyclic adenosine monophosphate (AMP). Stimulates cardiac muscle to increase flow rate | Shakiness, restlessness, insomnia, increased heart rate, mild diuresis | Theophylline has a low therapeutic index and a narrow therapeutic range of 10–20 $\mu$g/ml Monitor serum levels (see text) Give with food to avoid GI upset Do not crush or break extended relief forms Avoid caffeine (chocolate, cola drinks, coffee); increase fluids |

given in a loading dose, followed by a continuous infusion. Because aminophylline is a form of theophylline, serum theophylline levels are monitored. The therapeutic blood range is 10–20 µg/ml. Medications for drug interactions should be screened, as several drugs commonly prescribed for pediatric patients affect the rate of clearance. Steroids may be used in the oral or inhaled form. Prior to discharge, the patient is converted to oral medication. The nurse carefully monitors respirations during the transition from intravenous to oral or inhaled medications. Sedatives are not used because they may mask the signs of respiratory decline. Chest physical therapy is instituted when the acute attack subsides.

Asthma can generally be controlled sufficiently so that the child can lead a normal life with modest limitations. The condition sometimes disappears with puberty. Support groups for asthmatic patients are beneficial. Lung camps are also available in some states.

**Nursing Care.** General control of the environment is explained to the child and family. Certain pleasures must be eliminated—no pets or live Christmas trees or stuffed toys. Plants and aquariums, which harbor mold, are removed, and vaporizers are kept clean. Cellars or damp basements are not acceptable play areas. The child's bedroom is damp-dusted every day, and rugs, upholstered furniture, venetian blinds, and drapes, which collect dust, must be removed. A foam-rubber pillow is substituted for a feather pillow, and a plastic covering is placed on the mattress. The furnishings should consist of the necessities—bed, dresser, and wooden chair. The doors and windows to the bedroom are kept shut during the day. An air conditioner during the summer is advised. No woolen clothing is allowed to be worn, and cotton blankets are to be used. Foodstuffs detrimental to the child's health are avoided. These measures are also instituted during hospitalization.

If the child is in respiratory distress on admission, oxygen is administered per physician protocol, and the child is positioned comfortably. One method is to place a pillow on the overbed table and have the patient extend the arms over it, elbows bent. This is comfortable and allows maximum utilization of the accessory muscles of breathing. Lung sounds are assessed for rhonchi, wheezing, or rales. Arterial blood gases and vital signs are monitored. The child is evaluated for clinical improvement (quieter, slower respirations, relaxed facial expression, cessation of retractions). Oral fluids are encouraged, as

they help liquefy secretions and are needed to compensate for fluid loss from dyspnea and diaphoresis. Carbonated beverages, such as ginger ale and colas, are avoided when the patient is wheezing. Beverages are served at room temperature because cold liquids can trigger reflex bronchospasm. Milk products are avoided because they tend to increase the production of mucus. Record intake and output. The patient is observed for cracked lips, absence of tears, poor skin turgor, and decrease in urinary output, all of which signal dehydration.

A well-balanced diet is necessary for the patient's general health. Ample time is allowed for meals, as respiratory distress may intefere with eating. The nurse organizes tasks so that the child obtains sufficient rest. The child is assisted with the use of the nebulizer if this is required. With proper treatment, asthma attacks are not lengthy, and the child generally remains free of symptoms between attacks.

**Self-Care.** The child is gradually taught self-care. Patients are taught not to push themselves when they feel tightness in the chest, an early sign of difficulties. The importance of exercise to strengthen vulnerable lungs is emphasized. Swimming is an excellent sport for asthmatics. Children are taught to observe "personal triggers" that are forewarnings of an attack. They are taught how to use the peak expiratory flowmeter. Other aspects of care include how to administer metered-dose inhalers, and the monitoring and understanding of medications and their possible side effects. Specific information about how often and when to use inhalers is paramount. The child is encouraged to discuss daily school routines. The physician is seen regularly in order to evaluate progress and readjust medications as needed. *The nurse reviews the signs of respiratory infection and where, when, and whom to call for help.* Early attention to symptoms may prevent escalation of the disease. The nurse listens to and supports parents and siblings. Asthma is a chronic disease, and the stresses associated with such conditions apply. Family lifestyle is evaluated and proper referrals initiated when needed. The family is encouraged to contact the American Lung Association or the Asthma and Allergy Foundation of America for information on existing programs that could be of benefit. Patients with severe asthma should wear a Medic-Alert bracelet and are educated and provided with injectable epinephrine (EpiPen or EpiPen Jr.) for emergency use.

## NURSING CARE PLAN 26-2

### Selected Nursing Diagnoses for the Child with Bronchial Asthma

| Goals | Nursing Interventions | Rationale |
|---|---|---|
| **Nursing Diagnosis:** Ineffective breathing related to increased mucus production and narrowed respiratory passages evidenced by coughing and wheezing, restlessness. | | |
| Child's ventilation capacity will improve as evidenced by improved respirations and color, decrease in retractions, and stabilization of vital signs | 1. Remain calm; assist patient to a position that facilitates an open airway (infant seat or elevate head of bed); small child may sit on parent's lap<br>2. Provide aerosol treatments as ordered<br>3. Provide fluids at room temperature | 1. A calm presence may help diminish the anxiety-related increase in oxygen consumption; position and good posture promote ventilation<br>2. Aerosol therapy relaxes smooth muscles and provides for more effective airway clearance<br>3. Dehydration can occur from loss of fluids through dyspnea and diaphoresis; fluids aid in liquefying secretions; cold fluids can trigger reflex bronchospasm |
| **Nursing Diagnosis:** Impaired gas exchange related to inadequate respiratory function. | | |
| Child's respiratory distress decreases; arterial blood gases return to normal limits | 1. Provide oxygen as age-appropriate (hood, tent, cannula)<br><br>2. Monitor vital signs and chest sounds frequently<br><br><br>3. Monitor arterial blood gases<br><br>4. Monitor blood theophylline levels | 1. Oxygen reduces hypoxemia and corrects blood gas alterations; children may resist application of a mask<br>2. Increase in pulse and respiration indicate worsening condition and may require a change in medication; lung auscultation will evaluate air exchange<br>3. Arterial blood gas measurements assess carbon dioxide and oxygen levels and detect hypoxemia<br>4. Blood levels of theophylline greater than 20 µg/ml may lead to toxicity; watch for increased irritability, increase in pulse and respiration, arrythmias, nausea, vomiting, diarrhea, restlessness, headache, shakiness |
| **Nursing Diagnosis:** Knowledge deficit related to limited understanding of home care of child with asthma. | | |
| Parents and older child will verbalize increased knowledge about allergens, inhalers, self-management, and home care; they will know whom to contact with questions or for additional information | 1. Begin discharge teaching on day of admission, as teaching is extensive<br><br>2. Review precipitating allergens, and manifestations of an attack<br>3. Provide written instructions as to when to notify physician<br><br><br>4. Explain how to allergy-proof home as needed<br>5. Demonstrate proper use of metered-dose inhalers, including effects and side effects of medication<br>6. Discuss any physical restrictions<br><br><br>7. Assist parents in understanding importance of self-management to child's self-esteem | 1. Hospitalization is brief; too much information on day of discharge will overwhelm family<br>2/3. Knowing what to do helps provide control and reduces fear, as the family will understand initial appropriate action; may prevent hospitalization<br>4. This reduces environmental triggers<br>5. Correct use of inhalers and other equipment facilitates treatment<br><br>6. Regular exercise facilitates lung expansion; inappropriate exercise may overload respiratory system<br>7. Overprotectiveness can precipitate rebellion and stress that may lead to an attack |

## CYSTIC FIBROSIS

**Description.** Cystic fibrosis is the most common fatal genetic disease in the United States today. It affects approximately 30,000 children and adults. It occurs in approximately 1 in 25,000 live births. The diagnosis is usually made within the first 3 years of life.

The basic defect in cystic fibrosis is created by the faulty transport of sodium chloride (salt) from within the epithelial cells to their outer surfaces (Cystic Fibrosis Foundation, 1993). Epithelial cells line the surfaces of organs such as the lungs and pancreas. In healthy people, a protein called cystic fibrosis transmembrane regulator (CFTR) provides a channel by which sodium chloride can pass into and out of cells. Cystic fibrosis sufferers have a defective copy of the CFTR gene. As a result, salt accumulates in the cells lining the lungs and digestive tissues, turning the surrounding mucus into a sticky, suffocating paste (Cowley, 1993). In the pancreas, enzymes are prevented from reaching the intestine to digest food. Without treatment the body does not absorb enough nutrients.

Cystic fibrosis is an inherited disorder. Both parents must be *carriers* of the cystic fibrosis gene for the child to have the disease. When two *genes* for the disease combine at conception, cystic fibrosis results. The parents do not show any symptoms. The gene that causes cystic fibrosis was identified in 1989, and carriers can now be identified. Fetuses who have the disorder can be identified by amniocentesis. Clinical trials on humans are under way. It is hoped that by transferring a synthetic CFTR gene into the cells of a patient, the patient's cells might become healthy and function normally.

Meanwhile the survival rate for these children has increased, and many are living into adulthood. Better antibiotic control of pulmonary infection both at home and during hospitalization and increased numbers of cystic fibrosis centers have contributed to this success. Surgery, such as lung transplants, has also improved, as has nutritional control.

**Manifestations.** The manifestations of cystic fibrosis are illustrated in Figure 26–13.

*Lung Involvement.* Cystic fibrosis is considered the most serious lung problem in children in the United States. The air passages of the

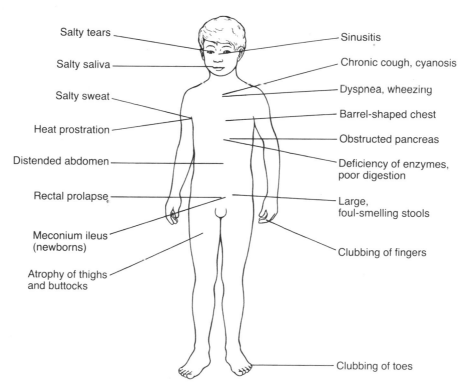

Salty tears

Salty saliva

Salty sweat

Heat prostration

Distended abdomen

Rectal prolapse

Meconium ileus
(newborns)

Atrophy of thighs
and buttocks

Sinusitis

Chronic cough, cyanosis

Dyspnea, wheezing

Barrel-shaped chest

Obstructed pancreas

Deficiency of enzymes,
poor digestion

Large,
foul-smelling stools

Clubbing of fingers

Clubbing of toes

**Figure 26–13.** Manifestations of cystic fibrosis.

lungs become clogged with mucus. There is a widespread obstruction of the bronchioles. It is difficult for the patient to breathe; expiration is especially difficult. More and more air becomes trapped in the lungs (obstructive emphysema), and small areas of collapse (atelectasis) may occur. Eventually, the chest assumes a barrel shape, with increased diameter across the front and back. The right ventricle of the heart, which supplies the lungs, may become strained and enlarged. Clubbing of fingers and toes, a compensatory response indicating a chronic lack of oxygen, may be present. *Staphylococcus* and *Pseudomonas* infections can easily occur in the lungs, which provide a suitable medium for the organisms' growth. This causes more thickening of the abnormal secretions, irritates and damages lung tissues, and further increases lung obstruction.

The time of onset of this disease varies. Symptoms may appear weeks, months, and years after birth. In general, the earlier the onset, the more severe is the disease. The symptoms range from mild to severe. Any or all symptoms may be present in varying degrees of severity in one individual. The patient develops a chronic cough that may produce vomiting. Dyspnea, wheezing, and cyanosis may occur. The child is irritable and tires easily. Gradually, there is a change in physical appearance. X-ray films of the chest reveal widespread infection. Evidence of obstructive emphysema, atelectasis, and fibrosis of lung tissue may also be present. The prognosis for survival depends on the extent of lung damage. However, this is only part of the picture, since cystic fibrosis also affects the pancreas and sweat glands.

*Pancreatic Involvement.* The pancreas lies behind the stomach. Some of its cells secrete pancreatic juice. This key digestive juice drains from the pancreatic duct into the duodenum at the same area in which bile enters. Changes occurring in the pancreas are due to obstruction by thickened secretions that block the flow of pancreatic digestive enzymes. As a result, foodstuffs, particularly fats and proteins, are not properly utilized by the body.

In infants, the stools may be loose. Gradually, because of impaired digestion and food absorption, the feces of the patient become large, fatty, and foul-smelling. They are usually light in color. The baby does not gain weight in spite of a good appetite and may look undernourished. The abdomen becomes distended, and the buttocks and thighs *atrophy* (waste away) as fat disappears from the main deposit sites. Laboratory tests show a deficiency of pancreatic enzymes (trypsin, lipase, amylase).

An oral pancreatic preparation, such as pancrelipase (Pancrease), is given to the child with each meal and snack in order to replace the pancreatic enzymes the child's body cannot produce. This medication is considered specific for the disease because it aids in the digestion and absorption of food, thus improving the condition of the stools. If the child is ill and not eating, the medication is withheld. When meals are erratic, such as during vacations, medication is given when the largest amount of food will be consumed.

A condition known as *meconium ileus* exists when the intestine of the newborn becomes obstructed with abnormally thick meconium while in utero. This is due to the absence of pancreatic enzymes that normally digest proteins in the meconium. The abnormal, putty-like stool sticks to the walls of the intestine, causing blockage. Rupture with signs of shock may occur. The presenting symptoms develop within hours after birth. Absence of stools, vomiting, and abdominal distention lead one to suspect intestinal obstruction. X-ray films confirm the diagnosis. The condition is surgically treated. The death rate is high, but the prognosis is more favorable when the obstruction is detected early. Most infants who survive will manifest cystic fibrosis. Fortunately, the incidence of meconium ileus is rare because the pancreatic enzyme deficiency is seldom complete. Nevertheless, the nurse assigned to the nursery must constantly be on guard for suspicious symptoms.

*Sweat Glands.* The sweat, tears, and saliva of the patient with cystic fibrosis become abnormally salty because of an increase in the sodium chloride levels. There is also an increase in the potassium level of sweat glands. Up to about 20 years of age, more than 60 mEq/liter of sodium chloride in sweat is diagnostic of cystic fibrosis when one or more criteria are present. Levels of 40–60 mEq/liter are highly suggestive. The analysis of sweat is a major aid in the diagnosis of the condition. The *sweat test*, using pilocarpine iontophoresis, is the best diagnostic study. A dilute solution of pilocarpine is applied to the arm, and a weak electric current is used to stimulate sweating. A positive test should be repeated for confirmation. Because these patients lose large amounts of salt through perspiration, they must be watched for heat prostration. Liberal amounts of salt should be given with food, and extra fluids and salt should be provided during the hot weather.

**Complications.** Cystic fibrosis is often responsible for rectal prolapse in infants and children. This is partly due to poor muscle tone in the rectal area and excessive leanness of the buttocks of the patient. However, surgery is almost never required, as the patient obtains relief by taking pancreatic medication.

As the disease progresses, the liver may become hard, nodular, and enlarged. There may be edema of the extremities. The retina of the eye may hemorrhage; there may be damage to the eye from swelling, and inflammation in part of the optic nerve may occur. Cor pulmonale (*cor*, "heart," and *pulmon*, "lung"), heart strain due to improper lung function, is frequently a cause of death. Osteoporosis (*osteo*, "bone," *pore*, and *osis*, "disease") may occur. When osteoporosis is caused by cystic fibrosis, the bones become porous because of poor utilization of fat-soluble vitamin D, which is necessary for proper calcium metabolism. There is a deficiency of vitamin A because the child is unable to absorb fats from which this vitamin is obtained. Sexual development may be delayed in these patients. Males are generally sterile; however, sexual function is unimpaired. Adolescent girls may experience secondary amenorrhea during exacerbations.

### Treatment and Nursing Care

*Respiratory Relief.* Antibiotics may be given as a preventive measure against respiratory infection; however, this treatment is subject to controversy. Full doses of antibiotics are given in an acute infection. The physician determines the particular antibiotic to be used by the results of throat and sputum cultures. The route may be oral, inhaled, intramuscular, or intravenous. Intravenous medication may be given via heparin lock or, in some cases, a Broviac catheter (see p. 587). This can successfully be employed in inpatients and outpatients.

Intermittent aerosol therapy is administered to provide medication and water to the lower respiratory tract and to promote evacuation of secretions. Expectorants, especially the iodides, are also employed in an effort to thin secretions. Bronchodilators are used to increase the width of the bronchi, allowing free passage of air into the lungs.

Postural drainage and chest-clapping exercises are also of value. These are performed by the physical or respiratory therapist during hospitalization. When postural drainage and chest clapping are done properly, the secretions in the chest are moved up and out. During latent periods or in mild cases, the patient may not raise sputum. This should be explained to the parents so that they will not discontinue this valuable procedure when the child comes home. Instructions may need frequent repetition in order to encourage full cooperation of the parents and child. These procedures are done following nebulization and at least 1 hour after eating. General exercise is good for the patient because it stimulates coughing. Somersaults, headstands, and wheelbarrow play within the child's endurance limits are therapeutic. In one 8-year study reported in *The New England Journal of Medicine*, patients with cystic fibrosis who achieved "aerobic fitness" had a significantly higher rate of survival (Cystic Fibrosis Foundation, 1993).

Breathing exercises may also be recommended for the older child. Pursed-lip breathing is one technique that is simple and effective. The patient is instructed to inhale through the nose, then to exhale through the mouth with the lips pursed as if whistling. Exhalation should be at least twice as long as inhalation. (If it takes 3 seconds to breathe in, 6 seconds are taken to allow all the air to escape.) The child is taught not to force the air out but to let it escape naturally.

Prevention of respiratory infections is essential. The child is isolated from patients and personnel who may harbor infections. The period of hospitalization is kept brief, if possible, in order to avoid cross-infection. This patient must be given the necessary immunizations against childhood diseases (see p. 434). Appropriate boosters are given, so if the child is hospitalized at the age when a booster is almost due, the schedule is reviewed with parents and they are reminded to keep up to date.

*Diet.* The maintenance of adequate nutrition is essential. The diet is high in calories, as much as 50% above normal. There should be increased protein and moderate amounts of fat in conjunction with pancreatic extracts. Simple sugars are easy to digest, and banana products are particularly good. Fruits, cottage cheese, vegetables, and lean meats, which are high in protein and low in fat and starches, are recommended. Restrictions on ice cream, peanut butter, butter, french fries, and mayonnaise are ad-

| NURSING CARE PLAN 26–3 | | |
| --- | --- | --- |
| **Selected Nursing Diagnoses for the Child with Cystic Fibrosis** | | |
| **Goals** | **Nursing Interventions** | **Rationale** |

**Nursing Diagnosis:** Ineffective airway clearance related to accumulation of mucus.

| Goals | Nursing Interventions | Rationale |
| --- | --- | --- |
| Child's aeration is improved as evidenced by decreased dyspnea and tachypnea | 1. Provide adequate hydration | 1. Helps liquefy secretions of lungs; fluid is lost through frequent stools; sweating may lead to dehydration, as excess sodium chloride is a manifestation of the disease |
| Child manages secretions with minimum distress; aeration improves | 2. Assist patient with aerosol therapy | 2. Inhalation therapy liquefies mucus and prevents or manages infections |
| | 3. Assist patient with postural drainage | 3. Postural drainage helps clear airways |
| | 4. Explain importance of breathing exercises | 4. Breathing exercises aerate lungs to maximum capacity |
| | 5. Administer medications and explain their use | 5. Careful explanation of medications, how much and when to take, avoids errors and increases compliance |
| Child shows no evidence of infection | 6. Prevent infection by maintaining a high level of suspicion and proper handwashing; review immunization schedule | 6. Early detection of lung infection may reduce or prevent exacerbations; flu immunizations are recommended yearly; immunizations of childhood require review and update |

**Nursing Diagnosis:** Altered nutrition related to enzyme deficiencies, anorexia, poor absorption of vitamins, excess sodium loss.

| Goals | Nursing Interventions | Rationale |
| --- | --- | --- |
| Child consumes a well-balanced diet as evidence by maintenance of weight or weight gain | 1. Administer pancreatic replacement enzymes; administer water-soluble vitamins | 1. Digestive and nutritional therapy consists of replacement of pancreatic enzymes, diet adjustment, and administration of water-soluble vitamins; water-soluble vitamins are suggested because of severe fat malabsorption |
| | 2. Monitor salt intake (will need to be increased during hot weather and increased exercise) | 2. Prevents NaCl depletion via sweat, especially in hot weather |
| | 3. Provide normal diet for age with supplemental protein, vitamins, minerals; modify fat intake if normal diet is not tolerated (breast milk or prescribed formula for infants) | 3. Digestion is impaired; maintaining adequate nutrition is essential, as child is growing; food needs to be age-appropriate; serve small, attractive portions |
| | 4. Anticipate anorexia and developmental issues surrounding food during adolescence | 4. Anorexia is common during adolescence; teenagers often rebel against food restrictions and medications as need to conform with peers increases |

**Nursing Diagnosis:** High risk for impaired skin integrity related to poor nutrition and acid stools.

| Goals | Nursing Interventions | Rationale |
| --- | --- | --- |
| Child's skin and mucous membranes remain intact; there will be no rectal abrasions | 1. Provide good skin care, change position frequently | 1. Child may be malnourished |
| | 2. In infants, cleanse diaper area, which becomes irritated by stool; observe for breakdown of skin | 2. Frequency of stools can lead to abrasions and infection in rectal area |
| | 3. Encourage good oral hygiene | 3. Patient raises sputum from postural drainage, may experience bad breath |

| NURSING CARE PLAN 26–3 *Continued* | | |
|---|---|---|
| **Selected Nursing Diagnoses for the Child with Cystic Fibrosis** | | |
| **Goals** | **Nursing Interventions** | **Rationale** |

**Nursing Diagnosis:** Knowledge deficit (parents) related to the cause and treatment of the disorder, prognosis, follow-up care.

| Goals | Nursing Interventions | Rationale |
|---|---|---|
| Parents will verbalize understanding of cystic fibrosis and care of child | 1. Assess level of understanding concerning diet, medication, respiratory therapy regimen, need for frequent follow-up care<br>2. Assess home environment | 1. Initial stage of diagnosis is bewildering to parents; thorough education increases family's confidence in caring for child<br>2. Home environment must be adequate to sustain child's growth and development plus demands of illness; visiting nurse services may be needed |
| | 3. Encourage parents' participation and acceptance of child's condition | 3. A chronic illness taxes entire family; involvement of individual members helps them feel included |
| | 4. Help parents understand and support child through various ages and stages | 4. Major stress of cystic fibrosis patient at all ages is fear of suffocation and dying; embarrassment over coughing, raising sputum, and flatulence is common |
| | 5. Initiate referrals; for example, school and community nurse, National Cystic Fibrosis Research Foundation, local chapter, social worker | 5. A social support network is important because of length and unpredictable course of disease |

**Nursing Diagnosis:** Disturbance in self-concept related to chronic disease, low self-esteem, loss of body image.

| Goals | Nursing Interventions | Rationale |
|---|---|---|
| Child is as self-sufficient as age-appropriate | 1. Promote self-care as appropriate | 1. Self-care increases self-esteem, independence, and confidence |
| | 2. Explain new procedures | 2. Careful explanations of new procedures decrease fear |
| | 3. Assist child in understanding disease and its treatment | 3. Education lessens stress |
| | 4. Encourage appropriate physical activities | 4. Daily exercises increase endurance, promote feelings of well-being, improve posture, and keep fluid from building up in lungs; swimming and hydrotherapy build muscles of respiration and promote good breathing habits |
| Child feels free to verbalize self-image concerns | 5. Draw body portrait (child lies on butcher paper on floor); draw around body; have child paint or color in features and clothes; cut out and hang up; discuss with child | 5. Having child draw a body portrait will assist nurse in communicating with child concerning feelings about body; children with this disease may have barrel chests and protruding abdomens |
| | 6. Educate peers | 6. Child feels different; may be ridiculed by other children; education of peers may assist child's entry into group |
| | 7. Promote involvement in self-help group | 7. Fosters independence, communication, identification with those who are living with disease |
| | 8. Listen emphatically to child | 8. A good listener learns a great deal about child |
| | 9. Encourage verbalization of feelings | 9. Verbalization of feelings of fear or sadness decreases their intensity |

vised. Extra salt may be provided by pretzels and salted bread sticks and crackers.

The doctor may allow exceptions in the diet in order to keep meals from becoming drab and to provide a more normal atmosphere. At such times, children are allowed to eat what they wish and are given extra digestive enzymes. Supplements of vitamins A, D, and E in a water-miscible base are given each day in double the recommended dosage. Vitamin K may also be given when indicated. Salt tablets may be given to the older child during hot weather. Forcing fluids may be ordered because larger amounts of fluid are lost in the stools. The nurse may be asked to weigh the child daily.

The nurse feeding the infant with cystic fibrosis must be calm and unhurried. The baby may cough, have difficulty breathing, and vomit. The baby needs careful bubbling in order to avoid abdominal distention. In general, the appetite is good. Older children need small amounts of food served attractively and frequently. Food piled high on a child's tray is discouraging. The patient may have eaten a meal adequate for body size, but the nurse who carries the remainder of the tray to the kitchen charts "poor appetite."

Because mealtime is a social time, the nurse remains with the child if the parents are not present. It is not necessary to hover over the child to see that every morsel is eaten with the proper utensil. Instead, the nurse tries to make the meal more satisfying by giving good companionship mixed with a little encouragement. The nurse records the fluid intake at the end of the meal. The child's reaction to new foods and any variations in stools resulting from the foods are noted. The food refused and the type, character, and amount of vomiting, if any, are recorded.

**General Hygiene.** The nurse must pay special attention to the skin of the child with cystic fibrosis. The diaper area is cleansed following each bowel movement. An ointment to protect the skin is advisable because the character of the stool subjects the diaper area to irritation. The buttocks are exposed to air when a rash occurs. Careful attention to bony areas is necessary in order to prevent decubitus ulcers. Because the patient has little fat and muscle, the position must be changed frequently, especially if the child is weak and cannot get out of bed. This also prevents pneumonia. When the patient's position is changed, the patient is not left staring at a blank wall. This can easily be remedied by turning the crib around.

Soiled diapers are immediately removed from the room to eliminate offensive odors. The patient wears light clothing in order to avoid becoming overheated; it should be loose to allow freedom of movement. Good oral hygiene is necessary, since the teeth may be in poor condition because of dietary deficiencies. Mouth care is given after postural drainage, as foul mucus may be raised, leaving an unpleasant taste in the patient's mouth.

**Long-Term Care.** Today the child with a lengthy illness spends most of the time at home. Hospitalization is mainly for diagnosis, relapses, and complications. This is extremely taxing financially, physically, and emotionally. Somehow, the parents must distribute their time and energy within the family yet give careful attention to their sick child or sometimes, in the case of cystic fibrosis, children. How do they keep from spoiling the child? Do they limit the normal activities of the remaining children in order to spare the sick one? What about birthday parties, camping, Scouts, pets, epidemics at school? What does a trip to the shore or mountains entail? When do the husband and wife find time for themselves?

These seemingly overwhelming problems are faced daily by many people in every community. Parent groups are helpful in promoting exchange of ideas and in providing support. The National Cystic Fibrosis Research Foundation disseminates useful information. The nurse becomes familiar with the local chapter in the area so that parents are guided to reliable sources of information.

Parents of these patients need encouragement and reassurance. When meeting them in the clinic or hospital, the nurse is kind and attentive. If a child looks obviously well cared for, this is mentioned to the parents. If asked direct questions about the illness, the nurse might say, "Doctor Parker is a fine pediatrician. What did she tell you about Bobby's illness?" This encourages the parents to express themselves and gives you an idea of what the patient has been told. Parents should not be overwhelmed with information that is difficult to absorb.

Parents need explicit instructions regarding diet, medication, postural drainage, prevention of infection, rest, and continued medical supervision. Many families require the assistance of a social worker in order to secure funds for equipment and drugs. Parents are told that help will be available as the need arises. The mother, who is usually more directly involved, may benefit from these added hints: (1) She needs rest herself; the family must take over some of the responsibilities of the household. Relatives may care for the child periodically so that she can "get away from it all." Respite care is another alternative; it is helpful if she can develop at least one outside interest of her own. (2) An alarm clock set for medication time will remind her of this task. (3) A downstairs bedroom for the child is preferable. (4) Extra spoons and a pitcher of water on the bedside stand save steps.

***Emotional Support.*** The child who is chronically ill finds it hard to accept restricted activity. The amount and kinds of diversion required vary in cystic fibrosis because the disease affects children of all ages, with variations in severity (see Table 19–3 for a list of suitable toys).

It is thought that children benefit from simple, straightforward answers to questions about their illness. An uncomplicated diagram might be helpful. Children who understand why they are being restricted from certain activities will be more cooperative. They should know why they must take medications with each meal, use the nebulizer, and have postural drainage. They should see and handle the unfamiliar equipment necessary for care.

The young child finds it more difficult to be separated from parents during hospitalization. Even when the prognosis is grave, a child's courage is sustained if parents are there. Visiting hours for parents must be flexible. Close contact by mail with school, church, and clubs is important for the child of school age. It is helpful for patients to develop an activity that they enjoy, for example, piano or art. This increases feelings of worth and provides outlets for feelings. Consideration must be given to ways of fostering love, acceptance, trust, fair play, security, freedom of choice, creativity, and maintenance of self-identity.

Nurses must learn the child's likes, dislikes, fears, and interests. They observe the child with the family and note the type of relationship that exists. They form their own impressions about the child and must not be misled by labels given by those with less understanding. The patient has to be allowed to communicate in a manner that is meaningful. Sometimes children can express feelings; sometimes they cannot. Drawing with the child may stimulate conversation. The nurse is aware of a child's facial expressions, posture, and eyes and of how the child plays. What is being said to toys or playmates? Observations of the child's behavior are incorporated into nursing care plans.

Nurses and parents must not show undue concern for the patient's illness. Overindulging children makes them demanding. The children's impressions of themselves and their illness are determined to a large extent by how they feel physically, how the family feels about their condition, and how others behave toward them. The actions of nurses and their interest or lack of it speak for themselves.

## KEY POINTS

- Congenital heart disease is the most common form of heart disease among children.
- The study of blood circulation is termed hemodynamics.
- Signs and symptoms of congenital heart abnormalities in infants include dyspnea, difficulty with feedings, choking spells, recurrent respiratory infections, cyanosis, poor weight gain, clubbing of fingers and toes, and heart murmurs.
- The nursing goals significant to the care of children with heart defects are (1) to reduce the work of the heart, (2) to improve respiration, (3) to maintain proper nutrition, (4) to prevent infection, (5) to reduce the anxiety of the patient, and (6) to support and instruct the parents.
- Rheumatic fever, an autoimmune disease, typically follows a streptococcal infection of the throat.
- The classic symptoms of rheumatic fever are polyarthritis, erythema marginatum, Sydenham's chorea, and rheumatic carditis.
- The symptoms of appendicitis in the young child are frequently obscure. Pain is often more generalized, and nausea and vomiting may occur.

- Hemorrhage is the most common postoperative complication of the removal of tonsils and adenoids. Because the bleeding is concealed, the nurse must watch carefully for evidence of bleeding.
- Status asthmaticus is a severe exacerbation of asthma, which usually requires hospitalization and can be life-threatening.
- Cystic fibrosis affects many parts of the body but particularly the lungs, sweat glands, and pancreas. Nursing care must be organized to prevent fatigue.

# Study Questions

1. Define the following: patent, anastomosis, polycythemia, and cardiac decompensation.
2. What modern methods are being used for the repair of congenital heart defects?
3. What are the signs of increasing respiratory distress in the infant or small child?
4. Roger, age 3, has been admitted with pneumonia. His orders include frequent observation, and he is to be placed in a mist tent. What psychological considerations would the nurse need to review for age-appropriate care?
5. What factors does the nurse need to consider when formulating the nursing care plan for Roger? List two nursing diagnoses.
6. Roger's mother expresses her concern that Roger, who is toilet-trained, has wet the bed. What is an appropriate response from the nurse?
7. Review the postoperative care of the child who has had a tonsillectomy. What instructions about home care are given to parents?
8. Describe the pathology and treatment of a child with asthma.
9. Jared is an 8-year-old with severe asthma. It is 7 PM, chilly, and he has been outdoors playing. You notice he is having difficulty breathing and complains of his neck itching. What is your response to this situation? Be prepared to discuss your answer and rationale in class.
10. List two tests important to the diagnosis of cystic fibrosis.
11. The nurse is instructing 8-year-old Heather's mother about the administration of pancreatic enzymes. When are these given? State the rationale for your answer.
12. List four problems that might arise in caring for the child with cystic fibrosis at home.

# Multiple Choice Review Questions

*Choose the most appropriate answer.*

1. The cardiovascular system develops during which stage of fetal life?
   a. between the 22nd and 30th weeks
   b. between the 3rd and 8th weeks
   c. between the 32nd and 40th weeks
   d. between the 12th and 20th weeks

2. Which of the following is a defect that decreases pulmonary blood flow?
   a. ventricular septal defect
   b. coarctation of the aorta
   c. tetralogy of Fallot
   d. patent ductus arteriosus

3. A common digitalis preparation used for patients with heart disease is
   a. Diuril
   b. Lanoxin
   c. Dilantin
   d. nitroglycerin

4. Albuterol, used in the treatment of asthma, is a member of which of the following drug groups?

   a. cholinergic
   b. xanthines
   c. beta-adrenergic
   d. corticosteroid

5. In cystic fibrosis, poor muscle tone and frequent stools can result in
   a. rectal prolapse
   b. volvulus
   c. intussusception
   d. hemorrhoids

## BIBLIOGRAPHY

American Academy of Pediatrics Committee on Nutrition. (1986). Prudent life-style for children: Dietary fat and cholesterol. *Pediatrics, 78,* 521–525.

Behrman, R.E. (1992). *Nelson textbook of pediatrics* (14th ed.). Philadelphia: W.B. Saunders.

Black, J.M., & Matassarin-Jacobs, E. (1993). *Luckmann and Sorensen's medical-surgical nursing: A psychophysiologic approach* (4th ed.). Philadelphia: W.B. Saunders.

Cowley, G. (1993, May). Closing in on cystic fibrosis. *Newsweek.*

Cystic Fibrosis Foundation. (1993, March). *Home line, home health and pharmacy services.* Bethesda, MD: Author.

Cystic Fibrosis Foundation. (1993, February). *Foundation facts.* Bethesda, MD: Author.

Cystic Fibrosis Foundation. (1993). *CF gene therapy.* Bethesda, MD: Author.

Daberkow-Carson, E., & Smith, P. (1994). Altered cardiovascular junction. In C. Betz, M. Hunsberger, & S. Wright (eds.), *Family-centered nursing care of children* (2nd ed.). Philadelphia: W.B. Saunders.

Frank G., et al. (1986). Dietary intake as a determinant of cardiovascular risk factor variables. In G. Berenson (Ed.), *Causation of cardiovascular risk factors in children: Perspectives on cardiovascular risk in early life.* New York: Raven.

Gellis, S.S., & Kagan, B.M. (1991). *Current pediatric therapy 13.* Philadelphia: W.B. Saunders.

Graef, J., & Cone, T. (1988). *Manual of pediatric therapeutics.* Boston: Little, Brown.

Green, M., & Haggerty, R.J. (1990). *Ambulatory pediatrics IV.* Philadelphia: W.B. Saunders.

Hayman, L., et al. (1988, November-December). Reducing risk for heart disease in children. *MCN: American Journal of Maternal Child Nursing,* pp. 442–448.

Hodgson, B.B., Kizior, R.J., & Kingdon R.T. (1993). *Nurse's drug handbook.* Philadelphia: W.B. Saunders.

Levine M.D., Carey, W.B., & Crocker, A.C. (1992). *Developmental-behavioral pediatrics* (2nd ed.). Philadelphia: W.B. Saunders.

Lockey, R.F., & Bakantz, S.C. (1987). *Principles of immunology and allergy.* Philadelphia: W.B. Saunders.

Mott, S., James, S.R., & Sperhac, A.M. (1991). *Nursing care of children and families* (2nd ed.). Reading, MA: Addison-Wesley.

Pillitteri, A. (1992). *Maternal and child health nursing: Care of the childbearing and childrearing family.* Philadelphia: J.B. Lippincott.

Rogers, F., & Head, B. (1983). *Mister Rogers talks with parents.* New York: Berkley.

Schwartz, R. (1984). Children with chronic asthma: Care by the generalist and the specialist. *Pediatric Clinics of North America, 31,* 84.

Thompson, E.D., & Ashwill, J.W. (1992). *Pediatric nursing: An introductory text* (6th ed.). Philadelphia: W.B. Saunders.

Whaley, L., & Wong, D. (1991). *Nursing care of infants and children* (4th ed.). St. Louis: C.V. Mosby.

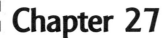

# Chapter 27

# The Child with a Condition of the Blood, Blood-Forming Organs, or Lymphatic System

**VOCABULARY**
cytochemistry (730)
hematemesis (735)
hypochromic (722)
infarct (724)
microcytic (722)
mutation (727)
petechiae (720)
purpura (720)
sickle cell crises (725)
splenomegaly (720)
thrombosis (724)

Iron-Deficiency Anemia
Sickle Cell Disease
Hemophilia
Idiopathic (Immunologic) Thrombocytopenic
  Purpura
The Leukemias
Hodgkin's Disease
Infectious Mononucleosis

# OBJECTIVES

*On completion and mastery of Chapter 27, the student will be able to*

■ Define each vocabulary term listed.
■ Summarize the components of the blood.
■ List two laboratory procedures commonly performed on patients with blood disorders.
■ List two manifestations of bleeding into the skin.
■ List the symptoms of iron-deficiency anemia.
■ Recommend four food sources of iron for Lorenzo, age 7 months, who is hospitalized for a herniorrhaphy and has been found to have an iron-deficiency anemia.
■ Devise a nursing care plan for a child with sickle cell disease.
■ Describe the symptoms of infectious mononucleosis.
■ Identify the pathologic changes that cause the following manifestations in a preschool child with leukemia: anemia, bone pain, proliferation of immature (blast) white cells, and petechiae.
■ Discuss the nursing care of a 14-year-old child receiving chemotherapy for cancer.

The blood and blood-forming organs make up the hematologic system. *Blood dyscrasias* or disorders occur when blood components fail to form correctly or when blood values exceed or fail to meet normal standards. Because the blood is vital to all body functions, disturbances can cause alterations that may be temporary or permanent. Plasma and blood cells are formed at about the 2nd week of life in the embryo. Blood forms in the liver at about the 5th week of development; later it forms in the spleen, thymus, lymph system, and bone marrow. The hematologic system along with the lymphatic system provides important information about the child's health. A large lymph node or lymphadenopathy may be the first sign of a disease. A number of diseases of the blood and lymph affect children. Figure 27–1 summarizes the differences between the child's and the adult's lymphatic system. Figure 27–2 depicts the main types of blood cells in the circulating blood.

Circulating blood consists of two portions: plasma and formed elements. The formed elements are erythrocytes (red blood cells), leukocytes (white blood cells), and thrombocytes (platelets). Erythrocytes primarily transport oxygen and carbon dioxide to and from the lungs and tissues. Leukocytes act as the body's defense against infections. Thrombocytes along with portions of blood plasma are involved with blood coagulation. In the young child, every available space in the bone marrow is involved with blood formation.

Lymphocytes, unlike other white blood cells, are produced in the lymphoid tissues of the body. They travel in the circulation but are more commonly found in the lymph tissue. They are released into the body to fight infection and provide immunity. Their numbers greatly increase in chronic inflammatory conditions. The spleen is the largest organ of the lymphatic system. One of the main functions of the spleen is to bring blood into contact with lymphocytes. Aside from trauma and rupture, the most frequently seen pathologic condition of the spleen is enlargement. This is termed *splenomegaly*. The spleen enlarges during infections, congenital and acquired hemolytic anemias, and liver malfunction.

Bone marrow aspiration is a procedure helpful in determining disorders of the blood. Numerous blood counts are utilized as well. Many are specific to a particular disease. The skin is sometimes an indicator of certain conditions of the blood. Purpura (black-and-blue bruises) and petechiae (pinpoint hemorrhagic spots) are often seen and should alert the nurse to the possibility of blood dyscrasia. The physician examines the liver and spleen by palpation and percussion to determine if they are enlarged. The following is a discussion of the child with iron-deficiency anemia, sickle cell disease, hemophilia, idiopathic (immunologic) thrombocytopenic purpura, leukemia, Hodgkin's disease, and mononucleosis. Hypocalcemia and hypoglycemia are discussed in Chapter 13. Acquired immunodeficiency syndrome (AIDS) and the thalassemias are discussed in Chapter 14.

## Iron-Deficiency Anemia

**Description.** The most common nutritional deficiency of children in the United States today is anemia due to insufficient amounts of iron in the body. The incidence is highest during infancy and adolescence, two rapid growth periods. Anemia (*an*, "without," and *emia*, "blood") is a condition in which there is a reduction in the amount and size of the red blood cells or in the amount of hemoglobin, or both. The clinical features are related to the decrease in the oxygen-carrying capacity of the blood. Iron is needed for the manufacture of red blood

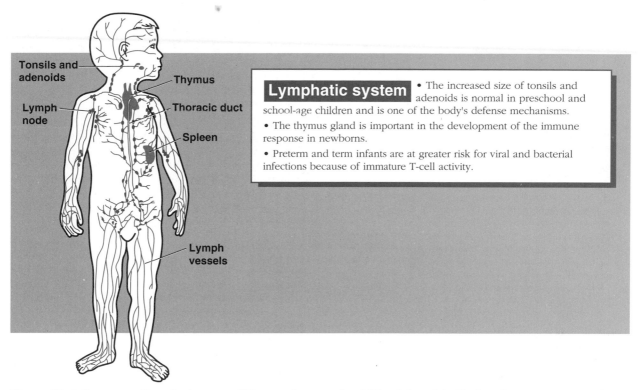

**Figure 27–1.** Summary of lymphatic system differences between the child and the adult. The lymphatic system is a subsystem of the circulatory system. It returns excess tissue fluid to the blood and defends the body against disease.

cells. Iron-deficiency anemia may be caused by severe hemorrhage, the child's inability to absorb the iron received, excessive growth requirements, or an inadequate diet. Researchers have also found that whole cow's milk can precipitate gastrointestinal bleeding (this is called lactose intolerance).

The prevention of iron-deficiency anemia begins with good prenatal care to ensure that the mother has a suitable intake of iron during pregnancy. During the first few months following birth the newborn relies on iron that was stored in the system during fetal life. Preterm infants may be deprived of a sufficient supply, since iron is obtained late in the prenatal period. Also, the iron stores of low-birth-weight babies and babies from multiple births are relatively small.

The highest incidence of this type of anemia occurs from the 9th month to the 24th month. During this rapid growth period, the baby outgrows the limited iron reserve that was in the body; in addition, iron-fortified formula and infant cereals may have been eliminated from the diet. Poorly planned meals or feeding problems also contribute to this deficiency. The mother

may sometimes rely too heavily on bottle feedings in order to avoid conflict at meals. Unfortunately, milk contains very little iron. Instead, the amounts of solid food should be increased, and the milk decreased. Boiled egg yolk, liver, leafy green vegetables, Cream of Wheat, dried fruits (apricots, peaches, prunes, raisins), dry beans, crushed nuts, and whole-grain bread are good sources of iron. Iron-fortified cereals eaten out of the box provide a nutritious snack. Unfortunately, not all the iron found in a food source is absorbed by the body. The bioavailability of iron in vegetables is less than that in meat.

**Manifestations.** The symptoms of iron-deficiency anemia are pallor, irritability, anorexia, and a decrease in activity. Some babies show no symptoms even when hemoglobin levels are quite low. Many babies are overweight because of excessive consumption of milk (so-called milk babies). Blood tests for anemia may include red blood cell count, hemoglobin, hematocrit, morphologic cell changes, and iron concentration. The stool may be tested for occult blood. A hemoglobin level of less than 11 gm/dl or a hema-

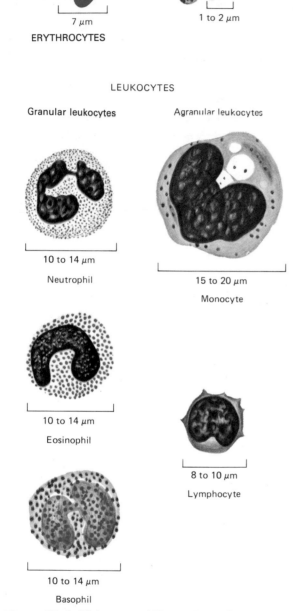

7 µm

**ERYTHROCYTES**

1 to 2 µm

LEUKOCYTES

Granular leukocytes

Agranular leukocytes

10 to 14 µm

Neutrophil

15 to 20 µm

Monocyte

10 to 14 µm

Eosinophil

8 to 10 µm

Lymphocyte

10 to 14 µm

Basophil

**Figure 27–2.** Main types of blood cells in the circulating blood. (From Solomon, E.P., & Phillips, G.A. [1987]. *Understanding human anatomy and physiology* [p. 200]. Philadelphia: W.B. Saunders.)

tocrit of less than 33% is usually considered definitive. However, this determination varies somewhat with the age of the patient. A dietary history is also obtained. Sometimes a slight heart murmur is heard. The spleen may be enlarged. Cells appear microcytic or hypochromic.

Untreated iron-deficiency anemias progress slowly, and in severe cases the heart muscle becomes too weak to function. If this happens, heart failure follows. Children with longstanding anemia may also show growth retardation and cognitive changes. Screening procedures are suggested at 9 and 24 months for full-term infants and earlier for low-birth-weight babies.

**Treatment.** This disease responds well to treatment. The physician must first differentiate it from other types of anemia. Iron, usually ferrous sulfate, is given orally two or three times a day between meals. Vitamin C aids in the absorption of iron; therefore, giving juice when administering iron is suggested. Therapy should be continued for 4–6 weeks after blood values are normal (Behrman, 1992). Liquid preparations are taken through a straw in order to prevent temporary discoloration of the teeth. (More recently available iron preparations do not have this disadvantage.) An iron-dextran mixture (Imferon) given intramuscularly is also highly effective. It must be injected deep in a large muscle using Z-track technique in order to minimize staining and irritation.

**Parent Education.** Parents need explicit instructions as to the proper foods for the infant. The nurse stresses the importance of breastfeeding for the first 6 months and the use of iron-fortified formula throughout the 1st year of life (the absorption of iron from human milk is much better than that from cow's milk). The amount of milk consumed during the day and night is determined. Consumption of over 1 qt/day is high. This should be limited to a more reasonable quantity, preferably to 1 pt/day or less (Behrman, 1992). The myth that milk is a perfect food should be dispelled. Solid food intake is reviewed and specific iron-enriched nutrients are suggested. The nurse considers financial, ethnic, and family preferences in discussions. Behavior concerns at mealtime may also need to be addressed.

The stools of babies placed on iron are tarry green. Absence of this finding may indicate poor

## Nursing Brief

Avoid iron poisoning in children by keeping preparations well out of reach. Educate parents about this hazard.

compliance with therapy by the parents. Oral iron preparations are not to be given with milk, which interferes with absorption. These preparations should be given between meals when digestive acid concentration is highest, in order to increase absorption. *It is important to emphasize that both dietary changes and supplemental iron therapy are necessary in order to eradicate iron-deficiency anemia.* Dietary changes must be lifelong in order to maintain good health and to prevent recurrence. Iron supplements are given until the prescription expires. Parents are encouraged to return for periodic evaluation of the child's blood status. They are also advised to remind new physicians of the condition, even though it may currently be rectified. During discussions, nurses attempt to support parents, who usually feel guilt or believe they are not successful parents. It may be comforting for the nurse to reiterate that most babies are in the process of "catching up on iron supplies" and that the condition is not uncommon.

Nursing Care Plan 27–1 specifies interventions for the child with iron-deficiency anemia.

| NURSING CARE PLAN 27–1 | | |
| --- | --- | --- |
| **Selected Nursing Diagnoses for the Child with Iron-Deficiency Anemia** | | |
| **Goals** | **Nursing Interventions** | **Rationale** |
| **Nursing Diagnosis:** Knowledge deficit (parents) related to cause and treatment of anemia. | | |
| Parents will verbalize understanding of the importance of dietary factors and iron supplements in the prevention and treatment of this condition | 1. Encourage breast feeding | 1. Absorption of iron from human milk is much better than that from cow's milk |
| Infant will ingest iron-rich formula plus two servings of iron-fortified cereal and iron supplement, if prescribed | 2. Encourage iron-rich formula for full 1st year | 2. Cow's milk contains little iron |
| | 3. Dispel myth that milk is a perfect food | 3. Parents often rely too heavily on milk because it is easier than preparing solid foods, which baby may initially dislike; ingestion of large amounts of milk may interfere with absorption of iron supplements |
| | 4. Give iron supplement between meals with juice | 4. Vitamin C aids in absorption of iron |
| **Nursing Diagnosis:** Altered nutrition: less than body requirements related to iron-poor diet. | | |
| Patient's hemoglobin level will improve with therapy; there will be no recurrence of anemia | 1. Review 24-hr dietary history | 1. Nurse can determine what foods are missing and quantities of food ingested; it can be used as a baseline for teaching |
| | 2. Review height and weight chart | 2. Determines child's status in relation to norms; compares patient's present measurements with former rate of growth and progress |
| | 3. Review solid food intake and suggest iron-rich foods as age-appropriate | 3. Solid foods high in iron need to be increased as age-appropriate (egg yolk, liver, leafy green vegetables, Cream of Wheat, dried fruits, whole-grain bread, iron-fortified cereal) |
| | 4. Educate parents as to how to administer iron supplement | 4. Usually given orally two or three times a day between meals; supplements are easily forgotten because evidence of improvement is slow and signs of disease may not be noticeable; poisoning can result from overdose |
| | 5. Stress importance of compliance with dietary regimen to prevent recurrence | 5. Dietary changes must be lifelong in order to maintain good health |

# Sickle Cell Disease

**Description.** Sickle cell disease is an inherited defect in the formation of hemoglobin. It occurs mainly in African-American populations, but it is also carried by some people of Arabian, Greek, Maltese, Sicilian, and other Mediterranean races. Many researchers believe that the gene for sickle cell anemia arose in these populations as protection against malaria. Sickling due to decreases in blood oxygen may be triggered by dehydration, infection, physical or emotional stress, or exposure to cold. Laboratory examination of the affected child's blood shows that the red blood cell has changed its shape to resemble that of a sickle blade, from which the name of the disorder is derived (Fig. 27–3).

Sickle cells contain an abnormal form of hemoglobin termed *hemoglobin S* (the sickling type). The membranes of these cells are fragile and easily destroyed. Their crescent shape makes it difficult for them to pass through the capillaries, causing a pile-up of cells in the small vessels. This clumping together may lead to a thrombosis (clot) and cause an obstruction.

*Infarcts*, or areas of dead tissue, may result when the tissue is denied proper blood supply. These generally develop in the spleen but may also be seen in other areas of the body, such as the brain, heart, lungs, gastrointestinal tract, kidneys, and bones. The patient feels pain in the affected area.

There are two types of sickle cell disorders: an asymptomatic (*a*, "without," and *symptoma*, "symptom") version, sickle cell trait, and a much more severe form requiring intermittent hospitalization, sickle cell disease.

**Sickle Cell Trait.** This form of the disease occurs in about 10% of the African-American population in the United States. The blood of the patient contains a mixture of normal (hemoglobin A) and sickle (hemoglobin S) hemoglobins. The proportions of hemoglobin S are low, since the disease is inherited from only one parent. The doctor can distinguish sickle cell trait from the more severe disease by studying the patient's red blood cells and hemoglobin. Sickling is more rapid and extreme in the disease. In sickle cell trait, the hemoglobin and red blood cell counts are normal.

Sickle cell trait does not develop into sickle

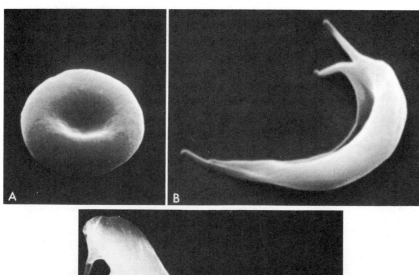
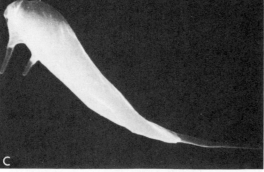

**Figure 27–3.** Scanning electron micrograph of erythrocytes. Comparison of a normal cell (*A*) with deoxygenated sickled cells (*B, C*). (Courtesy of Dr. James White. From Bunn, H.F., Forget, B.G., & Ranney, H.M. [1977]. *Human hemoglobins* [p. 240]. Philadelphia: W.B. Saunders.)

cell disease. Although there is no need for treatment of the patient with sickle cell trait, the patient *is* a carrier, and genetic counseling is important. Advice might be sought from a family physician, pediatrician, or genetic specialist. The nurse encourages and supports such efforts made by parents. The importance of regular visits to a well-child clinic or family-centered clinic is stressed. The nurse can also suggest organizations that help with transportation and baby-sitting problems that so often prevent parents from making maximum use of community facilities.

**Sickle Cell Disease.** This severe form of sickle cell disorder results when the abnormality is inherited from both parents (Fig. 27–4). *Each offspring* has one chance in four of inheriting the disease (not one of four children). The symptoms generally do not appear until the last part of the 1st year of life. There may be an unusual swelling of the fingers and toes. Damage to the kidney leads to increased urination. Patients tend to drink a lot of water. Small children are difficult to toilet train and may wet the bed for several years. When this is explained to parents as a side effect of the disease, they may be more able to accept the problem. Teenagers and adults with sickle cell disease may develop painful, slow-healing ulcers on the lower legs, particularly at the ankles.

There is chronic anemia. The hemoglobin level ranges from 6 to 9 gm/dl or lower. The child is pale, tires easily, and there is a loss of appetite. These manifestations of anemia are complicated by what is termed *sickle cell crises*, which can be fatal. A number of types of crises have been defined. They differ in pathology and

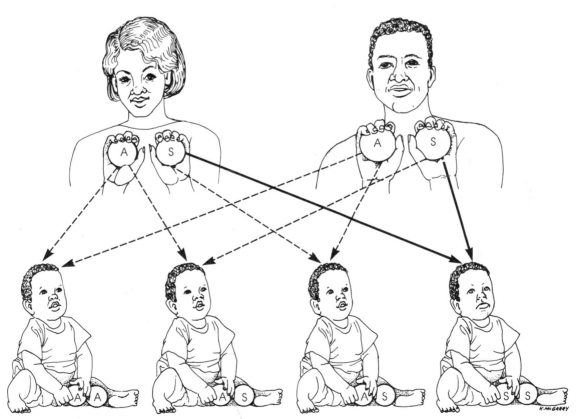

**Figure 27–4.** How sickle cell disease is transmitted from parents to children. Parents who are carriers of the sickle cell trait do not show symptoms of the disease because hemoglobin A (the normal form of hemoglobin) in their red blood cells protects them from hemoglobin S (the sickling form). However, when two carriers become parents, the possibilities are as follows: One child in four will inherit all normal hemoglobin (AA) and thus be free of the disease; two children in four will inherit both hemoglobin A and hemoglobin S and thus become carriers (AS) of the trait, like their parents; and one child in four will inherit all sickling hemoglobin (SS) and thus be affected by sickle cell anemia.

**Table 27–1.** TYPES OF SICKLE CELL CRISES

| Type | Comment |
| --- | --- |
| Vasoocclusive (painful crises) | Most common type, obstruction of blood flow by cells, infarctions, some degree of vasospasm |
| | Dactylitis, painful joints and extremities, abdominal pain (infarction or bleeding within liver, spleen, abdominal lymph node), central nervous system strokes, pulmonary disease, priapism |
| Splenic sequestration | Pooling of large amounts of blood in liver and spleen |
| | Spleen becomes massive |
| | Circulatory collapse, shock |
| | Children between 8 months and 5 years of age particularly susceptible |
| | Death may occur within hours of appearance of symptoms |
| | Minor episodes may resolve spontaneously |
| | Splenectomy may be indicated for children who have one or more severe crises |
| Aplastic crises | Bone marrow stops producing red blood cells, a number of infections may precipitate this (usually viral) |
| Severe anemia | Child may be transfused with fresh packed red cells |
| Hyperhemolytic | Rapid rate of hemolysis superimposed on already severe process, rare |
| Functional hyposplenism and overwhelming infection | Progressive fibrosis of spleen reduces its function, patient becomes more susceptible to infection |

Data from Dickerman, J., & Lucey, J. (1985). *Smith's the critically ill child* (3rd ed.). Philadelphia: W.B. Saunders.

may require somewhat different treatments (Table 27–1). Unfortunately, in some cases the sickle cell crisis is the first evidence of the condition. The patient appears acutely ill. There is severe abdominal pain. Muscle spasms, leg pains, or painful swollen joints may be seen. Fever, vomiting, hematuria, convulsions, stiff neck, coma, or paralysis can result, depending on the organs involved. The patient may be jaundiced. Cardiac enlargement and murmurs are not uncommon.

The sickle cell crises recur periodically throughout childhood; however, they tend to decrease with age. Between episodes, patients should be kept in good health. Immunizations of these children are particularly important. *Haemophilus influenzae* and hepatitis B are indicated. Pneumococcal vaccine may be given, although current forms of the vaccine are less beneficial in children under 5 years with this disease. Prophylactic penicillin G is highly effective in preventing serious pneumonia and should be administered to all children with

## Nursing Brief

During crises, anticipate the child's need for tissue oxygenation, hydration, rest, protection from infection, pain control, blood transfusions, and emotional support for life-threatening illness.

sickle cell disease (Behrman, 1992). Patients should refrain from becoming overly tired. They also should avoid situations such as flying in an unpressurized airplane or exercising at high altitude, because oxygen concentrations are already reduced in their blood. Extra stress and exposure to cold may lower resistance, causing additional problems. Overheating, which can lead to dehydration, is also to be avoided. Oral intake of iron is of no value.

**Treatment and Nursing Care.** When the infant or child is hospitalized during a crisis, the treatment is supportive and symptomatic. The patient is confined to bed. Analgesics are given for the relief of pain. Children in severe pain may need a continuous intravenous infusion containing a narcotic. If the patient has an infection, such as meningitis or pneumonia, antibiotics are given. Every effort is made to combat dehydration and acidosis. Small blood transfusions may be administered in an effort to increase the hemoglobin count, but the results are only temporary. Frequently, packed red blood cells are used for this purpose.

The nurse observes the overall appearance of the patient and assesses the developmental stage, body proportions, and relation of height and weight to age. Facial expressions, degree of restlessness, and areas of pain are noted and recorded. Elevated temperature; rapid, weak pulse; a sunken fontanel in infants younger than 18 months; weight loss; poor tissue turgor; dry skin, lips, and mucous membranes; and decrease in urination signal dehydration. If vomiting occurs, appropriate oral hygiene is given. The nurse observes and records infusions according to unit policy. An accurate record of intake and output is kept. Careful attention is given to the skin. Jaundice (icterus) can be detected by observing whether the skin (palms of the hands and soles of the feet) and whites of the eyes have taken on a yellowish tinge. The patient's body position is changed gently.

Because sickle cell disease can affect muscle tone, any rigidity of muscles should be reported. Eye movements, swallowing, or sucking is observed. The nurse notes if the child is uncomfortable when flexing the neck to have a gown changed. The nurse watches for twitching about the face or elsewhere. Sickle cell disease may take a wide variety of courses. As always, the individual patient's progress is followed. (Pocket-sized index cards containing nursing care plans may be helpful.) The nurse discusses and evaluates the child's progress with the team leader and instructor. The nurse uses the unit library to increase knowledge and effectiveness in order to anticipate problems that might occur in the patient with this disease.

The prognosis is guarded. Death may result from severe anemia or secondary infection. Pregnancy may increase the risk of death. There is also an increased likelihood of miscarriage, premature births, and stillborn infants in women with sickle cell disease. Ideally, all African-American women should be screened for the disease prior to pregnancy. Prenatal diagnosis is possible through amniocentesis. The sickling test (Sickledex) is commonly used for screening. When the result is positive, hemoglobin electrophoresis ("fingerprinting") is employed. This procedure separates and records the various peptide patterns of the blood. It distinguishes between patients with the trait and those with the disease (Whaley & Wong, 1991).

**Surgery.** The approach to splenectomy in children with sickle cell disease has been conservative. Recurrence of acute splenic sequestration becomes less likely after 5 years of age. Routine splenectomy is not recommended, as the spleen generally atrophies on its own because of fibrotic changes that take place in patients with sickle cell disease. However, splenectomy is indicated in selected patients. Because no form of prophylaxis is foolproof and since the duration of treatment is controversial, the child should continue to be carefully supervised for signs of infection. A sickle screening test should be performed on all African-American patients prior to elective surgery, as general anesthesia places these persons at greater risk for hypoxia. It is sometimes difficult to distinguish abdominal crises from appendicitis or peritonitis.

# Hemophilia

**Description.** Hemophilia is one of the oldest hereditary diseases known to humanity. In this disorder, the blood does not clot normally, and even the slightest injury can cause severe bleeding. It has been called the disease of kings because it has occurred in children of several royal families in Russia and Europe. This congenital disorder is confined almost exclusively to males but is transmitted by symptom-free females. Hemophilia is inherited as a sex-linked recessive trait. It is termed "sex-linked" because the defective gene is located on the X, or female, chromosome. Different combinations of genes account for the fact that some children inherit the disease, some become carriers, and others neither inherit nor carry the trait. New mutations do occur, and the reason for this is unclear. The sex of the fetus can be determined by amniocentesis. Fetal blood sampling detects hemophilia. Some carrier women can also be identified.

There are several types of hemophilia. For our purposes, this discussion is limited to classic hemophilia, or hemophilia A, which accounts for about 84% of cases. The incidence of hemophilia A is about 1 in 10,000 persons. The mechanism of blood formation is complex. Defects in the synthesis of protein may lead to deficiencies in any of the factors in blood plasma needed for clotting to occur. The various clotting factors in blood are numbered. The treatment of each type consists of replacing the deficient factor as it is isolated. The approaches to nursing care for all types are similar.

Hemophilia A is due to a deficiency of coagulation Factor VIII, or antihemophilic globulin (AHG). The severity of the disease depends on the level of Factor VIII in the plasma of the patient's blood. Some patient's lives are endangered by minor injury, whereas a child with a mild case of hemophilia might just bruise a little more easily than the normal person. The degree of severity tends to remain constant within a given family. The aim of therapy is to increase the level of Factor VIII in order to ensure clotting. It is possible to determine the level of Factor VIII in the blood by means of a test called the *partial thromboplastin time* (PTT). This aids in the diagnosis and assessment of the child's condition.

**Manifestations.** Hemophilia can be diagnosed at birth because maternal factor VIII is not transferred to the fetus. It is usually not apparent in the newborn unless abnormal bleeding occurs at the umbilical cord or following circumcision. As the child grows older and becomes more subject to injury, it is found that the slightest bruise or cut can induce extensive bleeding. Normal blood clots in about 3–6 minutes. In a patient with severe hemophilia, the time required for clotting may extend for 1 hour or longer. Anemia, leukocytosis, and a moderate increase in platelets may be seen in the hemorrhaging child. There may also be signs of *shock*. Spontaneous hematuria is seen. Death can result from excessive bleeding anywhere in the body, but particularly when hemorrhage into the brain or neck occurs. Severe headache, vomiting, and disorientation may reflect cranial bleeds. Bleeding into the neck can cause airway obstruction. Bleeding into the ears and eyes can affect hearing and vision. Bleeding into the spinal column can instigate paralysis.

The circumstances leading to diagnosis may be the inability of a parent to stop a child's bleeding from a cut about the mouth or gums. A deciduous tooth loss may precipitate problems in an unknown bleeder. Hematomas may develop following immunization. An injured knee, elbow, or ankle presents particular problems for this patient. Hemorrhage into the joint cavity, or hemarthrosis (*hema*, "blood," *arthron*, "joint," and *osis*, "condition of"), is considered a classic symptom of hemophilia. The effusion (*ex*, "out," and *fundere*, "to pour") into the joint is very painful because of the pressure build-up. Repeated hemorrhages may cause permanent deformities that could incapacitate the child. This deformity is sometimes referred to as an ankylosis (*ankyle*, "stiff joint," and *osis*, "condition of").

**Treatment.** The principal therapy for hemophilia is to prevent bleeding by replacing the missing factor. Currently this can be accomplished only by the use of fresh-frozen plasma or plasma concentrates. The clotting power of the blood is contained in its plasma, or liquid portion. This can be preserved by freezing. When fresh-frozen plasma came into use, it was considered a milestone for hemophiliacs.

Nevertheless, these transfusions present problems in that each unit contains little concentrate, which is not active in the body for more than a few days. Repeated transfusions create the risks of overloading the circulatory system, allergic reaction, acquired immunodeficiency syndrome (AIDS), and hepatitis.

In the 1960s, the development of plasma concentrates brightened the outlook for hemophiliacs. Several Factor VIII concentrates are now available. Because they are made from blood products, they are expensive. The most inexpensive, cryoprecipitate, can be prepared from single blood donors in the blood bank. It is then frozen. Patients or their parents are taught how to administer the prescribed concentrate so that treatment can be done at home. One of the major concerns in factor replacement is the risk of hepatitis and AIDS. All blood donors are now tested for blood-borne viruses, and all blood products are tested for hepatitis and human immunodeficiency virus (HIV). Heat treatments and pasteurization of blood products guard against the transmission of the virus that leads to AIDS. Children who receive the factor should be given hepatitis B vaccine. A new Factor VIII preparation made with recombinant deoxyribonucleic acid (DNA) is under investigation (Eckert, 1990). It is not derived from human blood, and researchers hope it will eliminate the risk of hepatitis and AIDS for this population.

**Nursing Care.** The most important factor in caring for the child with hemophilia is control of active bleeding episodes. This is accomplished by administering the missing factor and attending to the bleed. The longer a wound bleeds, the more damage is done. The child or parents can sometimes sense when a bleed is occurring. The patient may be restless and pale or may experience warmth in an area. An open wound is immediately treated by the application of cold, which causes vasoconstriction, and pressure. When possible, the bleeding area is elevated above heart level in order to decrease blood flow. Nosebleeds can often be controlled by application of pressure. However, nasal packing may also be required. The child is kept quiet to reduce the pulse until the bleed is stopped. Dental bleeds may need to be packed with epinephrine. Aminocaproic acid (Amicar), an antifibrinolytic agent, is specific for bleeding episodes of the mouth.

*Hemarthrosis* (bleeding into a joint) is common and may be disabling. It occurs most often in the elbows, knees, and ankles. When an injury does occur, the missing factor is given and ice packs are applied before the patient leaves for the hospital. The patient in pain may require sedation by the physician. Initially, immobilization of the area is needed to prevent contractures and further trauma to the bones and joints. A bivalve plaster cast may be used for this purpose. It provides support while allowing some movement. When the bleeding has ceased, the cast is removed and passive exercises are performed to prevent stiffness. When repositioning is required, the nurse must turn the patient gently and carefully. Even with the best of care, mobility of the joint may be impaired.

The nurse teaches the family how to care for the child without being overprotective. When the patient with hemophilia is an infant, the crib sides require padding, and all toys must be checked for sharp edges. It may be necessary for the toddler to wear a helmet, elbow protection, or knee pads. Floors should be carpeted and a fenced-in lawn area provided as feasible. Car seats are routinely utilized. Parents are instructed to observe the skin carefully at bath time for bruises or hematomas. The patient's nails are kept short.

Good oral hygiene is essential. The child's toothbrush should have soft bristles and should be wet before use. The dentist needs to be aware of the disease and how to handle bleeding should it occur. Parents consult the dentist early in the child's preschool years in order to establish a program of preventive therapy. The child requires well-balanced meals. Utensils and containers should be unbreakable. Excessive weight is to be avoided because it places additional strain on the joints. Exercise is healthy for this reason and because strong muscles help protect the joints from bleeding. Swimming, quiet ball games, golf, and bowling are some less traumatic activities. Skiing and tennis are not recommended because of the stress on the knees and ankles.

If the child is receiving medication by injection or if blood work has been ordered, the site is carefully observed in order to ensure that there is no bleeding. The patient's stools and urine are observed for blood. Patients with hemophilia are taught to avoid salicylates, antihistamines, and other drugs that interfere with platelet function. They are instructed to wear a Medic-Alert bracelet. They need to carry a supply of factor concentrate and infusion equipment when traveling.

Home-care programs are the treatment of choice. This greatly reduces the cost of treatment and decreases the risk of psychological trauma. Teaching is done by the physician and nurse in the clinic. Regional treatment centers are also becoming more numerous. Instruction includes an exact explanation of the illness, with emphasis on the signs and treatment of hemorrhage. Specific procedures include the storage and preparation of replacement factors, venipuncture, education about transfusion management and transfusion reactions, and record-keeping. Signs of complications are reviewed, and emergency numbers and other protocols are spelled out. Close supervision and support are maintained by a community nurse and the local physician.

Families require support for this lifelong disorder. It is difficult for parents not to be overprotective of these children. Children may resent being unable to participate in athletic activities with peers or may attempt to conceal their problem from others. Schooling is frequently interrupted, which makes it difficult to develop and maintain friendships. The struggle to protect them and still foster independence and a sense of autonomy may seem monumental. Allowing children to participate in decision-making about their care and focusing on their strengths are helpful.

Parent groups and professional counseling may provide support to enable children and parents to develop a healthy attitude toward the condition. Organizations that may be helpful are the National Hemophiliac Foundation and the American Red Cross. Genetic counseling and family planning services should be offered to the family and the adolescent. If an orthopedic deformity develops, surgery, braces, crutches, or other devices may be necessary. This is a drain on the family's finances, and avenues for financial assistance should be explored. Bleeding episodes tend to run in cycles and sometimes surface after the child has been under stress.

## Nursing Brief

Instruct parents of the hemophilic child to avoid administration of medications that inhibit platelet function, for example, aspirin. Explain the importance of contacting their physician or pharmacist before giving any over-the-counter drugs to the child.

# Idiopathic (Immunologic) Thrombocytopenic Purpura

**Description.** Idiopathic (immunologic) thrombocytopenic purpura (ITP) is an acquired platelet disorder that occurs in childhood. It is the most common of the purpuras, a group of disorders affecting the numbers of platelets or their function. The cause is unknown, but it is thought to be an autoimmune system reaction to a virus. Platelets become coated with antiplatelet antibody, are "perceived" as foreign material, and are eventually destroyed by the spleen. ITP occurs in all age groups, with the main incidence seen below the age of 8 years.

**Manifestations.** The classic symptoms of this disease include being easily bruised, which results in petechiae (pinpoint hemorrhagic spots beneath the skin) and purpura (hemorrhage into the skin). About 30% of the patients also have nosebleeds. There may have been a recent history of rubella, rubeola, or viral respiratory infection. The interval between infection and onset is about 2 weeks. The platelet count is reduced below 20,000/mm$^3$ (normals range between 150,000 and 400,000/mm$^3$). There is a preponderance of large platelets. Diagnosis is confirmed by bone marrow aspiration. This rules out leukemia. The bruises of ITP must be distinguished from those of child abuse.

**Treatment and Nursing Care.** Treatment is not indicated in most cases of ITP. Spontaneous remission occurs in about 6 weeks to 4 months. A few children go on to have chronic ITP. Drugs that interfere with platelet function should be avoided to prevent bleeding. These include aspirin, phenylbutazone (Butazolidin), and phenacetin, an ingredient of acetylsalicylic acid, phenacetin, and caffeine (APC). Activity is limited during the acute stage in order to avoid bruises from falls and trauma. Nursing considerations for the more acutely ill child focus on observing the patient for signs of bleeding. When there has been a large amount of blood loss, packed red blood cells may be administered. Platelets are usually not given because they are destroyed by the disease process. Steroids such as prednisone may be prescribed. Intravenous gamma globulin may be used to elevate platelet counts. Complications of ITP include bleeding from the gastrointestinal tract, hemarthrosis, and intracranial hemorrhage. Mortality in childhood ITP is less than 1%. All children need to be immunized against the viral diseases of childhood to prevent this complication.

# The Leukemias

**Description.** Leukemia (*leuko*, "white," and *emia*, "blood") is a malignant disease of the blood-forming organs of the body that results in an uncontrolled growth of immature white blood cells. The immature cells are termed *blasts*, or stem cells. This term comes from the Greek *blastos*, meaning "germ" or "formative cell." The nurse may see the terms lymphoblasts or myeloblasts referred to in descriptive histories. Leukemia is the most common form of childhood cancer. In the past it was considered fatal; however, the prognosis has improved greatly with modern treatments and medication.

In leukemia the white blood cell count fluctuates from 5000–10,000 to as high as 100,000 cells/mm$^3$. In some cases, the overall white blood cell count is normal, but the differential count may show a predominance of blast cells. Some cells are produced in the red marrow of the bone; others are produced in the spleen and lymph nodes. Except for differentiation, the following discussion refers to acute lymphocytic leukemia (ALL), which affects the body's lymphocytes as the name implies.

The classification of childhood leukemias has helped identify various prognostic factors and methods of treatment. Various subtypes are recognized on the basis of cell membrane markers and the reaction of body cells to different chemical agents. This science is termed *cytochemistry*. Two forms of leukemia in children are the *acute lymphocytic leukemias (ALL)*, which account for about 76% of childhood cases (Table 27–2), and the *acute nonlymphocytic (myelogenous) leukemia (ANLL or AML)*, which are less prevalent. The French, American, and British Working Group has also devised a classification based on the appearance of bone marrow leukemia cells at diagnosis. Three cytologic types have been identified. These are L1, L2, and L3. The L stands for lymphoblasts. In L1, the cells are relatively small and uniform. This type is associated with a good prognosis. L2 is associated with an intermediate prognosis, and L3 with a poor prognosis. L3 types are seen more frequently in adults.

Cellular destruction is by direct infiltration and competition for metabolic elements. The

**Table 27–2.** PROGNOSTIC FEATURES OF ACUTE LYMPHOCYTIC LEUKEMIA IN CHILDREN

| Factor | Favorable | Less Favorable |
|---|---|---|
| Age | 3–7 yr | <2 yr and >10 yr |
| Race | Caucasian | African American |
| Sex | Female | Male |
| Initial white blood cell count | <20,000/mm$^3$ | >50,000/mm$^3$ |
| Mediastinal mass | No | Yes |
| T-cell markers on lymphocytes | No | Yes |
| Morphology—lymphocyte type | L1 | L2, L3 |
| Central nervous system involvement (at diagnosis) | No | Yes |
| Massive adenopathy | No | Yes |
| Massive enlargement of liver and spleen | No | Yes |
| Early diagnosis | Yes | No |
| Length of first remission | Long | Short |

liver, spleen, and lymph glands are the organs most directly involved. The incidence of leukemia is highest between 3 and 4 years of age, and it occurs more commonly in boys than in girls. The cause of this disease is unknown. Current research on the relationship of viruses to leukemia is well under way. There seems to be a genetic correlation, as the incidence of leukemia is higher in children with Down syndrome and in twins. Investigators have associated leukemia with disorders of the immune mechanisms of the body.

All tissues of the body are affected, either by direct infiltration of cancer cells or by the change in the blood that is carried to them. There is a reduction in the number of red blood cells, which produces anemia. The platelet count is also reduced, and since platelets are essential for the clotting of blood, hemorrhage occurs. Intracranial bleeding is a common, immediate cause of death. Hemorrhage from other vital organs may occur. As cancer cells invade the bone marrow, bone and joint pain is experienced. Physiologic fractures may occur. Leukemia that occurs outside the bone marrow is referred to as *extramedullary* (*extra*, "outside," and *medulla*, "marrow"). The most common sites for this are the central nervous system (CNS) and the testicles. Increased evidence of extramedullary leukemia is being seen because children with this disorder are surviving longer.

**Manifestations.** The most common symptoms during the initial phase of the illness are low-grade fever, pallor, tendency to bruise, leg and joint pain, listlessness, abdominal pain, and enlargement of lymph nodes. These symptoms may develop gradually or may be sudden in onset. As the disease progresses, the liver and spleen become enlarged. The skin may be an unusual lemon-yellow. *Petechiae* and *purpura* may be early objective symptoms. Anorexia, vomiting, weight loss, and dyspnea are also common. The kidneys and testicles may enlarge, and the patient may develop hematuria.

Because the white blood cells are not functioning normally, bacteria easily invade the body. Ulcerations develop about the mucous membranes of the mouth and anal regions and have a tendency to bleed (Fig. 27–5). Anemia becomes severe despite transfusions. The child may die as a direct result of the disease or from secondary infection. The symptoms are the same regardless of the type of white blood cell affected, and they vary widely with each patient, depending on the parts of the body involved.

**Diagnosis.** The diagnosis of leukemia is based on the history and symptoms of the patient and the results of extensive blood tests that demon-

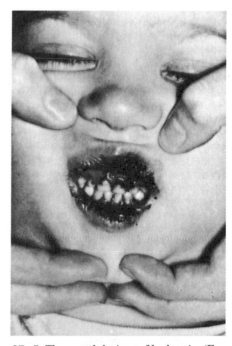

**Figure 27–5.** The mouth lesions of leukemia. (From Blake, F., Wright, F., and Waechter, E. [1970] *Nursing care of children* [8th ed.]. Philadelphia: J.B. Lippincott.)

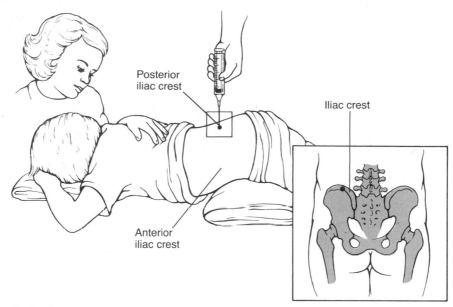

**Figure 27–6.** Bone marrow aspiration. Because many white and red blood cells are formed in the bone marrow, a bone marrow aspiration can determine the type and quantity of cells present and help rule out or confirm a serious disease.

strate the presence of leukemic blast cells in the blood, bone marrow, or other tissues. Because the bone marrow is where many white and red blood cells are formed, a bone marrow aspiration is commonly performed. A piece of the marrow of the bone is removed from the sternum or, more often in children, the iliac crest. A special needle is used and the marrow is studied in the laboratory (Fig. 27–6). X-ray films of the long bones show changes in the bones. After the diagnosis has been confirmed, a spinal tap determines CNS involvement. Kidney and liver function studies are also performed, because normal function of these organs is absolutely necessary for chemotherapy to be used in treating the disease.

**Treatment.** The development of specific chemotherapeutic agents for acute leukemia has significantly changed the survival time. In most cases of ALL, it is now possible to induce remissions that may be maintained for prolonged periods (longer than 3 years). There is mounting optimism that some patients may never relapse and that the chemotherapy may thus represent a complete cure. Other acute varieties show a less predictable response to therapy. Untreated leukemia results in death from infection or hemorrhage in about 6 months. Components of therapy include (1) an induction period, (2) CNS prophylaxis for high-risk patients, (3) maintenance, (4) reinduction therapy

(if relapse occurs), and (5) extra-medullary disease therapy.

The list of medications for treatment of this disease is growing. A combination of drugs used to induce remissions includes prednisone, vincristine sulfate, and daunorubicin or L-asparaginase. They work within 4–6 weeks in about 95% of children with ALL. The therapeutic effects of these drugs are of short duration, however, so it is necessary to use additional drugs that help maintain the remissions. The steroid prednisone has the side effects of masking the symptoms of infection, increasing fluid retention, inducing personality changes, and causing the child's face to appear moon-shaped. Methotrexate and 6-mercaptopurine are useful in maintaining remissions because they act against chemicals vital to the life of the white blood cell. These powerful medications produce side effects of varying degrees, such as nausea, diarrhea, rash, hair loss (alopecia), fever, anuria, anemia, and bone marrow depression. Peripheral neuropathy may be signaled by severe constipation due to decreased nerve supply to the bowel. Footdrop and difficulty with coordination may be seen. These complications are reversed once the offending drug is discontinued. The nurse should consult a pharmacology text for information about the particular drugs used for the patient in order to anticipate potential problems.

The various drugs used in treating leukemia may be given in cycles. Antibiotics are administered to prevent or control infection, and transfusions of whole blood or packed cells are given to correct anemia. Sedatives necessary for the patient's comfort are also administered. A pain reliever, such as oxycodone/aspirin (Percodan), codeine, meperidine hydrochloride (Demerol), acetaminophen, or morphine, may be ordered. Medications are administered before pain becomes too severe. Radiation therapy of the cranium is no longer administered routinely. Intrathecal chemotherapy may be utilized for central nervous system prophylaxis.

**Bone Marrow Transplants and Immunotherapy.** In recent years, patients with ALL who are in second remission have been treated by bone marrow transplant. The overall number of these patients is small, and the follow-up period is shorter than that for patients with ANLL who have been treated by this method. Patients treated by bone marrow transplants are often those considered to be at high risk for relapse. The purpose is to provide the child with healthy bone marrow that can produce normal blood cells. A number of problems in the use of this procedure remain unsolved.

Immunotherapy, although still in the research stages, is another area of therapeutics. Immunotherapy may be passive or active, specific or nonspecific. The main objective of treatment is to strengthen the patient's immune response to cancer cells and to attempt to prevent cancer by immunization.

**Nursing Care.** The child suffering from acute leukemia has many needs, both physical and psychological. They vary in intensity according to exacerbation and progression of the disease. The diagnosis has such an impact on the patient's family that they are unable to focus on anything other than the child and the illness. Suppression of their own needs mounts if the disease is prolonged, and this can lead to illness and broken marriages. Support groups such as those provided in Ronald McDonald Houses and various hospice programs aid parents in expressing and examining their concerns and give the child and family freedom to hurt but remain whole.

Children's anxiety often centers on their symptoms. They fear that the treatments necessary to correct their problems may be painful, as indeed some are, for example, venipunctures, bone marrow aspirations, and blood transfusions. Their trust in others is in a precarious balance. Nurses must inform children of what they are about to do and why it is necessary. The explanation is given in terms the patient will understand.

The child may ask the nurse the inevitable question, "Am I going to die?" One suggestion is to reply with a question, such as "Why do you ask that? Do you feel sick today?" This may encourage the child to verbalize feelings. The pediatric nurse who gives patients permission to discuss their concerns will find opportunities to clear up misconceptions and decrease children's feelings of isolation. Hope is conveyed because it is indispensable to continued functioning, although the nature of hope may change from that of cure to additional time to live. Further information on the holistic care of the dying child is presented in Chapter 34. The following discussion focuses on the intense physical care necessary for the child with leukemia.

**Remission Induction Period.** On diagnosis of leukemia, induction therapy is begun (Box 27–1). The goal is to reduce the number of leukemia cells and preferably to eradicate them. Careful explanations are given to the child and the family before any procedure is instituted. The disease and many of the necessary medications cause myelosuppression (*myelo*, "marrow," and *suppression*), which depresses the normal function of the bone marrow and destroys cancer cells. The patient becomes anemic, may hemorrhage, and is highly susceptible to infection (even from harmless environmental flora).

**Preventing Infection.** Some of the organisms that may be hazardous to the child with leukemia are listed in Table 27–3. The choice of medication used to combat these infections varies according to the physician's protocol and the causative organism. When fever occurs, broad-spectrum antibiotics are begun until the offending agent is identified. Trimethoprim (Proloprim or Trimpex) is helpful in preventing urinary tract infection (UTI). Sulfamethoxazole (Septra or Bactrim) are administered to prevent the development of *Pneumocystis carinii* pneumonia, which is life-threatening. White blood cell transfusions may also be used. Laminar-flow patient isolation rooms are available in some centers. They provide a protective environment for the highly susceptible patient.

In most hospitals, patients are placed in a private room. Reverse isolation may be instituted. The nurse limits visitors and any auxil-

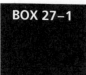

**An Effective Treatment Regimen for Standard-Risk Acute Lymphocytic Leukemia**

**Remission Induction (4–6 Weeks)**

Vincristine 1.5 mg/m² (max 2 mg) IV/wk
Prednisone 40 mg/m² (max 60 mg)/day by mouth
Asparaginase (*Escherichia coli*) 10,000 U/m²/day
   biweekly IM

**Intrathecal Treatment**

Triple therapy: Methotrexate*
             Hydrocortisone*
             Cytosine arabinoside*
             Weekly × 6 during induction, and
               then every 8 wk for 3 yr

**Systemic Continuation Treatment**

6-Mercaptopurine 50 mg/m²/day by mouth
Methotrexate 20 mg/m²/wk by mouth

**With Reinforcement**

Vincristine 1.5 mg/m² (max 2 mg) IV every 8 wk
Prednisone 40 mg/m²/day by mouth × 28 days every
   16 wk

---

*The dose of intrathecal medication is age-adjusted.
IV, intravenous; IM, intramuscular; max, maximum.
From Behrman, R.E. (1992). *Nelson textbook of pediatrics* (14th ed.). Philadelphia: W.B. Saunders.

iary or medical personnel who appear unhealthy. All persons must adhere to meticulous handwashing techniques. Teaching parents concurrently helps prepare them for home care,

**Table 27–3.** INFECTIOUS AGENTS HAZARDOUS TO THE CHILD WITH LEUKEMIA

| Type | Organism |
|------|----------|
| Bacterial | *Pseudomonas, Escherichia coli, Staphylococcus aureus, Klebsiella, Proteus* |
| Viral | Cytomegalovirus, varicella zoster (chickenpox) |
| Protozoan | *Pneumocystis carinii* |
| Fungal | *Candida albicans, Histoplasma* |

*Note:* Overwhelming infection can lead to death in children with leukemia. The possibility of infection is high during induction therapy, immediately following radiation therapy, and during maintenance.

that is, protecting the patient from children with communicable diseases, handwashing, and so on. The nurse explains to the child the purpose of the various procedures utilized.

The patient is frequently observed for signs of infection. Particular attention is paid to potential infected sites, such as the patient's mucous membranes and puncture breaks in the skin from laboratory or therapeutic procedures. Pierced ears are observed for inflammation. Vital signs are observed for subtle variances, as steroid therapy may mask these indicators. The patient is turned often and observed for skin breakdown, particularly in the perianal area. Nutritious meals and supplemental feedings that are high in protein and calories are offered. Parents and the child are taught what to look for and report. Chickenpox and other communicable diseases are a particular hazard to the child approaching school age. *Varicella zoster immune globulin* may lessen the severity of the disease on exposure. Open communication among the school nurse, family, clinic nurse, and physician is paramount.

**Hemorrhage.** Thrombocytopenic bleeding is a frequent complication of leukemia. The nurse observes the patient's skin for petechiae and ecchymosis. Nosebleeds are common and are treated by application of cold and pressure.

The mouth is inspected daily for ulcerations and hemorrhage from the gums. It may be rinsed with a prescribed solution. Commercial mouthwashes are used with caution because they may alter normal flora and may cause fungal overgrowth. A Water-Pik is helpful in massaging and toughening the gums. If the child is comatose, mouth-care supplies are kept at the bedside. A soft sponge toothbrush is helpful. The nurse may also clean food particles from the patient's teeth with a piece of gauze wrapped around the finger. Petroleum jelly or cold cream is applied to dry, cracked lips.

Hemorrhagic cystitis is not uncommon because some drugs irritate the mucosa of the bladder. The nurse is alert to complaints of burning on urination or feelings of pressure,

## Nursing Brief

Bleeding from the nose or mouth may be evidenced by a soiled pillowcase or sheet.

# Nursing Brief

If a blood transfusion reaction occurs, stop the infusion, keep vein open with normal saline solution, and notify charge nurse. Take patient's vital signs and observe closely.

---

which may indicate infection. Attention is given to providing plenty of fluids and encouraging frequent voiding. The physician is notified of complications immediately so that medications can be properly adjusted.

The nurse observes the patient for gastrointestinal bleeding. This is evidenced by hematemesis (*hema*, "blood," and *emesis*, "vomiting") and bloody or tarry stools. Hemarthrosis (*hema*, "blood," *arthron*, "joint," and *osis*, "condition of") may develop. This makes moving about painful; therefore, nursing intervention is necessary for the comfort of the patient when in or out of bed. The nurse manipulates catheters and suction drainage gently in order to avoid irritation of the sensitive mucosa. Scanning the patient's unit for environmental hazards is also important. Emergency procedures for control of bleeding are reviewed.

**Transfusions.** Platelets and packed red blood cells may be given to the patient. If student nurses are asked to assume responsibility for the leukemic child receiving a blood transfusion, they request explicit directions from the team leader or charge nurse. Hemolytic reactions caused by mismatched blood are rare. Nevertheless, the registered nurse should positively identify donor and recipient blood types and groups on labels and the patient's chart with another professional. Blood is infused through a blood filter to avoid impurities. Medications are *never* added to blood. Blood is administered *slowly*. The intravenous site is frequently checked for infiltration. The patient is observed for *signs of transfusion reaction*, which include chills, itching, rash, fever, headache, dyspnea, and pain in the back or elsewhere. If such a reaction occurs, the student nurse stops the infusion, keeps the line open with normal saline solution, and immediately notifies the nurse in charge. The nurse *does not* remove the needle unless specifically instructed to do so. Subsequently voided urine is saved for hemoglobin determination.

Transfusions with piggyback set-ups are com-mon. Blood and normal saline or other suitable intravenous solutions are connected by a stopcock. When blood must be stopped, tube patency can be maintained by opening the saline line. Necessary emergency medications can thus be administered, and the vein is preserved for future infusions. An *autosyringe* may be used to administer small amounts of blood. The line is flushed with normal saline before and after instillation.

Circulatory overload is always a danger with children. *An infusion pump is routinely used to regulate blood flow.* Dyspnea, precordial pain, rales, cyanosis, dry cough, and distended neck veins are indicative of this complication. Apprehension can also be a warning signal of air emboli or electrolyte disturbance. The nurse must maintain a high level of alertness for such signs, particularly in children whose conditions warrant repeated transfusions. If a reaction occurs, the blood bag and tubing are saved and returned to the blood bank. Most transfusion reactions occur within the first 10 minutes of administration; nevertheless, the patient is carefully monitored throughout this treatment. Diphenhydramine (Benadryl) may be ordered for allergic reactions. Aminophylline may be ordered for wheezing. Oxygen may be necessary to relieve dyspnea and cyanosis. Blood transfusions administered through central lines must be warmed in order to prevent cardiac arrhythmias. Establish baseline data (temperature, pulse, respiration, and blood pressure) before transfusion and monitor for changes. It is helpful if the parents remain with the child during this time. Suitable diversions minimize boredom.

**Skin and Hair Care.** The skin is bathed daily and whenever necessary. The nurse observes thoroughly for petechiae and bruising. Careful attention is given to the rectal mucosa, which is observed for fissures and ulcerations. The skin is cleansed well after each bowel movement. Use of a rectal thermometer is avoided. Stool softeners may be necessary for relief of constipation, which frequently accompanies chemotherapy. Sitz baths promote relaxation and may lessen discomfort. Dry heat promotes healing.

The child's hair is combed daily and whenever necessary. Hair loss due to drug therapy is not unusual. Psychological preparation of the child and family lessens the impact of hair loss. Hair will return in a period of time, and meanwhile a wig suitable to the child's preference and age may be worn. If this is not acceptable, a cap must be worn during cold weather.

**Positioning the Patient.** Repositioning of the patient is necessary in order to promote circulation and avoid pressure sores. Bone pain can be acute, and whenever possible, coordinating administration of pain relievers with posture change is helpful. The patient is handled gently. A beanbag chair, a water bed, or a flotation mattress may be employed for comfort. A footboard is used in case of footdrop due to peripheral neuropathy.

**Nutrition.** The patient is served well-balanced meals consisting of preferred foods. Because food may not be appealing to the child with leukemia, the individual nurse must use ingenuity to interest the patient. Mealtimes are kept pleasant. The companionship of a nurse or attendant is preferable. The nurse notes individual preferences and reports them to the dietitian. Food from home may be relished. When the child is too tired or irritable to eat, food is also offered between meals. When parents understand this, they are less anxious about what the child consumes at a particular meal. Steroid therapy often increases appetite, which is heartening but temporary. High-calorie commercial foods are tasty and can be used as an adjunct. A low-sodium diet may help reduce the side effects of steroids.

Small amounts of fluid are offered frequently. If the nurse places the fingers over the end of a drinking tube after it is in a glass of water, a suction can be created that holds the water in the tube until it is placed in the child's mouth. Removing the finger allows the water to flow out of the tube. In this way, the listless child can be given fluids. When parenteral fluids are given, they must be carefully observed (see p. 594). A record is kept of all fluid intake and output.

## Hodgkin's Disease

**Description.** Hodgkin's disease is a malignancy of the lymph system that primarily involves the lymph nodes. It may metastasize to the spleen, liver, bone marrow, lungs, or other parts of the body. The cell predominantly affected is the Reed-Sternberg cell, which contains two nuclei and is diagnostic of the disease (Fig. 27–7). Hodgkin's disease is rarely seen be-

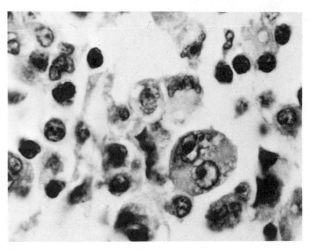

**Figure 27–7.** A Reed-Sternberg cell that contains two nuclei. This appearance in a lymph node is diagnostic of Hodgkin's disease. (From Behrman, R., & Kliegman, R. [1992]. *Nelson's textbook of pediatrics* [14th ed.]. Philadelphia: W.B. Saunders.)

fore 5 years of age, but the incidence increases during adolescence and early adulthood. It is twice as common in boys as in girls.

**Manifestations.** The presenting symptom of Hodgkin's disease is generally a painless lump along the neck. It occurs in older children and adolescents who are past the age at which infections in this area are more common. Occasionally, nodes of the supraclavicular, axillary, and inguinal areas are primary sites. Characteristically, there are few other manifestations. Generally the swelling is first noted by the patient or parents. In more advanced cases, there may be low-grade fever, anorexia, weight loss, night sweats, general malaise, rash, and itching of the skin. Blood counts may be nonspecific. Diagnosis is confirmed by x-ray films, body scan, and lymphangiogram. A laparotomy may be performed in order to determine the stage of the disease. At this time, the spleen may be removed, and biopsies of the liver, accessible nodes, and bone marrow are performed. The stages of Hodgkin's disease are defined in Table 27–4.

**Treatment.** Well-established treatment regimens are now being utilized to combat this illness. Both radiation therapy and chemotherapy are used in accordance with the clinical stage of the disease. The combination of nitrogen mustard, vincristine sulfate (Oncovin), procarbazine hydrochloride, and prednisone is a common pro-

**Table 27–4.** CRITERIA FOR STAGING OF HODGKIN'S DISEASE

| Stage | Criteria |
|-------|----------|
| I | Disease restricted to single site or localized in a group of lymph nodes; asymptomatic |
| II | Two or more lymph nodes in the area or on the same side of the diaphragm |
| III | Involves lymph node regions on both sides of the diaphragm, involves adjacent organ or spleen |
| IV | Diffuse disease, least favorable prognosis |

tocol. It is referred to as the MOPP regimen. Another drug combination currently being used is Adriamycin (doxorubicin hydrochloride), bleomycin, vinblastine sulfate, and dacarbazine (ABVD). The prognosis for remission is favorable. Cure is primarily related to the stage of the disease at diagnosis.

**Nursing Care.** Nursing care is mainly directed toward the symptomatic relief of the side effects of radiation therapy and chemotherapy. Education of the patient and family is paramount, as most patients are cared for in the home. A common side effect of radiation is malaise. The teenager tires easily and may be irritable and anorectic. The skin in the treated area may be sensitive and is protected against exposure to sunlight and irritation. During treatment the skin should not be exposed to sunlight. After treatment a sun-blocking agent containing paraaminobenzoic acid (PABA) should be used to prevent burning. The attending physician may prescribe an ointment to relieve itching of the skin. Nothing should be applied to the treatment area without the recommendation of the physician. There may be diarrhea after abdominal irradiation. The patient *does not* become radioactive during or after therapy.

Following splenectomy, the patient faces the long-term risk of serious infection. This risk is explained to the parents and teenager. Elevations of temperature need to be monitored carefully. There may also be infection with little or no fever as a result of masking by certain medications. In such cases, cultures of blood, urine, sputum, or stool may need to be taken. Parents or the adolescent is instructed to feel free to call the clinic, particularly if there is a change in the condition or apprehension or confusion about symptoms. Medication readjustments should not be attempted unless specifically advised by the physician. Emo-

tional support of the teenager is age-appropriate. Nurses must particularly be prepared for periods of anger, which may be directed at them. Suitable outlets, such as the use of a punching bag, allow for safe direction of anger. Routine use helps prevent a build-up of tension. Activity in general is regulated by the patient. The physician advises the patient if special precautions are necessary.

The appearance of secondary sexual characteristics and menstruation may be delayed in pubescent patients. This can be a source of anxiety. The nurse respects the patient concerns and can be most effective by listening empathetically. Sterility may result as a side effect of MOPP therapy in adolescent boys. Irradiation of the ovaries may induce sterility or early menopause in teenage girls and young women. "Girls who have had their ovaries repositioned prior to radiation may have no effect from the therapy" (Pillitteri, 1992).

# Infectious Mononucleosis

**Description.** Infectious mononucleosis is a global disease caused by a herpes-type Epstein-Barr virus (EBV). It occurs at almost all ages but is chiefly found in older children and adults, its peak incidence being in persons of age 17–25 years, or younger in low socioeconomic groups. The transmission occurs by exchange of saliva either through infected utensils or by kissing; however, its communicability is considered low. The incubation period is 2–6 weeks.

**Manifestations.** Symptoms vary from mild to moderately severe and may last for several weeks. They include low-grade fever, sore throat, headache, fatigue, skin rash, and general malaise. The cervical glands of the neck enlarge. Splenomegaly (*spleno*, "spleen," and *megas*, "large") develops in approximately half the patients. Liver involvement with mild jaundice occurs in a small number of persons and requires bed rest until serum bilirubin levels return to normal. Diagnosis is confirmed by the examination of peripheral blood. There are lymphocytosis and the presence of atypical lymphocytes. Rising titer of antibody to EBV is also indicative; the *monospot* test is rapid, can detect the infection earlier than the heterophile antibody test, and is now widely used. Complications, although uncommon, include rupture of

## Selected Nursing Diagnoses for the Adolescent Receiving Cancer Chemotherapy

| Goals | Nursing Interventions | Rationale |
|---|---|---|
| **Nursing Diagnosis:** Knowledge deficit concerning prevention of infection due to myelosuppression. | | |
| Patient will remain free of infection as evidenced by temperature of 36.5–37.6°C (99.7–99.6°F); skin and mucous membranes will show no signs of irritation or inflammation<br><br>Patient's hemoglobin level will improve with therapy; there will be no recurrence of anemia | 1. Instruct patient about body's immune system and immunotherapy as age-appropriate; use visual aids<br><br>2. Monitor white blood cell count and interpret blood values at patient's level of understanding<br><br><br><br><br><br>3. Place patient in private room, avoid crowds, practice proper handwashing and good personal hygiene, monitor temperature<br><br><br><br><br><br><br>4. Observe mouth and perianal area for infection<br><br><br><br><br><br><br><br><br>5. Use soft toothbrush, Water-pik, soothing mouthwashes<br><br>6. Limit exposure to direct sunlight | 1. Malignant process depresses immune system at onset of disease; chemotherapy further suppresses it and causes some physical changes that increase chances of infection<br><br>2. Leukopenia (decreased white blood cells), which predisposes patient to infection, and thrombocytopenia (decreased platelets), which predisposes patient to bruising and bleeding, are most serious side effects; anemia due to decreased erythrocyte count is also a side effect but is more easily treated<br><br>3. Bone marrow suppression as a side effect of chemotherapy or radiation predisposes child to anemia, infection, and bleeding; in addition to treatment effects, patients with leukemia are particularly vulnerable because their bone marrow is depressed as a result of disease; neutropenia may result; infection can be life-threatening<br><br>4. Ulcerations of mouth and anus are common; meticulous rectal care will prevent natural microbial flora (*Escherichia coli*) from being introduced by a break in mucosa; enemas and rectal temperatures are avoided because of this; stomatitis is a frequent side effect of chemotherapy<br><br>5. Protecting membranes decreases likelihood of capillary damage and mucous membrane breakdown<br><br>6. Photosensitivity is a side effect of some chemotherapeutic drugs |
| **Nursing Diagnosis:** High risk for hemorrhage due to platelet deficit from bone marrow suppression. | | |
| Patient shows no signs of bleeding, as evidenced by stable vital signs and absence of hematuria, petechiae, and ecchymosis | 1. Observe for hematuria, hematemesis, melena, epistaxis, petechiae, ecchymosis<br><br>2. Increase fluid intake<br><br><br><br><br><br><br>3. Use local measures if necessary to control bleeding<br><br><br><br><br><br>4. Monitor platelet counts and assist patient in types of safe activity when count is low | 1. Bleeding from these sites can occur because of myelosuppression<br><br>2. Patient may be febrile; a liberal fluid intake also prevents hemorrhagic cystitis; vomiting from chemotherapy may deplete fluid volume, and patient may become dehydrated<br><br>3. Direct pressure reduces small bleeds; avoid puncture wounds whenever possible; bandages and old blood are promptly removed, since they provide media for infection<br><br>4. Children with low platelet counts are advised to avoid temporarily activities that might cause bleeding or injury (skateboarding, contact sports, and so on); aspirin is avoided, because it destroys platelets |

## Selected Nursing Diagnoses for the Adolescent Receiving Cancer Chemotherapy

| Goals | Nursing Interventions | Rationale |
|---|---|---|
| **Nursing Diagnosis:** Altered nutrition due to stomatitis, nausea, and vomiting. | | |
| Patient is able to eat frequent small meals; caloric intake is adequate for age | 1. Inspect mouth daily for ulcerations | 1. Mouth lesions may lead to anorexia; early treatment is necessary |
| Nausea and vomiting will decrease; patient's weight will stabilize | 2. Serve bland, moist, soft diet | 2. Prevents trauma to mouth and lesions of the esophagus |
| | 3. Apply local anesthetics to ulcerated areas before meals | 3. Protects lesions and makes eating easier |
| | 4. Monitor weight | 4. Malnutrition may be present; weight loss is common owing to nature of treatments and side effects of medication, such as nausea and vomiting |
| | 5. Alert patient to expected reactions to treatment protocol | 5. Preparing patient in advance reduces anxiety |
| | 6. Give antiemetic prior to onset of nausea and vomiting | 6. Regularly scheduled antiemetics reduce discomfort of nausea and vomiting |
| | 7. Suggest appropriate relaxation techniques | 7. Symptoms can be controlled or lessened by relaxation techniques |
| **Nursing Diagnosis:** Disturbance in body image due to moon face, hair loss; patient may have amputation. | | |
| Patient verbalizes some satisfaction with appearance | 1. Allow teenager to ventilate feelings about body | 1. Accept all feelings |
| | 2. Provide continuity of care | 2. Teenagers need persons they can trust; continuity of care provides this |
| | 3. Utilize wigs, scarfs, eyebrow pencil, false eyelashes; stress that hair loss is temporary; suggest clothing that minimizes body changes and enhances appearance | 3. Looking and feeling attractive are morale boosters |
| | 4. Have patient draw "How it feels to be sick," "How it feels to be well"; discuss | 4. Indirect communication is helpful for self-conscious teenager; drawing provides an outlet for expression of feelings |
| **Nursing Diagnosis:** Disturbance in self-esteem and independence/dependence tasks. | | |
| Patient will participate in self-care and daily hygiene | 1. Involve patient in decision-making as age-appropriate | 1. Patients are less anxious if they can gain a measure of control over their lives; denial of this increases noncompliance |
| | 2. Set appropriate limits on disruptive behavior | 2. Limit-setting denotes caring; providing structure promotes security, particularly in a strange setting |
| | 3. Avoid overprotection, overattention, overanxiety; foster independence | 3. These behaviors may make patient feel different and not in control |

*Continued*

| NURSING CARE PLAN 27–2 *Continued* | | |
|---|---|---|
| **Selected Nursing Diagnoses for the Adolescent Receiving Cancer Chemotherapy** | | |
| **Goals** | **Nursing Interventions** | **Rationale** |

**Nursing Diagnosis:** Fear of sexual dysfunction due to treatment modalities.

| Goals | Nursing Interventions | Rationale |
|---|---|---|
| Patient expresses understanding of information | 1. Address sexuality issues and concerns | 1. Teenager is a teenager first and a cancer patient second; all normal longings and fears concerning sexuality, enticing opposite sex, and so on remain imprisoned unless someone is willing to listen and, more often than not, bring up subject |

**Nursing Diagnosis:** Social isolation related to interrupted schooling, rejection by peers.

| Goals | Nursing Interventions | Rationale |
|---|---|---|
| Patient remains in contact with peers | 1. Provide opportunity for group discussions with peers; encourage letter writing, telephone calls; suggest cancer camp; respect privacy with adolescent visitors; contact spiritual advisor, church youth groups, and the like | 1. Immersion into a peer group is one of the tasks of adolescence; long-term disease may disrupt this task and isolate patient |

**Nursing Diagnosis:** Fear of death due to treatment or nature of disease.

| Goals | Nursing Interventions | Rationale |
|---|---|---|
| Patient expresses two concerns regarding life expectancy | 1. Convey empathic understanding of patient's and family's worries, fears, and doubts | 1. Fear of death is like an elephant in living room that everyone pretends does not exist; by refusing to discuss it, family can pretend that it will not happen; because no feelings are shared, each member suffers in isolation; sharing threat lessens burden and brings members closer; nevertheless, this cannot be forced on persons who are not ready for it. |
| Patient expresses hope, although this may be changed from "hope" of cure to prolonged life | 2. Determine patient's perception of diagnosis, for example, "What are your concerns?"; "How can I help?" | 2. Misconceptions abound in life-threatening illness, as patient is in crisis |
| | 3. Support "hope" by clarifying and by educating patient about disease and side effects | 3. Hope is important to patient and family members; it may be hope of celebrating a birthday or seeing a special friend; it may be hope that suffering will end |
| | 4. Avoid discounting patient by making statements such as "I know exactly how you feel" or "You shouldn't feel that way" or by changing the subject | 4. Expression of feelings is basis for identifying effective coping methods |
| | 5. Draw and discuss "strongest feeling I've had today" | 5. Patient can distance self from feelings through drawings. This makes the feelings less threatening |

the spleen, secondary pneumonia, neurologic manifestations, and heart involvement. It must be differentiated from chronic fatigue syndrome.

**Treatment and Nursing Care.** Treatment is supportive because the disease is self-limiting. An antipyretic is given in order to reduce fever and discomfort. An initial period of rest and decreased activities is indicated. Gargling with warm saline solution and sucking throat lozenges are useful for pharyngitis. Adequate fluid intake is necessary, in particular, intake of bland, cool liquids that are not irritating to the throat. Smoking is discouraged. There is no special diet. Isolation is not necessary. The patient is alerted to signs of secondary infection. Steroid hormones are given when complications arise. Activities are increased as fever and fatigue diminish. The patient with an enlarged spleen is cautioned to avoid heavy lifting, trauma to the abdomen, and vigorous athletics. Severe abdominal pain is unusual except in the presence of splenic rupture and requires immediate attention.

Teenagers with mononucleosis may be discouraged and depressed. They worry about their jobs, school work, and ability to continue extracurricular activities. Open communications with school officials and classmates will help alleviate some of these anxieties. The prognosis for the patient with mononucleosis is good. It is no longer considered a prolonged debilitating disease. Many cases go unrecognized. Researchers are currently searching for a vaccine to prevent the disease.

## KEY POINTS

- Circulating blood consists of two portions: plasma and formed elements. Disorders associated with altered blood elements affect the function of these elements. For example, red blood cells carry oxygen, white blood cells fight infection, and platelets aid in coagulation.
- Bone marrow aspiration is one procedure that is helpful in determining disorders of the blood.
- The most common nutritional deficiency of children in the United States is iron-deficiency anemia.
- Sickle cell disease is an inherited defect in the formation of hemoglobin. The cells become crescent-shaped and clump together.
- Hemophilia A is due to a deficiency of coagulation Factor VIII. The child suffers from abnormal bleeding tendencies.
- The child with hemophilia who has an open bleeding wound is immediately treated by application of cold and pressure.
- Leukemia is the most common form of childhood cancer.
- Petechiae and purpura may be early objective symptoms in leukemia.
- In leukemia patients, myelosuppression resulting from the disease and certain drug regimens causes the patient to be highly subject to infections.
- Diagnostic procedures for patients with blood disorders are often invasive or painful. The nurse prepares and supports the patient and family during these procedures.

# Study Questions

1. Review the composition of blood. Name one function of red blood cells, one of white blood cells, and one of platelets.
2. Gown technique is being utilized for 6-month-old Tracy, whose immune system is depressed. Cassie, a 4-year-old, is visiting her and inquires, "Do you have ghosts in this hospital?" What fears predominate in the preschool years? How could the nurse assist Cassie to master her "ghostly" fears? (Refer also to Chap. 22.)
3. What is the cause of the bleeding from mucous membranes that is seen in leukemia? List two skin manifestations of bleeding.
4. Describe the nursing observations necessary for the child receiving a blood transfusion.
5. List the symptoms of iron-deficiency anemia.
6. Name three good food sources of iron.

7. How does sickle cell trait differ from sickle cell disease?

8. Troy, who is 5 years old, has sickle cell disease and is recovering from a crisis episode. What does this mean? Devise a nursing care plan for Troy.

9. Becky, age 11, has leukemia and has been in remission for 4 years. She is preparing to attend cancer camp. What, if any, precautions would you recommend to her parents?

10. Prepare a nursing care plan for Dennis, age 14, who is receiving chemotherapy.

# Multiple Choice Review Questions

*Choose the most appropriate answer.*

1. The most common nutritional deficiency of children in the United States is
   a. scurvy
   b. anemia
   c. rickets
   d. beriberi

2. Leukemia is a
   a. nutritional disease
   b. malignant disease
   c. collagen disease
   d. infectious disease

3. Pinpoint hemorrhages beneath the skin are termed
   a. petechiae
   b. ecchymoses
   c. purpura
   d. phagocytes

4. When the patient experiences apprehension and urticaria while receiving a blood transfusion, the nurse
   a. slows the transfusion and takes the patient's vital signs
   b. observes the child for further transfusion reactions
   c. stops the transfusion, lets normal saline run slowly, and notifies the charge nurse
   d. stops what he or she is doing and takes the patient's history

5. Symptoms of sickle cell disease generally occur at about age
   a. 1 month
   b. 11 months
   c. 5 months
   d. 8 months

## BIBLIOGRAPHY

Behrman, R.E. (1992). *Nelson textbook of pediatrics* (14th ed.). Philadelphia: W.B. Saunders.

Dickerman, J., & Lucey, J. (1985). *Smith's the critically ill child* (3rd ed.). Philadelphia: W.B. Saunders.

Eckert, E. (1990). *Your child and hemophilia.* New York: The National Hemophilia Foundation.

Eoff, M.J. (1990). Hematologic composition: Implications of altered blood elements. In S. Mott, et al. (Eds.), *Nursing care of children and families* (2nd ed., pp. 1282–1333). Redwood, CA: Addison-Wesley.

Gellis, S., & Kagan B. (1990). *Current pediatric therapy 13.* Philadelphia: W.B. Saunders.

Holbrook, T. (1985). The hematopoietic system. In L. Hayman & E. Sporing (Eds.), *Handbook of pediatric nursing.* New York: John Wiley & Sons.

Leonard, M. (1994). Altered hematologic function. In Betz, C., Hunsberger, M., & Wright, S., *Family-centered nursing care of children.* Philadelphia: W.B. Saunders.

Mahan, L., & Arlin, M. (1992). *Krause's nutrition and diet therapy* (8th ed.). Philadelphia: W.B. Saunders.

Mott, S., et al. (1991). *Nursing care of children and families* (2nd ed.). Reading, MA: Addison-Wesley.

Pierce, G.F., et al. (1989). The use of purified clotting factor concentrates in hemophilia; influence of viral safety, cost, and supply on therapy. *JAMA: Journal of the American Medical Association, 261,* 3434–3438.

Pillitteri, A. (1992). *Maternal and child health nursing.* Philadelphia: J.B. Lippincott.

Whaley, L., & Wong, D. (1991). *Nursing care of infants and children* (4th ed.). St. Louis: C.V. Mosby.

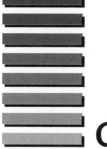

# Chapter 28

# The Child with a Gastrointestinal Condition

## VOCABULARY

endoscopy (744)
homeostasis (746)
incarcerated (759)
isotonic (746)
overnutrition (760)
peritonitis (758)
pica (767)
poisoning (766)
projectile vomiting (749)
sigmoidoscopy (744)
stenosis (748)

Vomiting
Fluid Imbalance
   Dehydration
   Overhydration
Gastroesophageal Reflux
Pyloric Stenosis
Diarrhea
   Rotavirus Infection
   Giardiasis
Enterobiasis (Pinworms)
Ascariasis (Roundworms)
Constipation
Hirschsprung's Disease (Aganglionic
   Megacolon)
Intussusception
Appendicitis
Meckel's Diverticulum
Inguinal Hernia
Umbilical Hernia
Obesity
Anorexia Nervosa
Bulimia
Acetaminophen Poisoning
Salicylate Poisoning
Lead Poisoning (Plumbism)
Corrosive Strictures

# OBJECTIVES

*On completion and mastery of Chapter 28, the student will be able to*

- Define each vocabulary term listed.
- List three procedures commonly used to diagnose problems of the gastrointestinal tract.
- Trace the route of the pinworm cycle and describe how reinfection takes place.
- Differentiate between umbilical and inguinal hernias.
- Discuss the postoperative nursing care of an infant with pyloric stenosis.
- Explain why infants and young children become dehydrated more easily than adults do.
- Identify the symptoms of and nursing care for gastroesophageal reflux, Meckel's diverticulum, and Hirschsprung's disease.
- Contrast anorexia nervosa and bulimia.
- List two measures being taken to reduce aspirin poisoning in children.
- Indicate the primary source of lead poisoning.

The gastrointestinal (GI) tract transports and metabolizes nutrients necessary for the life of the cell. It extends from the mouth to the anus. Nutrients are broken down into absorbable products by enzymes from various digestive organs. The anatomy of the digestive tract, along with differences between the child and adult, is depicted in Figure 28–1. The primitive digestive tube is formed by the yolk sac and is divided into the foregut, midgut, and hindgut. The foregut evolves into the pharynx, lower respiratory tract, esophagus, stomach, duodenum, and beginning of the common bile duct. The midgut elongates in the 5th week to form the primary intestinal loop. The remainder of the large colon is derived from the primitive hindgut. The liver, pancreas, and biliary tree evolve from the foregut. At 8 weeks, the anal membrane ruptures, forming the anal canal and opening. GI disorders may begin with acute pain in a specific organ or may reflect systemic involvement by such symptoms as failure to develop normally according to established growth parameters, that is, height, weight, and head circumference; vomiting; diarrhea; constipation; rectal bleeding; hematemesis; or jaundice. Pruritus in the absence of allergy may indicate liver dysfunction.

A number of procedures are available to determine GI disorders. Laboratory work, such as a complete blood count with differential will reveal anemia, infections, and chronic illness. An elevated erythrocyte sedimentation rate is indicative of inflammation. A sequential multiple analysis (SMA 12) will reveal electrolyte and chemical imbalances. X-ray films include GI series, barium enema, and flat plates of the abdomen. Endoscopy allows direct visualization of the GI tract through a flexible lighted tube. Upper endoscopy permits visualization and biopsy of the esophagus, stomach, and duodenum. It is also valuable in the removal of foreign objects and cauterization of bleeding vessels. Visualization of the bile and pancreatic ducts is also possible through endoscopy. The lower colon is inspected by sigmoidoscopy. Colonoscopy provides visualization of the entire colon to the ileocecal valve. Stool cultures and rectal biopsy are also important diagnostic tools. Ultrasonography is a noninvasive procedure useful in visualizing intestinal organs and masses, particularly of the liver and pancreas. Liver blood tests include serum glutamic-pyruvic transaminase (SGPT), serum glutamic-oxaloacetic transaminase (SGOT), prothrombin time, partial thromboplastin time, and others. Liver biopsy may also be indicated. Overall malabsorption tests, such as the 72-hour fecal fat test and the Schilling test, which can determine the absorption capacity of the lower ileum, are also useful.

Nursing intervention focuses on providing adequate nutrition and freedom from infection, which can result from malnutrition or depressed immune function. Developmental delays in children should be investigated to determine whether they are related to the GI system. Skin problems in these patients may be related to pruritus from liver disease or to irritation from frequent bowel movements, or to other disorders. Pain and discomfort may be related to acute episodes, but they may also be related to side effects of medication or referred pain. The following conditions reflect the more common conditions of the GI tract seen in children: vomiting, gastroesophageal reflux, pyloric stenosis, diarrhea, rotavirus, giardiasis, pinworms, roundworms, constipation, Hirschsprung's disease, intussusception, appendicitis, Meckel's diverticulum, inguinal hernia, umbilical hernia, obesity, anorexia nervosa, bulimia, acetaminophen and salicylate poisoning, lead poisoning, and corrosive strictures. Cleft lip and palate, thrush, and diarrhea in the newborn are

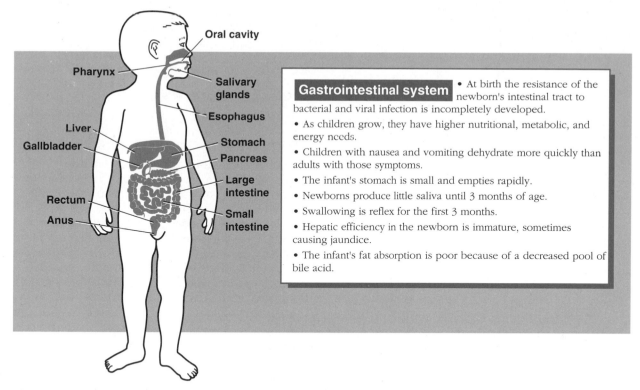

**Figure 28–1.** Summary of gastrointestinal system differences between the child and adult. The digestive system consists of the digestive tract and the glands that secrete digestive juices into the digestive tract. This system mechanically and chemically breaks down food and eliminates wastes.

discussed in Chapter 14. The relief of colic is described in Chapter 17 (see p. 419). Meconium ileus is discussed in Chapter 26 (see p. 710). Necrotizing enterocolitis is discussed on page 322.

# Vomiting

**Description.** Vomiting, a common symptom during infancy and childhood, results from sudden contractions of the diaphragm and muscles of the stomach. It must be evaluated in relation to the child's overall health status. Occasional vomiting is to be expected. Persistent vomiting requires investigation because it results in dehydration and electrolyte imbalance. The continuous loss of hydrochloric acid and sodium chloride from the stomach can cause *alkalosis*. In this condition, the acid-base balance of the body becomes disturbed because of a loss of chlorides and potassium. This can result in death if the patient is left untreated.

The well child vomits from various causes. Some stem from improper feeding techniques. The nurse should ask the following questions when the infant vomits: Was the baby fed too fast? Too much? Was the infant bubbled frequently and properly positioned following the feeding? Has there been a recent formula increase or change? Were any previous feedings vomited? Sometimes the difficulty lies with the formula. If the fat content is too high, it can slow down the emptying process of the stomach. The introduction of foods of a different consistency may also precipitate this symptom. Infants sometimes induce vomiting by gagging themselves with their fingers or objects of play.

Other causes of vomiting are ear, nose, and throat infections. Vomiting is seen in the primary stages of many communicable diseases. Specific disorders, such as Reye's syndrome, peptic ulcer disease, increased intracranial pressure, strangulated hernia, and various bowel obstructions, are also responsible. In these conditions, the vomiting is not necessarily associated with feeding. When the cause of the illness is discovered and properly treated, the symptom disappears. Aspiration and aspiration pneumonia are serious complications of vomiting. In aspiration, vomitus is drawn into the air passages on inspiration, causing immediate death in extreme cases. Health professionals and laypersons should become familiar with life-saving procedures such as the Heimlich maneuver for use in such emergencies (see Fig. 18–21).

**Treatment and Nursing Care.** To prevent vomiting, the nurse must carefully feed and bubble the baby. The nurse must be relaxed, and the surroundings peaceful. Treatments are avoided immediately following feedings. The baby is handled as little as possible at this time. To prevent aspiration of vomitus, the nurse places the infant on the right side following feedings. When an older child begins to vomit, the head is turned to one side, and an emesis basin and tissues are provided. The nurse can relieve some of the strain involved by firmly supporting the patient's head. When the vomiting has ceased, the basin is removed from sight. The nurse rinses the patient's mouth with cold water. The hands and face are bathed with warm water. In infants particular attention is given to cleansing the creases of the neck and the area behind the ears. To change position, the nurse turns the patient slowly and gently, because motion tends to increase nausea. A clean gown is applied, and the bed linen is changed if necessary.

The nurse may estimate the amount of material vomited by filling a similar basin with water to about the same level as the vomitus and measuring the water. Factors to be charted include time, amount, color (bloody, bile-stained), consistency, force, frequency, and whether or not vomiting was preceded by nausea. The diet following vomiting is prescribed by the doctor. In the hospital, intravenous fluids may be given (p. 588). Oral fluids are withheld for a short time to allow the stomach to rest. Gradually, sips of water are given according to the infant's tolerance and condition. The patient's intake and output are carefully recorded so that the physician is able to compare the kidney output with the total fluid intake.

When vomiting is persistent, drugs such as trimethobenzamide (Tigan) or promethazine (Phenergan) may be prescribed. They are available in rectal suppository form. The nurse lubricates the suppository and inserts it well into the rectum, where it dissolves. Slight pressure is exerted over the anus for a short time to ensure that the suppository is not expelled. Charting includes the time, name of suppository, and whether or not vomiting subsided.

## Fluid Imbalance

### DEHYDRATION

When a person is in good health, the intake and output of fluids are balanced and *homeostasis* (a uniform state) exists. This is accomplished by appropriate shifts of fluids and electrolytes across cellular membranes and by elimination of products of metabolism that are no longer needed or are in excess. The volume of blood plasma and interstitial and intracellular fluids remains relatively constant. Dehydration occurs whenever fluid output exceeds fluid intake, regardless of the cause.

Disorders of fluids and electrolytes—sodium (Na), potassium (K), calcium (Ca), and magnesium (Mg)—are more complex in growing children. A newborn's total weight is approximately 77% water, compared with 60% in adults (see Fig. 23–23). This varies with the amount of fat. Also, the daily turnover of water in infants is equal to almost 24% of total body water, compared with about 6% in adults. A baby's body surface in comparison with weight is three times that of the older child; therefore, the baby is subject to greater evaporation of water from the skin. The younger the patient, the higher the metabolic rate and the more unstable the heat-regulating mechanisms. (Elevations in temperature are also higher, increasing the rate of water loss.) Rapid respirations speed up this process, and when diarrhea is present, additional fluid is lost in the stools. Immaturity of the kidneys impairs the infant's ability to conserve water. Preterm and newborn infants are also more susceptible to dehydration from variations in room temperature and humidity. Cessation of intake alone can result insignificant depletion. When this is coupled with higher fluid losses, life-threatening deficits can ensue within a few hours.

Problems of fluid and electrolyte disturbance require evaluation of the type and severity of dehydration, clinical observation of the patient, and chemical analysis of the blood. The types of dehydration are classified according to the amount of serum sodium, which depends on the relative losses of water and electrolytes. These types are usually termed *isotonic* (the patient has lost equal amounts of fluids and elec-

**Table 28–1.** SIGNS OF ISOTONIC, HYPERTONIC, AND HYPOTONIC DEHYDRATION

| Area of Assessment | Signs of Dehydration | | |
| --- | --- | --- | --- |
| | *Isotonic* | *Hypertonic* | *Hypotonic* |
| Loss of body weight | Mild dehydration—up to 5% loss of body weight Moderate dehydration—5–10% loss of body weight Severe dehydration—over 10% loss of body weight | | |
| Behavior | Irritable and lethargic | Irritable when disturbed; lethargic | Lethargic to delirious; coma |
| Skin turgor | Dead elasticity | Good turgor; "foam rubber" feel | Very poor turgor; clammy |
| Mucous membranes | Dry | Parched | Clammy |
| Eyeballs and fontanel | Sunken and soft | Sunken | Sunken and soft |
| Tearing and salivation | Absent or decreased | Absent or decreased | Absent or decreased |
| Thirst | Present | Marked | Present |
| Urine | Decreased output; SG elevated | Normal to decreased output; SG elevated or decreased | Decreased output; SG elevated |
| Body temperature | Subnormal to elevated | Elevated | Subnormal |
| Respiration | Rapid | Rapid | Rapid |
| Blood pressure | Normal to low | Normal to low | Very low |
| Pulse | Rapid | Rapid | Rapid |
| Blood chemistry | BUN increased | BUN increased | BUN increased |
| | Na decreased | Na increased | Na decreased |
| | K normal or increased | K decreased | K varies or increased |
| | Cl decreased | Cl low during correction | Cl decreased |
| | pH usually decreased | Ca decreased | |

SG, serum globulin; BUN, blood urea nitrogen.
Courtesy of P. Chinn.

trolytes), *hypotonic*, and *hypertonic*, respectively, because plasma osmolality in large part reflects sodium concentrations (Table 28–1); however, in certain instances interchanging these terms may be technically inaccurate.

These classifications are important because each form of dehydration is associated with different relative losses from intracellular fluid (ICF) and extracellular fluid (ECF) compartments, and each requires certain modifications in treatment. *Maintenance* fluid therapy replaces normal water and electrolyte losses, and *deficit* therapy restores pre-existing body fluids and electrolyte deficiencies. Replacing a deficit may take several days, and the deficit will continue unless adequate maintenance therapy is also provided. The physician calculates the volume of fluids to be administered through the use of various formulas based on caloric expenditures because daily physiologic water losses are directly proportionate to caloric expenditure. The patient's temperature and activity (coma, restlessness) must also be considered. Basal calories are determined by the weight of the child. Volume is calculated on a 24-hour basis. Isotonic dehydration is the most common form in children.

The composition of intravenous fluids and the amount and rate of flow are important in preventing complications.

Fluid therapy is constantly adjusted according to the patient's condition. The higher daily exchange of water in infants leaves them a smaller-volume reserve when they are dehydrated. *Shock* (hypovolemia) is the greatest threat to life in isotonic dehydration. The electrolyte content of oral fluids is particularly significant in the care of infants and small children suffering from disorders of fluid balance and receiving infusions. Commercially prepared electrolyte solutions are available by bottle; however, the nurse should ascertain if they are to be given freely or only by doctor's order. Patients with hypotonic dehydration, that is, excess water with sodium electrolyte depletion, are at risk for water intoxication. This can also occur if tap water enemas are given to small children. Potassium is lost in almost all states of dehydration. Replacement potassium is administered only after normal urinary excretion is established.

## OVERHYDRATION

Overhydration results when the body receives more fluid than it can excrete. This can occur in patients with normal kidneys who receive intravenous fluids too rapidly. It also can occur in a patient receiving acceptable rates of fluid, especially when the patient's illness is related to disorders of fluid mechanism. These include kidney disease, burns, cardiovascular disease, protein deficiencies, and certain allergies. Hormonal therapy also may interrupt fluid mechanisms.

Edema is the presence of excess fluid in the interstitial (*interstitium*, "a thing standing between") spaces. Interstitial fluid is similar to plasma, but it contains little protein. In healthy persons, it responds well to shifts in fluid balance. Any factor causing sodium retention can cause edema. The flow of blood out of the interstitial compartments also depends on adequate circulation of blood and lymph. Low protein levels can also disturb osmotic cellular pressure, causing edema. This is seen in patients with nephrosis, in which large amounts of albumin are lost.

Trauma to or infections of the head can cause cerebral edema, which can be life-threatening. Constrictive dressing may obstruct venous return, causing swelling, particularly in dependent areas. Anasarca (*ana*, "throughout," and *sarx*, "flesh") is a severe generalized edema. Early detection and management of edema are essential. Taking accurate daily weights is indispensable, as is close attention to body weight changes. Vital signs, physical appearance, and changes in urine character or output are noted. Edema in infants may first be seen about the eyes and in the presacral, occipital, or genital areas. In pitting edema, after exerting gentle pressure with the finger, the nurse notices an impression in the skin that lasts for several seconds.

# Gastroesophageal Reflux

**Description.** Gastroesophageal reflux (GER, or chalasia) results when the lower esophageal sphincter is relaxed or not competent. This allows stomach contents to be easily regurgitated into the esophagus.

The term *chalasia* is derived from the Greek word *chalasis*, which means "relaxation." Although many infants have this condition to a small degree, about 1 in 300 to 1 in 1000 have significant reflux and associated complications (Behrman, 1992). The exact cause of this condition is uncertain. It is associated with neuromuscular delay and is seen frequently in preterm infants and children with neuromuscular disorders, such as cerebral palsy and Down syndrome. In many infants, the symptoms decrease around 12 months, when the child stands upright and eats more solid foods.

**Manifestations.** The symptoms include vomiting, weight loss, bleeding, and respiratory problems. The vomiting occurs within the 1st and 2nd week of life. It may be forceful at times. The baby is fussy and hungry. Aspiration pneumonia may occur if the contents of the esophagus enter the pharynx. Periods of apnea may be observed. Blood may be vomited or evident in the stools. This finding is due to repeated irritation of the lining of the esophagus by gastric acid. Anemia and failure to thrive sometimes accompany this disorder.

**Treatment and Nursing Care.** A careful history is taken. Of particular interest are when the vomiting started, type of formula, type of vomiting, feeding techniques, and the baby's eating in general. Tests used to determine the presence of GER include a barium swallow under fluoroscopy or esophagoscopy. Esophageal sphincter pressure may also be measured. Prolonged esophageal pH monitoring is one of the most definitive diagnostic tests and helps determine the acuity of the disease and the course of treatment.

Therapy depends on the severity of symptoms. Some parents need only reassurance and education about feeding the baby. The routine includes careful burping, supplying sufficient calories without overfeeding (which distends the stomach), and proper positioning. In infants with more complicated GER, medication and surgical intervention may be required. Parents are instructed to burp the baby well. Feedings are thickened with cereal (although there is controversy over its effectiveness). After being fed, the baby is placed in an upright prone position. The body is inclined about 30–40 degrees, and the baby is held in place by a harness (Fig. 28–2). Sitting upright in an infant seat is not recommended because it increases intraabdominal pressure. Medications that relax the pyloric sphincter and promote stomach emptying may be utilized. Metoclopramide (Reglan) or bethanechol chloride (Urecholine) are two such medications. A trial of medical management usually precedes surgery. The postoperative nursing care is similar to that for other types of abdominal surgery.

# Pyloric Stenosis

**Description.** Pyloric stenosis (narrowing) is a disorder of the digestive tract. The pylorus, the lower end of the stomach, becomes partially blocked so that food does not empty properly into the duodenum. Pyloric stenosis is caused

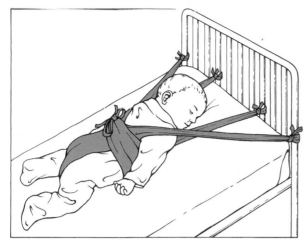

**Figure 28–2.** Position for the infant with gastroesophageal reflux.

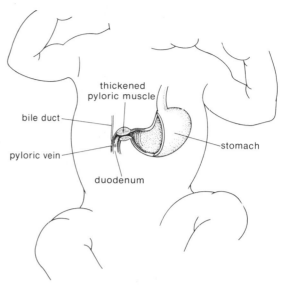

**Figure 28–3.** Pyloric stenosis. Hypertrophy or thickening of the pyloric sphincter blocks the stomach contents, causing the infant to regurgitate forcefully. Serious electrolyte imbalances ultimately occur, and surgery is necessary to correct the condition. (From Betz, C., Hunsberger, M., & Wright, S. [1994]. *Family-centered nursing care of children* [2nd ed.]. Philadelphia, W.B. Saunders.)

by an overgrowth of the circular muscles of the pylorus or by spasms of the sphincter. The stomach muscles above the obstructed area also enlarge in their attempt to force material through the narrowed passage. Such abnormal enlargement of an organ (or organ part) is called *hypertrophy*. This condition is commonly classified as a congenital anomaly; however, its symptoms do not appear until the baby is 2 or 3 weeks old. Pyloric stenosis is the most common surgical condition of the digestive tract in infancy (Fig. 28–3). Its incidence is higher in boys than in girls, and it has a tendency to be inherited. Miniepidemics of this condition sometimes occur. The reason for this is unknown (Behrman, 1992).

**Manifestations.** Vomiting is the outstanding symptom of this disorder. The force progresses until most of the food is ejected a considerable distance from the mouth. This is termed *projectile vomiting*, and it occurs before and after feeding. The vomitus contains mucus and may be blood-streaked. The baby is constantly hungry and will eat again immediately after vomiting. Dehydration—as evidenced by sunken fontanel, inelastic skin, and decreased urination—and malnutrition are present. In severe cases, the fat pads of the cheeks disappear, giving the patient a withered "old man" look. An olive-shaped mass may be felt in the right upper quadrant of the abdomen. X-ray films confirm an enlarged stomach. It is difficult for the barium to pass into the duodenum. Ultrasonography is commonly used today for diagnostic purposes, as it is noninvasive and accurate. In severe cases, the outline of the

distended stomach and peristaltic waves are visible during feeding. The urine and blood are alkaline because the fluid being lost from the body is mostly hydrochloric acid from the stomach juices. Bowel movements gradually diminish, since little or no food passes into the intestine.

**Treatment.** There are two methods of treating pyloric stenosis, one medical and the other surgical. Medical treatment today is rare, since the results from surgery are excellent. The operation performed for pyloric stenosis is called a pyloromyotomy (*pylorus*, *myo*, "muscle," and *tomy*, "incision of"). The surgeon incises the pyloric muscle to enlarge the opening so that food may easily pass through it again. This is done as soon as possible if the infant is not dehydrated.

**Nursing Care.** The dehydrated infant is given intravenous fluids preoperatively in order to restore fluid and electrolyte balance. If this is not done, shock may occur during surgery. Thickened feedings may be given until the time of operation in hopes that some nutrients will be retained. The physician prescribes the degree of thickness of the formula, which is given by teaspoon or through a nipple with a large hole. The infant is bubbled *before* as well as during feedings in order to remove any gas accumulated in the stomach. The feeding is done slowly, and the baby is handled gently and as little as possible. The infant is placed on the right side following feedings. The pylorus is on the right side of the abdomen; thus, drainage into the intestine is facilitated. If vomiting occurs, the nurse may be instructed to refeed the infant. Charting of the feeding includes time, type, and amount offered; amount taken and retained; and type and amount of vomiting. The nurse also notes whether the baby appeared hungry after the feeding.

The nurse obtains and records a baseline weight and weighs the patient at about the same time each morning. Other factors to be charted include the type and number of stools and the color of urine and frequency of voiding. Position is changed frequently because the infant is weak and vulnerable to pneumonia. All procedures designed to protect from infection must be strictly carried out.

The care of the patient following surgery includes such procedures as careful observation of vital signs and administration of intravenous fluids. The wound site is inspected frequently for bleeding. Signs of shock are an increase in the rate of pulse and respiration; pale, cool skin; and restlessness. Most infants have a nasogastric tube in place, which is removed soon after surgery in order to begin oral feedings. On removal of the nasogastric tube, the baby is observed for vomiting. The position of the patient is changed gently. When indicated, the doctor prescribes oral feedings of small amounts of sugar and water that gradually increase until a regular formula can be taken and retained. As soon as intravenous feedings are discontinued and oral fluids are tolerated, the baby is held and fed from a bottle or is breast fed by the mother. The nurse must avoid overfeeding the patient. Vomiting is seen following surgery; however, it is not as severe as before the operation and gradually diminishes. The diaper is placed low over the abdomen in order to prevent infection of the wound.

# Diarrhea

An in-depth discussion of diarrhea is found in Chapter 14. Please review it at this time. Infants under age 1 year are frequently admitted to the hospital because this condition can quickly become serious. All children with diarrhea are initially isolated and presumed infectious. Nursing Care Plan 14–2 describes the care of an infant with diarrhea.

## ROTAVIRUS INFECTION

**Description.** A virus that causes diarrhea in children and is seen frequently in the winter months is the rotavirus. The incubation period is 2–3 days. It affects all age groups, but infants of 6–25 months are more susceptible. Symptoms are low-grade fever, nausea and vomiting, and mild abdominal pain. Diarrhea caused by rotavirus may be preceded by an upper respiratory infection. It generally affects the small bowel. Stools are green and watery. Treatment is symptomatic. The rotavirus is highly contagious, particularly in newborn nurseries, hospitals, and day-care centers. Stool precautions are taken. The infection is generally self-limited.

## GIARDIASIS

**Description.** *Giardia lamblia* is an intestinal protozoan that causes diarrhea. It became noticeable in the United States during the 1970s, when outbreaks of the disease were reported by groups of American travelers returning from the Soviet Union. Since then, studies have shown *G. lamblia* to have a high incidence in day-care centers and in family contacts of infected children. The child ingests the cysts, which are activated by stomach acid and passed into the duodenum. They eventually develop into trophozoites (active, feeding parasites), which colonize in the intestinal epithelium of the duodenum and proximal jejunum. As the cycle continues, cysts emerge and are passed in the feces of the victim. These infected cysts can survive in the environment for varying periods of time. Giardiasis is spread from person to person, by contaminated water (mountain streams, swimming pools that diapered babies frequent), by food, by puppies, and by fecal contamination of the environment.

**Manifestations.** Infants who are infected may be asymptomatic but more often have symptoms of acute or chronic diarrhea, anorexia, and failure to thrive. Older children may evidence abdominal cramps with intermittent diarrhea and constipation. The stools are foul-smelling and greasy and may float. The child may also complain of headaches and stomachaches. Most infections resolve in 4–6 weeks. Giardiasis should be considered in any patient who has come in contact with an infected person, in a young child attending day care, or in a person who has a history of recent travel to an endemic area.

**Treatment and Nursing Care.** The diagnosis of giardiasis becomes complicated because *G. lamblia* is not easily seen in the stools. The organisms are excreted in highly variable patterns; therefore, it is easy to obtain a false-negative result. Medications, including antibiotics, antacids, antidiarrheal compounds, and certain enema and laxative preparations, can interfere with identification of the organisms by altering the morphology or by causing a temporary disappearance of parasites from stool specimens. Patients should not receive these compounds for 48–72 hours prior to collection of stool for identification of *G. lamblia*. The method of stool collection is important. The specimens should be examined within 1 hour of passage or preserved in vials containing polyvinyl alcohol or 10% formalin. Two methods of more rapid detection of *G. lamblia* are counterimmunoelectrophoresis and the enzyme-linked immunosorbent assay.

Three drugs that have shown effectiveness in the treatment of giardiasis are quinacrine hydrochloride (Atabrine), metronidazole (Flagyl), and furazolidone (Furoxone). Atabrine appears to have the highest cure rate and is less expensive, but it also has side effects of vomiting and yellow staining of the skin, sclera of the eye, and urine. It should be taken with meals in order to decrease stomach upset. There is debate as to whether asymptomatic persons should receive treatment. Recurrence is not uncommon.

Prevention of giardiasis is paramount. Cleanliness of community diaper areas in daycare centers and public restrooms and disinfection of toilet seats with dilute household bleach or Lysol are necessary. Soiled diapers are placed in a plastic bag and discarded in a closed container. Fruits and vegetables are washed before eaten. Parents are educated about the importance of *handwashing*. One should avoid drinking untreated water when camping. Animals are kept away from playgrounds and sandboxes.

# Enterobiasis (Pinworms)

**Description.** Of the several varieties of worms that affect humans, the most common is the pinworm—*Enterobius vermicularis* (*en-*

*teron*, "intestine," *bios*, "life," and *vermis*, "wormlike"). It is seen more often in toddlers but can develop in older children and adults. The pinworm looks like a white thread about $\frac{1}{3}$ inch long. It lives in the lower intestine but comes out of the anus to lay its eggs, generally during the night. These eggs become infective a few hours after they have been deposited. This type of parasite spreads from one person to another, particularly where there are large groups of children in close contact with one another. The child becomes infected by inhaling the eggs or by handling contaminated toys, toilet seats, doorknobs, food, or soiled linen. The route of entry is the mouth. Reinfection takes place by way of the rectum to the fingers to the mouth or by way of the rectum to the clothing to the fingers to the mouth.

**Manifestations.** The nurse or parent may notice that the child scratches the anal area and may complain of itchiness. There may be associated irritability and restlessness. Weight loss, poor appetite, and fretfulness during the night may develop. The rectal area may become irritated from scratching. Worms may be seen on the surface of stools or around the anus. A special pinworm diagnostic tape or paddle or a tongue blade covered with cellophane tape, sticky side out, may be placed against the anal region to obtain pinworm eggs. This is done early in the morning, before the child has a bowel movement or bathes. The tape is put on a glass slide and examined under a microscope. The eggs are typical of pinworms.

**Treatment and Nursing Care.** Several effective anthelmintics (*anti*, "against," and *helminth*, "worms") are available. Mebendazole (Vermox) is a single-dose, chewable tablet and is the drug of choice for children over age 2. Pyrantel pamoate (Antiminth) also controls the infestation. Pyrvinium pamoate (Povan) suspension, a one-dose treatment, is an alternative drug; nurses advise parents that Povan stains and turns the stools red.

If it is determined that a hospitalized child has pinworms, linen and stool precautions are taken. The child must be taught to wash the hands well following bowel movements. The child's fingernails are kept short. A soothing ointment is applied to the rectal area. The patient should wear clean underwear that fits snugly. It is changed daily.

All symptomatic members of the family should be treated for this condition in order to prevent reinfection. Pregnant women should not take Vermox and should consult a physician before taking any alternative drug. In the home, the toilet seat is scrubbed daily. Diapers and bed linens are washed in hot water.

## Ascariasis (Roundworms)

*Ascaris lumbricoides* is a roundworm infestation that can be asymptomatic or can cause abdominal pain. The infestation is estimated to affect 1 billion persons world wide. It thrives in warm climates and among the impoverished. In the United States, it is seen more often in the southern states and among immigrants and migratory workers living below poverty levels. It is caused by the unsanitary disposal of human feces and poor hygiene practices. An egg from an infected person can survive for weeks in the soil. The child ingests eggs from contaminated soil. The eggs develop into larvae in the intestine, penetrate the intestinal wall, and enter the liver, from which they circulate to the lungs and heart. The patient is generally without symptoms until the larvae reach the glottis, are swallowed, and enter the small intestine. There they develop into adult male and female species. They survive on undigested food in the canal and produce eggs that are expelled in the child's feces. The adult worms can migrate along the intestinal tract and sometimes are regurgitated or passed in the stool. Nausea, vomiting, and weight loss can occur when infestation is heavy. Diagnosis is made by confirmation of the eggs in the patient's stool. The treatment of ascariasis is the same as that for enterobiasis (pinworms). Nursing considerations are outlined in Nursing Care Plan 28–1.

## Constipation

**Description.** Constipation is difficult or infrequent defecation with passage of hard, dry fecal material. There may be associated symptoms, such as abdominal discomfort or blood-streaked stools.

The frequency of bowel movements varies widely in children. There may be periods of diarrhea or *encopresis* (constipation with fecal soiling). Constipation may be a symptom of other disorders, particularly obstructive conditions. Diet, culture, and social, psychological, and familial patterns may also influence its oc-

---

**NURSING CARE PLAN 28–1**

**Selected Nursing Diagnoses for the Preschool Child with Ascariasis (Roundworm Infestation)**

| Goals | Nursing Interventions | Rationale |
|---|---|---|
| **Nursing Diagnosis:** High risk for altered nutrition; less than body requirements related to anorexia, nausea, deprivation of host nutrients by parasites. | | |
| Child maintains adequate growth and development parameters for age as evidenced by weight and growth charts | 1. Administer appropriate antiparasitic medication as prescribed: mebendazole (Vermox) single-dose, chewable tablet; pyrantel pamoate (Antiminth) | 1. Several drugs are effective against ascariasis; none is useful during the pulmonary phase of the infection |
| | 2. Offer light diet until digestive symptoms subside | 2. Child may experience anorexia, stomach pain |
| | 3. Observe child for nausea, diarrhea, regurgitation, or passage of adult worms in stool | 3. Larvae rise to oropharynx and are swallowed; obstruction of the intestine by adult worms can occur |
| | 4. Observe for signs of associated anemia | 4. Children with few resources may have poor eating habits; anorexia may accompany disorder |
| | 5. Monitor child's growth with growth grid | 5. To ascertain growth and development parameters for comparison |
| | 6. Assess child's behavior—is it age-appropriate? | 6. Child may come from dysfunctional family; pica maybe present |

| NURSING CARE PLAN 28–1 *Continued* |
|---|

## Selected Nursing Diagnoses for the Preschool Child with Ascariasis (Roundworm Infestation)

| Goals | Nursing Interventions | Rationale |
|---|---|---|
| **Nursing Diagnosis:** Knowledge deficit (parents) regarding mode of transmission. | | |
| Parents verbalize knowledge of transmission of roundworm | 1. Draw picture for parents showing life cycle of roundworm | 1. Visualization helps promote understanding; disease is caused by soil contaminated by human feces or subsequently by eating raw fruits and vegetables contaminated by flies |
| | 2. Point out that these worms have high outputs of eggs | 2. Eggs also remain infective in soil for weeks |
| | 3. Explain roundworms only live in human hosts | 3. Dispelling misinformation is of importance in education |
| | 4. Emphasize strict handwashing practices; preschool child is taught to wash hands before meals and is supervised | 4. Handwashing removes eggs and other organisms |
| | 5. Emphasize washing of all raw fruits and vegetables before eating | 5. These foods may be contaminated by flies and infested soil |
| | 6. Stress necessity of laundering towels, sheets, underwear, and night clothing | 6. Eggs may be found on articles contaminated by soil; disease is perpetuated by poor sanitary facilities and poor hygiene practices |
| | 7. Advise of necessity of treating all family members | 7. This will prevent transmission and reinfection |
| | 8. Suggest services of public health nurse if this appears warranted | 8. Proper referrals will ensure follow-through |
| **Nursing Diagnosis:** Knowledge deficit (parents) regarding growth and development parameters of preschooler that predispose child to infestation from parasites. | | |
| Parents verbalize knowledge of growth and development of preschool child | 1. Review growth and development of preschooler | 1. Many parents have little knowledge of growth and development |
| Parents verbalize necessity for hygienic practices in order to prevent parasitic infection from various sources | 2. Emphasize need for all members of family to use frequent and thorough handwashing | 2. Handwashing is most effective method of preventing disease transmission; remind small child |
| | 3. Stress need for child to wear shoes when outdoors | 3. Going barefoot is discouraged because of danger of hookworm, which penetrates bare feet |
| | 4. Explain necessity for keeping dogs and cats away from sandboxes | 4. Sandboxes contaminated by dog or cat feces may lead to *Toxocara canis* or *Toxocara cati* |
| | 5. Advise periodic cleansing of toys in order to avoid pinworms and other parasites | 5. Children often play with community toys; they are chewed on, dropped on ground, and so on |
| | 6. Remind parents to teach preschool child not to put dirt and other contaminated objects into mouth | 6. Prevention of parasitic and other diseases may be accomplished by these simple measures |
| | 7. Suggest that child's fingernails be trimmed frequently | 7. This prevents larvae from accumulating under nails |
| | 8. Suggest parents wash hands well before and after handling raw meats | 8. Raw meats often contain disease organisms, which can cause food poisoning and other conditions |
| | 9. Emphasize need to cook beef and pork adequately | 9. This prevents tapeworm infestation |

currence. The overuse of laxatives and enemas may contribute to the problem. Most children use the bathroom every day, but they may be hurried and have an incomplete bowel movement. Some children are embarrassed or even afraid to use school or public bathrooms.

**Treatment and Nursing Care.** Evaluation begins with a thorough history of dietary and bowel habits. It is not uncommon for parents to be unaware of these patterns in their child. The frequency, color, and consistency of the stool are noted. The nurse inquires about any medication the child may be taking. The parents are asked to define what they mean by constipation. Some children are constipated but pass soft stools every other day or irregularly. If there are no indications of pathology, the nurse begins educating the parents.

Dietary modifications include adding more roughage foods. Foods high in fiber include whole-grain breads and cereals, raw vegetables and fruits, bran, and popcorn for older children. Increasing fluid intake is also important. The physician may suggest an enema as initial therapy, but its continuous use is discouraged because it is intrusive and may not be effective. See Chapter 23 for enema procedure. A stool softener such as docusate sodium (Colace) may be prescribed. Both enemas and stool softeners are intended to be temporary, and this is carefully explained to parents. The child is encouraged to try to move the bowels at the same time each day to establish a routine. The child should not be hurried. Increased exercise may help sedentary children. Shifting the focus away from the problem may be helpful.

# Hirschsprung's Disease (Aganglionic Megacolon)

**Description.** Hirschsprung's disease occurs when there is an absence of ganglionic innervation to the muscle of a segment of the bowel. This usually happens in the lower portion of the sigmoid colon. Because of the absence of nerve cells, there is a lack of normal peristalsis. This results in chronic constipation. Ribbon-like stools are seen as feces pass through the narrow segment. The portion of the bowel nearest to the obstruction dilates, causing abdominal distention (Fig. 28–4). It is seen more often in boys than girls and has familial tendencies. The incidence is approximately 1 in 5000 live births. There is a higher incidence in children with

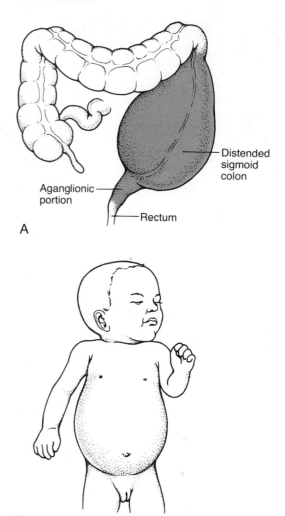

Figure 28–4. *A and B*, Hirschsprung's disease (megacolon). There is no ganglionic nerve innervation or peristalsis in the narrowed section. The adjacent bowel becomes enlarged, causing distention of the abdomen.

Down syndrome. The condition may be acute or chronic.

**Manifestations.** In the newborn, failure to pass meconium stools within 24–48 hours may be a symptom. In the infant, constipation, ribbon-like stools, abdominal distention, anorexia, vomiting, and failure to thrive may be evident. If the patient is untreated, other signs of intestinal obstruction and shock are seen. The development of *enterocolitis* (inflammation of the small bowel and colon) is a serious complication. It may be signaled by fever, explosive stools, and depletion of strength. Diagnostic evaluation usually includes a barium enema and rectal biopsy, which shows a lack of innervation. Anorectal manometry tests the strength of the internal rectal sphincter. In this procedure, a balloon catheter is placed into the rectum, and the pressure exerted against it is measured.

**Treatment and Nursing Care.** Megacolon is treated by surgery. The impaired part of the colon is removed, and an anastomosis of the intestine is performed. In newborns a temporary colostomy may be necessary, and more extensive repair may follow at about age 12–18 months. Closure of the colostomy follows in a few months.

Nursing care is age-dependent. In the newborn, detection is a high priority. As the child grows older, careful attention to a history of constipation and diarrhea is important. Signs of undernutrition, abdominal distention, and poor feedings are suspect.

On occasion when a child is given an enema at home, normal saline—not tap water—is used. Tap water enemas in infants and small children can lead to water intoxication and death. Parents can obtain normal saline solution from the pharmacy without prescription, or they can make it at home by using ½ teaspoon of noniodized salt to 1 cup of lukewarm tap water. The amount of fluid administered should be determined by the health-care provider. The nurse stresses to parents the importance of adding salt to water.

Preoperative assessment of the patient's nutritional, hydration, and serum electrolyte status is important. Oral antibiotics may be administered in conjunction with antibiotic enemas. The abdomen is measured daily at the largest diameter. An accurate record of intake and output is kept. Axillary temperatures prevent further irritation to the rectum. Postoperative assessment following anastomosis includes observation of the nasogastric tube, intravenous infusions, and urinary catheter. Bowel sounds are assessed, as is the presence of flatus and stools. If surgery is a temporary colostomy, the services of the ostomy nurse to educate the family are valuable. Several disposable infant stoma appliances are available to facilitate care.

# Intussusception

**Description.** Intussusception (*intus*, "within," and *suscipere*, "to receive") is a slipping of one part of the intestine into another part just below it (Fig. 28–5). It is frequently seen at the

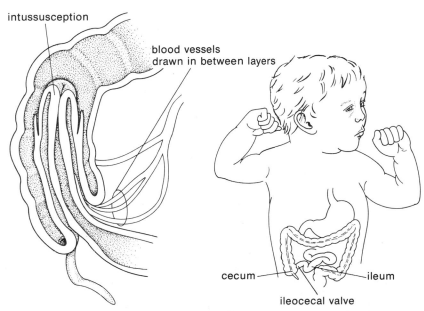

**Figure 28–5.** Intussusception. The most common type begins at or near the ileocecal valve, pushing into the cecum and onto the colon. At first the obstruction is partial, but as the bowel becomes inflamed and edematous, complete obstruction occurs. (From Betz, C., Hunsberger, M., & Wright, S. [1994]. *Family-centered nursing care of children* [2nd ed.]. Philadelphia: W.B. Saunders.)

ileocecal valve, where the small intestine opens into the ascending colon. The *mesentery*, a double fan-shaped fold of peritoneum that covers most of the intestine and is filled with blood vessels and nerves, is also pulled along. Edema occurs. At first this telescoping of the bowel causes intestinal obstruction, but as peristalsis forces the structures more tightly, strangulation takes place. This portion may burst, causing peritonitis.

Intussusception generally occurs in boys between 3 months and 6 years of age who are otherwise healthy. Its frequency decreases after 36 months of age (Behrman, 1992). The exact cause is still in question. Predisposing factors, such as a correlation with adenovirus, acute enteritis, Meckel's diverticulum (see p. 758), polyps, cysts, or lymphosarcoma, have been cited. Occasionally the condition corrects itself without treatment. This is termed a spontaneous reduction. However, because the patient's life is in danger, the doctor does not waste time waiting for this to occur. The prognosis is good when the patient is treated within 24 hours.

**Manifestations.** In typical cases, the onset is sudden. The infant feels severe pain in the abdomen, evidenced by loud cries, straining efforts, and kicking and drawing of the legs toward the abdomen. At first there is comfort between pains, but the intervals shorten and the condition becomes worse. The child vomits. The stomach contents are green or greenish-yellow; this is due to bile stain, and the contents are described as bilious. If the condition is left untreated, fecal vomiting ensues. Bowel movements diminish, and little flatus is passed. Movements of blood and mucus that contain no feces are common about 12 hours after the onset of the obstruction; these are termed *currant jelly stools*. The child's fever may run as high as 106°F (41.1°C), and signs of shock, such as sweating, weak pulse, and shallow, grunting respirations, are evident. The abdomen is rigid.

**Treatment.** Intussusception is an *emergency*, and because of the severity of symptoms, most parents contact a doctor promptly. The diagnosis is determined by the history and physical findings. The doctor may feel a sausage-shaped mass in the right upper portion of the abdomen during bimanual rectal and abdominal palpation. Abdominal films also may indicate the mass. A barium enema is the treatment of choice, with surgery scheduled if reduction is not achieved. The recurrence rate following barium enema re-

duction is about 10%; therefore, the child is held for observation following treatment.

During the operation, a small incision is made into the abdomen, and the wayward intestine is "milked" back into position. The intestine is inspected for gangrene, and if all is well, the abdomen is sutured. Barring complications, recovery is straightforward. If the intestine cannot be reduced or if gangrene has set in, a resection is done and the affected bowel is removed. The cut end of the ileum is joined to the cut end of the colon; this is called an *anastomosis*.

### Nursing Care

*Preoperative Care.* The patient is admitted to the hospital for procedures done to prepare for surgery and to prevent postoperative complications. Treatment is aimed at combating shock and restoring blood, fluids, and electrolytes. The doctor or charge nurse obtains written consent for surgery from the parents or guardians. It is wise for the admitting nurse to confirm this by checking the appropriate sheet in the patient's chart. This procedure takes on even greater importance in emergencies.

Gastric suction is necessary to prevent stomach distention. It may be continued for some time following surgery, particularly if a resection is done. The nurse applies elbow restraints to the patient in order to prevent dislodging of the nasal tube, if this has not already been done for intravenous therapy. The child's identification band is checked to ensure that it is secure. Voidings before surgery are recorded. Preoperative medication is given to relax the patient and to prevent the aspiration of secretions. Once the child has been medicated, activity should be kept at a minimum. En route to the operating room, the patient is covered with a light cotton blanket. The medical record accompanies the child. Proper safety precautions are taken during transit. The parents might appreciate the services of the mental health clinician at this time.

*Postoperative Care.* Following surgery, care is mainly symptomatic. Vital signs are checked frequently, the child's position is changed often, and careful attention is given to the skin. Mouth care is essential, as the patient will receive little or nothing by mouth for a while. The nostrils require cleaning and lubricating, as the nasal tube can be irritating. If a urinary catheter has been inserted in the operating room, it is observed for kinks that could hamper flow of urine. The drainage from the catheter is measured and described in the nurses' notes. The operative site is kept clean and dry. The nurse promptly reports any odor from the incision and is alert for abdominal distention. Clear fluids are given when bowel sounds are heard. The passage of gas, liquids, or solids through the rectum is of particular significance, as it indicates peristalsis.

As in all nursing care, the patient and family are given support throughout this ordeal. A pacifier may soothe the young child who is deprived of feeding by mouth. Some of these patients are at an age when fear of strangers is prevalent; thus, their need for the security of the parents is paramount. Parents need assurance that their child is in good hands and that their presence is not a hindrance to the hospital staff.

# Appendicitis

**Description.** Appendicitis occurs when the opening of the appendix into the cecum becomes obstructed. This may be due to a number of conditions: fecaliths (blockage by fecal matter), infection, or allergy. Diet has also been implicated. Appendicitis is rare in children younger than 2 years of age, but it is the most common cause of abdominal surgery during childhood. The incidence is higher among boys.

**Manifestations.** The symptoms in older children are similar to those in adults and include nausea, vomiting, abdominal tenderness, fever, constipation or diarrhea, and elevated blood count. Pain, which is initially about the umbilicus, localizes in the right lower quadrant, midway between the umbilicus and the iliac crest (the McBurney point). Absent or diminished bowel sounds and rigid abdomen are also indicative of appendicitis. Rectal examination elicits evidence of tenderness. Diarrhea may be present in retrocecal appendicitis. A chest film may be ordered to rule out lower-lobe pneumonia, which sometimes mimics appendicitis. A careful history and physical examination are paramount. The presence of vomiting and the degree of change in the child's behavior are considered particularly significant. The child may "guard" the abdomen or voluntarily lie down. One position frequently seen in the child with pain of appendicitis is lying on the side with the knees flexed toward the abdomen.

The symptoms of appendicitis in the young child are more obscure. The diagnosis requires carefully observing the patient over a period of time. The child cries and is restless. There is low-grade fever. Pain is more generalized and harder to pinpoint, and nausea and vomiting may occur. Because these symptoms are indicative of many childhood upsets, the diagnosis is more difficult to establish than in adolescents or adults.

**Treatment.** The patient with appendicitis is treated by a surgical operation called an appendectomy. This is performed soon after diagnosis unless the child is dehydrated. Antibiotics may be given preoperatively if the appendix has ruptured. *Heat is never applied, as it might cause a rupture, leading to the possibility of peritonitis.*

Oral fluids and feedings are withheld pending surgery. As in other emergency situations, the nurse gives emotional support to the patient and family. Cathartics are withheld when a patient has abdominal pain in order to prevent rupture of the appendix. The prognosis for the child with uncomplicated appendicitis is good.

**Nursing Care.** A recovery bed is prepared to receive the child on return to the unit. The furniture is arranged so that the stretcher can easily be wheeled to the bedside. The bed should be equipped with side rails. An emesis basin and tissues are placed on the bedside table, and an intravenous pole is brought into the room. The patient is gently transferred from the stretcher to the bed. Temperature, pulse, respiration, and blood pressure are taken on arrival, and the dressing is observed for drainage. If an intravenous line is running, the type, amount, and rate are observed. The nurse records observations, including the time the patient arrived on the unit, the state of consciousness (e.g., alert, groggy), the presence of nausea or vomiting, and the appearance of any drainage. The student nurse reports to the team leader or head nurse in order to review the postoperative orders left by the physician.

During the course of the day, the following nursing measures are carried out. The patient's position is changed frequently. The patient is taught to take deep breaths and to cough. The hands and face are washed, and the patient is assisted in putting on a clean gown. An accurate record of intake and output is kept. The nurse reports the first voiding to the head nurse. If the child has not voided during the shift, the nurse should report this too. The physician's orders will indicate whether or not the child with nausea may have sips of water or ice chips.

As soon as the child is able to take and retain

water and other fluids by mouth, intravenous feedings are discontinued. Vital signs and bowel sounds are monitored as ordered or according to institution policies. The patient is encouraged to move about in bed; reluctance to move and anorexia may be early signs of complications. Evidence of pain is reported, and analgesics are administered as ordered.

Pediatric patients recuperate quickly from uncomplicated surgery. Ambulation is generally not a problem. Children can usually return to school in 1 or 2 weeks, but specific instructions about restriction of activity should be reviewed before hospital discharge.

**Ruptured Appendix.** Early recognition of appendicitis decreases the danger of perforation. Because diagnosis in children is difficult, the nurse may come in contact with more patients with a ruptured appendix in the pediatric unit than in adult divisions. In addition, the body systems of a child are less mature; thus, the condition progresses rapidly. Parents may also be confused by the symptoms and hesitate to obtain medical attention. If the appendix ruptures, the infected contents spill into the abdominal cavity, and a generalized infection called *peritonitis* results. It is often seen in younger children. Progression is rapid because the child's omentum is smaller and less effective in localizing the infection. In the older child, a walled-off abscess may occur. Accessory organs of the digestive tract and the reproductive organs may also become infected. The child is acutely ill, and the recovery period prolonged.

***Preoperative Care.*** Medical management to prevent shock, dehydration, and infection is instituted. This usually includes intravenous administration of fluids and electrolytes, blood volume replacement with plasma or albumin, systemic antibiotics, oxygen, nasogastric suctioning, and positioning in the semi-Fowler position to facilitate drainage into the pelvic area. The patient is given nothing by mouth. Intermittent suction is maintained at appropriate negative pressure, and irrigations are carried out as ordered to ensure patency of the tube. When a perforated appendix is suspected, triple antibiotic therapy of gentamicin, ampicillin, and clindamycin or cefoxitin may be ordered (Behrman, 1992).

***Postoperative Care.*** Penrose drains are placed in the incision to drain exudate or abscess. Care is taken not to dislodge drains while changing soiled dressings. Wound precautions are instituted according to universal precau-

## Nursing Brief

In explaining sterile dressings to children, use the term *bandage*, which may be more easily understood.

tions and hospital procedure. The area about the drains is kept clean and dry. The semi-Fowler position reduces the spread of infection. Analgesics are administered for pain relief. Intake, output, and bowel sounds are monitored. Nutritious foods are supplied as the diet is increased. Nursing care is given as described for the child with simple appendicitis, including appropriate modifications and interventions in nursing care plans.

## Meckel's Diverticulum

**Description.** During fetal life the intestine is attached to the yolk sac by the vitelline duct. If this duct fails to disappear completely, a small blind pouch may form. This condition is termed Meckel's diverticulum (Fig. 28–6). It usually occurs near the ileocecal valve. It may be connected to the umbilicus by a cord. A fistula may also form. This sac is subject to inflammation, much like the appendix. This disorder is the most common congenital malformation of the gastrointestinal tract. It is seen more frequently in boys.

**Manifestations.** Symptoms may occur at any age but appear most often before age 2. Painless bleeding from the rectum is the most common sign. Bright-red or dark-red blood is more usual than tarry stools. Abdominal pain may or may not be present. In some persons it may exist without causing symptoms. Sometimes this condition can predispose one to an intussusception. Barium enema and radionuclide scintigraphy are useful in diagnosing Meckel's diverticulum. X-ray films are not helpful because the pouch is so small it may not appear on the screen.

**Treatment and Nursing Care.** The diverticulum is removed by surgery. Nursing care is the same as for the patient undergoing exploration of the abdomen. Because this condition appears suddenly and bleeding causes parental anxiety, emotional support is of particular importance.

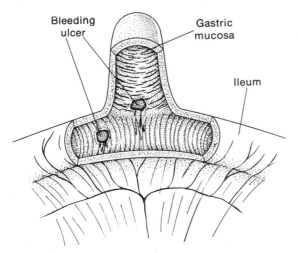

**Figure 28–6.** Meckel's diverticulum is a congenital anomaly characterized by an outpouching of the ileum. (From Betz, C., Hunsberger, M., & Wright, S. [1994]. *Family-centered nursing care of children* [2nd ed.]. Philadelphia: W.B. Saunders.)

# Inguinal Hernia

**Description.** An inguinal hernia is a protrusion of part of the abdominal contents through the inguinal canal in the groin. It is more common in boys than in girls. It is also seen frequently in preterm infants. Hernias may be present at birth (congenital) or may be acquired, and they can vary in size. A hernia is termed reducible if it can be put back into place by gentle pressure; if this cannot be done, it is called an irreducible or an incarcerated (constricted) hernia. Incarceration occurs more often in infants under 10 months of age. Hernias may be bilateral.

**Manifestations.** The infant with a hernia may be relatively free of symptoms. Irritability, fretfulness, and constipation are sometimes evident. The diagnosis is made when physical examination shows a mass in the inguinal area that reappears from time to time, particularly when the child cries or strains. A *strangulated* hernia occurs when the intestine becomes caught in the passage and the blood supply is diminished. This happens more frequently during the first 6 months of life. Vomiting and severe abdominal pain are present. Emergency surgery is necessary if strangulation occurs, and in some cases a bowel resection is performed.

**Treatment and Nursing Care.** Inguinal hernias are successfully repaired by the surgical operation called a herniorrhaphy. This is a relatively simple procedure that is tolerated well by the child. Most patients are scheduled for same-day surgery units. The benefits of this method are both economic and psychological. Parents are instructed to bring the fasting child to the hospital about 1 hour before surgery. Parents remain with the child during the entire time except during the actual procedure. They are encouraged to assist in routine postoperative care if they choose.

Often no dressing is applied to the wound. Sometimes a waterproof collodion dressing, which looks like clear nail polish, is applied. Postoperative care is directed toward keeping the wound clean. Diapers are left open for this purpose. Wet diapers are changed frequently. The circulation in the leg below the site of the hernia is assessed, as edema of the groin may compress blood vessels.

The child is discharged in about 2–3 hours, when fluids are tolerated. Sponge baths for 1 week are suggested. Activity is not limited. Parents are provided with written instructions as to home management. Follow-up telephone calls are made by nursing personnel, and return appointments are scheduled.

Patients who experience incarcerated hernias are hospitalized. Following surgery, vital signs are carefully monitored. Nasogastric suctioning and intravenous fluids are maintained until bowel function returns. The nurse measures and records the patient's intake and output. The patient's gown and linen are changed when necessary. The patient is turned frequently in order to avoid respiratory complications. The nurse carefully observes the child for signs of peritonitis or bowel obstruction.

# Umbilical Hernia

**Description.** An umbilical hernia is a protrusion of a portion of intestine through the umbilical ring (an opening in the muscular area of the abdomen through which the umbilical vessels pass) (Fig. 28–7). This type of hernia appears as a soft swelling covered by skin, which protrudes when the infant cries or strains. Most of the small umbilical hernias disappear spontaneously during the 1st year of life.

**Treatment.** The treatment of the patient with an umbilical hernia is controversial. In general, surgery is not advised unless the hernia causes symptoms, becomes enlarged, or persists until the child is 3–5 years of age.

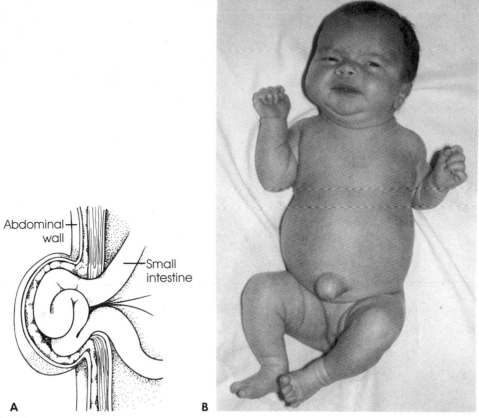

**Figure 28–7.** *A*, Diagrammatic representation of an umbilical hernia. *B*, Infant with an umbilical hernia. (From Marlow, D.R., & Redding, B.A. [1988]. *Textbook of pediatric nursing* [6th ed.]. Philadelphia: W.B. Saunders.)

# Obesity

**Description.** Obesity, or overnutrition, is the accumulation of excess body fat. It is the most common nutritional disorder in Western society today, and its treatment record is dismal. Obesity is difficult to define during adolescence because of height and age variations within this age group. Some definitions include the criteria of body weight 20% or more over ideal body weight based on weight tables and triceps skin folds exceeding 85% (Behrman, 1992). The problem with weight-for-age or weight-for-height measurements is that they do not distinguish the truly fat child from the child whose weight is increased because of increased lean body mass, as in a very muscular or a very tall child with advanced skeletal development. An increase in lean body mass and fat is characteristic of this age group; therefore, one must know the teenager's stage of puberty and whether or not growth is completed.

Weight gain may occur at any age but appears most frequently during the 1st year of life, at 5–6 years of age, and during adolescence. Most children stay plump during puberty and then return to a normal weight.

**Self-Concept.** Obesity is particularly troublesome for school children and adolescents, when feelings of inadequacy are pronounced. Obese children are concerned about their appearance but are unable to conform to the standards of the group. They are often the subject of cruel ridicule. For instance, fat boys frequently appear to have developed breasts, white striae may appear on the abdomen, and the penis appears disproportionately small. Obese teenagers date less often and may feel rejected, unattractive, and unloved. Accompanying the mental anxieties are the more obvious physical handicaps. They may be unable to participate in sports or other school activities and are more accident-prone. Their choice of careers is more limited. They may find it difficult to obtain youthful-looking clothes.

**Causes.** There are many theories about the causes of obesity. In reality the etiology is complex. The onset of obesity can be traced to excess food or reduced physical activity, or both. Contrary to popular belief, obesity due to abnormal function of the glands is rare. Genetic studies show an increased incidence of obesity in twins, even if they are raised in separate homes. Children born to obese parents are more likely to become obese. However, environmental factors such as ethnic diet, family eating practices, and psychological factors also operate and are difficult to isolate from genetic factors. The prevalence of obesity in childhood is difficult to ascertain, but it appears that 5–15% of infants and preschoolers and 10–35% of adolescents are obese. The prevalence is greater in adolescent females and in disadvantaged groups (Levine, Carey, & Crocker, 1992).

**Prevention.** The prevention of obesity in children is a matter of great importance. The earlier in life this begins, the better the outcome will be. The infant or child at risk must be identified while still under parental control and before eating and activity patterns are firmly established. Breast feeding is desirable for infants, in that sufficient quantities of milk are obtained and there is less chance of overfeeding. Mothers are informed that a baby's food requirements diminish greatly because growth slows at about the 1st year. Overfeeding should be discouraged, as *fat babies are not necessarily healthy babies*. Parents should foster activities that promote freedom of movement and exercise during the first few years of life. Any questions about weight gain are voiced during well-baby conferences.

During the school years, nutritious snacks, rather than junk foods, are kept in the home. TV viewing should be restricted, and walking and other exercise encouraged. Parents need to promote participation in a regular exercise program. Sound nutritional practices are of particular importance during puberty, when there is an increase in fat cells. The teenager is capable of assuming responsibility for what she or he eats. If a weight problem exists at this time, realize that unlike for adults, "a reasonable goal is not always weight loss but may be just a slowing down of the weight gain or mainte-

nance of body weight until linear growth occurs" (Neuman & Jenks, 1992).

Helping obese children to feel good about themselves by encouragement, praise, and support is essential. The depressed young person may turn toward food as an outlet for emotions. One should be generous and specific with praise. Conversation can be sprinkled with such comments as "I knew you could do it"; "That's quite an improvement"; "You make it look easy"; "I couldn't have done better myself." A positive approach may help children or young persons to feel better about themselves and decrease the need to overeat. Parents who eat properly are good role models.

**Treatment and Nursing Care.** Weight reduction is difficult. When the problem begins in early childhood, a person is faced with a lifetime of fighting calories. This is complicated by the ready availability of food in the United States and advertisers' bombardment of the public with tempting treats. Many obese children have obese parents. Parents must be keenly interested in helping their child lose weight if the diet is to be successful. Sometimes it is necessary for the entire family to go without some of the richer dishes. They should refrain from buying cookies and cakes, and fresh fruits should be substituted as between-meal snacks. The nurse emphasizes that food plans must be nutritious. Adolescents are apt to invent diets that are dangerous to their health. The great satisfaction of eating must be replaced with something equally satisfying and rewarding, such as new social activities, hobbies, friends, or sports.

Behavior modification techniques show promise, although their long-term value is not yet established. This approach helps a person identify and control poor eating patterns. Such techniques include eating only at the table, using a smaller plate, eating only at specific times, and recording food intake and feelings at the time of eating. A point system or system of rewards is established on initiation of this technique. Support groups, such as Weight Watchers, Overeaters Anonymous, or diet workshops, although helpful, consist mostly of adults. A few parents accompany their teenagers and participate themselves, which is to be commended.

Support groups for adolescents are more acceptable. These are usually found in teenage clinics, schools, and specialized summer camps. Diet pills are not recommended. Their long-

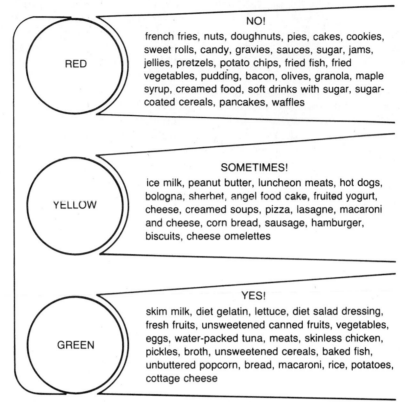

**Figure 28–8.** The "traffic light" theme helps adolescents become aware of their eating patterns. (From Cecere, M.E. [1983]. PIP [Positive Image Program]: A group approach for obese adolescents [questionnaire]. *Nursing Clinics of North America*, *18*, 254.)

term effectiveness is minimal, and the potential for misuse is great. At this time, surgery such as gastric stapling is reserved for the seriously obese youngster. Other techniques, such as jejunoileal bypass, are subject to many complications and are seldom advised. The long-term consequences of these procedures have yet to be established.

The nurse interested in helping children in weight reduction can play an important role. Many nurses are or have been personally involved with losing weight and know how frustrating it can be. Motivating others requires ingenuity and patience (Fig. 28–8). A sense of hope must be instilled. The nurse involves the individual and tries to recognize achievements and increase self-esteem. The dignity of the individual should always be foremost. Family therapy may be necessary in order to alleviate tension and promote understanding; nurses can assist in the referral process, including referral to a registered nutritionist.

## Anorexia Nervosa

**Description.** Anorexia nervosa (*anorexia*, "want of appetite," and *nervosa*, "nervous") is a form of self-starvation seen mostly in girls of age 10–25, with a mean age of 13.75 years (Neinstein, 1984). The criteria for this disorder are well outlined in the *Diagnostic and Statistical Manual of Mental Disorders* (DSM-III R). It is characterized by severe weight loss and an intense fear of obesity. The incidence of anorexia nervosa and bulimia has increased over the last 2 decades (Behrman, 1992). The disorder was first described in 1689 but was not widely recognized until 1873. Its name is somewhat misleading because many patients do not suffer from a lack of appetite. Instead they experience intense hunger, which they deny or they satisfy during eating binges.

The etiology of anorexia nervosa is unclear. There appears to be a combination of factors, including psychosomatic disorders, dysfunctional family life, societal influences, and genetics. Endocrine abnormalities are also under investigation. Patients with anorexia were thought to come from model middle- to upper-class families. However, it is now appearing in lower socioeconomic levels and in a variety of ethnic and racial groups (Behrman, 1992). It is seen in boys and young men but much less frequently than in girls and women. The patients have average to superior intelligence and are generally overachievers who expect to be perfect in all areas. For young people with the disorder, their own emerging sexuality is very threatening. They experience anxiety and guilt over imagined or real fear of intimacy.

It has been suggested that families of these young people are dysfunctional. They may exhibit such behaviors as overprotectiveness, rigidity, lack of privacy, and inability to resolve conflicts. In addition, the patient's illness may serve to maintain family balance, as the parents focus on the needs of the child and thus avoid other internal and relationship conflicts.

**Manifestations.** The primary symptom of anorexia nervosa is severe weight loss. However, early symptoms may be ambiguous. Nevertheless, the patient has much energy and may exercise strenuously in order to reduce weight. The onset can often be pinpointed to the young girl's inability to wear some of her clothes or to life changes, such as a move, parental divorce, or death of a relative or close friend. On physical examination, some of the following conditions may be evident: dry skin, amenorrhea, lanugo hair over the back and extremities, cold intolerance, low blood pressure, abdominal pain, and constipation. Persistent vomiting can cause erosion of the enamel of the teeth and eventually tooth decay and loss of the teeth. Electrolyte imbalance may be noticeable in the patient who induces vomiting or uses laxatives or diuretics.

Teenagers with anorexia experience feelings of helplessness, lack of control, low self-esteem, and depression. Socialization with peers diminishes. Mealtime becomes a family battleground. The patient feels guilty and may go on an eating binge, which is followed by self-induced vomiting as the fear of gaining weight returns. The body image becomes increasingly disturbed (Fig. 28–9), and there is a lack of self-identity. The young person remains egocentric and unable to complete normal adolescent tasks. The relentless pursuit to be thin may lead to shoplifting of laxatives and other associ-

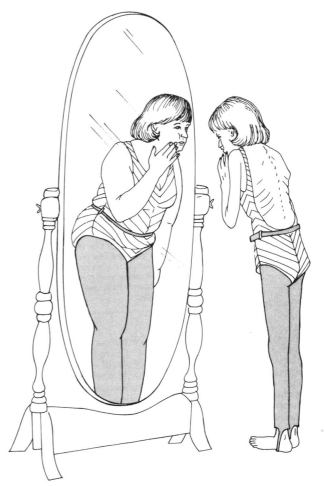

**Figure 28–9.** Patients with eating disorders often have a disturbance in self-image.

ated items. Although eating less, the anorexic individual is preoccupied with food and its preparation. Hunger is denied. The patient complains of bloating and abdominal pain after ingesting small amounts of food.

**Treatment and Nursing Care.** The treatment of anorexia nervosa is complex and involves several modalities. Some hospitals have eating disorder units. A brief period of hospitalization may be necessary in order to correct electrolyte imbalance, establish minimum restoration of nutrients, and stabilize the patient's weight. It also provides "time out" from a dysfunctional home environment.

Therapies include individual and family psychotherapy, behavioral therapy, and pharmacologic therapy. Hyperalimentation may be required in severe cases. Antidepressant medications are a more recent addition to therapy. The nurse plays an important role in ensuring that the atmosphere is relaxed and nonpunitive. Follow-up after discharge from the unit is essential. Individual and family therapy are continued.

Nurses working with adolescents in any capacity need to be alert to the symptoms of this disease, a lack of recognition is one of the biggest obstacles to treatment. In the early stages, dissatisfaction with body image, amenorrhea, and social isolation are suspect. Young people need to be educated abut the seriousness of the disorder. Educational materials, referral sources, and counseling are available from the National Association of Anorexia Nervosa and Associated Disorders. Encouragement and support from self-help groups are also valuable.

**Prognosis.** Most patients gain weight in the hospital, regardless of the type of therapy. This may not, however, predict future success. Complications include gastritis, cardiac arrhythmias, inflammation of the intestine, and kidney problems. Fatalities do occur, particularly in untreated persons. Both anorexia and bulimia are chronic disorders; therefore, periods of relapse and remission are to be anticipated.

## Bulimia

Bulimia, or compulsive eating, is recognized by the Diagnostic and Statistical Manual of Mental Disorders as a separate eating disorder. It has been estimated that as many as 20% of college women have this condition (Krause & Mahan, 1992). Bulimics binge periodically, usually on easily accessible high-calorie food items. These episodes are generally carried out in private. They may be followed by self-induced vomiting or the use of cathartics. The person is aware that the eating is out of control. Binging periods are followed by feelings of dejection, guilt, and self-deprecation. Table 28–2 presents a comparison summary of anorexia and bulimia. The principles of nursing care are similar to those mentioned for the anorexic patient.

## Acetaminophen Poisoning

Acetaminophen overdose is listed along with other poisons commonly encountered in pediatrics in Box 28 1.

**Description.** Acetaminophen (Tylenol) has now replaced aspirin as the most commonly ingested drug that causes toxicity. This is because it is so widely used and because aspirin associated with Reye's syndrome is no longer recommended for fever in children with flu-like symptoms. Acetaminophen poisoning occurs mainly from acute overdose rather than from the cumulative effects seen with aspirin. Because acetetaminophen is metabolized in the liver, overdose results in hepatic destruction. With early treatment most children recover without complications. Adolescents have a higher incidence of toxicity than do younger children (Behrman, 1992).

**Manifestations.** Four stages of toxicity are seen in untreated acetaminophen poisoning. Within 30 minutes to 24 hours, anorexia, nausea, vomiting, and sweating appear. In the second stage (24–48 hours), these symptoms resolve and the patient's condition appears to improve, but there may be upper-quadrant abdominal pain, oliguria, and elevated liver enzymes. In the third stage (72–96 hours), the liver becomes seriously affected and associated jaundice, pain in right upper quadrant, confusion, and general malaise are seen. In the final stage, from 4 days to 2 weeks, recovery takes

**Table 28–2.** COMPARISON OF ANOREXIA NERVOSA AND BULIMIA

| Factor | Anorexia Nervosa | Bulimia |
|---|---|---|
| Age range | 10–25 yr (mean, 13 yr) | Older (average 18 yr) |
| Weight | Fear of normal weight | Many are of normal weight or overweight prior to onset, wider weight fluctuations |
| Impulse control | Normal to slight variations | More prone to substance abuse, shoplifting |
| Vomiting | Varies | More prevalent |
| Starvation | Yes | Seldom |
| Severity | More severe | Usually not as devastating |

| BOX 28–1 | **Poisons Commonly Encountered in Pediatrics** |
|---|---|

**Acids**

Toilet bowl cleaners
Swimming pool pH adjustment solutions
Concentrated acids in hardware and paint stores

**Alkalines**

Clinitest tablets
Drain-cleaning crystals
Dishwasher soaps
Industrial cleaners (brought home in unlabeled containers)

**Medications**

Diet pills
Sleeping pills
Sedatives
Cold remedies
Birth control pills
Vitamin supplements, iron
Diarrhea remedies (Lomotil)
Menstrual pain relievers
Antipyretics (aspirin, acetaminophen)
Oil of wintergreen

**Cyanide**

Pesticides
Metal polishes
Photographic solutions
Fumigating products

**Ethanol**

Alcoholic beverages
Cold remedies
Perfumes
Mouthwashes
Aftershave lotions

**Petroleum Distillates**

Heavy greases, oils
Turpentine
Furniture polishes
Gasoline, kerosene
Lighter fluid

**Insecticides**

Home gardening products
Recently sprayed lawns

**Carbon Monoxide**

Accidental
Suicidal

**Lead**

Paint
Air
Food
Ant poison
Unglazed pottery
Colored newsprint
Curtain weights
Fishing sinkers
Lead water pipes
Acid juices in leaded pottery

**Arthropods, Insect Stings**

Spiders (brown recluse, black widow)
Certain scorpions
Insects (bees, wasps, hornets)

**Snakes**

Rattlesnakes
Moccasins
Copperheads
Others

**Poisonous Plants**

Boston ivy
Split-leaf philodendron
Umbrella plant
Azalea
Daffodil
Foxglove
Mistletoe
Tulip
Others

place unless fatality occurs. Manifestations and treatment modalities that the nurse might anticipate in patients with acute poisoning are shown in Box 28–2.

**Treatment and Nursing Care.** The stomach is emptied by lavage or induced emesis from syrup of ipecac. Depending on the serum aceta-

minophen level, this may be followed by the N-acetylcysteine (Mucomyst) antidote. In small children, it may be administered directly into the nasogastric tube following lavage. Otherwise it is generally given orally every 4 hours for 72 hours. This medicine has a bad smell and taste and the patient needs coaxing and sup-

| BOX 28–2 | **Nursing Alert for Poisoning** |
| --- | --- |

**Anticipate:**

Emptying (lavage, ipecac, activated charcoal)
Central nervous system: restlessness, agitation, seizures, coma
Respiratory: airway obstruction, hypoventilation, hypoxia, oxygen therapy, respiratory arrest, cardiopulmonary resuscitation (keep artificial airway handy), chemical pneumonitis
Cardiovascular: difficulties with electrolytes, blood urea nitrogen, creatinine, glucose; need for electrocardiogram monitor
Gastrointestinal: difficulty swallowing, abdominal pain, possible gastrostomy
Kidneys: urine specific gravity, intake and output, intravenous tubes
Methods to increase elimination: cathartic, forced diuresis, dialysis, hemoperfusion
Hypo- or hyperthermia: sponge baths, cooling blanket
Child: physical and psychological crises
Parents: guilt, anger, family dysfunction

port to assist with compliance. The medicine may be mixed with a soft drink or juice. If the patient is admitted to the hospital, the nurse records vital signs and intake and output. Jaundice and tenderness of the liver are assessed. Liver enzymes (SGOT and SGPT) are monitored. Prevention of overdose is of utmost importance. Even in uncomplicated cases, the child is subject to unpleasant, stressful procedures. Because parents are often informed that acetaminophen is "safer" than aspirin, they may be more careless in storing it.

## Salicylate Poisoning

**Description.** Aspirin (acetylsalicylic acid) poisoning is seen less frequently than in the past because of safety packaging and the increase in use of acetaminophen. Nevertheless, aspirin is often used in most homes and may be stored carelessly on bedside stands or in mother's purse. This drug acts rapidly but is excreted slowly. Ingestion of 150 mg/kg causes symptoms. Although most cases of aspirin poisoning are emergencies, a child may unknowingly be poisoned by aspirin's cumulative effect. The use of several aspirin-containing products at once, for example, over-the-counter cold remedies and aspirin, can be hazardous. Time-release aspirin is especially dangerous, because the symptoms of poisoning are delayed and aspiration of the stomach is of little avail. It is wise, therefore, to read labels carefully and to administer aspirin sparingly. It is even better to use it only under a physician's direction.

Oil of wintergreen (methyl salicylate) is also extremely hazardous when mistakenly administered as cough medicine or swallowed by the curious child. It is sometimes used as a home remedy for arthritic pain. Even a dose as small as 1 teaspoon can cause a child's death.

**Manifestations.** The symptoms of salicylate poisoning are varied. The peak action occurs about 2–4 hours after a single toxic dose. *In general, the younger the child, the more serious is the overdose.* Mild poisoning may consist of ringing in the ears, dizziness, anorexia, sweating, nausea, vomiting, and diarrhea. Hyperpnea (*hyper*, "above," and *pnea*, "breathing") is an early symptom of more serious trouble. The patient's respirations are faster and deeper than usual, much like the breathing after exercise. This change occurs because the respiratory center is stimulated by the drug. When carbon dioxide is eliminated, respiratory alkalosis quickly follows. Dehydration, metabolic acidosis, high fever, convulsions, and coma may ensue. Bleeding is sometimes seen because excessive levels of aspirin inhibit the formation of prothrombin, which is necessary for normal blood clotting. Hypokalemia often accompanies this condition because salicylates directly affect the renal tubular mechanism.

**Treatment and Nursing Care.** There is no specific antidote for salicylate poisoning; therefore, treatment is aimed at relieving the patient's symptoms. In mild cases of poisoning, the drug is discontinued and fluids are forced. When a child has swallowed an unspecified amount, gastric lavage is performed. A blood sample is taken in order to detect the level of poisoning. A positive ferric chloride urine test result is highly indicative of poisoning. The doctor may request that the child be admitted to the hospital for observation. A sponge bath may be given in order to reduce fever. The patient's vital signs are closely observed and recorded. The nurse also determines the pH of the urine. When intravenous fluids are necessary to correct electrolyte imbalance and rid the body of toxins, the child's intake and output of fluid are charted hourly.

Vitamin K is administered to control bleeding. Peritoneal dialysis (*peritoneum* and *dialysis*, "passing of a solute through a membrane") is a therapeutic measure used in acute renal failure. The therapy utilizes the principles of osmosis and diffusion through the semipermeable peritoneal membrane, with the purpose of removing toxic substances from the blood. The artificial kidney is another method used for essentially the same purpose. An exchange transfusion may also be given. In cases of severe poisoning, the latter procedures are executed in an attempt to save the life of the child.

The nurse must realize the danger of drug poisoning and must constantly practice and teach safety measures to prevent tragedies. Treatment, utility rooms, and drug baskets are scrutinized to ensure that nothing harmful is within reach of ambulatory patients.

## Lead Poisoning (Plumbism)

**Description.** Lead poisoning results when a child repeatedly ingests or absorbs substances containing lead. The primary source is paint from old, deteriorating buildings. Lead contents of food, water, and air have decreased substantially during the past decade. Lead poisoning is most common in children between the ages of $1\frac{1}{2}$ and 3 years. The incidence is increased in tenement areas of large cities. Although the incidence is highest among the poor, lead poisoning is also found among suburban and middle-class children. It is more common during the summer months.

The patients chew on windowsills and stair rails. They ingest flakes of paint, putty, or crumbled plaster. Food, particularly fruit juices consumed from improperly glazed earthenware, is another source. Lead poisoning among Mexican Americans may be due to azarcon, a bright-orange powder containing approximately 93.5% lead. Azarcon is used as a folk remedy to treat empacho and other digestive problems in infants. Lead poisoning among Hmong Laotian refugees may be due to Paylooah, a bright orange-red powder, which may be used for fever or rash. Unwashed fresh fruit sprayed with insecticides and dust from enclosed shooting galleries are also culprits. Lead intoxication from retained bullets has been reported. Another source is dust in homes near lead processing plants or lead dust on the clothes of working parents.

Lead can have a lasting effect on the nervous system, especially the brain. The incidence is high among siblings of an affected child, and recurrence is common. Mental retardation may occur in severe cases. In much of the United States, lead poisoning is a reportable disease. The Agency for Toxic Substances and Diseases Registry (ATSDR) provides information on this condition.

**Manifestations.** The symptoms occur gradually and range from mild to severe. Because the infant's or young child's central nervous system is extremely vulnerable, acute symptoms of encephalitis may follow a relatively short period of exposure. The lead settles in the soft tissues and bones and is excreted in the urine. In the beginning, weakness, weight loss, anorexia, pallor, irritability, vomiting, abdominal pain, and constipation may be seen. In the later stages, signs of anemia and nervous system involvement—muscular incoordination, neuritis, convulsions, and encephalitis—are seen.

**Treatment, Nursing Care, and Education of Parents.** Blood and urine tests are performed in order to determine the amount of lead in the system. Lead is especially toxic to the synthesis of *heme* in the blood; heme is necessary for hemoglobin formation and for functioning of renal tubules. Blood lead levels are the primary screening test gradually replacing the free erythrocyte protoporphyrin test as a definitive diagnostic tool. X-ray films of the long bones show further deposits of lead. The history of the patient may reveal *pica*. This is a condition in which the child has a distorted appetite and eats a variety of things that most persons consider unpalatable, such as sand, grass, wool, glass, plaster, coal, animal droppings, and paint from furniture. This tendency is sometimes seen in neurotic children and is common in mentally retarded children. An underlying nutritional disturbance and family dysfunction may also account for it.

Treatment is aimed at reducing the concentration of lead in the tissues and blood. First, the child is removed from the source of lead and is closely supervised. The entire family should be tested, especially any pregnant members, as the fetus is especially sensitive to lead. In children with mild cases, periodic rescreening may

| NURSING CARE PLAN 28–2 | | |
| --- | --- | --- |
| **Selected Nursing Diagnoses for the Child with Lead Poisoning** | | |
| **Goals** | **Nursing Interventions** | **Rationale** |
| **Nursing Diagnosis:** Pain related to multiple injections. | | |
| Child experiences minimal pain as evidenced by vocalization, facial expression, and body language<br>Child engages in play and sleeps well | 1. Prepare child for injection through needle play; anticipate frustration and anger<br>2. Rotate sites of injection; when an intravenous route cannot be used chelation therapy is given intramuscularly into a large muscle mass<br>3. Move painful areas slowly and gently | 1. Preparation reduces anxiety levels, helps patient feel more in control<br>2. Rotation of sites prevents formation of painful fibrotic areas; EDTA is so painful that physician may order combining local anesthetic procaine with the drug; it is drawn into syringe last so that it enters child first |
| **Nursing Diagnosis:** Knowledge deficit (parents) related to the dangers of lead ingestion. | | |
| Parents can list the environmental sources of lead<br>Parents verbalize early symptoms of poisoning | 1. Obtain a careful history concentrating on possible exposure to lead<br>2. Discuss common environmental sources of lead: peeling paint from dilapidated housing, and other areas such as day care, folk remedies, occupations of household adults<br>3. Assess child's nutritional status<br>4. Review early signs and symptoms of disease for detection<br>5. Enlist services of public health nurse and social services | 1. A careful history will provide a course of direction<br>2. Information increases understanding and compliance<br>3. These children may be malnourished or may have a history of pica<br>4. Patients may experience behavior changes of irritability, hyperactivity, being easily distracted<br>5. Environment must be modified before child returns; child must have lead blood levels regularly monitored |

be all that is required. Chelating agents that render the lead nontoxic and increase its excretion in the urine are given in more severe cases. Calcium disodium edetate (CaEDTA) and dimercaprol are commonly used. CaEDTA may be given intravenously or as a deep intramuscular injection. A drug more recently approved by the Food and Drug Administration for treatment of asymptomatic and mild symptomatic lead poisoning is meso-2,3,-dimercaptosuccinic acid (DMSA). It can be given orally, has not been associated with serious side effects, and does not cause zinc depletion as does CaEDTA (Behrman, 1992). Complete de-leading takes several months, and retreatment may be neces-

sary when the child has an acute infection or other metabolic disturbance. The prognosis depends on the extent of poisoning. All children with elevated lead blood levels need to be followed to evaluate developmental and intellectual capacities.

The nurse stresses the importance of continued treatment to prevent recurrence of lead poisoning symptoms. Infectious disease in these youngsters must be treated promptly in order to avoid reactivation of the process. Parents are taught to be suspicious of changes in the child's disposition. Siblings and playmates should also be screened. Children should be removed from homes being de-leaded in order to avoid accidental exposure. Parents living in apartments owned by uncooperative landlords may need assistance in communicating with the housing authority. Appropriate literature and explanations are provided at the "therapeutic moment" and thereafter.

Prevention of this condition is foremost. Lead paint should not be used on children's toys or furniture. Instead, one should use paint marked for indoor use. Close observation of children in this age group is also a deterrent. The nurse and parents should provide opportunities for the toddler to suck and chew on safe objects, such as a teething ring or wash cloth, during the oral stage of development; this will meet the normal sucking and chewing needs.

Nursing Care Plan 28–2 presents a summary of interventions for the child experiencing lead poisoning. Nursing care is mainly symptomatic. Unnecessary handling of the patient is avoided in order to prevent stimulating the central nervous system. Injection sites are rotated, and the skin is evaluated for thickness or fibrous lumps. Therapeutic needle play is advised. Observation and charting of convulsions are discussed on page 640. Indications of respiratory distress are immediately reported. The services of the public health nurse are valuable in investigating the physical and emotional environment of the child and in continuing the education of the parents.

## Corrosive Strictures

**Description.** Children who have ingested toxic substances such as lye, bleach, ammonia, and drain cleaners are frequently seen in hospital emergency rooms. The destruction varies from slight pharyngitis and esophagitis to death.

**Manifestations.** The first mouthful that is swallowed is painful and acts as a deterrent to some children; however, the damage is done. Swelling of the lips, chin, tongue, throat, and esophagus occurs. Ulcerations appear on the mucous membranes. The patient is unable to swallow. Edema may interfere with breathing; in this case, a tracheotomy is necessary. If the

patient survives, an esophageal stricture generally develops within a short time. This is evidenced by anorexia and difficulty in swallowing.

**Treatment.** If the child will swallow it, water is given to dilute the chemical. The poison control center is immediately called for information on how to proceed. The child is taken to the nearest emergency room. Vomiting is *not* induced because the corrosive substance will cause further damage as it comes up. Edema of the airways may require endotracheal intubation or tracheostomy. The patient is given nothing by mouth and intravenous fluids are given initially. Analgesics are given intravenously. A gastrostomy (*gastro*, "stomach," and *stoma*, "opening") may be necessary for continued feedings. Early detection and dilatation of developing strictures are part of ongoing care. Surgery may also be necessary. Long-term complications in addition to strictures include the rare development of esophageal cancer.

**Nursing Care.** Nurses stress prevention through education of the public. Toxic substances should never be placed in food containers such as soda pop bottles or water glasses. Children should not be allowed to play in the family garage unless it is child-proof or an adult is closely supervising the activity. The nurse also stresses the potential danger of furniture polish, kerosene, ant traps, insecticides, and toilet bowl cleaners.

A gastrostomy is made for the purpose of introducing food directly into the stomach through the abdominal wall. This is done by means of a surgically placed tube. It is used in patients who cannot have food by mouth because of anomalies or corrosive strictures of the esophagus or who are severely debilitated or in a coma. The nurse may be asked to administer such feedings. This procedure is presented on page 596.

Good oral hygiene is essential. It is administered gently in order to prevent injury to damaged tissues. The psychological needs of these patients are important because these children do not have the satisfaction of eating foods. They are given additional attention and love by cuddling and other forms of contact whenever feasible.

## KEY POINTS

- Problems of fluid and electrolyte disturbance require evaluation of the type and severity of dehydration, clinical observation of the patient, and chemical analysis of the blood.
- Nursing care for the child with pyloric stenosis involves frequent assessment, careful feeding, positioning on the right side following feedings, and education and support of the parents.
- The higher daily exchange of water that occurs in infants leaves them less volume reserve when they are dehydrated.
- In gastroesophageal reflux, the stomach contents are easily regurgitated into the esophagus. Nursing management is directed toward proper feeding and positioning.
- Children infect themselves with pinworms by inhaling the eggs or by handling contaminated toys, toilet seats, doorknobs, food, or soiled linens. The route of entry is the mouth. Education of the family includes emphasizing the importance of handwashing.
- Nursing care for congenital inguinal hernia or hydrocele is directed toward assessment and management of fluids, observation for bowel obstruction, and prevention of postoperative complications.
- Hirschsprung's disease occurs when there is an absence of ganglionic innervation of the muscle of a segment of the bowel. Nursing care may include preoperative bowel care and postoperative ostomy care.
- The primary symptom of anorexia nervosa is severe weight loss.
- The main source of lead poisoning in children occurs from ingestion of paint from old, deteriorating buildings. Blood and urine tests are performed to determine the amount of lead in the body.
- The nurse stresses to parents that toxic substances are never placed in food containers such as soda pop bottles or water glasses.

# Study Questions

1. What measures can be taken to reduce aspirin poisoning in the home?
2. List the symptoms of pyloric stenosis. Why must infants with pyloric stenosis be fed so carefully?
3. You are working the evening shift with Mrs. Green, the charge nurse, who is assisting the doctor in the treatment room. Lee, a 2-year-old who was brought in for vomiting, has an intravenous infusion running. What would you observe about the baby and the intravenous line as you make rounds?
4. Describe how a preschool child might contract pinworms. Include the routes of entry and exit from the body.
5. Differentiate between an inguinal hernia and an umbilical hernia.
6. List the symptoms of intussusception.
7. What is meant by maintenance fluid therapy?
8. What measure would you teach parents to reduce acetaminophen poisoning?
9. Contrast anorexia nervosa and bulimia.
10. List three ways to prevent childhood obesity.
11. Describe the treatment and nursing care for Todd, age 2, who has a corrosive stricture of the esophagus from swallowing ammonia.

# Multiple Choice
# Review Questions

*Choose the most appropriate answer.*

1. In the infant with pyloric stenosis, the pathology is due to
   a. edema of the pyloric muscle
   b. ischemia of the pyloric muscle
   c. hypertrophy of the pyloric muscle
   d. neoplastic obstruction
2. Vigorous preoperative treatment of infants with pyloric stenosis will help prevent
   a. infection during surgery
   b. shock during surgery
   c. asphyxia during surgery
   d. dehydration during surgery
3. An eating disorder characterized by severe weight loss and self-starvation is
   a. anorexia
   b. anorexia nervosa
   c. nervosa mania
   d. anuresis
4. Lead is chiefly eliminated from the body via
   a. the urinary tract
   b. the skin
   c. the intestinal tract
   d. the respiratory tract
5. Pinworms common in children are caused by
   a. bacteria
   b. amebae
   c. parasites
   d. protozoa

## BIBLIOGRAPHY

Behrman, R.E. (1992). *Nelson textbook of pediatrics* (14th ed.). Philadelphia: W.B. Saunders.

Centers for Disease Control. (1983). Folk remedy–associated lead poisoning in Hmong children in Minnesota. *Morbidity and Mortality Weekly Report, 32*, 555.

Gellis, S.S., & Kagan, B.M. (1990). *Current pediatric therapy 13*. Philadelphia: W.B. Saunders.

Grey, M. (1993). Stressors and children's health. *Journal of Pediatric Nursing, 8*, 85–91.

Golden, N., & Sacker, I. (1984). An overview of the etiology, diagnosis, and management of anorexia nervosa. *Clinical Pediatrics, 23*, 209.

Graef, J., & Cone, T. (1988). *Manual of pediatric therapeutics*. Boston: Little, Brown.

Hay, P. (1992). Bone loss in patients with anorexia nervosa. *American Journal of Psychology, 149*, 415–416.

Levine, M.D., Carey, B.W., & Crocker, A.C. (1992). *Developmental-behavioral pediatrics* (2nd ed.). Philadelphia: W.B. Saunders.

Mahan, L.K., & Arlin M.T. (1992). *Krause's food, nutrition, & diet therapy* (8th ed.). Philadelphia: W.B. Saunders.

Marcos, A., et al. (1993). Evaluation of immunocompetence and nutritional status in patients with bulimia nervosa. *American Journal of Clinical Nutrition, 57*, 65–69.

Neinstein, L. (1984) *Adolescent health care*. Baltimore: Urban & Schwarzenberg.

Neumann, C., & Jenks, B. (1992). Obesity. In M.D. Levine, B.W. Carey, & A.C. Crocker (Eds.), *Developmental-behavioral pediatrics* (2nd ed.). Philadelphia: W.B. Saunders.

Mott, S., James, S.R., & Sperhac, A.M. (1992). *Nursing care of children and families* (2nd ed.). Reading, MA: Addison-Wesley.

Pickering, L., & Engelkirk, P. (1988). Giardia lamblia. *Pediatric Clinics of North America, 35*, 565.

Pillitteri, A. (1992). *Maternal and child health nursing*. Philadelphia: J.B. Lippincott.

Whaley, L., & Wong, D. (1991). *Nursing care of infants and children* (4th ed). St. Louis: C.V. Mosby.

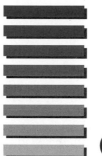

# Chapter 29

# The Child with a Urinary Condition

## VOCABULARY

Anomalies of the Urinary Tract
   Phimosis
   Hypospadias
   Exstrophy of the Bladder
Obstructive Uropathy
Acute Urinary Tract Infection
Nephrotic Syndrome (Nephrosis)
Acute Glomerulonephritis
Wilms' Tumor

# OBJECTIVES

*On completion and mastery of Chapter 29, the student will be able to*

■ Define each vocabulary term listed.
■ Differentiate between nephrosis and acute glomerulonephritis.
■ Name the functional unit of the kidney.
■ List four urologic diagnostic procedures.
■ Discuss the skin care pertinent to the child with nephrosis.
■ Explain any alterations in diet applicable to the child with nephrosis.
■ Outline the nursing care for 2-year-old Cecilia, who is diagnosed as having Wilms' tumor.

The urinary system consists of two kidneys, two ureters, the urinary bladder, and the urethra. Figure 29–1 depicts these structures and how they differ in the developing child from in the adult. The function of the kidneys is to rid the body of waste products and maintain body fluid homeostasis (Fig. 29–2). The kidneys also produce substances important in stimulating red blood cell formation in the bone marrow and in regulating blood pressure. Microscopically, the functional unit of the kidneys is the nephron. Each kidney contains over 1 million nephrons. Although the newborn's kidneys are immature, they function quite effectively. Nevertheless, the functional limitations must be considered carefully when the newborn is premature or ill. This applies especially to the administration of medications, formulas, and parenteral fluids.

Soon after implantation, the embryonic mass differentiates into three distinct layers of cells. These layers are called the ectoderm, mesoderm, and endoderm. The urinary and reproductive organs originated from the mesoderm. At about the 3rd month of gestation, the fetal kidney begins to secrete urine. The amount gradually increases as the fetus matures, and it contains an increased portion of amniotic fluid volume. An absence or small amount of amniotic fluid may indicate genitourinary difficulties.

Urologic diagnostic procedures include urinalysis, ultrasonography, intravenous pyelogram, and computed tomographic (CT) scan of the kidneys. Renal biopsy is used to diagnose

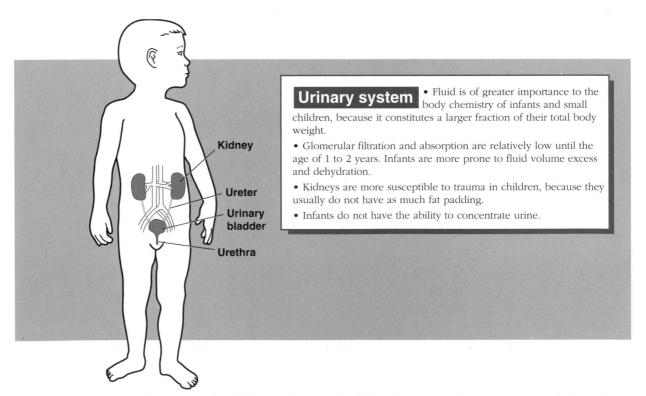

**Urinary system**
• Fluid is of greater importance to the body chemistry of infants and small children, because it constitutes a larger fraction of their total body weight.
• Glomerular filtration and absorption are relatively low until the age of 1 to 2 years. Infants are more prone to fluid volume excess and dehydration.
• Kidneys are more susceptible to trauma in children, because they usually do not have as much fat padding.
• Infants do not have the ability to concentrate urine.

**Figure 29–1.** Summary of urinary system differences between the child and the adult. The urinary system is the main excretory system. The kidneys remove wastes and excess materials from the blood and produce urine. This system helps regulate blood chemistry.

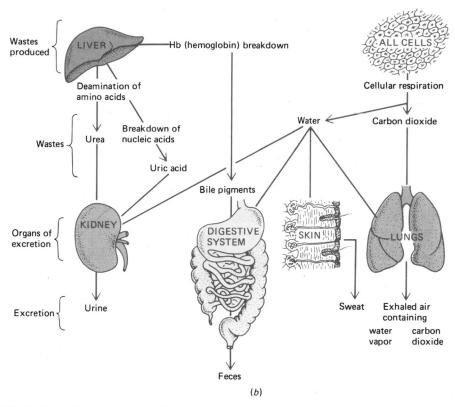

**Figure 29–2.** The kidneys, lungs, skin, and digestive system participate in the disposal of metabolic wastes. Nitrogenous wastes are produced by the liver and transported to the kidneys. The kidneys excrete these wastes in the urine. All cells produce carbon dioxide and some water during cellular respiration. (From Solomon, E.P., & Phillips, G.A. [1987]. *Understanding human anatomy and physiology* [p. 310]. Philadelphia: W.B. Saunders.)

the extent of kidney disease. Uroflow is an assessment procedure used to determine the rate of urine flow. The child voids into a receptacle, and a uroflowmeter graphs the volume. This is useful in diagnosing stricture or scarring. Cytoscopy is useful for investigating congenital abnormalities or acquired lesions in the bladder and lower urinary tract or for catheterization. X-ray examination of the bladder and urethra before and during micturition is called voiding cystourethrography. The cystometrogram and urethral pressure profile assess bladder capacity and function. Both tests require catheterization and infusion of sterile water.

The following is a discussion of phimosis, hypospadias, exstrophy of the bladder, obstructive uropathy, acute urinary tract infection, nephrotic syndrome, acute glomerulonephritis, and Wilms' tumor. Congenital and acquired conditions of the urinary and reproductive systems requiring surgical correction are listed in Table 29–1. Hydrocele and cryptorchidism are discussed in Chapter 30 (see p. 800).

Enuresis is discussed in Chapter 19 (see p. 486). Reproductive disorders are discussed in Chapter 30.

# Anomalies of the Urinary Tract

## PHIMOSIS

**Description.** Phimosis is a narrowing of the preputial opening of the foreskin, which prevents the foreskin from being retracted over the penis (Fig. 29–3). This is normal in newborns and usually disappears with growth. In some children this narrowing may obstruct the stream of urine, cause dribbling or irritation. The condition is corrected by circumcision, preferably at an early age.

When circumcision is performed on an older boy, careful explanations and reassurance are provided. The nurse is sensitive to the child's embarrassment and fear. Postoperatively the

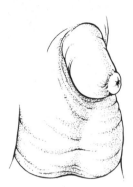

**Figure 29–3.** Phimosis. The foreskin is advanced and fixed; it cannot be retracted over the glans.

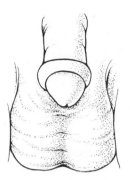

**Figure 29–4.** Paraphimosis. The foreskin is retracted and fixed; it cannot be returned to its original position. Constriction impedes circulation.

penis is covered with a petrolatum gauze. It is tender and may burn on urination.

Cleansing of the uncircumcised penis and retraction of the foreskin are discussed in Chapter 12 (see p. 304). Forcible retraction of a tight foreskin is avoided because it can lead to *paraphimosis* (Fig. 29–4). When this occurs, the foreskin cannot be returned to its normal condition. There may be swelling due to the constriction. This condition requires immediate evaluation by a physician.

## HYPOSPADIAS

**Description.** Hypospadias is a congenital defect in which the urinary meatus is not at the end of the penis but on the lower shaft. In mild cases it is just below the tip of the penis, but it may be found at the midshaft or near the penal-scrotal junction. This deformity, unlike *epispadias*, is fairly common, occurring in 1 in 250–500 newborn boys. In epispadias the opening of the urinary meatus is on the upper surface of the penis (Fig. 29–5). Hypospadias may be accompanied by *chordee*, a downward curvature of the penis caused by a fibrosis band of tissue. Undescended testes may also be present (see p. 800).

**Treatment and Nursing Care.** The alert nurse may discover hypospadias or epispadias in the nursery during neonatal assessment. In many mild cases, surgery is not necessary for either condition unless the location and extent of the defect is such that the child will not be able to stand to void, the defect would cause embarrassment in the growing child, or the defect is extensive. In these instances, treatment consists of surgical repair, usually performed before 18 months of age. It is sometimes done in stages, depending on associated defects. Most techniques can be performed during same-day surgery. Surgery is technically demanding and is best done by a specialist in these disorders. Routine circumcision of the newborn is to be avoided in these patients, as the foreskin may be useful in the repair. Following uncomplicated surgery, patients are normal in both urinary and reproductive functions. Postoperatively a urinary catheter may be required. Parents are instructed in the home care of the catheter. Medication for bladder spasms may be required.

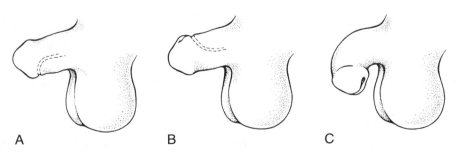

A          B          C

**Figure 29–5.** *A*, Hypospadias. *B*, Epispadias. *C*, Chordee.

As this condition is corrected at a time in childhood when fears of separation and mutilation are great, attention is directed to psychological considerations (see Chap. 22). In more complex conditions and as the child grows older, questions about virility and reproduction may surface and need to be addressed.

## EXSTROPHY OF THE BLADDER

**Description.** In exstrophy of the bladder, the lower portion of the abdominal wall and anterior wall of the bladder are missing. As a result, the bladder lies open and exposed on the abdomen (Fig. 29–6). Exstrophy is due to failure of the midline to close during embryonic development. Other congenital anomalies may also be present. This rare anomaly occurs more often in boys than in girls.

**Manifestations.** This disorder is noticeable by fetal sonogram. The defect may range from a small cutaneous fistula in the abdominal wall to complete exstrophy (the turning inside out of an organ). Urine leaks continually from the bladder. The skin around the bladder becomes excoriated. Other anomalies, such as epispadias and hernias, are common.

**Treatment and Nursing Care.** The bladder is covered with a plastic shield or appropriate dressing to protect the bladder mucosa but allow for urinary drainage. This also protects the bladder from irritation by bedclothes or diapers. The skin is protected by a suitable ointment. Diapers are generally placed under rather than around the infant. The baby is positioned so that urine drains freely. Antibiotics are given to prevent infection. Surgical closure is ideally performed during the first 48 hours of life, to preserve the function of the bladder. Other repairs may be necessary as the child grows. Some children may require urinary diversion surgery if reconstruction is not possible or effective.

# Obstructive Uropathy

**Description.** Many conditions, such as exstrophy of the bladder, calculi (stones), tumors, strictures, and scarring of valves, may cause an obstruction of the normal flow of urine (Fig. 29–7). These conditions may be congenital or acquired. Blockage may be either partial or complete. One or both kidneys may be affected. The pathologic changes depend on the nature and location of the problem. *Hydronephrosis* (*hydro*, "water," and *nephro*, "kidney") is the distention of the renal pelvis because of an obstruction. In children it generally occurs in the first 6 months (King & Hatcher, 1990). Regardless of the cause, the pelvis of the kidney becomes enlarged and cysts form. This may eventually damage renal nephrons, resulting in deterioration of the kidneys. *Polycystic kidney* refers to a condition in which large, fluid-filled cysts form in place of healthy kidney tissue in the fetus. This is inherited as an autosomal recessive trait.

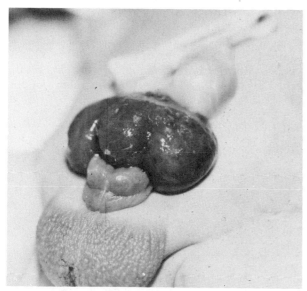

**Figure 29–6.** Bladder exstrophy. (From Behrman, R. [1992]. *Nelson's textbook of pediatrics* [14th ed., p. 1373]. Philadelphia: W.B. Saunders.)

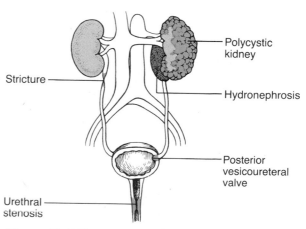

**Figure 29–7.** Frequent sites of urinary obstruction.

**Urinary Diversion.** Urinary diversion is necessary in certain conditions, and it may be accomplished by several procedures (Table 29–2). This type of surgery is a source of great apprehension for parents. The physical care of the child with a urinary stoma (artificially created opening or passage) presents hygiene problems, skin problems, and difficulties in leaving the infant in the care of others. Frequent trips to the clinic add to the strain of everyday life.

Stress from the urinary diversion is age-related. The toddler may be unable to attain independence in toilet training. The school-age child suffers from being different and may have a distorted body image. The adolescent may have lowered self-esteem and is concerned about sexuality. Parents with affected newborns grieve for the loss of a perfect child and experience concerns about the length and quality of the infant's life. The nurse anticipates the impact of this type of diagnosis and incorporates suitable psychological interventions into daily care.

**Table 29–2.** SURGICAL PROCEDURES USED IN URINARY DIVERSION

| Procedure | Definition |
| --- | --- |
| Ureterostomy | Surgical implantation of ureters to outside abdominal wall; allows urine to drain into collection device |
| Ileal or colon conduit (artificial channel) | Diverts urine at ureter, bypassing bladder and urethra; ureters are removed from bladder and attached to ileum or colon, which then acts as a bladder without voluntary control of voiding; patient has stoma, which is larger and not as prone to stenosis as ureterostomy; child wears ileostomy appliance (*Note:* Urine from a conduit may appear cloudy from the secretions of the bowel conduit; this is not a sign of urinary tract infection) |
| Nephrostomy | Tube passes through flank into pelvis of kidney, allowing urine to be drained from pelvis (bypassing ureter, bladder, and urethra; drains into ostomy bag) |
| Suprapubic tube placement | Suprapubic tube is placed above pubis into bladder to provide urinary drainage |
| Vesicostomy (*vesico,* "bladder," *stoma,* "passage") | Surgical opening into bladder between umbilicus and pubis; bladder wall brought to surface of abdomen |

# Acute Urinary Tract Infection

**Description.** Urinary tract infections are common in children. They are more common in girls (except during the neonatal period) than in boys and occur predominantly in the 7–11 age group. Of all infections, 75–90% are caused by *Escherichia coli,* followed by *Klebsiella* and *Proteus* (Behrman, 1992). The nurse will see the following terms used to describe the location and problem of urinary tract disturbances:

**urethritis:** infection of the urethra
**cystitis:** inflammation of the bladder
**bacteriuria:** bacteria in the urine
**pyelonephritis:** infection of the kidney substance and pelvis
**ureteritis:** infection of the ureters
**vesicoureteral reflux:** backward flow of urine into the ureters.

Several factors account for the preponderance in girls. These include the shorter urethra in girls, location of urethra closer to anus, wearing of nylon underwear, use of bubble bath, retention of urine, and vaginitis. In young girls with repeated infections, incest or other sexual abuse should be considered.

Certain chemical and physical factors are important. Normal urine is acidic. Alkaline urine favor pathogens. Urine that remains in the bladder for a period of time serves as an excellent medium for bacterial growth. In certain conditions, such as *vesicoureteral reflux,* the urine actually flows backward from the bladder into the ureters during urination (Fig. 29–8). This condition may be either congenital (primary) or ac-

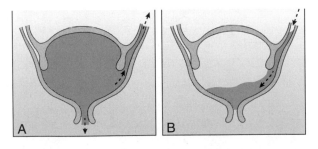

**Figure 29–8.** Congenital abnormalities of the ureters and/or infection can cause urine to flow backward into the ureters during voiding (*A*). After voiding, residual urine from the ureter remains in the bladder (*B*).

quired (secondary). In congenital reflux, the ureters are short or improperly positioned in the bladder. Acquired reflux occurs when frequent infections cause edema and blocking of the passageway, which can lead to pyelonephritis.

**Manifestations.** Signs and symptoms of urinary infection are age-dependent. Infants frequently present with fever, weight loss, failure to thrive, nausea, vomiting, and increased voiding. Foul-smelling urine and persistent diaper

---

**NURSING CARE PLAN 29–1**

### Selected Nursing Diagnoses for the Child with a Urinary Tract Infection

| Goals | Nursing Interventions | Rationale |
|---|---|---|
| **Nursing Diagnosis:** Altered patterns of urinary elimination related to dysuria, incontinence. | | |
| Child does not complain of frequency, urgency, or pain on urination<br>Infant does not strain or fret before voiding<br>Child verbalizes reasons for frequent bladder emptying | 1. Administer antibiotics as prescribed<br><br>2. Encourage complete bladder emptying; explain necessity for this, as age appropriate<br>3. Remind child to void frequently; anticipate incontinence<br><br><br><br><br><br>4. Encourage fluids<br><br><br>5. Keep accurate intake and output records<br><br><br>6. Teach child how to collect urine specimens, if age appropriate<br><br>7. Provide privacy | 1. Antibiotics are chosen according to urine culture and sensitivity; Pyridium may be given to decrease dysuria<br>2. Standing urine in the bladder is very susceptible to the growth of organisms<br>3. Under normal conditions the bladder flushes away organisms by regularly ridding itself of urine; this prevents organisms from accumulating and invading nearby structures; the convalescent bladder is less resistant to invasion than is a healthy bladder<br>4. Child may be febrile; increasing fluids decreases concentration of solutes and alleviates urinary stasis<br>5. This is essential to determine the progress of treatment since the kidneys and bladder play an important part in fluid balance<br>6. Education ensures that specimen will be correctly obtained without contamination<br>7. Children must be given same courtesy as adults, as they are sensitive and embarrassed by body exposure |
| **Nursing Diagnosis:** Knowledge deficit concerning hygiene measures useful in prevention of urinary tract infection. | | |
| Girl demonstrates on doll how to wipe herself after voiding<br>Child verbalizes methods to accomplish this | 1. Instruct girl in importance of wiping self from front to back<br>2. Emphasize need to avoid bubble baths, water softeners<br>3. Encourage use of showers<br><br>4. Explain need for cotton underwear<br>5. Suggest juices such as apple or cranberry to maintain acidity of urine<br><br><br><br>6. Recommend frequent pad change for menstruating girls and proper genital cleansing during period | 1. Good perineal hygiene avoids fecal contamination of urethra<br>2. Oils in these products are known to irritate urethra<br>3. These hygienic measures are helpful in preventing infection<br>4. Cotton underwear is more absorbent<br>5. Acidifying urine decreases rate of bacterial multiplication; an acid-ash diet of meats, cheese, prunes, cranberries, plums, and whole grains is also beneficial<br>6. Old pooled blood fosters growth of organisms; proper cleansing helps prevent irritation |

*Continued*

| NURSING CARE PLAN 29–1 *Continued* | | |
| --- | --- | --- |
| **Selected Nursing Diagnoses for the Child with a Urinary Tract Infection** | | |
| **Goals** | **Nursing Interventions** | **Rationale** |

**Nursing Diagnosis:** Knowledge deficit (parents) concerning follow-up care.

| | | |
| --- | --- | --- |
| Parents verbalize necessity for continued supervision and medication | 1. Instruct parents to administer medication as prescribed and to continue for length of time recommended by the physician | 1. Typical course of antibiotic treatment is 7–10 days; emphasize need to complete prescribed dosage |
| | 2. Suggest patient avoid hot tubs or whirlpool baths | 2. May be potential sources of infection |
| | 3. Remind parents of necessity of adequate hydration for child | 3. Children dehydrate very quickly |
| | 4. Instruct parents that recurrence is most likely within 3–12 mo following infection, often asymptomatic | 4. Emphasize the need for routine office visits to pick up asymptomatic infections |
| | 5. Explain necessity for periodic follow-up urine cultures | 5. Recurrence is common; a urine culture obtained approximately 1 wk after medicine is discontinued will determine if medication has eradicated bacteria |

rash may also be indicators. In the older child, urinary frequency, pain during micturition, onset of bedwetting in a previously "dry" child, abdominal pain, and hematuria may be present. When the kidney is involved, there may be fever, chills, and flank pain. Many children show no symptoms.

Diagnosis depends on the culture of bacteria from the urine. In toilet-trained children, a midstream urine specimen obtained after cleansing the urethral meatus with a povidone-iodine solution and rinsing with sterile water is usually satisfactory. In girls, the labia are spread in order to avoid contamination. In uncircumcised boys, the prepuce must be retracted. Catheterization may be necessary in certain instances. An intravenous pyelogram, cystogram, or sonogram may be indicated.

**Treatment and Nursing Care.** Acute cystitis is treated promptly in order to avoid pyelonephritis. Sulfonamides or broad-spectrum antibiotics are usually commenced. If anatomic defects are present, surgical correction may be suggested. Methods of preventing urinary tract infections are taught to parents and to the patient, as age-appropriate. The nurse stresses the need for proper amounts of fluid to maintain the sterility and flushing of the bladder. Nursing Care Plan 29–1 presents the nursing considerations appropriate for these patients. The prognosis is excellent with prompt treatment.

Some patients develop chronic pyelonephritis and experience recurring infections. More seriously ill children may require hospitalization. Blood pressure, weight, and fever are important parameters to observe in detecting early complications in such patients. Anticipatory guidance by explaining procedures helps decrease the child's and the parents' stress levels.

# Nephrotic Syndrome (Nephrosis)

**Description.** Nephrotic syndrome refers to a number of different types of kidney conditions that are distinguished by the presence of marked amounts of protein in the urine. Minimal change nephrotic syndrome (MCNS), found in approximately 85% of cases, is discussed here.

Nephrosis is more common in boys than in girls and is seen most often in children 2–7 years of age. The cause is not known. The prognosis is good in steroid-responsive patients. Most patients have periods of relapse until the disease resolves itself. Other forms of the syndrome are less predictable.

**Manifestations.** The characteristic symptom of nephrosis is *edema*. This occurs slowly; the child does not appear to be sick. It is first noticed about the eyes and ankles and later becomes generalized. The edema shifts with the position of the child during sleep. The patient gains weight because of the accumulation of fluid. The abdomen may become so distended that *striae*, or stretch marks similar to those that appear on the skin of a pregnant woman, may occur. The child is pale, irritable, and listless and has a poor appetite.

Urine examination reveals albumin (protein). The glomeruli, the working units of the kidneys that filter the blood, become damaged and allow albumin and blood cells to enter the urine. The level of protein in the blood falls; this is termed hypoalbuminemia (*hypo*, "below," *albumin*, and *emia*, "blood"), and the cholesterol content rises; this is termed hyperlipidemia (*hyper*, "above," *lipos*, "fat," and *emia*, "blood"). Vomiting and diarrhea may also be present. Renal biopsy and examination of the tissue under light and electron microscopes provide valuable information.

### Treatment

*Control of Edema.* The child with nephrosis is given medications designed to reduce proteinuria and consequently edema. Steroid therapy is currently used for this purpose. Oral prednisone is initially given. The dosage is reduced for maintenance therapy, which continues for 1–2 months. Because steroids mask the signs of infection, the patient must be watched closely for more subtle symptoms of illness. Study blood reports carefully. Children are prone to infection when absolute granulocyte counts fall below 1000 cells mm$^3$. This is called *neutropenia*.

The child's skin is examined at sites of punctures, wounds, pierced ears, catheters, and the like. The nurse watches for temperature variations and changes in behavior. Suspicions are promptly reported, as septicemia is life-threatening. Prompt antibacterial therapy is begun when an acute infection is recognized. Diuretics have not generally been effective in reducing nephrotic edema. Immunosuppressive therapy (i.e., cyclophosphamide [Cytoxan] and chlorambucil) has shown promise for some steroid-resistant children.

*Diet.* A well-balanced diet high in protein is desirable because protein is constantly being lost in the urine. The carbohydrate and fat content of the diet should be high enough to prevent protein from being used for energy. If either dietary protein or body protein is used for energy, the waste product urea is excreted through the kidneys, which increases their workload. Low-sodium diets may be ordered for

short periods during the course of the disease, but they are generally not appealing to the child. Normal amounts of water are given unless otherwise ordered.

*Care of Ascites.* Ascites, an abnormal collection of fluid in the peritoneal cavity, is seen in advanced cases of nephrosis. This fluid can also cause pressure on the heart and the organs of respiration. The doctor removes some of this fluid by a procedure known as an abdominal paracentesis (*para*, "beside," and *kentésis*, "puncture"). Fluid may also accumulate in the chest. This is termed hydrothorax (*hydro*, "water," and *thorax*, "chest"). The procedure used to remove fluid from the chest is called thoracentesis (*thorax*, "chest," and *kentésis*). The advent of corticosteroid diuresis has greatly reduced the need for these procedures.

*Mental Hygiene.* The physician provides supportive care to the parents and child through the long course of this disease. Whenever possible the child is treated at home and brought to the hospital for special therapy only. Parents are instructed to keep a daily record of the child's weight, urinary proteins, and medications. Signs of infection, such as abnormal weight gain, and increased protein in the urine must be reported promptly. The child is allowed up and about after the acute stage of the illness subsides, to participate in normal childhood activities.

**Nursing Care.** The nursing care of the patient with nephrosis is of the greatest significance because the disease requires long-term therapy. The patient is periodically hospitalized and becomes a familiar personality to hospital personnel. The following factors are important in creating nursing care plans for each child.

*Skin Care.* Good skin care is especially important during periods of marked edema. The skin is bathed daily and whenever necessary. Special attention is given to the neck, underarms, groin, and other moist areas of the body. The patient is handled gently in order to prevent injury to the skin. The male genitals may become edematous; they are bathed and dusted with a soothing powder. A scrotal support increases the patient's comfort during ambulation. Cotton is used to separate the skin surfaces in order to prevent the formation of a rash. Children who are not toilet trained require meticulous care of the diaper area because urine acidity predisposes them to breakdown of the skin.

*Positioning.* The patient is turned frequently in order to prevent respiratory infection. A pillow placed between the knees when the patient is lying on the side prevents pressure on edematous organs. The child's head is elevated from time to time during the day in order to reduce edema of the eyelids and to make the patient more comfortable. Swelling impairs the circulation of the lacrimal secretions. It may therefore be necessary to bathe the eyes to prevent the accumulation of exudate.

*Diet.* The appetite of the patient is poor. Small quantities of food are attractively arranged and served on brightly colored dishes. The child's favorite foods are served if they are nutritious. Colored straws may also be used. The nurse sits by the patient during feedings, is relaxed, and allows plenty of time. Self-feeding is encouraged if the child is able to do it. The nurse's presence during meals makes them more enjoyable, particularly if the patient is in a private room. If the parents are available, the child can enjoy their company during meals.

The child's intake and output are strictly charted. This is the responsibility of the nurse, regardless of who feeds the patient. Parents are instructed to inform the nurse of how much fluid has been taken. If the nurse does not obtain this information, the fluid balance of the day will not be accurate. The importance of keeping *proper fluid balance sheets* (i.e., intake and output records) for patients with diseases of the kidneys cannot be overemphasized.

*Urine Assessment.* As stated previously, the patient's urine must be carefully measured. This is difficult to do for the toddler who is not toilet-trained or whose urinary habits have regressed. Diapers may be weighed on a gram scale before application and after removal (1 gm = 1 ml). The weights are marked on the diaper. A careful check of the number of voidings is of particular value. The character, odor, and color of the urine are also important. If a 24-hour urine collection is ordered, *every* voided specimen within that time must be saved or the test will not be valid. The specimens are collected in a large bottle or container that is correctly labeled. Some tests require that certain preservatives be added to the container; this matter is clarified before the procedure begins.

If a specimen is discarded by accident, the nurse notifies the team leader at once. The procedure for a 24-hour urine collection is outlined in Chapter 23 (see p. 576).

The specific gravity of the urine is measured, and the urine is also examined for albumin (protein). Normally, little or no albumin is found in the urine of a healthy child. Reagent strips especially intended for this purpose are available. The nurse dips the end of the strip into urine and compares it with a special color chart. Specific instructions accompany test materials.

*Weight, Protection from Infection.* The patient is weighed two or three times a week in order to determine changes in the degree of edema. The child is weighed on the same scale each time, and at about the same time of day. Abdominal girth (circumference) should also be measured every day.

Nurses make every effort to protect the patient from exposure to upper respiratory tract infections. They carefully wash their hands before caring for the patient. Children who are up and about must not be allowed to wander into areas where they would be in danger of contracting an infection. *No vaccinations or immunizations should be administered while the disease is active and during immunosuppressive therapy.*

The vital signs of a patient with nephrosis are taken regularly. Ordinarily there is no elevation of temperature unless an infection is present. Blood pressure remains normal. Any increase in blood pressure must be reported. A reading that remains high over a period of time is a grave sign.

Parental guidance and support are given by all members of the nursing team. Family education as to weighing, measuring abdominal girth, and determining urine specific gravity and urine albumin is necessary. Rooming-in is desirable but not always possible. The parents should be allowed to visit the patient as often as they can. The child with nephrosis is kept under close medical supervision over an extended period. Prognosis is considered favorable but depends on the patient's response to drug therapy.

## Nursing Brief

Remember to measure and record urine specimens sent to the laboratory.

## Acute Glomerulonephritis

**Description.** Acute glomerulonephritis, formerly called Bright's disease, seems to be an allergic reaction (antigen-antibody) to an in-

allergic reaction (antigen-antibody) to an infection in the body. The infection is generally caused by a nephritogenic strain of group A beta-hemolytic streptococci infecting the throat. It may appear after the patient has had scarlet fever or skin infections. The body's immune mechanisms appear to be important in its development. Antibodies produced to fight the invading organisms also react against the glomerular tissue. Glomerulonephritis is the most common form of nephritis in children, and it occurs most frequently in boys 3–7 years of age. It has a seasonal incidence with peaks in winter and spring. Both kidneys are affected.

The nephron is the working unit of the kidneys. Nephrons number in the millions. Within the bulb of each nephron lies a cluster of capillaries called the glomerulus. It is these structures that are affected, as the name implies. They become inflamed and sometimes blocked, permitting red blood cells and protein, which are normally retained, to enter the urine. The kidneys become pale and slightly enlarged.

The prognosis is excellent. Patients with mild cases of the disease may recover within 10–14 days. Patients with protracted cases may show urinary changes for as long as 1 year but have complete recovery. Chronic nephritis is seen in a small number of children, and death is generally the result of kidney or heart failure. These severe complications plus hypertensive changes in the blood supply of the brain necessitate careful observation and care of each patient.

**Manifestations.** Symptoms range from mild to severe. From 1 to 3 weeks after a streptococcal infection has occurred, the parent may notice that the child's urine is smoky brown or bloody. This is frightening to the parent and child; most parents immediately seek medical advice. Periorbital edema (mild swelling about the eyes) may also be present, with fever (high at first but gradually leveling off to about 37.8°C [100°F]), headache, diarrhea, and vomiting. Urinary output is decreased. The urine specific gravity is high, and albumin, red and white blood cells, and casts may be found on examination. The blood urea nitrogen level is elevated, as are the serum creatinine and sedimentation rate. The serum complement level is usually reduced. Hyperkalemia (excessive potassium in the blood) may produce cardiac toxicity. Hypertension may occur. Chest x-ray films may reveal cardiac enlargement or pulmonary changes.

**Treatment.** Although children may feel well, they are confined to bed until gross hematuria subsides. The urine is regularly examined. Every effort is made to prevent children from becoming overtired, chilled, or exposed to infection. As renal function is impaired, there is danger of accumulation of nitrogenous wastes and sodium in the body. Sodium is restricted until symptoms disappear; then the patient is returned to a regular diet. Protein restriction is not usually required. Fluid restriction may be necessary for some patients. A liquid diet is instituted and is followed by a soft to full diet as tolerated. Penicillin is given during the acute phase and may be continued orally for a period of time in order to prevent renewed activity before healing is complete. Second attacks of glomerulonephritis are rare.

**Nursing Care.** The nurse tries to make the period of bed rest as pleasant as possible for the patient by providing quiet diversions. The child is protected from being chilled in bed, during baths, and during trips to various departments. Sufficient blankets are provided at night. When the child is allowed to get up, the nurse observes frequently for signs of fatigue. The patient is protected from contact with persons with infections.

The patient's vital signs are regularly taken, preferably with the same apparatus. A rise in blood pressure is immediately reported. Between readings the nurse should be alert for symptoms such as headache, drowsiness, vomiting, and blurring of vision. If any of these are noticed, the child is returned to bed and the crib sides or rails are raised. Because convulsions can occur, someone should remain with the child until medication is given. Hypotensive drugs may be ordered by the physician. These rapidly reduce the blood pressure, and the cerebral symptoms subside. If cardiac failure is evidenced by an electrocardiogram or chest radiograph, sedation, oxygen, and digitalis may be required.

An *accurate* record is kept of the patient's fluid intake and urine output. Fluids may be restricted, especially if the urine output is scant. The physician orders the oral intake allowed, for example, 650 ml daily. This must be distributed throughout the 24-hour period. The nurse on each shift should know the specific amount of fluids the patient is to receive so that an excessive amount is not given. The greater amounts of fluid are allotted to the day and evening shifts, when thirst is more pronounced. The individual needs of the child should be observed and incorporated into the day's events. Daily weighing of the patient also helps determine progress. Persistent anuria may require dialysis by the artificial kidney.

Although glomerulonephritis is generally benign, it can be a source of anguish for parents and child. If the patient is treated at home, the parents must plan activities to keep the child occupied while confined to bed. They must understand the importance of continued medical supervision, as follow-up urine and blood tests are necessary to ensure that the disease has been eradicated.

## Wilms' Tumor

**Description.** Wilms' tumor, or nephroblastoma (*nephro*, "kidney," *blasto*, "bud," and *oma*, "tumor"), is one of the most common malignancies of early life. It is an embryonal adenosarcoma (*adeno*, "glandular," and *sarcoma*, "cancer of connective tissue") that is now known to be associated with certain congenital anomalies, particularly of the genitourinary tract. It is thought to have a genetic basis.

About two-thirds of these growths occur before the child is 3 years old. During the early stages of growth, as with some other malignancies, there are few or no symptoms. A mass in the abdomen is discovered generally by a parent or by the physician during a routine checkup. X-rays of the kidneys (most importantly, intravenous pyelograms) indicate a growth and verify the fact that the remaining kidney is normal. Chest x-ray films, ultrasound, bone surveys, liver scan, and CT may also be indicated. Wilms' tumor seldom affects both kidneys.

**Treatment and Nursing Care.** Treatment of the Wilms' tumor patient consists of a combination of surgery, radiation therapy, and chemotherapy. The kidney and tumor are removed as soon as possible after the diagnosis has been confirmed. It is important to prepare the parents and the child for the extent of the incision, which is considerable. Radiation therapy is given before and after surgery. The

National Wilms' Tumor Study (NWTS) lists several categories of effective treatment. Five states of tumor activity are cited, and appropriate refinements in radiation therapy and chemotherapy are suggested. Two drugs currently shown by the NWTS to be effective are actinomycin D and vincristine sulfate. A third drug, doxorubicin hydrochloride (Adriamycin), has also shown usefulness, particularly when there is metastasis. Children with localized tumors (stage I and stage II) have a 90% chance of cure. Prognosis also depends on the histologic character of the tumor and evidence of recurrence. Patients younger than 2 years of age have a higher rate of response to therapy.

General nursing measures for the comfort the patient are carried out. One factor pertinent to this condition is that all unnecessary handling of the abdomen is to be avoided, as it can cause the disease to spread. The doctor explains this to the parents, and in the hospital a sign is placed on the crib or child: "Do not palpate abdomen." The nurse considers this extremely important. Drugs and irradiation may cause toxic reactions, such as nausea, vomiting, anorexia, and general malaise. Ulceration of the mouth, hair loss, and peeling of the skin may also be seen. The student anticipates such problems and immediately reports their appearance to the team leader or the nurse in charge of the unit. Follow-up care is essential, as these patients survive with only one kidney.

The lungs are the most common site of metastasis for this disease. Observations of bloody urine, elevated blood pressure, and symptoms of infection, especially during chemotherapy, are immediately reported. Helping the family and patient face the possibility of a fatal illness is discussed in Chapter 34 (see p. 889). Nursing Care Plan 29–2 outlines care for a child undergoing surgery of the renal system.

## Nursing Brief

Most newborns urinate within the first 24 hours of life. The nurse's recording and reporting presence or absence of urination is highly important.

| NURSING CARE PLAN 29–2 |
| :--- |
| **Selected Nursing Diagnoses for the Child Undergoing Surgery of the Renal System** |

| Goals | Nursing Interventions | Rationale |
| :--- | :--- | :--- |

**Nursing Diagnosis:** Anxiety related to surgical experience.

| Goals | Nursing Interventions | Rationale |
| :--- | :--- | :--- |
| Parents state two ways they are coping with the stress of this surgery<br>Child verbalizes understanding of procedure, as age appropriate | 1. Provide surgical tour, include wake-up room<br><br>2. Encourage parents to remain with child, as appropriate<br>3. Explain mask and anesthesia equipment<br><br>4. Determine small child's words for penis, urination<br>5. Provide support and reassurance | 1. Explanations and familiarity with physical surroundings may decrease apprehension<br>2. Child is more secure when parents are close by<br>3. It is frightening to have something placed over face; equipment is intimidating<br>4. This will promote understanding postoperatively<br>5. Urinary surgery may raise anxiety about sexual function, which parents or patients are often unable to express |

**Nursing Diagnosis:** High risk for ineffective airway clearance related to poor cough effort associated with postanesthesia, postoperative immobility, pain.

| Goals | Nursing Interventions | Rationale |
| :--- | :--- | :--- |
| Patient maintains airway patency as evidenced by clear lung sounds, vital signs within normal range | 1. Assist child to turn, cough, deep breathe; reposition infants<br><br><br><br><br><br><br><br><br>2. Monitor vital signs frequently<br><br>3. Teach splinting of incision preoperatively<br>4. Teach incentive spirometry preoperatively<br><br><br><br><br>5. Assess and medicate for bladder spasm and incisional pain | 1. Prolonged postoperative immobility leads to decreased chest expansion, pooling of mucus in bronchi, and hypostatic pneumonia; in nephrectomy patients, incision is close to diaphragm, making breathing painful; allow infants to cry for a few seconds to ensure deep breathing; if secretions are present, coughing will generally follow; ambulate as ordered<br>2. Monitoring vital signs will assess cardiovascular function and tissue perfusion<br>3. Splinting incision lessens pain<br><br>4. Spirometry promotes alveolar inflation, restores and maintains lung capacity, and strengthens respiratory muscles; it also provides immediate feedback as to effectiveness of deep breathing<br>5. Postoperative pain and discomfort may make patients reluctant to turn, cough, and deep breathe |

*Continued*

| NURSING CARE PLAN 29–2 *Continued* | | |
|---|---|---|
| **Selected Nursing Diagnoses for the Child Undergoing Surgery of the Renal System** | | |
| **Goals** | **Nursing Interventions** | **Rationale** |

**Nursing Diagnosis:** High risk for fluid volume deficit related to patient's age, surgery, catheters, refusal to drink.

| Goals | Nursing Interventions | Rationale |
|---|---|---|
| Vital signs remain within normal limits<br>Patient's hydration and acid-base balance remain stable as evidenced by laboratory reports | 1. Regulate intravenous fluids | 1. Child will probably take nothing by mouth for a brief period prior to and following surgery; intravenous fluids maintain hydration and replace lost electrolytes |
| | 2. Keep accurate intake and output records | 2. Careful monitoring of fluid intake and output will identify early renal complications |
| | 3. Weigh infants daily | 3. Daily weights in infants will assist in monitoring under- or overhydration; comparison with preoperative weight will assess infant's nutritional progress |
| | 4. Record separate output for each drainage tube | 4. An unexpected reduction in urine flow requires prompt intervention; each catheter drains into its own collection bag, so that source of reduced flow will be immediately noticed |
| | 5. Observe fontanels of infants for depression | 5. Depressed fontanels, sunken eyeballs, lack of tears, dark circles around eyes, and poor skin turgor denote dehydration, which can occur quickly in infants and children |
| | 6. Begin clear oral fluids gradually | 6. Replacement of fluids and electrolytes by mouth is generally considered to be safest method; clarify ambiguous orders, such as "force fluids," "restrict fluids," particularly in infants and small children with urologic disorders, cardiac conditions, and so on |
| Child's temperature will remain at or below 38°C (100.4°F); incision site will not be erythematous or foul-smelling | 1. Assess for signs of infection | 1. Fever, incisional tenderness, redness, drainage from incisions, lethargy indicate infection |
| | 2. Observe and record patency, color, amount, and consistency of drainage | 2. Catheters can become plugged by mucous shreds, blood clots, and chemical sediment; plugging of conduits can lead to infection of urinary tract, urine stasis, and if obstruction persists, hydronephrosis |
| | 3. Obtain urine cultures as indicated | 3. Pathogens in urine are most specifically determined by culture; goal is to obtain urine that is uncontaminated by organisms outside urinary tract |
| | 4. Maintain aseptic closed drainage system | 4. Maintaining a closed drainage system aids in preventing infection; careful handwashing before and after handling of catheter or drainage system is also of importance |

**Selected Nursing Diagnoses for the Child Undergoing Surgery of the Renal System**

| Goals | Nursing Interventions | Rationale |
|---|---|---|
| | | |

**Nursing Diagnosis:** Health-seeking behaviors regarding ostomy care.

| Goals | Nursing Interventions | Rationale |
|---|---|---|
| Parents and child (as age appropriate) demonstrate ostomy care before discharge<br>Parents verbalize ability to care for ostomy | 1. Explain need to keep skin dry and odor free | 1. Breakdown of skin can result from poor appliance fit, frequent leakage, appliance changes, and sensitivity to products or tape used |
| | 2. Demonstrate procedures to parents or child as age appropriate | 2. Careful demonstration of procedures will reduce anxiety |
| | 3. Provide written instructions to parents | 3. Written instructions can be reviewed at less stressful times |
| | 4. Provide contact number should problems occur | 4. Department telephone numbers reassure patient and family and denote continued interest and support; provide a name to contact in order to avoid confusion |
| | 5. Provide telephone number of local ostomy support group | 5. A local support group can answer many questions for family, exchange information, and provide socialization |

# KEY POINTS

- The functional unit of the kidney is the nephron.
- Children with hypospadias are born with the urethral opening located on the undersurface of the penis.
- Bladder exstrophy is a serious congenital defect in which the bladder lies exposed on the lower portion of the abdominal wall. Surgical correction of this defect is lifesaving.
- Obstruction along the urinary tract may lead to hydronephrosis, a distention of the kidney pelvis. This is a serious condition because it could eventually lead to kidney failure if untreated.
- To avoid fecal contamination of the urinary tract, girls are taught to wipe the perineal area from front to back after urination.
- Ascites is an abnormal collection of fluid in the peritoneal cavity. It is seen in advanced cases of nephrosis and other conditions.
- The accurate charting of intake and output on patients with kidney problems is absolutely essential to their treatment and recovery. This includes ostomy and urinary drainage.
- Accurate blood pressure measurements will detect hypertension, a condition frequently associated with kidney problems.
- Plugging of catheters by mucus, clots, and sediment can lead to infection.
- Normally urine flows from the ureters into the bladder, and almost no flow reenters the ureters. Repeated urinary tract infections causing edema or improper position of the ureters in the bladder at birth may result in reflux of urine into the ureters.

# Study Questions

1. Define acute glomerulonephritis. What nursing measures are specific for this disease?
2. What is the characteristic symptom of nephrosis?
3. Define the following: diuretic, hypoalbuminemia, hyperlipidemia, and paracentesis.
4. How does the nurse test for albumin in the urine?
5. Discuss the proper care of the uncircumcised penis in a child of age 4.
6. What is the pathophysiology of hydronephrosis?
7. What specific nursing measures are indicated for the child with Wilms' tumor?
8. Plan a day's menu for the toddler with nephrosis. Include your rationale for the various foods suggested.
9. Six-year-old Larry has ascites. Discuss the cause of this condition.
10. Discuss the psychological considerations inherent in the care of the child with a urinary diversion device.

# Multiple Choice Review Questions

*Choose the most appropriate answer.*

1. The functional unit of the kidneys is the
   a. neuron
   b. dendrite
   c. nephron
   d. synapse
2. The administration of prednisone to children with nephrosis creates the problem of
   a. intolerance of foods
   b. increased risk of infection
   c. increased periorbital edema
   d. weight loss
3. The reason for daily weights in children with nephrosis is to monitor
   a. weight loss from low-protein diet
   b. accuracy of fluid balance sheets
   c. changes in the amount of edema
   d. percentile on growth grid
4. Wilms' tumor is categorized as a
   a. benign tumor
   b. malignant tumor
   c. neurologic tumor
   d. tumor of the bone
5. Accurate fluid intake and output records are particularly important in patients with kidney disease because
   a. they aid in assessing kidney damage
   b. they help to determine nutritional adequacy
   c. they are important in assessing hypertension
   d. they provide a reliable method of determining infection

# BIBLIOGRAPHY

Behrman, R.E. (1992). *Nelson textbook of pediatrics* (14th ed.). Philadelphia: W.B. Saunders.

Gellis, S., & Kagan, B. (1990). *Current pediatric therapy 13.* Philadelphia: W.B. Saunders.

Burroughs, A. (1992). *Maternity nursing* (6th ed.). Philadelphia: W.B. Saunders.

Graef, J., & Cone, T. (1985). *Manual of pediatric therapeutics.* Boston: Little, Brown.

Hayman, L., & Sporing, E. (1985). *Handbook of pediatric nursing.* New York: John Wiley & Sons.

King, L., & Hatcher, P. (1990). The natural history of fetal and neonatal hydronephrosis. *Urology, 35,* 433.

Mahan, L., & Arlin, M. (1992). Krause's food, nutrition & diet therapy (8th ed.). Philadelphia: W.B. Saunders.

Mott, S., et al. (1991). *Nursing care of children and families* (2nd ed.). Reading, MA: Addison-Wesley.

Petrillo, M., & Sanger, S. (1980). *Emotional care of hospitalized children.* Philadelphia: J.B. Lippincott.

Pillitteri, A. (1992). *Maternal and child health nursing.* Philadelphia: J.B. Lippincott.

Skoog, S., & Belman, A. (1991). Primary vesicoureteral reflux in the black child. *Pediatrics, 87,* 538.

Snow, B., et al. (1990). Techniques for outpatient hypospadias surgery. *Urology, 35,* 327.

Vignoux, A., Hunsberger, M. (1994). Altered genitourinary/renal function. In Betz, C., Hunsberger, M., Wright, S. *Family-centered nursing care of children.* Philadelphia: W.B. Saunders.

Thompson, E.D., & Ashwill, J.W. (1992). *Introduction to pediatric nursing* (6th ed.). Philadelphia: W.B. Saunders.

Whaley L., & Wong, D. (1991). *Nursing care of infants and children.* (4th ed.). St. Louis: C.V. Mosby.

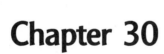

# Chapter 30

# The Child with a Reproductive Condition

## VOCABULARY
Cinderella disease (799)
encopresis (792)
gonad (792)
lues (799)
orchipexy (801)
ovaries (792)
Papanicolaou smear (792)
premenstrual syndrome (792)
serologic (799)
sexually transmitted disease
   (794)

Primary Dysmenorrhea
Sexually Transmitted Diseases
   Nursing Care
   Gonorrhea
   Nongonococcal Urethritis
   Syphilis
   Genital Herpes
Hydrocele
Undescended Testes (Cryptorchidism)

# OBJECTIVES

*On completion and mastery of Chapter 30, the student will be able to*

- Define each vocabulary term listed.
- List four tests helpful in diagnosing conditions of the reproductive tract.
- List the grades of primary dysmenorrhea and provide two suitable nursing interventions for each grade.
- Discuss four ways to prevent sexually transmitted diseases.
- Differentiate among the three stages of syphilis.
- Discuss a sensitive approach to Larry, a 17-year-old who just learned he has contracted a sexually transmitted disease.
- Outline the treatment for genital herpes.
- Discuss the clinical manifestations and treatment for a child with undescended testes.

Figure 30–1 shows the female and male reproductive systems and lists the differences between child and adult systems. The reproductive system provides for perpetuation of the human species. Each sex is equipped with a gonad, which provides a reproductive cell, and a set of accessory organs. The gonads (ovaries in the female and testes in the male) produce sex cells and hormones, which affect the reproductive organs and other body systems.

Sex is genetically determined at the time of fertilization. The presence of a Y chromosome is essential for the development of the testes and their hormones. Sex differentiation occurs early in the embryo. The organs specific to the male or female child develop. Before this, the embryo has neither male nor female characteristics. The development of the ovaries occurs later than that of the testes. By the 12th week, the external genitals of the fetus are recognizably male or female.

Several tests are helpful in diagnosing conditions of the reproductive tract. These include a Papanicolaou (Pap) smear, serologic blood tests, gonococcal cultures, ultrasound procedures, pregnancy tests, and routine blood and urine tests. Sexual abuse in children may be manifested by such behaviors as urinary frequency, excessive masturbation, encopresis (fecal soiling beyond 4 years), severe nightmares, bedwetting, irritation or pain in the genital area, and a decrease in physical or emotional development. Suggestive posturing by young children or explicit knowledge of sex acts shown by children under 8 years old needs further investigation. The following is a discussion of conditions of the reproductive system that affect children. They include dysmenorrhea, gonorrhea, nongonococcal urethritis, syphilis, and genital herpes. Acquired immunodeficiency syndrome (AIDS) and sexual abuse of the child are discussed in more detail in Chapters 14 and 34, respectively. Sexually transmitted disease during pregnancy is discussed on page 108.

## Primary Dysmenorrhea

**Description.** *Primary dysmenorrhea*, or painful menstruation, refers to pain associated with the menstrual cycle in the absence of organic pelvic disease. It is distinguished from *secondary dysmenorrhea*, in which the patient may have an underlying condition, such as endometriosis, pelvic inflammatory disease, ovarian cysts, adhesions, or congenital abnormalities. *Mittelschmerz* refers to midcycle pain during ovulation. For many years, dysmenorrhea was thought to be psychological. It is now recognized that painful menses results from myometrial stimulation by prostaglandins E and F produced in the endometrium (Litt, 1990). Prostaglandins are a group of fatty acid derivatives present in many tissues including the prostate gland, menstrual fluid, brain, kidney, thymus, seminal fluid, and pancreas. The concentration of these prostaglandins is higher in women suffering from dysmenorrhea than in controls.

**Prevalence and Manifestations.** About two-thirds of postpubescent teenagers in the United States experience some degree of dysmenorrhea. Approximately 10% are incapacitated 1–3 days each month. Dysmenorrhea is the greatest single cause of lost school and work days in teenage girls and women. Its onset is usually before age 20. Symptoms include cramping, abdominal discomfort, and leg aches. Systemic symptoms such as nausea, vomiting, dizziness, diarrhea, backache, and headache may occur. Dysmenorrhea is graded from mild to severe (Table 30–1). *Premenstrual syndrome* (PMS) is more common in adults than in teenagers. Although the symptoms may overlap with those of dysmenorrhea, weight gain, breast tenderness, irritability, and insomnia are also shown. PMS does not generally occur before ovulatory cycles begin (see p. 26).

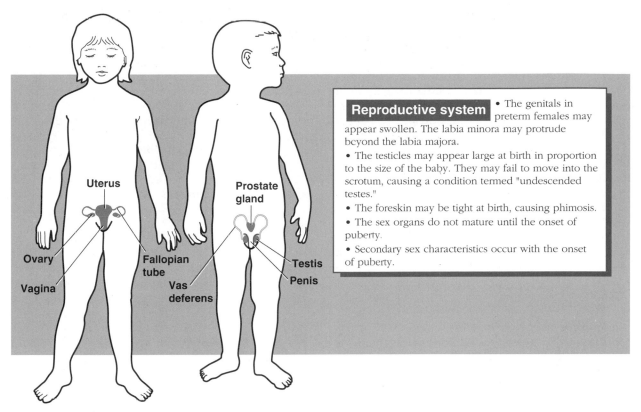

**Reproductive system**  • The genitals in preterm females may appear swollen. The labia minora may protrude beyond the labia majora.
• The testicles may appear large at birth in proportion to the size of the baby. They may fail to move into the scrotum, causing a condition termed "undescended testes."
• The foreskin may be tight at birth, causing phimosis.
• The sex organs do not mature until the onset of puberty.
• Secondary sex characteristics occur with the onset of puberty.

Uterus

Prostate gland

Ovary

Fallopian tube

Vagina

Vas deferens

Testis

Penis

**Figure 30–1.** Summary of reproductive system differences between the child and the adult male and female. Each reproductive system consists of gonads and associated structures. The reproductive system maintains sexual characteristics and perpetuates the species.

**Treatment and Nursing Care.** Psychological factors are no longer considered the sole cause of dysmenorrhea, and one must consider a holistic approach to this disorder. Principles of proper menstrual hygiene need to be reviewed with the adolescent. Factors that may aggravate the condition include lack of exercise, poor posture, lack of sleep, constipation, and unbalanced meals. Improving the health status of patients is always a consideration of care. The perceptive nurse also recognizes that a complaint of cramps in a young girl often masks other concerns, and intervenes accordingly.

A warm beverage, acetaminophen, and application of a heating pad to the lower abdomen may be sufficient. When these measures fail, a thorough history and pelvic examination by a gynecologist should be performed in order to rule out organic disorders. Patients with dysmenorrhea who also need contraception may be candi-

**Table 30–1.** NURSING INTERVENTIONS FOR VARIOUS GRADES OF PRIMARY DYSMENORRHEA

| Grade | Severity | Nursing Interventions |
|---|---|---|
| I | Mild: does not interfere with daily activities | Educate patient in menstrual physiology, good hygiene, exercise |
| II | Moderate: may interfere with some activities, minimum of systemic symptoms | Recommend warm fluids, heating pad, or acetaminophen as directed |
| III | Severe discomfort: interferes with daily activities, systemic symptoms | Consult physician; if patient is on antiprostaglandin medication, administer after eating in order to avoid stomach irritation |

dates for combination (estrogen-progesterone) oral contraceptives. Grade III patients benefit from the use of prostaglandin inhibitors such as ibuprofen (Motrin), naproxen sodium (Anaprox), and mefenamic acid (Ponstel). These medications decrease myometrial contractions. Some side effects that the nurse must be aware of include gastric irritation (pain, nausea, and vomiting), headache, pruritus, and fluid retention.

## Sexually Transmitted Diseases

**Overview.** Sexually transmitted disease (STD) is the general name given to infections that are spread through direct sexual activity. This term replaces venereal disease, which was used in the past. The two most common types of STD are gonorrhea and syphilis; however, over 20 other diseases are now considered prevalent. Some of these are scabies, pediculosis pubis, herpes progenitalis, genital warts, chlamydial infection, cytomegalovirus, and AIDS. Gonorrhea occurs far more frequently than does syphilis, but the effects of untreated syphilis are more debilitating. One may contract both diseases at the same time. Each can be transmitted by a pregnant woman to her unborn child, causing serious problems in the fetus, such as blindness, birth defects, and death.

The earliest record of STDs appears in the Bible and was written about 1500 BC. It was thought that with the advent of penicillin, STDs would be eradicated, but there has been a widespread resurgence, particularly among teenagers. The United States Public Health Service is calling it "an epidemic" and a "national health emergency." The incidence of STDs surpasses that of all other communicable diseases combined, except the common cold.

The reasons for this resurgence are many. They involve cultural, economic, social, and moral factors that are intertwined. Specific reasons cited include changing values and lifestyles of society; an increase in sexual contacts; the increase in the mobility of society and surges in population; the reluctance of many persons to seek medical help (particularly adolescents); inadequate education about venereal disease; widespread apathy among professionals; social equality of the sexes; and change in common methods of contraception. The occurrence of an STD in a prepubertal patient should always prompt investigation into the possibility of sexual abuse.

Human immunodeficiency virus (HIV) is discussed on pages 360–365. Its incidence continues to increase; therefore, education of the public as to its sexual transmission is crucial. HIV has been isolated from lymphocytes of patients, making it possible to detect victims and carriers of the disease. A great deal of controversy exists over the identification of carriers. The disease is seen in children, who acquire it in utero or perinatally; in those who have received infected blood from transfusions; and in sexually abused children (see p. 898). Nursing care is focused on management of symptoms.

### NURSING CARE

Regardless of the medical professional's feelings about the changes in society and sexual permissiveness, the consequences of these changes must be recognized and managed (Nursing Care Plan 30–1). Nurses who wish to help teenagers with STDs must create an environment in which they will feel safe and at ease. What adolescents need at this point is ego support, which the nurse is able to provide through listening and through a nonjudgmental attitude.

**Approach.** The nurse approaches the patient with sensitivity and recognizes that the teenager is embarrassed and in need of privacy, especially during examinations. Girls are often afraid and always nervous about a pelvic examination. This is true even when their outward manner may seem otherwise. Careful explanations are needed. The patient is draped appropriately, and the nurse remains during the examination in order to provide reassurance. The findings are discussed with the patient, and questions are encouraged. Most teenagers need help in being drawn out and do not readily ask questions, even when they do not understand.

The legal requirement to report sexual contacts is an emotionally charged topic that often prevents patients from seeking help. The person who is assured of confidentiality and who has been treated in a dignified manner is more apt to cooperate. Girls who are sexually active must be taught to take responsibility for their own health and are encouraged to request a gonorrhea culture as a routine part of their physical examination. This is especially important if they suspect that their partner has an STD. Medical attention should be sought immediately, even if they are menstruating. Young people need to be made aware of the fact that sex with only one partner does not eliminate the risk, as this person may have had con-

| | NURSING CARE PLAN 30–1 | |
|---|---|---|
| | **Selected Nursing Diagnoses for the Adolescent with a Sexually Transmitted Disease (STD)** | |
| **Goals** | **Nursing Interventions** | **Rationale** |

**Nursing Diagnosis:** Knowledge deficit regarding genital hygiene.

| Goals | Nursing Interventions | Rationale |
|---|---|---|
| Adolescent verbalizes understanding of general hygiene measures related to the genitals | 1. Assess patient's knowledge of cleansing genitals | 1. Patient education is an ongoing responsibility of entire health-care team; it communicates interest and concern for adolescent's welfare; both formal and informal teaching are necessary |
| | 2. Educate as to effective genital care | 2. Adolescent girls need to wipe themselves from front to back in order to avoid spreading bacteria from anus to vagina |
| | 3. Stress importance of drinking lots of fluids and voiding regularly in order to avoid cystitis and other infections | 3. Good fluid intake prevents stagnation of urine in the bladder; frequent voiding cleanses urethra |
| | 4. Suggest that teenage girls wear loose-fitting cotton underwear | 4. Cotton underwear is absorbent; tight-fitting garments restrict perineal ventilation and may contribute to vaginitis |
| | 5. Recommend that bubble baths, hygiene sprays, and douching be avoided | 5. These products and procedures may cause irritation; douching is unnecessary, and some believe it is detrimental, as it washes away normal protective mucus and bacterial flora of vagina and may introduce bacteria; tampons need to be changed at least three to four times a day during menses; wash hands before and after changing |
| | 6. Uncircumcised boys need to retract foreskin and cleanse penis regularly | 6. This prevents smegma from collecting under foreskin and causing irritation |
| | 7. Suggest importance of daily baths and showers with particular attention to cleansing of genital area | 7. Soap and water are all that are necessary for keeping perineal and perianal areas clean; thorough drying of genitals prevents irritation |
| | 8. Educate as to normal secretions of genital area | 8. All adolescent girls have normal, nonbloody, asymptomatic vaginal discharge called leukorrhea; this discharge is secreted by endocervical glands; this keeps mucous membranes of vagina moist and clean; urethra in a boy should show no signs of discharge, infection, or abnormal tissue growth |
| | 9. Suggest that adolescents become aware of their personal anatomy and seek health care for any deviations or abnormal secretions | 9. Patients who are familiar with their own anatomy can identify abnormal changes |

*Continued*

tact with others; the partner needs only one sexual experience with one infected person in order to transmit the disease.

Changes in methods of contraception have been cited as one reason for the increased incidence of STDs. As more women used birth control pills and intrauterine devices (IUDs), fewer men used condoms ("rubbers"), which helped reduce the spread of infection by protecting the partner from direct contact with the organisms. This is changing because of AIDS. The proper use of male and female condoms is described on

| | NURSING CARE PLAN 30–1 *Continued* | |
|---|---|---|

### Selected Nursing Diagnoses for the Adolescent with a Sexually Transmitted Disease (STD)

| Goals | Nursing Interventions | Rationale |
|---|---|---|
| **Nursing Diagnosis:** Knowledge deficit regarding transmission of STDs | | |
| Patient verbalizes understanding of transmission of STDs<br>Patient does not evidence symptoms of rash, pain, itching, odor, or discharge<br>Patient verbalizes knowledge that some infections may have no symptoms | 1. Encourage limitation of partners, preferably limiting sex to one partner<br>2. Discourage sex with strangers (a pickup or prostitute)<br>3. Instruct adolescents that use of oral contraceptive does not protect against STDs<br>4. Emphasize importance of using latex condoms when having intercourse<br><br>5. Suggest that vaginal sprays, douches, and lubricants that lower vaginal pH may protect against some STDs but are *not* effective against HIV<br>6. Educate as to importance of avoiding anal intercourse, particularly with a person who injects drugs<br><br>7. Dispel misinformation<br><br>8. Stress importance of keeping clinic appointments and taking all medications prescribed should one become infected | 1. Limiting partners reduces exposure to STDs<br><br>2. These persons are more apt to be infected; there is little way of knowing their health history<br>3. The pill actually raises the pH of the vagina, increasing the susceptibility to infection<br>4. Lambskin and natural-membrane condoms are not as effective against virus that leads to AIDS (human immunodeficiency virus [HIV]) because of pores in material; on package look for words *latex* and *5% nonoxynol 9* (a spermicide)<br>5. HIV is carried in body secretions of infected person, particularly in blood and semen; mixing of body secretions is to be avoided<br>6. Drug users are a very high-risk group for AIDS and other STDs; rectal intercourse is particularly contraindicated because even small breaks in the rectal mucosa provide a direct route to blood stream<br>7. There is a great deal of misinformation concerning STDs<br>8. Follow-up care is essential for health and welfare of patient and patient's contacts |

pages 276–278. The use of foam and other local agents prior to intercourse lowers the pH of the vagina and decreases (but does not eliminate) the risk of infection. The pill actually raises the pH of the vagina, increasing the susceptibility to infection. Disease organisms may also travel along the wick of an intrauterine device. Douching is not an effective means of birth control and may force disease organisms into the uterus. Some means of reducing the risk of STDs include bathing the external genitals and perianal area with soap and water and urinating before and after intercourse. There is no immunity to STDs; one can be infected repeatedly. The best way to prevent these disorders is to avoid sexual contact with diseased persons.

The percentage of patients hospitalized with STDs is small because of adequate outpatient treatment measures. Patients with diagnosed cases are isolated. Nevertheless, because of the insidious nature of these disorders, nurses

## Nursing Brief

The use of condoms to prevent STDs, although recommended, is not considered 100% effective because they are apt to slip or break during intercourse.

## Nursing Brief

Sex education is not limited to the mechanics of intercourse, but rather includes the feelings involved in a sexual experience—the expectations, fantasies, fulfillments, and disappointments.

---

must practice scrupulous techniques of universal precautions and handwashing when assisting with vaginal and rectal examinations on new admissions and when handling equipment such as rectal thermometers and douche nozzles. Hands should be kept away from the face in order to prevent gonorrheal conjunctivitis.

An illness of this nature, which affects the reproductive organs, is a serious threat to the self-image and creates a great deal of anxiety. The nurse has to assess the person's level of knowledge and provide information at an understandable level. Many young people have lit-

tle knowledge of their bodies and their developing sexuality. Others have mild to deep-seated emotional problems that need to be addressed. They may be using sex to escape from reality, to express hostility or rebellion, or to call attention to themselves. They may be involved in relationships they no longer desire, so they need help in formulating positive attitudes toward themselves. They also need help understanding their behavior and that of others. In particular, adolescents need to learn that they are responsible for their own actions if they choose to be sexually active.

The prevention of STDs is everyone's concern and demands individual initiative and responsibility. Table 30–2 describes age-appropriate interventions. Nurses must keep themselves informed about the latest techniques in diagnosis and treatment. Education of the public, particularly young people, is paramount. Nurses who work in settings frequented by teenagers can distribute some of the many excellent health pamphlets available. Structured courses

**Table 30–2.** NURSING CARE IN THE PREVENTION AND TREATMENT OF STDs

**Nursing Goals**

To provide anticipatory guidance concerning sexuality at a level that the child or young person can comprehend throughout developmental cycle
To prevent infection
To identify early symptoms and provide prompt treatment if infection occurs
To prevent sequelae

| Assessment | Nursing Interventions |
|---|---|
| Children under age 12 | Provide age-appropriate instruction concerning sexuality; also explore expected patterns that might occur before next visit |
| Puberty and adolescence | Review structure and function of reproductive systems; review personal hygiene; discuss values and decision-making, possible sexual behavior and consequences, prevention of pregnancy and STDs |
| Self-concept: anticipate evidence of fear, embarrassment, anger, and decreased self-esteem upon suspicion of infection | Create nonjudgmental atmosphere, listen, assess level of knowledge, observe nonverbal behavior, establish confidentiality; provide privacy when assisting with pelvic or genital examination; provide appropriate draping of patient; realize anger is often a mask for depression, grief—do not take personally |
| Skin and hair | It is not uncommon to see skin rashes, "crabs" (pubic lice) or scabies (mites) Clothing is disinfected by washing in hot water |
| Sexual partners | Determine sexual preference; investigate and direct to treatment; persons with multiple sexual partners, homosexuals, persons with new partners, and those with history of prior STD are at particular risk |
| Sexual intercourse | Abstain during treatment; use condom in order to prevent reinfection |
| Medication | Take all of prescribed medication; if on tetracycline, advise to take 1 hr before or 2 hr after meals (on empty stomach); avoid dairy products, antacids, iron, and sunlight |
| Compliance with treatment | Stress importance of follow-up, routine Pap smears |
| Sequelae | Discuss possible complications of specific disorders such as birth defects, infertility |

STD, sexually transmitted disease; Pap, Papanicolaou.

in sex education should include presentations on STDs (there are also excellent audiovisual aids) and discussion of how one establishes healthy sexual behavior patterns. The community health or school nurse is involved in case finding and referral. Delays due to fear of disclosure have tragic results. Legislation in all 50 states permits physicians to treat infected minors without first obtaining parental consent.

## GONORRHEA

**Description.** The infectious agent that causes this highly communicable disease is *Neisseria gonorrhoeae*. It is an anaerobic bacterium that penetrates the mucous membrane surfaces that line the genital tract, rectum, and mouth. These bacteria thrive in warm, moist areas of the body and can also survive in the tissues around the eyes of the newborn and in the immature vulvular tissues of prepubescent girls. They quickly die outside the human body. The street names for this disease include "GC," "clap," "a dose," "strain," or "the drip."

**Manifestations.** The symptoms in males appear within 3–5 days after sexual contact with an infected person (although some males are asymptomatic). The germs invade the urethral canal, causing a painful burning sensation during urination. Pus that gradually becomes thin and watery is discharged from the penis. Increased burning, urinary frequency, and urgency are signs of bladder infection. The disease may spread to the prostate gland, seminal vesicles, and testes. The scrotum when inflamed is hard, swollen, painful, and heavy. Scarring of the tubules and of the epididymides can result in permanent sterility. The disease can be transmitted by homosexual practices in both males and females. Anal gonorrhea is increasing in prevalence and causes no symptoms.

Of female patients with gonorrhea, 80–90% are asymptomatic; therefore, they may spread the infection without knowing it. Those who have symptoms experience mild burning or smarting in the genital area, with or without discharge. When discharge is present, it is light-yellow and purulent. There may be slight inflammation and swelling of the Bartholin glands, which makes sitting or walking painful. The patient may also complain of a feeling of pelvic heaviness and discomfort in the abdomen. Anal itching and urinary symptoms may prevail. After one or more menstrual periods, the disease may invade the reproductive organs—including the fallopian tubes and ovaries—or may spread to the pelvis, causing pelvic inflammatory disease. Scar tissue may cause sterility. Adhesions of the abdomen and fibroids (leiomyofibroma: *leios*, "smooth," *mys*, "muscle," *fibra*, "fiber," and *oma*, "tumor") may also occur. The incidence of gonococcemia appears to be increasing in association with pimple-like lesions on the extremities that were once seldom seen. In both sexes, arthritis, endocarditis, and death may occur if gonorrhea is untreated.

**Treatment.** The diagnosis of gonorrhea is based on medical history, symptoms, and laboratory test results. In male patients, a smear of the discharge from the penis is taken with a cotton swab and transferred to a special culture plate or bottle where the organisms are grown for identification. The physician may want to take separate cultures 1 or 2 weeks apart. In female patients, the doctor usually takes a culture from within the vagina. Fluorescent-tagged antibody methods are the most accurate laboratory tests in female patients. Procedures are simple and painless, and the results are confidential. The patient who is a minor can still receive free, confidential treatment without parental consent from the city or state health department or most physicians. If the test results are positive, sexual contacts are traced so that those persons may be treated before complications arise.

Antibiotics, particularly penicillin, have been the drugs of choice in the past. Today broad-spectrum antibiotics may be given for penicillin-resistant strains or to allergic patients. A single intramuscular injection of ceftriaxone may be the choice for urethral, rectal, and endocervical gonorrhea due to insensitive or resistant gonococci (Behrman, 1992). For nonresistant strains, the initial treatment may be an injected single dose of 4.8 million units of aqueous procaine penicillin G for adults or children who weigh more than 45 kg (100 pounds). Probenecid may be given to prolong antibiotic activity. Efforts to develop a vaccine to prevent gonorrhea have been unsuccessful as of this writing.

Gonorrhea during pregnancy must be identified because it has been associated with spontaneous abortion, preterm delivery, and endometritis in the postpartum period. If the infection is present at birth, it may cause blindness in the newborn (see discussions of ophthalmia neonatorum, p. 234, and of STD during pregnancy, p. 108).

## NONGONOCOCCAL URETHRITIS

Nongonococcal urethritis (NGU), also known as "Cinderella disease," is an inflammation of the urethra, which carries urine from the bladder. The incidence of NGU is increasing at epidemic rates, particularly among young college students and single whites from the upper and middle classes. In many cases, *Chlamydia trachomatis* has been cited as the organism responsible for the infection. The symptoms include painful urination and a watery mucoid discharge. In women the disease may be asymptomatic. When untreated, the infection can cause sterility. It can also be transmitted to the newborn during birth and cause eye infections and pneumonia. NGU currently is diagnosed by the process of elimination. A culture of the discharge is examined for gonococci; if none is present, a diagnosis of NGU is made. Treatment consists of the administration of tetracycline or ceftriaxone (Rocephin). If tetracycline is prescribed, the patient is advised to take it 1 hour before or 2 hours after meals and to avoid dairy products, antacids, iron, and sunlight. The patient is instructed to return for evaluation 4–7 days after therapy is finished, or earlier if symptoms recur. Sexual relations are to be avoided until the patient and partners are cured. Condoms should be used in order to prevent further infection. It is important to educate the public to the seriousness of this infection, as the symptoms may be minimal.

## SYPHILIS

**Description.** Syphilis, also known as *lues*, causes destruction throughout the body. It was also a major cause of stillbirths, prematurity, and neonatal infection before the use of penicillin. The disease is caused by the spirochete *Treponema pallidum*, a spiral organism that reproduces rapidly in warm, moist areas of the body and quickly invades other tissues and organs. The organisms enter the body during coitus or through cuts or other breaks in the skin and mucous membranes. The incubation period is usually 3 weeks but may be anywhere from 7 to 90 days.

**Manifestations.** The symptoms of syphilis occur in three stages: primary, secondary, and tertiary (third). The primary stage consists of the appearance of a painless sore called a *chancre* (pronounced "shanker"), which appears where the spirochete enters the body—at genital, anal, or oral membranes. The chancre resembles a pimple, which ulcerates and forms a crater-like depression. It is highly infectious. In female patients, the chancre may go unnoticed when it is located around the cervix or in the vagina. It disappears without treatment in about 6 weeks. During this time, the serologic blood test result is negative, but the organism can be identified by examination of the scrapings from the sore under the dark-field microscope. Although the chancre disappears, the destructive work of the spirochete continues as it invades various body systems.

The symptoms of secondary syphilis vary among individuals and can begin from 6 weeks to 6 months after the infection. A rose-colored skin rash may be evident. Wartlike lesions called mucous patches, or *condylomata lata*, may also appear on the skin and mucous membranes. These are highly infectious. *Alopecia* (the loss of hair) may occur, usually in patches. The patient complains of general malaise, sore throat, and fever. The lymph glands may swell. Symptoms subside and reappear intermittently. If left untreated, the disease enters a latent period, in which there are no symptoms, that may last for many years. The disease remains contagious during the first 2 years, after which it is generally not communicable. Serologic test results are positive.

The tertiary stage occurs after the 4th year. The disease is noninfectious at this time, but very serious. The spirochetes attack the heart, blood vessels, brain, and spinal cord, in any of which the infection can cause death. Insanity and blindness can result. Destruction of bone tissue and severe crippling or paralysis are seen.

**Transmission to the Fetus and Newborn.** A mother who has syphilis can infect her unborn child. A serologic test called a "VDRL," for Venereal Disease Research Laboratory, is performed at the first prenatal visit. This has been successful in preventing congenital syphilis. Some physicians repeat these tests later in pregnancy in order to detect syphilis contracted after the original test. When the result is positive, the mother is treated with penicillin, which effectively permeates the placenta, regardless of the stage of pregnancy, and protects the fetus. If the syphilitic mother is untreated, miscarriage, stillbirth, or congenital syphilis may result. Young unwed mothers and their babies are in jeopardy, particularly when early prenatal care is neglected. Case-finding in adults is furthered by means of pre-employment physicals, required by many companies, and by preinduction physicals by the armed services. The adolescent who has been raped and is at risk may need prophylactic treatment.

### GENITAL HERPES

Herpes simplex virus type II is a sexually transmitted organism that infects the genitals. Its frequency among teenagers appears to be increasing. Of all cases of herpes, 5–10% are caused by herpes simplex virus type I. Type I virus is isolated most frequently from lesions above the umbilicus, whereas type II is generally isolated from genital lesions (Green & Haggerty, 1990). In male patients, the herpetic blisters or ulcers appear on the glans penis, prepuce, or penile shaft. In female patients, the vulva and vagina may be involved, although the cervix is the primary site. Recurrence of herpes is common.

The incubation period is 5–10 days, and the lesions may persist 3–6 weeks. The infection can be extremely painful, especially if the urethra and bladder are involved. The virus can be identified by tissue culture (Tzanck test). Systemic symptoms include fever, headache, malaise, and anorexia. Patients are advised to abstain from sex while symptomatic, as both initial and recurring lesions shed the virus in high concentrations.

Acyclovir (Zovirax) ointment used topically appears to shorten the initial infection period and relieve discomfort. It should be initiated as early as possible following onset. Zovirax does not prevent recurrences.

Sitz baths, heat lamps, and local compresses of aluminum acetate (Burow) solution may also bring relief. Herpes simplex virus type II, which can be fatal to the newborn, is acquired from the mother during passage through the birth canal. Overwhelming infection involving many of the body systems occurs. A cesarean delivery is performed on mothers known to have this virus.

Herpes is thought to be a predisposing factor in cancer of the cervix. Regular follow-up Pap smears will detect early carcinoma.

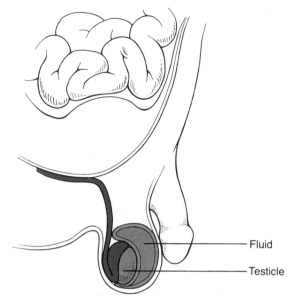

**Figure 30–2.** Hydrocele.

## Hydrocele

**Description.** A hydrocele (*hydro*, "water," and *cele*, "tumor") is an excessive amount of fluid in the sac that surrounds the testicle, which causes the scrotum to swell (Fig. 30–2). When the testes descend into the scrotum in utero, the *processus vaginalis*, a fold of tissue, precedes them. This tissue ordinarily fuses, separating the peritoneal cavity from the scrotum. When this fusion does not take place, peritoneal fluid may enter the inguinal canal. Its appearance in the newborn is not uncommon, and in many cases the condition corrects itself as the baby grows.

**Treatment.** If a chronic hydrocele persists in the older child, it is corrected by surgery. Routine postoperative nursing care is given. This is outlined in Chapter 23 (see p. 604). Same-day surgery may be arranged.

## Undescended Testes (Cryptorchidism)

**Description.** The testes are the male sex glands. These two oval bodies begin their development in the abdominal cavity below the kidneys of the embryo. Their function is to produce spermatozoa (male sex cells) and male hormones, particularly testosterone. Toward the end of the fetal period, they begin to descend along a pathway into the scrotum. If, for reasons that are yet unclear, this descent does not take place normally, the testes may remain in the abdomen or inguinal canal. This condition is common in about 30% of low-birth-weight infants. When one or both testes fail to lower into the scrotum, the condition is termed cryptorchidism (*kryptos,* "hidden," and *orchi,* "testis"). The unilateral form is more frequently seen.

Because the testes are warmer in the abdomen than in the scrotum, the sperm cells begin to deteriorate. If both testes are affected, sterility results. Other complications include increased exposure to injury, increased risk of tumor formation, and emotional problems, particularly in the school-age boy, who may be ridiculed by his peers. *Inguinal hernia* often accompanies this condition. Secondary sex characteristics, such as voice change and growth of facial hair, are not affected, since the testes continue to secrete hormones directly into the blood stream.

**Treatment and Nursing Care.** Occasionally, a testis or the testes spontaneously descend during the 1st year of life. If this does not happen, the patient may first be treated medically. Hormonal management before surgery consists of the administration of human chorionic gonadotropin (HCG). This hormone is useful as a diagnostic aid, and it may also precipitate descent of the testes. If this does not occur, an operation called an orchiopexy (*orchio,* "testicle," and *pexy,* "fixation") is performed. The optimal time at present (although controversial) is about 2–3 years of age. Although it is not known whether surgery at this age improves testicular function, it is thought that early scrotal placement and the use of a prosthesis for congenital absence are psychologically important for the growing boy.

Although orchiopexy improves the condition, the fertility rate among these patients, even when only one testis is undescended, may be reduced. In addition, the incidence of testicular tumors is increased in these patients during adulthood. Parents are told to teach the growing child the importance of self-examination of the testes.

When the child returns from surgery, his testicle will be held in position by an internal suture that is placed in the testis and attached to a rubber band. The band is fastened to the thigh by adhesive tape. This remains in place for about 1 week. Care is taken to prevent contamination of the suture line.

The psychological approach of the nurse to the patient and his family is important because of the embarrassment they may feel. People may ask the child why he is being operated on when there is no visible evidence of trauma. This problem is frequently compounded by the fact that the older child has been told not to discuss his condition; in addition, his understanding of his problem and just what is going to happen in surgery may be vague. Therefore, the nurse caring for the child should know what he has been told and how he feels about his operation in order to give emotional support. Terminology is clarified. The nurse assures the child that his penis will not be involved in the surgery.

The parents, too, may have anxieties that they cannot verbalize. It is difficult for many of them to communicate with their child about such matters. They may also fear that the child will become homosexual or less virile. A thoughtful, sensitive nurse who tries to anticipate these and other related feelings and fears promotes the patient's adjustment.

## KEY POINTS

- Good health habits include assessing one's body, including the genitals.
- Tests helpful in diagnosing conditions of the reproductive tract include the Papanicolaou (Pap) smear, serologic blood tests, gonococcal cultures, ultrasound, pregnancy tests, and routine blood and urine assessment.
- Mittelschmerz refers to midcycle pain during ovulation.
- For patients with moderate discomfort during menstruation, warm fluids, a heating pad, and acetaminophen are suggested.
- To prevent the transmission of sexually transmitted disease, suggest limitation of partners, discourage sex with strangers, emphasize importance of using latex condoms when having intercourse, educate the client, and dispel misinformation.

■ The symptoms of syphilis occur in three stages: primary, secondary, and tertiary.
■ The VDRL is a serologic test for syphilis performed on pregnant women to prevent congenital syphilis in the newborn.
■ Herpes simplex type II blisters appear on the glans penis, prepuce and penile shaft in men. The cervix is the primary site in women, although lesions may also appear on the vulva and vagina.
■ A hydrocele is an excessive amount of fluid in the sac that surrounds the testicle, which causes the scrotum to swell.
■ Undescended testes (cryptorchidism) refers to a condition in which the testes do not lower into the scrotum during the fetal period but remain in the abdomen or inguinal canal.

# Study Questions

1. What disease organism causes acquired immunodeficiency syndrome (AIDS)?
2. How is AIDS spread?
3. When do the symptoms of gonorrhea appear?
4. List the grades of primary dysmenorrhea.
5. Describe three methods of preventing sexually transmitted diseases (STDs).
6. Discuss the treatment for genital herpes.
7. With what disease is a chancre associated?
8. Why are expectant mothers tested for venereal disease?
9. What STD is also known as Cinderella disease?
10. Mel, who is 15, disclosed to you that he has a friend who has "clap." What knowledge do you need in order to discuss this with Mel? What immediate suggestions might you offer?
11. Discuss the treatment for hydrocele.
12. Outline the postoperative care for the child with an undescended testis.

# Multiple Choice Review Questions

*Choose the most appropriate answer.*

1. The reproductive organs of the fetus are recognizable as male or female by the
   a. 3rd week
   b. 6th week
   c. 12th week
   d. 24th week
2. Lues is another name for
   a. gonorrhea
   b. syphilis
   c. genital herpes
   d. STD
3. A painless sore associated with syphilis is termed
   a. chalazion
   b. chancroid
   c. cheloid
   d. chancre

4. The VDRL test is used to diagnose
   a. gonorrhea
   b. erythroblastosis
   c. syphilis
   d. genital herpes
5. A type of skin cancer seen in AIDS is
   a. epithelioma
   b. Kaposi's sarcoma
   c. Keith-Flack node
   d. keratiasis

## BIBLIOGRAPHY

Behrman, R.E. (1992). *Nelson textbook of pediatrics* (14th ed.). Philadelphia: W.B. Saunders.

Gellis, S.S. & Kagan, B.M. (1990). *Current pediatric therapy 13*. Philadelphia: W.B. Saunders.

Graef, J., & Cone T. (1988). *Manual of pediatric therapeutics* (4th ed.). Boston: Little, Brown.

Levine, M.D., Carey, W.B., & Crocker, A.C. (1992). *Developmental-behavioral pediatrics* (2nd ed.). Philadelphia: W.B. Saunders.

Litt, I. (1990). Adolescent health care. In M. Green & R.J. Haggerty (Eds.), *Ambulatory pediatrics IV*. Philadelphia: W.B. Saunders.

Mott, S., James, S.R., & Sperhac, A.M. (1992). *Nursing care of children and families* (2nd ed.). Reading, MA: Addison-Wesley.

Pillitteri, A. (1992). *Maternal and child health nursing*. Philadelphia: J.B. Lippincott.

Thompson, E.D., & Ashwill, J.W. (1992). *Introduction to pediatric nursing* (6th ed.). Philadelphia: W.B. Saunders.

Whaley, L., & Wong, D. (1991). *Nursing care of children* (4th ed.). St. Louis: C.V. Mosby.

# Chapter 31

# The Child with a Skin Condition

## VOCABULARY

allergens (813)
débridement (823)
dermabrasion (812)
emollient (814)
eschar (823)
hives (807)
heterografts (824)
homografts (824)
pediculosis (818)
pruritus (807)

Miliaria
Intertrigo
Seborrheic Dermatitis (Cradle Cap)
Diaper Dermatitis (Diaper Rash)
Strawberry Nevus
Acne Vulgaris
Herpes Simplex Type I (Cold Sore)
Infantile Eczema (Atopic Dermatitis)
Staphylococcal Infection
Impetigo
Folliculitis (Furuncle, Carbuncle)
Fungal Infections (Tinea Capitis, Corporis,
    Pedis, Cruris)
Pediculosis
    Pediculosis Capitis
Scabies
Burns

# OBJECTIVES

*On completion and mastery of Chapter 31, the student will be able to*

- Define each vocabulary term listed.
- Describe the skin of the fetus.
- List two diagnostic tests useful for patients with conditions of the skin.
- Describe two topical agents used in the treatment of acne.
- Summarize the nursing care for 15-month-old Peter, who has infantile eczema. State the rationale for each nursing measure.
- Discuss the symptoms and treatment of pediculosis.
- Differentiate among first-, second-, and third degree burns in anatomic structures involved, appearance, level of sensation, and first aid required.
- List five objectives of the nurse caring for the burn patient.
- Discuss the emotional considerations of importance when caring for the child with burns.
- Describe how caring for the child with burns differs from caring for the adult.
- Prepare a nursing care plan for 2-year-old Mendez who has received second- and third-degree coffee burns to his chest.

The main function of the skin is protection. It acts as the body's first line of defense against disease. It prevents the passage of harmful physical and chemical agents and prevents the loss of water and electrolytes. It also has a great capacity to regenerate and repair itself. The skin and the structures derived from it, such as hair and fingernails, are known as the integumentary system. Figure 31–1 depicts these structures and how they differ in the developing child from in the adult.

Maintaining skin integrity is important to self-esteem and therefore has a psychological as well as a physiologic component. This is particularly evident in patients with facial disfiguration. Four basic skin sensations—pain, temperature, touch, and pressure—are felt by the skin in conjunction with the nervous system. The skin also secretes sebum, which helps protect and maintain its texture. The outer surface of the skin is acidic, with a pH of 4.5–6.5. This may protect the skin from pathologic bacteria, which thrive in an alkaline environment.

The skin is composed of two layers: the epi-

dermis, derived from the ectoderm, and the dermis, derived from the mesenchyma. Vernix caseosa, a cheeselike substance, covers the fetus until birth. This protects the fetus from maceration as it floats in its watery home. The fetal skin is at first so transparent that blood vessels are clearly visible. Downy lanugo hair begins to develop at about 13–16 weeks, especially on the head. At 21–24 weeks, the skin is reddish and wrinkled, with little subcutaneous fat. Adipose tissue forms during later weeks. At birth, the subcutaneous glands are well developed, and the skin is pink and smooth with a polished look. It is thinner than the skin of an adult. Figure 31–2 is an electron micrograph of human skin with a hair follicle.

Certain skin conditions in children may be associated with age, as in the case of milia in babies and acne in adolescents. A skin condition may be a manifestation of a systemic disease, such as chickenpox. Some lesions, such as strawberry nevi and mongolian spots, are congenital. Other skin conditions, such as rubella and fifth disease, are self-limited and do not require treatment.

There are great individual differences in skin texture, color, pH, and moisture. Skin color is an important diagnostic criterion in cases of liver disease, heart conditions, and child abuse and for overall assessment. Complete blood counts and serum electrolyte levels are helpful in diagnosing skin conditions, particularly burns. Skin tests are used in diagnosing allergies. The tine test is useful in screening for tuberculosis. Skin scrapings are used for microscopic examination. The Wood light is an instrument used to diagnose certain skin conditions. It reflects a particular color according to the organism present.

Hair condition is important to observe. Hair is inspected for color, texture, quality, distribution, and elasticity. The hair of individuals of different races varies. African-American children have hair that is generally curlier and coarser that that of Caucasian children. Hair may become dry and brittle and may lack luster owing to inadequate nutrition. Hair may begin to fall out or even change color during illness.

Skin conditions may be acute or chronic. The nurse should describe the lesions with regard to size, color, configuration (e.g., butterfly rash), presence of pain or itching, distribution (e.g., arms, legs, behind ears), and whether the rash

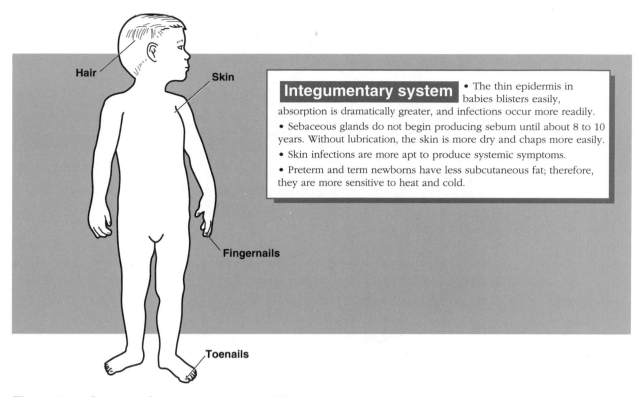

Hair

Skin

**Integumentary system** • The thin epidermis in babies blisters easily, absorption is dramatically greater, and infections occur more readily.

• Sebaceous glands do not begin producing sebum until about 8 to 10 years. Without lubrication, the skin is more dry and chaps more easily.

• Skin infections are more apt to produce systemic symptoms.

• Preterm and term newborns have less subcutaneous fat; therefore, they are more sensitive to heat and cold.

Fingernails

Toenails

**Figure 31–1.** Summary of integumentary system differences between the child and the adult. The integumentary system consists of the skin and the structures derived from it. This system protects the body, helps regulate body temperature, and receives stimuli such as pressure, pain, and temperature.

is general or local. Hives, a general rash that appears abruptly, is frequently a medication reaction. The condition of the skin around the lesions is also significant, as is the skin turgor. Managing itching is a key component in preventing secondary infection from scratching. Dressings and ointments are applied as prescribed. Preventing tetanus is a consideration in open wounds.

The following skin conditions frequently seen in children are discussed: miliaria, intertrigo, seborrhea, diaper dermatitis, strawberry nevus, acne, herpes simplex, eczema, staphylococcal infections, impetigo, folliculitis, fungal infections, pediculosis, scabies, and burns. Mongolian spots and physiologic jaundice are covered in Chapter 12. The communicable diseases are discussed in Chapter 34.

**Skin Lesions: Overview.** Many childhood infectious diseases, such as measles (see Color Plate Fig. 3), German measles (see Color Plate Fig. 4), and chickenpox (see Color Plate Fig. 5), involve the presence of an *exanthem* (a rash).

Box 31–1 identifies several conditions of the skin that the nurse may witness. Some rashes begin as one lesion and evolve into others. For example, the pattern of chickenpox rash is macule, papule, vesicle, and crust.

## Miliaria

**Description.** Miliaria (prickly heat) refers to a rash caused by excess body warmth. There is retention of sweat in the sweat glands, which have become blocked or inflamed. Rupture or leakage into the skin causes the inflamed response. It appears suddenly as tiny pinhead-sized reddened papules with occasional vesicles and pustules. It may be accompanied by *pruritus* (itching). It is seen in infants during hot weather or in newborns who sleep in overheated rooms. It can also result from wearing too much clothing. It usually starts on the neck and face but may spread downward into the

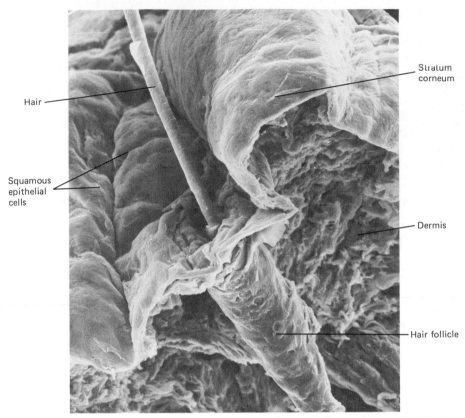

Hair

Stratum corneum

Squamous epithelial cells

Dermis

Hair follicle

**Figure 31–2.** Scanning electron micrograph of human skin showing hair follicle, approximately 250 times life size. (Courtesy of Dr. Karen A. Holbrook. From Solomon, E.P., & Phillips, G.A. [1987]. *Understanding human anatomy and physiology* [p. 62]. Philadelphia: W.B. Saunders.)

trunk or diaper area. This harmless condition may be reversed by removing extra clothing, finding a shady spot, or having a tepid bath.

## Intertrigo

**Description.** Intertrigo (*in*, "into," and *terere*, "to rub") is the medical term for chafing (see Color Plate Fig. 6). It is a dermatitis that occurs in the folds of the skin. The patches are red and moist and are usually along the neck and in the inguinal and gluteal folds. This condition is aggravated by urine, feces, heat, and moisture. Prevention consists of keeping the affected areas clean and dry. The child is allowed to be out of diapers for periods of time to expose the area to air and light (Fig. 31–3). A nonmedicated powder is helpful. The parents are instructed to shake a small amount of powder into the hand

and apply. This prevents particles of powder from entering baby's lungs.

## Seborrheic Dermatitis (Cradle Cap)

**Description.** Seborrheic dermatitis is an inflammation of the skin (see Color Plate Fig. 7). It is characterized by thick, yellow, oily, adherent, crustlike scales on the scalp and forehead. The skin beneath the patches may be red. Less often it may involve the eyelids, external ear, and inguinal area. Secondary bacterial and yeast infections may occur. *Pityrosporum ovale* has been implicated as a causative agent (Behrman, 1992). It is seen in newborns, in infants, and at puberty. In newborns it is commonly known as "cradle cap." It is seen in ba-

## BOX 31–1    Terms Used to Describe Conditions of the Skin

**Ecchymosis:** black and blue-purple mark (bruise)

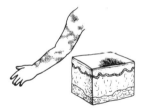

**Crust:** scab

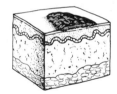

**Macule:** flat rash (freckles)

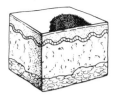

**Papule:** elevated area (pimple)

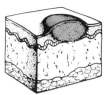

**Pustules:** elevated, pus filled (impetigo, acne)

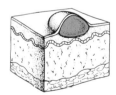

**Stye:** infection of eyelash follicle

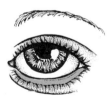

**Vesicle:** elevated fluid-filled blister (cold sore, chickenpox)

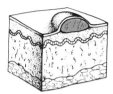

**Wheal:** raised red, irregular (mosquito bite, allergic reactions)

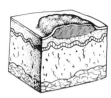

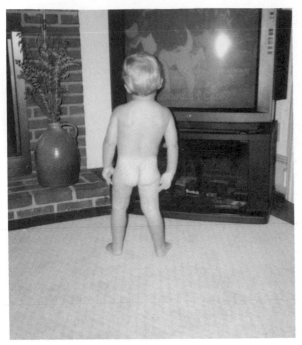

**Figure 31–3.** The child with chafing or a rash in the diaper area benefits from periods of exposure to air and/or sunlight.

bies with sensitive skin, even when the head and hair are washed frequently. Seborrhea resembles eczema; however, it usually does not itch and there is a negative family history. In adolescence it is more localized, usually confined to the scalp. A condition resembling seborrheic dermatitis is common in human immunodeficiency virus (HIV)-infected children and adolescents (Behrman, 1992).

**Treatment.** Treatment consists of shampooing the hair on a regular basis. In newborns if the scales are particularly stubborn, they may be softened by applying baby oil to the head the evening before and shampooing the hair in the morning. The scalp is rinsed well. A soft brush is helpful in removing loose particles from the hair. Some parents may be afraid to wash the newborn's head because of possible injury to the fontanels. The nurse demonstrates the football hold (see p. 562) and assures parents that the soft spots are really rather tough and are not injured by ordinary care. In adolescents a dandruff-control shampoo is used. Medications such as sulfur, salicylic acid, or hydrocortisone

may be prescribed. Topical antifungal agents effective against *Pityrosporon* have also been suggested.

## Diaper Dermatitis (Diaper Rash)

**Description.** Diaper dermatitis is a frequently seen condition that results when the skin becomes irritated by prolonged contact with urine, feces, retained diaper soaps, and friction. It may be seen with the addition of solid foods or with a change in breast or bottle feedings. Changes in detergent, water softeners, or other household substances may precipitate the irritation. The rash may appear as a simple erythema (redness) (see Color Plate Fig. 8) or may be evidenced by scales, blisters, and ulcerations. Perianal involvement may be apparent if the baby has loose stools.

**Treatment and Nursing Care.** It is easier to prevent diaper rash than to cure it. This is accomplished by frequent diaper changes to limit the exposure to moisture. The diaper is periodically removed to expose the skin to light and air. With each diaper change, the perineal area is thoroughly cleansed (preferably with warm water) and gently dried. Plastic pants are avoided. After bowel movements, the area is cleansed with mild soap and water. *The skin folds are thoroughly washed, rinsed, and dried.* The use of powder is controversial, as it may irritate the respiratory tract. If a medicated powder is used, it should be applied to hands first rather than shaken from the container. This helps protect the infant from inhaling particles. A thin film is applied because excessive powder accumulates in skin folds, causing irritation. If a rash is persistent, the pediatrician may apply a light application of a mild hydrocortisone ointment.

## Strawberry Nevus

The strawberry nevus is a common *hemangioma*, which may not become apparent for a few weeks after birth. Although it is harmless and disappears without treatment, it is disturbing to parents, especially when it appears on

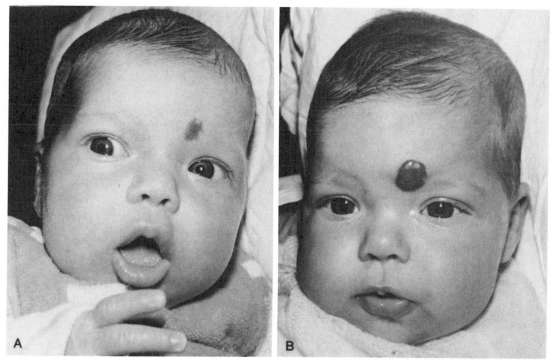

**Figure 31–4.** Strawberry nevus. *A,* Appearance 4 days after birth. *B,* Appearance 6 weeks later; the nevus has enlarged and become raised above the skin. This minor lesion can result in major psychological problems. (From Beischer, N.A., & MacKay, E.B. [1986]. *Obstetrics and the newborn* [2nd ed., p. 637]. Philadelphia: W.B. Saunders/Bailliere Tindall.)

the head or face (Fig. 31–4). At first it is flat, but it gradually becomes raised. Parents are frequently quizzed about the growth by insensitive persons and may be advised of various unorthodox treatments. These marks gradually fade as the child grows. The nurse offers support and reassurance to parents and corrects misinformation.

## Acne Vulgaris

**Description.** Acne is an inflammation of the sebaceous glands and hair follicles in the skin (see Color Plate Fig. 9). At puberty, owing to hormonal influence, the sebaceous follicles enlarge and secrete increased amounts of a fatty substance called *sebum.* Genetic factors and stress are also thought to play a part. The course of acne may be brief or prolonged (lasting 10 years or longer). Premenstrual acne in girls is not uncommon. The principal lesions

include comedones, papules, and nodulocystic growths.

A *comedo* (plural, *comedones*) is a plug of keratin, sebum, and bacteria. Keratin is a protein substance that is the main constituent of epidermis and hair. There are two types of comedones, open and closed. In the open comedo, or blackhead, the surface is darkened by melanin. Closed comedones, or whiteheads, are responsible for the inflammatory process of acne. With continued build-up, the walls of the follicle rupture, releasing their irritating contents into the surrounding skin. A pustule may appear when this develops near the exterior. This process occurs no matter how carefully the teenager washes because surface bacteria are not involved in the pathogenesis. Acne is usually seen on the chin, cheeks, and forehead. It can also develop on the chest, upper back, and shoulders. It usually is more severe in winter.

**Treatment.** The basic treatment of acne has changed considerably over the past few years. It is no longer thought that certain foods trigger the condition: therefore, restriction of chocolate, peanuts, and cola drinks is unwarranted unless the patient is convinced of a correlation between a specific item and the condition. A regular, well-balanced diet is encouraged. Patients who are not taking tetracycline or vitamin A benefit from sunshine. General hygienic measures of cleanliness, rest, and avoidance of emotional stress may help prevent exacerbations.

The physician may prescribe a special soap, such as Fostex. Excessive cleansing of the skin can be harmful, however, since it irritates and chaps the tissues. Squeezing pimples ruptures intact lesions and causes local inflammation. The topical preparations recommended include benzoyl peroxide gels, such as Benzagel, Panoxyl, or Desquam-X, which dry and peel the skin and suppress fatty acid growth. Vitamin A acid (Retin-A) aids in the elimination of keratinous plugs. Vitamin A acid can increase sensitivity to the sun, so precautions should be taken when it is used. Tetracycline or erythromycin may be given in conjunction with topical medications in more serious cases. Monilial vaginitis is a secondary complication sometimes seen when these drugs are used, and this should be explained to the unsuspecting teenage girl. Topical antibiotics such as clindamycin (Cleocin T) or erythromycin (T-Stat, A/T/S) are also available (Behrman, 1992).

Isotretinoin (Accutane) is given to patients with severe pustulocystic acne who have been unable to benefit from other types of treatment. It has many side effects; thus the patient must be carefully monitored. *It is not prescribed during pregnancy or to those at risk for pregnancy because of the possibilities of fetal deformity.* The long-term effects of this medication have not been established. *Dermabrasion* (planing of the skin in order to minimize scarring) is done selectively, as it is not always successful.

Acne is distressing to the adolescent, particularly when the face is extensively involved. Sometimes even a minimum problem is seen as disastrous when it happens before an important event. The self-conscious young person feels different and embarrassed. The nurse who is attuned to the feelings of individuals can provide understanding support. Although the teenager is educated to assume responsibility for the regimen, including the parents helps prevent conflict surrounding it.

# Herpes Simplex Type I (Cold Sore)

**Description.** Herpes simplex type I, a viral infection, is commonly known as a cold sore or fever blister. It may begin by a feeling of tingling, itching, or burning on the lip. Vesicles and crusts form (see Color Plate Fig. 10). Spontaneous healing occurs in about 8–10 days. Communicability is highest early in the formation and is spread by direct contact. Recurrence is common because the virus lies dormant in the body until it is activated by stress, sun exposure, menstruation, fever, and other causes. Patients need to become familiar with their own personal triggers. Herpes can be serious in newborns and in patients who are immunocompromised.

**Treatment and Nursing Care.** Topical acyclovir may reduce viral shedding and hasten healing. In the hospital, ointments are applied with gloved hands. Contagiousness is reduced by frequent handwashing. Patients are instructed not to pick at lesions, as this may cause spreading to other sites. They should not share lipstick and should avoid kissing while lesions are active. The lips are protected by sunscreen during sunbathing. Sensitivity to the self-conscious teenager who has a cold sore is important. Genital herpes caused by the herpes virus type II and spread by sexual intimacy are discussed on page 800. The distinction between the two types has become less clear because of an increase in the practice of oral-genital sex (Betz, 1994).

# Infantile Eczema (Atopic Dermatitis)

**Description.** Infantile eczema, or atopic dermatitis, is an inflammation of genetically hypersensitive skin. The pathophysiology is characterized by local vasodilatation in affected areas. This progresses to *spongiosis*, or the breakdown of dermal cells and the formation of intradermal vesicles. Chronic scratching produces weeping and results in lichenification, or coarsening of the skin folds. The exact cause of this condition is difficult to pinpoint, as it is believed to be mainly due to allergy. Infantile eczema is rarely seen in breast-fed babies until they begin to eat additional food. It seems to have a definite familial tendency; emotional factors are often involved.

Eczema actually is a symptom rather than a disorder. It indicates that the infant is oversensitive to certain substances called *allergens*, which enter the body via the digestive tract (food), by inhalation (dust, pollen), by direct contact (wool, soap, strong sunlight), and by injections (insect bites, vaccines). In most cases, the skin heals by age 2 or 3 years, and the eczema does not occur again. Some children develop the triad of atopic dermatitis, asthma, and hay fever. Manifestations of allergy, by age group, are listed in Table 31–1.

**Manifestations.** Although infantile eczema can occur at any age, it is more common during the first 2 years. The lesions form vesicles that weep and develop a dry crust. They are more severe on the face but may occur on the entire body, particularly in the skin folds (see Color Plate Fig. 11). Eczema is worse in the winter than in the summer and has periods of tempo-

**Table 31–1.** MANIFESTATIONS OF ALLERGY BY AGE GROUP

| Age | Allergen | Sex | Distribution |
|---|---|---|---|
| Neonatal period to 6 mo | Primary foods | Male > female 2:1 | Pylorospasm, colic, projectile vomiting<br>Chronic diarrhea<br>Atopic eczema<br>Persistent nasal congestion with recurrent respiratory infection |
| 6 mo to 1 yr | Food (66%)<br>Environmental inhalants (34%) | Male > female 2:1 | Atopic eczema<br>Chronic diarrhea with or without growth failure<br>Chronic nasal congestion<br>Asthma |
| 1–5 yr | Food (25%)<br>Environmental inhalants (70%)<br>Pollens (5%) | Male > female 2:1 | Atopic eczema (spontaneous improvement in 75% by age 3 yr)<br>Chronic respiratory infections<br>Chronic nasal congestion without fever<br>Asthma<br>Persistent middle ear fluid |
| 5–12 yr | Food (5%)<br>Environmental inhalants (25%)<br>Pollens (20%)<br>Combined inhalants (environmental and pollens) (50%) | Male > female 2:1 | Chronic nasal congestion, eustachian tube dysfunction, and hearing loss (serous otitis, secretory otitis)<br>School problems (poor attendance, poor attention span)<br>Hay fever<br>Asthma—extrinsic > intrinsic<br>Exercise-induced asthma<br>Urticaria |
| 12–21 yr | Food (>5%)<br>Environmental inhalants and pollens (95%) | Male = female 1:1 | Nasal congestion (perennial)<br>Hay fever (seasonal)<br>Exercise-induced asthma<br>Asthma—extrinsic > intrinsic<br>Chronic sinus disease<br>Allergic bronchitis<br>Urticaria |
| 21–40 yr | Food (<5%)<br>Environmental inhalants and pollens (60%)<br>Unknown (intrinsic factors) (35%) | Male = female 1:1 | Asthma—extrinsic > intrinsic<br>Nasal allergy<br>Nasal polyps and sinus disease<br>Drug reactions<br>Contact dermatitis<br>Occupational lung disease |
| 40+ yr | Inhalants (25%)<br>Infection (50%)<br>Unknown (25%) | Male < female 1:2 | Asthma—extrinsic < intrinsic<br>Nasal allergy<br>Nasal polyps and sinus disease<br>Chronic bronchitis<br>Urticaria<br>Occupational lung disease<br>Drug reaction |

From Smith, D. (1977). *Introduction to clinical pediatrics* (2nd ed.). Philadelphia: W.B. Saunders.

rary remission. Foods to which these infants are sensitive include egg white, wheat cereal, cow's milk, and citrus juices.

The baby scratches because the itching is constant, and is irritable and unable to sleep. The lesions become easily infected by bacterial or viral agents. Infants and children with eczema should not be exposed to adults with "cold sores" because they may develop a systemic reaction with high fever and multiple vesicles on the eczematous skin. Eczema may flare up following immunization. Laboratory studies may show an increase in immunoglobulin E and eosinophil rates.

**Treatment.** Treatment of the child with infantile eczema is aimed at promoting comfort by relieving symptoms. Dermatologists disagree about what types of ointments and solutions are most effective. The patient's reaction to an ointment or solution is the best guide. Frequently, the doctor applies an ointment to a small area of the skin as a trial in order to determine sensitivity to it. If redness and itching occur within a short time, the doctor is notified and the medication is removed. Different types of medications may be used on the various parts of the body at the same time. For example, lesions on the face may be of the type that requires ointment, whereas those on the extremities may require wet soaks.

An emollient bath is sometimes ordered for its soothing effect on the skin. Oatmeal and a mixture of cornstarch and baking soda are examples of substances prescribed. The baby's hair is washed with a soap substitute rather than a shampoo. Some dermatologists believe that bathing should be kept to a minimum. The physician may suggest that a bath oil such as Alpha-Keri be used as the lesions begin to heal. This prevents the skin from becoming too dry. To be correctly used, bath oils should be added after the patient has soaked for a while and the skin is hydrated. In this way, moisture is sealed rather than excluded, as it is when oil is added before the patient gets into the tub. Whenever possible, patients are treated at home because of the danger of infection in the hospital.

Corticosteroids may be administered systemically or locally. Antibiotics are needed if infection is present. Medication to help relieve itching is ordered for the patient. A child who is uncomfortable and unable to sleep should receive sedation.

**Nursing Care.** The nurse plays a vital role in the treatment of patients with skin problems; the doctor's prescribed therapy is of little value if ointments and wet soaks are not applied. It is a rewarding experience for the nurse, who can see the direct results of these efforts more vividly than in other types of nursing.

Hospitalized infants with eczema are sometimes isolated for their own protection, and therefore they must receive as much attention as possible. They are unhappy and irritable. Little fingers can dig and scratch a week's good treatment to ruins in a matter of minutes, so out of necessity they are restrained. They can tolerate such frustration more easily when they are frequently cuddled in the nurse's lap and their attention is diverted from their discomfort. This also shows the parents that the nurse is not repulsed by the baby's appearance and increases their confidence in the type of care received.

The kind of restraint used varies with the size and condition of the infant. Combinations of the elbow cuff, abdominal jacket, and ankle restraint are sometimes necessary. The least amount of restraint that accomplishes its purpose is devised. The fingernails must be kept short. Cotton socks or mittens may be placed over the hands and feet to prevent scratching. The restraints are observed frequently in order to make sure that they are not interfering with normal circulation. They are removed periodically, one at a time, to enable the baby to move about. The child's position must be changed at short intervals in order to prevent pneumonia.

Medicated baths may be part of the treatment. Towels and needed clothing are obtained in advance. The tub is filled and then cold water is run through the faucets before they are closed so that they are cool if the baby grasps them. The bath water should be 35°C (95°F). The infant is placed in the tub for 15–20 minutes. Floating toys amuse the infant. *One must remain with the baby for the entire time spent in the tub.* Children with eczema should not be overdressed because undue warmth adds to their discomfort.

Wet dressings are applied in order to cool the body and, in some cases, to remove crusts. A gauze bandage is dipped into the prescribed solution, squeezed gently to remove excess fluid, and applied to the involved area. The bandage must cover the entire rash. Soaks are usually ordered to be done continuously, and their effectiveness is measured only in terms of their being *wet.* When they are left on too long and become dry, itching increases. This type of bandage is *not* covered with towels or rubber sheeting in an effort to protect the bed linens, because the itching is relieved by the cooling effect of the medication, and covering the bandage would prevent evaporation.

Wet compresses may also be applied to the face by means of a mask, which consists of a square piece of gauze material in which holes for the eyes, nose, and mouth have been cut. It is held in place by strings attached to the four corners. When it is necessary to change wet bandages, they are completely removed, soaked in the solution, and reapplied. The nurse charts the following observations regarding the application of wet soaks: time of application, name of solution, strength of solution, area to which it was applied, length of time, general condition of the involved area (changes in the appearance or area of the rash), and comfort and tolerance of the patient during and following the procedure.

Ointment is usually applied to the skin by a gloved hand rather than by a tongue depressor. It is applied evenly and must be kept constantly on the skin to be effective. Because some of these ointments are expensive, the nurse must not be wasteful in using them. Most hospitals provide special linen for their dermatology patients, because many ointments leave a permanent stain on the sheets.

The physician may prescribe an elimination diet. Initially, a basic diet consisting of only hypoallergenic foods is given to the child. One new food at a time is added to determine the infant's reaction to it. When the baby is allergic to cow's milk, a substitute such as soybean milk can be used. Vitamin supplements are needed, particularly if the infant is not taking enough of the prescribed fruits and vegetables. The nurse charts the kind and amount of food taken at each meal and any allergic reactions that may have occurred. The time is planned so that treatments do not interfere with mealtime. Elbow restraints are removed from the toddler who is able to eat alone. The nurse assists with the patient's meals and prevents the scratching of irritated skin. Infants are held and shown love during feedings, as an emotional climate that discourages tension is important to their recovery.

The nurse tries to establish a good working relationship with the parents. They need encouragement, as the course of eczema is unstable and they provide much of the care at home. The nurse listens in order to make sure that they understand the doctor's instructions and

clarifies matters as needed. Nursing Care Plan 31–1 describes interventions for the child with eczema.

## Staphylococcal Infection

**Description.** The genus of bacteria called *Staphylococcus* comprises common bacteria that are found in dust and on the skin. Under normal conditions, they do not present a problem to the healthy body's defenses. If the number of organisms increases in preterms and newborns, whose general resistance is low, skin infections may occur. An abscess may form, and infection may enter the blood stream. This condition is called *septicemia*. Pneumonia, osteomyelitis, or meningitis may result. Primary infection of the newborn may develop in the umbilicus or circumcision wound. It may occur while the newborn is in the hospital or after discharge. This infection spreads readily from one infant to another. Small pustules on the newborn must immediately be reported.

**Treatment and Nursing Care.** Antibiotics effective against the appropriate strain of *Staphylococcus* are administered. Ointments may be locally applied.

In past years, the staphylococci that invade the body developed resistance to the drugs in current use. In some hospitals, serious epidemics have occurred in the newborn nursery and among surgical patients. It is difficult to control the spread of this infection because personnel act as carriers. The chief reservoir is the nose. The incidence of staphylococcal infections in newborn nurseries appears to have subsided. The reasons for this are not clearly understood.

To prevent staphylococcal infections, no one with a skin infection should be allowed to visit mothers or enter the nursery. Mothers or newborn infants who have acquired this infection must be isolated. Strict standards must be upheld in the nursery; adequate space must be provided for each bassinet to avoid overcrowding, and each baby should have individual equipment. The number and quality of personnel and their health status are also important factors. All personnel must thoroughly scrub their hands with a bactericide before they enter the nursery. Washing the hands before and after touching each patient and before and after handling equipment is *essential*. Medical supervision of all discharged babies must be continued to detect latent cases.

| NURSING CARE PLAN 31–1 |
| --- |
| **Selected Nursing Diagnoses for the Child with Eczema** |

| Goals | Nursing Interventions | Rationale |
| --- | --- | --- |
| **Nursing Diagnosis:** Skin integrity impaired related to inflammation. | | |
| Child's skin does not show signs of irritation or infection | 1. Describe types of lesions, configuration and location | 1. Eczema has a typical pattern of distribution; vesicles, oozing, and crusting may denote infection |
| | 2. Provide supervision rather than restraints whenever possible | 2. Elbow restraints may assist in avoiding self-inflicted skin damage due to scratching and picking; restriction of movement in infants has been related to learning difficulties and other problems, therefore, judicious application of any restraint is necessary |
| | 3. Keep fingernails short | 3. Trimming fingernails and covering hands with "sock mittens" will reduce excoriation from scratching |
| | 4. Administer medicated baths such as Aveeno | 4. Medicated baths soothe and rehydrate the skin |
| | 5. Apply wet dressings | 5. Wet dressings promote cooling of the skin, which decreases inflammation and itching (pruritus) |
| | 6. Administer oral antibiotics and sedatives as prescribed | 6. Systemic antibiotics such as erythromycin may be prescribed if there is an infection; sedatives reduce itching |
| | 7. Apply steroid ointments as prescribed | 7. Steroid creams reduce inflammation |
| **Nursing Diagnosis:** High risk for altered nutrition, less than body requirements, related to irritability, sensitivity to certain foods. | | |
| Child will eat portions of each meal and maintain weight<br>Child receives adequate nutrition as evidenced by growth charts and other parameters | 1. Serve hypoallergenic diet if prescribed | 1. This is a basic diet in which only one new food is added at a time to determine whether the infant is allergic to it |
| | 2. Determine specific food sensitivities from parents if child not on diet | 2. Parents have the most knowledge from experience with their child |
| | 3. Observe child for food sensitivities | 3. Any food can produce allergic symptoms, but some are thought to be highly allergenic; certain antigens (foreign protein) may enter the bloodstream and activate antibody formation of immune system; one reason this takes place during infancy is that baby's gastrointestinal tract is immature; allergy may be outgrown as body systems mature |
| | 4. Administer vitamins and mineral supplements as prescribed | 4. Child may be deficient in nutrients owing to irritability and food restrictions; adequate intake of vitamins and minerals is essential to the maintenance of healthy skin (particularly vitamins A, B, and C) |
| | 5. Provide adequate fluids | 5. Adequate hydration prevents drying of the skin and pruritus, and it makes the skin less prone to breaks, which can become infected |

**Selected Nursing Diagnoses for the Child with Eczema**

| Goals | Nursing Interventions | Rationale |
|---|---|---|
| **Nursing Diagnosis:** Knowledge deficit (parents) related to nature of disorder. | | |
| Parents verbalize understanding of potential allergens<br>Parents state that they have an understanding of disease process | 1. Advise parents to remove articles that irritate skin, for example, wool, and to provide loose cotton clothing | 1. Clothing with rough and tightly woven fibers will prevent natural evaporation from skin; wool may cause an allergic reaction; sweating increases itching |
| | 2. Encourage parents to use mild detergents, rinse clothes thoroughly | 2. Avoiding strong detergents and rinsing clothing thoroughly will prevent skin flare-ups |
| | 3. Expose infant to sunlight but monitor carefully | 3. Although sunlight is beneficial, overexposure to ultraviolet rays can seriously damage the skin; infants and young children require special protection from the sun because their epidermis is thin; exposure time should be brief, even on hazy days |
| | 4. Help parents identify products in which wheat, milk, eggs may not be readily apparent | 4. Food labels are read carefully to determine content |
| | 5. Advise parents to expect exacerbations and remissions | 5. Eczema is a chronic disease that takes time and energy to control |

# Impetigo

**Description.** Impetigo is an infectious disease of the skin caused by staphylococci or by group A beta-hemolytic streptococci. It results when the organism comes in contact with a break in the skin, such as an insect bite. The bullous form seen primarily in infants is usually staphylococcal, whereas nonbullous types are more commonly seen in children and young adults. Both organisms can usually be cultivated in the latter. The newborn is susceptible to this infection because resistance to skin bacteria is low. Impetigo tends to spread from one area of skin to another and is contagious.

**Manifestations.** The first symptoms of a bullous lesion are red papules (pimples) (see Color Plate Fig. 12). These eventually become small vesicles or pustules surrounded by a reddened area. When the blister breaks, the surface beneath is raw and weeping. The lesions may occur anywhere but are most often found around the nose and mouth and in moist areas of the body, such as the creases of the neck, axilla, and groin. In older children, a crust may form, and scratching may cause further infection.

**Treatment and Nursing Care.** Systemic antibiotics are administered either orally or parenterally. Parents are instructed to wash the lesions with soap and water three or four times a day to remove crust. Ointments such as mupirocin (Bactroban) may be applied topically. Prevention of the disease by prompt treatment of small cuts is important.

The prognosis with proper treatment is good. The nursing care consists primarily of preventing this disease. Education of parents includes reminding them of the necessity for prompt attention to minor cuts and bites. In diagnosed cases, compliance with the treatment regimen is needed to prevent the spread of infection to other children and family members. If the diagnosis is made in the newborn nursery, the baby is isolated in order to prevent other newborns from becoming infected. Nephritis may occur as a complication of beta-hemolytic streptococcal infections.

# Folliculitis (Furuncle, Carbuncle)

**Description.** Folliculitis refers to infection of the hair follicle. It is uncommon in infants but is widely seen during adolescence. White pustules occur on the forehead, back, neck and other areas. They are usually caused by *Staphylococcus aureus*. They may appear alone or in clusters. *Furuncle* is another name for a *boil*, which is more deep-seated. If several run together, the lesion is called a *carbuncle*. Carbuncles (multiple boils) are characterized by a painful node at first covered by tight, reddened skin that later becomes filled with purulent exudate (pus). There may be several draining points. They form most often on the nape of the neck, the upper back, or the buttocks. There may be systemic symptoms, such as fever and leukocytosis. They are *autoinoculable* (spread from one part of the body to another) and contagious.

**Treatment and Nursing Care.** Localized folliculitis is treated with warm compresses, gentle washing, and topical antibiotics. Adolescents are instructed not to squeeze the lesions. Carbuncles are treated with systemic antibiotics. Incision and drainage may be performed when the lesion is about to come to a head. Sterile technique is used when dressings are changed. Contaminated dressings are disposed of per universal precautions. Adolescents are taught to use disposable razors. The spread of infection is reduced by careful handwashing and by separate laundering of bed linens.

## Fungal Infections (Tinea Capitis, Corporis, Pedis, Cruris)

**Description.** Fungal infections are caused by closely related fungi that have a preference for invading the stratum corneum, hair, and nails. The word *tinea* comes from the Latin "worm." The common name for this infection is *ringworm*. Fungi are larger than bacteria. Some fungi may be transmitted from person to person and others from animal to person. The name denotes the part of the body involved.

*Tinea Capitis.* Tinea capitis (ringworm of the scalp) is seen in school children. It is characterized by patches of *alopecia* (hair loss). The hair loses pigment and may break off. The papules become pustules, which progress to red scales. There are areas of circular balding (see Color Plate Fig. 13).

Diagnosis is made by history and appearance. Some strains of tinea capitis glow green under a Wood light. This condition is treated with griseofulvin (Fulvicin, Grisactin), which is administered by mouth. It is given with or after meals to avoid gastrointestinal irritation and increase absorption. Suspensions should be well shaken. Parents are instructed to continue therapy as long as ordered and not to miss a dose. Exposure to sun is avoided. Treatment may be necessary for 8–12 weeks. Children may go to school but are warned not to exchange hats, combs, or other personal items. This can be a stubborn infection and may take several weeks to clear.

*Tinea Corporis.* Tinea corporis, ringworm of the skin, is evident as a scaly inflamed ring with a clear center. It is seen on the face, neck, arms, and hands (see Color Plate Fig. 14). It can be transmitted by infected pets. Treatment consists of local application of an antifungal preparation such as clotrimazole, or haloprogin twice daily for 2–4 weeks. More severe cases may require oral griseofulvin.

*Tinea Pedis.* Tinea pedis refers to athlete's foot. Lesions are located between the toes, on the instep, and on the soles (see Color Plate Fig. 15). There is accompanying pruritus. It occurs more often in preadolescents and adolescents. It is diagnosed by direct microscopic scrapings of the lesions. Treatment consists of topical therapy with clotrimazole (Mycelex) or haloprogin (Halotex). Oral griseofulvin therapy may also be given. Adolescents are cautioned to avoid alcohol when taking this medicine, as it may cause tachycardia and flushing.

Because this condition is aggravated by heat and moisture, feet need to be carefully dried, especially between the toes. An absorbent antifungal powder, such as zinc undecylenate, may suffice for mild infections (Behrman, 1992). Clean socks are worn. Shoes need to be well ventilated. Plastic shoes that retain heat are avoided. Recurrences are common.

*Tinea Crurus.* Tinea crurus ("thigh") affects the groin area and is commonly referred to as "jock itch." It occurs on the inner aspects of the thighs and scrotum. The initial lesion is small, raised, and scaly. It spreads, and tiny vesicles occur at the margins of the rash. Local application of tolnaftate liquid (Tinactin, Aftate) or powder is effective. Stinging may occur when spray solution is applied.

## Pediculosis

The infestation of humans by lice is termed pediculosis. There are three types: pediculosis capitis, head lice; pediculosis corporis, body lice;

and pediculosis pubis, crabs or pubic lice. The various types usually remain in the part of the body designated by their name. They are transmitted from person to person or by contact with contaminated articles. Their survival depends on the blood they extract from the infected person. Severe itching in the affected area is the main symptom. Treatment in all cases is aimed at ridding the patient of the parasite, treating the excoriated skin, and preventing the infestation of others. The most common form seen in children is head lice.

## PEDICULOSIS CAPITIS

**Description.** Pediculosis capitis, known commonly as head lice, affects the scalp and hair. The louse lays eggs, called nits, which attach to the hair, and hatch within 3 or 4 days (Fig. 31–5). Head lice are more common in girls than in boys because of hair length. The parasite may be acquired from hats, combs, or hairbrushes. It is easily transferred from one child to another and is seen most frequently in the school-age child and in preschool children who attend day-care centers.

**Manifestations.** Children with pediculosis capitis suffer from severe itching of the scalp. They scratch their heads frequently and often cause further irritation. The hair becomes matted. Pustules and excoriations may be seen about the face. Nurses admitting patients to pediatric units should be on the alert for head lice. In particular, the nurse inspects the hairline at the back of the neck and about the ears. Crusts,

pediculi, nits, and dirt may cause matting of the hair and a foul odor. When the condition is discovered, it is handled with discretion so as not to embarrass the child or parents.

**Treatment and Nursing Care.** Treatment is directed toward killing the lice, getting rid of the nits, and managing any infections of the face and scalp. Family members and playmates of the child should be examined and treated as necessary. Prescription shampoos, such as pyrethrin, are commonly used. Retreatment may be necessary in 1 week to 10 days. Lindane (Kwell) has also been used; however, it has more reported side effects (consult circular). Nonprescription remedies are also available. The manufacturer's directions should be carefully followed. One should watch for an allergic response, particularly in children with a history of skin problems.

If the eyebrows and eyelashes are involved, a thick coating of petroleum jelly (Vaseline) is applied, followed by removal of remaining nits. Nits on the head are removed by combing the hair with a fine-tooth comb dipped in a 1:1 solution of white vinegar and water. The hair is then washed. In some cases, recovery is hastened by cutting the hair.

Nurses protect themselves during these procedures by wearing gloves and a cap. Charting includes date, time, condition of scalp and hair prior to treatment, odor (if noticeable), type of shampoo used, how the patient tolerated the procedure, and the amount of relief obtained. Any signs of systemic infection are also documented.

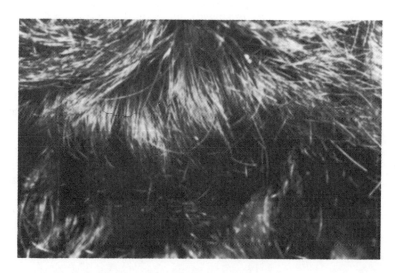

**Figure 31–5.** Pediculosis. White nits or eggs of head lice attached to hair. (From Levy, M. [1991]. Disorders of the hair and scalp in children. *Pediatric Clinics of North America, 38,* 917.)

In the home, clothing or bedding is laundered in hot water and dried for 20 minutes or aired in sunlight. Mattresses may be sprayed with a disinfectant. Wool clothing requires dry cleaning. Children should be cautioned against swapping caps, head scarfs, and combs. Parents are instructed to inspect the child's head regularly. Parents are encouraged to report infestations to the school nurse, as widespread outbreaks are periodically encountered.

## Scabies

**Description.** Scabies is a parasitic infection caused by the itch mite *Sarcoptes scabiei*. It is seen worldwide. It is caused by the adult female mite, who burrows under the skin and lays eggs. The mite has a round body and four pairs of legs and is visible by microscopic examination. A characteristic burrow is sometimes seen under the skin, particularly between the fingers. Burrows contain eggs and feces of the mite. Itching is intense, especially at night.

Scabies may occur anywhere on the body but is seldom seen on the face. It thrives in moist body folds, but in young children the lesions may appear on the head, palms, and soles of the feet. It is spread by close personal contact, including sexual relations. It is rarely transmitted by fomites because the isolated mite dies within 2–3 days.

**Treatment and Nursing Care.** Treatment consists of the application of permethrin (Elimite). This is a newer remedy with less toxicity than lindane (Kwell), which was the mainstay of treatment in the past. It can be used for children older than 2 months of age. Parents are instructed to follow the directions carefully. All family members, baby-sitters, and close associates require treatment. The nurse wears gloves when caring for these patients and adheres to careful handwashing. Bedding and clothing are treated as precaution linens.

## Burns

**Description.** Burns occur frequently during childhood. They are the leading cause of accidental death in the home for children between the ages of 1 and 4 years. The incidence is higher among boys than among girls. Sometimes burns are a result of child abuse and neglect. The two times of day in which burns are

## Nursing Brief

The small child is taught to *stop, drop, and roll,* should the clothes become ignited.

most likely to occur are the early morning hours before parents awaken and after school. Burns may be caused by many factors, such as a stove, heater, vaporizer, radiator, iron, fireplace, bath water, curling irons, coffee pot or cup, defective wiring, unguarded outlets, strong acids, and strong alkalis such as lye or ammonia. The fillings of pastries placed in the microwave can become very hot and cause mouth burns. Electrical burns carry the risk of thrombosis in other parts of the body. Burns acquired in an enclosed area or facial burns may lead to inhalation complications, such as airway obstruction and hypoxia.

Major burns to the face, hands, feet, or groin are considered critical. Immediate and long-term management to reduce scarring and disfiguration and to prevent limitation of motion is essential. Minor burns are those of first or second degree, partial-thickness types that cover less than 15% of the body and do not involve critical areas. They are treated on an outpatient basis. Children younger than 2 years are at risk because they are subject to greater and to more rapid fluid loss and because their immune systems are immature and not as effective in fighting infection. Children under 4 years of age have a higher mortality rate than do children of other age groups with a similar-size injury, because of their smaller body mass and other factors (Jones & Feller, 1989).

**Classification.** The severity of a burn depends on the area, extent, and depth of involvement. The size of the burn is calculated as a percentage of total body surface (Fig. 31–6). In children, age-related charts are used because their body proportions differ from those of adults and the standard (rule of nines) cannot be applied. The extent of destruction of the skin is described as partial-thickness or full-thickness. In partial-thickness burns, only part of the skin is damaged. These burns heal in time. Full-thickness burns are more extensive and require skin grafting. The classification of and first-aid treatment for burns are summarized in Table 31–2. One can survive a rather extensive su-

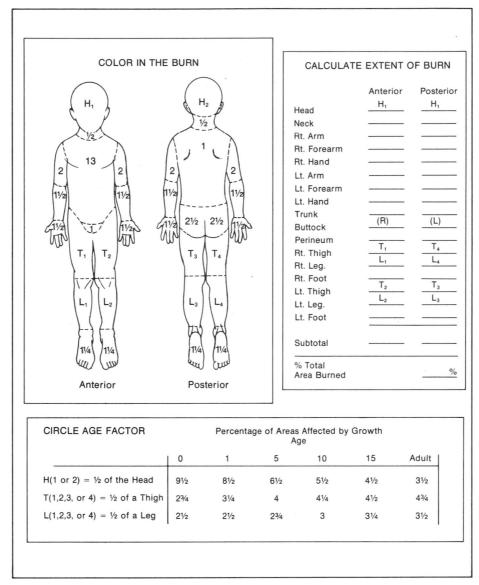

**Figure 31–6.** Estimation of size of burn by percentage. (1) Shade in the diagram to represent the extent of the burn as viewed anteriorly and posteriorly. (2) Circle the age closest to that of the patient and use the percentages in the table for the head, thigh, and leg to identify the extent of the burn. The areas that vary with age are marked with H (head), T (thigh), and L (leg). For areas that do not vary with age, the percentage of total body surface is printed on the diagram. (3) Calculate the extent of the burn by adding the percentages of each affected area. If a portion of a body part is burned, an approximate fraction of the percentage should be used. (From Betz, C., Hunsberger, M., & Wright, S. [1994]. *Family-centered nursing care of children* [2nd ed., p. 2076]. Philadelphia: W.B. Saunders. Redrawn from Fuller, I., & Jones, C.A. [1977]. *Emergency care for the burn victim.* Ann Arbor, MI: National Institute for Burn Medicine.)

perficial burn, whereas a deep burn involving a smaller surface area can threaten the patient's life.

Burns can also be complicated by fractures, soft tissue injury, or preexisting conditions such as diabetes, obesity, epilepsy, and heart or re- nal disease. Moderate burns are (1) partial-thickness burns involving 15–30% of body surface or (2) full-thickness burns involving less than 10% of body surface. Major burns are (1) partial-thickness types involving 30% or more of body surface or (2) full-thickness burns in-

**Table 31–2.** CLASSIFICATION AND FIRST-AID TREATMENT OF BURNS

| Degree | Anatomy and Depth | Appearance and Sensation | First-Aid Treatment |
|---|---|---|---|
| First | Epidermis only; partial thickness | Skin red but blanches easily on pressure and refills quickly; painful, indicating tissue viability | Immerse in cold water to halt burning process; apply petroleum jelly (Vaseline) or other suitable sterile ointment |
| Second | | | |
| Superficial | Epidermis and much of dermis; partial thickness | Blistered, moist, pink or red; painful, indicating tissue viability | If area is small, treat as for first-degree burn; otherwise, treat as for deep dermal burn |
| Deep dermal | Extends deep into dermis; partial thickness but can become full thickness with infection, trauma, or poor blood supply | Mottled; red, tan, or dull white; blisters; painful, indicating tissue viability | Immerse in cold water to halt burning process; cover with sterile dressing or clean cloth to prevent contamination and decrease pain from contact with air; avoid breaking blisters; seek medical attention immediately |
| Third | Subdermal; involves entire skin and all its structures; full thickness | Tough, leathery, dry; does not blanch or refill; dull brown, tan, black, or pearly white; painless to touch, indicating death of tissue | Halt burning process by immersing in cold water or rolling in blanket or rug; wrap in clean sheet or other sterile dressing; provide blanket for warmth; have victim lie down; DO NOT apply ointment or any other substance to burned area; take patient to nearest emergency treatment center immediately |

## Nursing Brief

A severe burn can cause loss of function in two of the most important properties of the skin: the ability to protect against infection and the ability to prevent loss of body fluid.

volving 10% or more of body surface. Second- and third-degree burns must be regarded as open wounds having the added danger of infection.

The chief cause of death from burns is the toxic condition that arises from shock. Toxicity results from the sudden loss of large amounts of plasma, the liquid portion of the blood, when fluid passes from the blood vessels into the tissues. There is a decrease in blood volume, a concentration of red blood cells, and eventually an increase in hematocrit. Circulation becomes sluggish. All organs suffer from lack of oxygen and nutrients. Waste products accumulate in the blood. Burned children are prone to congestive heart failure, pulmonary edema, and renal failure.

The symptoms of shock are increased pulse and respirations; decreased blood pressure; decreased temperature; pallor; cold, clammy skin; prostration; and dilated pupils.

**Treatment.** The immediate treatment of shock in cases of severe burns is handled by the physician, nurse, and respiratory therapist and other specialists in the emergency room or in some instances the operating room. Priorities include establishing an airway in patients with facial burns or smoke inhalation, instituting intravenous lifelines, and assessing burn wounds and other, perhaps initially unrecognized, injuries. At times, some of these procedures are carried out simultaneously.

*Establishing an Airway.* Cyanosis, singed nasal hairs, charred lips, and stridor are indications of an inhalation problem. An endotracheal tube is inserted in order to maintain an adequate airway, although this is not required for all patients. This permits delivery of humidified air with oxygen, easy removal of secretions from respiratory passages, and use of a pressure ventilator if needed. Sedation is administered with caution in order to avoid further respiratory embarrassment.

If eschar (*eschara*, "scab") from burns on the trunk inhibits respirations, an incision called an *escharotomy* is made in order to prevent restriction of chest movement. Blood gas levels, including level of carbon monoxide, are ascertained. Clothing is carefully removed, by cutting along the seams of the material if possible. The child is placed on sterile sheets. Attendants wear face masks, sterile gown, and gloves.

Intravenous infusions are begun in order to prevent intravascular dehydration and electrolyte imbalance. A cutdown may be performed, particularly in small children. Although the composition of fluids to be administered to burn victims is a subject of controversy, Ringer's lactate solution is often used initially. Within 24–48 hours, when capillary permeability is restored, albumin or plasma may be used.

Laboratory studies include hematocrit and sodium chloride, potassium, carbon dioxide, blood urea nitrogen, creatinine, and serum protein levels. Blood typing and cross-matching are performed. Fluid therapy is complicated and requires close monitoring throughout hospitalization. Other criteria that help to determine individual fluid therapy include state of consciousness, body weight, vital signs, urine volume and characteristics, central venous pressure, and skin turgor. To determine urine volume and characteristics, a urinary catheter is inserted.

The loss of fluid causes renal vasoconstriction, leading to depressed glomerular filtration and oliguria. Without adequate therapy, acute renal failure can develop. Urine output is observed hourly. It varies considerably, but on the average 20–30 ml/hr for patients older than 2 years is considered adequate during the resuscitative stage. The patient's present weight is recorded and is used as baseline data for determining adequacy of treatment.

A nasogastric tube is inserted and is attached to low Gomco suction. This empties the stomach and prevents complications such as gastric dilatation, vomiting, and paralytic ileus. The patient has nothing by mouth for the first 24 hours. Sporadic bleeding as a result of Curling's or stress ulcer is not uncommon in patients with severe burns; the administration of antacids, such as magnesium hydroxide (Maalox), has helped to reduce its incidence.

***Wound Care.*** Immediate care of the wound itself includes cleansing and débridement (removal of dried crusts) of necrotic tissue. The loss of skin increases the threat of infection, and fluid loss due to evaporation can be significant. The immune system is depressed. Strict asepsis is maintained, and the wound site is treated in accordance with the physician's instruction. A tetanus immunization history is obtained, and tetanus prophylaxis is administered as required. Low doses of penicillin may be prescribed in order to prevent streptococcal infection.

A semiopen method of burn dressing is currently favored as treatment, although exposure methods may be useful on accessible areas such as the face. The wound is covered by a few layers of sterile gauze that has been saturated with antibacterial ointment or cream. The gauze is held in place by elastic netting (Fig. 31–7). When the wound is being dressed, *no two burn surfaces should touch*. A sterile blanket may be used in order to prevent chilling. The wound is cleansed by povidone-iodine (Betadine) tub baths, or in many cases, hose or whirlpool baths are utilized to soften necrotic

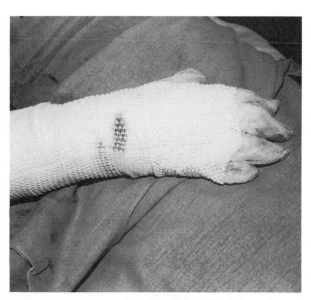

**Figure 31–7.** Occlusive dressing applied to a burned hand. (Courtesy of the Burn Center at St. Agnes Medical Center, Philadelphia, PA. From deWitt, S.C. [1992]. *Essentials of medical-surgical nursing* [2nd ed., p. 641]. Philadelphia: W.B. Saunders.)

## Nursing Brief

Electrical burns of the mouth are common in small children who put everything into their mouths. Biting into electrical cords is not unusual. Such wounds are usually deep and leave an entrance and exit burn. They are subject to bleeding for several weeks.

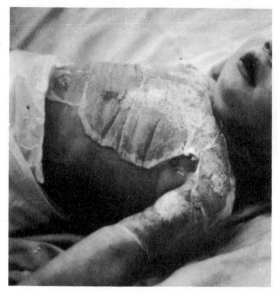

**Figure 31–8.** Porcine dressing. (Courtesy of St. Agnes Medical Center Photography Department, Philadelphia, PA. From Marlow, D.R., & Redding, B. A. [1988]. *Textbook of pediatric nursing* [6th ed., p. 801]. Philadelphia, W.B. Saunders.)

areas and débride the wound. Débridement is done in all methods when needed to cleanse the wound and prepare the new granulation tissue for grafting. The use of enzymes such as Travase may be prescribed. Granulation tissue is fragile and bleeds easily. Small children may need to be restrained in order to protect the area from trauma. The burn area is closed and resurfaced by grafting.

***Skin Grafts.*** Temporary grafts are used during the acute stage of recovery. They protect the wound from infection and reduce fluid loss but are eventually rejected by the body. Temporary grafts include homografts, usually tissue from cadavers free from disease, and heterografts, tissues obtained from different species. Heterografts are also referred to as xenografts (*xeno*, "foreign," and *graft*, "slice of skin").

Today most grafts are derived from pigskin, which is available commercially either fresh or frozen; these biologic dressings are frequently used in children and are called porcine xenografts (Fig. 31–8). They are particularly useful in partial-thickness or deep dermal burns and have greatly improved burn management. Deep dermal wounds may be preceded by tangential (merely touching) excision, which is a surgical technique of removing burned eschar with a dermatome. Thin layers are shaved down to the live tissues, and temporary porcine grafts are applied.

There are two types of permanent grafts, autografts and isografts. An autograft (*auto*, "self") is healthy tissue obtained from another part of the patient's body. An isograft (*iso*, "equal") is obtained from the patient's identical twin. Permanent grafts are done during the rehabilitative stage of the patient's illness in order to improve appearance and function. The site from which the tissue has been removed is called the donor area.

Advances in grafting techniques have improved the overall prognosis in burn patients and have helped minimize scarring. A split-thickness skin graft can be prepared with the use of a dermatome. In extensive burns, it is sometimes difficult to find enough intact skin for use. Special methods such as the Tanner mesh graft may be used. In this method, a strip of split-thickness skin is run through a special cutting machine that makes multiple slits to expand the skin in order to provide more coverage, in some cases as much as nine times the original area of the skin. The graft is sutured in place to maintain tension.

The postage-stamp graft consists of small pieces of donor skin placed on the granulation tissue. Spaces between grafts allow for drainage and healing. Full-cover grafts are sheets of skin placed intact over the wound. These are cosmetically more effective than patch and mesh grafts but are not always available. The donor site is covered with xenograft or fine mesh gauze; it heals in about 2 weeks. Newly grafted areas are covered with sterile dressings. Every effort is made to prevent *bleeding* and *infection*. The areas surrounding the wound are observed for edema and impaired circulation.

**Nursing Care.** Children who have suffered extensive burns and survive the early dangers face a long period of hospitalization and require specialized care. Unlike with other traumatic injuries, complications are the rule rather than the exception with most severe burns, especially with burns treated in nonspecialized facilities (Jones & Feller, 1989). The various aspects of nursing care differ with the age of the patient, the area of the burn, and the type of treatment used. Nursing Care Plan 31–2 lists some interventions for children with burns.

***Preventing Wound Infection.*** Every effort must be made to prevent the injured area from becoming infected. Dead tissue and exudate furnish fertile ground for bacterial growth. In addition, the decrease in blood supply to the area diminishes phagocytic activity. The burn is treated according to the protocol of the patient's

---

### NURSING CARE PLAN 31–2

#### Selected Nursing Diagnoses for the Child with Burns (Subacute Phase)

| Goals | Nursing Interventions | Rationale |
| --- | --- | --- |
| **Nursing Diagnosis:** High risk for infection related to loss of protective layer of skin secondary to burn. | | |
| The child's rectal temperature will remain below 37°C (98.6°F) <br> Skin around wound remains intact and is not red or warm to touch | 1. Wash hands for 1 full minute before touching patient | 1. Handwashing is essential to prevent introducing pathogens; the immune system of a child is immature, which results in an increased susceptibility to infection and organ failure |
| | 2. Wear sterile gown and mask when handling burn wound | 2. Necrotic tissue serves as an excellent breeding ground for microorganisms, which multiply rapidly in a burn wound |
| | 3. Use sterile bed linens if exposure method is utilized | 3. When wound is exposed to air, nurse must constantly observe patient for signs of infection; serous fluid that exudes from wound hardens and forms a covering, but bacteria may enter through breaks in dried exudate |
| | 4. Cleanse wound as ordered | 4. Hydrotherapy is often used to cleanse burned area; children lose heat more rapidly than adults do; therefore, nurse must maintain warmth of water and room temperature |
| | 5. Apply prescribed antibacterial ointments | 5. Antibacterial ointments reduce number of organisms in wound; after 18–24 hours, if left untreated, a wound becomes colonized with pathogenic bacteria |
| | 6. Obtain wound cultures as ordered | 6. Cultures provide baseline data; antibiotics are prescribed to treat specific organisms |
| | 7. Screen visitors for infections | 7. Child needs to be protected from infected persons |
| | 8. Check vital signs, especially temperature | 8. Decrease excessive metabolic expenditures (child should not become overheated or chilled); temperature readings can determine early signs of general sepsis, wound infection, or bacterial pneumonia |
| | 9. Observe wound for purulent, foul drainage | 9. Purulent, foul drainage indicates wound infection |
| | 10. Handle child gently | 10. Gentle handling will prevent injury to wound or donor site |

*Continued*

| NURSING CARE PLAN 31–2 *Continued* |
| :---: |
| **Selected Nursing Diagnoses for the Child with Burns (Subacute Phase)** |

| Goals | Nursing Interventions | Rationale |
| --- | --- | --- |

**Nursing Diagnosis:** Altered nutrition, less than body requirements, related to hypermetabolism as the body attempts to restore tissue.

| Goals | Nursing Interventions | Rationale |
| --- | --- | --- |
| Child ingests sufficient calories to compensate for catabolism as evidenced by normal healing and stable body weight | 1. Provide high-calorie, high-protein meals and snacks | 1. Although edema usually accompanies a severe burn, a gradual weight loss follows because of increased energy and protein requirements |
| | 2. Avoid painful procedures around mealtime | 2. Discomfort decreases child's appetite |
| | 3. Cater to child's food preferences as feasible | 3. Children frequently lack appetite; poor nutritional status impairs wound healing, compromises immune response, and increases chance of infection |
| | 4. Provide nourishing between-meal feedings | 4. Child's metabolic demands may require two to three times normal calorie intake for age |
| | 5. Administer supplementary vitamins and minerals | 5. Anorexia may lead to vitamin deficiencies |
| | 6. Anticipate total parenteral nutrition | 6. If caloric requirements cannot be met, supplemental feedings may be required |
| | 7. Provide companionship at meals | 7. Parents understand child's food preferences; they may bring food from home if feasible; presence of nurse may distract child from discomfort and promote socialization |

**Nursing Diagnosis:** High risk for altered skin integrity, pressure ulcers related to immobility.

| Goals | Nursing Interventions | Rationale |
| --- | --- | --- |
| Child's skin is not erythematous and shows no signs of breakdown | 1. Turn patient frequently, rub skin | 1. Frequent repositioning prevents pressure necrosis |
| | 2. Check peripheral areas for color, capillary refill, pulse, sensation, motion | 2. Burns that encompass whole circumference of extremities (circumferential burns), such as fingers and toes, and chest require careful attention, particularly in first few hours following injury; edema puts pressure on underlying blood vessels and nerves; children's fingers and toes are very small and thin, and circulation can be cut off very easily |
| | 3. Keep child from picking and scratching; restrain if necessary | 3. Itching is common with burns; scratching can cause infection |

**Nursing Diagnosis:** High risk for impaired physical mobility related to burn.

| Goals | Nursing Interventions | Rationale |
| --- | --- | --- |
| Child demonstrates full range of motion<br>Child does not develop contractures | 1. Explain and perform range-of-motion exercises | 1. Contractions that limit function can develop from scar formation and immobility of unaffected limbs |
| | 2. Encourage water play | 2. Water soothes the stressed child; other games that encourage use of limbs are also beneficial |
| | 3. Observe for constricting eschar, particularly over joints | 3. Early intervention prevents or minimizes contractures |

| NURSING CARE PLAN 31–2 *Continued* | | |
| --- | --- | --- |
| **Selected Nursing Diagnoses for the Child with Burns (Subacute Phase)** | | |
| Goals | Nursing Interventions | Rationale |

**Nursing Diagnosis:** High risk for fluid volume deficit related to loss of fluids via open wound.

| | | |
| --- | --- | --- |
| Fluids and electrolytes are maintained as evidenced by laboratory data and clinical signs<br><br>Skin turgor and urinary output are adequate | 1. Monitor electrolyte levels<br>2. Encourage fluid intake<br>3. Observe urinary output<br>4. Monitor IV fluids<br>5. Keep *accurate* intake and output records<br>6. Observe patient for evidence of fluid overload, such as altered behavior or sensorium<br>7. Test tissue turgor | 1 to 7. Throughout recovery process, fluid and electrolyte balance fluctuates with surgical procedures, sepsis, and evaporative losses; careful monitoring is needed until wound is healed; errors in fluid therapy in children can be life-threatening, as infants, in particular, have high rates of heat exchange relative to size and weight, high rates of water exchange in relation to total body water, and significant differences in muscle, water, and electrolyte composition; they also require relatively larger volumes of urine for excretion of waste products than do adults, and insensible water losses when expressed in terms of body weight are significantly greater in children than in adults |

**Nursing Diagnosis:** Pain related to burn, nature of treatment.

| | | |
| --- | --- | --- |
| Patient is comfortable as evidenced by nonirritable behavior and absence of crying | 1. Avoid drafts or overheating by adjusting room temperature | 1. Body responds to a large burn area by increasing metabolic rate; oxygen consumption increases as temperature, respirations, and heart rate rise; controlled environment reduces water evaporation and heat losses from the wound; increases comfort of patient |
| | 2. Administer pain relievers before dressing changes | 2. Adjust time of dressing change to coincide with peak action of pain reliever |
| | 3. Observe for hostility, irritability, depression, guarding of body parts, which may indicate pain in nonverbal child | 3. Children do not understand necessity for treatments; they protest loudly and are afraid; dressing changes are painful and difficult for nurse and child; determining child's level of pain tolerance during a procedure is helpful in assisting child to stay in control; allowing pauses when tension escalates is of importance |
| | 4. Allow child to express feelings | 4. Expression of feelings is necessary for a healthy personality |
| | 5. Use distraction techniques | 5. Distraction may take child's mind off pain |
| | 6. Provide tactile contact | 6. Appropriate touch is an important aspect of human communication, especially with nonverbal child |

*Continued*

### Selected Nursing Diagnoses for the Child with Burns (Subacute Phase)

| Goals | Nursing Interventions | Rationale |
|---|---|---|
| **Nursing Diagnosis:** High risk for disturbance of self-concept related to scars, disfigurement, isolation. | | |
| Child maintains healthy self-concept during rehabilitation period as evidenced by a sense of humor, absence of depression, and increased acceptance of body disfigurement. | 1. Reassure child and parents | 1. A calm and straightforward manner promotes confidence |
| | 2. Help alleviate guilt | 2. Acknowledging guilt feelings validates reality and facilitates problem solving |
| | 3. Explore feelings concerning physical appearance by having patients draw themselves before and after burn | 3. Patient may gain insight from drawing; aids in expression of feelings; a series of drawings provide more information than does one drawing |
| | 4. Discuss ways to camouflage disfigurement | 4. Often families have false hope about plastic repair; plastic surgery may restore function, but evidence of burn may still need to be camouflaged |
| | 5. Anticipate regressive behavior | 5. Regression often occurs in patients in crisis as patient tries to return to a safer time of life |
| | 6. Incorporate developmental aspects into nursing care plans | 6. Incorporating developmental aspects is particularly relevant for accident prevention and nursing intervention |
| | 7. Encourage contact with peers | 7. Reentry into social life can be problematic, particularly with disfigurement of face and neck; child may need to "test the waters" gradually; burn camps are available at major treatment centers |
| **Nursing Diagnosis:** High risk for dysfunctional grieving related to appearance. | | |
| Child is able to observe burn wound and feels free to express negative as well as positive feelings to nurse | 1. Support patient in expressing grief concerning "imperfect appearance" | 1. Verbalization of grief reduces its impact |
| | 2. Anticipate grief reflected as anger and fear as well as sadness | 2. Anger, fear, and grief are normal responses to loss |
| **Nursing Diagnosis:** Knowledge deficit in child and family regarding accident prevention. | | |
| Family verbalizes understanding of the importance of installing smoke detectors, and sheltering children from strong sunlight, hot liquids, electrical outlets, etc. | 1. Assess knowledge of accident prevention in this and other areas | 1. Accidents and injuries are major cause of death in children over 1 yr of age |
| | 2. Provide ongoing education as required | 2. Ongoing education is necessary, as child is constantly developing new motor and cognitive skills that may carry risks |
| | 3. Assess parenting skills, suggest classes if needed | 3. Many adults have not had good role models for parenting; they may under- or overestimate child's capabilities |

**Table 31–3.** TOPICAL AGENTS USED IN TREATING BURN PATIENTS

| Agent | Comment |
|---|---|
| Silver sulfadiazine cream 1% (Silvadene) | Effective against gram-negative and gram-positive bacteria and yeast (Candida albicans) |
| | Do not use if patient is allergic to sulfa drugs |
| | Cream does not sting, softens eschar |
| | Do not waste (expensive) |
| | Gently remove old cream before reapplying |
| Mafenide acetate 10% (Sulfamylon) | Effective against gram-positive and gram-negative organisms |
| | Painful because it draws water out of the tissues; pain may last 15–30 min or longer |
| | Remain with child after application for comfort and diversion |
| | Allergic rash common |
| | Tendency to cake, best used with hydrotherapy |
| | Potential for metabolic acidosis |
| Silver nitrate 0.5% (AgNO₃) | Effective against gram-negative organisms |
| | Dressings must be kept *wet* and changed frequently |
| | Stains unburned skin, linen, and most surfaces a dark brown or black |
| | Eschar becomes light brown |

physician. Table 31–3 lists topical agents used in treating burn patients.

Protective isolation is instituted. The nurse wears sterilized gown, cap, mask, and gloves when dressing the wound. All instruments that come in contact with the wound must be sterile. Ointments are applied with a gloved hand or a sterile tongue depressor. Care must be taken to avoid injury to granulation tissue. If the wound is to be covered, a layer of fine mesh gauze is secured with sterile fluffs, followed by Kling bandages and a stockinette or elastic tubular netting. Nurses carefully wash their hands before caring for the patient and assisting with dressing changes.

With young children, restraints may be required to keep their fingers away from the wound. When enemas are given, waterproof materials must be used in order to prevent contamination of the dressing. The patient is protected from persons with upper respiratory infections. Drafts are avoided. Wound, nose, and throat cultures are taken periodically. Areas ad-

jacent to the burn are observed for signs of infection or pressure. Vitamins and medications are administered as ordered.

The nurse reports signs of infection immediately. These are elevation of temperature, pulse, and respiration; restlessness and confusion; pain; purulent drainage; and odor of wound dressing. A careful description of the wound in nurse's notes facilitates daily comparison and determination of progress. All infection must be cleared before skin grafting can be performed.

***Fluids and Nourishment.*** The physician prescribes the amount of fluids to be given on the basis of blood test results. Loss of plasma in the blood results in an increase in the concentration of red blood cells. A simple hemoglobin count or a hematocrit (which indicates the proportion of red blood cells in a specific amount of blood) provides the necessary information. Typing and cross-matching of the blood for possible transfusions are also done. Parenteral therapy is given in order to replace fluids and electrolytes.

The nurse remains alert for signs of fluid overload, in particular, behavioral changes and altered sensorium. Oral fluids, although initially restricted in order to prevent nausea and vomiting, are necessary during the convalescent stages to aid the body in getting rid of poisons, to prevent kidney damage, and to maintain body fluid requirements. The nurse must use ingenuity in order to persuade the child to take sufficient amounts of fluids. An accurate record of intake and output of fluids is kept.

There is an increase in demands on the metabolism as it deals with this trauma, and more calories are spent as water evaporates from the wound site. Frequent feedings of foods high in calories, protein, and iron are therefore necessary. A high-protein diet, a normal diet with added amounts of meat, milk, eggs, fish, or poultry, is usually prescribed. Iron therapy may be initiated if anemia begins to develop. Eggnogs are nourishing between-meal drinks for burn patients with such needs. Small amounts are offered frequently. Vitamins A, B, and C and zinc sulfate are given to hasten healing and to stimulate the appetite. Gavage feedings may be necessary. Accurate daily records of foods consumed, calorie count, and patient's weight will help determine the nutritional status.

*Positioning the Patient.* The foot of the crib is raised at first if the child appears to be in shock. The doctor designates the positions to be used later. If the doctor applies a dressing to an extremity, the extremity is placed in correct alignment before the bandage is applied; a splint may also be used to maintain correct position.

The nurse bears in mind that other parts of the body that are not affected need exercise and proper positioning in order to prevent painful contractures. The child's position is changed every 2–4 hours unless contraindicated. A footboard is used to prevent footdrop. Support should be given by means of pillows, sandbags, and rolled towels as necessary. The nurse is gentle when positioning the patient in order to prevent injury to the delicate skin that is healing beneath the bandages.

The physical therapist attends the child regularly to exercise and keep the joints limber and healthy. The child begins to ambulate as soon as possible. Self-help activities and mobility are encouraged. Pressure splints or elasticized garments help reduce scar tissue and are sometimes worn for months following discharge (Fig. 31–9).

The room is kept well-ventilated in order to prevent offensive odors. A deodorizer is used when necessary. The patient's unit is kept neat, clean, and adequately lighted. The use of a bed cradle prevents the weight of the covers from touching the affected areas. The urinal is emptied as necessary, and the amount of urine is recorded. The child's hair is combed and arranged neatly. Back rubs are given, and good oral hygiene is maintained.

Signs of abdominal discomfort such as nausea, vomiting, and abdominal distention may be early indications of a stress ulcer. Signs of bleeding include bloody stools, dark brown urine, and blood in the nasogastric tube. In addition, the nurse assesses the patient's vital signs in order to detect early symptoms of pneumonia, hypertension, and renal impairment. Measurements of the amount, color, and specific gravity and periodic laboratory evaluations of urine may detect low-grade irregularities. The

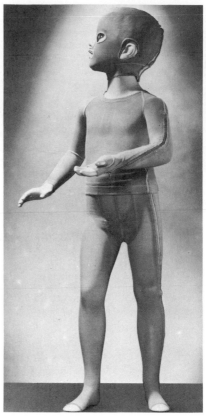

**Figure 31–9.** Pressure garments for various body parts. (Courtesy of Jobst Institute, Inc., Toledo, OH.)

patient may complain of pruritus, in which case the nurse inspects all areas of the skin for medication rash.

*Emotional Support.* A burn injury is taxing to the child and parents. It requires long periods of hospitalization and frequent readmissions. The accident itself is terrifying for the child, but it is made even worse if it was caused by disobedience. Nurses encourage children to express their feelings. Patients may scream during dressing changes or take out their frustrations on the nurse. The nurse maintains a calm but firm manner and refrains from showing a reaction to the wound, since children are quick to recognize an expression of alarm or disgust. Assistance and support by other persons are ideal because the second person may be able to distract the patient. Analgesics are administered *prior* to painful procedures. See page 542 for methods of detecting pain in children.

The long-term patient requires diversions of

various types. Toys are kept within easy reach in order to prevent excessive movement. The crib is placed near the door so that the child may observe the outside activities. As the condition improves, the patient is permitted the companionship of other children. Older patients enjoy helping with routine unit functions, which gives them a feeling of accomplishment.

Nurses give constant support to the parents, who usually feel guilty if their child was injured in an accident. They indicate by their manner that they do not blame them for what has happened. Preparation for discharge begins early. Instructions are given as to wound care, diet, exercise, and rest. Return appointments are made, and referral agencies are contacted. Methods to improve the physical appearance of the patient are discussed. This can sometimes be accomplished through clothing, make-up, and other disguise techniques.

The importance of prevention of burns cannot be overemphasized.

## KEY POINTS

- The skin is the body's first line of defense against disease.
- Certain skin conditions are symptoms of systemic disease.
- Common skin problems in infants are diaper dermatitis, seborrheic dermatitis, and atopic dermatitis (eczema).
- A strawberry nevus is an example of a hemangioma.
- Pediculosis is the term for lice. Lice may occur in the head, body, or pubic area.
- Tinea pedis, or athlete's foot, is prevented by drying the feet well, particularly between the toes, and wearing well-ventilated footwear.
- A severe burn can cause loss of function in two of the most important properties of the skin: the ability to protect against infection and the ability to prevent the loss of body fluid.
- Electrical burns carry the risk of thrombosis in other parts of the body.
- The severity of a burn depends on the area, extent, and depth of involvement.
- Preventing infection is an important nursing intervention for patients with burns.

## Study Questions

1. List two functions of the skin.
2. Name the two layers of the skin.
3. Name the cheeselike layer that covers the skin of the newborn at birth.
4. Name the generalized rash that appears abruptly and is often a reaction to medication.
5. Wanda, age 14, has severe acne on her forehead and cheeks. Discuss the psychological implications for this teenager.
6. Discuss the nursing care of the infant with eczema. Include the rationale for each measure. What factors must the nurse chart in regard to this condition?
7. Five-year-old Perez has pediculosis. Write a brief paragraph discussing the detection and management of this infestation.
8. How do burns interfere with the normal functioning of the skin?
9. Compare and contrast first-, second-, and third-degree burns.
10. Discuss the nutritional considerations of a severely burned toddler.

# Multiple Choice
# Review Questions

*Choose the most appropriate answer.*

1. Which of the following is to be avoided in babies with eczema?
   a. rice cereal
   b. cotton mittens
   c. herpes simplex
   d. coal tar preparations

2. The relief of pain is important in the burn patient because
   a. it prevents discomfort
   b. the child must be kept from crying
   c. parents become upset
   d. pain contributes to shock

3. Which of the following would be contraindicated in a patient with infantile eczema?
   a. wrapping the baby in a wool blanket
   b. covering hands with cotton mittens
   c. the use of elbow restraints to prevent scratching
   d. open, wet dressings

4. Head lice is termed
   a. scabies
   b. pediculosis corporis
   c. pediculosis capitis
   d. pediculus

5. A characteristic of third-degree burns not present in second-degree burns is
   a. lack of pain
   b. blisters, warmth
   c. redness
   d. pain

## BIBLIOGRAPHY

Behrman R.E. (1992). *Nelson textbook of pediatrics* (14th ed.). Philadelphia: W.B. Saunders.

Betz, C., Hunsberger, M., & Wright, S. (1994). *Family-centered nursing care of children* (2nd ed.). Philadelphia: W.B. Saunders.

Dickerman, J., & Lucey, J. (1985) *Smith's the critically ill child* (3rd ed.). Philadelphia: W.B. Saunders.

Graef, J., & Cone, T. (1988). *Manual of pediatric therapeutics* (4th ed.). Boston: Little, Brown.

Green, M., & Haggerty, R. (1990). *Ambulatory pediatrics 3.* Philadelphia: W.B. Saunders.

Hayman, L., & Spring, E. (1985). *Handbook of pediatric nursing.* New York: John Wiley & Sons.

Jarvis, C. (1992). *Physical examination and health assessment.* Philadelphia: W.B. Saunders.

Jones, C., Simmons, F., & Feller, I. (1994). The child with burns. In Betz, C., Hunsberger, M., & Wright, S. *Family-centered nursing care of children* (2nd ed.). Philadelphia: W.B. Saunders.

Levy, M. (1991). Disorders of the hair and scalp in children. *Pediatric Clinics of North America*, 38, 905.

Mott, S., et al. (1991). *Nursing care of children and families* (2nd ed.). Reading, MA: Addison-Wesley.

Neinstein, L. (1984). *Adolescent health care.* Baltimore: Urban & Schwarzenberg.

Pillitteri, A. (1992). *Maternal and child health nursing.* Philadelphia: J.B. Lippincott.

Thompson, E.D., & Ashwill, J.W. (1992). *Introduction to Pediatric Nursing* (6th ed.). Philadelphia: W.B. Saunders.

Whaley, L., & Wong, D. (1991). *Nursing care of children* (4th ed.). St. Louis: C.V. Mosby.

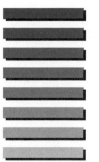

# Chapter 32

# The Child with a Metabolic Condition

## VOCABULARY
Autolet (841)
galactosemia (836)
glucagon (847)
glycosuria (838)
hormone (847)
hyperglycemia (838)
hypotonia (851)
lipoatrophy (846)
Somogyi phenomenon (848)
target organ (834)

Inborn Errors of Metabolism
    Maple Syrup Urine Disease
    Galactosemia
    Tay-Sachs Disease
Endocrine Disorders
    Diabetes Mellitus
    Hypothyroidism
Nutritional Deficiencies
    Kwashiorkor (Protein Deficiency)
    Rickets (Vitamin D Deficiency)
    Scurvy (Vitamin C Deficiency)

# OBJECTIVES

*On completion and mastery of Chapter 32, the student will be able to*

- Define each vocabulary term listed.
- Relate why growth parameters are of importance to patients with a family history of endocrine disease.
- List four tests pertinent to the patient with a metabolic condition.
- Differentiate between type I and type II diabetes.
- List a predictable stress that the disease of diabetes has on children and families during the following periods of life: infancy, toddlerhood, preschool age, elementary school age, puberty, and adolescence.
- Outline the educational needs of the diabetic child and parents in the following areas: nutrition and meal planning, exercise, urine tests, administration of insulin, and skin care.
- List three precipitating events that might cause diabetic ketoacidosis.
- List three possible causes of insulin shock.
- Explain the Somogyi phenomenon.
- Discuss the preparation and administration of insulin to a child, highlighting any differences between pediatric and adult administration.
- List two benefits of exercise for the diabetic teenager.
- List the symptoms of hypothyroidism in infants.
- Identify a vitamin deficiency seen in children. Include the food sources of the vitamin and its function in the body.
- Determine the average daily requirement of vitamin C for infants.

The two major control systems that monitor the functions of the body are the nervous system and the endocrine system. These systems are interdependent. The endocrine, or ductless, glands regulate the body's metabolic processes. They are primarily responsible for growth, maturation, reproduction, and response of the body to stress. Figure 32–1 depicts the organs of the endocrine system and outlines how this system in children differs from that in adults. Hormones are chemical substances produced by the glands. They pour their secretions directly into the blood that flows through them. An organ specifically influenced by a certain hormone is called a target organ. Too much or too little of a given hormone may result in a disease state.

Most of the glands and structures of the endocrine system develop during the 1st trimester of pregnancy.

Maternal endocrine dysfunction may affect the fetus; therefore, an in-depth maternal history is a valuable tool in nursing assessment. Because endocrine dysfunction can lead to growth problems, the developmental history is important. The average child grows in height and weight in a fairly predictable pattern. Variance from the pattern requires further investigation.

Radiographic studies to determine bone age are a valuable diagnostic tool. Serum electrolytes and glucose, hormonal, and calcium level tests may be indicated. Phenylketonuria testing of newborns is an important screening device for identifying an enzyme deficiency. Chromosomal studies and tissue biopsy are other diagnostic tools. Sexual maturation and skin texture, pigment, and temperature may be indicators of specific disorders. Thyroid function tests may be indicated. Ultrasound is helpful in determining the size and character of the adrenal glands and ovaries as well as other organs. A 24-hour urine specimen may reveal important data. The glucose tolerance test is commonly performed in order to detect and monitor diabetes. Genetic counseling can help prevent some disorders.

The following is a discussion of the disorders related to metabolic, endocrine, and nutritional deficiencies. These include maple syrup urine disease, galactosemia, Tay-Sachs disease, diabetes mellitus, hypothyroidism, kwashiorkor, rickets, and scurvy. Cystic fibrosis is discussed in Chapter 26; phenylketonuria is discussed in Chapter 14.

# Inborn Errors of Metabolism

The term *inborn errors of metabolism* was coined at the turn of the century by Garrod. There are literally hundreds of these hereditary biochemical disorders that affect body metabolism. They are continually being discovered (Behrman, 1992). Most of these disorders are caused by a lack of or deficiency in a particular enzyme and impair the body's ability to metabolize food (i.e., protein, carbohydrate, and fat). The pattern of inheritance is generally

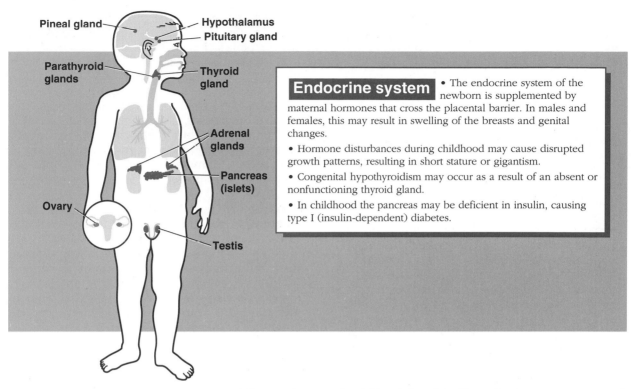

Pineal gland

Hypothalamus

Pituitary gland

Parathyroid glands

Thyroid gland

Adrenal glands

Pancreas (islets)

Ovary

Testis

**Endocrine system**
- The endocrine system of the newborn is supplemented by maternal hormones that cross the placental barrier. In males and females, this may result in swelling of the breasts and genital changes.
- Hormone disturbances during childhood may cause disrupted growth patterns, resulting in short stature or gigantism.
- Congenital hypothyroidism may occur as a result of an absent or nonfunctioning thyroid gland.
- In childhood the pancreas may be deficient in insulin, causing type I (insulin-dependent) diabetes.

**Figure 32–1.** Summary of endocrine system differences between the child and the adult. The endocrine system consists of the ductless glands that release hormones. It works with the nervous system to regulate metabolic activities.

autosomal recessive. These conditions range from mild to severe. They are usually detected during the newborn period. Prenatal diagsis of certain conditions is possible. Individually, inborn errors of metabolism are rare, but in combination they account for significant morbidity and mortality. Phenylketonuria, which results from a lack of phenylalanine, is discussed on pages 349–351.

## MAPLE SYRUP URINE DISEASE

**Description.** Maple syrup urine disease is caused by a defect in the metabolism of the branched-chain amino acids. It causes marked serum elevations of leucine, isoleucine, and valine. This results in acidosis, cerebral degeneration, and death if left untreated.

**Manifestations.** The infant appears healthy at birth but soon develops feeding difficulties, loss of Moro reflex, hypotonia, and irregular respirations. The urine, sweat, and cerumen (ear wax) have a characteristic sweet or maple syrup odor. This is due to ketoacidosis, a

process similar to that which may occur in diabetic children, and cause a fruity odor of the breath. However, the condition does not resolve with correction of blood glucose levels. The urine contains high levels of leucine, isoleucine, and valine.

**Treatment and Nursing Care.** Early detection in the newborn period is extremely important. The nursery nurse should report any newborn whose urine has a sweet aroma. Initial treatment consists of removal of these amino acids and their metabolites from the tissues of the body. This is accomplished by hydration and peritoneal dialysis to decrease serum levels. It is recommended that plasma leucine levels be maintained between 2 and 5 mg/dl. A level above 10 mg/dl is associated with symptoms (Mahan & Arlin, 1992). The patient is placed on a lifelong diet low in the amino acids leucine, isoleucine, and valine. Several formulas specifically for this disease are available. Exacerbations are most often related to the degree of abnormality of the leucine level. These exacerbations are frequently related to infection and can be life-threatening. The nurse must frequently assess the patient and instruct parents about the need to prevent infections.

## GALACTOSEMIA

**Description.** In galactosemia the body is unable to use the carbohydrates galactose and lactose. In the healthy person, the liver converts galactose to glucose. In the galactosemia patient, because an enzyme is defective or missing, there is a disturbance in a normally occurring chemical reaction. The result is an increase in the amount of galactose in the blood (galactosemia) and in the urine (galactosuria). This can cause cirrhosis of the liver, cataracts, and mental retardation if left untreated. Because galactose is present in milk sugar, early diagnosis is necessary so that a milk substitute can be used.

**Manifestations.** Early signs of galactosemia consist of lethargy, vomiting, hypotonia, diarrhea, and failure to thrive. These commence as the newborn begins breast feeding or ingesting formula. Jaundice may be present. Diagnosis is made by observing galactosuria, galactosemia, and evidence of decreased enzyme activity in the red blood cells. Screening tests are available.

**Treatment and Nursing Care.** Milk and lactose-containing products are eliminated from the diet of the patient with galactosemia. The nursing mother must discontinue breast feeding. Lactose-free formulas and those with a soy-protein base are frequently substituted. The length of time required for the restrictions in diet is not definite at this writing. The nurse must realize the frustration and anxiety that this diagnosis creates. Parents experience periods of feeling overwhelmed and inadequate. They can also becoming totally absorbed in the dietary program. When a disease is rare, it creates feelings of isolation and uncertainty. Because surveillance is ongoing, some of the emotional characteristics of the family with a child who has a chronic disease are pertinent.

## TAY-SACHS DISEASE

**Description.** In Tay-Sachs disease, there is a deficiency of *hexosaminidase*, an enzyme necessary for the metabolism of fats. Lipid deposits accumulate on nerve cells, causing both physi-cal and mental deterioration. This is a disease that is found primarily in the Ashkenazic Jewish population.

**Manifestations.** The infant with Tay-Sachs disease is normal until about 5–6 months of age, when physical development begins to slow. There may be head lag or inability to sit. The disease progresses, and when deposits occur on the optic nerve, blindness may result. Mental retardation eventually develops, as the brain cells become damaged. Most children die before the age of 5 from secondary infection or malnutrition.

**Treatment and Nursing Care.** There is no treatment for this devastating disease. The nursing care is mainly palliative. Most care is done in the home with periodic hospitalization for complications such as pneumonia. Chapter 34 discusses the care of the dying child. Carriers can be identified by screening tests. Genetic and prenatal counseling have markedly decreased the frequency of Tay-Sachs disease among Jewish couples (Behrman, 1992).

# Endocrine Disorders

## DIABETES MELLITUS

**Description.** Diabetes is a chronic metabolic condition in which the body is unable to utilize carbohydrates properly because of a deficiency of insulin, an internal secretion of the beta cells of the pancreas. Insulin deficiency leads to impairment of glucose transport (sugar cannot pass into the cells). The body is also unable to store and utilize fats properly. There is a decrease in protein synthesis. When the blood glucose level becomes dangerously high, glucose spills into the urine and diuresis occurs. Incomplete fat metabolism produces ketone bodies that accumulate in the blood. This is termed *ketonemia*. Untreated diabetes can lead to coma and death.

Type I diabetes is the most common endocrine-metabolic disorder of childhood. It is found worldwide, affects every organ of the body, and is unique in that it requires a great deal of self-management by the person affected. Patient education and compliance are essential. Morbidity and mortality are associated with chronic complications that affect small and large blood vessels, resulting in retinopathy, nephropathy, ischemic heart disease, and obstruction of large vessels.

**Classification.** It is now clear that diabetes is not a single entity but rather a syndrome. In order to help eliminate confusion in terminology, the National Institutes of Health appointed an international committee, the National Diabetes Data Group, to classify the carbohydrate intolerance syndromes. As more is learned about diabetes, further refinements in classification will be necessary. Three of the categories pertinent to this discussion of pediatric diabetes are described here.

*Type I, Insulin-Dependent Diabetes Mellitus (IDDM).* This was formerly termed juvenile-onset diabetes, or brittle diabetes. It is characterized by absolute or complete insulin deficiency. Childhood diabetes is usually of this type. Although there may be some insulin production during certain phases of the disease, patients eventually become insulin-deficient. They are prone to ketosis. Type I diabetes has been associated with an increased incidence among persons with certain human leukocyte antigen (HLA) haplotypes. Environmental as well as genetic factors are strongly implicated. Apparently, IDDM is sometimes set off by seemingly harmless viruses believed to provoke the immune system into mistakenly destroying its own beta cells of the islets of Langerhans. The presence of islet cell antibodies and reports associating IDDM with juvenile rheumatoid arthritis would appear to support an autoimmune etiology. Mumps, congenital rubella, and coxsackie B4 virus have also been implicated.

*Type II, Non–Insulin-Dependent Diabetes Mellitus (NIDDM).* This was formerly called adult-onset diabetes. These persons are not usually dependent on insulin and rarely develop ketosis. Although NIDDM may occur at any age, it generally develops after the age of 40. There is no association with HLA, autoimmunity, or islet cell antibodies. When type II diabetes is seen in young adults, it is sometimes called maturity-onset diabetes of youth. Table 32–1 lists clinical features of type I and type II diabetes.

*Secondary Diabetes.* Secondary diabetes may be caused by diseases of the pancreas, such as cystic fibrosis or cancer; hormonal causes; drug-induced causes; or other syndromes. Secondary diabetes is often reversed by treating the underlying cause. *Gestational diabetes* is the appearance of symptoms for the first time during pregnancy.

**Incidence.** Approximately 12 million Americans have diabetes. In the United States, the annual incidence is about 12–15 new cases per 100,000 children (Behrman, 1992). The frequency is increasing. Some factors contributing to this are (1) patients with diabetes are living into their reproductive years and having children; (2) life expectancy has increased; (3) obesity has increased; and (4) good prenatal care has decreased the mortality rates of mothers and babies.

Symptoms of IDDM may occur at any time in childhood, but the rate of occurrence of new cases is highest among 5- and 7-year-old children and pubescent children 11–13 years of age. In the former group, the stress of school and the increased exposure to infectious diseases may be responsible. During puberty, increased growth, increased emotional stress, and insulin antagonism of sex hormones may be implicated. It occurs in both sexes with equal frequency. Socioeconomic correlations have not been seen. The disease is more difficult to manage in childhood because the patients are growing, they expend a great deal of energy, their nutritional needs vary, and they have to face a lifetime of diabetic management. Young children with IDDM often do not demonstrate the typical "textbook" picture of the disorder; the initial diagnosis may be determined when the child presents with ketoacidosis. Therefore,

**Table 32–1.** CLINICAL FEATURES OF TYPE I AND TYPE II DIABETES

| Feature | Type I (IDDM) | Type II (NIDDM) |
|---|---|---|
| Onset | Abrupt, frequently can date week of onset | Insidious, often found by screening tests |
| Body size | Normal or thin | Frequently obese |
| Blood glucose | Fluctuates widely with exercise and infection | Fluctuations are less marked |
| Ketoacidosis | Common | Infrequent |
| Sulfonylurea-responsiveness | Rare | Greater than 50% |
| Insulin required | Almost all | Less than 25% |
| Insulin dosage | Increases until total diabetes occurs | May remain stable |

IDDM, insulin-dependent diabetes mellitus; NIDDM, non–insulin-dependent diabetes mellitus.

the nurse must be particularly astute in subjective and objective observations.

**Manifestations.** Children with diabetes present a classic triad of symptoms: polydipsia, polyuria, and polyphagia. The symptoms appear more rapidly in children. The patient complains of excessive thirst (polydipsia), excretes large amounts of urine frequently (polyuria), and is constantly hungry (polyphagia). An insidious onset with lethargy, weakness, and weight loss is also common. Anorexia may be seen. The child who is toilet-trained may begin wetting the bed or have frequent "accidents" during play periods, may lose weight, and is irritable. The skin becomes dry. Vaginal yeast infections may be seen in the adolescent girl. Abdominal cramps are common. There may be a history of recurrent infections. The symptoms may go unrecognized until an infection becomes apparent or coma results. Laboratory findings indicate glucose in the urine (glycosuria or glucosuria). Hyperglycemia (*hyper*, "above," *gly*, "sugar," and *emia*, "blood") is also apparent.

### Diagnostic Blood Tests

*Blood Glucose.* A random blood glucose may be drawn at any time and requires no preparation of the client. The results should be within normal limits for both nondiabetics and diabetics in good control.

*Fasting Blood Glucose.* Fasting blood glucose is a standard and reliable test for diabetes. The blood glucose level is measured in the fasting patient, usually first thing in the morning. If the patient has a dextrose intravenous solution running, the results of the test will not be accurate. If the child is known to have diabetes, food and insulin are withheld until after the test. If a person's blood glucose is greater than 140 mg/dl on two separate occasions and the history is positive, the patient is considered to have diabetes and requires treatment. In nondiabetics the results are usually less than 115 mg/dl. A high blood glucose level before eating is a clear sign of diabetes.

*Glucose Tolerance Test.* Another test to determine the amount of sugar in the blood is the glucose tolerance test. Results are plotted on a graph (Fig. 32–2). An intravenous glucose tolerance test is preferred in children, as oral glucose tolerance tests have had low detection rates. Glucose is administered intravenously over several minutes to the fasting child. Blood samples are taken at 30, 60, 90, 120, and 180 minutes. Generally, small amounts of water are allowed. Parents and teenagers are advised to bring reading material, homework, headsets, and so on to the physician's office or laboratory, as the procedure is time-consuming. A blood glucose concentration greater than 200 mg/dl is considered positive. Normal values may not return for over 3 hours.

*Glycosylated Hemoglobin Test.* The glycosylated hemoglobin test (GHb) reflects glycemic

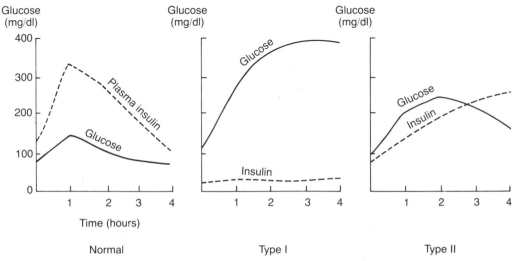

**Figure 32–2.** The glucose tolerance test: *left*, normal; *center*, type I diabetes; *right*, type II diabetes. The graphs show the relationship between the ingestion of glucose and the level of plasma insulin over 4 hours in a normal person and in persons with type I and type II diabetes. (Adapted from Waechter, E.H. & Blake, F.G. [1976]. *Nursing care of children* [9th ed.]. Philadelphia: J.B. Lippincott.)

levels over a period of months. Values are found to be elevated in virtually all children with newly diagnosed diabetes. This study also helps confirm the results of blood and urine tests done either at home or by the doctor. Glucose in the blood stream is constantly entering red blood cells and linking with, or glycosylating, molecules of hemoglobin. The more glucose is in the blood, the more hemoglobin becomes coated with glucose. The red blood cells carry this glucose until they are replaced by cells with fresh hemoglobin. This process takes about 3–4 months. Values vary according to measurement used. Values of 6–9% represent very good metabolic control. Values above 12% indicate poor control (Behrman, 1992). One clinic awards an "under 9" badge to their patients who achieve this value and reports that a low glycosylated hemoglobin test can be a tremendous psychological boost.

Glycosylated albumin (fructosamine) is a newer test used to measure blood glucose control over the preceding 7–10 days. C-peptide (connecting chains of insulin peptides) may also be measured to determine how much insulin the body is producing (endogenous). This is of particular value during the "honeymoon" period of the disease.

**Diabetic Ketoacidosis (DKA).** Diabetic ketoacidosis is also referred to as *diabetic coma*, although a person may have diabetic ketoacidosis with or without being in a coma. It may result if a diabetic patient contracts a secondary infection and does not follow proper self-care. It may also result, as occurs fairly often in diabetic children, if the disease proceeds unrecognized. Even minor infections, such as a cold, increase the body's metabolic rate and thereby change the body's demand for insulin and the severity of diabetes.

The symptoms range from mild to severe and occur within hours to days. The skin is dry and the face flushed. Patients appear dehydrated. They are thirsty but may vomit if fluids are offered. They perspire and are restless. There may be generalized pain in the abdomen and throughout the body. A characteristic *fruity odor* of the breath is apparent because the patient expels acetone from the respiratory tree, and the lips are cherry-red. As the condition becomes worse, the patient becomes weak and drowsy. Breathing patterns are peculiar in that there is no normal period of rest between inspiration and expiration; this is termed *Kussmaul* breathing. The patient becomes unconscious. Death results unless insulin, fluids, and electrolytes are administered.

The replacement of depleted fluids, frequent checking of vital signs, urine tests, blood chemistry measurements, and close observation of consciousness are necessary. Baseline studies include venous blood glucose, serum acetone, pH, total carbon dioxide, blood urea nitrogen, electrolytes, calcium, phosphate, white blood cell count, urinalysis, and appropriate cultures. Glucose levels in the blood and urine, electrolytes, and any abnormal laboratory values are monitored carefully until the child stabilizes. Low doses of regular insulin both intravenously and subcutaneously are administered, and the patient is observed. If the patient has an infection, this is treated. Cerebral edema, although rare, can be life-threatening. A diabetic flow chart at the bedside registers all pertinent information. Response to treatment is gradual.

**Treatment and Nursing Care.** The aims of treatment in type I diabetes are (1) to ensure normal growth and development through metabolic control, (2) to enable the child to have a happy and active childhood and to be well integrated into the family, and (3) to prevent complications. Teaching ideally begins when the diagnosis is confirmed. An algorithm for diagnosis and treatment of diabetic ketoacidosis is presented in Figure 32–3. A planned educational program is necessary to provide a consistent body of information, which can then be individualized. The patient's age and financial, educational, cultural, and religious background must be considered. Many hospitals hold group clinics for diabetic patients and their relatives. These sessions are conducted by various professionals, such as the diabetes nurse educator, dietitian, and pharmacist. Patients who are living with the disease provide encouragement and help by sharing concerns. Health professionals become directly involved with the patient's progress and can offer necessary feedback and support. Continuous follow-up is essential.

Because diabetic children are growing, additional dimensions of the disorder and its treatment become evident. Growth is not steady but occurs in spurts and plateaus that affect treatment. Infants and toddlers may have hydration problems, especially during illness. Preschool children have irregular activity and eating patterns. School-age children may grieve over the diagnosis and ask, "Why me?" They may use their illness to gain attention or to avoid responsibilities. The onset of puberty may require adjustments in insulin as a result of growth and the antagonistic effect of the sex hormones on insulin. Adolescents often resent this condi-

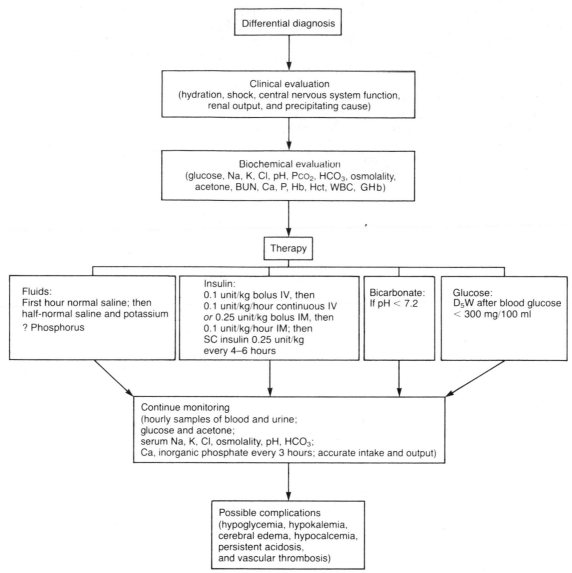

**Figure 32–3.** Algorithm for the diagnosis and treatment of diabetic ketoacidosis. (Adapted from Dickerman, J., & Lucey, R. [1985]. *Smith's the critically ill child* [3rd ed., p. 122]. Philadelphia: W.B. Saunders.)

tion, which deviates from their conception of the "body ideal." They have more difficulty in resolving their conflict between dependence and independence. This may lead to rebellion against parents and treatment regimens.

The impact of the disease on the rest of the family must also be considered. One mother commented, "I was so scared. I felt very strongly that whether my child lived or died depended on me. It was overwhelming. I couldn't allow myself mistakes. This was reinforced by all the do's and don'ts of the instructions." Almost all of the par-

ents of young diabetics whom I have met have these strong initial emotions of fear. Parents may also feel guilty for having passed on the disease. Siblings may feel jealous of the patient. The sharing of responsibility by parents is ideal but not necessarily a reality. Everyone may have difficulty accepting the diagnosis and the more regimented lifestyle it imposes. Family members must cope with their individual reactions to the stress of the illness.

Children must assume responsibility for their care gradually and with a minimum of pressure. Overprotection can be as detrimental as neglect. Parents who have received satisfaction from their child's dependence on them may need help "letting go." Diabetic camp experience is helpful in this respect.

The nursing management of childhood diabetes requires knowledge of growth and development, pathophysiology, blood glucose self-monitoring, nutritional management, insulin management, insulin shock, exercise, skin and foot care, infections, effects of emotional upsets, and long-term care. Nursing Care Plan 32–1 lists interventions for the child with diabetes mellitus.

**Pathophysiology of Diabetes.** The patient and family are instructed about the location of the pancreas and its normal function. The nurse explains the relationship of insulin to the pancreas, differentiating between type I and type II diabetes.

All information is given gradually and at the level of understanding of the child and family. Audiovisual aids and pamphlets are incorporated into the session. If the patient is newly diagnosed, hospitalization offers opportunities for instruction.

**Blood Glucose Self-Monitoring.** Blood glucose self-monitoring has dramatically changed the approach to diabetes. Previously, blood tests for glucose could be carried out only in a doctor's office or laboratory. The patient had to rely on urine tests, which often presented a confusing picture, particularly when the urine had been in the bladder for several hours (glucose might turn up in the urine when the diabetic's blood glucose level was actually low). Only a blood check can show the actual amount of glucose in the blood at the time of the test. Technology has made it possible for patients to test their own blood glucose in the home. While still being supervised by and consulting with the physician, the patient can nonetheless make rational changes in insulin dosage, nutritional requirements, and daily exercise. This is of great psychological value to the child, teenager, and parents, as it reduces feelings of helplessness and complete dependence on medical personnel. Home glucose monitoring should be taught to all young patients or their caretakers. The patient must not only be skilled in the techniques but also understand the results and how to incorporate them into daily regimens. This means involving the entire health-care team in ongoing supervision, demonstrations, and support. Although instruc-

tions come with the various products, patients need individual training.

Newer glucometer systems provide read-outs and automatically store data by time and date. Some also keep track of diet and the amount of exercise for the day. This can be connected to a computer or computer printer for review. Records can be transmitted over the telephone to the physician.

Obtaining blood specimens has been simplified by the use of capillary blood-letting devices, such as the Glucolet. This device automatically controls the depth of penetration of the lancet into the skin. Other brands include the Hamalet, Autoclix, Monoject, and Autolet. The sides of the fingertips are recommended testing sites, as there are fewer nerve endings and more capillary beds in these areas. The best finger to use is the middle, ring, or little finger on either hand. If the child washes the hands in warm water for about 30 seconds, the finger will bleed more easily. To perform the test, a drop of blood is put on a chemically treated reagent strip. The test strip with a drop of blood is inserted into the glucometer, and the blood glucose reading appears (Fig. 32–4).

Cost, convenience, and portability are factors to consider when selecting devices. Most products can be obtained at the local pharmacy. Newer and more precise instruments are being developed constantly. Frequency of use is determined by the amount of diabetes control required by the particular patient.

**Nutritional Management.** The triad of management of diabetes comprises a well-balanced diet, insulin, and regular exercise. The importance of glycemic control (tight blood sugars) in decreasing the incidence of symptoms and complications of the disease has been established. The advent of blood glucose self-monitoring is affecting food intake, in that diets can be fine-tuned and more flexible while the cornerstone of *consistency* (in amount of food and time of feeding) is maintained. Contrary to popular belief, there is no scientific evidence that persons with diabetes require special foods. In fact, if it is good for the diabetic, it is good for the entire family. The nutritional needs of diabetic children are essentially no different from those of nondiabetic children, with the exception of the elimination of concentrated carbohydrates (simple sugars). These cause a marked increase in blood glucose and should generally be avoided.

The goals of nutritional management in children are to ensure normal growth and develop-

| NURSING CARE PLAN 32–1 |
| :-: |
| **Selected Nursing Diagnoses for the Child with Diabetes Mellitus** |

| Goals | Nursing Interventions | Rationale |
| --- | --- | --- |

**Nursing Diagnosis:** High risk for injury related to hypoglycemia or diabetic ketoacidosis (hyperglycemia).

| Goals | Nursing Interventions | Rationale |
| --- | --- | --- |
| Child is able to measure blood glucose with glucometer, as age appropriate<br>Child is adequately hydrated as evidenced by good tissue turgor and intake and output records<br>Child is asymptomatic of hypoglycemia or hyperglycemia | 1. Teach child home glucose monitoring<br>2. Record vital signs regularly | 1. Self-care increases feelings of control<br>2. Vital signs detect infection and illness, which affect diabetes; in ketoacidosis, Kussmaul respirations may be seen until blood pH and serum bicarbonate normalize |
| | 3. Monitor fluid intake and output | 3. Dehydration may occur as a result of vomiting, polyuria, and hyperglycemia |
| | 4. Serve meals and snacks on time | 4. Serving meals on time prevents hypoglycemia and minimizes hyperglycemia |
| | 5. Administer or have patient administer insulin as ordered | 5. Insulin is individualized to meet the response of patients. It cannot be taken by mouth, as stomach juices would destroy it before it could be used |
| | 6. Assess level of consciousness | 6. Both hypoglycemia and hyperglycemia affect sensorium, depending on stage of reaction |
| | 7. Carefully observe patient for signs of hypoglycemia or hyperglycemia | 7. Many factors such as diet, increased exercise, or illness can contribute to the body's balance of insulin and glucose; changes in hormone levels that accompany menstruation can cause swings of high or low blood sugar |

**Nursing Diagnosis:** Knowledge deficit regarding exercise.

| Goals | Nursing Interventions | Rationale |
| --- | --- | --- |
| Child describes physical exercise program<br>Child is prepared for hypoglycemia, should it occur | 1. Assess child's activity level as age-appropriate<br>2. Explain that exercise lowers the blood sugar and in this respect acts like more insulin<br>3. Instruct as to symptoms of hypoglycemia such as irritability, shakiness, hunger, headache, altered levels of consciousness<br>4. Teach child importance of carrying extra sugar when exercising or playing sports<br>5. Teach child dangers of swimming alone | 1. Exercise increases glucose utilization<br>2. Patient may need to adjust insulin for days when involved in high-impact exercise<br>3. Early recognition and prompt treatment will prevent injury<br><br>4. Taking sugar reverses symptoms of hypoglycemia<br><br>5. Child could drown if symptoms occur |

**Nursing Diagnosis:** Knowledge deficit regarding identification.

| Goals | Nursing Interventions | Rationale |
| --- | --- | --- |
| Child states understanding of importance of wearing proper identification in regards to condition<br>Family acquires identification bracelet | 1. Child demonstrates proper identification<br>2. Encourage purchase of means of identification | 1. Diabetes symptoms may be mistaken for other conditions, such as flu<br>2. Child may be unconscious or too young to inform others of condition |

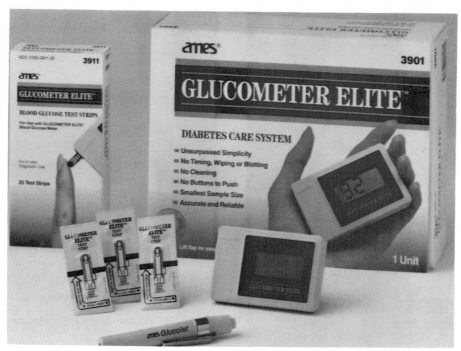

**Figure 32–4.** Glucometer used to determine blood glucose values. (Courtesy of Miles, Inc., Diagnostics Division, Tarrytown, NY.)

ment, to distribute food intake so that it aids metabolic control, and to individualize the diet in accordance with the child's ethnic background, age, sex, weight, activity, family economics, and food preferences. Once a diet order is received from the physician, the dietitian calculates the distribution of carbohydrates, protein, and fat. Portion size is demonstrated by the use of food models and measuring cups and spoons. Regularly spaced meals and snacks are planned and the family is taught how to read labels and the differences among carbohydrates, protein, and fat. The dietitian also explains the use of exchange lists.

Education of the patient is ongoing. Too much information given at one time may overwhelm the parents and discourage the child. Well-informed nurses can offer much reinforcement and support. They can clarify such terms as dietetic, sugar-free, juice-packed, water-packed, and unsweetened. Meal trays in the hospital provide an excellent opportunity for teaching. Children should bring their lunch to school. Teenagers need to be advised that alcohol lowers the blood sugar. It suppresses gluconeogenesis and is high in calories. Most cocktail mixes contain sugar; however, water, sugar-free pop, club soda, and tomato juice do not. Although the consumption of alcohol is discouraged, the young person who wishes to drink should do so after dinner or should consume the beverage with some type of food.

***Constant Carbohydrate Diet.*** The constant carbohydrate diet is an approach to meal planning. The goal is to maintain a consistent amount of carbohydrate at each meal and snack. Regularity of meals is stressed. The amount of carbohydrate may, and usually does, vary from meal to meal. The initial carbohydrate pattern is determined by the individual's current food intake. In order to calculate the number of grams of carbohydrate in food, exchange lists that divide food into six categories are used. This food plan appeals to young diabetics because it is easy to use and flexible.

***Fiber.*** The importance of fiber in diets is well documented. In the diabetic patient, soluble fiber has been shown to reduce blood sugar levels, lower serum cholesterol values, and sometimes reduce insulin requirements. Fiber appears to slow the rate of absorption of sugar by the digestive tract. Raw fruits and vegetables, bran cereals, wheat germ, beans, peas, and lentils are good sources of soluble fiber.

***Glycemic    Index,    Cholesterol,    Artificial***

*Sweeteners.* The glycemic index for selected foods suggested by Jenkins will no doubt have an impact on the manipulation of dietary needs. Because persons with diabetes have an increased risk for atherosclerosis, the reduction of serum cholesterol is another concern. These persons (like most of the general public) need to reduce their intake of animal fats or substitute vegetable fat for animal fat. This is accomplished by consuming less beef and pork and more lean meat, chicken, turkey, fish, low-fat milk (depending on age of patient), and vegetable proteins. The use of polyunsaturated fats in cooking is advised. The form of the food is also significant. An apple, apple juice, and applesauce may precipitate different blood sugar responses. Portions, the type of processing, cooking, and combinations of foods have also been shown to have a bearing on these responses.

Aspartame (NutraSweet) was approved by the Food and Drug Administration in 1981. It is used in items that do not require cooking. Aspartame is made of two amino acids. Both contain insignificant amounts of carbohydrate. One granulation form is called Equal. Sorbitol, mannitol, and xylitol are sugars commonly found in foods called "sugar-free." These substances are absorbed more slowly into the blood stream. They are carbohydrates and must be calculated in the food plan.

*Role of the Nurse.* The student nurse has a number of responsibilities as a member of the team concerned with the patient and food management. These begin with preparing the child for meals. The child is asked to void if a urine specimen is needed. Blood glucose is generally checked before meals, at snack time, and before bed. The child's face and hands are washed, and distracting toys are removed for the time being. The child is served the meal tray in the crib on a bed table or at the regular table suited to the size of the child. Small children require bibs. The tray is served *on time*. Patients who receive regular insulin before meals may have an insulin reaction if food is not eaten within 20 minutes. If nurses are scheduled for their own lunch break when meals are served the child, they notify the team leader and do not assume that others will feed the child. No foods or liquids, except water, are given between meals unless authorized by the physician or dietitian. The nurse must be sure that the tray is served to the *right patient*. A mistake can occur, particularly if several children are on special diets.

This can happen more easily on the pediatric unit, where patients roam about freely. Food is cut into small pieces as age-appropriate. Toast or muffins are buttered, and eggs are removed from their shells. A child who is able to eat independently is encouraged to do so. The nurse uses powers of observation to determine when help is needed. Foods that the child especially enjoys or dislikes are noted.

When the child has finished eating, the tray is removed. The nurse observes the types and amounts of foods that the patient refused, charts them in the nurses' notes, and informs the nurse in charge. These observations are brought to the attention of the dietitian, who determines the number of calories that need to be made up and orders a between-meal snack, such as orange juice, to compensate. Anorexia or vomiting is reported promptly. After the meal, the nurse washes the child's hands and face, straightens the crib, and returns toys.

**Insulin Management.** Insulin is used principally as a specific drug for the control of diabetes mellitus. When injected into the diabetic patient, it enables the body to burn and store sugar.

Current data emphasize the importance of tight blood glucose control in the prevention of microvascular disease. Insulin pumps are used in certain patients (Fig. 32–5). More highly purified insulins are being developed to reduce complications. *Human insulin*, which is not made from humans but is produced bio-synthetically in bacteria using recombinant DNA technology, is widely used. It is reported to be very

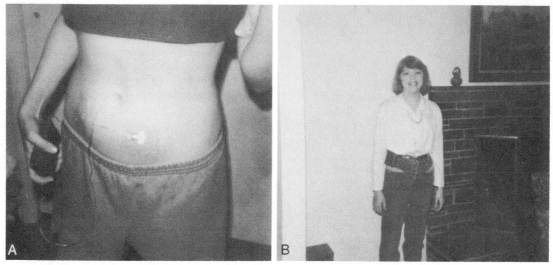

**Figure 32–5.** The insulin pump offers continuous subcutaneous insulin infusion without the need for frequent injections.

similar to the body's natural insulin. One example is Humulin, manufactured by the Eli Lilly Company.

The dose of insulin is measured in units, and special syringes are used in its administration. U-100 (100-unit) insulin is the standard form. Each marking on the 1-ml (100-unit) syringe represents 2 units of insulin. The 50-unit disposable syringe is intended for small doses. All vials of U-100 insulin have color-coded orange caps, and all labels bear black printing on a white background. Bold letters indicate type: "R" for regular, "P" for protamine zinc insulin (PZI), "N" for neutral protamine Hagedorn (NPH) insulin, "L" for lente, "U" for ultralente, and "S" for semilente.

It is important to teach the parents and child about the administration of insulin. Insulin cannot be taken orally because it is a protein and would by broken down by the gastric juices. The usual method of administration is *subcutaneously* (Fig. 32–6). When injected at a 90-degree angle, the short needle enters the subcutaneous space. This technique may be easier for the child to learn because it takes less coordination to administer than a 45-degree-angle technique. Automatic injection devices (Fig. 32–7), the insulin pump, and needle-free injectors such as Medi-Jector, EZ, or Tendertouch are fairly easy to use and promote independence in the child. A child can generally be taught to perform self-injection after the age of 7. The doctor prescribes the type and amount of insulin and specifies the time of administration.

The site of the injection is rotated in order to prevent poor absorption and injury to tissues (Fig. 32–8). Injection model forms made from construction paper and site rotation patterns are useful. One suggested site rotation pattern is to use one area for 1 week. For each injection, a different site within that area is used.

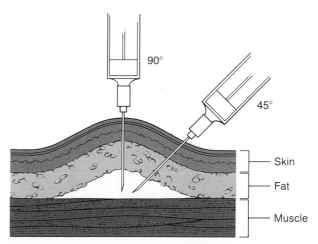

**Figure 32–6.** Subcutaneous injection of insulin. (From Betz, C., Hunsberger, M., & Wright, S. [1994]. *Family-centered nursing care of children* [2nd ed.]. Philadelphia: W.B. Saunders.)

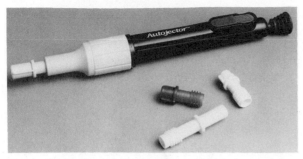

**Figure 32–7.** The Autojector delivers the predrawn dosage at the pre-set depth by a button control. It has four depth adjusters. (Courtesy of Ulster Scientific, New Paltz, NY.)

Injections should be about 1 inch apart. The young child can use a doll to practice self-injection. Parents usually find the experience of injecting their own child difficult. One mother stated that for the first few months she gave the injection in the child's hips so that her daughter could not see the expression on her face.

Allergic responses to insulin can be divided into those that occur locally at the injection site, rare systemic sensitivities (true insulin allergy), and immunologic reactions. Lipoatrophy (*lipo,* "fat," and *atrophy,* "loss of") and lipohypertrophy (*lipo,* and *hypertrophy,* "increase of")

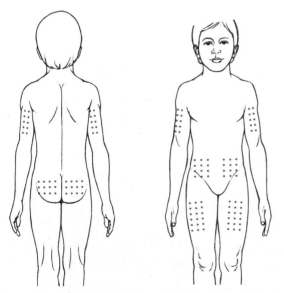

**Figure 32–8.** Sites of injection of insulin. (From Betz, C., Hunsberger, M., & Wright, S. [1994]. *Family-centered nursing care of children* [2nd ed.]. Philadelphia: W.B. Saunders.)

refer to changes in the subcutaneous tissue at the injection site. Proper rotation of sites and the availability of the newer purified insulins have helped eliminate these conditions. The child is taught to "feel for lumps" every week and to avoid using any sites that are suspicious.

The nurse ascertains what brand of insulin the patient is using. In general it is not wise to switch brands of insulin (e.g., Lilly, Squibb) because they may be slightly different. Questions should be directed to the hospital pharmacist. It is no longer necessary to refrigerate insulin to prevent deterioration. However, one should avoid exposing insulin to extremes in temperature and should check expiration dates.

The various types of insulin and their action are listed in Table 32–2. The main difference is in the amount of time required for it to take effect and the length of protection time. The values listed in Table 32–2 are only *guidelines.* The response of each diabetic child to any given insulin dose is highly individual and depends on many factors, such as site of injection, local destruction of insulin by tissue enzymes, and insulin antibodies.

Regular or crystalline insulin is a purified form of regular insulin and is less likely to cause allergic reactions. Both NPH, an intermediate type, and PZI, a long-lasting insulin, have had small amounts of chemicals added in order to prolong their action and to make them more stable. They offer protection over a period of hours, enabling the patient to do without repeated injections of unmodified insulin. They are cloudy and require mixing before being withdrawn from the vials. This is done by gently rolling the bottle between the palms of the hands. Insulin is not used if it is discolored.

Frequently the physician orders a combination of a short-acting insulin and an intermediate-acting one; for example, "Give 10 units of NPH insulin and 5 units of regular insulin at 7:30 A.M." This offers the patient immediate and longer-lasting protection. NPH or Lente insulin may be given in the same syringe as regular or crystalline insulin (Fig. 32–9). Long-acting types of insulin are seldom given to children because of the danger of hypoglycemia during sleep. Stable premixed insulins are now being introduced by some manufacturers.

***Insulin Shock.*** Insulin shock, also known as hypoglycemia (*hypo,* "below," *glyco,* "sugar," and *emia,* "blood"), occurs when the blood sugar level becomes abnormally low. This condition is caused by too much insulin. Factors that may

**Table 32–2.** HYPOGLYCEMICS: INSULIN

| | Brand Name(s) | Hypoglycemic Effect | | |
|---|---|---|---|---|
| | | *Onset (Hours)* | *Peak (Hours)* | *Duration (Hours)* |
| Rapid-acting | | 0.5–1 | — | 6–8 |
| Regular insulin | Humulin R Novolin R Velosulin | | | |
| Semilente insulin | Semilente | 1–1.5 | 5–10 | 12–16 |
| Intermediate-acting | | | | |
| Lente insulin | Humulin L Novolin L | 1–2.5 | 7–15 | 24 |
| Neutral protamine Hagedorn (NPH) insulin | Humulin N Insulintard Novolin N | 1–1.5 | 4–12 | 24 |
| Long-acting | | | | |
| Protamine zinc insulin (PZI) | PZI | 4–8 | 14–24 | 36 |
| Ultralente insulin | Humulin U Ultralente | 4–8 | 10–30 | >36 |

From Hodgson, B.B., Kizior, R.J., & Kingdon, R.T. (1993). *Nurse's drug handbook.* Philadelphia: W.B. Saunders.

## Nursing Brief

A period of remission or the "honeymoon" phase of the disease may occur within a few weeks of beginning insulin administration. There is a decline in insulin need and improved metabolic control. This, however, is temporary.

account for this imbalance include poorly planned exercise, reduction of diet, improvement of the condition so that the patient requires less insulin, and errors made because of improper knowledge of insulin and the insulin syringe.

Children are more prone to insulin reactions than adults because (1) the condition itself is more unstable in young people, (2) they are growing, and (3) their activities are more irregular. *Poorly planned exercise* is frequently the cause of insulin shock during childhood. Hospitalized patients who are being regulated must be observed frequently during naptime and at night. The nurse becomes suspicious of problems if unable to arouse the patient or if the child is perspiring heavily.

The symptoms of an insulin reaction, which range from mild to severe, are generally noticed and treated in the early stages. They appear suddenly in the otherwise well person. Examination of the blood would reveal a lowered blood sugar level. The child becomes irritable and may behave poorly, is pale, and may complain of feeling hungry and weak. Sweating occurs. Symptoms related to disorders of the nervous system arise because glucose is vital to the proper functioning of nerves. The child may become mentally confused and giddy, and muscular coordination is affected. If insulin shock is left untreated, coma and convulsions can occur.

The immediate treatment consists of administering sugar in some form, such as orange juice, cola beverages, ginger ale, hard candy, or a commercial product such as Glutose. The patient begins to feel better within a few minutes and at that time may eat a small amount of protein or starch (sandwich, milk, cheese) in order to prevent another reaction.

*Glucagon* is recommended for the treatment of severe hypoglycemia. It quickly restores the child to consciousness in an emergency; the child can then consume some form of sugar. Glucagon is a hormone produced by the pancreatic islets that also produce insulin. Normally, a fall in blood glucose makes the body release this substance. It causes a rapid breakdown of glycogen to glucose in the liver. Glucagon is packaged commercially in individual-dose units that are very stable in powdered form. When it is diluted, it can be given subcutaneously, intramuscularly, or intravenously. Families of patients on insulin can be instructed to administer glucagon subcutaneously or intramuscularly. If the patient does not respond rapidly,

1. Wash your hands.
2. Gently rotate the intermediate insulin bottle.
3. Wipe off the tops of the insulin vials with an alcohol sponge.
4. Draw back an amount of air into the syringe equal to the total dose.
5. Inject air equal to the NPH dose into the NPH vial. Remove the syringe from the vial.

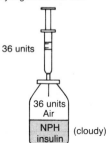

36 units

36 units
Air

NPH insulin (cloudy)

6. Inject air equal to the regular dose into the regular vial.

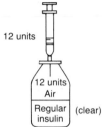

12 units

12 units
Air

Regular insulin (clear)

7. Invert the regular insulin bottle and withdraw the regular insulin dose.

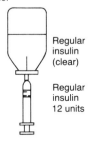

Regular insulin (clear)

Regular insulin 12 units

8. Without adding more air to the NPH vial, carefully withdraw the NPH dose.

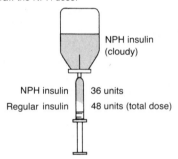

NPH insulin (cloudy)

NPH insulin   36 units
Regular insulin   48 units (total dose)

the physician is contacted. The unconscious patient is kept warm by covering with a blanket. The patient is given nothing by mouth; medical attention is immediately sought.

The Somogyi phenomenon (rebound hyperglycemia) occurs when blood glucose levels are lowered to a point at which the body's counterregulatory hormones (epinephrine, cortisol, glucagon) are released. Glucose is released from muscle and liver cells, which precipitates a rapid rise in blood glucose (Black & Matassarin-Jacobs, 1993). It is generally the result of chronic insulin use, especially in patients who require fairly large doses of insulin to regulate their blood sugar. Hypoglycemia during the night and high glucose levels in the morning are suggestive of the phenomenon. The child may awaken at night or have frequent nightmares and experience early morning sweating and headaches. The child actually needs *less* insulin, not more, to rectify the problem.

The Somogyi phenomenon differs from the *dawn phenomenon*, in which early morning elevations of blood glucose occur *without* preceding hypoglycemia. Together the Somogyi and dawn phenomena are the most common causes of instability in diabetic children. Testing blood glucose around 3 AM helps differentiate the two conditions and assists in regulation of insulin dosage.

**Exercise.** Exercise is important for the patient with diabetes because it causes the body to use sugar and promotes good circulation. It lowers the blood glucose, and in this respect it acts like more insulin. The diabetic patient who has planned vigorous exercise should carry extra sugar in order to avoid insulin reactions. The patient should also carry money for candy or a drink or to use a telephone. The blood glucose level is high directly after meals, so the child can participate in active sports at such times. Games enjoyed directly before meals should be less active. The diabetic child is able to participate in almost all active sports. Poorly

**Figure 32–9.** Mixing insulin. This step-order process avoids the problem of contaminating the regular insulin with the intermediate insulin. If contamination of the regular insulin does occur, the rapid-acting effect of this drug would be dampened, and it would be unreliable as a quick-acting insulin in an acute situation such as diabetic ketoacidosis. (From Price, M.J. [1983]. Insulin and oral hypoglycemic agents. *Nursing Clinics of North America, 18,* 687–706.)

planned exercise, however, can lead to difficulties. The diabetic child, like any child, is not allowed to swim unsupervised.

**Skin Care.** The patient is instructed to bathe daily and dry well. Cleansing of the inguinal area, axillae, perineum, and inframammary areas is especially important, as yeast and fungal infections tend to occur there. Skin is inspected for cuts, rashes, abrasions, bruises, cysts, or boils. These lesions are managed promptly. If skin is very dry, an oil such as Alpha-Keri may be used in the bath water. Adolescents are taught to use electric razors. Exposing the skin to extremes in temperatures is avoided. Injection sites are inspected for lumps.

**Foot Care.** Although circulatory problems of the feet are less common in children, proper habits of foot hygiene need to be established. The patient is instructed to wash and dry the feet well each day. The feet are inspected for interdigital cracking, and the condition of the toenails is checked. Nails are trimmed straight across. Corn remedies, iodine, or alcohol should not be used. Socks are changed daily, and tight socks or large ones that bunch up are avoided. Shoes are replaced often as the child grows. Boots are worn for short periods to minimize sweating. The patient should not go barefoot. If problems arise, consult a physician or podiatrist.

**Infections.** Immunizations against communicable diseases are obtained. Cystitis, subcutaneous nodules, and monilial vulvitis occur with greater frequency in diabetic patients. During late adolescence, female patients should see a gynecologist yearly.

**Emotional Upsets.** Emotional upsets can be as disturbing to the patient as an infection and may require food or insulin adjustments, or both. Early detection of and intervention in deteriorating personal relationships and rebellion against diabetic management will decrease the severity of the effects on the diabetic. The nurse is attuned to little problems, which frequently are veiled requests for help. Family therapy and other forms of psychotherapeutic help may be required. Support by caretakers aids in prevention. Table 32–3 lists nursing interventions for stress on child and family related to type I diabetes.

**Urine Checks.** Routine urine checks for sugar are being replaced by the more accurate glucose blood monitoring. However, this procedure does not test for acetone, which the patient may need to determine, particularly when the blood glucose level is high and during illness. Daily urine checks may be advocated for some patients. Saying urine "check" rather than "test" is less confusing to young children.

During hospitalization, urine testing may be ordered. The two-drop method using a second voided specimen is frequently performed. It is not always possible to obtain a second specimen from a child; therefore, it may be prudent to test the one already obtained. If this is done, it is recorded as the first or second voiding. The nurse reads the manufacturer's directions and reviews the directions with the child. Regardless of which method is used, *exact timing* is important. Clinitest tablets are poison and must be kept away from children and confused adults. Test results may be affected by large doses of aspirin, antibiotics, and other medications.

Expiration dates on the carton or bottle are checked. The child is instructed to wash the hands before and after the procedure. Results are recorded. Quantitative urine collection is sometimes ordered. All voided specimens over a period of time are collected in a receptacle. The results show how many grams of glucose are eliminated during the time allocated (generally 24 hours).

**Glucose-Insulin Imbalances.** The patient is taught to recognize the signs of insulin shock and ketoacidosis. Early attention to change and daily record-keeping are stressed. Many excellent teaching films and brochures are available. The child should wear an identification bracelet. Wallet cards are also available. Teachers, athletic coaches, and guidance personnel are informed about the disease and should have the telephone numbers of the patient's parents and physician.

**Travel.** With planning, children can enjoy travel with their families, and older adolescents can travel alone. Before leaving, the child should be seen by the physician for a checkup and prescriptions for supplies. A written statement and a card identifying the child as diabetic should be carried. Time changes may affect meals. Additional supplies of insulin, sugar, and food are kept with the child. These are never checked with luggage, especially on an airplane, as they may be lost. If foreign travel is planned, parents need to become familiar with the food in the area so that dietary requirements can be met. Local chapters of the American Diabetes Association or the Juvenile Diabetes Foundation can help vacationing families in an emergency.

**Table 32–3.** NURSING INTERVENTIONS FOR PREDICTABLE TYPES OF STRESS ON A CHILD WITH TYPE I DIABETES AND THE FAMILY

| Age | Issue | Nursing Interventions |
|---|---|---|
| Infant | Trust versus mistrust<br>Onset and diagnosis particularly difficult during infancy; anxiety can be transmitted to baby | Stress consistency in need fulfillment<br>Involve both parents in education<br>Avoid information overload<br>Instill hope and confidence<br>Focus on child rather than disease<br>Review normal growth and development of infancy<br>Assist in problem-solving (baby-sitters, difficulty in obtaining specimens, baby food exchange lists, and so on) |
| Toddler | Autonomy versus shame and doubt<br><br><br>Is this a temper tantrum or high or low blood sugar? | Prepare child for procedures or separations<br>Encourage exploration of environment<br>Stress limit setting as a form of love<br>Admit it is difficult to distinguish temper tantrums from symptoms<br>If behavior worsens or is prolonged or if physical symptoms appear, check blood sugar<br>Provide 24-hr telephone number |
| Preschool | Initiative versus guilt<br>May view injections as punishment<br><br>May view denial of sweets as lack of love<br><br><br><br>"Picky eater" | Foster sense of competence<br>Educate parents to provide consistent warmth, reassurance, and love<br>Discuss feelings about child's life and diabetes<br>Avoid negative connotation by words, for example, "bad blood test," "cheating"<br>Help parents sort out child's fantasies<br>Plan favorite party dishes on occasion<br>Invite a playmate for lunch<br>Suggest alternative nutritious snacks |
| Elementary school | Industry versus inferiority<br><br>Patients may feel they will be cured by hospitalization<br>Grief over lack of cure<br>Rebellion over treatment regimen<br><br><br>Rebellion over food plan<br>Anxiety about disclosure of condition to friends<br>Embarrassed about reactions in school, missed days<br>Unpredictable effects of exercise | Assist child in how to respond to teasing from peers ("Yecch, needles")<br>Explain "honeymoon" stage of disease<br><br>Accept child's disappointment<br>Gradually assume self-management of insulin and specimen tests; this increases feelings of mastery and control<br>Provide lists of fast-food exchanges<br>Group-related education with diabetic peers<br>Promote open dialogue among health personnel and teachers, school nurse, fellow students<br>Continually reinforce treatment principles with specific regard to hypoglycemia or hyperglycemia and emergencies |
| Puberty | "Bouncing" blood sugars may make child feel out of control<br><br><br><br><br>Anger at the disease: "Why must I be different?"<br><br><br>More frequent hospitalizations | Explain that growth and sex hormones affect blood sugars<br>Girls, in particular, experience difficulties about the time of menstruation<br>Adjustments in insulin and food are common for most diabetics at this stage<br>Assist patient in acceptable ways of expressing anger; discuss anger with parents, as they are often its target<br>Provide encouragement and support; be alert to marital stress and sibling deprivation |

**Table 32–3.** NURSING INTERVENTIONS FOR PREDICTABLE TYPES OF STRESS ON A CHILD WITH TYPE I DIABETES AND THE FAMILY *Continued*

| Age | Issue | Nursing Interventions |
|---|---|---|
| Teenage | Threatens sexual identity and body image | Encourage teenager to meet other adolescents with diabetes (camps, support groups, if not tried earlier); this helps to decrease isolation |
| | Surge toward independence, risk-taking, or greater than usual need for security | Provide consistency with limit setting, avoid over control—listen, listen, listen |
| | Worries about health, prospects for marriage and family | Adolescents need to have full instruction about pregnancy risk or male potency; provide a safe environment for discussion; make appropriate referrals |
| | | Encourage patient's interest in diabetic research |
| | Alcohol and drug abuse | Share concerns and dangers with teenager |

**Follow-up Care.** The child needs to see the physician regularly and have a physical examination every 3–4 months. The patient should also be taught to visit the dentist regularly for cleaning of teeth and gums; appointments are scheduled for right after meals. Brushing and flossing daily are essential. Eyes should be examined regularly; blurry vision must not be disregarded. Magazines such as *Diabetes Forecast* and *Diabetes in the News* offer excellent suggestions and guidance.

**Surgery.** The diabetic usually tolerates surgery well. Insulin may be given before or after the operation. If the patient is restricted to nothing by mouth, calories may be supplied by intravenous glucose. Details vary according to the procedure and the patient's treatment for diabetes. Careful review of the patient's history helps in formulating nursing care plans and provides a basis for teaching.

**Prospects for the Future.** Diabetic research is being conducted on many fronts. Geneticists are helping to determine how diabetes is inherited so that one day they will be able to predict who will inherit the disease. If a virus is involved, a vaccine may help prevent diabetes. Pancreas transplantation has been performed, and the success rate is improving. Beta cell transplantation in animals has resulted in their cure. An artificial pancreas is another possibility; its precursors might be the insulin pumps being refined today. The laser beam has aided in treatment for complicated eye conditions. Such advances hold promise for resolving or eradicating the dilemma of diabetes.

## HYPOTHYROIDISM

**Description.** Hypothyroidism occurs when there is a deficiency in the secretions of the thyroid gland. It may be congenital or acquired. It is one of the more common disorders of the endocrine system in children. The thyroid gland controls the rate of metabolism in the body by the production of thyroxine ($T_4$) and triiodothyronine ($T_3$). In congenital hypothyroidism, the gland is absent or not functioning. The symptoms of hypothyroidism may not be apparent for several months.

*Juvenile hypothyroidism* is acquired by the older child. It may be caused by a number of conditions, the most common being lymphocytic thyroiditis. Often it appears during periods of rapid growth. Infectious disease, irradiation for cancer, certain medications containing iodine, and lack of dietary iodine (uncommon in the United States) may predispose one to its onset. Symptoms, diagnosis, and treatment are similar to those mentioned for congenital hyperthyroidism. Because brain growth is nearly complete by 2–3 years of age, mental retardation and neurologic complications are not seen in the older child.

**Manifestations.** The baby is very sluggish and sleeps a lot. The tongue becomes enlarged, causing noisy respiration (Fig. 32–10). The skin is dry, there is no perspiration, and the hands and feet are cold. The infant feels floppy when handled. This *hypotonia* also affects the intestinal tract, causing chronic constipation. The hair eventually becomes dry and brittle. If left un-

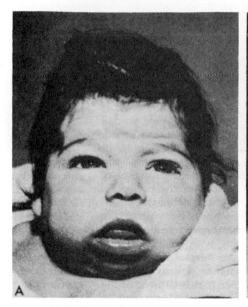
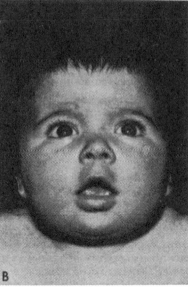

**Figure 32–10.** *A,* Congenital hypothyroidism in a 6-month-old infant. The infant fed poorly and was constipated. She had a large tongue, poor head control, puffy face, and persistent nasal discharge. *B,* Same infant four months after treatment. Note the decreased facial puffiness and the alert expression. (From Behrman, R., & Kliegman, R. [1992]. *Nelson textbook of pediatrics* [14th ed.]. Philadelphia: W.B. Saunders.)

treated, irreversible mental retardation and physical disabilities result.

**Treatment and Nursing Care.** Early recognition and diagnosis are essential to prevent the developing sequelae. A screening test for hypothyroidism is mandatory at birth. It consists of $T_4$ measurement supplemented by thyroid-stimulating hormone when $T_4$ is low. This is generally part of an overall screen for other metabolic defects. Treatment involves administration of the synthetic hormone sodium levothyroxine (Synthroid or Levothroid). Hormone levels are monitored regularly. Therapy reverses the symptoms and prevents further mental retardation but does not reverse existing retardation. This is why early detection of congenital hypothyroidism is so important. Medication is taken at the same time each day, preferably in the morning. Parents are cautioned not to interchange brands. Children may have reversible hair loss, insomnia, and aggressiveness, and their school work may decline during the first few months of therapy. This is temporary. Full therapeutic effect may take 1–3 weeks. Medication is not to be discontinued because replacement for hypothyroidism is lifelong. Parents are instructed about these measures and advised to consult their physician before giving other medications.

# Nutritional Deficiencies

Because infancy is a period of rapid growth, poor nutrition is particularly dangerous at this time. Severe vitamin deficiencies are rare in prosperous countries; those that do occur are caused by poverty, ignorance, or neglect. Figure 32–11 shows a child, from the United States, with general, moderate malnutrition. Severe malnutrition is still rampant in many underdeveloped countries. Every person must be concerned with the plight of the starving child. Sometimes the baby's body is unable to utilize food even though the diet is adequate. An example of this is celiac disease, in which the intestines are unable to handle fats and starches. Severe malnutrition may also be seen in failure to thrive (see pp. 893–894). See also Chapter 27 for a discussion of iron-deficiency anemia.

## KWASHIORKOR (PROTEIN DEFICIENCY)

In many parts of the world, children still starve to death. There are no well-planned maternal and child health programs to elevate health standards in these localities. In some areas, superstition and ignorance prevent children from utilizing nutritious foods found in their environment. In kwashiorkor, also known

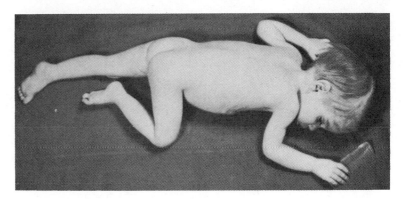

**Figure 32–11.** This child has general malnutrition of moderate degree, frequently seen in the United States. (Courtesy of University of Rochester, Rochester, NY.)

by various other names depending on the country in which it is found, there is a severe deficiency of protein in the diet in spite of the fact that the number of calories consumed may be nearly adequate. It belongs to a class of disorders termed protein-energy malnutrition. In these disorders, there are various degrees of protein and energy deficiencies. They may be accompanied by vitamin deficiencies and infection.

Kwashiorkor occurs in children 1–4 years of age who have been weaned from the breast. It was first described in 1933 by Cicely Williams, a pediatrician working with native children on the African Gold Coast (Ghana). Kwashiorkor means, in native dialect, "the disease of the deposed baby when the next one is born" (Krause & Mahan, 1992). The child fails to grow normally. Muscles become weak and wasted. There is edema of the abdomen that may become generalized. Diarrhea, skin infections, irritability, anorexia, and vomiting may be present. The hair becomes thin and dry. The child looks pathetic and miserable.

Treatment for kwashiorkor is mainly preventive. Although hunger may never be completely erased in the world, many private, public, and world health agencies sponsor programs in an effort to alleviate such suffering. Early dietary treatment in established cases may prevent more serious retardation of growth.

## RICKETS (VITAMIN D DEFICIENCY)

Rickets is a disease of infancy and childhood caused by deficient amounts of vitamin D.

Vitamin D is necessary for the proper absorption and metabolism of calcium and phosphorus, which are needed for normal growth of bones. The classic symptoms of rickets are bowlegs; knock-knees; beading of the ribs, called the *rachitic rosary*; and improper formation of the teeth.

The widespread use of vitamin supplements and fortification of foods have largely eliminated the problem of rickets in North America. When the condition is observed, it usually results from poverty, ignorance, or unusual diet patterns within small groups. It is apt to be seen in preterm infants and in infants receiving unenriched cow's milk or infants on total parenteral nutrition.

Some overzealous mothers may give additional vitamin D supplements to infants already receiving the minimum daily requirement. This is to be discouraged, as it can lead to hypercalcemia. The recommended daily allowance is estimated to be 7.5 μg for infants birth to 6 months and 10 μg for infants 6–12 months. Good sources of vitamin D are fish liver oils, sunlight, and vitamin D–enriched milk. It is a stable vitamin in heat and during storage. Yogurt does not contain vitamin D and is not intended to be a milk substitute.

## SCURVY (VITAMIN C DEFICIENCY)

Scurvy is a disease caused by insufficient fruits, vegetables, and vitamin C in the diet. The symptoms of scurvy include joint pains, bleeding gums, loose teeth, and lack of energy. Good sources of vitamin C are citrus fruits and raw, leafy vegetables. Vitamin C is easily destroyed by heat and exposure to air. Small amounts of water should be used for cooking vegetables in order to prevent vitamin C from being destroyed, since it is also water-soluble. It may be given to infants in the form of orange juice, which should not be boiled. The daily requirement for infants is 30 mg for the first 6 months and 35 mg for the second 6 months. Because some babies are allergic to orange juice, the doctor may prefer the use of vitamin drops. Older children require 40–45 mg of ascorbic acid per day, whereas adolescents require 50–60 mg/day.

## KEY POINTS

- The two major systems that control and monitor the functions of the body are the nervous system and the endocrine system.
- The term inborn error of metabolism refers to a group of inherited biochemical disorders that affect body metabolism.
- Phenylketonuria, galactosemia, maple syrup urine disease, and Tay-Sachs disease are examples of inborn errors of metabolism.
- Screening programs for early detection of inborn errors is important because some conditions can cause irreversible neurologic damage.
- Diabetes mellitus type I (IDDM) is the most common endocrine disorder of children. The body is unable to utilize carbohydrates properly because of a deficiency of insulin, an internal secretion of the pancreas.
- The symptoms of diabetes appear more rapidly in children. Three symptoms are polydipsia, polyuria, and polyphagia.
- The mainstays of the management of diabetes are insulin replacement, diet, and exercise.
- Diabetic ketoacidosis is a serious complication that may become life-threatening.
- Self-management to maintain glucose control and to prevent complications is a major goal of education of the child with diabetes.
- A deficiency in the secretion of the thyroid gland is termed hypothyroidism. It may be congenital or acquired and requires lifelong treatment by oral administration of a synthetic thyroid hormone.

## Study Questions

1. Gloria, age 3, is diabetic. What is the action of insulin in the body? How does Gloria's disease affect this?

2. What are the clinical manifestations of type I diabetes?

3. Gloria is receiving a combination of regular insulin and lente insulin. Compare these two insulins in terms of onset, peak, and duration of action. What implications does this have for Gloria's nursing care plan?

4. Gloria is having lunch with her grandmother, who is also diabetic. Plan a meal for their lunch. Explain how the meals are similar. Explain how they are different.

5. How do the onset, treatment, and nursing care of diabetes in the child differ from those in the adult?

6. Describe the important dietary factors for the child with diabetes.

7. What factors would you consider in determining whether Melinda, age 11, should sterilize her insulin syringe at home? If you determine that she should do so, what would your instructions consist of?

8. Evaluate your dietary pattern for foods high in vitamins A and D, ascorbic acid, and iron. Make suggestions for improvement.

9. What effect do the cooking and handling of foods have on their nutritional value?

10. Search the literature for a current article on infant nutrition. Report to the class on your findings.

# Multiple Choice Review Questions

*Choose the most appropriate answer.*

1. The secretions of the endocrine glands are called
   a. islets
   b. luteals
   c. homogeneous
   d. hormones

2. Insulin is secreted by the
   a. pancreas
   b. gallbladder
   c. liver
   d. adrenal gland

3. The term denoting sugar in the urine is
   a. polyphagia
   b. glycosuria
   c. polyuria
   d. hyperglycemia

4. Kussmaul respirations are seen in diabetic children with
   a. neuropathy
   b. ketoacidosis
   c. hypoglycemia
   d. retinopathy

5. Deficient amounts of vitamin D may result in
   a. scurvy
   b. kwashiorkor
   c. rickets
   d. beriberi

## BIBLIOGRAPHY

Behrman, R.E. (1992). *Nelson textbook of pediatrics* (14th ed.). Philadelphia: W.B. Saunders.

Betz, C., Hunsberger, M., & Wright, S. (1994). *Family-centered nursing care of children* (2nd ed.). Philadelphia: W.B. Saunders.

Gellis, S.S., & Kagan, B.M. (1990). *Current pediatric therapy 13*. Philadelphia: W.B. Saunders.

Germak, J., & Folley, T. (1990). Longitudinal assessment of L-thyroxine therapy for congenital hypothyroidism. *Journal of Pediatrics, 117*, 211.

Hodgson, B.B., Kizior, R.J., & Kingdon, R.T. (1993). *Nurse's drug handbook*. Philadelphia: W.B. Saunders.

Mahan, L., & Arlin, M. (1992). *Krause's food, nutrition & diet therapy* (8th ed.). Philadelphia: W.B. Saunders.

Murphy, G.H., et al. (1990). Congenital hypothyroidism: Physiologic and psychological factors in early development. *Journal of Child Psychology and Psychiatry, 31*, 711.

Mott, S., James, S.R., & Sperhac, A.M. (1991). *Nursing care of children and families* (2nd ed.). Reading, MA: Addison-Wesley.

Pillitteri, A. (1992). *Maternal and child health nursing*. Philadelphia: J.B. Lippincott.

Thompson E.D., & Ashwill, J.W. (1992). *Introduction to pediatric nursing* (6th ed.). Philadelphia: W.B. Saunders.

Whaley, L., & Wong, D. (1991). *Nursing care of infants and children* (4th ed.). St. Louis: C.V. Mosby.

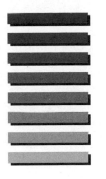

# Chapter 33

# The Child with an Emotional or Behavioral Condition

# OBJECTIVES

*On completion and mastery of Chapter 33, the student will be able to*

- Define each vocabulary term listed.
- Discuss the impact of early childhood experience on a person's adult life.
- List four symptoms of potential suicide in children and adolescents.
- Discuss immediate and long-range plans for the suicidal client.
- Differentiate among the following terms: psychiatrist, psychoanalyst, clinical psychologist, and counselor.
- List five criteria for referring a child to a mental health counselor or agency.
- List four behaviors that may indicate substance abuse.
- Name two programs for members of families of alcoholics.
- Discuss problems facing children of alcoholics.
- List four symptoms of attention-deficit hyperactivity disorder.

## Origins of Emotional and Behavioral Conditions

Early childhood experiences are critical to personality formation. Situations that disrupt family patterns can have a lasting impact on the child. Children who come from dysfunctional families may suffer from any of the following: failure to develop a sense of trust (in their caretakers and environment), excessive fears, misdirected anger manifested as behavior problems, depression, low self-esteem, lack of confidence, and feelings of lack of control over themselves and their environment. These and other manifestations may make children feel negative about themselves and the world. They experience guilt and may blame themselves when confronted with disappointment and failure.

Growing up can be painful even under the best circumstances. It is difficult for the child in the early school years to live up to so many rapidly developing standards. Guilt and anxiety develop. Finger-sucking, nail-biting, excessive fears, stuttering, and conduct problems are reflections of nervous tension. Disorders that may or may not be traced to emotional problems include constipation, diarrhea, stomachache, der-

matitis, obesity, frequent urination, enuresis, and the common cold.

The current trend toward prevention by identification of risk factors and intervention is a major goal of children's mental health services. The term *psychosomatic* has come to refer to the bodily dysfunctions that seem to have emotional and organic bases. Each person has a different potential for coping with life. Truancy, lying, stealing, failure in school, and a crisis such as death or divorce of parents are but a few of the difficulties that may require intervention. Box 33–1 summarizes some of the disorders that can affect behavior and appear during infancy, childhood, and adolescence.

## The Nurse's Role in Care

The nurse is often the person who has the greatest amount of contact with the family. Assessing child-parent relations is an important and ongoing aspect of care. In order for nurses to work effectively with the disturbed child, they first must understand the types of behavior considered within normal range. They are a valuable member of the health-care team in that they work closely with the hospitalized

---

**BOX 33–1** **Summary of Disorders Usually First Evident in Infancy, Childhood, and Adolescence**

Mental retardation
Autistic disorder
Attention-deficit hyperactivity disorder
Developmental disorders (e.g., language, math)
Conduct disorder
Oppositional disorder
Substance induced
Anxiety disorders (separation, obsessive-compulsive)
Major depression
Bipolar depression
Schizophrenia
Eating disorders (anorexia, bulimia, pica)
Stereotyped movement disorders (tics, Tourette's syndrome)
Stuttering
Enuresis
Encopresis
Sleep disorders
Adjustment disorders

Data adapted from *Diagnostic and statistical manual of mental disorders* (4th ed.), 1994. Washington DC: American Psychiatric Association.

child, the long-term patient in particular. They keep a careful record of behavior and note relationships with members of the family. Such notations are meaningful to the physician and other staff members who are as concerned with preventing problems from arising as they are with treating them. Is 4-year-old Janice wetting the bed? What about Bobby who continually bangs his head against the crib during naptime? What does Manuel do in the playroom? Is he sitting alone in a corner? Does he hit the other children? Is he constantly in motion? Does Eric seem indifferent to attempts to establish rapport? Is there a physical cause for his behavior?

An action in itself might be considered within the normal limits of behavior, but carried to extremes it may interfere with the child's experience of and reaction to reality and should be investigated further. Nurses must bear in mind that behavior one might describe as "bratty" may be a call for intervention. They feel free to discuss the conduct problems of their patients with other members of the staff and do not consider these problems a threat to their own abilities.

One might ask where else nurses see children with emotional and behavioral problems. They see them wherever children are—in the home, in nursery school, in residential institutions, at child health conferences, in special clinics, in the doctor's office. Perhaps they are their own children. Everyday, everywhere, children are trying to cope with stress. Many succeed and grow stronger; some do not. Early childhood intervention programs are becoming more numerous and helpful in preventing problems. Parenting classes teach what to expect at various ages and stages. They also stress the importance of age-appropriate discipline and guidance. Parent groups provide education, socialization, and support. Other agencies provide a variety of services. The names include the National Alliance for the Mentally Ill (NAMI),

Family Service Association of America, Inc., Toughlove, and Youth Suicide National Center. Nurses need to be aware of such resources in order to guide parents appropriately.

When parents request guidance, the nurse encourages them to seek help from their family physician or pediatrician or from a community mental health center (Box 33–2). In the hospital, a psychiatric clinical nurse specialist (CNS) is an excellent resource. If the child is in school, the services of the school psychologist or guidance counselor may prove valuable. Some churches employ counselors who are available free of charge to parishioners. Families who lack adequate financial resources can be directed to appropriate agencies. Some agencies not only provide emergency funds but can also set up a budgeting system for those receiving meager wages. This is particularly helpful when parents are young teenagers.

No matter how dysfunctional the parent-child relationship, most children consciously and unconsciously identify with parental values. Discrediting parents threatens the child's security and creates anxiety. The nurse reas-

## Nursing Brief

Parents provide important assessment data about the child that the young child cannot provide. They are also important in bringing the child to therapy. Discrediting parents threatens the child and is not therapeutic.

---

**BOX 33–2    Criteria for Referral to a Mental Health Resource**

Life-threatening behavior (e.g., suicide attempt, homicide attempt, drug abuse, poisoning in children over 10 yr old)

Chronic aggressive or antisocial behavior (e.g., juvenile delinquency, running away, fire setting, repeated stealing, extreme cruelty to animals)

Bizarre behavior (e.g., autism, thought disorder)

Chronically withdrawn behavior (e.g., chronic depression)

Academic failure on emotional basis

Victim of repeated physical or sexual abuse

Rejected child (i.e., parent can describe no good points)

Previous psychiatric hospitalization

Previous unsuccessful psychotherapy

Multiple problems, dysfunctional families

Inadequate progress after six or more sessions of pediatric counseling

From Levine, M.D., Carey, W.B., Crocker, A.C., & Gross, R.T. (1992). *Developmental-behavioral pediatrics* (2nd ed.). Philadelphia: W.B. Saunders.

sures parents and helps them regain or maintain confidence in their parenting role. In addition, because children do not seek treatment on their own, the nurse assists parents in becoming invested in the treatment modality.

Finally, as a professional, the nurse supports organizations concerned with mental health, votes on issues that are pertinent to the welfare of children in the community, and offers services when they are needed.

## Types and Settings of Treatment

The first psychiatric clinic for children in the United States was established in Chicago in 1909 in order to serve delinquents. The basic staff of the modern child guidance clinic is composed of a psychiatrist, a psychologist, and a social worker; frequently a pediatrician is also a member of the staff. Usually the child guidance clinic provides diagnostic and treatment services. It may be part of a hospital, a school, a court, or a public health or welfare service, or it may be an independent agency.

The various psychiatric specialties may be confusing to the average person. The psychiatrist is a medical doctor who has specialized in mental disorders. The psychoanalyst is usually a psychiatrist but may be a psychologist (lay analyst); all psychoanalysts have advanced training in psychoanalytic theory and practice. The clinical psychologist should have a doctorate of philosophy in clinical psychology from a recognized university. Many of these specialists work in the school system with children, teachers, and families in an attempt to prevent or resolve problems.

A counselor is a professional with a master's degree from an accredited institution. Many counselors specialize in a specific area, such as substance abuse or counseling of children. In most states, counselors have to be licensed. Parents are instructed to interview several mental health professionals to see which one might be appropriate for the personality of their child. Suggestions from former clients or a referral from another mental health professional or from the child's physician may also be helpful.

Children who do not respond well to individual outpatient therapy may require the type of care provided in residential treatment centers. Their home situations may be so disruptive that they benefit from a change of environment. This alternative also provides a cooling-down period for the family. Family therapy is begun. The length of stay varies from 1 to 3 weeks. Partial hospitalization programs in which the child attends therapy during the day and returns home at night are gaining popularity.

Intervention may involve individual, family, or group therapy; behavior modification; or milieu therapy; or it may involve a combination of these. Behavior modification focuses on modifying specific bothersome behaviors by means of stimulus and response conditioning. *Milieu therapy* refers to the physical and social environment provided for the child. Art therapy, music therapy, and play therapy are particularly helpful in dealing with younger children who have difficulties expressing themselves. Recreation therapy is also valuable. *Bibliotherapy*, the reading of stories about children in a situation similar to the child's, is also therapeutic. Creating an emotionally *safe environment* is basic to all forms of therapy.

Residential care or hospitalization is a source of anxiety and stress for children and their families. There remains a discrepancy between what we know and what is being done to meet the child's and family's needs during this time of disruption in their lives. Therefore, the nurse sets short- and long-term goals and re-evaluates them at regular intervals.

## Conditions That May Require Treatment

The following conditions or situations may require treatment: depression, suicidal ideation, alcohol and marijuana abuse, children living in a home with alcoholic parents, and attention-deficit disorder. Anorexia, bulimia, and obesity are discussed in Chapter 28. Child abuse is discussed in Chapter 34.

### DEPRESSION AND SUICIDE

**Description.** Suicide is one of the leading causes of death among persons aged 15–19 years. It ranks third as the cause of death of adolescents and college students. The incidence increases during the spring. Completed suicide is more common in boys than in girls, but girls make more attempts. Many adolescent suicides are not intended to result in death but are cries for help. The risk of death increases when there is a definite plan of action, the means are readily available (e.g., pills, guns), and the person has few resources for help and support.

**Manifestations.** Adolescents who do not have socially acceptable ways to express their frustration may turn their anger and hostility inward. Their self-esteem is low, and they feel trapped, rejected, and abandoned. Often there is a family history of depression. Failed relationships and high-school pressures are also significant. Although each experience is individual, a group of teenagers who had attempted suicide had these common feelings: emptiness and loss, inability to experience pleasure, lack of concentration, confusion, inability to make decisions, and feeling that there was no meaning or purpose to life. Physical problems revolved around eating and sleeping disturbances. Patients experienced lack of appetite and insomnia or the reverse (they slept all day). Hyperactivity was yet another symptom. Behavioral problems surfaced; these included a drop in school grades, truancy, running away, promiscuity, and other forms of acting out (Fig. 33–1). Alcoholism and drug abuse were significant contributing factors, as were the breakdown of family ties and the pressure to succeed. Some felt that their own expectations and those of others significant to them were too high.

Over half of suicide attempts are directly pre-

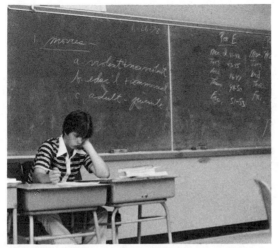

**Figure 33–1.** A drop in school grades may be a signal of inner turmoil.

ceded by conflict with parents, ranging from misunderstanding to long-term, deep-seated problems. Some teenagers are loners, isolated from their peers and family and unable to communicate their distress. Because the symptoms are difficult to distinguish from healthy adolescent reactions to stress, they may go unrecognized. However, if the manifestations are uncharacteristic and interfere with the person's ability to function daily, further investigation is imperative. In assessing the situation, questions asked of the patient must be direct and specific: "Are you planning to kill yourself? How? When?" Determine what coping skills the individual has used in the past to solve problems. If there were previous serious suicide attempts, the current suicidal situation should be considered more dangerous.

Depression may be defined as an overall feeling of sadness and hopelessness. It is not always a negative experience. *Often it is a reaction to a real or fancied loss.* Although it is painful, it can lead to personal growth. Risk factors for depression may be genetic or environmental. Depression in children under 15 years of age is becoming more common. Withdrawal is frustrating to those close to the young person, and they experience a feeling of helplessness. It is futile to bombard the depressed person with platitudes such as "Cheer up" and "Nothing can be that bad."

Nurses accept adolescents as they are and help them examine and externalize feelings. They ask how they can help and remain available to listen. Activities that promote physical exercise provide "hostility outlets" and are highly therapeutic. Some days nurses may not feel very effective and need to retreat. They assure the young person that they will return. This helps minimize feelings of abandonment. Nurses need to keep in touch with their own feelings in order to avoid burnout. As the teenagers begin to feel more secure, they will "reach out" and progress at their own rate.

Adults are disturbed when, for example, a 15-year-old boy takes his life. Many adults view adolescence as a carefree time and forget the pain of their own adolescence. Suicide is unacceptable in Judeo-Christian society, and many persons find it difficult to console the grieving family members, who carry a heavy burden of guilt, anger, and sorrow. Self-help groups for survivors are available in most cities. The nurse needs assistance in identifying feelings toward the patient who expresses suicidal intentions.

It is preferable that the responsibility for a suicidal patient be shared by as many people as possible. A combined effort indicates to the young person that others care, are interested, and are ready to help. It is beneficial for the team in that concerns and interventions can be discussed, and grief shared should the suicidal intent be carried out. In the hospital, the nurse is often the person most accessible and least threatening to the patient. Frequent brief visits provide surveillance and serve to break destructive thought chains.

**Treatment.** Treatment is multidimensional. When possible, individual, group, and family therapies are provided in an outpatient setting, such as a community mental health agency. Group therapy seems to be especially helpful for adolescents. The adolescent mental health or behavioral unit of a hospital provides a structured environment with peers. It has the additional advantages of separating the adolescent from the stressful surroundings and providing support and protection. Crisis intervention is required for acute and repeated episodes. One resource for problems of this nature is the National Mental Health Association, telephone number 1-800-969-6642. Other voluntary services, such as hotlines, drop-in centers, runaway houses, and free clinics, focus on the immediate needs of the patient and are usually accepted by troubled youngsters. Unfortunately, there are not enough of these resources.

Professionals need to be alert for warning signals of destructive behavior so that prompt intervention can be initiated; this might include earlier consideration of placement in a foster home. Community training courses for parenthood are becoming more popular and may be another means of resolving the complex problem of teenage suicide. Nursing Care Plan 33–1 lists interventions for the depressed adolescent.

## SUBSTANCE ABUSE

**Description.** The problem of substance abuse is serious, complex, and of great magnitude. Government efforts to control the supply and distribution of dangerous drugs have generally failed. Adult society, through its widespread acceptance of self-administered pills and alcohol, has compounded the problem; in particular, the drinking patterns of teenagers appear to reflect directly those of their parents and the community.

Numerous reasons have been cited for adolescents' resorting to drug use. Some are curiosity; peer pressure; rebellion; need to escape from loneliness, boredom, or family problems; and desire to become more sociable and to relax. The single most predictive variable for drug use by an adolescent is drug use by that person's closest friend (Neinstein, 1984). Teenagers differ from adults in a preference for polypharmacy (use of several drugs together), a sense of invulnerability, and a delay in psychosocial maturation with chronic drug use. Drug-seeking behavior may include stealing—shoplifting in particular, drug dealing, sexual promiscuity, and prostitution. In addition, a disproportionately high number of suicides are related to substance abuse. Sex-related differences have narrowed, particularly in the use of alcohol (more teenage girls are experimenting with drugs and alcohol).

Four levels of substance abuse have been established: experimentation, controlled use, abuse, and dependence. Although there is often a fine line between controlled use and abuse, frequency may be a major signal. This is especially true when accompanied by inappropriateness, for example, "getting stoned" at the weekend party versus on the way to school. There are two kinds of dependence, *psychological* and *physical*. Psychological dependence includes craving for and a compulsive need to use a substance. Physical dependence occurs with drugs such as heroin and alcohol. People become hooked on the drug, and in addition to psycho-

## Nursing Brief

It has been estimated that over 2 million people are using cocaine on a regular basis. "Crack" is a popular form that can be extremely addictive.

### Selected Nursing Diagnoses for the Depressed Adolescent

| Goals | Nursing Interventions | Rationale |
|---|---|---|
| **Nursing Diagnosis:** High risk for violence: self-directed, related to depression and stress. | | |
| Adolescent states whether suicide is contemplated<br>Adolescent does not harm self and states two healthy coping measures<br>Adolescent verbalizes acceptance of protective measures<br>Family verbalizes seriousness of suicidal threats | 1. Ask adolescent if suicidal thoughts are present | 1. This information is important to know, as it will determine intervention; most depressed teenagers are filled with contradictory feelings; talking honestly about them helps clarify them |
| | 2. Inquire as to precipitating event: broken romance, poor grades, and so on | 2. Suicidal reactions are associated with feelings of hopelessness often related to loss of a significant or valued relationship or a disappointment |
| | 3. Determine if adolescent has specific suicidal plan | 3. How person plans to take life is one of most significant criteria of assessing suicidal potential; more specific plans are a more dangerous threat |
| | 4. Determine if person has a history of suicidal attempts | 4. If patient has made serious attempts in past, situation is considered more critical |
| | 5. Determine if person has history of emotional instability | 5. History of emotional instability is more dangerous |
| | 6. Determine if adolescent has means available | 6. If the means to commit suicide are available (i.e., pills, gun), threat is imminent and more serious |
| | 7. Provide supervision as outlined by physician or institution | 7. Surveillance and support by staff and family are important |
| | 8. Determine if safe contract has been signed | 8. This is a written agreement that person will contact a nurse, counselor, or crisis line or go to an emergency room before harming self |
| | 9. Attend team conferences | 9. It is wise to have available as many persons as possible to support one another and share stress of situation |
| | 10. Administer antidepressants if ordered | 10. Antidepressants elevate the mood of the client; unfortunately, most antidepressants must be taken for 3–4 wk before a therapeutic response is evident; some require monitoring of blood values |
| | 11. Monitor room for potentially dangerous articles | 11. Belts, glasses, rope, and other materials may be used to self-destruct |
| | 12. Explain precautions to adolescent and family members | 12. Explanations will lessen fear and increase compliance |
| | 13. Reinforce the seriousness of adolescent's suicidal threat to parents | 13. *All* suicidal threats need to be taken seriously |

*Continued*

| NURSING CARE PLAN 33–1 *Continued* | | |
| --- | --- | --- |
| **Selected Nursing Diagnoses for the Depressed Adolescent** | | |
| **Goals** | **Nursing Interventions** | **Rationale** |

**Nursing Diagnosis:** Ineffective individual coping related to poor self-esteem, isolation, inability to deal with painful feelings.

| Goals | Nursing Interventions | Rationale |
| --- | --- | --- |
| Adolescent makes positive statement about self | 1. Have client list two positive things about self | 1. Determines adolescent's strengths so that nurse can build on them |
| Adolescent accepts positive statements from others | 2. Instruct adolescent to draw "how I see myself" and "how others see me" | 2. Provides valuable information about person's self-esteem; self-destructive behavior reflects underlying depression related to low self-esteem and anger directed inward; drawing offers a release from feelings, helps clarify emotions, and is a vehicle for discussion between client and nurse |
| Adolescent accepts presence of nurse, peers, or significant others | | |
| Adolescent gradually deals with painful feelings by sharing and expressing them either verbally or nonverbally | | |
| Adolescent speaks in future terms | | |
| | 3. Build extra time into visits so that adolescent does not feel rushed; give your undivided attention | 3. This indicates that you are truly interested; ringing telephone and personal interruptions devalue visit |
| | 4. Instruct adolescent to draw a box and put things that bring happy feelings in the box; then instruct to draw another box and place things that cause sadness in that box; encourage adolescent to verbalize feelings about drawings; respect adolescent's wish not to talk should this occur | 4. Drawings help clients distance themselves from problem and see it more clearly |
| | 5. Review methods of coping | 5. Discovering how he/she coped in the past when the patient was less distressed is of importance so that these methods can be reinforced |
| | 6. Suggest healthy methods of coping such as exercise, relaxation tapes, talking things out with parents or peers | 6. Many teenagers are not aware of healthy coping methods |

logical dependence they experience physical withdrawal symptoms. *Tolerance* develops when a user's body becomes accustomed to certain drugs. The person must then increase the dose each time in order to maintain its effect. Table 33–1 summarizes the characteristics of some of the more commonly abused drugs and the adolescent's reactions to them. Table 33–2 lists street names for some of these drugs.

## Teenage Alcoholism

**Description.** Alcohol abuse is the number-one drug problem of American teenagers and even children. Experimentation with alcohol has traditionally been accepted as a normal part of growing up. Although nearly all states have legal drinking ages of 21 years, these laws have not prevented most teenagers from drinking.

The first drinking experience generally occurs at about 12 years of age. The amount and frequency of drinking increase with age. In 1992 10 million people had five or more alcoholic drinks more than once a week, and there has been no decrease since 1988.

The American Medical Association, the American College of Physicians, the American Psychiatric Association, and other professional bodies have accepted the concept of alcoholism as a disease for some time. Unfortunately, this has not been true of the general public. Many people still consider the alcoholic a derelict or moral degenerate who does not have enough "will power" to control the drinking. Others consider it a laughing matter. Nurses working with adolescents need to emphasize that alcoholism is a disease with established criteria and that it is treatable.

**Table 33–1.** CHARACTERISTICS OF ABUSED DRUGS AND THEIR ACUTE REACTIONS IN ADOLESCENTS

| Class | Example | Route | Behavioral Signs | Physical Signs | Medical Complications |
|---|---|---|---|---|---|
| Opiates | Heroin, methadone, morphine | Subcutaneous, intranasal, intravenous | Euphoria, lethargy to coma | Constricted pupils, respiratory depression, cyanosis, rales, needle marks | Injection site infection, hepatitis, bacterial endocarditis, amenorrhea, peptic ulcer, pulmonary edema, tetanus |
| Hypnotics sedatives | Barbiturates, glutethimide | Oral, intravenous | Slurred speech, ataxia, short attention span, drowsiness, combativeness, violence | Constricted pupils (barbiturates), dilated pupils (glutethimide), needle marks | Injection site infection, hepatitis, endocarditis |
| | Alcohol | Oral | As above | Hypertension, weight loss, dilated pupils | Gastritis, central nervous system infection, depression |
| Stimulants | Amphetamines | Oral, subcutaneous, intravenous | Hyperactivity, insomnia, anorexia, paranoia, personality change, irritability | Hypertension, weight loss, dilated pupils | Injection site infection, hepatitis, endocarditis, psychosis, depression |
| | Cocaine | Intravenous, intranasal | Restlessness, hyperactivity, occasional depression or paranoia | Hypertension, tachycardia | Nausea, vomiting, inflammation or perforation of nasal septum |
| Hallucinogens | LSD, THC, PCP, STP (DOM), mescaline, DMT | Oral | Euphoria, dysphoria, hallucinations, confusion, paranoia | Dilated pupils, occasional hypertension, hyperthermia, piloerection | Primarily psychiatric with high risk to individuals with unrecognized or previous psychiatric disorder |
| Hydrocarbons, fluorocarbons | Glue (toluene) | Inhalant | Euphoria, confusion, general intoxication | Nonspecific | Secondary trauma, asphyxiation from plastic bag used to inhale fumes |
| | Cleaning fluid (trichloroethylene) | Inhalant | Euphoria, confusion, general intoxication, vomiting, abdominal pain | Oliguria, jaundice | Hepatitis, renal injury |
| | Aerosol sprays Freon | Inhalant | Euphoria, dysphoria, slurred speech, hallucinations | Nonspecific | Psychiatric |
| Cannabis | Marijuana, hashish, THC | Smoke, oral | Mild intoxication and simple euphoria to hallucination (dose-related) | Occasional tachycardia, delayed response time, poor coordination | Occasionally psychiatric, with depressive or anxiety reactions |

LSD, lysergic acid diethylamide; THC, tetrahydrocannabinol; PCP, phencyclidine piperidine; STP (DOM), 2,5-dimethoxy-4-methylamphetamine; and DMT, dimethyltryptamine.

From Vaughan, V., McKay, R., & Behrman, R. (1979). *Nelson textbook of pediatrics* (11th ed.). Philadelphia: W.B. Saunders.

**Table 33–2.** STREET NAMES* FOR COMMONLY ABUSED DRUGS

| Street Name | Drug |
| --- | --- |
| A's | Amphetamines |
| Acid | Lysergic acid diethylamide (LSD) |
| Angel dust | Dimethyltryptamine (DMT) or phencyclidine piperidine (PCP) sprinkled over parsley or tobacco |
| Barbs | Barbiturates |
| Bennies | Benzedrine (amphetamine sulfate) |
| Black | LSD |
| Bullets | Secobarbital (Seconal) |
| Charlie | Cocaine |
| Coke | Cocaine |
| Crack | A form of cocaine |
| Crap | Heroin |
| Downers | Barbiturates or tranquilizers |
| Goofballs | Barbiturates |
| Hash | Hashish |
| Horse | Heroin |
| Joint | Marijuana cigarette |
| Mickey | Combination of alcohol and chloral hydrate |
| Pot | Marijuana |
| PG | Paregoric |
| Rainbows | Tuinal (secobarbital sodium and amobarbital sodium) |
| Smack | Heroin |
| Speed | Methamphetamine |
| Uppers | Central nervous system stimulants |
| Yellow jackets | Pentobarbital |

*These names change frequently and vary within subcultures.

Alcohol is a mind-altering drug that works as a depressant. Because of the small size of the ethyl alcohol molecule, alcohol begins to oxidize immediately and is absorbed into the stomach and small intestine virtually unchanged. It is carried by the blood to the liver, which is not able to handle large amounts. The excess is pumped back into the circulation in relatively pure form. It reaches every part of the body, including the brain, and eventually returns to the liver. This process continues until the alcohol is completely oxidized. Alcohol has no food value but contains calories, which accounts for the weight gain seen in some persons.

Excessive alcohol consumption over a period of time can cause problems such as vomiting, diarrhea, ulcers, cirrhosis of the liver, pancreatitis, and brain damage. Although teenagers are seldom impressed by these remote consequences, the abusive effects on immature body systems are being seen earlier. This is particularly significant because a substantial number of alcoholics are preadolescents whose smaller bodies are affected more quickly by the drug. Studies have shown that even a low concentration of alcohol in the blood is a factor in teenage accidents. Because body weight strongly influences the effect of the drug, adults should not encourage small children to sample their drinks.

Alcohol dependence adversely affects the mental health of adolescents. Although the scope of the problem cannot be covered here, a few facts bear mentioning. Alcoholism prevents the teenager from mastering crucial developmental tasks. Self-deception replaces self-esteem. Normal feelings of inadequacy, which are first masked by the drug, are then intensified by it. Social awkwardness is concealed, retarding growth in this area. Sexual inhibitions are lowered; thousands of unmarried adolescents are bearing children each year. Research shows that girls who drink heavily before pregnancy is detected and during pregnancy run a greater risk of having smaller or deformed babies. Sexual performance decreases with continued use, which can shatter the adolescent's emerging sexuality. Serious emotional problems may be camouflaged by alcohol use and abuse.

**Treatment.** Although the exact cause of alcoholism is unknown, several theories have been proposed. Investigations have revealed that genetics may play a part, as may biochemical, nutritional, psychological, and sociologic factors.

Treatment programs vary. Alcoholics Anonymous (AA), a worldwide, nonprofit organization, has had the highest success rate. Its approach is based on abstinence "one day at a time" with the help of a "higher power." Its leaders are recovering alcoholics who offer group counseling and answering services throughout the world. In the United States, AA's telephone number is listed in the local directory. AA programs for young people are available in some cities; however, because these programs are not as developed, young alcoholics are also welcomed at regular adult meetings. The concept of alcoholism as a family disease is well established.

Two programs closely related to AA are Al-Anon and Alateen. Their inclusion in any treatment program for the adolescent is important. Al-Anon offers guidance to nonalcoholic family members who have their own problems resulting from living with the disease, and it teaches them how changes in their attitudes best help the alcoholic. Alateen, a fellowship for teenage sons and daughters of alcoholics, provides a setting in which youngsters can exchange experiences and learn to cope with problems that may be related to the drinking adult in their family.

Some communities also have public and private alcoholism rehabilitation centers. As the magnitude of the problem increased and more monies became available, general hospitals established detoxification units and counseling for these patients. One such model program was dedicated to 13–19-year-old alcohol users. Unfortunately these programs have been scaled down or have dwindled because of emphasis on brief therapy and managed care. Other kinds of help include family therapy, alcohol clinics, and physicians specializing in the disease. Often patients use AA in combination with other treatments.

**Prevention and Nursing Goals.** The prevention of alcohol and other types of substance abuse begins by helping expectant parents to develop good parenting skills. It is imperative that children learn to feel good about themselves very early in life. They need a safe environment and adults whom they can trust and who serve as good role models. As orderly development proceeds, the growing child learns to interact with others and develops a sense of identity (Fig. 33–2). A positive self-image and feelings of self-worth help adolescents to fine-tune their adaptive coping skills. In time they will rely on their own problem-solving abilities and ideally will not need chemicals to manage the complexities of life. Nurses in their various

settings can contribute to this process. They can also educate their clients about the seriousness of substance abuse.

Although it is generally true that the problem drinkers cannot be helped unless they want to be, more *intervention* is now being done. Most adolescents involved in substance abuse do not choose to enter treatment but are coerced by family members or the juvenile justice system. Although this is a controversial issue, clinical experience in substance abuse treatment settings has shown that many adolescents become interested in treatment and make behavioral changes after they have been required to enter a treatment program.

**Nursing Care.** How the nurse views the disease and responds during a crisis may significantly affect the adolescent. Assessment of the patient includes finding out what alcoholic beverage was taken and what has happened to the patient since its consumption. Behavior and mood, level of consciousness, vital signs, pupil size, and any gastrointestinal disturbance are noted. The patient is placed on the abdomen when possible in order to prevent aspiration of fluids. Time is the only way to sober the patient, and the amount of time it takes depends on the patient's body weight and the amount of alcohol consumed. The treatment plan of abstinence is especially difficult for adolescents, whose developmental patterns for conformity are at their peak. The motivational phase of treatment has the goal of establishing in the

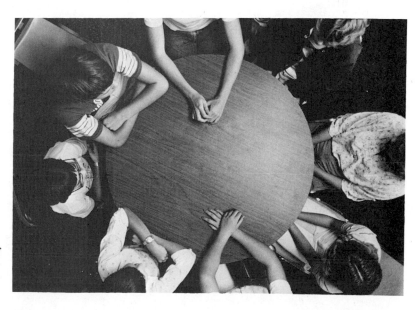

**Figure 33–2.** Talking with groups of peers is an important therapeutic modality for adolescents with various addictions or mental health problems.

adolescent both a sense of self-worth and a commitment to self-help. The rehabilitative phase requires the readiness to substitute dependence on oneself for dependence on alcohol.

### Children of Alcoholics

**Description.** Until recently, little attention has been given to children of alcoholics. This trend is changing, and support groups such as Adult Children of Alcoholics are more numerous. This discussion is directed to young children of alcoholics, although unresolved issues are similar in adults. Pediatric nurses are in an excellent position to recognize and intervene in cases in which physical or emotional neglect exists because of parental alcoholism. These problems stem from the parents' preoccupation with the disease. It is not unusual for both parents to be users.

Children of alcoholics are often confused by the unpredictability of family life. They do not understand why their needs are not being met. In some families, there is a role reversal with the child being forced to act maturely and make decisions ordinarily assumed by a parent. Often these children feel that they are responsible for the disruptive environment. They are at high risk for physical abuse, including sexual abuse. Children of alcoholics are also strong candidates for developing alcoholism as adults. Role models are distorted or lacking. A parent may try to cover up for the drinking partner by lying to employers and relatives but may punish the child for the same behavior. The child may become isolated from peers while trying to avoid embarrassment at home. Four predominant coping patterns of these children are flight, fight, the perfect child, and the super coper or family savior (Fig. 33–3).

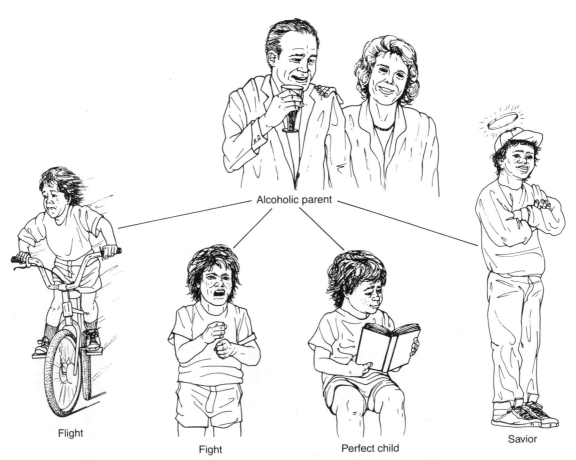

Alcoholic parent

Flight

Fight

Perfect child

Savior

**Figure 33–3.** Some defense patterns of children of alcoholics.

The child who flees may do so literally or emotionally. The goal is to get away, and as the child grows older, more and more time is spent away from home. Feelings are buried and left unexpressed. The child fighter is aggressive and displays acting-out behavior. The perfect child tries to gain love by never causing any trouble. The child is obedient and generally a good student. The savior or super coper feels overly responsible, often has a job to help out, and tries to do everything perfectly.

**Manifestations, Nursing Care, and Treatment.** Early recognition of and intervention for children of alcoholics are paramount. The astute nurse with heightened awareness of alcoholism can expand admission observations and nursing history. Some clues that may or may not be related to this problem include refusal to talk about family life, poor school grades or overachievement, unusual need to please, fatigue, passive or acting-out behavior, or maturity beyond the child's years. Treatment is multifold. One immediate priority is to teach the child how to get help in an emergency and to put the youngster in touch with someone from the extended family, school, or other suitable agency. Cultural diversities need to be incorporated into treatment plans.

### Marijuana Abuse

**Description.** Marijuana, also known as "pot" or "grass," is a drug found in the plant *Cannabis sativa*, which grows wild in almost any temperate climate. The dried tops and leaves are usually chopped up like tobacco and rolled and smoked in cigarettes known as "joints." Marijuana produces a state of relaxation when smoked or eaten. The drug quickly enters the blood stream and acts on the nervous system. The physical effects include tachycardia and reddening of the eyes. Patients may also experience an acute increase in appetite ("the munchies"). The psychological effects vary with the individual. The patient may feel excited or depressed. There may be distortions in the sense of time, perception of color, and hearing. Memory and reaction time are impaired (Fig. 33–4). The inexperienced user may develop "pot panic" and paranoia.

The active ingredient of marijuana is tetrahydrocannabinol (THC), which is primarily metabolized by the liver. The drug is fat-soluble and can accumulate for long periods of time in the body. There has been an increase in

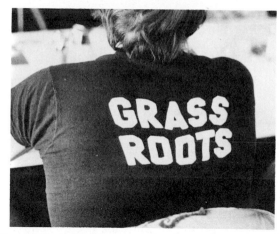

**Figure 33–4.** Marijuana remains in popular use, particularly among male adolescents. Driving under the influence of the drug is extremely hazardous.

potency in THC, leading to more side effects. The young person who smokes frequently is at greater risk than the adult who smokes occasionally. Marijuana should not be used by those with seizure disorders, as it is known to cause convulsions in animals and interferes with anticonvulsant medication. Cardiopulmonary and endocrine problems have also been cited (Neinstein, 1984). Driving an automobile while under the influence of the drug is extremely hazardous.

Nothing in this drug causes a person to go on to use harder drugs, but the *personality of the user* may lead to use of other drugs. Studies show that users also tend to drink alcohol and smoke cigarettes more heavily than nonusers do; alcohol is often used along with pot. The Marijuana Tax Act of 1937 made possession of the drug a criminal offense. In spite of this, it has been widely available. More information is required to determine the long-term consequences of using the drug.

## Nursing Brief

The incidence of cigarette smoking by teenage girls is increasing. Nurses can attempt to discourage this habit by education and example. Tobacco chewing, as well as smoking, by teenage boys is to be discouraged because of its link to gum disease and cancer.

## ATTENTION-DEFICIT HYPERACTIVITY DISORDER

**Description.** The term attention-deficit hyperactivity disorder (ADHD) refers to a developmentally inappropriate degree of gross motor activity, impulsivity, and inattention in the school or home setting (Greenhill, 1990). It is more common in boys than in girls. It occurs more frequently in some families, which suggests a genetic connection. The Diagnostic and Statistical Manual of Mental Disorders IV (DSM-IV) has defined the condition precisely and established specific criteria for diagnosis.

*Learning disability* is an educational term; however, learning disabilities occur frequently in children with ADHD. Although these children may have average or above-average intellectual ability, they experience difficulties in such areas as perception, language, comprehension, conceptualization, memory, and control of attention. Dyslexia (reading difficulties) and dysgraphia (writing difficulties) may be apparent. These children may transpose letters, for example, may read "pot" for "top." They may be unable to express themselves.

**Manifestations.** The symptoms of ADHD as defined by the DSM-IV are summarized as follows:

- Inattention (at least three): is easily distracted, needs calm atmosphere in which to work, fails to complete work, does not appear to listen, has difficulty concentrating unless instruction is one-to-one, needs information repeated
- Impulsivity (at least three): is disruptive with other children, talks out in class, is extremely excitable, cannot wait turn, is overtalkative, requires a lot of supervision
- Hyperactivity (at least two): climbs on furniture, fidgets, is always "on the go," cannot stay seated, does things in a loud and noisy way

Other diagnostic criteria include onset before age 7 years; duration of at least 6 months; and determination that disorder is not caused by mental retardation, schizophrenia, disorders of sensory organs (particularly deafness), or seizure disorders.

**Treatment and Nursing Care.** The cause of these difficulties is not thoroughly understood. Proponents of biochemical factors suggest that hyperactive children have a total lack or diminished amount of norepinephrine, a neurotransmitter in the brain. Others attribute the problem to an alteration of the reticular activating system of the midbrain that causes the child to react to every stimulus in the environment rather than to selected ones. Newer evidence indicates that genetic factors may play an important role. These disorders have also been linked to fetal alcohol syndrome and lead toxicity.

The specific medications used for the treatment of behavior problems in ambulatory ADHD patients are listed in Table 33–3. They are believed to act directly on the reticular activating system or to stimulate the release of norepinephrine from the brain stem. Although the use of drugs to modify behavior in children is controversial, extensive experience has demonstrated their effectiveness, particularly in children with disorders of attention, activity, and organization. There is no evidence that these drugs are addictive; abuse is unlikely because the effect on the patient is the opposite of that on persons without the problem. More controversial therapies include diet (particularly elimination of food additives, such as preservatives, artificial flavors, and artificial colors) and megavitamins.

Initially, a careful medical history and neurologic examination are indicated. Intelligence and psychological tests may aid in determining the specific assets and liabilities of the child so that an individual learning plan can be outlined. Today many schools have special learning disability classes in which children are helped to establish self-discipline by consistent controls, elimination of distractions, and recognition and appreciation of accomplishments. The nurse reinforces these methods when the child is hospitalized.

A priority in the care of ADHD patients is a thorough nursing admission history, which is a most useful tool. Nurses observe the patient's behavior alone and with the family. They document what they see but do not interpret it, for example, "Eric threw four crayons on the floor," not "Eric appeared distraught and misbehaved this morning." Careful attention is given to the child's attitude toward school. Other responsibilities might include dietary counseling if ordered, education in parenting, and assisting with screening and psychological tests. Functions pertinent to the nurse's work setting might also include referral to appropriate agencies and assessing the home and school environments.

Listening to the child and parents and pro-

**Table 33–3.** MEDICATIONS USEFUL IN ATTENTION-DEFICIT HYPERACTIVITY DISORDER

| Drug | Dosage (mg) | Dosage Interval | Side Effects | Nursing Implications |
|---|---|---|---|---|
| Methylphenidate (Ritalin, Ritalin-SR) | 2.5–20 20–40 | 8 AM, noon 8 AM | Anorexia, weight loss, nervousness, insomnia, occasional dizziness, headache | Frequently used because of rapid and predictable onset, few side effects CBC, differential, and platelet count should routinely be performed during therapy Give 30–45 min before meals Do not give drug in afternoon or evening to avoid insomnia Monitor growth parameters Teach family to avoid tasks that require alertness until response to drug is established Give sugarless gum for dry mouth, or sips of water |
| Dextroamphetamine (Dexedrine) | 2.5–20 | 8 AM, noon | Temporary suppression of weight and height patterns Increased motor activity, talkativeness, mild euphoria, insomnia Dry mouth | Avoid tasks that require alertness, motor skills until response to drug is established |
| Pemoline (Cylert) | 18.75–112.5 | 8 AM | Anorexia, insomnia, occasional abdominal discomfort, diarrhea | Liver function tests should be performed before therapy begins and periodically during therapy Teach family that the therapeutic response is gradual and may take 3–4 wk Insomnia and anorexia usually disappear during continued therapy Presence of a tic disorder (muscle spasm) or appearance of tics while on stimulant medication is a contraindication to its use or continued use |

viding support are particularly important. If the child is hyperactive, opportunities for gross motor play and screaming in order to externalize feelings, which must be encouraged at home, are limited in the hospital. The use of puppets, finger paints, and singing may be employed in order to offset this imbalance. One nurse on each shift is assigned to a particular child in order to provide continuity of care. Nursing care plans should include short- and long-term goals.

When medications are necessary, the child and family must understand the reasons for their use and their possible side effects. Periodic evaluation by the physician is essential. It is helpful if a behavior chart is kept and is submitted to the doctor before prescriptions

are renewed. The child with a learning disability should not become a "sacrificial lamb" of the educational process: the emphasis on education should not be disproportionate to the child's innate capabilities. Personal growth and self-esteem are emphasized. Parents should be aware that other opportunities exist that can be adjusted to the child's abilities. ADHD may extend into adulthood.

# Divorce: Impact on Children and Families

**Description.** Divorce is a difficult event for the people involved. The California Children of Divorce Project studied 131 children and their divorcing parents over a 10-year period. The following is based on a summary by Judith Wallerstein, titled "Separation, Divorce and Remarriage" (1992).

According to the 1993 Census Bureau report, the divorce rate fell slightly after peaking in the late 1970s. By the end of the 1980s, there were 37 divorces for every 1000 married women of age 15–44, compared with 40 of every 1000 in 1979. This remains a significant number. Estimates suggest that marriages last an average of 6.6 years. This means that children of divorcing parents are younger, in the infant, toddler, and preschool age groups (Wallerstein, 1992).

Families going through divorce face issues of custodial care, decrease in finances, stress, and disruption of routine. Parents experience feelings of failure, open hostility, and depression. These feelings affect their capacity to parent during this transitional period. The need for the custodial parent to work often leaves children alone more often, and they may experience loneliness and anxiety (Box 33–3). As the parent begins to form new relationships, children may feel replaced by others. Parents also fear rejection by their children, which can lead to less discipline. Decision-making is complicated by psychosocial pressures. The child's loss of a parent may also mean the loss of grandparents, and the child needs to grieve for these losses.

**Guidance.** Children need to be prepared for the divorce before one of the parents leaves the house. Several discussions are necessary because the impact is overwhelming. Children must not be made a pawn of the feuding parents, and they need to understand that this was not a spur-of-the-moment decision. Children need to know what they can expect in their living arrangements and daily routine and where the noncustodial parent will live. Parents need to make it clear that the children did not cause the divorce and that neither parent expects them to take sides. Children need permission to experience their anger, sadness, and fear. They need to know that they will continue to be cared for in the future (see Nursing Care Plan 33–2).

Following a divorce, the family experiences a change in roles. The visiting parent's influence may be strengthened or weakened. The custodial parent must assume additional responsibilities. Both parents must adjust to life as a single parent. The oldest child may be given the message or may perceive that he or she must now become more mature in managing family matters. The child may become a confidant for the custodial parent. The period of disequilibrium may last for several years. The eventual outcome depends not only on what has been lost but on what has been constructed to replace the failed marriage (Wallerstein, 1992).

---

| BOX 33–3 | Issues Affecting Children of Divorcing Parents |
| --- | --- |

Continued fighting between the parents
Abandonment by one parent
Continued litigation over custody and visitation
Emotional or mental disturbances in parents
Diminished parenting
Poor relationships with step-parents
Little support from outside nuclear family
Economic hardships

From Levine, M.D., Carey, W.B., & Crocker, A.C. (1992). *Developmental-behavioral pediatrics.* (2nd ed.). Philadelphia: W.B. Saunders.

---

# Nursing Brief

The disruption of the family because of marital conflict may result in a decrease in attention to the children's physical health.

| NURSING CARE PLAN 33–2 | | |
| --- | --- | --- |
| **Selected Nursing Diagnoses for the Family Experiencing a Divorce** | | |
| **Goals** | **Nursing Interventions** | **Rationale** |

**Nursing Diagnosis:** High risk for ineffective family coping related to disruption in lifestyle, separation, and divorce.

| | | |
| --- | --- | --- |
| Family members will state their chief concern<br>Parents will designate two resources for support | 1. Ask each member to state chief concern at the moment | 1. Stating chief concern helps family prioritize problems, rather than tackling everything at once |
| | 2. Encourage parents to include children in discussion as age-appropriate | 2. This helps decrease feelings of loneliness and isolation |
| | 3. Develop a written daily routine for 2 days with the parent | 3. Writing down routine may help lessen confusion; individuals tend to repeat patterns of behavior when coping with stress and frustration; assistance in problem solving can help parent to think of new ways to approach situation |
| | 4. Determine parents' knowledge of community resources | 4. Parents are not usually aware of resources; remember that health-care provider may also be a source of support |

**Nursing Diagnosis:** Health-seeking behaviors (parents) related to developmental needs of children during divorce.

| | | |
| --- | --- | --- |
| Parents will express one behavior of each child that they think may need attention | 1. Determine what parents know about growth and development and what problems they may see for children | 1. This approach builds on current knowledge; it provides baseline information about general patterns of growth and assists in anticipatory guidance; it helps parents understand what is normal behavior |
| | 2. Suggest that household routines be maintained and child's routine be as stable as possible | 2. This helps to provide a safe and secure environment for child who is under stress |
| | 3. Discuss possibility of regression in small children (return to thumb-sucking, security blankets, sleep and separation disturbances) | 3. Young children are most likely to show regression, particularly on separation; they may also exhibit irritable and demanding behavior |
| | 4. Discuss ways of handling hostility and grief in older child and adolescent | 4. Often latency-age children and adolescents deny their feelings; they may be worried about their own future; offer reassurance, support, and provide opportunities for private discussion |
| | 5. Maintain confidentiality | 5. Confidentiality is vital for establishing trust |

# KEY POINTS

- Early childhood experiences are critical to personality formation.
- The child's environment must be safe and one in which the child can trust caretakers.
- Nurses play an important role in the mental and emotional assessment of children because they often have the most contact with the hospitalized child and family.
- Talk of suicide must always be taken seriously.
- The risk of suicide increases when there is a definite plan of action, the means are available, and the person has few resources for help and support.

- Alcohol abuse is the number-one problem of American teenagers.
- Al-Anon and Alateen are two excellent resources for family members of alcoholics.
- Pediatric nurses must maintain a high index of suspicion and intervene in cases in which physical or emotional neglect exists because of parental alcoholism.
- The Diagnostic and Statistical Manual of Mental Disorders IV (DSM-IV) lists specific criteria for various mental conditions seen in children and adults.
- Greenhill defines attention-deficit hyperactivity disorder as a developmentally inappropriate degree of gross motor activity, impulsivity, and inattention in school or at home.

# Study Questions

1. Suicide among the teenage population and among younger children has become recognized as a serious problem. What factors increase the risk of death in suicide attempts?
2. List four levels of substance abuse.
3. Differentiate between psychological and physical dependence on drugs.
4. In what ways does alcoholism in the teenager differ from alcoholism in the adult?
5. Discuss the treatment for alcoholism.
6. How might nurses, in their work setting, recognize the child of alcoholic parents?
7. List the physical effects of marijuana.
8. Define the following: psychiatrist, psychoanalyst, clinical psychologist, and art therapist.
9. Monica, age 6, has been diagnosed as having attention-deficit hyperactivity disorder. List four symptoms of this disorder. What medications and therapy are useful in its treatment?
10. List six criteria for referring a child to a mental health resource.

# Multiple Choice Review Questions

*Choose the most appropriate answer.*

1. Suicide is most prevalent during
   a. preadolescence
   b. adolescence
   c. ages 7 to 12
   d. none of the above

2. Suicide is considered more likely if
   a. the patient has made previous attempts
   b. the patient is depressed or agitated
   c. the patient has insomnia and anorexia
   d. the patient has no previous history of attempts

3. One of the most common untoward reactions to marijuana is
   a. a feeling of persecution
   b. a feeling of exuberance
   c. hypochondria
   d. hyperactivity
4. Alcohol is a mind-altering drug that works as a
   a. stimulant
   b. depressant
   c. antidepressant
   d. antipsychotic
5. A medical doctor who specializes in mental disorders is called a
   a. clinical psychologist
   b. psychiatrist
   c. philosopher
   d. psychoanalyst

## BIBLIOGRAPHY

Behrman, R.E. (1992). *Nelson textbook of pediatrics* (14th ed.). Philadelphia: W.B. Saunders.

Diagnostic and Statistical Manual of Mental Disorders IV (DSM-IV) (1994). Washington, DC: American Psychiatric Association.

Graef, J., & Cone, T. (1988). *Manual of pediatric therapeutics* (4th ed.). Boston: Little, Brown.

Greenhill, L. (1990). Attention-deficit hyperactivity disorder in children. In: B.D. Garfinkel, G.A. Carlson, & E.B. Weller (Eds.), *Psychiatric disorders in children and adolescents* (pp. 149–191). Philadelphia: W.B. Saunders.

Levine, M.D., Carey, W.B., & Crocker, A.C. (1992). *Developmental-behavioral pediatrics* (2nd ed.). Philadelphia: W.B. Saunders.

Neinstein, L. (1984). *Adolescent health care*. Baltimore: Urban & Schwarzenberg.

Pillitteri, A. (1992). *Maternal and child health nursing*. Philadelphia: J.B. Lippincott.

Snyder, R. (1990). Attention deficit disorder. In: S.S. Gellis & B.M. Kagan (Eds.), *Current pediatric therapy 13* (pp. 44, 45). Philadelphia: W.B. Saunders.

Stuart, G., & Sundeen, S. (1991). *Principles and practice of psychiatric nursing* (4th ed.). St. Louis: Mosby–Year Book.

Thompson, E.D., & Ashwill, J.W. (1992). *Introduction to pediatric nursing*. Philadelphia: W.B. Saunders.

Triplett, J., & Arbeson S. (1983). Working with children of alcoholics. *Pediatric Nursing 9*, 317.

Wallerstein, J. (1992). Separation, divorce and remarriage. In: M.D. Levine, W.B. Carey, & A.C. Crocker (Eds.). *Developmental-behavioral pediatrics* (2nd ed.) Philadelphia: W.B. Saunders.

Whaley, L., & Wong, G. (1991). *Nursing care of children* (4th ed.). St. Louis: C.V. Mosby.

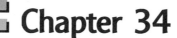

# Chapter 34

# Special Topics

## OBJECTIVES

*On completion and mastery of Chapter 34, the student will be able to*

- Define each vocabulary term listed.
- Identify the type of test devised by Stanford and Binet.
- List four causes of mental retardation.
- List six symptoms that may be indicative of mental retardation.
- Differentiate between natural and acquired immunities.
- Discuss the more common communicable diseases during childhood.
- Define sudden infant death syndrome (SIDS).
- List three nursing interventions appropriate for the family of a SIDS baby.
- Discuss the concept of death as experienced by the following: toddler, preschool child, school-age child, and adolescent.
- Summarize the nursing goals significant to the care of the dying child and the family.
- Identify five symptoms of abuse or neglect in children.
- Discuss the nurse's role in intervention of abuse and neglect.

In this chapter, consideration is given to several topics that are unrelated but deserve special attention. Most of these topics do not fit neatly into a certain system or age group. They can nevertheless be individually selected and placed in the curriculum at any point. The fact that they are discussed in the last chapter does not minimize their importance but instead reflects the author's attempt to organize content for the student.

## Mental Retardation

Mental retardation, or cognitive impairment, is defined as significantly subaverage general intellectual functioning, resulting in impaired adaptive behavior and manifested during the developmental period. Tests to measure intelligence are numerous. One test that is frequently given to children and adolescents is the Stanford-Binet. Alfred Binet of France was a pioneer in the field of intelligence measurement. His work was modified and revised in America by Lewis Terman of Stanford University. These tests differ somewhat depending on the age of the subject.

Intelligence of children is difficult to evaluate and is best tested on an individual basis. Personality tests such as picture story tests, inkblot tests, drawing tests, and sentence completion tests may also be administered. All such tests have their limitations, and of course their accuracy is subject to the abilities of the person interpreting them. Nonetheless, the tests are of value when used in conjunction with a thorough study of the child's physical, mental, emotional, and social development.

There are many causes of mental retardation. Some conditions that can develop during the prenatal period are phenylketonuria, hypothyroidism, fetal alcohol syndrome, Down syndrome, malformations of the brain (such as microcephaly, hydrocephalus, craniostenosis), and maternal infections. Birth injuries or anoxia during or shortly after delivery may also cause mental retardation. Diseases such as meningitis, lead poisoning, neoplasms, and encephalitis can cause mental retardation in a child or adult of any age. Heredity is a factor in mental retardation. It is also possible that living in a physically and emotionally deprived environment will cause the child to become mentally retarded.

The diagnosis is determined after a thorough study is made. The DSM-IV lists the criteria for mental retardation to aid in determination. Conditions such as epilepsy, cerebral palsy, severe malnutrition, emotional disturbances, blindness, deafness, and speech disorders must be ruled out. Severe mental retardation may be noticeable at birth. The nursery nurse must be alert for the following symptoms: failure to suck, feeding difficulties, spasticity, listlessness, twitching or convulsions, vomiting, jaundice, unusual-looking stools, unusual odor of urine, enlarged tongue, and Oriental appearance in a non-Asian child (Box 34–1). In certain cases, early recognition can lessen or prevent brain damage.

Other symptoms of mental retardation are associated with landmarks of the growth process. Children who do not smile, sit, climb stairs, stand, or walk within the usual age limits may be cognitively impaired (Fig. 34–1.) These children may also be slow in speech, in learning to help themselves, or in toilet training. Unusual clumsiness and failure to respond to stimuli are early indications. Sometimes this disorder is not discovered until the child enters school.

For purposes of clarification, mental retardation is classified in groups (Table 34–1). Each case must be frequently reevaluated according

| BOX 34–1 | Signs Suggesting a Cognitive Handicap in the Newborn Period and During Early Infancy |
|---|---|

Failure to suck
Feeding difficulties
Spasticity
Convulsions
Listlessness, irritability
Floppy, hypotonic muscles
Decreased alertness
Unresponsiveness to eye contact
Unusual clumsiness
Jaundice
Unusual-looking stools
Unusual odor of urine
Enlarged tongue
Upslanting eyes
Stubby fingers or toes
Failure to master milestones of development (smile, roll over, sit, and so on)

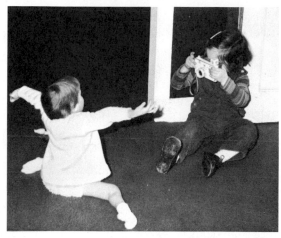

**Figure 34–1.** The 4-year-old child with her back to the camera is mentally retarded. She was born with a meningomyelocele and a dislocated hip. She enjoys playing with Mary, age 2 ½.

to the child's individual progress. No patients should be kept stagnant merely because they happen to fall within a certain category.

**Management and Nursing Goals.** For nurses to be of substantial help to the retarded child

**Table 34–1.** CHARACTERISTICS OF THE MENTALLY RETARDED FROM BIRTH TO ADULTHOOD

| Type of Retardation (IQ) | Age (Years) | | |
|---|---|---|---|
| | *Birth to 5* | *6–21* | *Over 21* |
| Mild (53–69) | Often not noticed as retarded by casual observer but is slower to walk, feed self, and talk than most children | Can acquire practical skills and useful reading and arithmetic to a 3rd- to 6th-grade level with special education; can be guided toward social conformity | Can usually achieve social and vocational skills adequate to self-maintenance; may need occasional guidance and support when under unusual social or economic stress |
| Moderate (36–52) | Noticeable delays in motor development, especially in speech; responds to training in various self-help activities | Can learn simple communication, elementary health and safety habits, and simple manual skills; does not progress in functional reading or arithmetic | Can perform simple tasks under sheltered conditions; participates in simple recreation; travels alone in familiar places; usually incapable of self-maintenance |
| Severe (20–35) | Marked delay in motor development; little or no communication skill; may respond to training in elementary self-help—for example, self-feeding | Usually walks, barring specific disability; has some understanding of speech and some response; can profit from systematic habit training | Can conform to daily routines and repetitive activities; needs continuing direction and supervision in protective environment |
| Profound (below 20) | Gross retardation; minimum capacity for functioning in sensorimotor area; needs nursing care | Obvious delays in all areas of development; shows basic emotional responses; may respond to skillful training in use of legs, hands, and jaws; needs close supervision | May walk, need nursing care, have primitive speech; usually benefits from regular physical activity; incapable of self-maintenance |

Courtesy of United States President's Panel on Mental Retardation.

## Nursing Brief

The retarded child needs to develop a sense of accomplishment. Do not "take over" projects because of your own need to assist or speed up the process.

and family, they must face their own feelings and develop a positive attitude toward the problem. It is not unusual for a person to feel repelled and uneasy on seeing a severely retarded child for the first time. It is helpful for the student to discuss these feelings in a group where ideas can be exchanged and support provided. They should realize that experienced personnel who work with and understand these children as individuals have a view of them entirely different from that of the casual observer.

The parents of a retarded child need support, compassion, and understanding, not pity. It should be clear to them that the nurse does not regard the child's condition as a disgrace. Usually the problems confronting parents become greater as the child develops physically and chronologically but continues to require constant supervision. The decision to institutionalize the patient is a difficult one. Many factors must be considered, such as the health of the parents, the effect on other children in the family, the community services available, and the financial status of the family. Even when the decision is made, few institutions are available. Facilities are overcrowded, and they tend to take the most severely retarded children first.

The trend in dealing with retarded people is toward deinstitutionalization and admittance or full inclusion in society. In 1975, the United States Congress passed the Education for All Handicapped Children Act X (PL 94-142), which ensures that retarded individuals and other persons who are physically challenged have the right to receive education at public expense. The child has the right to the least restrictive environment possible. New or expanded programs must be developed to satisfy this legislative requirement.

Nurses must be familiar with the resources of the community so that they can direct the family to them. The local chapter of the National Association for Retarded Citizens may provide information and support. Summer camps, such as those run by the Easter Seal Society, provide stimulation and opportunities for socialization to children with mental and physical disabilities. The child guidance clinic or the psychological services of a nearby college or hospital may be tapped. The visits of the public health nurse are often invaluable. Arrangements for proper dental health must be made because some patients may be unable to cooperate with the necessary procedures. Patients may also be eligible to obtain help from their local vocational and rehabilitation agency. Respite care workers afford needed rest and increased mobility for parents. In some communities, parent groups meet to discuss mutual problems.

The training of retarded children is similar to that of children with normal intelligence, only slower. Early infant stimulation may help increase awareness and alertness. However, these children lack the ability to think abstractly, so they cannot transfer learning from one situation to another. They must learn by habit formation, which involves routine, repetition, and relaxation. The nurse working with these patients must have a good understanding of the growth and development process. Children must show a *readiness* for the task, whether it is toilet training, eating, or dressing. The atmosphere is one of friendliness, and directions are kept simple. Limits must be set on behavior. The adult must be firm and consistent. Correction must directly follow the offense. Love, liberal praise, respect, and infinite patience are essential in helping these children to develop to their capacity.

The nurse caring for retarded children in the hospital needs to know their stage of maturation and ability. A detailed history, including a habit and care sheet, is completed. Self-help activities are documented. Communicating with the patient may be difficult. Home routines are to be followed as closely as possible to avoid reversal of gains already made. Good communications between parents and nurse help make the transition from home to hospital as smooth as possible for the child. In obtaining information about the child from the parents, a positive approach is recommended. A request such as "Tell me about Carla's eating habits" is preferable to "Does she feed herself?" and is likely to yield more helpful information.

**Prevention.** The outlook is good for continued success in the prevention of mental retardation. Nurses can contribute to this by the promotion of genetic counseling, immuniza-

**Table 34–2.** INTERVENTIONS CURRENTLY AVAILABLE TO PREVENT MENTAL RETARDATION

| Factor | Intervention |
|---|---|
| *Nearly Total Elimination* | |
| Congenital rubella | Early immunization, antibody screening |
| Phenylketonuria, galactosemia, congenital hypothyroidism | Newborn screening, dietary management, replacement therapy |
| Kernicterus | Reduction of sensitization via globulin therapy |
| *Major Reduction* | |
| Tay-Sachs disease | Carrier screening, prenatal diagnosis in high-risk persons |
| Morbidity from prematurity | Newborn intensive care nurseries |
| Measles encephalitis | Early vaccination |
| *Significant Current Efforts* | |
| Neural tube defects | Maternal serum alpha-fetoprotein screen, prenatal diagnosis |
| Down syndrome | Prenatal diagnosis, counseling of older women |
| Lead intoxication | Screening for lead levels, improvement in environment, chelation when necessary |
| Fetal alcohol syndrome | Public education |
| Morbidity from head injury | Automobile child restraints, safety helmets |
| Child neglect and abuse | Parenting classes and family life education through the schools |
| *Special Assistance and Relief* | |
| Multiple handicaps, hearing, speech, Down syndrome | Early identification |
| | Support for families |
| | Genetic counseling of special risks |

Data from Levine, M.D., Carey, W.B., & Crocker, A.C. (1992). *Developmental-behavioral pediatrics*. Philadelphia: W.B. Saunders.

tions, newborn screening, and good prenatal care (Table 34–2). Comprehensive programs for early assessment and treatment of the mentally retarded must also be promoted. The nurse may serve as an advocate for the child and/or adolescent to help ensure that their rights are upheld.

# Communicable Disease

There have been only a few brief periods in history when infectious disease did not dominate the attention of health-care professionals. In spite of immunization, sanitation, antibiotics, and other controls, the world again faces infectious agents such as human immunodeficiency virus (HIV) and *Legionella*. Hepatitis, tuberculosis, rheumatic fever, and sexually transmitted diseases continue to persist. In spite of our knowledge of immunizations, many children still suffer from common communicable diseases. Antibiotic resistance organisms increase, and immunocompromised

patients are threatened by nonpathogenic organisms. Prevention and control are key factors in the management of infectious disease.

## REVIEW OF TERMS

A communicable disease is one that can be transmitted, directly or indirectly, from one person to another (Table 34–3). Organisms that cause disease are called *pathogens*.

The *incubation* period is the time between the invasion by the pathogen and the onset of symptoms. The *prodromal* period refers to the initial stage of a disease: the interval between the earliest symptoms and the appearance of the rash or fever. Children are frequently contagious during this time, but because the symptoms are not specific they may attend preschool or another group program and spread the disease. A *fomite* is any material that absorbs and transmits infection. The *chain of infection* refers to the way in which organisms spread and infect the individual (Fig. 34–2). Preventing the spread of infection depends on breaking the chain. The principles of medical asepsis and isolation precautions for specific diseases are discussed on page 606. Universal precautions are found in Appendix F. Careful handwashing is essential to the containment of infection.

## HOST RESISTANCE

Many factors contribute to the virulence of an infectious disease. The age, sex, and genetic makeup of the child have a bearing. The nutritional status of the person, as well as physical and emotional health, is also important. The efficiency of the blood-forming organs and the immune systems has an effect on resistance. The child who has an underlying condition, such as diabetes, cystic fibrosis, burns, or sickle cell disease, may be more susceptible to certain organisms.

Children with acquired immunodeficiency syndrome (AIDS) or cancer often have depressed immune systems. This makes them very susceptible to *opportunistic* infections as well as to pathogens. Patients with cerebrospinal fluid shunts, prolonged intravenous regimens, tracheostomies, respiratory life support systems, and indwelling urinary catheters may also be predisposed to this type of infection. Nurses must fine-tune their detection abilities when caring for such persons. An infection acquired in a health-care facility during hospitalization is termed a *nosocomial* infection.

**Types of Immunity.** Immunity is *natural* or *acquired* resistance to infection. In natural immunity, resistance is inborn. Some races apparently have a greater natural immunity to certain diseases than others. Immunity also varies from person to person. If two people are exposed to the same disease, one may become very ill and the other may have no indications of the disease. However, a person who is immune to one disease is not necessarily immune to another.

Acquired immunity is not due to inherited factors but is acquired as a result of having the disease or is artificially acquired by receiving vaccines and immune serums. Vaccines are not strong enough to cause the disease, but they stimulate the body to develop an immune reaction. Live or dead organisms may be used for this purpose. The Salk poliomyelitis vaccine is an example of the type in which dead viruses are used. In contrast, the Sabin oral polio vaccine is made with live, attenuated

viruses (see the immunization schedules in Tables 17–2 and 17–3).

If a person needs immediate protection from a disease, antibodies are obtained in immune serums from other sources; most are from animals, but some are from humans. For example, tetanus serum, used to prevent lockjaw, is procured from the horse, but gamma globulin, which is rich in antibodies and is particularly effective against measles, is obtained from human blood. This type of immunity, known as passive immunity, acts immediately but does not last as long as immunity that the body actively produces.

A *carrier* is a person who is capable of spreading a disease but does not show evidence of it. Typhoid is an example of a disease spread by a carrier.

Tests are available to determine whether an individual is susceptible to a particular disease. Examples are the Schick test for diphtheria, the Dick test for scarlet fever, and the tuberculin test for tuberculosis; the nurse may commonly see the last done by the tine test or the Mantoux intradermal skin test.

**Resurgence of Tuberculosis.** Active pulmonary tuberculosis (TB) in children is still seen in immigrants, Native-American populations, and patients with AIDS. Tuberculosis is one of the few diseases associated with HIV infection that is transmissible, treatable, and preventable. *Miliary TB*, which is a *disseminated* form, is seen in infants and small children. Disseminated means that large numbers of the tubercle bacilli have been spread throughout the blood stream to many parts of the body. TB represents a potential hazard to health-care workers but only if it is not recognized and not treated. All patients with HIV infection and undiagnosed pulmonary disease should be suspected of having TB. Appropriate universal precautions to prevent airborne transmission are taken until TB is diagnosed and treated or ruled out. The Public Health Department keeps records of patients and determines which family members may be candidates for prophylaxis.

## RASHES

Many infectious diseases begin with a rash (see Color Plate Figs. 3 to 6). Regardless of cause, rashes tend to be itchy (pruritus) and uncomfortable. Acetaminophen (Tylenol) may

*Text continued on page 887*

**Table 34–3.** FEATURES OF COMMUNICABLE DISEASES

| Disease | First Signs | Incubation Period | Prevention | How Long Contagious | What You Can Do |
|---|---|---|---|---|---|
| Chickenpox (varicella) | Mild fever followed in 36 hr by small raised pimples that become filled with clear fluid; scabs form later; successive crops of pox appear | 2–3 wk usually, 13–17 days | None: immune after one attack; vaccine now available for children at high risk; used with caution in general public at present | 6 days after appearance of rash | Not a serious disease; trim fingernails to prevent scratching; a paste of baking soda and water may ease itching; premature removal of scabs may cause scars; dangerous to children receiving immunosuppressive therapy |
| Fifth disease (Erythema infectiosum) | Child has "slapped cheek" appearance; rash appears and progresses from face to upper and lower extremities; it subsides but reappears if skin is irritated by, e.g., sun or heat | 4–14 days | None | Uncertain | Benign condition unless child is immunocompromised; isolation not required; no treatment needed; may last 1–3 wk |
| German measles, 3-day measles (rubella) | Mild fever, sore throat, or cold symptoms may precede tiny, rose-colored rash; enlarged glands at back of neck and behind ears | 2–3 wk, usually 18 days | Vaccine may be given at 15 mo as measles-rubella, rubella-mumps, or measles-mumps-rubella combined vaccines; priority immunization should be given to children in kindergarten and elementary school; all children should receive vaccine | Until rash fades, about 5 days | Generally not a serious disease in childhood, complications rare; give general good care and rest; avoid exposing any woman who is or might be in early months of pregnancy |
| Hepatitis (type A) | Symptoms develop rapidly; may be mild with few symptoms or accompanied by fever, anorexia, headache, abdominal pain, nausea, diarrhea, general weariness; later, skin and white of eyes are yellow (jaundice), urine is dark, and bowel movements are chalklike | 2–6 wk, commonly 25 days | Injection of gamma globulin gives temporary immunity if child is exposed | Uncertain | Caused by ingestion of fecally contaminated water or shellfish from such water, local flooding, swimming in contaminated water; may be spread from contaminated changing tables; enteric precautions; ensure proper handwashing; wear gloves when handling fecal materials |

*Continued*

**Table 34–3.** FEATURES OF COMMUNICABLE DISEASES *Continued*

| Disease | First Signs | Incubation Period | Prevention | How Long Contagious | What You Can Do |
|---|---|---|---|---|---|
| Hepatitis (type B) | Symptoms same as type A but more insidious onset and more serious | 50–180 days, average 120 days | Hepatitis B vaccine (HBV) during newborn period | Uncertain, may persist in carrier state | Caused by direct contact with secretions of blood contaminated with HBV; more common in children on hemodialysis or receiving blood products; drug use, fetal transfer in last trimester places newborns at risk |
| Infectious mononucleosis (glandular fever) | Sore throat, swollen glands of neck and elsewhere; sometimes a rash over whole body and jaundiced appearance; low persistent fever | Probably 4–14 days or longer | None | Probably 2–4 wk but mode of transmission is not clear; Monospot test for detection | Keep in bed while feverish; restrict activity thereafter |
| Lyme disease | Skin lesion at site of tick bite; macule forms, then a large papule with a raised border and clear center; may be described as burning; may be accompanied by fever, headache, arthralgia, stiff neck; may involve joints, heart, and neurologic systems in late stages | 3–32 days | Protective clothing in wooded areas; inspect child following play in these areas; light-colored clothing makes tick more noticeable; remove visible tick with tweezers; inspect family pets | Spread only by infected tick | Antibiotics prescribed by physician; prednisone and antiinflammatory drugs may provide relief |
| Measles (rubeola) | Mounting fever; hard, dry cough; running nose and red eyes for 3 or 4 days before rash, which starts at hair line and spreads down in blotches; small red spots with white centers in mouth (Koplik's spots) appear before rash | 1–2 wk, usually 10 or 11 days | All children should receive measles vaccine at 15 mo of age; if an unvaccinated child is exposed to measles, gamma globulin given shortly after exposure may minimize or prevent the disease | Usually 5–9 days, from 4 days before to 5 days after rash appears | May be mild or severe with serious complications; follow doctor's advice in caring for a child with measles, as it is a most treacherous disease |

| Disease | Symptoms | Incubation period | Immunization | Isolation | Treatment |
|---|---|---|---|---|---|
| Meningitis | May be preceded by a cold, headache, stiff neck, vomiting, high temperature with convulsions or drowsy stupor; fine rash with tiny hemorrhages into skin | 2–10 days | *Haemophilus influenzae* B Conjugate vaccine (HbCV) during infancy | Until recovery | Immediate treatment is necessary; take child to hospital if doctor unavailable; continue treatment with antibiotics as long as doctor advises |
| Mumps (parotitis) | Fever, headache, vomiting, glands near ear and toward chin at jaw line ache and develop painful swelling; other parts of body may be affected | 11–26 days, usually around 18 days | Live mumps vaccine may be used at any age after 15 mo; combination measles-mumps-rubella, rubella-mumps may be used | Until all swelling disappears | Child kept in bed until fever subsides; stays indoors unless weather is warm; observe tenderness of testes |
| Polio (infantile paralysis or poliomyelitis) | Slight fever, general discomfort, headache, stiff neck, stiff back | 1–4 wk, commonly 1–2 wk | Be sure to complete series of Sabin vaccine | 1 wk from onset or as long as fever persists | Hospital care is usually advised |
| Rocky Mountain spotted fever | Muscle pains, nosebleed occasionally, headache, rash on 3rd or 4th day | About 1 wk after bite by infected tick | Injections can be given to a child who lives in heavily infested area (see Lyme disease above) | Spread only by infected ticks | New drugs have improved treatment |
| Roseola | High fever that drops before rash or large pink blotches covering whole body appear; child may not seem very ill despite high fever (103–105°F) but may convulse | About 2 wk | None; usually affects children from 6 mo to 3 yr of age | Until seems well | No special measures except rest and quiet |
| Smallpox | Sudden fever, chills, headache and backache; rash that becomes raised and hard, later blisters and scabs | 6–18 days, commonly 12 days | Routine smallpox vaccination is no longer recommended | Until all scabs disappear | Doctor's care necessary; vaccinate if traveling to areas to which disease is endemic |
| Strep throat (septic sore throat) and scarlet fever (scarlatina) | Sometimes vomiting and fever before sudden and severe sore throat; if followed by fine rash on body and limbs, it is called scarlet fever | 1–7 days, usually 2–5 days | Antibiotics may prevent or lighten an attack if doctor thinks it wise | 7–10 days; when all abnormal discharge from nose, eyes, throat has ceased | Frequently less severe than formerly; responds to antibiotics, which should be continued for full course in order to prevent serious complications |

*Continued*

**Table 34–3.** FEATURES OF COMMUNICABLE DISEASES *Continued*

| Disease | First Signs | Incubation Period | Prevention | How Long Contagious | What You Can Do |
|---|---|---|---|---|---|
| Tuberculosis | Fever, malaise, anorexia, weight loss, cough, night sweats; may be asymptomatic, symptoms extremely variable in children; immunocompromised patients, such as persons with AIDS are at increased risk | Approximately 2–10 wk; spread by droplet infection, airborne | Early detection by tuberculin skin test (PPD); examination of contacts for disease, chest x-ray film, pasteurization of milk; in hospital utilize universal precautions for persons with undiagnosed pulmonary disease | Once child is on medication, risk of transmission is greatly reduced; young children with primary tuberculosis are generally not considered infectious because they have minimal pulmonary involvement and little or no cough or sputum | Teach children to cover their nose and mouth when coughing; physician treats with specific medicines such as isoniazid (INH) and rifampin, which stops growth of bacilli; INH may also be administered to children with a high probability of exposure to prevent the disease; duration of treatment varies–*child continues to take medication until* physician discontinues |
| Whooping cough (pertussis) | At first seems like a cold with low fever and cough, which changes at end of 2nd wk to spells of coughing accompanied by a noisy gasp for air that creates "whoop" | 5–21 days, usually around 10 days | Give injections of vaccine to all children in infancy; if an unvaccinated child has been exposed, doctor may want to give a protective serum promptly | Usually no longer after 4th wk | Child needs careful supervision of doctor throughout this taxing illness |

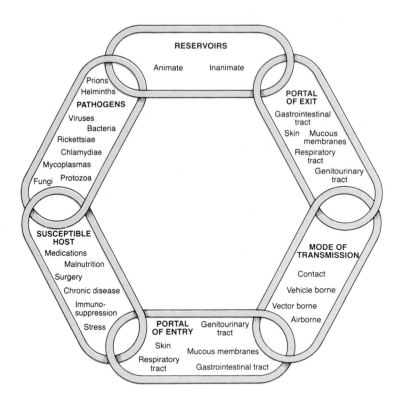

**Figure 34–2.** The chain of infection. The process by which pathogens are transmitted from the environment to a host, invade the host, and cause infection. (From Ignatavicius, D., & Bayne, M. [1991]. *Medical-surgical nursing*. Philadelphia: W.B. Saunders.)

be given to reduce pruritus and decrease fever. A lukewarm bath (not hot) and lotions such as calamine may reduce discomfort. The child is dressed in light clothing. The child is not bundled up, as this increases itching and fever. The physician may prescribe an antihistamine such as diphenhydramine (Benadryl) in an age-related dose. Aspirin is to be avoided because of the danger of Reye's syndrome.

## PSYCHOLOGICAL CONSIDERATIONS

The majority of children with common communicable diseases are cared for at home. The child is admitted to the hospital when complications arise. As soon as the patient's condition improves and the dangers of cross-infection are over, the child is removed from isolation.

Isolation is psychologically taxing for the child. Toddlers, in particular, need company because their attention span is short. When confined to a crib, they become anxious and cry. They cannot amuse themselves in play because they are afraid. They may cling, demand attention, or simply refrain from contact with anyone. These and other displays of anxiety must not be mistaken for "spoiled" behavior.

School-age children can cope better with isolation, for their attention span is longer. Nevertheless, life soon becomes dreary without visitors. Radio and TV are no substitute for friends and play. Nursing Care Plan 34–1 specifies the interventions appropriate for the child with a communicable disease.

# Sudden Infant Death Syndrome

Sudden infant death syndrome (SIDS) is clinically defined as the sudden, unexpected death of an apparently healthy infant between 2 weeks and 1 year, for which a routine autopsy fails to identify the cause. It is also referred to as "crib death" or "cot death." Although precise data are not available, it is estimated that in the United States, SIDS kills about 7000 infants each year, or about 2 of every 1000 babies born. SIDS Europe, a coalition of research groups, estimates that 10,000 babies fell victim to cot death across Europe in 1992. In industrialized countries, SIDS is one of the leading causes of death in early infancy; the peak incidence is between 2 and 4 months of age. It is more common in low-birth weight babies, in baby boys, in families with crowded living conditions, and during winter. Autopsy may reveal slight respiratory infection or otitis media, petechiae over the pleurae, and pulmonary edema. Two clinical features of the disease remain constant: (1) death occurs during sleep, and (2) the infant does not cry or make other sounds of distress. It has occurred even when the parents were sleeping in the same room. In some cases, the baby is found in one corner of the crib with blood-tinged froth coming from the nose.

Although there appears to be an increased incidence of SIDS among siblings, no genetic pattern has been determined. The risk of SIDS is increased in twins. Native-American populations are more susceptible to SIDS.

Theories about the cause of SIDS are numerous. Those implicating suffocation, aspiration allergy, and hormone deficiency have been disproved, and the exact cause is not known. Such researchers propose that SIDS results from an interruption of some basic function in the central or autonomic nervous system that causes apnea. Carotid bodies located in the neck and involved in the control of breathing have been found to be abnormal in SIDS victims. Research shows that only about 60% die in respiratory failure and that 30% or more succumb to circulatory failure. More recent research suggests that low-birth-weight babies, those who become overheated, and those whose mothers smoked during pregnancy are at greater risk. In England the number of cot deaths has halved since doctors advised putting babies to sleep on their backs instead of on their stomachs. Some physicians believe that this finding may lead to a sense of false security

---

| NURSING CARE PLAN 34–1 | | |
|---|---|---|
| **Selected Nursing Diagnoses for the Child with a Communicable Disease** | | |
| **Goals** | **Nursing Interventions** | **Rationale** |

**Nursing Diagnosis:** Pain (pruritus) related to rash.

| Goals | Nursing Interventions | Rationale |
|---|---|---|
| Infant will be less fussy, older child will verbalize relief; there will be no signs of excess scratching or bleeding | 1. Administer acetaminophen (Tylenol) | 1. Helps relieve itching and fever |
| | 2. Place child in lukewarm bath | 2. Tepid rather than hot water is used, as hot water may intensify rash and itching |
| | 3. Dress in lightweight clothing | 3. Less irritating, prevents overheating, which increases itching and fever |
| | 4. Administer topical medications as prescribed | 4. Relieves pruritus |
| | 5. Force fluids | 5. Prevents dehydration that may accompany fever |
| | 6. Keep fingernails short | 6. Prevents problems of secondary infection from scratching |

**Nursing Diagnosis:** Impaired social interaction related to isolation.

| Goals | Nursing Interventions | Rationale |
|---|---|---|
| Child will understand need for isolation, as age appropriate | 1. Prepare child for isolation | 1. Preparing child for sights of gown and masks decreases anxiety |
| | 2. Anticipate loneliness by providing toys | 2. Child may feel he or she is being punished |
| | 3. Provide telephone for older child | 3. Promotes socialization |
| | 4. Allow time to sit and visit with child as condition permits | 4. Denotes you care, that you are not repelled by patient's appearance and are not afraid of catching anything |
| | 5. Encourage parents to remain with child | 5. Provides support and socialization; reassures parents of care |

and stress that *vulnerable* babies need continuing, close observation.

Babies with infantile apnea (also called "near miss" infants) and subsequent siblings of SIDS babies are often monitored at home until they are past the age of danger. Monitors can be leased. Parents are provided with ongoing education and support during this period. They should receive appropriate training in cardiopulmonary resuscitation.

In talking with grieving parents after the death of their infant, the nurse must convey some important facts: that the baby died of a disease entity called sudden infant death syndrome, that currently the disease cannot be predicted or prevented, and that they are *not* responsible for the child's death. Grieving parents need time to say good-bye to their child. They are encouraged to hold and rock the infant, shed tears, and assist in burial preparations. This process, not common in the past, is conducive to the resolution of grief. One mother who was denied this experience stated that *5 years later*, while visiting a florist shop, she noticed a heart-shaped wreath intended for an infant. She unexpectedly burst into tears and wept.

Parents experience much guilt and are catapulted into a totally unexpected bereavement requiring numerous explanations to relatives and friends. Often, needless blame has been placed on one parent by the other or by relatives. The family baby-sitter and physician may also be targets of attack. Emergency room personnel need to be especially sensitive and supportive during this crisis. There have been crib deaths for which parents have been charged with child abuse and have even been jailed because of lack of public knowledge about the disease.

SIDS can occur in the hospital, and many nurses and physicians have personal experience of the suffering that losing a child to SIDS can cause. Nurses can recommend group therapy with other parents of SIDS victims. Two nationally supported organizations are The Compassionate Friends Inc. and The National Sudden Infant Death Syndrome Foundation. These groups have local chapters in most states.

## Facing Death

Facing death with a child and the family is not an easy task, but it can be rewarding. We learn from each patient. Each provides us

## Nursing Brief

The American Academy of Pediatrics recommends that healthy newborns and infants be placed on their backs or side to sleep, to help reduce the likelihood of SIDS.

with the opportunities to aid another human being through suffering, to grow in gentleness and patience, and to deal more effectively with the losses in our personal lives. We also develop a greater appreciation for life and for enjoying the moment. Nurses who do become involved with dying patients often express gratitude for the privilege of the experience; however, it is not glamorous. It can be tiring, discouraging, and sad, and it requires profound acceptance.

### SELF-EXPLORATION

One important, if not the most important, task to prepare for working with the dying patient is self-exploration. Our own attitudes about life and death affect our nursing practice. Emotions buried deep within us can form barriers to effective communication unless they are recognized and released. How we have or have not dealt with our own losses affects our present lives and our ability to relate to patients. Nurses must recognize that *coping is an active and ongoing process*. At times we need loving detachment from patients and their families in order to become revitalized. We must find constructive outlets, such as exercise and music, in order to maintain our equilibrium. An active support system consisting of nonjudgmental people who are not threatened by natural expressions of feelings is crucial. Proper channeling of these emotions can be a valuable part of our empathetic response to others. *It is vital that nurses support one another in the work environment.*

### THE CHILD'S REACTION TO DEATH

*Each child, like each adult, approaches death in an individual way,* drawing on limited experience. Nurses must become well acquainted with patients and view them within the context of the family and social culture. Their anxiety often centers on symptoms. They fear that the treatments necessary to alleviate their problem may be painful, as indeed some are. Their sense

## Nursing Brief

Brothers and sisters often feel neglected and lonely. They are frustrated because they are unable to comfort their parents and loved ones.

of trust is in a precarious balance. Nurses must be honest and inform them of what they are about to do and why it is necessary. This is done in terms that the patients understand. Expression of feelings is encouraged: "You seem angry." Sufficient time for a response is allowed. Children should be allowed to have as much control over what happens to them as possible. This is fostered by including them in decisions that concern their welfare. However, the child should not be offered a choice when there is none. Children often communicate symbolically. The nurse *listens* to what they say to adults, to their toys, and to other children. Crayons and paper are provided.

Although age is a factor, the child's level of cognitive development, rather than chronologic age, affects the response to death (Table 34–4). Children younger than 5 years are mainly concerned with separation from their parents and abandonment. (Even adults are threatened by thoughts of dying alone.) Preschool children respond to questions about death by relying on their experience and by turning to fantasy. They may believe death is reversible or that they are in some way responsible. Children do not develop a realistic conception of death as a permanent biologic process until the age of 9 or 10.

Dying adolescents face conflicts between their treatment regimens and their need to establish independence from their parents and conformity with their peers. This leads to anger and resentment, which are frequently displaced onto hospital staff members. An atmosphere of acceptance and nonjudgmental listening allows patients freedom to ventilate their hostility in a nonthreatening environment.

Nursing Care Plan 34–2 specifies nursing interventions for the dying child.

### THE CHILD'S AWARENESS OF HIS/HER CONDITION

Surprising as it may seem, many investigators have shown that terminally ill children are generally aware of their condition, even when it

**Table 34–4.** THE CHILD'S CONCEPT OF DEATH AT VARIOUS AGES

| Age | Concept |
|---|---|
| Infant-toddler | Little understanding of death |
| | Fear and anxiety over separation |
| Preschooler | Something that happens to others |
| | Not permanent |
| | Curious about dead flowers and animals |
| | Magical thinking |
| | Feel "bad thought" may come true, harbor guilt |
| Early school years | Death is final |
| | Feel they might die but only in the distant future |
| | May understand death as a "person" |
| | Death is universal |
| | Suspect parents will die "some day" |
| | Fear of mutilation |
| Preadolescent-adolescent | Able to understand death in a logical manner |
| | Understand it is universal |
| | Understand it is permanent |
| | Fear of disfigurement and isolation from peers |

is carefully concealed. This is reflected in their drawings and play and can be detected through psychological testing. Failure to be honest with children leaves them to suffer alone, unable to express their fears and sadness or even to say good-bye. "It is better to address the issue of the seriousness of the child's illness from the time of diagnosis. In this way, energy that would be wasted in maintaining deceit can be applied to the real problem of living with a life-threatening illness" (Spinetta et al., 1983).

### PHYSICAL CHANGES OF IMPENDING DEATH

Physical changes that take place when death is impending include cool, mottled, cyanotic skin and the slowing down of all body processes. There may be loss of consciousness, although hearing is intact. Rales in the chest may be heard, which result from increased secretions pooling in the lungs. Movement and neurologic signs lessen. If thrashing or groaning occurs, the patient is assessed for pain.

## NURSING CARE PLAN 34-2

### Selected Nursing Diagnoses for the Dying Child

| Goals | Nursing Interventions | Rationale |
|---|---|---|
| **Nursing Diagnosis:** Anxiety, anticipatory (family members) due to potential death of child. | | |
| Parents will express two anxieties to nurse<br>Communications among parents, other children, patient, and nurse remain open | 1. Remain available to family as child grows weaker<br>2. Give parents permission to talk and grieve about upcoming death and to think about funeral arrangements if they choose<br>3. Involve siblings in plans and progress of brother or sister<br>4. Provide permission for laughter, play, friends (make every day count)<br>5. Suggest that overprotection and attention, even when provided out of love, can be detrimental to dying child<br>6. Encourage family to maintain as normal a lifestyle as possible, and each member to take time for own needs (continue to go to hairdresser, a movie—whatever they previously enjoyed)<br>7. Facilitate honesty about child's imminent death among family members and patient<br>8. Explain that family members often cannot support one another, as each grieves in his or her own way<br>9. Recognize that grief is often expressed as anger<br><br>10. Provide for ventilation of guilt ("If only I had taken her to the doctor sooner" and the like)<br>11. Suggest meditation, progressive relaxation, guided imagery | 1. Nurse's presence provides support<br>2. Helps prepare family for inevitable; sorts out and identifies actual sources of feelings<br><br>3. Siblings will feel less isolated<br><br>4. Laughter and play are tension reducers<br>5. Child will feel more in control if not overprotected<br><br>6. When all members are taking care of themselves, they will have more energy to cope with crises<br><br><br><br>7. Information helps relieve anxiety<br><br>8. Explanation of this to family helps relieve guilt stemming from irritability or anger<br>9. Anger is a natural emotion; it is not fearsome in itself, although its expression may be; family has a right to all feelings<br>10. Prevents accumulation or repression of guilt<br><br>11. Helps reduce stress |
| **Nursing Diagnosis:** Anxiety (dying child) due to pain, isolation, lack of information. | | |
| Child verbalizes feelings of comfort; if nonverbal, child rests comfortably, no crying<br>Child is not isolated<br>Child verbalizes understanding of treatment, procedures, outcome as age-appropriate | 1. Administer pain relievers as necessary<br>2. Encourage parents to hold, cuddle, touch child as condition permits<br>3. Encourage visits from friends and siblings as age-appropriate<br>4. Decorate hospital room with cards, pictures, mementos; provide telephone as age-appropriate<br>5. Investigate possibility of home or hospice care<br><br>6. Explain all procedures | 1. Child may deny pain because of fear of treatment<br>2. Reduces anxiety, which contributes to pain<br>3. Provides emotional support and distraction from disease<br>4. Attractive environment promotes mental health<br><br>5. Familiar and stable environment may facilitate child's emotional healing<br>6. Information relieves anxiety |

*Continued*

| NURSING CARE PLAN 34–2 *Continued* |||
|---|---|---|
| Selected Nursing Diagnoses for the Dying Child |||
| **Goals** | **Nursing Interventions** | **Rationale** |
| **Nursing Diagnosis:** Anxiety (dying child) due to pain, isolation, lack of information. |||
|  | 7. Assess child's knowledge about impending death | 7. Nurse can determine level of understanding as age-appropriate; this assists in communication |
|  | 8. Answer all questions about death honestly, use open-ended questions to assist patient in expression of feelings | 8. Conveys that all feelings are acceptable |
|  | 9. Listen to what child says in play | 9. Children work through many fears in play |
|  | 10. Assist child in drawing "a wish," "yesterday, today, tomorrow" | 10. Drawings promote release of feelings and a means of communication |
|  | 11. Allow child to grieve (behavior may be sulky, cranky, withdrawn) | 11. Therapeutic grieving prevents depression |
| **Nursing Diagnosis:** Grieving, actual: related to death of child. |||
| Family members have an opportunity to say good-bye | 1. Provide time for family to be alone with dead child as desired | 1. Family needs to say good-bye |
| Family members express feelings of grief, fear, anger, loss, guilt | 2. Remain available, express your own loss and grief | 2. Parents derive comfort from knowing others loved their child |
|  | 3. Assist parents in making decisions | 3. Even a simple decision such as when to telephone relatives becomes monumental at this stage |
|  | 4. Offer a beverage | 4. Denotes concern |
|  | 5. Assess spiritual need; refer to pastoral counseling if desired | 5. A belief in God provides strength for many persons; pastoral counselors are effective in this area |
|  | 6. Respect family's beliefs, world view, philosophy | 6. Many beliefs may be unconventional |
|  | 7. Listen to expressions of grief | 7. Family needs to repeat story in order to work through grief |

## STAGES OF DYING

The stages of dying as detailed by Kübler-Ross (1969)—denial, anger, bargaining, depression, and acceptance—can be applied to parents and siblings as well as to the sick child. (Nurses may also respond with similar feelings.) It is important to accept and support each participant at whatever stage has been reached and not to try to direct progress. Nurses should be available and make their availability known.

Parents are encouraged to assist in the care of their child (Fig. 34–3). This is facilitated by hospice and the movement toward supervised home care. It is therapeutic for children to be in their own surroundings whenever possible. Siblings involved in the patient's care feel less neglected, and the sacrifices they must make become more meaningful. Discussions before death allow them to make amends for their hostilities toward the sick child (Petrillo & Sanger, 1980). The family's religious and spiritual philosophy can be a source of strength and support, as can caring neighbors and friends.

Statistics show a high correlation between the death of a child and divorce. Nurses must observe signs of tension between parents so that suitable intervention may be established. Each parent grieves in an individual time and way, often making it impossible for spouses to

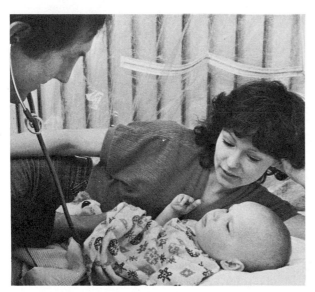

**Figure 34–3.** Close contact between caregivers and family is of great importance for a child who has a potentially life-threatening disease. (Courtesy of Blank Memorial Hospital for Children, Des Moines, IA.)

be supportive of each other. The suppression of strong feelings of guilt, helplessness, and outrage can be devastating. The father can easily be overlooked because some men think the expression of feelings is unmasculine. Feelings left unexpressed can cause depression and/or physical illness.

Kübler-Ross (1969) reminds us that dying is the easy part. Helping our patients to live until they die is the real challenge. She discusses this beautifully in *A Letter to a Child with Cancer*, which she wrote in response to Dougie's request, "What is life, what is death, and why do little children have to die?" Copies may be purchased from the Elisabeth Kübler-Ross Center, South Rt. 616, Head Waters, VA 24442.

There are several hospices in the United States that limit their services to children. St. Mary's Hospice in Bay Side, New York, is credited with being the first. The trend today is for

### Nursing Brief

Grandparents, teachers, and friends are also grieving. Be alert for all significant others.

### Nursing Brief

Organ donation for transplantation is a consideration in today's world. Most hospitals have organ procurement nurses that handle this process.

existing hospices to extend their care to children.

## Failure to Thrive

Failure to thrive describes infants and children who, without superficially evident cause, fail to gain and often lose weight. Although this condition can be caused by organic abnormalities, this discussion is limited to environmental etiologies. Infants who fail to thrive are frequently admitted to the hospital for evaluation with presenting symptoms of weight loss or failure to gain, irritability, and disturbances of food intake, such as anorexia, pica, or abnormal consumption of food. Vomiting, diarrhea, and general neuromuscular spasticity sometimes accompany the condition. Patients fall below the 3rd percentile (some authorities suggest the 5th) in weight and height on standard growth charts. Their development as ascertained by the Denver Developmental Screening Test and other means is delayed. Children who fail to thrive seem apathetic. Some have a "ragdoll limpness" (hypotonia), and often they appear wary of their caretakers. Others appear stiff and unresponsive to cuddling. The personality of the baby may not foster maternal attachment. Failure to thrive with malabsorption has been reported with frequency among autistic children and among institutionalized retarded patients.

Although causality is sometimes obscured, there appears to be a disturbance in the mother-child or caretaker-child relationship. The situation is complex and often associated with marital discord, economic pressures, parental immaturity and low stress tolerance, and single parenthood. Alcohol and drug abuse are often present. Many mothers feel deprived and unloved and have conflicting needs. Infants suffer from the inability to establish a sense of trust in their caretakers. Their coping abilities are affected by a lack of nurturing.

Outward neglect and physical abuse are not uncommon.

Prevention of environmental failure to thrive consists chiefly of social measures, such as parenting classes, family planning, and early recognition and support of families at risk. All children should receive routine health assessments. The pregnancy history may detect circumstances that may contribute to lack of bonding, such as an unplanned pregnancy or desertion by the child's father. Additional research is necessary to develop standardized tools for observing behaviors, teaching, and planning interventions that will enhance parent-infant interaction.

Treatment involves a multidisciplinary approach in accordance with the circumstance; that is, physician, nurse, social worker, family agency, and counselor may all participate. If no progress can be made, temporary or permanent placement of the child or children in a foster home may be required. During hospitalization one nurse per shift is selected to increase nurturing and interaction with the infant.

Treatment of the child who fails to thrive requires maturity on the part of the nurse. It is vital to support rather than reject the mother. Maternal attachment can be facilitated by listening and helping the mother to understand her feelings and frustrations and to explore her choices. The nurse encourages her to assist with the daily care of her child. The patient's uniqueness and responses to mother are stressed. The nurse points out developmental patterns and provides anticipatory guidance in this area. Lecturing is avoided. The nurse tries to understand the mother's situation. Frequently the mother's "lack of interest" stems from her own insecurities and feelings of rejection by hospital staff who seem critical of her. Parents are given a 24-hour telephone number and encouraged to use it when stress mounts. Parents Anonymous and parent aides are other resources. Nursing Care Plan 34–3 lists nursing interventions for the infant who fails to thrive.

The prognosis of this condition is uncertain. Emotional starvation, particularly in the early years, can be psychologically traumatic. Inadequacies in intelligence, language, and social behavior have been documented in children who fail to thrive. A small but significant number of children die later under suspicious circumstances (Behrman, 1992).

# Family Violence

Family violence consists primarily of child abuse or spouse abuse.

## CHILD ABUSE

**Description.** The term *battered child syndrome* was coined by Kempe in his landmark paper published in 1962 by the Journal of the American Medical Association. It refers to "a clinical condition in young children who have received serious physical abuse, generally from a parent or foster parent." The impact of Kempe's research was considerable and focused the attention of physicians on unexplained fractures and signs of physical abuse (Fig. 34–4).

Today, most authorities consider Kempe's definition narrow and have broadened it to include neglect and maltreatment. Because of the scope of the problem, no one definition seems entirely satisfactory, but efforts are being made to reduce ambiguity. Differences of opinion about what constitutes child abuse exist from state to state, as do differences in the criteria of various agencies concerned with this problem. Nurses must become aware of the mandates of the states and institutions in which they practice.

Approximately 1 million cases of child abuse occur each year. The exact number is unknown, as many cases go unreported. However, the incidence and reports of cases have increased.

The victims are most often between the ages of 3 months and 3 years. The younger the child, the greater the risk of death. Preterm babies have a greater risk of abuse. Adolescent abuse and neglect are also common.

The temperament of the child as well as that of the parent can be a causal factor. Children who are different from others in any way become particular risks. This includes preterm infants; sick, retarded, or disabled children; and merely unattractive children. Unwanted or illegitimate babies and stepchildren are particularly vulnerable. Often one child in the family is singled out to be the target of abuse. Ordinal position (e.g., oldest child, youngest child) may also have a bearing.

There are many myths about families who maltreat children. Research indicates that only a small percentage of child abusers suffer from psychosis. Not a phenomenon peculiar to the poor, child abuse crosses economic and social

| NURSING CARE PLAN 34–3 |
| :---: |
| **Selected Nursing Diagnoses for the Infant Who Fails to Thrive (Nonorganic)** |

| Goals | Nursing Interventions | Rationale |
| --- | --- | --- |

**Nursing Diagnosis:** Altered nutrition, less than body requirements, related to feeding difficulties.

| Goals | Nursing Interventions | Rationale |
| --- | --- | --- |
| Infant's nutritional status will improve as determined by height and weight parameters | 1. Assess behavior of infant and parents during feeding | 1. Often there is a history of feeding difficulties, such as poor sucking, vomiting, rumination following feedings; parent may appear indifferent to baby's needs (handles only when necessary, is disgusted with diaper change, props bottle, leaves infant unattended) |
| | 2. Provide age-appropriate diet | 2. Formula first year, followed by gradual increase of solids; watch for opportunities to teach parents about nutrition and feeding |
| | 3. Weigh daily and record | 3. Daily weights will assess progress; weigh naked on same scale and record; report a weight loss |
| | 4. Provide consistency of personnel | 4. Ensures continuity and consistency of care for baby and parents |
| | 5. Provide cuddling before and after feeding | 5. Infants who are nurtured very little may show signs of apathy, passivity, or absence of stranger anxiety; they may be watchful and do not smile; the nurse demonstrates caring by role modeling and by providing appropriate developmental stimulation |
| | 6. Encourage parents to cuddle baby | 6. Parents may not be aware of importance of touch to personality and health of child; parents may not have received loving attention themselves and therefore have difficulty expressing love and tenderness to baby |

**Nursing Diagnosis:** High risk for altered parenting related to (specify age of parents, knowledge deficit, depressed mother, etc.).

| Goals | Nursing Interventions | Rationale |
| --- | --- | --- |
| Mother states she feels more secure with baby <br><br> Mother holds and feeds baby appropriately | 1. Encourage mother (parents) to visit child and become involved in daily care | 1. Provides teaching opportunities; do not lecture, as this only intensifies parents' feelings of inadequacy; ideally, they will become more comfortable in caring for infant |
| | 2. Document teaching and parents' ability to comprehend instructions | 2. Documentation provides for continuity of care |
| | 3. Discuss developmental milestones | 3. Provides anticipatory guidance |
| | 4. Point out positive feedback from baby | 4. Parents may not notice baby's response to tender, loving care; stressing positive measure parents are taking helps them see progress |

boundaries and can exist in any neighborhood. It has been noted that people are often reluctant to report occurrences in middle- and upper-income families or when the incident involves friends or relatives. Many children suffer from the unrealistic expectations of their caretakers and the lack of knowledge concerning the developmental process in children.

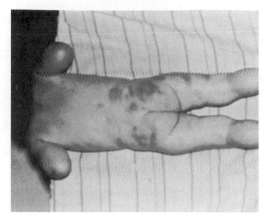

**Figure 34–4.** Child abuse. Inflicted bruises of the lower back, buttocks, and upper thighs. (From Reece, R.M., & Grodin, M.A. [1985]. Recognition of nonaccidental injury. *Pediatric Clinics of North America*, *32*, 44.)

Studies indicate that child abusers are more likely to be women.

**Federal Laws and Agencies.** By 1963 the United States Children's Bureau drafted a model mandatory state reporting law, which has been adopted in some form in all 50 states. This law aids in establishing statistics and is based on the need to provide therapeutic help to both child and family. Immunity from liability is provided for persons reporting suspected cases. Most states have penalties for failure to report child abuse. Originally, only physicians were held responsible for reporting suspected

## Nursing Brief

*Reporting suspected abuse or neglect*: A citizen can report suspected child abuse or neglect by contacting the Children's Protective Services in the yellow pages of the telephone directory under "Social Service Organizations." This can be done with or without the use of the caller's name. After obtaining the facts, the agency will inform the parents that a report is being filed and will check the condition of the child. A visit must be initiated within 72 hours. In most cases, this is accomplished within 48 hours, or earlier if the situation is life-threatening. All persons who report suspected abuse or neglect are given immunity from criminal prosecution and civil liability if the report is made in good faith. Many professionals, such as physicians, nurses, and social workers, are mandatory reporters of child abuse.

cases; however, many states now include all professionals who are in contact with children, for example, nurses, social workers, teachers, and clergy. Other laws state specifically that anyone may report an offense. Referrals usually are made to Child Protective Services, and a case worker is assigned.

**Identification and Types.** The kinds of child abuse and means of identification are listed in Table 34–5. In the past, much of the treatment of child abuse has been after-the-fact. Current literature stresses the necessity for prevention and early intervention.

Gil and others suggest three manifestations of abuse: collective, institutional, and individual. Collective abuse refers to characteristics of a society, including the nature of its social, economic, and political institutions; the amount of discrimination and violence in general; and the society's priorities. Institutional abuse occurs in day-care centers, schools, courts, child-care agencies, welfare departments, and correctional and other residential care settings. Individual abuse refers to abusive interaction between children and their caretakers in homes. Of these, Gil considers abuse at the collective level to be most severe, "for what happens at this level determines not only how children fare on the institutional level, but also, by way of complex interactions, how they fare in their own homes" (Gil, 1979).

**Nursing Care and Intervention.** The prevention of child abuse is of utmost importance (Box 34–2). One approach currently taken is identification of high-risk infants and parents during the prenatal and perinatal periods. Predictive questionnaires are being used as screening tools in some clinics. Many hospitals also provide closer follow-up of mothers and newborns. Maternal-infant bonding and its significance to later parent-child relationships have been explored.

Nurses in obstetric clinics have the opportunity to observe parents and their abilities to cope. The history of the patient, the desirability of the pregnancy, the number of children already in the family, the financial and personal stability of the family, their types of support systems, and other factors may have a bearing on how the parents accept the new offspring. Pertinent observations include a description of parent-newborn interaction. Both verbal and nonverbal communications are important, as is the level of body and eye contact. Lack of interest, indifference, or negative comments about

**Table 34–5.** HOW TO RECOGNIZE CHILD ABUSE AND NEGLECT

| Type | Child's Appearance | Child's Behavior | Parent's or Caretaker's Behavior |
|------|-------------------|------------------|----------------------------------|
| Physical abuse | Unusual bruises, welts, burns, or fractures<br>Bite marks<br>Frequent injuries, always explained as "accidents" | Reports injury by parents<br>Is unpleasant, hard to get along with, and demanding; often does not obey; frequently causes trouble or interferes with others; often breaks or damages things<br>OR<br>Is unusually shy; avoids other people, including children; seems too anxious to please; seems too ready to let other people say and do things to without protesting<br>Is frequently late for or absent from school; often comes to school much too early; hangs around after school is dismissed<br>Avoids physical contact with adults<br>Wears long sleeves or other concealing clothing to hide injuries<br>Story of how a physical injury occurred is not believable or does not seem to fit type or seriousness of injury<br>Shows little or no distress at being separated from parents<br>Seems frightened of parents<br>Is apt to seek affection from any adult | Has a history of abuse as a child<br>Uses harsh discipline that does not seem right for the age, condition, or offense of child being punished<br>Offers an explanation of child's injury that does not seem to make sense or to fit type and seriousness of injury, or offers no explanation at all<br>Seems unconcerned about child<br>Sees child as "bad," "a monster"<br>Misuses alcohol or other drugs<br>Attempts to conceal child's injury or to protect identity of person responsible |
| Neglect (physical, emotional) | Often is not clean, is tired, and has no energy<br>Comes to school without breakfast, often does not have lunch or lunch money<br>Clothes dirty or wrong for the weather<br>Seems to be alone, for long periods of time<br>Needs glasses, dental care, or other medical attention | Is frequently absent from school<br>Begs or steals food<br>Causes trouble in school; often has not done homework<br>Uses alcohol or drugs<br>Engages in vandalism or sexual misconduct | Misuses alcohol or other drugs<br>Has a disorganized, upset home life<br>Seems not to care much about what happens; gives impression of feeling nothing is going to make much difference anyway<br>Lives very much isolated from friends, relatives, neighbors<br>Does not seem to know how to get along well with others<br>Has a long-term or chronic illness<br>Has a history of neglect as a child |

*Continued*

the sex, looks, or temperament of the baby could be significant.

In other areas, a cooperative team approach is necessary. This includes providing a wide range of services, such as family planning, protective services, day-care centers, homemakers, education for parenthood classes, hotlines, self-help groups, family counseling, emergency shelters for children, child advocates, and a massive effort to reduce the incidence of preterm birth. Other related areas include financial assistance, employment services, transportation,

**Table 34–5.** HOW TO RECOGNIZE CHILD ABUSE AND NEGLECT *Continued*

| Type | Child's Appearance | Child's Behavior | Parent's or Caretaker's Behavior |
|---|---|---|---|
| Emotional abuse (often verbal) | Signs are less obvious than in other forms of mistreatment<br>Behavior is best indication | Is unpleasant, hard to get along with, and demanding; frequently causes trouble; will not let others alone<br><center>OR</center>Is unusually shy; avoids others; is too anxious to please; puts up with unpleasant acts or words from others without protesting<br>Is either unusually adult in actions or overly young for age (for example, sucks thumb, rocks constantly)<br>Is "behind" for age in physical, emotional, or intellectual development | Blames or belittles child<br>Is cold and rejecting<br>Withholds love from child<br>Treats children in family unequally<br>Does not seem to care much about child's problems |
| Sexual abuse | Has torn, stained, or bloody underclothing<br>Experiences pain or itching in genital area<br>Has venereal disease | Appears withdrawn or engages in fantasy or baby-like behavior<br>Has poor relationships with other children<br>Is unwilling to participate in physical activities<br>Is engaging in delinquent acts or runs away<br>States that she/he has been sexually assaulted by parent or caretaker | Is very protective or jealous of child<br>Encourages child to engage in prostitution or sexual acts in his or her presence<br>Misuses alcohol or other drugs<br>Is frequently absent from home |

Data from *New light on an old problem: 9 questions and answers about child abuse and neglect* (1978, pp. 6–11). (DHEW Publication No. OHDS 79-31108). Washington, DC: Head Start and National Center on Child Abuse and Neglect.

emotional support and encouragement, and long-term follow-up. More research and data services are required, as are an evaluation and reduction of violence generally occurring in our society.

Individual nurses can help detect child abuse by maintaining a high level of suspicion in their work settings. Record-keeping should be factual and objective. Pediatric nurses should make a point of reviewing old records of their patients, which may reveal repeated hospitalizations, x-ray films of multiple fractures, persistent feeding problems, history of failure to thrive, and chronic absenteeism in school. Neglect or delay in seeking medical attention for a child or failure to obtain immunization and well-child care is sometimes significant. Children who seem overly upset about being discharged need to be brought to the attention of the physician. Runaway teenagers are frequently victims of abuse.

The abused child is approached quietly, and preparation for treatments is carefully explained in advance. The number of caretakers should be kept to a minimum. The child may be able to express some hostility and fear through play or drawing (Fig. 34–5). It is not unusual for these patients to be either unresponsive or openly hostile or to show affection indiscriminately. Direct questioning is kept to a minimum. Praise is used when appropriate. Activities that promote physical and sensory development are encouraged. The nurse avoids speaking to the child about the parents in a negative manner. Other professionals are consulted about setting limits for poor behavior.

The nurse must acknowledge that in cases of child abuse there are always two victims: the child *and* the abuser. Because of personal problems, the abuser often leads an isolated life. Some have been battered or neglected children themselves. Many have unrealistic expectations

| BOX 34–2 | Ideas for Informing Children About Sexual Abuse and Preventive Measures |
|---|---|

A "good touch" is nice, like a hug, whereas a "bad touch" makes a person uncomfortable. Children need to be told, "Your body belongs to you: you can decide who touches it. Private areas are those covered by a bathing suit. If you are touched by someone and you don't like it, tell the person to stop and tell someone else about it."

Secrets and surprises are not the same. Secrets sometimes are not fair to keep. Surprises are fun; secrets are not fun if they make you feel funny or uncomfortable.

Strangers can be dangerous. Never go with someone you don't know who says anything like, "Your mother is ill and sent me to get you." or "Will you help me look for my lost puppy in the woods?"

Do not let others undress you, even if they promise to give you something such as candy or new clothes.

Do not listen when an older person tells you that they are going to help you grow up by showing you what big people do.

If you feel uncomfortable with someone, do not allow yourself to be left alone with that person.

From Mott, S., James, S.R., & Sperhac, A.M. (1992). *Nursing care of children and families:* (2nd ed.). Reading, MA: Addison-Wesley.

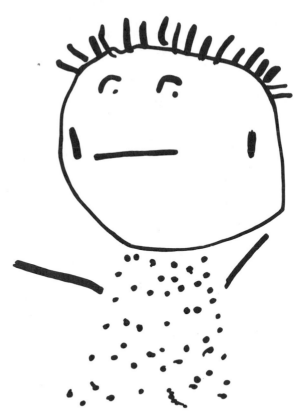

**Figure 34–5.** A 5-year-old girl's self-portrait. The child was sexually abused, and the portrait shows fear (hair standing on end), helplessness (no hands, legs, or feet), shame (bright red cheeks), and reluctance to talk of experience (tightly closed mouth). (Courtesy of Iowa Children's and Family Services, Des Moines, IA.)

about the child's intelligence and capabilities. There may be a role reversal in which the child becomes the comforter. Although removing the child from the home is one answer, many authorities believe that this can be more detrimental in the long run.

Being open to parents during this type of crisis is difficult but essential if the nurse wishes to be part of the solution rather than part of the problem. When placement in a foster home is necessary, parents experience grief, loss, and remorse. The child also mourns the loss of the family, even though there has been abuse. The nurse should be aware of the child's needs and facilitate expression of feelings of loss. The nurse who recognizes the potential for violence within us all is better able to respond to this complex problem.

## SPOUSE ABUSE

**Description.** Spouse abuse is the physical and/or emotional battering of one partner, typically the woman, by the other (Olds et al., 1992). The exact incidence is unknown. In a study of over 7000 women, 51% reported that abuse occurred at least once a week (Shaw, 1990). Such actions stem from the fact that his-

## Nursing Brief

Bruises heal in various stages that are indicated according to color (1–2 days, swollen, tender; 0–5 days, red; 5–7 days, green; 7–10 days, yellow; 10–14 days, brown; 14–28 days, clear). Does the bruise match the caretaker's explanation of what happened?

torically women and children were considered the "property" of the male. In some socioeconomic or ethnic groups, the husband is still expected to "keep his family in line." Battering tends to escalate gradually, sometimes leading to murder or suicide. It is estimated that a woman is beaten in her home every 15 seconds. Wife abuse is the most common and least reported crime in the United States. The power and control wheel (Fig. 34–6) depicts the various forms of abuse.

It is commonly thought that battering is a problem of lower-income, uneducated persons with few resources. This is a myth. Wife abuse occurs in all age groups, socioeconomic classes, races, and religions, and it is not related to educational background. However, unemployment and/or alcoholism may be precipitating factors. Many husbands lack respect for women and are described by their wives as having "a very short fuse." Some men have witnessed abuse in their families of origin.

Battered women may be reluctant to leave a bad situation because of poor self-esteem, lack of finances, and guilt feelings. They are often led to believe that they are at fault, inadequate, or stupid. Often the abuser has isolated them from family and friends. The wife may need permission to go anywhere. Many have no skills to earn a living. They may fear for their lives and the lives of their children. Such concerns frequently leave them immobilized, particularly if there is no assurance of support from their family or community.

The cycle of violence occurs in three phases. In phase one, there is increased tension, anger, blaming, and arguing. In phase two, battering occurs. There may be verbal threats and sexual

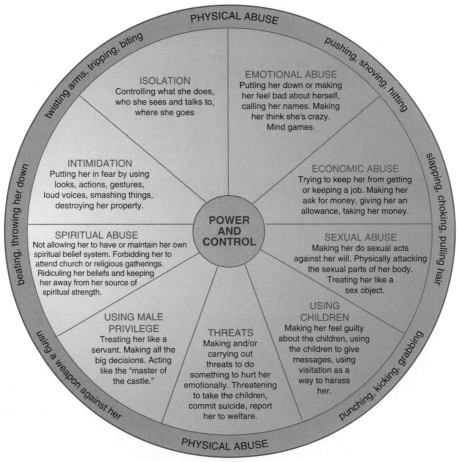

**Figure 34–6.** The power and control wheel outlining forms of abuse. (From Domestic Violence: A Guide for Health Care Providers. Section III-32. Adapted from Domestic Abuse Intervention Project, Duluth, MN.)

abuse. In phase three, a calm stage returns; however, the length of this stage may diminish over time. The abuser is contrite (e.g., vows never to do it again). Phase one redevelops and the cycle continues.

Violence in families affects children in many ways. They are exposed to violence as an acceptable method of handling aggression and of solving problems. Their role models are poor. The children learn to bully, to hit, to break things. They may evidence a lot of manipulation and control. Others become withdrawn or overly good. They learn the caretaking role early in life. Many eventually become batterers or victims. In wife-abusing families, the children are often battered as well. Therapy must be directed toward all family members.

**Nursing Interventions.** Battered women may be seen in many different settings, such as the prenatal clinic, emergency room, or outpatient clinic. Battering frequently begins during a pregnancy, when stress is heightened. These women are difficult to recognize because they often hide their bruises and are afraid to admit their problem. Some have a history of codependency, alcohol abuse, and drug abuse.

Because battering is so prevalent, the admitting nurse should maintain a high level of suspicion for the possibility of domestic violence. A detailed history of the accident may reveal pertinent information. Head injury is common, as are burns and lacerations. Often the latter are in areas of the body that are concealed by clothing. The woman may appear hesitant to provide facts about what happened. There may be a delay in reporting of symptoms, poor eye contact,

and self-deprecating comments. If the man is present, he may interrupt, answer for the patient, and remain in close proximity.

The woman is taken to a quiet, safe place, away from anyone suspected of causing the injuries. Assessment is made of specific injuries and any evidence of previous bruises in various healing stages. Any lapse between accident and arrival time is noted. The nurse also notes whether the woman is more disturbed than usual for the type of injury (e.g., uncontrollable crying, fearful affect). It is important to determine the woman's strengths and sources of support. Documentation should be specific. The nurse notes whether the injuries involve the face, head, neck, chest, or abdomen. If the nurse suspects abuse and questions the patient, an entry might read, "Patient denies physical abuse," "Patient states significant other 'flew off the handle' and pushed her against coffee table," "Woman states she was beaten," or "Woman has a history of being battered."

Other aspects of care include active listening, encouraging verbalization, pointing out strengths, acknowledging the love-hate relationships that may exist, and assisting with clarification of events. *Above all, the nurse does not blame the victim.* Educating the woman about community resources, such as shelters, counseling, financial aid, legal aid, and job training, may instill hope. Eventually such assistance may help the victim choose a direction that is more healthy for herself and her children (Nursing Care Plan 34–4). The National Domestic Violence Hotline is 1-800-333-SAFE.

---

### NURSING CARE PLAN 34–4

#### Selected Nursing Diagnoses for the Battered Woman

| Goals | Nursing Interventions | Rationale |
| --- | --- | --- |
| **Nursing Diagnosis:** Ineffective individual coping related to physical abuse evidenced by fractured wrist, bruises on head and face. | | |
| Woman will demonstrate decreased anxiety as evidenced by body language | 1. After patient's fractured wrist and bruises are treated, take to physically safe, quiet area | 1. Physical injuries are priority; it is essential to promote a sense of safety for these frightened, confused patients |
| | 2. Encourage verbalization of event | 2. Verbalization of crisis will help to diffuse feelings; nurse can clarify information by such statements as "If I understand you correctly [etc.]" or "You say he pushed you [etc.]" |

*Continued*

| | NURSING CARE PLAN 34–4 *Continued* | |
| --- | --- | --- |
| | **Selected Nursing Diagnoses for the Battered Woman** | |
| **Goals** | **Nursing Interventions** | **Rationale** |

**Nursing Diagnosis:** Ineffective individual coping related to physical abuse evidenced by fractured wrist, bruises on head and face.

| | | |
| --- | --- | --- |
| | 3. Listen nonjudgmentally | 3. Acceptance of patient is extremely important in establishing trust; patient feels highly vulnerable |
| | 4. Identify victim's strengths | 4. Helps empower patient: "Look, you came to the hospital—that took a lot of courage" |
| Patient will state telephone number of woman's shelter | 1. Contact social services to discuss community resources | 1. Social services can also provide follow-up |
| | 2. Determine support system of patient | 2. Patients with few supports will require closer supervision |
| | 3. Provide shelter number | 3. Woman needs to have an alternate plan for family safety in case abuse recurs; other family members may have witnessed crisis and need shelter and counseling; it may not be safe to call woman at home |
| | 4. Inquire about children | 4. If mother is distraught, information concerning condition of children may be haphazard or left out |

# KEY POINTS

- The American Association on Mental Deficiency defines mental retardation as "significantly subaverage general intellectual functioning existing concurrently with deficits in adaptive behavior and manifested during the developmental period."
- One intelligence test frequently given to children and adolescents is the Stanford-Binet test.
- In 1975 the United States Congress passed the Education for All Handicapped Act, which ensures that retarded persons as well as others who are physically or mentally challenged have the right to an education at public expense.
- In natural immunity, resistance is inborn. Acquired immunity results from having the disease or is artificially acquired through immunizations.
- A carrier is a person who is capable of spreading a disease but does not show evidence of it.
- The exact cause of sudden infant death syndrome is unknown.
- Nurses must deal with their own feelings of grief when caring for the dying child to avoid burnout. It is important that nurses support one another.
- The stages of dying as originally described by Elisabeth Kübler-Ross include denial, anger, bargaining, depression, and acceptance. Patients do not always go through this in a linear fashion but may go back and forth or stay fixed in one area. Patients must be allowed to proceed at their own pace.
- Child abuse may be physical, emotional, or sexual, or it may involve neglect.
- Failure to thrive may be classified as organic when there is an underlying physical problem or nonorganic when it is primarily the result of psychosocial factors involving the infant and parents.

# Study Questions

1. You are assigned to a child with a fatal illness. What responsibilities do you have to the child? The parents? Yourself? Be prepared to discuss your answer in class.
2. What facilities are available in your community for mentally retarded children?
3. List the symptoms of the following diseases: mumps, chickenpox, measles, German measles, and roseola.
4. Anthony, age 4, has chickenpox. What comfort measures might you use for Anthony? Discuss age-appropriate diversional activities and your rationale for using them.
5. Review two theories concerning crib death. How can the nurse assist grieving parents?
6. What clues might lead the nurse to suspect child abuse?
7. List four persons who are mandatory reporters of child abuse.

# Multiple Choice Review Questions

*Choose the most appropriate answer.*

1. One cause of mental retardation is
   a. meningitis
   b. scoliosis
   c. hemophilia
   d. malabsorption syndrome
2. A person who is capable of spreading a disease but does not show evidence of it is termed a
   a. carrier
   b. host
   c. fomite
   d. parasite
3. A yellow bruise is approximately
   a. 2 days old
   b. 5–7 days old
   c. 7–10 days old
   d. 10–14 days old
4. Children do not develop a realistic conception of death as a permanent biologic process until the ages of
   a. 5–7 years
   b. 9–10 years
   c. 14–15 years
   d. 3–4 years
5. Mrs. Rodriguez has just been told that 4-year-old Juan has died. He has been hospitalized for a week and has been in a coma from a head injury. Which of the following would be the most appropriate initial action for the nurse?
   a. checking to see if there will be an organ donation
   b. assuring Mrs. Rodriguez that he is in a good place
   c. calling her priest
   d. encouraging Mrs. Rodriguez to hold Juan

## BIBLIOGRAPHY

Behrman, R.E. (1992). *Nelson textbook of pediatrics* (14th ed.). Philadelphia: W.B. Saunders.

Black, J.M., & Matassarin-Jacobs, E. (1993). *Luckmann &*

*Sorensen's medical-surgical nursing* (4th ed.). Philadelphia: W.B. Saunders.

Burgess, A., et al. (1990). Assessing child abuse. The TRI-

ADS checklist. *Journal of Psychosocial Nursing and Mental Health Services, 28,* 6.

Davern, L., & Schnorr, R. (1991). Public schools welcome students with disabilities as full members. *Children Today, 20.*

Gil, D. (1979). *Child abuse and violence.* New York: AMS.

Gil, F.T. (1989). Caring for abused children in the emergency department. *Holistic Nursing Practice, 4,* 37.

Grossman, H. (1977). *Manual on terminology and classification in mental retardation.* Washington, DC: American Association on Mental Deficiency.

Hammer, M., Nichols, D., & Armstrong, L. (1992). A ritual of remembrance. *MCN: American Journal of Maternal Child Nursing, 17,* 310.

Ignatavicius, D., & Bayne, M. (1991). *Medical-surgical nursing.* Philadelphia: W.B. Saunders.

Kempe, C., & Kelfer, R. (1962). The battered child syndrome. *JAMA: Journal of the American Medical Association, 181,* 17.

King, M.C., & Ryan, J. (1989). Abused women: Dispelling myths and encouraging intervention. *Nursing Practice, 14,* 47.

Kübler-Ross, E. (1983). *On children and death.* New York: Macmillan.

Kübler-Ross, E. (1969). *On death and dying.* New York: Macmillan.

Levine, M.D., Carey, W.B., & Crocker, A.C. (1992). *Developmental-behavioral pediatrics* (2nd ed.). Philadelphia: W.B. Saunders.

Lobo, M., Barnard, K., & Coombs, J. (1992). Failure to thrive: A parent-infant interaction perspective. *Journal of Pediatric Nursing, 7,* 251.

Mott, S., James, S.R., & Sperhac, A.M. (1992). *Nursing care of children and families* (2nd ed.). Reading, MA: Addison-Wesley.

New Hampshire Coalition Against Domestic and Sexual Violence. (1989). A fact sheet on domestic violence. Concord, NH: Author.

NiCarthy, G. (1982). *Getting free. A handbook for women in abusive relationships* (2nd ed.). Seattle: The Seal Press.

Olds, S., London, M., & Ladewig, P. (1992). *Maternal-newborn nursing* (4th ed.). Reading, MA: Addison-Wesley Nursing.

Petrillo, M., & Sanger, S. (1980). *Emotional care of hospitalized children.* Philadelphia: J.B. Lippincott.

Pillitteri, A. (1992). *Maternal and child health nursing.* Philadelphia: J.B. Lippincott.

Shaw, B. (1990). Woman abuse: Frequent and severe. Springfield, IL: Illinois Coalition Against Domestic Violence.

Spinetta, J., et al. (1983). *Emotional aspects of childhood leukemia.* New York: Leukemia Society of America.

Thompson, E.D., & Ashwill, J.W. (1992). *Pediatric nursing: An introductory text* (6th ed.). Philadelphia: W.B. Saunders.

Varvaro, F., & Lasko, D. (1993). Physical abuse as cause of injury in women: Information for orthopaedic nurses. *Orthopaedic Nursing, 12.*

Warda, M. (1992). The family and chronic sorrow: Role theory approach. *Journal of Pediatric Nursing, 7,* 205.

Whaley, L., & Wong, D. (1991). *Nursing care of infants and children* (4th ed.). St. Louis: C.V. Mosby.

Zylke, J. (1989, September). Sudden infant death syndrome. *JAMA: Journal of the American Medical Association.*

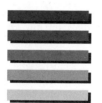

# Glossary

**abdominal:** pertaining to the abdomen.

**abdominal delivery:** cesarean birth.

**abortion:** end of a pregnancy before the fetus is viable (20 weeks' gestation), whether spontaneous or elective.

**abruptio placentae:** premature separation of a normally implanted placenta.

**abuse:** to attack or cause injury—physical, emotional, or spiritual.

**acme:** peak, or period of greatest strength, of a uterine contraction.

**acrocyanosis:** peripheral blueness of the hands and feet, which is normal in newborns.

**adolescence:** period of human development beginning with puberty and ending with young adulthood.

**afterbirth:** placenta and membranes delivered during the third stage of labor.

**afterpains:** painful contractions of uterus that occur for several days after delivery; occur most often in multiparas and are more painful during breast feeding.

**AIDS:** acquired immunodeficiency syndrome, caused by HIV; characterized by depression of the immune system and opportunistic infection; seen in newborns and infants who live in high-risk populations and in children with hemophilia and other conditions who have received contaminated blood products.

**amenorrhea:** absence or suppression of menstruation; normal before puberty, during pregnancy and lactation, and after menopause.

**amniocentesis:** transabdominal puncture of the amniotic sac (fetal membranes) to obtain a sample of fluid for study.

**amnioinfusion:** infusion of warmed saline into the uterus to relieve cord compression or to wash meconium out of the cavity to prevent aspiration at birth.

**amnion:** the inner of the two fetal membranes; thin and transparent; holds fetus suspended in amniotic fluid.

**amniotic fluid:** transparent, almost colorless fluid contained in the fetal membranes/amnion; protects fetus from injury, maintains even temperature, and allows fetal movement.

**amniotic sac:** the sac formed by the amnion and chorion that contains fluid and the fetus.

**analgesic:** a drug that relieves pain but does not produce unconsciousness.

**androgen:** a substance that stimulates masculinization, such as the male hormones testosterone and androsterone.

**android pelvis:** a female pelvis with masculine size and shape.

**anesthesia:** partial or complete loss of sensation, especially of pain, with or without loss of consciousness.

**angioma:** a tumor, usually benign, that is made up chiefly of blood and lymph vessels.

**animism:** a period of cognitive development in which the child attributes life to inanimate objects.

**anomaly:** not normal in form, structure, or position; birth defect or congenital abnormality.

**anorexia nervosa:** a syndrome most often seen in adolescent girls, characterized by an extreme form of poor appetite or self-starvation. Although its onset may be acute, the underlying emotional problem develops over a relatively long period of time.

**anoxia:** absence of oxygen.

**antenatal:** before birth.

**antepartum:** before the onset of labor.

**anterior:** pertaining to front.

**anterior fontanel:** diamond-shaped area between the two frontal and the two parietal bones of the newborn's head; the soft spot.

**anthropoid pelvis:** a female pelvis with a transverse diameter that is equal to or smaller than the anteroposterior diameter.

**antibody:** specific protein substance, formed in the body in response to antigens, that restricts or destroys the antigens.

**antigen:** a substance that induces formation of antibodies that interact specifically with it. This antigen-antibody reaction forms the basis for immunity.

**Apgar score:** an evaluation tool with a maximum score of 10, used to assess a newborn at 1 minute and 5 minutes after delivery. Five signs, scored 0, 1, or 2, are heart rate, color, muscle tone, reflex irritability, and respiratory effort.

**aplastic anemia:** anemia caused by deficient red blood cell production because of bone marrow dysfunction.

**apnea:** cessation of respirations.

**areola:** pigmented circle of tissue around the nipple of the breast.

**AROM:** artificial rupture of (amniotic) membranes with a sterile instrument, such as an Amnihook or Allis clamp.

**arthroscopy:** direct visualization of a joint by means of an arthroscope.

**artificial insemination:** mechanical injection of viable semen into the vagina for the purpose of impregnation.

**ascariasis:** roundworm infestation.

**asphyxia:** reduced amount of oxygen or an increased amount of carbon dioxide in the body.

**asynchrony:** lack of concurrence in time. The appearance of a growing child may be gangling because of asynchrony of growth, i.e., different body parts maturing at different rates.

**atelectasis:** incomplete expansion of the lungs or a collapse after expansion due to mucous plug, tumor, pressure from organs, and other causes.

**atresia:** a congenital anomaly in which a normal opening is absent, e.g., atresia of the esophagus.

**augmentation of labor:** stimulation of labor after it has begun.

**autism:** a severe type of pervasive developmental disorder in which the child becomes absorbed in himself or herself, excluding reality.

**autoimmunity:** a condition in which the body produces antibodies against its own tissues.

**autonomy:** functioning independently; self-control.

**bacteriuria:** presence of bacteria in the urine.

**bag of waters:** the membrane containing the amniotic fluid and the fetus.

**ballottement:** In obstetrics, the fetus, when pushed, floats away and then returns to touch the examiner's fingers.

**barrier technique:** a method of medical asepsis using various types of isolation. In contraception, a method in which sperm are prevented from entering the cervix.

**Bartholin's glands:** two small mucous glands situated on each side of the vaginal orifice that secrete small amounts of mucus during coitus (intercourse).

**bilirubin:** orange or yellowish pigment in bile; a breakdown product of hemoglobin carried by the blood to the liver, where it is chemically changed and excreted in bile or is conjugated and excreted in the stools.

**bleb:** an irregularly shaped elevation of the epidermis; a blister or bulla.

**bonding:** attachment; the process whereby a unique relationship is established between two people; used in conjunction with parent-newborn ties.

**bone marrow transplant:** transplantation of bone marrow from one person to another; currently used to treat aplastic anemia and leukemia.

**booster injection:** administration of a substance in order to renew or increase the effectiveness of a prior immunization injection, e.g., a tetanus booster.

**bougie:** a thin flexible tube used to dilate a body cavity (may be used to dilate the esophagus in corrosive strictures).

**Bradford frame:** a special oblong frame made of 1-inch pipe, covered with canvas strips, and supported by blocks to raise it from the mattress. The canvas strips are movable; thus the patient can urinate and defecate without moving the spine.

**Braxton Hicks contractions:** intermittent contractions of the uterus; they occur more frequently toward the end of pregnancy and are sometimes mistaken for true labor contractions.

**breech presentation:** a birth in which the buttocks or feet, or both, present instead of the head; occurs in approximately 3% of all deliveries.

**Broviac catheter:** a central venous line used in small children who require total parenteral or continuous intravenous infusion.

**brown fat:** also called "brown adipose tissue"; forms in the fetus around the kidneys, adrenals, and neck; between the scapulae; and behind the sternum. Its dark brown hue is due to its density, enriched blood supply, and abundant nerve supply. Its main purpose is heat production in the neonate.

**Bryant traction:** a type of traction apparatus commonly used for toddlers suffering from a fractured femur. Vertical suspension is used.

**bulimia:** a neurotic disorder seen in female adolescents and young women who wish to remain thin; characterized by overeating and induced vomiting, fasting, and use of purgatives.

**café-au-lait spots:** light brown patch spots on the skin characteristic of neurofibromatosis (condition of tumors of various sizes on peripheral nerves).

**caput:** the head; the occiput of the fetal head, which appears at the vaginal introitus prior to delivery of the head.

**caput succedaneum:** swelling or edema occurring in the fetal scalp during labor; usually simply called "caput."

**cardiac decompensation:** heart failure.

**catecholamines:** a group of compounds, including epinephrine and dopamine, that have a marked effect on nervous, cardiovascular, and other systems.

**celiac disease:** an inability to absorb fats, which results in malnutrition, vitamin deficiency, foul bulky stools, and a distended abdomen.

**cephalohematoma:** subcutaneous swelling containing blood, found on the head of an infant several days after delivery; usually disappears within a few weeks to 2 months.

**cephalic presentation:** birth in which the fetal head is presenting against the cervix.

**cephalocaudal:** the orderly development of muscular control, which proceeds from head to foot.

**cephalopelvic disproportion (CPD):** a condition in which the fetus cannot pass through the maternal pelvis. Also called fetopelvic disproportion.

**cerebral palsy:** a group of nonprogressive disorders that affect the motor centers of the brain.

**certified nurse-midwife (CNM):** registered nurse who has received special training and education in the care of the family during childbearing and the prenatal, labor and delivery, and postpartum periods. After a period of formal education, the nurse-midwife takes a certification test to become a CNM.

**cerumen:** ear wax.

**cervical os:** the small opening of the cervix that dilates during the first stage of labor.

**cervix:** the lower part of the uterus.

**cesarean birth:** delivery of the fetus by means of an incision into the abdominal wall and the uterus; abdominal delivery.

**Chadwick's sign:** violet-bluish color of vaginal mucous membrane caused by increased vascularity; visible about the 4th week of pregnancy.

**chickenpox:** a communicable disease of childhood; varicella. It is caused by the varicella virus and is characterized by successive crops of macules, papules, vesicles, and crusts.

**chignon:** newborn scalp edema created by vacuum extractor.

**chloasma:** brownish pigmentation over the bridge of the nose and cheeks during pregnancy and in some women who are taking oral contraceptives; mask of pregnancy.

**chordee:** a congenital anomaly in which a fibrous strand of tissue extends from the scrotum to the penis, preventing urination with the penis in the normal elevated position; commonly associated with hypospadias.

**chorion:** the fetal membrane closest to the interior uterine wall; it gives rise to the placenta and continues as the outer membrane surrounding the amnion.

**chorionic villi:** threadlike projections on the chorionic surface of the placenta; they help form the placenta and secrete human chorionic gonadotropin.

**chromosome:** structure composed of tightly packed DNA found in the nuclei of plant and animal cells, responsible for the transmission of hereditary characteristics.

**chronic ulcerative colitis:** a serious chronic inflammatory disease of the large intestine.

**circumcision:** the surgical removal of the foreskin of the penis.

**cleft lip and palate:** congenital anomalies due to failure of the embryonic structures of the face to unite; characterized by an opening in the upper lip and/or palate.

**clitoris:** female organ homologous to male penis; a small oval body of erectile tissue situated at the anterior junction of the vulva.

**clubfoot:** a congenital orthopedic anomaly, characterized by a foot that has been twisted inward or outward.

**coarctation of the aorta:** a constriction of the aortic arch or of the descending aorta.

**coccyx:** a small bone at the base of the spinal column.

**coitus:** sexual intercourse.

**colostrum:** secretion from the breast before onset of true lactation; it has a high protein content, provides some immune properties, and cleanses the newborn's intestinal tract of mucus and meconium.

**comedo:** a skin lesion caused by a plug of keratin, sebum, and bacteria; there are two types, blackheads and whiteheads.

**conception:** union of male sperm and female ovum; fertilization.

**congenital:** present at birth.

**congenital anomaly:** a malformation present at birth.

**contraception:** prevention of conception or impregnation.

**contraction:** tightening and shortening of uterine muscles during labor, causing effacement and dilation of the cervix; contributes to downward and outward movement of fetus.

**contraction stress test (CST):** a method for assessing the reaction (or response) of the fetus to stress of uterine contractions. This test may be utilized when contractions are occurring spontaneously or when contractions are artificially induced by oxytocin challenge test (OCT) or breast self-stimulation test (BSST).

**couvade:** a syndrome in which the father experiences the symptoms of the pregnant partner.

**craniosynostosis:** premature closure of the cranial sutures that produces a head deformity and damage to the brain and eyes; craniostenosis.

**cretinism:** a congenital defect in the secretion of the thyroid hormones, characterized by physical and mental retardation.

**Crohn's disease:** regional enteritis; inflammation is most often found in the anus and ileum.

**crowning:** appearance of presenting fetal part at vaginal orifice during labor.

**cryptorchidism:** failure of the testicles to descend into the scrotum.

**cystic fibrosis:** a generalized disorder of the exocrine glands, especially the mucous and sweat glands. The lungs and pancreas in particular are involved.

**cystic hygroma:** a lymphangioma most frequently seen in the neck and axillae.

**DDST:** Denver Developmental Screening Test. Assesses the developmental status of a child during the first 6 years of life in five areas: personal, social, fine motor adaptive, language, and gross motor activities.

**deceleration:** periodic decrease in baseline fetal heart rate.

**decidua basalis:** the part of the decidua that unites with the chorion to form the placenta. It is shed in lochial discharge after delivery.

**deciduous teeth:** baby teeth.

**decrement:** decrease or stage of decline, as of contraction.

**delivery:** expulsion of infant with placenta and membranes from the woman at birth.

**Denis Browne splint:** two separate footplates attached to a crossbar and fitted to a child's shoes, used in the correction of clubfeet.

**developmental task:** a skill that occurs at a particular time and when accomplished provides the basis for future tasks.

**diaphoresis:** profuse sweating.

**diploid:** containing a set of maternal and a set of paternal chromosomes. In humans, the diploid number of chromosomes is 46.

**disseminated intravascular coagulation (DIC):** a secondary disease characterized by abnormal overstimulation of the coagulation process.

**dizygotic twins:** fetuses that develop from two fertilized ova; fraternal twins.

**DNA (deoxyribonucleic acid):** a complex molecule that is the storehouse of hereditary information. It is present in the chromosomes of cell nuclei.

**Down syndrome:** a form of mental retardation caused by chromosomal defects.

**Duchenne's muscular dystrophy:** a genetically determined progressive muscular disorder.

**ductus arteriosus, patent:** see patent ductus arteriosus.

**dyscrasia:** a disease that is usually undefined and associated with blood disorders.

**dysfunctional:** inadequate, abnormal.

**dysfunctional uterine bleeding:** abnormal bleeding from uterus for reasons that are not readily established.

**dyspareunia:** painful sexual intercourse.

**dystocia:** difficult labor due to mechanical factors produced by the fetus or the maternal pelvis, or due to inadequate uterine or other muscular activity.

**eclampsia:** pregnancy-induced hypertension complicated by one or more seizures.

**ectoderm:** outer layer of cells in the developing embryo that give rise to the skin, nails, and hair.

**cctopic pregnancy:** implantation of fertilized ovum outside uterine cavity; most common ectopic site is the fallopian tube.

**eczema:** an inflammation of the skin, frequently associated with an allergy to food protein or environment.

**effacement:** thinning and shortening of the cervix that occurs late in pregnancy and during labor.

**egocentrism:** a kind of thinking in which a child has difficulty seeing anyone else's point of view; this self-centering is normal in young children.

**embryo:** early stage of development. In humans, the period from about 2 to 8 weeks' gestation, characterized by cellular differentiation and predominantly hyperplastic growth.

**empyema:** pus, especially in the chest cavity.

**encephalitis:** an inflammation of the brain.

**encopresis:** the passage of stools in a child's underwear or other inappropriate places after the age of 4 years. Some children display concurrent behavioral problems.

**endoderm:** inner layer of cells in a developing embryo that give rise to internal organs such as the intestines.

**endometrium:** the mucous membrane that lines the inner surface of the uterus.

**engagement:** entrance of fetal presenting part into the pelvis; the leading edge of the fetal head is at the level of the maternal ischial spines in a vertex presentation.

**engorgement:** vascular congestion or distention. In obstetrics, the swelling of breast tissue brought about by an increase in blood and lymph supply to breast, preceding true lactation.

**enuresis:** abnormal inability to control urine; may be due to organic, allergic, or psychological problems.

**epidural block:** regional anesthetic block achieved by injecting local anesthetic agent in the space overlying the dura of the spinal cord.

**epilepsy:** a convulsive disease, characterized by seizures and loss of consciousness.

**episiotomy:** incision of the perineum to facilitate delivery and to avoid laceration of perineum.

**epispadias:** a congenital anomaly in which the urethral meatus is located on the upper (dorsal) surface of the penis.

**erythroblastosis fetalis:** pathologic he-
molytic anemia due to blood incompatibility. Associated with babies born of Rh-positive fathers and Rh-negative mothers.

**estimated date of delivery (EDD):** "due date."

**estrogen:** the hormones estradiol and estrone, produced by the ovaries.

**Ewing's sarcoma:** endothelioma that occurs in long bones and in flat bones such as the pelvis, ribs, and scapulae.

**external os:** lower cervical opening.

**facies:** pertaining to the appearance or expression of the face; certain congenital syndromes typically present with specific facial appearance.

**fallopian tubes:** tubes that extend from the uterus to the ovaries. They serve as a passageway for ova from the ovary to the uterus and for spermatozoa from the uterus toward the ovary; oviducts; uterine tubes.

**false labor:** contractions of the uterus, regular or irregular, that may be strong enough to be interpreted as true labor but do not dilate the cervix.

**family Apgar:** screening test that reveals how a member of the family perceives its function.

**fertility rate:** number of births per 1000 women age 15–44 in a given population per year.

**fertilization:** union of an ovum and a sperm.

**fetal:** pertaining or relating to the fetus.

**fetal alcohol syndrome (FAS):** syndrome caused by maternal alcohol ingestion and characterized by microencephaly, intrauterine growth retardation, short palpebral fissures, and maxillary hypoplasia.

**fetal death:** death of developing fetus after 20 weeks' gestation; fetal demise.

**fetal heart rate (FHR):** the number of times the fetal heart beats per minute; normal range is 110–160 beats/min at term.

**fetal heart tones (FHTs):** the fetal heartbeat as heard through the mother's abdominal wall.

**fetoscope:** a stethoscope specially adapted to facilitate listening to the fetal heart.

**fetus:** term used for the developing structure from the 8th week after fertilization until birth.

**first stage of labor:** stage beginning with the first contractions of true labor and completed when the cervix is fully dilated to 10 cm.

**flexion:** in obstetrics, a situation that occurs when resistance to the descent of the infant down the birth canal causes its head to flex or bend, the chin approaching the chest, thus reducing the diameter of the presenting part.

**follicle-stimulating hormone (FSH):** hormone produced by the anterior pituitary gland during the first half of the menstrual cycle, stimulating development of the graafian follicle.

**fontanels:** openings at the point of union of skull bones, often referred to as "soft spots."

**footling:** a breech presentation in which one foot or both feet present.

**forceps:** obstetric instruments occasionally used to aid in birth by assisting fetal rotation and/or descent.

**foreskin:** the fold of loose skin covering the end of the penis; prepuce.

**Friedman graph:** a method of describing and recording the progress of labor.

**fulminating:** occurring rapidly; usually said of a disease.

**fundus:** the upper portion of the uterus between the fallopian tubes.

**gamete:** a mature germ cell; an ovum or sperm.

**gavage:** feeding the patient by means of a stomach tube or with a tube passed through the nose, pharynx, and esophagus into the stomach.

**gene:** smallest unit of inheritance; genes are located on the chromosomes.

**genetics:** the study of heredity.

**geographic tongue:** unusual patterns of papilla formation and denuded areas on the tongue.

**gestation:** period of intrauterine development from conception through birth; pregnancy.

**glioma:** sarcoma involving the support tissue or glial cells of the brain.

**glucometer:** a meter used to measure blood glucose.

**gonad:** sex gland; ovaries in the female and testes in the male.

**Goodell's sign:** softening of cervix that occurs during 2nd month of pregnancy.

**graafian follicle:** the ovarian cyst containing the ripe ovum; it secretes estrogens.

**gravid:** pregnant.

**gravida:** the number of times a woman has been pregnant; a pregnant woman.

**haploid:** one member of each pair of chromosomes. In humans there are 23 chromosomes, the haploid number, in each germ cell (ovum or sperm).

**Hegar's sign:** softening of the lower uterine segment found upon palpation in the 2nd or 3rd month of pregnancy.

**hemangioma:** a benign tumor of the skin that consists of blood vessels.

**hemophilia:** a hereditary disease characterized by an abnormal tendency to bleed.

**hemorrhoids:** varicose veins of the rectum; may be external or internal.

**Henoch-Schönlein purpura:** an allergic purpura seen in children generally between the ages of 2 and 8 years. Can be caused by medication, insect bites, or other factors.

**herpesvirus:** a family of viruses characterized by the development of clusters of small vesicles. The infection is recurring and is frequently found about the lips and nares; a genital form also exists that is primarily sexually transmitted.

**Hickman catheter:** a tiny catheter that is inserted into a chest vein to establish a long- or short-term central venous line. Used mainly in adults and teen-agers.

**Hirschsprung's disease:** megacolon; enlargement of the colon without evidence of mechanical obstruction. There is a congenital absence of ganglionic cells in the distal segment of the colon.

**holism:** an approach to caring for a person that recognizes and adapts to her physical, intellectual, emotional, and spiritual nature; a way of relating to the patient as a whole or biopsychosocial individual rather than just a person with an ailment.

**hormone:** substance produced in an organ or gland and conveyed by blood to another part of the body in order to exert an effect.

**human chorionic gonadotropin (hCG):** hormone produced by chorionic villi and found in the urine of pregnant women.

**human immunodeficiency virus (HIV):** the organism that causes AIDS.

**hyaline membrane disease:** respiratory distress often seen in preterm infants, in which a membranous substance lines the alveoli of the lungs, preventing the exchange of gases.

**hydatidiform mole:** degenerative process in chorionic villi, giving rise to multiple cysts and rapid growth of the uterus with hemorrhage.

**hydramnios:** an excess of amniotic fluid, leading to overdistention of the uterus. Frequently seen in diabetic pregnant women even if there is not coexisting fetal anomaly; polyhydramnios.

**hydrocele:** an abnormal collection of fluid

surrounding the testicles, causing the scrotum to swell.

**hydrocephalus:** a congenital anomaly characterized by an increase of cerebrospinal fluid in the ventricles of the brain, which results in an increase in the size of the head and in pressure changes in the brain.

**hymen:** membranous fold that normally partially covers the entrance to the vagina.

**hypercapnia:** increased amount of carbon dioxide in the blood.

**hyperemesis gravidarum:** excessive vomiting during pregnancy, leading to dehydration and starvation.

**hypernatremia:** excess sodium in the blood.

**hypokalemia:** potassium deficit in the blood.

**hypospadias:** a developmental anomaly in which the urethra opens on the lower surface of the penis.

**icterus neonatorum:** jaundice in the newborn.

**imperforate anus:** a congenital anomaly in which there is no anal opening.

**impetigo:** an infectious disease of the skin caused by staphylococci or streptococci.

**implantation:** embedding of fertilized ovum in uterine mucosa 6 or 7 days after fertilization.

**impregnate:** to make pregnant or to fertilize.

**incarcerated:** confined, constricted.

**incest:** sexual activities among family members. Often seen in father-daughter relationships, less frequently in mother-son or sibling relationships.

**incompetent cervix:** a mechanical defect in the cervix, making it unable to remain closed throughout pregnancy.

**increment:** increase or addition; to build up, as of a contraction.

**induction:** artificial initiation of labor.

**infant mortality:** the ratio between the number of deaths of infants less than 1 year of age during any given year and the number of live births occurring in the same year.

**infanticide:** the killing of an infant.

**infectious mononucleosis:** a generalized disease causing enlargement of the lymph tissues throughout the body. There is an increase in the number of mononuclear leukocytes in the blood. It occurs mainly in older children and adolescents.

**inlet of the pelvis:** the upper opening into the pelvic cavity.

**innominate bone:** the hip bone, ilium, ischium, and pubis.

**interatrial septal defect:** an abnormal opening between the right and left atria of the heart. Blood that contains oxygen is forced from the left to the right atrium.

**intertrigo:** a chafe of the skin that occurs when two skin surfaces come together.

**interventricular septal defect:** an opening between the right and the left ventricles of the heart. Blood passes directly from the left to the right ventricle.

**intussusception:** the slipping of one part of an intestine into another part just below it, often noted in the ileocecal region.

**in vitro fertilization:** test tube fertilization in which the ripe ovum is collected and fertilized in vitro (in glass) by sperm from the woman's husband. The embryo is then transferred to the woman's uterus.

**involution:** rolling or turning inward; reduction in the size of the uterus following delivery.

**karyotype:** the chromosomal makeup of a body cell, arranged from largest to smallest. The normal number of chromosomes in humans is 46.

**kernicterus:** a grave form of jaundice of the newborn, accompanied by brain damage.

**kwashiorkor:** extreme protein malnutrition seen in infants and children living in poverty.

**labia:** in obstetrics, the external folds of skin on either side of the vulva.

**labia majora:** the larger outer folds of skin on either side of the vulva.

**labia minora:** the smaller inner folds of skin on either side of the vulva.

**labor:** the process by which the fetus is expelled from the uterus; childbirth; confinement; parturition.

**laceration:** in obstetrics, a tear in the perineum, vagina, or cervix.

**lactase:** the enzyme that breaks down lactose.

**lactation:** process of producing and supplying breast milk.

**lactiferous ducts:** tiny tubes within the breast that conduct milk from the acini cells to the nipple.

**lactogenic hormone:** hormone produced by the anterior pituitary gland to promote growth of breast tissue and to stimulate production of milk.

**lanugo hair:** fine, downy hair seen on all parts of the fetus, except the palms of the hands and soles of the feet, by the end of 20 weeks of gestation.

**laryngotracheobronchitis:** inflammation of the larynx, trachea, and bronchi.

**Legg-Calvé-Perthes disease:** inadequate blood supply to the head of the femur characterized by pain in the hip joint; flat hip.

**letdown reflex:** pattern of stimulation, hormone release, and muscle contraction that forces milk into the lactiferous ducts, making it available to the infant; milk ejection reflex.

**lightening:** moving of the fetus and uterus downward into the pelvic cavity.

**linea nigra:** line of darker pigmentation extending from the pubis to the umbilicus noted in some women during later months of pregnancy.

**lochia:** maternal discharge of blood, mucus, and tissue from the uterus that may last for several weeks after birth.

**lochia alba:** white vaginal discharge that follows lochia serosa and that lasts from about the 10th to the 21st day after delivery.

**lochia rubra:** red, blood-tinged vaginal discharge that occurs following delivery and lasts 2–4 days.

**lochia serosa:** pink, serous, and blood-tinged vaginal discharge that follows lochia rubra and lasts until the 7th–10th day after delivery.

**L/S ratio:** the ratio of the phospholipids lecithin and sphingomyelin produced by the fetal lungs; useful in assessing fetal lung maturity.

**lunar month:** a 28-day cycle corresponding to the phases of the moon. A normal pregnancy lasts 10 lunar months.

**lupus erythematosus:** a chronic inflammatory disease of collagen or connective tissue that may be life-threatening.

**luteinizing hormone (LH):** anterior pituitary hormone responsible for stimulating ovulation and for development of the corpus luteum.

**mammary glands:** compound glandular elements of the breast that in the female secrete milk to nourish the infant.

**maternal mortality:** number of deaths from any cause during the pregnancy cycle per 100,000 live births.

**McDonald's sign:** a probable sign of pregnancy, in which the examiner can easily flex the body of the uterus against the cervix.

**mechanisms (cardinal movements) of labor:** the positional changes of the fetus as it moves through the birth canal during labor and delivery.

**Meckel's diverticulum:** a congenital blind pouch, sometimes seen in the lower part of the ileum. A cord may continue to the umbilicus or a fistula may open at the umbilicus. An intestinal obstruction may occur if the cord becomes strangulated. Corrected by surgery.

**meconium:** the first stool of the newborn; a mixture of amniotic fluid and secretions of the intestinal glands.

**meconium ileus:** a deficiency of pancreatic enzymes in the intestinal tract in which the meconium of the fetus becomes excessively sticky and adheres to the intestinal wall, causing obstruction. Occasionally seen in babies born with cystic fibrosis.

**meconium-stained fluid:** amniotic fluid that contains meconium.

**megacolon:** Hirschsprung's disease.

**meiosis:** cell division to halve number of chromosomes in the ova and sperm to 23.

**menarche:** beginning of menstrual and reproductive function in girls.

**meningocele:** a congenital anomaly caused by a protrusion of the meninges or membranes through an opening in the spinal column.

**meningomyelocele:** a congenital anomaly characterized by a protrusion of the membranes and spinal cord through an opening in the spinal column.

**menopause:** the permanent cessation of menses.

**menstrual cycle:** cyclic build-up of uterine lining, ovulation, and sloughing of the lining occurring approximately every 28 days in nonpregnant females.

**menstruation (menses):** shedding of uterine lining at the end of the menstrual cycle, resulting in a bloody discharge from the vagina.

**mesoderm:** intermediate layer of germ cells in embryo that gives rise to connective tissue, bone marrow, muscles, blood, lymphoid tissue, and epithelial tissue.

**microcephaly:** a congenital anomaly in which the head of the newborn is abnormally small.

**miliaria:** prickly heat; inflammation of the skin caused by sweating.

**miscarriage:** lay term for spontaneous abortion.

**mitosis:** cell division in all body cells other than the gametes (ova and sperm).

**molding:** shaping of fetal head to facilitate movement through birth canal during labor.

**monozygotic twins:** two fetuses that develop from a single divided fertilized ovum; identical twins.

**mons veneris:** fleshy tissue over the female symphysis pubis, from which hair develops at puberty.

**Montgomery's glands:** small nodules located around the nipples that enlarge during pregnancy and lactation. They produce moisturizing secretion.

**morbidity:** pertains to illness, disease.

**morning sickness:** nausea and vomiting occurring during the 1st trimester of pregnancy; may occur at any time during the day.

**Moro reflex:** when a newborn is jarred, the legs draw up and the arms fold across the chest.

**mortality:** pertains to death.

**mucous plug:** a collection of thick mucus that blocks the cervical canal during pregnancy.

**mucoviscidosis:** cystic fibrosis.

**multifactorial:** the result of many factors, such as a disease resulting from the combined action of several conditions.

**multifetal pregnancy:** a pregnancy in which the woman is carrying two or more fetuses; also called multiple gestation.

**multigravida:** a woman who has been previously pregnant.

**multipara:** a woman who has had more than one pregnancy in which the fetus(es) was viable ($\geq 20$ weeks' gestation).

**murmur:** a sound heard when listening to the heart, caused by blood leaking through openings that have not closed before birth, as is normal.

**muscular dystrophy:** wasting away and atrophy of muscles. There are several forms, all having some common characteristics.

**mutation:** a change in genetic material.

**Nägele's rule:** a method of determining the estimated date of delivery (EDD): after obtaining the 1st day of the last menstrual period, subtract 3 months and add 7 days.

**neonatal mortality rate:** number of deaths of infants in the first 28 days per 1000 live births.

**nevus (pl, nevi):** a congenital discoloration of an area of the skin, such as a strawberry mark or mole.

**Niemann-Pick disease:** a hereditary disease in which there is a disturbance in the metabolism of lipids (substances resembling fats), causing physical and mental retardation.

**NST:** nonstress test. An assessment method by which the reaction (or response) of the fetal heart rate to fetal movement is evaluated.

**nuchal:** pertaining to the neck.

**nuclear family:** family group consisting of one or more adults and one or more children.

**nulligravida:** a female who has never been pregnant.

**nullipara:** a female who has not delivered a live fetus.

**obstetrics:** the branch of medicine concerned with the care of women during pregnancy, childbirth, and the postpartum period.

**occiput:** the posterior part of the skull.

**oligohydramnios:** decreased amount of amniotic fluid.

**oliguria:** decrease in urine secretion by the kidney.

**omphalocele:** a herniation of abdominal contents at the umbilicus.

**ophthalmia neonatorum:** acute conjunctivitis of the newborn, often caused by the gonococci of gonorrhea.

**orthopnea:** a disorder in which the patient has to sit up in order to breathe.

**Osgood-Schlatter disease:** tendinitis of the knee seen in adolescents who participate in sports.

**osteochondroma:** benign tumor composed of cartilage and bone.

**osteogenesis imperfecta:** a congenital bone disease in which the bones fracture easily.

**osteosarcoma:** the malignant bone tumor most frequently encountered in children.

**otitis media:** inflammation of the middle ear.

**ovary:** female sex gland in which the ova are formed and in which estrogen and progesterone are produced. Normally there are two ovaries, located in the lower abdomen on each side of the uterus.

**ovulation:** normal process of discharging a mature ovum from an ovary approximately 14 days prior to the onset of menses.

**ovum:** female reproductive cell; egg.

**oxytocics:** drugs that intensify uterine contractions to hasten birth or control postpartum hemorrhage.

**oxytocin challenge test (OCT):** see contraction stress test (CST).

**para:** a woman who has borne offspring who reached the age of viability (>20 weeks' gestation).

**paraphimosis:** impaired circulation of the uncircumcised penis due to improper retraction of the foreskin.

**parity:** the condition of having borne offspring who attained the age of viability. The number of pregnancies that ended after 20 weeks' gestation.

**parturient:** pertaining to the act of childbirth. A woman giving birth.

**parturition:** the process of giving birth.

**patent ductus arteriosus:** one of the most common cardiac anomalies, in which the ductus arteriosus fails to close. Blood continues to flow from the aorta into the pulmonary artery.

**pectus excavatum:** a variation in the normal configuration of the chest in which the lower portion of the sternum is depressed.

**pelvis:** the lower portion of the trunk of the body, bounded by the hip bones, coccyx, and sacrum.

**penis:** the male organ of copulation, reproduction, and urination.

**perineum:** the area of tissue between the anus and the scrotum in males or between the anus and the vagina in females.

**phenotype:** the whole physical, biochemical, and physiologic makeup of an individual as determined both genetically and environmentally.

**phenylalanine:** a naturally occurring amino acid essential for optimum growth and nitrogen balance in humans.

**phenylketonuria (PKU):** a recessive hereditary metabolic error that causes the build-up of phenylalanine, leading to mental retardation, brain damage, light pigmentation, and other characteristics. Can be treated with a low-phenylalanine diet.

**phimosis:** a tightening of the prepuce of the uncircumcised penis.

**phocomelia:** absence of or incomplete formation and development of arms, forearms, thighs, and legs. Hands and feet are present but may be abnormally developed.

**phototherapy:** the treatment of disease by exposure to light. Used frequently to treat physiologic jaundice in the newborn.

**pica:** the eating of substances not ordinarily considered edible or to have nutritive value.

**PIH:** pregnancy-induced hypertension, characterized by hypertension, albuminuria, and edema.

**placenta:** specialized disk-shaped organ that connects the fetus to the uterine wall for gas, nutrient, and waste exchanges; afterbirth.

**placenta previa:** abnormal implantation of the placenta in the lower uterine segment.

**placental souffle:** soft blowing sounds produced by blood coursing through the placenta; has the same rate as the maternal pulse.

**poliomyelitis:** an acute infectious disease of the brain stem and spinal cord.

**polydactyly:** a developmental anomaly characterized by the presence of extra fingers or toes.

**positive signs of pregnancy:** indications that confirm the presence of pregnancy.

**postpartum:** after childbirth.

**postpartum hemorrhage:** loss of blood greater than 500 ml following delivery. The hemorrhage is classified as early or immediate if it occurs within the first 24 hours and late or delayed after the first 24 hours.

**precipitate birth:** a birth that occurs without a trained attendant present.

**precipitate labor:** rapid progression of labor, one that lasts less than 3 hours.

**pregnancy:** the condition of having a developing embryo or fetus in the body after fertilization of the female egg by the male sperm.

**prehension:** use of hands to pick up small objects; grasping.

**prenatal:** before birth.

**presentation:** the fetal body part that enters the maternal pelvis first.

**presenting part:** the fetal part that first enters the maternal pelvis.

**presumptive signs of pregnancy:** symptoms that suggest pregnancy but that do not confirm it, such as cessation of menses, quickening, Chadwick's sign, and morning sickness.

**primigravida:** a woman who is pregnant for the first time.

**primipara:** a woman who has given birth to her first child (past the point of viability), whether or not that child is living or was alive at birth.

**probable signs of pregnancy:** manifestations that strongly suggest the likelihood of pregnancy, such as positive pregnancy test, enlarging abdomen, and positive Goodell's, Hegar's, and Braxton Hicks signs.

**progesterone:** a hormone produced by the corpus luteum, adrenal cortex, and placenta, whose function it is to stimulate proliferation of the endometrium to facilitate growth of the embryo.

**prolapsed cord:** umbilical cord that becomes trapped between the fetal presenting part and maternal pelvis.

**PROM:** premature rupture of amniotic membranes. Rupture of the membranes before the onset of labor.

**pseudocyesis:** a condition in which the woman has symptoms of pregnancy but in which hormonal pregnancy test results are negative; false pregnancy.

**psychoprophylaxis:** psychophysical training aimed at preparing the expectant parents to cope with the processes of labor and to avoid concentration on the discomforts associated with childbirth.

**puberty:** the period of time during which the secondary sexual characteristics develop and the ability to procreate is attained.

**pudendal block:** injection of an anesthetizing agent at the pudendal nerve to produce numbness of the external genitals and the lower one-third of the vagina.

**puerperium:** the period of time after delivery until involution of the uterus is complete, usually 6 weeks.

**pyloric stenosis:** a congenital narrowing of the pylorus of the stomach due to an enlarged muscle.

**quickening:** first fetal movements felt by the pregnant woman, usually between 16 and 18 weeks' gestation.

**rapport:** harmonious relation.

**rectal prolapse:** a dropping or protrusion of the mucosa of the rectum through the anus.

**relaxin:** a water-soluble protein secreted by the corpus luteum that causes relaxation of the symphysis pubis and facilitates cervical dilation during birth.

**retrolental fibroplasia:** blindness usually found in the preterm infant that is associated with oxygen concentrations and in which the blood vessels of the retina become damaged.

**Reye's syndrome:** acute encephalopathy with fatty degeneration of the liver, characterized by fever and impaired consciousness.

**Rh factor:** antigen present on the surface of blood cells that make the blood cell incompatible with blood cells that do not have the antigen.

**rhabdomyosarcoma:** extremely malignant neoplasm originating in skeletal muscle.

**rickets:** a disease of the bones, caused by lack of calcium or vitamin D.

**ROM:** rupture of (amniotic) membranes.

**rooting reflex:** an infant's tendency to turn the head and open the lips to suck when one side of the mouth or cheek is touched or stroked.

**roscola:** self-limited infection manifested by high fever followed by maculopapular rash. The child appears well otherwise and usually remains active.

**rubella:** German measles.

**rubeola:** measles.

**sacrum:** five fused vertebrae that form a triangle of bone just beneath the lumbar vertebrae and between the hip bones.

**scoliosis:** lateral curvature of the spine.

**scurvy:** a disease caused by a lack of vitamin C in the diet and characterized by joint pains, bleeding gums, loose teeth, and lack of energy.

**second stage of labor:** stage lasting from complete dilation of the cervix to expulsion of the fetus.

**semen:** thick, whitish fluid ejaculated by the male during orgasm, which contains the spermatozoa and their nutrients.

**sex chromosomes:** the X and Y chromosomes, which are responsible for sex determination; women have two X chromosomes; men have one X and one Y chromosome.

**sexually transmitted disease (STD):** refers to diseases ordinarily transmitted by direct sexual contact with an infected individual.

**shunt:** a bypass.

**sickle cell anemia:** a disease associated with an inherited defect in the structure of hemoglobin.

**SIDS:** sudden infant death syndrome. The sudden and unexpected death of an apparently healthy infant, typically occurring between the ages of 3 weeks and 5 months, and not explained by careful postmortem studies; crib or cot death.

**small for gestational age (SGA):** inadequate weight or growth for gestational age; birth weight below the 10th percentile.

**Snellen alphabet chart:** a device used to measure near and far vision; a variation of the Snellen E chart.

**spermatogenesis:** process by which mature spermatozoa are formed, during which the number of chromosomes is reduced by half.

**spermatozoa:** mature sperm cells produced by the testes.

**spina bifida:** a congenital defect in which

there is an imperfect closure of the spinal canal.

**spinnbarkeit:** elasticity seen in cervical mucus at the time of ovulation.

**station:** relationship of the presenting fetal part to an imaginary line drawn between the pelvic ischial spines.

**stillbirth:** the delivery of a dead fetus.

**striae gravidarum:** stretch marks; shiny reddish lines that appear on the abdomen, breasts, thighs, and buttocks of pregnant women as a result of stretching the skin.

**subarachnoid block:** injection of local anesthetic drug beneath the dura and arachnoid membranes of the spinal cord.

**surfactant:** a surface-active mixture of lipoproteins secreted in the alveoli and air passages that reduces the surface tension of pulmonary fluids and contributes to the elasticity of pulmonary tissue.

**talipes equinovarus:** clubfoot.

**Tay-Sachs disease:** A degenerative, fatal brain disease caused by a lack of hexosaminidase A in all body tissues; seen mostly in Eastern European Jews and is genetically transmitted.

**teratogen:** a nongenetic factor that can produce malformations of the fetus.

**term infant:** a live-born infant of 38-42 weeks' gestation.

**testes:** the male gonads, in which sperm and testosterone are produced.

**testosterone:** the male hormone; responsible for the development of secondary male characteristics.

**tetralogy of Fallot:** a congenital heart defect involving pulmonary stenosis, ventricular septal defect, dextroposition of the aorta, and hypertrophy of the right ventricle.

**thalassemia:** a hereditary blood disorder in which the patient's body cannot produce sufficient hemoglobin.

**third stage of labor:** the time from the delivery of the fetus to the time when the placenta has been completely expelled.

**thrush:** an infection of the mucous membranes of the mouth or throat caused by the fungus *Candida albicans*.

**tinea:** a contagious fungal infection; ringworm.

**tocodynamometer:** external device that can be used to identify the pressure of uterine contractions during labor.

**tocolytic:** a drug that inhibits uterine contractions.

**TORCH:** acronym used to describe a group of infections that represent potentially severe fetal problems if infection occurs during pregnancy. TO, toxoplasmosis; R, rubella; C, cytomegalovirus; and H, herpesvirus.

**torticollis:** wryneck; a condition in which the head inclines to one side because of a shortening of either sternocleidomastoid muscle.

**TPN:** total parenteral nutrition. Providing for all nutritional needs by administration of liquids into the blood; used in life-threatening conditions; hyperalimentation.

**tracheoesophageal fistula:** the esophagus, instead of being an open tube from the throat to the stomach, is closed at some point. A fistula between the trachea and the esophagus is common.

**transition:** the period during labor when the cervix is approximately 8 cm dilated, contractions are very strong, and the laboring woman feels the urge to push.

**trimester:** one-third of the gestational time for pregnancy.

**truncus arteriosus:** a single arterial trunk that leaves the ventricular portion of the heart and supplies the pulmonary, coronary, and systemic circulations.

**turgor:** good elasticity of the skin.

**tympanometry:** measurement of mobility of the tympanic membrane of the ear and estimation of middle ear pressure.

**ultrasound:** high-frequency sound waves that may be directed, through use of a transducer, into the maternal abdomen. The ultrasonic sound waves reflected by the underlying structures of varying densities allow maternal and fetal tissues, bones, and fluids to be identified.

**umbilical cord:** the structure connecting the placenta to the umbilicus of the fetus through which nutrients from the woman are exchanged for wastes from the fetus.

**uterus:** hollow muscular organ in which the fertilized ovum is implanted and the developing fetus is nourished until birth.

**vacuum extractor:** device to assist birth of fetal head using suction.

**vagina:** the musculomembranous tube or passageway located between the external female genitals and the uterus.

**varicella:** chickenpox.

**varicose veins:** permanently distended veins.

**variola:** smallpox.

**VBAC:** an acronym for vaginal birth after cesarean.

**ventriculography:** x-ray examination of the ventricles of the brain following the injection of air into the ventricles.

**vernix caseosa:** a protective cheeselike whitish substance made up of sebum and desquamated epithelial cells that is present on fetal skin and skin of newborn.

**vertex:** top or crown of the head.

**viable:** capable of living.

**volvulus:** a twisting of the loops of the small intestine, causing obstruction.

**vulva:** the external structure of the female genitals, lying between the mons veneris and anus.

**Wharton's jelly:** yellow-white gelatinous material that surrounds and protects the vessels of the umbilical cord.

**wheal:** large, slightly raised red or blistered area of skin; may itch.

**Wilms' tumor:** a malignant tumor of the kidneys.

**X chromosome:** female sex chromosome.

**Y chromosome:** male sex chromosome.

**zygote:** a fertilized ovum.

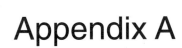

# Appendix A

# Some Factors with Known or Possible Teratogenic Effects on the Fetus*

| Agent | Potential Fetal Effects |
|---|---|
| | *Environmental Factors* |
| Agent Orange | Possible weak mutagenic (producing changes in the genes) effects, although not proven |
| Heavy metals (lead, arsenic, cadmium) | Incomplete data; possible increased spontaneous abortions |
| Mercury | Central nervous system damage, including cerebral palsy, seizures, and mental retardation |
| Naphthalene (mothballs) | Hemolysis (breakdown) of erythrocytes, leading to anemia |
| Polychlorinated biphenyls (PCBs, most likely to be found in sport fish from contaminated waters) | IUGR (intrauterine growth retardation); skin discoloration |
| Radiation | No evidence of human malformations caused by diagnostic levels of radiation; high doses associated with abnormalities of the brain, spinal cord, palate, skeleton, internal organs, and with mental retardation |
| | *Maternal Infection* |
| Human immunodeficiency virus (HIV) | Development of acquired immunodeficiency syndrome (AIDS) after birth in about 30% of infants |
| Human papillomavirus (HPV) | Nodules on the larynx |
| TORCH infections | |
| Toxoplasmosis | Spontaneous abortion; blindness, seizures, mental retardation, hydrocephaly, microcephaly (small head), enlarged spleen and liver, jaundice, and rash |
| Rubella (German measles) | Effects vary according to time of infection; IUGR, failure to thrive, seizures, cataracts and other eye abnormalities, deafness, congenital heart defects, enlarged liver and spleen, mental retardation, or developmental delay; preventable with immunization before pregnancy |
| Cytomegalovirus (CMV) | IUGR, enlarged liver and spleen, jaundice, "blueberry muffin" rash (petechiae), microcephaly, severe mental retardation, eye abnormalities, and seizures; infant may shed virus for a prolonged time after birth |
| Herpesvirus | Microcephaly, microphthalmia (small eyes) and other eye abnormalities, mental retardation, and death |
| Varicella (chickenpox) | Skin scarring, muscle atrophy, and mental retardation |
| | *Maternal Substance Use* |
| Alcohol | Spontaneous abortion; *fetal alcohol syndrome (FAS)*, which includes growth retardation before and after birth, facial and cranial abnormalities, mental retardation and developmental delay; *fetal alcohol effects* are a milder version of FAS |

*Teratogen: An agent that can cause defects in a developing baby if it is taken by the pregnant woman.
Food and Drug Administration Pregnancy Risk Categories:

*Continued*

| Agent | Potential Fetal Effects |
|---|---|
| Amphetamines ("speed" or "ice") | IUGR, abstinence effects (lethargy), cardiac abnormalities, and cleft palate |
| Caffeine | Stimulates fetus; increased risk for spontaneous abortion; women are presently advised to limit caffeine consumption, ideally before conceiving. |
| Cocaine, including "crack" | Fetal death, prematurity, IUGR, irritability, poor feeding, vomiting, diarrhea, mental retardation, and absent abdominal muscles (prune-belly syndrome) |
| Marijuana ("grass" and "pot") | Effects not clear; possibly associated with prematurity, IUGR, neonatal tremors, and light sensitivity |
| Narcotics (heroin, methadone, morphine) | IUGR, asphyxia, mental retardation, neonatal abstinence syndrome, neonatal infections, and sudden infant death syndrome (SIDS) |
| Sedatives, tranquilizers | Neonatal abstinence syndrome, seizures, and delayed lung maturation |
| Tobacco | Prematurity, IUGR, developmental delay, increased incidence of SIDS, pneumonia |
| | ***Prescribed Drugs*** |
| Anticonvulsants | |
| Carbamazepine (Tegretol) | Minor cranial and facial abnormalities, underdeveloped fingernails, and developmental delay; risk category C |
| Phenobarbital | Possible neonatal abstinence effects with high doses, but rare at usual therapeutic doses; risk category D |
| Phenytoin or diphenylhydantoin (Dilantin) | Fetal hydantoin syndrome, which includes IUGR, microcephaly, mental retardation, cranial and facial abnormalities, and underdeveloped nails and fingers; risk category D |
| Trimethadione (Tridione) | Fetal risk is greater than with other anticonvulsants; associated with developmental delay, cranial and facial abnormalities, and cardiovascular and other internal abnormalities; risk category D |
| Valproic acid (Depakene) | Neural tube defects (such as spina bifida or anencephaly) and other cranial and facial abnormalities; risk category D |
| Antihistamines | Varies with specific drug; little risk is apparent with brompheniramine, chlorpheniramine, diphenhydramine, triprolidine (risk category B); slightly increased risk with astemizole and terfenadine (risk category C) |
| Antimicrobials | |
| Aminoglycosides (gentamicin, kanamycin, neomycin, streptomycin) | Hearing loss |
| Chloramphenicol | If given near birth, "gray syndrome" in newborn (rapid respiration, pallor, poor feeding, abdominal distention, vascular collapse, death); risk category C |
| Tetracyclines | Abnormal tooth enamel; discolored teeth; risk category D |
| Antitussives (cough preparations) | Dextromethorphan and guaifenesin are risk category C |
| Antivirals | |
| Acyclovir | Risk category C; often used to treat herpes infections |
| Ribavirin | Risk category X; drug should not be administered to a woman of childbearing age |
| Decongestants | Most should not be used during 3rd trimester; pseudoephedrine is risk category B; most others are risk category C |
| Hormones | |
| Adrenocorticotropins | Risk category C; prednisone is preferred for the pregnant asthmatic woman; betamethasone and dexamethasone may be used therapeutically to speed fetal lung maturation |
| Estrogens | Risk category X; diethylstilbestrol (DES) is associated with vaginal cancer in female offspring; male and female genital tract abnormalities may occur |
| Oral contraceptives | Risk category X; doses much higher than those used for contraception are associated with masculinization of a female fetus's genitalia |
| Oral hypoglycemic agents | Prolonged neonatal hypoglycemia, other adverse effects; insulin is the only antidiabetic agent that should be used during pregnancy; risk category X |
| Psychoactive drugs | |
| Benzodiazepines (such as alprazolam [Xanax], diazepam [Valium]) | Alprazolam and diazepam are risk category D; several are risk category X |
| Lithium | Cardiac abnormalities; risk category D |
| Meprobamate | Contraindicated because of a significant increase in abnormalities; the combination drug Equagesic contains meprobamate |
| Phenothiazines | Risk category C; risk of malformations is unclear; continued use during pregnancy should be evaluated |
| Tricyclic antidepressants | Risk varies according to drug, either B, C, or D; definite association with birth defects is unclear |

| Agent | Potential Fetal Effects |
|---|---|
| Thyroid medications | |
|   Antithyroids (methimazole, propylthiouracil) | Neonatal goiter or hypothyroidism, scalp defects |
|   Iodine | Massive thyroid enlargement, which interferes with swallowing and compresses the trachea |
|   Thyroid replacement hormone | Risk category A; little transfer to fetus |
| Vitamins and related drugs | |
|   Acne medications (etretinate [Tegison] and isotretinoin [Accutane]) | Risk category X; severe fetal malformations, including microcephaly, ear abnormalities, cardiac defects, and CNS defects; drugs are related to vitamin A |
|   Vitamin A | Risk category A unless dose exceeds recommended daily allowance (RDA), then category X |
|   Vitamin D | Risk category C (D if dose exceeds RDA); high intake associated with aortic stenosis, facial abnormalities, and mental retardation |
| Warfarins (Coumadin) | Abnormal development of nose, skeleton, and eyes; microcephaly, mental retardation; risk category X |
| | Heparin is the only acceptable anticoagulant for use during pregnancy |

A—No evidence of risk to the fetus.

B—Animal reproduction studies have not demonstrated a risk to the fetus. There are no adequate and well-controlled studies in pregnant women.

C—Animal reproduction studies have shown an adverse effect on the fetus, but there are no adequate and well-controlled studies in humans. Potential benefits may warrant use of the drug in pregnant women despite fetal risks.

D—Positive evidence of human fetal risk, but potential benefits may warrant use of the drug in pregnant women despite fetal risks. Essentially, there are no safer alternatives.

X—Positive evidence of human fetal risk based on animal or human studies and/or adverse reaction data. Risks of using drug in pregnant women clearly outweigh potential benefits. There may be safer alternatives for some drugs.

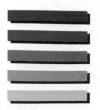

# Appendix B

# Drugs Used During Antepartum, Intrapartum, Postpartum, and Neonatal Care

| Drug | Common Obstetric Uses | Usual Routes of Administration | Usual Dosage, Remarks |
|------|----------------------|-------------------------------|-----------------------|
| *Antacids and Antiflatulents* | | | |
| Aluminum hydroxide, magnesium hydroxide (Gelusil, Maalox, milk of magnesia) | Relieves heartburn, indigestion, flatulence ("gas") | PO | 2 teaspoons or 2 tablets 1 hr after meals |
| Simethicone (Mylicon) | Relieves flatulence | PO | 40–80 mg after meals and at bedtime; must be chewed |
| *Antifungals* | | | |
| Clotrimazole (Lotrimin) | Vaginal candidiasis ("yeast") infections | PO Intravaginally | 10 mg 5 times a day<br>Cream: 1 applicator at bedtime for 7–14 days<br>Vaginal tablets: 100 mg at bedtime for 7 days; 200 mg at bedtime for 3 days; or 500-mg tablet at bedtime once |
| Metronidazole (Flagyl) | *Trichomonas vaginalis* infections | PO | *Not recommended during the 1st trimester of pregnancy*<br>2 gm in a single dose or 2 divided doses, or 250 mg 3 times a day for 7 days |
| Miconazole nitrate (Monistat) | Vaginal candidiasis | Intravaginally | 200-mg suppository at bedtime for 3 days; or 100-mg suppository or 1 applicator at bedtime for 7 days |
| *Analgesics, Antipyretics, and Antiinflammatories* | | | |
| Acetylsalicyclic acid (aspirin) | Relieves mild pain and inflammation (nonsteroidal); reduces fever; decreases platelet aggregation, interfering with blood coagulation; investigational for prevention of pregnancy-induced hypertension | PO | 325–650 mg every 4–6 hr; should be avoided in adolescents with viral infections, such as influenza or varicella (chickenpox), because of association with Reye's syndrome (see p. 623); may be combined with a narcotic (see acetaminophen) |

PO, oral; IM, intramuscular; IV, intravenous. Note: this chart serves as a summary and should not replace the use of a more detailed reference.

| Drug | Common Obstetric Uses | Usual Routes of Administration | Usual Dosage, Remarks |
|------|----------------------|-------------------------------|----------------------|
| *Analgesics, Antipyretics, and Antiinflammatories (Continued)* | | | |
| Acetaminophen (Tylenol) | Relieves mild pain; no antiinflammatory or blood coagulation effects; reduces fever | PO | 325–650 mg every 4–6 hr; often combined with a narcotic analgesic such as codeine (Empirin No. 3), hydrocodone (Vicodin, Lortab), or oxycodone (Percocet, Tylox) |
| Ibuprofen (Advil, Motrin) | Relieves mild to moderate pain and inflammation; nonsteroidal | PO | 200–400 mg every 4–6 hr |
| *Narcotic (Opiate) Analgesics* | | | |
| Butorphanol (Stadol) | Reduces labor pain; has some narcotic-antagonist effects | IV | 1 mg every 3–4 hr (range 0.5–2 mg). *Should not be given to the opiate-addicted woman or after a dose of a pure narcotic, such as meperidine or morphine*; observe newborn for respiratory depression |
| Meperidine (Demerol) | Reduces labor pain and moderate-to-severe pain postpartum | IM | Labor, 50–100 mg every 2–3 hr (not preferred route) Postpartum, 50–100 mg every 3–4 hr |
| | | IV | Labor (preferred route), 12.5–50 mg every 2–4 hr |
| Morphine sulfate | Relieves severe postoperative pain (cesarean birth); epidural morphine (Duramorph) may be given through epidural catheter to provide long-lasting pain relief after cesarean birth | IM | 10 mg every 4 hr |
| | | Epidural | Given by anesthesiologist or nurse-anesthetist; observe for respiratory depression, which may be late in onset (up to 24 hr), and itching |
| Nalbuphine (Nubain) | Relieves labor pain | IV | 10 mg every 3–6 hr; has some narcotic-antagonist effects (see butorphanol) |
| Narcotic combinations Acetaminophen with codeine (Tylenol or Empirin with codeine) | Relieves postpartum pain, including postoperative pain | PO | Acetaminophen with codeine: 1–2 tablets every 4 hr |
| Acetaminophen with hydrocodone (Vicodin, Lortab) | | | Acetaminophen with hydrocodone: 1 tablet every 4 hr or 2 tablets every 6 hr |
| Acetaminophen with oxycodone (Percocet, Tylox) | | | Acetaminophen with oxycodone: 1 tablet or capsule every 6 hr |
| *Analgesic Adjunct Drugs* | | | |
| Promethazine (Phenergan) | Enhances analgesic effects of narcotics and counteracts nausea that may occur when they are given | IM, IV | 12.5–25 mg every 4–6 hr |
| Diphenhydramine (Benadryl) | See Antihistamines | | |
| Hydroxyzine (Vistaril) | Relieves nausea and vomiting occurring with narcotic use and postoperatively | IM | 25–100 mg; infrequently used during labor |

*Continued*

| Drug | Common Obstetric Uses | Usual Routes of Administration | Usual Dosage, Remarks |
|------|----------------------|-------------------------------|------------------------|
| *Narcotic Antagonists* | | | |
| Naloxone (Narcan) | Reverses respiratory depression caused by narcotics; relieves itching caused by epidural narcotics; does not affect respiratory depression caused by other drugs, such as barbiturates | Adult: IV<br>Newborn: IV (umbilical vein) or intratracheal | 0.4–2 mg<br>0.1 mg/kg |
| Naltrexone (Trexan) | Relieves pruritus from epidural narcotics (investigational) | PO | 6 mg (1 dose) |
| *Anticoagulants* | | | |
| Heparin | Decreases clotting ability of blood in thromboembolic disease | SC, IV | Doses individualized based on coagulation studies; *protamine sulfate is the antagonist for heparin* |
| Warfarin (Coumadin) | Same as heparin; *contraindicated during pregnancy* | PO | 2–25 mg, based on evaluations of prothrombin time; *vitamin K is the antagonist for warfarin* |
| *Anticonvulsants* | | | |
| Phenytoin (also called hydantoin or diphenylhydantoin [Dilantin]) | Prevents epileptic seizures; *associated with birth defects (fetal hydantoin syndrome), so benefits of use during pregnancy are weighed against potential fetal harm* | PO | 300–400 mg daily in divided doses |
| Magnesium sulfate | Prevention or relief of seizures associated with pregnancy-induced hypertension; inhibition of preterm labor or excessive uterine contractions (investigational) | IM | 2–4 gm IV loading dose, followed by 10 gm IM; continued with 5 gm IM every 4 hr; *IM injection must be given deeply into gluteus maximus and is quite painful* |
| | | IV (preferred) | 2–4 gm initially, followed by continuous infusion of 1–2 gm/hr |
| *Antidote for Magnesium* | | | |
| Calcium gluconate | Reverses toxicity (particularly respiratory depression) caused by magnesium | IV | 1 gm (10 ml of 10% solution) |
| *Antihistamines and Decongestants* | | | |
| Diphenhydramine (Benadryl) | Relieves allergies; relieves itching caused by epidural narcotics | PO | 25–50 mg every 4–6 hr (3–4 times a day total) |
| | | IV | 25–50 mg 4 times a day to relieve itching from epidural narcotics |
| Pseudoephedrine (Sudafed) | Relieves nasal congestion | PO | 60 mg every 4–6 hr |
| Terfenadine (Seldane) | Relieves allergies | PO | 60 mg 2 times a day |

| Drug | Common Obstetric Uses | Usual Routes of Administration | Usual Dosage, Remarks |
|------|----------------------|-------------------------------|----------------------|
| | ***Antihypertensives*** | | |
| Hydralazine (Apresoline) | Reduces dangerously high blood pressure in pregnancy-induced hypertension | IV | 5–20 mg, repeated as necessary |
| | ***Antimicrobials*** | | |
| Amoxicillin (Amoxil) | Respiratory, gastrointestinal, and genitourinary tract infections | PO | 500 mg every 8 hr |
| Ampicillin (Polycillin) | Used for gram-positive and some gram-negative infections | PO, IM, IV | 250–500 mg every 6–8 hr |
| Cephalexin (Keflex) | Respiratory, urinary tract, and soft tissue infection | PO | 250–500 mg every 6 hr |
| Chloramphenicol (Chloromycetin) | Serious infections that are unresponsive to other antibiotics | PO, IV | 50 mg/kg in divided doses every 6 hr. *Not recommended near term or during labor because it is associated with "gray syndrome," a potentially fatal toxic reaction in the infant* |
| Clindamycin (Cleocin) | Respiratory tract, skin or soft tissue, septicemia, and urinary tract infections | PO<br><br>IM, IV | 150–300 mg (up to 450 mg for serious infections) every 6 hr<br>600–1200 mg/day in 2–4 divided doses (1.2–2.7 gm/day in 3 or 4 divided doses for serious infections) |
| Erythromycin | Prevents neonatal eye infections caused by gonorrhea or chlamydia; respiratory, ear infections; prophylaxis for women with heart abnormalities or artificial implants before dental or other invasive procedures; alternate antimicrobial for syphilis if woman is allergic to penicillin | Ophthalmic ointment<br><br>PO<br><br>IV | 1 ribbon in the lower conjunctiva of each eye 1 time after birth<br>250 mg every 6 hr; 500 mg every 12 hr; or 333 mg every 8 hr<br>15–20 mg/kg/day in divided doses; maximum of 4 gm/day |
| Penicillin G | Syphilis and gonorrhea infections (see also p. 110); prophylaxis for women with heart abnormalities or artificial implants | IM | For syphilis: 2.4 million units; alternate, 600,000 units daily for 8 days (total of 4.8 million units)<br>For gonorrhea: 4.8 million units in 2 divided doses |
| Silver nitrate | Prevents neonatal eye infection caused by gonorrhea; *ineffective against eye infections caused by chlamydia* | Ophthalmic drops | 2 drops of 1% solution into each conjunctival sac; do not irrigate eyes after application |
| Sulfonamides (Bactrim, Septra, AVC) | Treats bladder infections and some vaginal infections | PO | Varies with specific sulfonamide drug |
| Tetracycline (Achromycin) | Prevents neonatal eye infection caused by gonorrhea or chlamydia; *not recommended for use during pregnancy* | Ophthalmic ointment | Same as erythromycin ophthalmic ointment |

*Continued*

| Drug | Common Obstetric Uses | Usual Routes of Administration | Usual Dosage, Remarks |
|---|---|---|---|
| *Expectorants and Antitussives* | | | |
| Dextromethorphan (many brand names) | Decreases coughing (nonnarcotic) | PO | 10–20 mg every 4–8 hr, or 30 mg every 6–8 hr |
| Guaifenesin (Robitussin, many other brands) | Expectorant—expulsion of mucus | PO | 200–400 mg every 4 hr |
| *Hypoglycemics* | | | |
| Insulin | Lowers blood glucose levels in women who have diabetes mellitus, including gestational diabetes | SC, IV (regular insulin only) | Individualized according to gestation and blood glucose levels |
| *Immunologic Agents* | | | |
| Rh$_o$(D) immune globulin (RhoGAM, Gamulin Rh, HypRho-D) | Given to Rh-negative woman to prevent sensitization to Rh-positive erythrocytes, thus preventing fetal hemolytic disease in a subsequent pregnancy | IM | After abortion: 50–300 µg (depending on gestation) within 72 hr<br>Antepartum: 300 µg at 28 wk gestation<br>Postpartum: 300 µg within 72 hr of birth of Rh-positive infant |
| Rubella vaccine | Prevents infection with rubella; *do not administer during pregnancy* | SC | 1 single-dose vial; *caution woman to avoid pregnancy for 3 mo;* should not be given if the woman is sensitive to neomycin or if she has had a transfusion within the last 3 mo |
| *Laxatives and Rectal Drugs* | | | |
| Fecal wetting agents<br>  Docusate calcium (Surfak)<br>  Docusate sodium (Colace) | Softens feces to prevent or relieve constipation | PO | 240 mg/day (docusate calcium)<br>50–500 mg/day (docusate sodium) |
| Bisacodyl (Dulcolax) | Stimulant laxative to promote expulsion of feces | PO<br>Rectal | 10–15 mg<br>1 suppository |
| *Oxytocins* | | | |
| Methylergonovine (Methergine) | Prevents or controls postpartum hemorrhage | PO, IM | 0.2 mg every 6–12 hr; *may be given IM, but this route is associated with significant, and possibly severe, blood pressure elevations* |
| Oxytocin (Pitocin) | Induces or augments labor; prevents or controls postpartum hemorrhage | IV | Induction or augmentation of labor (see p. 189); control of postpartum bleeding: 10–40 units in 1000 ml IV solution at a rate to control bleeding<br>Before birth, oxytocin is given only in a dilute IV solution controlled by an infusion pump |
| | | IM (control of postpartum bleeding only) | 10 units |

| Drug | Common Obstetric Uses | Usual Routes of Administration | Usual Dosage, Remarks |
|------|----------------------|-------------------------------|------------------------|
| *Tocolytics and Related Drugs* | | | |
| Magnesium sulfate | See Anticonvulsants | | |
| Ritodrine (Yutopar) | Stops preterm labor; only drug with FDA approval for this purpose; however, ritodrine's significant side effects have led to use of several other drugs as tocolytics on an investigational basis | IV | Start at 0.5–1.0 mg/min; increase by 0.05 mg/min every 30 min until contractions stop or significant side effects (maternal or fetal tachycardia) develop; maintain on oral drug |
| | | PO | 10 mg every 2 hr, gradually shifting to maintenance dose of 10–20 mg every 4–6 hr; *give first PO dose 30 min before IV drug is stopped* |
| Terbutaline (Brethine) | Stops preterm labor; also may be given to reduce excessive contractions (tetanic) during labor. | IV | Start at 0.01 mg/min, increase by 0.005 mg/min at 10–20 min intervals until contractions stop (maximum of 0.080 mg/min); maintain by SC or PO route |
| | | SC | 0.25 mg every 1–3 hr |
| | | Continuous SC infusion pump | Basal rate of 0.02–0.9 mg/hr, with individualized boluses |
| | | PO | 2.5–5 mg every 2–4 hr |
| *Corticosteroids* | | | |
| Betamethasone Dexamethasone | Accelerates maturation of fetal lungs if preterm birth cannot be avoided | IM | 12 mg, repeated in 12–24 hr; repeat treatment weekly until 34 wk gestation; *concurrent administration with drugs such as terbutaline or ritodrine has been associated with development of maternal pulmonary edema;* may worsen conditions such as diabetes |
| *Topical Pain Relievers* | | | |
| Benzocaine (Americaine) | Relieves perineal pain from episiotomy or lacerations | Topical | After doing perineal care following urination or bowel movement, spray on affected area |
| Hydrocortisone acetate (Epifoam) | Relieves localized perineal pain and inflammation | Topical | After perineal care, apply a small amount to perineal pad and apply to affected area |
| *Vitamins and Minerals* | | | |
| Folic acid | Prevents or treats folic-acid deficiency during pregnancy | PO | 300 μg (0.3 mg) daily (prevention of deficiency); 0.7–1.0 mg/day (treatment of deficiency) |
| Iron | Prevents or treats iron-deficiency anemia during pregnancy | PO | 30–60 mg/day (prevention); 180–200 mg/day (treatment of deficiency); take with vitamin C food; do not take with milk or calcium |
| Vitamin K (AquaMEPHYTON, Konakion) | Prevents hemorrhagic disease of the newborn due to temporary lack of vitamin K production in gastrointestinal tract | IM | 0.5–1 mg in either anterior thigh 1 time after birth |

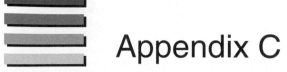

# Appendix C

# Effects of Drugs During Breast Feeding

| Drug | Comments |
|------|----------|
| *Analgesics* | |
| Aspirin | Possibility of blood clotting abnormalities; rash or metabolic acidosis may occur with high doses |
| Narcotic analgesics | Most are compatible with breast feeding when used in therapeutic doses; infant lethargy or poor feeding may occur; prolonged use may result in dependence with possible abstinence symptoms when the mother stops taking the drug |
| *Anticonvulsants* | |
| Phenobarbital | Use cautiously; sedation and infantile spasms after weaning may occur |
| Trimethadione (Tridione) | Safety has not been established |
| Valproic acid (Depakene) | Excreted in breast milk; use cautiously |
| *Antidiabetic Agents* | |
| Insulin | Safe; breast feeding may decrease woman's insulin requirements |
| Oral hypoglycemics | Infant hypoglycemia may occur |
| *Antihistamines and Decongestants* | |
| Cyclizine; promethazine | Contraindicated; may reduce milk supply |
| Pseudoephedrine | Compatible with breast feeding |
| *Antihypertensives* | |
| Calcium channel blockers | Nicardipine and nifedipine are contraindicated; Verapamil compatible |
| Hydralazine (Apresoline) Methyldopa (Aldomet) Propranolol (Inderal) | No adverse effects reported |
| *Antimicrobials and Antivirals* | |
| Aminoglycosides (gentamicin, kanamycin, neomycin, streptomycin) | Safety not established; preterm infants and newborns may be especially susceptible to toxicity |
| Chloramphenicol (Chloromycetin) | Contraindicated; may cause bone marrow depression |
| Erythromycins and penicillins | Considered safe for breast feeding, although it may alter gastrointestinal bacteria, or cause allergies |
| Metronidazole (Flagyl) | Contraindicated; breast feeding may be discontinued for 12–24 hr after the last dose to allow the mother to excrete the drug |
| Nitrofurantoin (Macrodantin) | May cause hemolytic anemia in an infant with a certain enzyme deficiency (G6-P-D) |
| Sulfonamides | Should not be given to nursing mothers or infants younger than 2 mo |
| Ribavirin | Contraindicated; not known if excreted in breast milk |
| *Hormones* | |
| Estrogens | Contraindicated; excreted in breast milk |
| Oral contraceptives | May decrease milk production if taken before lactation is well established |
| *Psychoactive Drugs* | |
| Benzodiazepines | May cause sedation; some are concentrated in breast milk |
| Lithium | Present in breast milk; contraindicated |
| Meprobamate | Concentrations in milk are higher; may cause sedation |

Effects of drugs used during lactation have not always been studied. In general, if a drug is safe for use in infants, it is usually safe for use in the nursing mother. Other drugs may not be excreted in breast milk, or may be excreted in very low concentrations, and thus be safe.

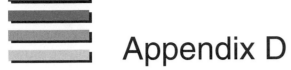

# Appendix D

# Conversion of Pounds and Ounces to Grams for Newborn Weights*

|  | **Ounces** | | | | | | | | | | | | | | | |  |
|---|---|---|---|---|---|---|---|---|---|---|---|---|---|---|---|---|---|
|  | **0** | **1** | **2** | **3** | **4** | **5** | **6** | **7** | **8** | **9** | **10** | **11** | **12** | **13** | **14** | **15** |  |
| **0** | — | 28 | 57 | 85 | 113 | 142 | 170 | 198 | 227 | 255 | 283 | 312 | 336 | 369 | 397 | 425 | 0 |
| **1** | 454 | 482 | 510 | 539 | 567 | 595 | 624 | 652 | 680 | 709 | 737 | 765 | 794 | 822 | 850 | 879 | 1 |
| **2** | 907 | 936 | 964 | 992 | 1021 | 1049 | 1077 | 1106 | 1134 | 1162 | 1191 | 1219 | 1247 | 1276 | 1304 | 1332 | 2 |
| **3** | 1361 | 1389 | 1417 | 1446 | 1474 | 1503 | 1531 | 1559 | 1588 | 1616 | 1644 | 1673 | 1701 | 1729 | 1758 | 1786 | 3 |
| **4** | 1814 | 1843 | 1871 | 1899 | 1928 | 1956 | 1984 | 2013 | 2041 | 2070 | 2098 | 2126 | 2155 | 2183 | 2211 | 2240 | 4 |
| **5** | 2268 | 2296 | 2325 | 2353 | 2381 | 2410 | 2438 | 2466 | 2495 | 2523 | 2551 | 2580 | 2608 | 2637 | 2665 | 2693 | 5 |
| **6** | 2722 | 2750 | 2778 | 2807 | 2835 | 2863 | 2892 | 2920 | 2948 | 2977 | 3005 | 3033 | 3062 | 3090 | 3118 | 3147 | 6 |
| **7** | 3175 | 3203 | 3232 | 3260 | 3289 | 3317 | 3345 | 3374 | 3402 | 3430 | 3459 | 3487 | 3515 | 3544 | 3572 | 3600 | 7 |
| **8** | 3629 | 3657 | 3685 | 3714 | 3742 | 3770 | 3799 | 3827 | 3856 | 3884 | 3912 | 3941 | 3969 | 3997 | 4026 | 4054 | 8 |
| **9** | 4082 | 4111 | 4139 | 4167 | 4196 | 4224 | 4252 | 4281 | 4309 | 4337 | 4366 | 4394 | 4423 | 4451 | 4479 | 4508 | 9 |
| **10** | 4536 | 4564 | 4593 | 4621 | 4649 | 4678 | 4706 | 4734 | 4763 | 4791 | 4819 | 4848 | 4876 | 4904 | 4933 | 4961 | 10 |
| **11** | 4990 | 5018 | 5046 | 5075 | 5103 | 5131 | 5160 | 5188 | 5216 | 5245 | 5273 | 5301 | 5330 | 5358 | 5386 | 5415 | 11 |
| **12** | 5443 | 5471 | 5500 | 5528 | 5557 | 5585 | 5613 | 5642 | 5670 | 5698 | 5727 | 5755 | 5783 | 5812 | 5840 | 5868 | 12 |
| **13** | 5897 | 5925 | 5953 | 5982 | 6010 | 6038 | 6067 | 6095 | 6123 | 6152 | 6180 | 6209 | 6237 | 6265 | 6294 | 6322 | 13 |
| **14** | 6350 | 6379 | 6407 | 6435 | 6464 | 6492 | 6520 | 6549 | 6577 | 6605 | 6634 | 6662 | 6690 | 6719 | 6747 | 6776 | 14 |
| **15** | 6804 | 6832 | 6860 | 6889 | 6917 | 6945 | 6973 | 7002 | 7030 | 7059 | 7087 | 7115 | 7144 | 7172 | 7201 | 7228 | 15 |
|  | **0** | **1** | **2** | **3** | **4** | **5** | **6** | **7** | **8** | **9** | **10** | **11** | **12** | **13** | **14** | **15** |  |
|  | **Ounces** | | | | | | | | | | | | | | | |  |

(Left and right margins labeled **Pounds**.)

*To convert the weight known in grams to pounds and ounces, for example, of a baby weighing 3717 gm, glance down columns to find the figure closest to 3717, which is 3714. Refer to the number to the far left or right of the column for pounds and the number at the top or bottom for ounces to get 8 pounds, 3 ounces.

*Conversion formulas:*
Pounds × 453.6 = grams
Ounces × 28.35 = grams
Grams ÷ 453.6 = pounds
Grams ÷ 28.35 = ounces

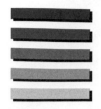

# Appendix E

# Temperature Equivalents

| Celsius | Fahrenheit | | Celsius | Fahrenheit |
|---|---|---|---|---|
| 34.0 | 93.2 | | 38.4 | 101.1 |
| 34.2 | 93.6 | | 38.6 | 101.4 |
| 34.4 | 93.9 | | 38.8 | 101.8 |
| 34.6 | 94.3 | | 39.0 | 102.2 |
| 34.8 | 94.6 | | 39.2 | 102.5 |
| 35.0 | 95.0 | | 39.4 | 102.9 |
| 35.2 | 95.4 | | 39.6 | 103.2 |
| 35.4 | 95.7 | | 39.8 | 103.6 |
| 35.6 | 96.1 | | 40.0 | 104.0 |
| 35.8 | 96.4 | | 40.2 | 104.3 |
| 36.0 | 96.8 | | 40.4 | 104.7 |
| 36.2 | 97.1 | | 40.6 | 105.1 |
| 36.4 | 97.5 | | 40.8 | 105.4 |
| 36.6 | 97.8 | | 41.0 | 105.8 |
| 36.8 | 98.2 | | 41.2 | 106.1 |
| | | | 41.4 | 106.5 |
| 37.0 | 98.6 | | 41.6 | 106.8 |
| | | | 41.8 | 107.2 |
| 37.2 | 98.9 | | 42.0 | 107.6 |
| 37.4 | 99.3 | | 42.2 | 108.0 |
| 37.6 | 99.6 | | 42.4 | 108.3 |
| 37.8 | 100.0 | | 42.6 | 108.7 |
| 38.0 | 100.4 | | 42.8 | 109.0 |
| 38.2 | 100.7 | | | |

*Conversion formulas:*
  Fahrenheit to Celsius ($°F - 32$) $\times$ (5/9) = $°C$
  Celsius to Fahrenheit ($°C$) $\times$ (9/5) + 32 = $°F$

# Appendix F

# Universal Precautions

The U.S. Department of Health and Human Services, Centers for Disease Control and Prevention (CDC), in Atlanta, Georgia, issues "Recommendations for Prevention of HIV Transmission in Health-Care Settings," known as "CDC Guidelines."

Human immunodeficiency virus (HIV), which causes acquired immunodeficiency syndrome (AIDS), is transmitted through sexual contact and exposure to infected blood or blood components and perinatally from mother to newborn. HIV has been isolated from blood, semen, vaginal secretions, saliva, tears, breast milk, cerebrospinal fluid, amniotic fluid, and urine and is likely to be isolated from other body fluids, secretions, and excretions. However, epidemiologic evidence has implicated only blood, semen, vaginal secretions, and possibly breast milk in transmission of the virus.

The increasing prevalence of HIV increases the risk that health-care workers will be exposed to blood from patients infected with HIV, especially when blood and body fluid precautions are not followed for all patients. The CDC emphasizes the need for health-care workers to consider *all* patients as potentially infected with HIV or other bloodborne pathogens (e.g., hepatitis B). Health-care workers are defined as persons, including students and trainees, whose activities involve contact with patients or with blood or other body fluids from patients in a health-care setting.

Recent studies indicate that the incubation period for AIDS may be as long as 5–7 years after exposure; therefore, the use of *universal precautions* in all areas in which body fluids are encountered is advisable.

## Summary of Universal Precautions in CDC Guidelines

1. All health-care workers should routinely use appropriate barrier precautions to prevent skin and mucous membrane exposure when contact with blood or other body fluids of any patient is anticipated.
   - *Gloves* should be worn for touching blood and body fluids, mucous membranes, or nonintact skin of all patients; for handling items or surfaces soiled with blood or body fluids; and for performing venipuncture and other vascular access procedures. Gloves should be changed after contact with *each* patient.
   - *Masks* and *protective eyewear* or *face shields* should

be worn during procedures that are likely to generate droplets of blood or body fluids.
   - *Fluid resistant gowns* or *aprons* should be worn during procedures that are likely to generate splashes of blood or body fluids.
2. Hands and other skin surfaces should be *washed immediately* and *thoroughly* if contaminated with blood or body fluids.
3. All health-care workers should take precautions to prevent injuries caused by needles, scalpels, and other sharp instruments. To prevent needlestick injuries, needles should *not* be recapped, bent, broken, removed from disposable syringes, or otherwise manipulated by hand. After sharp items are used, they should be placed in nearby *puncture-resistant containers* for disposal or, in the case of large-bore reusable needles, for transport to the reprocessing area.
4. To minimize the need for emergency mouth-to-mouth resuscitation, mouthpieces, resuscitation bags, or other ventilation devices should be available for use in areas in which the need for resuscitation is predictable.
5. Health-care workers who have exudate (oozing) lesions or weeping dermatitis (inflammation of the skin) should refrain from all direct patient care and from handling patient-care equipment until the condition resolves.
6. Pregnant health-care workers should be especially familiar with precautions to minimize the risk of HIV transmission and should strictly adhere to such precautions.
7. Health care workers exposed to breast milk may wear gloves.
8. Gloves are worn when handling materials soiled with blood such as linens, Chux, soiled pads, etc.

## Precautions for Invasive Procedures

The following precautions for invasive procedures, combined with the preceding *universal precautions*, are recommended as the minimum precautions for invasive procedures on *all* patients.

Invasive procedures include surgical entry into tissues, cavities, or organs; repair of major traumatic injuries, cardiac catheterization, and angiographic procedures; vaginal or cesarean deliveries or other invasive obstetric procedures during which bleeding may occur; or manipulation, cutting, or removal of any oral or perioral tissues during which the potential for bleeding exists.

1. All health-care workers who participate in invasive procedures must routinely use appropriate barrier precautions to prevent skin and mucous-membrane contact with blood or other body fluids of *all* patients.
   - *Gloves* and *surgical masks* must be worn for all invasive procedures.
   - *Protective eyewear* or *face shields* should be worn for procedures that commonly result in the generation of droplets, splashing of blood or other body fluids, or the generation of bone chips.
   - *Gowns* or *aprons* made of materials that provide an effective barrier should be worn during invasive procedures likely to result in the splashing of blood or other body fluids.
   - All health-care workers who perform or assist in *vaginal or cesarean deliveries* should wear *gloves and gowns* when handling the placenta or the infant until blood and amniotic fluid have been removed from the infant's skin and should wear *gloves during postdelivery care of the umbilical cord.*
2. If a glove is torn or a needlestick or other injury occurs, the glove should be removed and a new glove used as promptly as patient safety permits. The needle or other instrument involved in the incident should also be removed from the sterile field.

## Implementation of Precautions

The CDC Guidelines state that employers of health-care workers should ensure that policies exist for
1. *Initial orientation and continuing education and training* of all health-care workers on the epidemiology, modes of transmission, and prevention of HIV and other bloodborne infections, *and routine use of universal precautions for all patients.*
2. *Provision of equipment and supplies* necessary to minimize the risk of infection with HIV and other bloodborne pathogens.
3. *Monitoring adherence to recommended protective measures.* When monitoring reveals a failure to follow recommended precautions, counseling, education, or retraining should be provided, and, if necessary, appropriate disciplinary action should be considered.
4. If the health-care worker is exposed to blood and body fluids,
   - Wash exposed area immediately.
   - Save sharps or other items involved for possible testing.
   - Report to supervisor incidents of needlestick or other cut or puncture; splashing blood or other body fluids into eyes, nose, or mouth; direct contact with a large amount of blood or body fluids or contact for a prolonged period of time.
   - Follow procedure recommended for testing.

## National Resources

- AIDS Hotline 1-800-342-2437
- National AIDS Information Clearing House (for printed materials) 1-800-458-5231
  P.O. Box 6003
  Rockville, MD 20850

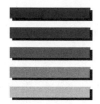

Appendix G

# Drugs Commonly Used in Pediatric Nursing

| Drug | Route* and Form | Dosage | Some Indications for Use | Nursing Considerations |
|---|---|---|---|---|
| Acetaminophen (Tylenol, Liquiprin, Tempra) | PO<br>Tablets, drops, syrup, elixir | Infants and children—PO: 30–40 mg/kg/24 hr divided every 4–6 hr prn | Analgesic and antipyretic | See label<br>In general, do not use for more than a few days unless under care of a physician<br>Keep away from children; overdose may cause liver failure; contact poison control center immediately for advice |
| Albuterol (Proventil, Ventolin) | PO<br>Inhalation, tablets, solution for nebulizer | Children 2–6 yr—PO: 0.1 mg/kg 3 times per day<br>Children over 12 yr—2 inhalations, 4–6 times per day | Relaxes bronchospasm of asthma, cystic fibrosis | Teach patient use of inhaler<br>Increase fluid intake<br>Avoid excess use of cola, chocolate, other caffeine derivatives |
| Amoxicillin (Amoxil, Larotid) | PO<br>Capsules, oral suspension, pediatric drops | 20–40 mg/kg/24 hr divided every 8 hr | Broad-spectrum antibiotic | Hypersensitivity may cause anaphylactic reaction<br>Shake suspension well |
| Ampicillin (Omnipen, Penbritin) | PO, IM, IV<br>Capsules, oral suspension, pediatric drops | 50–100 mg/kg/24 hr divided every 6 hr (PO), 100–200 mg/kg/24 hr divided every 4 hr (IV), every 6 hr (IM) | Septicemia, meningitis | May cause agranulocytosis, rash, stomatitis; contraindicated in patients with a history of hypersensitivity to penicillins; take on empty stomach |
| Aspirin (acetylsalicylic acid) | PO, R<br>Tablets, suppositories | Infants and children—PO: 30–65 mg/kg/24 hr divided every 4–6 hr prn | Rheumatic fever | Do not use in children with chickenpox or influenza-like symptoms<br>Ringing in ears, gastrointestinal upsets, disturbance in acid-base balance of body<br>Keep out of reach of children |
| Cephalexin (Keflex) | PO<br>Capsules, tablets, suspension | Infants and children—PO: 25–50 mg/kg/24 hr divided every 6 hr | Antibiotic, antibacterial | Contraindicated in patients with known allergies to cephalosporin group of antibiotics<br>Observe for rash, diarrhea<br>Evaluate glycosuria with Tes-Tape to avoid false-positive tests |
| Cephalothin sodium (Keflin) | IM, IV<br>Ampules | Infants and children—IM, IV: 80–160 mg/kg/24 hr every 4 hr | Broad-spectrum antibiotic for most infections, particularly of urinary tract or by resistant staphylococci | Anaphylaxis, diarrhea<br>Rotate injection sites, chart exact site<br>Administer punctually to maintain blood levels |

| Drug | Route/Form | Dosage | Use | Comments |
|---|---|---|---|---|
| Digoxin (Lanoxin) | PO, IV, IM<br>Tablets, elixir, solution for injection | Individualized regimens; consult pharmacopeia | Frequently used for newborns and children with heart conditions | Check apical pulse before administering<br>If anorexia, dizziness, or irregular or slow heartbeat develops, withhold additional doses and consult physician |
| Epinephrine (Adrenalin, Sus-Phrine) | SC, IM, inhalation<br>Ampules, vials | In acute asthmatic attack—children—SC: 0.01 mg/kg/dose, repeat prn every 20 min, 2 times | Antispasmodic for use in patients with asthma<br>Local hemostat in surgery | Causes blood pressure to rise; use with caution in cardiac patients<br>Massage well after injection<br>Do not use discolored solution |
| Erythromycin (Pediamycin, Ilotycin), Erythromycin estolate (Ilosone) | PO, IV<br>Tablets, drops, suspension, ampules | Infants and children—PO: 30–50 mg/kg/24 hr divided every 6 hr<br>IV: 15–20 mg/kg/24 hr divided every 6 hr | Rheumatic fever prophylaxis<br>Useful if child is sensitive to penicillin | Gastrointestinal irritation, rash<br>Administer punctually to maintain blood levels<br>Take careful history to determine allergies |
| Ferrous sulfate (Feosol, Fer-In-Sol) | PO<br>Tablets, capsules, syrup, elixir, drops | For prophylaxis: 0.5–1 mg/kg/24 hr, single or divided doses<br>For treatment: 6 mg/kg/24 hr divided into 3 doses | Iron-deficiency anemia | Gastrointestinal distress, diarrhea, constipation<br>Administer after meals or use coated tablets<br>Administer oral liquid through straw to avoid discoloration of teeth<br>Keep out of reach of children; overdose may be fatal<br>As oral iron products tend to interfere with the absorption of oral tetracycline antibiotics, these products should not be taken within 2 hr of each other |
| Glucagon | SC, IM, IV<br>Ampules | 0.025 unit/kg; may repeat in 20 min | Emergency treatment of severe hypoglycemia reactions in diabetes | Rare; when the patient responds, give supplemental carbohydrate to restore liver glycogen and prevent secondary hypoglycemia; this is particularly important for juvenile diabetics who may not have as great a response in blood glucose levels as adults have |
| Hydralazine (Apresoline) | PO, IM, IV<br>Tablets | Children—0.75 mg/24 hr (PO), every 6 hr, maximum dosage 3.5 mg/kg/24 hr | Antihypertensive in glomerulonephritis | Diarrhea, nausea, vomiting, rapid pulse, headache, sodium retention<br>When renal function is reduced, monitor blood pressure closely |
| Hydroxyzine hydrochloride (Atarax), Hydroxyzine (Vistaril) | PO, IM<br>Tablets, syrups, solutions for injection | Children—PO: 2 mg/kg/24 hr divided every 6–8 hr | Mild tranquilizer for problems of behavior<br>Preoperative medication | Drowsiness, dry mouth, tremors<br>May potentiate central nervous system (CNS) depressants |

*Continued*

| Drug | Route* and Form | Dosage | Some Indications for Use | Nursing Considerations |
|---|---|---|---|---|
| Ipecac syrup | PO<br>Syrup | Emetic (for children older than 1 yr): 15 ml (PO) in single dose; may repeat once in 20 min<br>Expectorant: 1–2 ml taken with glass of water | To induce vomiting in poisoning | Follow with water<br>Always order by complete name (other preparations are toxic)<br>Store in dry, cool place<br>Do not give to unconscious patients<br>Do not induce vomiting for poisoning with substances such as petroleum distillates, strong alkali or acid, or strychnine |
| Iron dextran (Imferon) | IM<br>Solution for injection | Dose calculated by formula using weight of child + hemoglobin | Iron-deficiency anemia; used when oral administration is unsatisfactory or impossible | Arthralgias, anaphylactoid reactions, rash, itching<br>Test dose of 0.5 ml should be given on first day<br>Use Z-track technique, inject deeply, observe for tissue staining |
| Isoproterenol (Isuprel) | Sublingual, R, IV<br>Inhalation, tablets, vials, mist | By nebulizer; pressurized mist, 1:400, 3 or 4 times a day | Bronchodilator in treatment of asthma, bronchitis | Tachycardia, flushing of skin, restlessness<br>Use with care in patients with heart complications |
| Methylphenidate hydrochloride (Ritalin) | PO | Patients over 3 yr; 5 mg (PO) before breakfast and lunch | CNS stimulant, used in treatment of minimum brain dysfunction and hyperkinetic behavior | Elicit child's cooperation<br>Nervousness, weight gain, anorexia, insomnia<br>Last dose is given several hours before bedtime<br>Contraindicated in convulsive disorders |
| Methylprednisolone sodium succinate (Solu-Medrol) | PO, IM, IV, R | PO: 0.4–1.67 mg/kg/day in 3–4 divided doses<br>IV: 1.6 mg/kg/day every 6 hr | Corticosteroid with antiinflammatory | Take with food<br>Do not end abruptly; must taper off under supervision<br>Avoid immunization with live viruses<br>Watch for infection<br>Incompatible with aminophylline |
| Nystatin (Mycostatin) | PO, topical<br>Tablets, suspension, powder, ointment, vaginal tablets | Suspension, PO, and topical: 100,000 units/ml, 3 or 4 times a day, swabbed in mouth of newborn | Antifungal antibiotic for thrush, diaper rash, other types of skin lesions caused by *Candida albicans* | Gastrointestinal distress<br>Virtually nontoxic, well tolerated by all age groups |
| Oxacillin sodium (Prostaphlin) | PO, IM, IV<br>Capsules, solutions for injection | Infants and children—PO: 50–100 mg/kg/24 hr divided every 6 hr | Mild to moderate infections of skin, soft tissues, or upper respiratory tract and resistant staphylococcal infections | See penicillin G<br>Take careful history to determine allergies<br>Chart exact site of IM injection<br>Administer punctually to maintain blood level<br>Give oral preparations 1–2 hr before meals |

| Drug | Form/Route | Dosage | Use | Nursing Considerations |
|---|---|---|---|---|
| Pancreatic enzymes (Cotazym, Viokase) | PO; Granules, tablets, capsules | Individualized dose | Aid to digestion in cystic fibrosis | Contraindicated in persons hypersensitive to beef or pork products; May be taken with water or milk or sprinkled on foods |
| Penicillin G (benzyl penicillin G) (Pentids) | PO, IM, IV; Many forms and preparations | Older children—25,000–50,000 units/kg/24 hr divided into 4–6 doses | Antibiotic used for many types of infection | Take careful history to determine allergies; May cause anaphylactic reactions; Many other warnings—consult pharmacopeia; Chart exact site of injection, administer on time |
| Phenobarbital (Luminal) | PO, IM; Tablets, capsules, elixir, solution for injection | Sedation: 2 mg/kg/24 hr in divided doses every 8 hr (PO) | CNS depressant, epilepsy, convulsions associated with high fever | May be habit-forming; avoid sudden withdrawal; reactions uncommon with small doses |
| Phenytoin (Dilantin) | PO, IM, IV; Tablets, capsules, suspension, solution for injection | As anticonvulsant—infants and children—PO: 3–8 mg/kg/24 hr divided every 8–12 hr | Anticonvulsant for seizures, epilepsy | Confusion, slurred speech, blood dyscrasias, ataxia, rash, nausea, vomiting; Give with at least a half glass of water with or after meals to minimize gastric distress; Avoid abrupt withdrawal; Instruct patients to adhere strictly to prescribed dosage routine; call physician if skin rash develops; stress good oral hygiene to prevent gingivitis |
| Promethazine hydrochloride (Phenergan) | PO, R, IM, IV; Tablets, syrup, ampules, vials, suppositories | Children—PO: 1 mg/kg/24 hr divided into half dose at bedtime and quarter doses every 6 hr of the remaining day | As treatment for nausea, vomiting, or motion sickness or as antihistamine | Causes drowsiness; When giving IM, aspirate carefully before injecting; Rotate injection sites |
| Pyrivinium pamoate (Povan) | PO; Tablets, suspension | 5 mg/kg single dose (PO) | Anthelmintic used in treating pinworms | Colors stools red, nausea, vomiting; Avoid chewing tablets—will stain teeth; Not for aspirin-sensitive patients |
| Sodium methicillin (Staphcillin) | IM, IV; Solution for injection | Infants and children—200–400 mg/kg/24 hr divided every 4 hr IV, every 6 hr IM | Treatment of respiratory and skin infections caused by susceptible organisms; Form of penicillin | Superimposed infections, blood changes, nausea, vomiting, diarrhea; Use with care in patients with allergies (especially to other penicillins); may cause anaphylactic reactions; Administer punctually; chart exact site of IM injection |

*Continued*

| Drug | Route* and Form | Dosage | Some Indications for Use | Nursing Considerations |
|---|---|---|---|---|
| Sulfadiazine (a sulfonamide) | PO, SC, IV Tablets, suspension, solution for injection | Infants and children—PO, IV: 120–150 mg/kg/24 hr divided into 4–6 doses | Rheumatic fever prophylaxis, urinary tract infections, meningococcal meningitis | Record intake and output<br>Sore throat, fever, and rash may indicate blood dyscrasia; report immediately<br>Crush tablets if large<br>Report oliguria, hematuria<br>Observe for mouth sores |
| Tetracycline (Achromycin) | PO, IM, IV Tablets, capsules, syrup | Children—PO: 25–50 mg/kg/24 hr divided every 8 hr; IM: 15–25 mg/kg/24 hr divided every 8–12 hr; IV: 10–20 mg/kg/24 hr divided every 12 hr | Broad-spectrum antibiotic | Diarrhea; limit in children under 8 to avoid staining and pitting of teeth, photosensitivity, gastric distress, superimposed infection<br>Do not give with milk or antacids<br>Take careful history to determine allergies<br>Give 1 hr before meals |
| Theophylline (Slo-phyllin) | PO, R Tablets, elixir, suppositories | According to weight of child | Bronchodilator used for asthmatics and patients with chronic bronchitis | Nausea, vomiting, irritability, convulsions<br>Contraindicated in patients with peptic ulcers, diabetes, hypertension<br>Monitor vital signs |

Adapted from Behrman, R.E. (1992). *Nelson textbook of pediatrics* (14th ed.). Philadelphia: W.B. Saunders; and other sources.
*IM, intramuscular injection; IV, intravenous injection; PO, oral; R, rectal; SC, subcutaneous; prn, as necessary. Note: This chart serves as a summary, and should not replace the use of a more detailed reference.

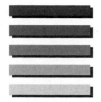

# Appendix H

# NANDA-Approved Nursing Diagnoses

This list represents the NANDA-approved nursing diagnoses for clinical use and testing (1992).

## Pattern 1: Exchanging

| | |
|---|---|
| *1.1.2.1 | Altered nutrition: more than body requirements |
| 1.1.2.2 | Altered nutrition: less than body requirements |
| 1.1.2.3 | Altered nutrition: potential for more than body requirements |
| 1.2.1.1 | High risk for infection |
| 1.2.2.1 | High risk for altered body temperature |
| 1.2.2.2 | Hypothermia |
| 1.2.2.3 | Hyperthermia |
| 1.2.2.4 | Ineffective thermoregulation |
| 1.2.3.1 | Dysreflexia |
| *1.3.1.1 | Constipation |
| 1.3.1.1.1 | Perceived constipation |
| 1.3.1.1.2 | Colonic constipation |
| *1.3.1.2 | Diarrhea |
| *1.3.1.3 | Bowel incontinence |
| 1.3.2 | Altered urinary elimination |
| 1.3.2.1.1 | Stress incontinence |
| 1.3.2.1.2 | Reflex incontinence |
| 1.3.2.1.3 | Urge incontinence |
| 1.3.2.1.4 | Functional incontinence |
| 1.3.2.1.5 | Total incontinence |
| 1.3.2.2 | Urinary retention |
| *1.4.1.1 | Altered (specify type) tissue perfusion (renal, cerebral, cardiopulmonary, gastrointestinal, peripheral) |
| 1.4.1.2.1 | Fluid volume excess |
| 1.4.1.2.2.1 | Fluid volume deficit |
| 1.4.1.2.2.2 | High risk for fluid volume deficit |
| *1.4.2.1 | Decreased cardiac output |
| 1.5.1.1 | Impaired gas exchange |
| 1.5.1.2 | Ineffective airway clearance |
| 1.5.1.3 | Ineffective breathing pattern |
| †1.5.1.3.1 | Inability to sustain spontaneous ventilation |
| †1.5.1.3.2 | Dysfunctional ventilatory weaning response (DVWR) |
| 1.6.1 | High risk for injury |
| *1.6.1.1 | High risk for suffocation |
| 1.6.1.2 | High risk for poisoning |
| 1.6.1.3 | High risk for trauma |
| 1.6.1.4 | High risk for aspiration |
| 1.6.1.5 | High risk for disuse syndrome |
| 1.6.2 | Altered protection |
| 1.6.2.1 | Impaired tissue integrity |
| *1.6.2.1.1 | Altered oral mucous membrane |
| 1.6.2.1.2.1 | Impaired skin integrity |
| 1.6.2.1.2.2 | High risk for impaired skin integrity |

## Pattern 2: Communicating

| | |
|---|---|
| 2.1.1.1 | Impaired verbal communication |

## Pattern 3: Relating

| | |
|---|---|
| 3.1.1 | Impaired social interaction |
| 3.1.2 | Social isolation |
| *3.2.1 | Altered role performance |

*Categories with modified label terminology.
† New diagnostic categories approved 1992.

| | |
|---|---|
| 3.2.1.1.1 | Altered parenting |
| 3.2.1.1.2 | High risk for altered parenting |
| 3.2.1.2.1 | Sexual dysfunction |
| 3.2.2 | Altered family processes |
| † 3.2.2.1 | Caregiver role strain |
| † 3.2.2.2 | High risk for caregiver role strain |
| 3.2.3.1 | Parental role conflict |
| 3.3 | Altered sexuality patterns |

## Pattern 4: Valuing

| | |
|---|---|
| 4.1.1 | Spiritual distress (distress of the human spirit) |

## Pattern 5: Choosing

| | |
|---|---|
| 5.1.1.1 | Ineffective individual coping |
| 5.1.1.1.1 | Impaired adjustment |
| 5.1.1.1.2 | Defensive coping |
| 5.1.1.1.3 | Ineffective denial |
| 5.1.2.1.1 | Ineffective family coping: disabling |
| 5.1.2.1.1 | Ineffective family coping: compromised |
| 5.1.2.2 | Family coping: potential for growth |
| † 5.2.1 | Ineffective management of therapeutic regimen (individuals) |
| 5.2.1.1 | Noncompliance (specify) |
| 5.3.1.1 | Decisional conflict (specify) |
| 5.4 | Health-seeking behaviors (specify) |

## Pattern 6: Moving

| | |
|---|---|
| 6.1.1.1 | Impaired physical mobility |
| † 6.1.1.1.1 | High risk for peripheral neurovascular dysfunction |
| 6.1.1.2 | Activity intolerance |
| 6.1.1.2.1 | Fatigue |
| 6.1.1.3 | High risk for activity intolerance |
| 6.2.1 | Sleep pattern disturbance |
| 6.3.1.1 | Diversional activity deficit |
| 6.4.1.1 | Impaired home maintenance management |
| 6.4.2 | Altered health maintenance |
| *6.5.1 | Feeding self-care deficit |
| 6.5.1.1 | Impaired swallowing |

| | |
|---|---|
| 6.5.1.2 | Ineffective breast feeding |
| † 6.5.1.2.1 | Interrupted breast feeding |
| 6.5.1.3 | Effective breast feeding |
| † 6.5.1.4 | Ineffective infant feeding pattern |
| *6.5.2 | Bathing/hygiene self-care deficit |
| *6.5.3 | Dressing/grooming self-care deficit |
| *6.5.4 | Toileting self-care deficit |
| 6.6 | Altered growth and development |
| † 6.7 | Relocation stress syndrome |

## Pattern 7: Perceiving

| | |
|---|---|
| *7.1.1 | Body image disturbance |
| *7.1.2 | Self-esteem disturbance |
| 7.1.2.1 | Chronic low self-esteem |
| 7.1.2.2 | Situational low self-esteem |
| *7.1.3 | Personal identity disturbance |
| 7.2 | Sensory/perceptual alterations (specify) (visual, auditory, kinesthetic, gustatory, tactile, olfactory) |
| 7.2.1.1 | Unilateral neglect |
| 7.3.1 | Hopelessness |
| 7.3.2 | Powerlessness |

## Pattern 8: Knowing

| | |
|---|---|
| 8.1.1 | Knowledge deficit (specify) |
| 8.3 | Altered thought processes |

## Pattern 9: Feeling

| | |
|---|---|
| *9.1.1 | Pain |
| 9.1.1.1 | Chronic pain |
| 9.2.1.1 | Dysfunctional grieving |
| 9.2.1.2 | Anticipatory grieving |
| 9.2.2 | High risk for violence: self-directed or directed at others |
| † 9.2.2.1 | High risk for self-mutilation |
| 9.2.3 | Post-trauma response |
| 9.2.3.1 | Rape-trauma syndrome |
| 9.2.3.1.1 | Rape-trauma syndrome: compound reaction |
| 9.2.3.1.2 | Rape-trauma syndrome: silent reaction |
| 9.3.1 | Anxiety |
| 9.3.2 | Fear |

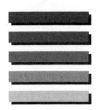

# Answers to Multiple Choice Review Questions

**Chapter 1**
1. b
2. a
3. b
4. c
5. b

**Chapter 2**
1. b
2. d
3. c
4. a
5. b

**Chapter 3**
1. c
2. b
3. a
4. d
5. c
6. c
7. c

**Chapter 4**
1. c
2. c
3. c
4. c
5. b
6. b
7. c
8. a
9. d
10. a

**Chapter 5**
1. a
2. d
3. b
4. a
5. d
6. b
7. a

8. c
9. b
10. c

**Chapter 6**
1. b
2. d
3. c
4. a
5. b
6. a
7. b
8. c
9. c
10. b
11. c

**Chapter 7**
1. b
2. c
3. d
4. b
5. a
6. b
7. c
8. d
9. b
10. d
11. a

**Chapter 8**
1. b
2. c
3. d
4. a
5. c
6. b
7. d
8. a
9. c
10. b
11. d

**Chapter 9**
1. c
2. a
3. c
4. a
5. d
6. b
7. c
8. d
9. c
10. a

**Chapter 10**
1. b
2. d
3. b
4. c
5. a
6. c
7. b
8. d
9. a
10. c

**Chapter 11**
1. c
2. c
3. a
4. c
5. b

**Chapter 12**
1. d
2. b
3. b
4. c
5. a

**Chapter 13**
1. b
2. d
3. b
4. a
5. c

**Chapter 14**
1. a
2. a
3. c
4. c
5. b

**Chapter 15**
1. c
2. a
3. b
4. b
5. c

**Chapter 16**
1. b
2. b
3. a
4. d
5. b

**Chapter 17**
1. a
2. c
3. a
4. b
5. b

**Chapter 18**
1. c
2. b
3. d
4. c
5. d

**Chapter 19**
1. c
2. a
3. b
4. a
5. b

**Chapter 20**
1. c
2. b
3. a
4. d
5. c

**Chapter 21**
1. a
2. d
3. a
4. d
5. d

**Chapter 22**
1. a
2. b
3. c
4. a
5. c

**Chapter 23**
1. b
2. a
3. b
4. b
5. b

**Chapter 24**
1. b
2. a
3. c
4. a
5. c

**Chapter 25**
1. d
2. a
3. a
4. d
5. a

**Chapter 26**
1. b
2. c
3. b
4. c
5. a

**Chapter 27**
1. b
2. b
3. a
4. c
5. b

**Chapter 28**
1. c
2. b
3. b
4. a
5. c

**Chapter 29**
1. c
2. b
3. c
4. b
5. a

**Chapter 30**
1. c
2. b
3. d
4. c
5. b

**Chapter 31**
1. c
2. d
3. a
4. c
5. a

**Chapter 32**
1. d
2. a
3. b
4. b
5. c

**Chapter 33**
1. b
2. a
3. a
4. b
5. b

**Chapter 34**
1. a
2. a
3. c
4. b
5. d

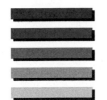

# Index

Page numbers in *italics* refer to illustrations.
Page numbers followed by the letter b refer to boxed material; page numbers followed
by the letter t refer to tables.